LEXIKON

JOINT COMMISSION

LEXIKON

Dictionary of
Health Care Terms,
Organizations,
and Acronyms for
the Era of Reform

Margaret R. O'Leary, MD
and a team of Joint Commission experts

Joint Commission on Accreditation of Healthcare Organizations
One Renaissance Boulevard•Oakbrook Terrace, Illinois

JOINT COMMISSION MISSION

The mission of the Joint Commission on Accreditation of Healthcare Organizations is to improve the quality of care provided to the public.

TABLE OF CONTENTS

FOREWORD

No, we didn't misspell the title of this book. *Lexikon* is taken directly from the Greek term meaning "word book," and this is a book of health care words, phrases, organizations and acronyms. It is the stuff—the language—that we in health care use, sometimes with difficulty, to communicate with ourselves and with others less familiar with our lexicon.

The use of language to express thought and feelings is as old as man. From that beginning, we have progressively elaborated our words and how we use them. Today, we draw upon our armamentarium of language to provide direction, state an opinion, convey an intent, express humor, articulate an expectation, or simply share information.

These varied uses of language to communicate cut across multiple fields of endeavor. But we take the biased view that the lexicon of the health care field is special. It is certainly special for the individual patient whose increasingly complex care commonly requires careful coordination and communication among care-givers. And it has now become special to public policymakers and a wide spectrum of other interested parties who—with health care reform on their minds—have placed the entire American health care delivery system under their collective dissecting microscope.

Communication would be easier if words were always spelled the same way, their meanings remained constant, new words and phrases were not coined, and older words and phrases did not fall into disuse. Unfortunately, language and its usage are constantly changing, and health care, in particular, is serving as a generous contributor to the diversity, vitality, and rapid evolution of American English. In addition, the American penchant for abbreviating has found particularly fertile ground in health care. Now in the era of reform, the language of health care is burgeoning with new definitions of old terms, new terms, and new acronyms.

We should not be surprised by the rich and varied contributions of health care to the American language. Health care accounts for more than 12% of the U.S. gross domestic product. That translates into an extensive array of people—patients, purchasers, professionals, interest groups, media, providers, policymakers, consumers, and just plain spectators—who communicate with each other every day. Neither all of the health care costs nor all of the health care communications lie any longer within the dominant realm of providers. Economists, lawyers, engineers, ethicists, legislators, computer scientists, statisticians, businessmen, social scientists, educators, environmentalists, public welfare workers, labor leaders, and other groups each have their own language, definitions of terms, and vernacular. Within their own individual worlds, that undoubtedly facilitates communication. But when they all come together at the common table of health care, there is often more noise than communication, especially when the language *within* health care is itself also rapidly changing.

For an American public having a greater need than ever before to understand health care issues, the media of communication can no longer be the languages of insiders. We thus face the real risk of a "tower of babble" in a critically important arena in a critically important time. Words do mean different things to different people, and we frequently find ourselves trying to understand familiar words in a new context. For instance, we may know the definition of health care and the definition of alliance. But what is a "health care alliance?" It is different things to different people. Although there is not always one right definition for a term, there is usually a range of understanding. It is essential that we capture, synthesize, and translate this understanding if we are to be able to communicate effectively with each other. The stakes are high—for patients and for all of us—and they will get higher.

The *Lexikon* offers concise explanations and examples—not merely definitions—of the terms, organizations, and abbreviations used in the new public discourse of American health care. *Lexikon: Dictionary of Health Care Terms, Organizations and Acronyms for the Era of Reform* has its origins in the Joint Commission's efforts to research and define measurement and evaluation of organizational performance. In these initial efforts, we found that the degree of variation in meanings in the language of health care quality had become so extreme that many individuals, ostensibly using the same language, were having significant difficulties in understanding each other. This was an important object lesson that two parties communicating purely through word labels can easily be deluded into believing there is an understanding, despite the fact that each of the parties literally does not know what the other is talking about. This book is first and foremost meant to help those who are seeking to communicate in a common language, with the objectives of better patient care and a better health care delivery system.

The *Lexikon* also has roots in the Joint Commission's Agenda for Change. Like the functional emphasis of the new standards framework in the *Accreditation Manual for Hospitals*, the *Lexikon* is meant to break down barriers—here of miscommunication and misunderstanding—and hence to diminish the mystique and obfuscation of health care "jargon." The *Lexikon's* purposes are straightforward:

- Document the language of health care.
- Clarify its meanings.
- Identify the key organizations that are part of, or relate to, the health care field.
- Decipher health care's myriad acronyms and abbreviations.
- Mold a common language that facilitates communication and consensus across health care.
- Support the daily transactions of all those within, affected by, or having an interest in health care.

Spanning the horizons of all professional disciplines, the *Lexikon's* intent is to make accessible health care's complex vocabulary. And in describing the diverse national organizations whose activities contribute to the fabric of the health care environment, the *Lexikon* provides a "scorecard" of the key players and their roles in the new world of health care.

The timing of this important book is exquisite. As the nation's leaders work to reach agreement on how best to address the health care needs of the American people, clarity and consensus of language must be achieved before there can be clarity and consensus of ideas. Now, as different groups having different backgrounds and different perspectives work towards a common goal of accessible, high-quality, cost-effective health care for every American, a comprehensive and authoritative reference, inclusive of and accessible by all of the parties of interest, is essential.

The content of the *Lexikon* is exhaustive, but not meant to be prescriptive or unyielding with respect to its definitions and descriptions of the words, phrases, acronyms, or organizations contained therein. Different, even competing, definitions are provided, along with extensive cross and comparative referencing. The carefully selected terms are intended to give definitions a context and framework for understanding. This *Lexikon* presents a description—a record—of a living, changing language.

It has been said that the only certainty ahead is change. And certainly the language of health care will continue to change. New terms will be coined even as this book goes to press, and other terms will drop from common usage. The *Lexikon* is, like the language itself, a work in progress. Subsequent editions will continue to capture and document the words, acronyms, abbreviations, and organizations that make up the health care lexicon. Like health care reform, this is only the beginning.

Dennis S. O'Leary, MD

GUIDE TO THE LEXIKON

The *Lexikon: Dictionary of Health Care Terms, Organizations, and Acronyms for the Era of Reform* has been designed to serve as a reference book of health care language for the 1990s. Its itemized and cross-referenced content reflects the many complex, interrelated elements that comprise health care. These range from health professions to business, from computer science to law, from government and politics to ethics, and from epidemiology to statistics. This guide explains the conventions used in presenting the terms, acronyms, and organizations contained in the *Lexikon*.

Overview of Entries

American health care language is rich in multiple word phrases such as nursing audit, drug usage evaluation, and prospective pricing system. As a result, the reader will find numerous multiple word entries in the *Lexikon*. Multiple word entries occur in the text according to the first letter of the first word of the multiple word phrase. The definition for **outcome assessment**, for example, is located in the **O** section of the *Lexikon* under **outcome assessment**, rather than in the **A** section under assessment.

Cross References

Multiple word entries, including names of health care organizations and associations, are frequently cross referenced. For example, the reader can find following the entry **audit, medical**: *See* medical audit, and following the entry **executive, nursing**: *See* nursing executive. There are two reasons for this approach. First, a reader can easily locate an entry knowing only one or two key words. For example, to locate information about therapeutic recreational health care organizations and associations, a reader can look in the T

section for the entry **therapeutic . . .**, and find **therapeutic recreation** and several relevant organization entries including:

> **Therapeutic Recreation Association, American** *See* American Therapeutic Recreation Association;
>
> **Therapeutic Recreation Certification, National Council for** *See* National Council for Therapeutic Recreation Certification; and
>
> **Therapeutic Recreation Society, National** *See* National Therapeutic Recreation Society.

A second reason for cross referencing multiple word entries is that a reader interested in a topic can find a cluster of entries sharing a common first word that bears on that topic. A reader interested in engineering in health care, for example, will find most of the entries offered throughout the *Lexikon* simply by looking under **engineering**. Although a strong effort was made to provide numerous cross references for each entry in the *Lexikon*, the reader should always check all possible locations for a term.

More on Cross References

A cross reference *after* a definition signals that additional information can be found at another entry. In these cases the additional term or terms is printed following *See also* at the conclusion of a definition; for example:

> **megalomania** Unreasonable conviction of one's own extreme greatness, goodness, or power. The ideas of a megalomaniac are called delusions of grandeur. *See also* delusions of grandeur.

When additional information can be found at another entry that is the exact or near exact opposite in meaning to the first entry (that is, an antonym), the term or terms is printed following *Compare* at the conclusion of a definition; for example:

> **deduction**   Reasoned argument proceeding from the general to the particular. *Compare* induction.

Sometimes a definition may contain, where appropriate, both *Compare* and *See also* references. In these cases, the *Compare* cross reference precedes the *See also* cross reference; for example:

> **deduction**   Reasoned argument proceeding from the general to the particular. *Compare* induction. *See also* deduce.

When an entry is fully defined at another location, a reference rather than a definition is provided. This applies to abbreviations and synonyms; for example:

> **CO**   *See* carbon monoxide.
> **cold sore**   *See* herpes simplex.

Alphabetization

All entries, including abbreviations (acronyms and initialisms) and multiple word phrases, are alphabetized letter by letter rather than word by word. Abbreviations and multiple word phrases are thus treated as single words; for example, de facto follows *deemed status*. This approach is also used for cross referenced multiple word phrases; for example:

> **assay, bio-**   *See* bioassay.
> **assay, ligand**   *See* ligand assay.

The prepositions *for* and *of* are alphabetically ignored in entries containing them. For example, American Board for Certification in Orthotics appears between American Board of Cardiovascular Perfusion and American Board of Certified and Registered Encephalographic Technicians.

All abbreviations are alphabetized within, not separately from, the main text of the *Lexikon*; for example, ASSE (American Society of Safety Engineers; American Society of Sanitary Engineering) is alphabetized between AS-Score Index and Assembly of Hospital Schools of Nursing, **not** in an appendix (or

separate section) consisting solely of abbreviations as is sometimes the custom.

Proper names are listed according to an individual's surname. Thus, the entry for W Edwards Deming is listed under **Deming, W Edwards**.

Abbreviations

The *Lexikon* contains entries for hundreds of acronyms and initialisms. After each entry, the reader is provided with the term (or terms) to which the abbreviation refers and is referred to the appropriate entry (or entries) for a definition; for example:

> **ASSE**   *See* American Society of Safety Engineers; American Society of Sanitary Engineering.

> **ONS**   *See* Oncology Nursing Society.

Health Care Organizations and Associations

The *Lexikon* contains entries for hundreds of health care organizations and associations. Most, but not all, of these entries were drawn from the 1993 edition of *Encyclopedia of Associations*, a comprehensive source of detailed information containing over 23,000 nonprofit American membership organizations of national scope, nonmembership organizations, and other categories of organizations. This source has been continuously updated and published for over 30 years. The information provided for each organizational entry in the *Lexikon* typically consists of its name, acronym (if any), founding date, number of members (for membership organizations), and a short description of its objectives and services.

Organizations were selected for inclusion in the *Lexikon* based on three main criteria: relevance to health care, geographic scope, and size. Organizations to which these three criteria were applied were initially identified through examination of each listing in over 3,600 pages of the Index volume of the *Encyclopedia of Organizations*. When potential relevant organizations were identified, examination of individual expanded entries followed to confirm relevance to health care, and to assess individual organizations for geographic scope, and size.

Relevance to health care was broadly interpreted for inclusion in the *Lexikon*, and included the following categories of organizations:

- Health and medical organizations, such as American Hospital Association, American

Association of Certified Orthoptists, and Association for Health Services Research;

- Trade, business, and commercial organizations, such as Contact Lens Manufacturers Association, National Association of Medical Equipment Suppliers, and Public Relations Society of America;
- Environmental organizations, such as Hazardous Materials Control Research Institute;
- Legal, governmental, public administration, and military organizations, such as Association of Food and Drug Officials, American Academy of Forensic Psychology, and National Health Law Program;
- Engineering, technological, and natural and social sciences organizations, such as Association of Cytogenetic Technologists, IEEE Engineering in Medicine and Biology Society, and National Society of Biomedical Equipment Technicians;
- Educational organizations, such as American Association of Dental Schools, Council for Medical Affairs, and Association of Professors of Medicine;
- Cultural organizations, such as Interagency Council on Library Resources for Nursing, Medical Library Association, and Hospital Audiences;
- Social welfare organizations, such as National Association of Public Child Welfare Administrators, National Committee for Prevention of Child Abuse, and National Organization of Adolescent Pregnancy and Parenting;
- Public affairs organizations, such as Council for Responsible Genetics, National Council Against Health Fraud, National Health Policy Forum, and Intergovernmental Health Policy Project;
- Religious organizations, such as American Baptist Homes and Hospitals Association, American Association of Pastoral Counselors, and Association for Clinical Pastoral Education;
- Athletic and sports organizations, such as American Medical Athletic Association, North American Society for the Psychology of Sport and Physical Activity, and American Fitness Association; and
- Labor unions, associations, and federations, such as National Federation of Housestaff

Organizations and Federation of Nurses and Health Professionals.

United States health-related organizations, most North American health-related organizations (for example, North American Society of Pacing and Electrophysiology), and a few important international health-related organizations (for example, World Health Organization) met criteria for inclusion in the *Lexikon*. Local and regional, and most international organizations were not included in this edition of the *Lexikon*.

It is not unusual for organizations to change their names over time. Any name by which an organization has been known between 1980 and 1993 has been listed in the *Lexikon* with a cross reference to the organization's current (1993) name. For example, the Joint Commission on Accreditation of Healthcare Organizations was formerly (1987) known as the Joint Commission on Accreditation of Hospitals. There is an entry for Joint Commission on Accreditation of Hospitals that refers the reader to the Joint Commission on Accreditation of Healthcare Organizations. Names by which organizations have been known prior to 1980 are not listed in the *Lexikon*.

There are many small organizations (less than 100 members) that contribute to the quality of health care today but could not be included in this first edition of the *Lexikon* because of space limitations. Exceptions were organizations for which the population from which members are drawn is limited. For example, the 50 member American Society for Pediatric Neurosurgery is drawn from a small total population of pediatric neurosurgeons in the United States.

Every effort was made to include accurate and timely information for each organization mentioned in the *Lexikon*. Hence, organizations listed in the *Encyclopedia of Associations* as inactive, defunct, or untraceable are not included. As change is inevitable, readers interested in the Lexikon are referred to the *Encyclopedia of Associations*, carried by most libraries. Addresses, telephone numbers, and other information listed for each organization in the *Encyclopedia of Associations* enables readers to contact organizations directly.

Revisions or Additions

Readers are encouraged to send suggestions for revision or additions to Publications Director; Joint Commission on Accreditation of Healthcare Organizations; One Renaissance Boulevard; Oakbrook Terrace, IL 60181.

Acknowledgment

The preparation of the *Lexikon* involved much research and review of valuable materials. These resources included numerous books, newspaper and magazine articles, brochures, pamphlets, journals, reports, statutes, fact sheets, dictionaries, and glossaries. Through many of these specialized sources, the reader can pursue, in more depth, subjects suggested by the entries. A bibliographical list of such materials follows.

A Discursive Dictionary of Health Care. Committee on Interstate and Foreign Commerce; US House of Representatives, 94th Congress, 2nd Session; Washington, DC; Feb 1976.

A Health-Care Glossary. *The Wall Street Journal*. Mar 11, 1993; A12.

American Board of Medical Specialties. *Medical Specialty Certification and Related Matters* (booklet). Evanston , IL; 1991.

American Board of Medical Specialties. *Which Medical Specialist for You* (booklet). Evanston, IL; 1992.

American College of Emergency Medicine. Policy Forum looks at future of emergency medicine. *ACEP News*. Dec 1993; 6.

American College of Physician Executives. *The ACPE Medical Management Glossary Series*. Tampa, FL; 1994.

American Dental Association. *Have You Considered Dentistry?* (folder of information). Chicago; 1993.

American Dental Association. *Referral to a Dental Specialist* (brochure). Chicago; 1989.

American Dietetic Association. *Set Your Sights: Your Future in Dietetics* (brochure). Chicago; 1991.

American Health Care Consultants Inc. *An Executive's Pocket Guide to QI/TQM Terminology*. 1992.

American Heritage Dictionary of the English Language, 3rd ed. Boston: Houghton Mifflin Co; 1992.

American Hospital Association. *Guidelines: Role and Functions of the Hospital Nurse Executive*. Chicago; 1985.

American Medical Association. *Twenty Eight Allied Health Careers*. Chicago; 1992.

American Osteopathic Association. *Osteopathic Medical Education* (brochure). Chicago; 1991.

American Osteopathic Association. *What is a DO?* (brochure). Chicago; 1991.

American Osteopathic Association. *American Osteopathic Medicine* (brochure). Chicago; 1991.

American Physical Therapy Association. *A Future in Physical Therapy* (brochure). Alexandria, VA.

American Podiatric Medical Association. *A Point of Reference* (brochure). Bethesda, MD.

American Podiatric Medical Association. *The Physician; The Profession; the Practice* (brochure). Bethesda, MD.

American Society for Quality Control. Quality glossary. *Quality Progress*. Feb 1992; 26.

American Society for Quality Control. *American National Standard Quality Systems Terminology*. Milwaukee, WI; 1987.

Armey D. Your future health plan. *The Wall Street Journal*. Oct 13, 1993.

Batalden PB. Building Knowledge for Quality Improvement in Healthcare: An Introductory Glossary. *Journal of Outcomes Assessment*. 1991; 13:9-12.

Berry ZS, Lynn J. Hospice medicine. *Journal of the American Medical Association*. 1993; 270; 221-222.

Boothe R. Who defines quality in service industries? *Quality Progress*. Feb 1990.

Bradford Hill, A. *Principles of Medical Statistics*. New York: Oxford University Press; 1971.

Burek DM (Ed). *Encyclopedia of Associations*. 27th ed. Detroit: Gale Research Inc; 1992.

Commission for Accreditation of Freestanding Birth Centers. *American Journal of Public Health*. 1989; 79:1067.

DeAngelis CD. Nurse Practitioner Redux. *Journal of the American Medical Association*. 1994; 271:868-871.

Dorland's Illustrated Medical Dictionary. 27th ed. Philadelphia: WB Saunders Co; 1988.

Faucher AD. Glossary. *Journal of the American Medical Association*. 1993; 269:1715.

Felsenthal E. No-fault for medical cases gains support. *The Wall Street Journal*. July 28, 1993; B2.

The Foundation Center. *1993 Foundation Directory*. New York; 1992.

Friedman JP. *Dictionary of Business Terms*. Hauppauge, NY: Barron's Educational Series, Inc; 1987.

Gifis SH. *Law Dictionary*. Hauppauge, NY: Barron's Educational Series, Inc; 1991.

Gitlow HS, Gitlow SH, Oppenheim A, Oppenhiem R. *Tools and Methods for the Improvement of Quality*. Homewood, IL: Irwin; 1989.

Glossary of Terms Relating to Managed Care and Capitalization. *The Quality Letter for Healthcare Leaders*. 1993; (4):25-27.

Goal/OPC: *The Memory Jogger: A Pocket Guide for Continuous Improvement*. 2nd ed. Methuen, MA: Goal/OPC; 1988.

Grzybowski DM. The transition from signature to authorship. *Journal of American Health Information Management Association*. 1993; 64:80-90.

Health Security Act. 103rd Congress 1st Session; Washington, DC; 1993.

Herbert V, Subak-Sharpe GJ, Hammock DA. *The Mount Sinai School of Medicine Complete Book of Nutrition*. New York: St. Martin's Press; 1990.

Joint Commission on Accreditation of Healthcare Organizations. *Introduction to Quality Improvement in Health Care*. Oakbrook Terrace, IL; 1991.

Joint Commission on Accreditation of Healthcare Organizations. *The Measurement Mandate*. Oakbrook Terrace, IL; 1992.

Joint Commission on Accreditation of Healthcare Organizations. *Primer on Indicator Development and Application*. Oakbrook Terrace, IL; 1990.

Journal of the American Medical Association: Instructions for preparing structured abstracts. *Journal of the American Medical Association*. 1993; 270:34-39.

Juran JM, Gryna FM (eds). *Juran's Quality Control Handbook*. 4th ed. New York: McGraw-Hill Book Co; 1988.

Katz J, Green E. *Managing Quality: A Guide to Monitoring and Evaluating Nursing Services*. St Louis: Mosby Year Book; 1992.

Kriger AF. *Acronyms and Initialisms in Health Care Administration*. American Hospital Association Resource Center; Chicago. 1986.

Kriger AF. *Hospital Administration Terminology*. 2nd ed. American Hospital Association Resource Center; Chicago. 1986.

Last JM. *A Dictionary of Epidemiology*. New York: Oxford University Press; 1988.

Lisella FS (ed). *The VNR Dictionary of Environmental Health and Safety*. New York: Van Nostrand Reinhold; 1994.

Lohr KN. *Medicare: A Strategy for Quality Assurance*. Vol I. Washington, DC: National Academy Press; 1990.

Lohr KN. *Medicare: A Strategy for Quality Assurance, Vol II Sources and Methods*. Washington, DC: National Academy Press; 1990.

Lord JT (ed). *The Physician Leader's Guide*. Rockville, MD: Bader & Associates; 1992.

Lutz W. *Double-Speak*. NY: Harper & Row, Publishers; 1981.

Maloney P. Clinical Laboratory Improvement Amendments of 1988 (CLIA '88). *Physician's Practice Digest.* Spring 1993; 30-33.

McKusick VA. Medical genetics: a 40-year perspective on the evolution of a medical specialty from a basic science. *Journal of the American Medical Association* 1993; 270:2351-2356.

Midwest Bioethics Center, Kansas City, MO *Glossary of Terms.*

Nolan J, Nolan-Haley JM. *Black's Law Dictionary.* St. Paul, MN: West Publishing Co; 1990.

Paxson WC. *The New American Dictionary of Confusing Words.* New York: Signet; 1990.

Picker/Commonwealth Program for Patient-Centered Care. *Through the Patient's Eyes: Understanding and Promoting Patient-Centered Care.* San Francisco: Jossey-Bass Publishers; 1993.

Plaster M. Positive predictive value. *Emergency Department Law.* Washington, DC: Buraff Publications; 1993; 8.

Presson EW. Differences in multihospital systems, health systems, networks. *AHA News.* Chicago; Aug 30, 1993.

Rhea JC, Ott JS, Sharfitz JM. *Facts on File Dictionary of Health Care Management.* New York: Facts on File Publications; 1988.

Rice T, Brown R, Wyn R. Holes in the Jackson Hole approach to health care reform. *Journal of the American Medical Association.* 1993; 270:1357-1362.

Rothenberg MA, Chapman CF. *Dictionary of Medical Terms for the Nonmedical Person.* Hauppauge, NY: Barron's Educational Series, Inc; 1989.

Sagin T. *A Glossary of Legal Terms.* Tampa, FL: American College of Physician Executives; 1993.

Slee VN, Slee DA. *Health Care Reform Terms.* St Paul, MN: Tringa Press; 1993.

Slee VN, Slee DA. *Health Care Terms.* 2nd ed. St Paul, MN: Tringa Press; 1991.

Snook D. *Opportunities in Hospital Administration Careers.* Lincolnwood, IL: VGM Career Horizons; 1989.

Stedman's Medical Dictionary. 22nd ed. Baltimore: The Williams & Wilkins Co; 1972.

Toward a National Health Information Infrastructure: Report of the Work Group on Computerization of Patient Records. To the Secretary of the US Department of Health and Human Services. Washington, DC; April 1993.

Tullock S. *The Oxford Dictionary of New Words.* New York: Oxford University Press; 1992.

Office of the Federal Register, National Archives and Records Administration. *United States Government Manual 1992/1993.* Lanham, MD: Bernan Press; 1992.

US Congress, Office of Technology Assessment. *The Quality of Medical Care: Information for Consumers,* OTA-H-386. Washington, DC: US Government Printing Office; 1988.

Walton J, Beeson PB, Scott RD (eds). *The Oxford Companion to Medicine. Volumes I-II.* New York: Oxford University Press; 1986.

Walton M. *The Deming Management Method.* New York: Putnam; 1986.

Washington Information Directory 1993-1994. Congressional Quarterly, Inc; 1993.

What Do These Words Mean? *Chicago Medicine.* 1993; 96:21-24.

Wieseltier L. Total quality meaning. *The New Republic.* July 19 & 26, 1993; 16-26.

Words to live by: a reader's guide: decoding the lingo in the brave new world of healthspeak. *Newsweek.* April 5, 1993; 33.

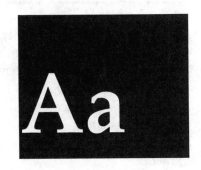

AA *See* Alcoholics Anonymous World Services; anesthesiologist's assistant.

AAA *See* American Academy of Actuaries; American Acupuncture Association; American Ambulance Association; American Association of Anatomists.

AAAAPSF *See* American Association for Accreditation of Ambulatory Plastic Surgery Facilities.

AAAHC *See* Accreditation Association for Ambulatory Health Care.

AAAI *See* American Academy of Allergy and Immunology; American Association for Artificial Intelligence.

AAALAC *See* American Association for Accreditation of Laboratory Animal Care.

AAAM *See* Association for the Advancement of Automotive Medicine.

AAANA *See* American Academy of Ambulatory Nursing Administration.

AAAOM *See* American Association for Acupuncture and Oriental Medicine.

AAAS *See* American Association for the Advancement of Science.

AAB *See* American Association of Bioanalysts.

AABB *See* American Association of Blood Banks.

AABR *See* Association for Advancement of Blind and Retarded.

AABT *See* Association for Advancement of Behavior Therapy.

AAC *See* Association for Assessment in Counseling.

AACA *See* American Association of Certified Allergists.

AACAP *See* American Academy of Child and Adolescent Psychiatry.

AACBP *See* American Academy of Fixed Prosthodontics.

AACC *See* American Association for Clinical Chemistry; American Association for Continuity of Care.

AACDP *See* American Association of Chairmen of Departments of Psychiatry.

AACE *See* American Association for Cancer Education.

AACI *See* American Academy of Crisis Interveners; Association of American Cancer Institutes.

AACN *See* American Association of Colleges of Nursing; American Association of Critical-Care Nurses.

AACO *See* American Association of Certified Orthoptists.

AACOM *See* American Association of Colleges of Osteopathic Medicine.

AACP *See* American Academy of Clinical Psychiatrists; American Association of Colleges of Pharmacy; American Association of Community Psychiatrists; American Association for Correctional Psychology.

AACPDM *See* American Academy for Cerebral Palsy and Developmental Medicine.

AACPM *See* American Association of Colleges of Podiatric Medicine.

AACR *See* American Association for Cancer Research.

AACRC *See* American Association of Children's Residential Centers.

AACS *See* American Academy of Cosmetic Surgery.

AACT *See* American Academy of Clinical Toxicology.

AACU *See* American Association of Clinical Urologists.

AACVPR *See* American Association of Cardiovascular and Pulmonary Rehabilitation.

AAD *See* American Academy of Dermatology.

AADA *See* Association for Adult Development and Aging.

AADC *See* American Association of Dental Consultants.

AADE *See* American Academy of Dental Electrosurgery; American Association of Dental Editors; American Association of Dental Examiners; American Association of Diabetes Educators.

AADEP *See* American Academy of Disability Evaluating Physicians.

AADGP *See* American Academy of Dental Group Practice.

AADPA *See* American Academy of Dental Practice Administration.

AADPRT *See* American Association of Directors of Psychiatric Residency Training.

AADR *See* American Association for Dental Research.

AADS *See* American Association of Dental Schools.

AAE *See* American Association of Endodontists.

AAED *See* American Association of Entrepreneurial Dentists.

AAEE *See* American Academy of Environmental Engineers.

AAEEH *See* American Association of Eye and Ear Hospitals.

AAEH *See* Association to Advance Ethical Hypnosis.

AAEM *See* American Academy of Environmental Medicine; American Association of Electrodiagnostic Medicine.

AAFO *See* American Association for Functional Orthodontics.

AAFP *See* American Academy of Family Physicians; American Academy of Forensic Psychology.

AAFPRS *See* American Academy of Facial Plastic and Reconstructive Surgery.

AAFS *See* Academy of Ambulatory Foot Surgery; American Academy of Forensic Sciences.

AAGFO *See* American Academy of Gold Foil Operators.

AAGL *See* American Association of Gynecological Laparoscopists.

AAGO *See* American Academy of Gnathologic Orthopedics.

AAGP *See* American Association for Geriatric Psychiatry.

AAGUS *See* American Association of Genito-Urinary Surgeons.

AAH *See* Alliance for Alternatives in Healthcare.

AAHA *See* American Academy of Hospital Attorneys; American Association of Homes for the Aging.

AAHC *See* American Association of Healthcare Consultants.

AAHCC *See* American Academy of Husband-Coached Childbirth.

AAHD *See* American Academy of the History of Dentistry; American Association of Hospital Dentists.

AAHE *See* Association for the Advancement of Health Education.

AAHM *See* American Association for the History of Medicine.

AAHN *See* American Association for the History of Nursing.

AAHP *See* American Association of Homeopathic Pharmacists; American Association of Hospital Podiatrists.

AAHS *See* American Association for Hand Surgery.

AAHSLD *See* Association of Academic Health Sciences Library Directors.

AAI *See* American Association of Immunologists.

AAID *See* American Academy of Implant Dentistry.

AAIH *See* American Academy of Industrial Hygiene.

AAIM *See* American Academy of Insurance Medicine; American Association of Industrial Management.

AAIP *See* American Academy of Implant Prosthodontics; Association of American Indian Physicians.

AAISW *See* American Association of Industrial Social Workers.

AALAS *See* American Association for Laboratory Animal Science.

AALIM *See* American Society of Legal and Industrial Medicine.

AALNC *See* American Association of Legal Nurse Consultants.

AAM *See* American Academy of Microbiology.

AAMA *See* American Academy of Medical Administrators; American Association of Medical Assistants.

AAMC *See* American Association of Medico-Legal Consultants; Association of American Medical Colleges.

AAMFT *See* American Association for Marriage and Family Therapy.

AAMHPC *See* American Association of Mental Health Professionals in Corrections.

AAMI *See* Association for the Advancement of Medical Instrumentation.

AAMLA *See* American Academy of Medical-Legal Analysis.

AAMMC *See* American Association of Medical Milk Commissions.

AAMN *See* American Assembly for Men in Nursing.

AAMP *See* American Academy of Maxillofacial Prosthetics.

AAMR *See* American Academy on Mental Retardation; American Association on Mental Retardation.

AAMS *See* Association of Air Medical Services.

AAMSE *See* American Association of Medical Society Executives.

AAMT *See* American Association for Medical Transcription; American Association for Music Therapy.

AAN *See* American Academy of Neurology; American Academy of Nursing.

AANA *See* American Association of Nurse Anesthetists; Arthroscopy Association of North America.

AANC *See* American Association of Nutritional Consultants.

AANFA *See* African-American Natural Foods Association.

AANFP *See* American Academy of Natural Family Planning.

AANN *See* American Association of Neuroscience Nurses.

AANP *See* American Academy of Nurse Practitioners; American Association of Naturopathic Physicians; American Association of Neuropathologists.

AANS *See* American Association of Neurological Surgeons.

AAO *See* American Academy of Ophthalmology; American Academy of Optometry; American Academy of Osteopathy; American Association of Orthodontists.

AAOA *See* American Academy of Otolaryngic Allergy.

AAOE *See* American Association of Osteopathic Examiners.

AAOGP *See* American Academy of Orthodontics for the General Practitioner.

AAOHN *See* American Association of Occupational Health Nurses.

AAO-HNS *See* American Academy of Otolaryngology - Head and Neck Surgery.

AAOM *See* American Academy of Oral Medicine; American Association of Orthomolecular Medicine.

AAOMR *See* American Academy of Oral and Maxillofacial Radiology.

AAOMS *See* American Association of Oral and Maxillofacial Surgeons.

AAON *See* American Association of Office Nurses.

AAOP *See* American Academy of Oral Pathology; American Academy of Orthotists and Prosthetists.

AAOrthMed *See* American Association of Orthopedic Medicine.

AAOS *See* American Academy of Orthopaedic Surgeons; American Association of Osteopathic Specialists.

AAP *See* American Academy of Pediatrics; American Academy of Periodontology; American Academy of Psychoanalysis; American Academy of Psychotherapists; American Association for Parapsychology; American Association of Pathologists; American Association of Psychiatrists from India; Association of Academic Physiatrists; Association for Advancement of Psychology; Association for the Advancement of Psychotherapy; Association of American Physicians; Association for Applied Poetry; Association for Applied Psychoanalysis; Association of Aviation Psychologists.

AAPA *See* American Academy of Physician Assistants; American Academy of Podiatric Administration; American Association of Pathologists' Assistants; American Association of Psychiatric Administrators; Asian American Psychological Association.

AAPAA *See* American Academy of Psychiatrists in Alcoholism and Addictions.

AAPB *See* Association for Applied Psychophysiology and Biofeedback.

AAPC *See* American Association of Pastoral Counselors; American Association for Protecting Children.

AAPCC *See* American Association of Poison Control Centers.

AAPD *See* American Academy of Pediatric Dentistry.

AAPH *See* American Association for Partial Hospitalization; American Association of Professional Hypnotherapists.

AAPHD *See* American Association of Public Health Dentistry.

AAPHP *See* American Association of Public Health Physicians.

AAPHR *See* American Association of Physicians for Human Rights.

AAPL *See* American Academy of Psychiatry and the Law.

AAPM *See* American Association of Physicists in Medicine.

AAPMR *See* American Academy of Physical Medicine and Rehabilitation.

AAPOR *See* American Association for Public Opinion Research.

AAPPO *See* American Association of Preferred Provider Organizations.

AAPPS *See* American Association of Podiatric Physicians and Surgeons.

AAPS *See* American Association of Pharmaceutical

Scientists; American Association of Plastic Surgeons; Association of American Physicians and Surgeons.

AAPSC *See* American Association of Psychiatric Services for Children.

AAPSM *See* American Academy of Podiatric Sports Medicine.

AAR *See* Alliance for Aging Research; Association for Automated Reasoning.

AARC *See* American Association for Respiratory Care.

AARD *See* American Academy of Restorative Dentistry.

Aaron Diamond Foundation, The *See* The Aaron Diamond Foundation, Inc.

AARP *See* American Association of Retired Persons.

AARS *See* American Association of Railway Surgeons.

AART *See* American Association for Rehabilitation Therapy; American Association of Religious Therapists.

AAS *See* American Academy of Sanitarians; American Academy of Somnology; American Apitherapy Society; American Association of Suicidology; American Auditory Society; Association for Academic Surgery.

AASA *See* American Association of Surgeon Assistants.

AASCIN *See* American Association of Spinal Cord Injury Nurses.

AASECT *See* American Association of Sex Educators, Counselors and Therapists.

AASH *See* American Association for the Study of Headache.

AASLD *See* American Association for the Study of Liver Diseases.

AASND *See* American Association for the Study of Neoplastic Diseases.

AASP *See* American Academy of Sports Physicians; American Association of Senior Physicians; American Association for Social Psychiatry.

AASS *See* American Academy of Spinal Surgeons.

AASSWB *See* American Association of State Social Work Boards.

AAST *See* American Association for the Surgery of Trauma.

AAT *See* American Academy of Thermology.

AATA *See* American Art Therapy Association; American Athletic Trainers Association and Certification Board.

AATB *See* American Association of Tissue Banks.

AATH *See* American Association for Therapeutic Humor.

AATM *See* American Academy of Tropical Medicine.

AATP *See* American Association of Testifying Physicians.

AATS *See* American Association for Thoracic Surgery.

AAUAP *See* American Association of University Affiliated Programs for Persons with Developmental Disabilities.

AAWD *See* American Association of Women Dentists.

AAWH *See* American Association for World Health.

AAWR *See* American Association for Women Radiologists.

ABA *See* American Bar Association; American Board of Anesthesiology; American Burn Association; Association for Behavior Analysis.

ABACPR *See* American Bar Association Center for Professional Responsibility.

ABAI *See* American Board of Allergy and Immunology.

abandonment Desertion or willful forsaking, as in child abandonment or patient abandonment. *See also* patient abandonment.

abandonment, patient *See* patient abandonment.

ABAS *See* American Board of Abdominal Surgery.

ABB *See* American Board of Bioanalysis.

abbreviated injury scale (AIS) In trauma care, a scoring instrument that uses an anatomic scale in which the body is divided into seven regions: external, head and face, neck, thorax, abdomen and pelvis, spine, and extremities. Six levels of possible severity are assigned to each anatomic injury, resulting in more than 500 separate injury descriptions. The AIS is used retrospectively and was originally designed (1971) for rating tissue damage in automobile accident research. Its most important use today is in injury severity score (ISS) calculations. *See also* injury severity score; trauma; traumatology.

abbreviated new-drug application (ANDA) An application filed by a pharmaceutical company requesting marketing and sales authority for a new drug for which the conditions of its use (as indicated in the labeling) were previously approved (for a different but similar drug) under the standard Food and Drug Administration approval process for prescription drugs, and whose active ingredients are the same as those of a drug that previously was approved by the Secretary of Health and Human Services. The Secretary is required to approve or disapprove an ANDA within 180 days of its submittal. *See also* drug; Drug Price Competition and Patent Term Restoration Act of 1984; Food and Drug Administration; "me too" drug; new-drug application.

abbreviation Any shortened form of a word or phrase used chiefly in writing to represent the complete form, such as Dr for doctor. *See also* acronym; initialism.

ABBRP *See* American Board of Bionic Rehabilitative Psychology.

ABC *See* American Blood Commission; American Board for Certification in Orthotics and Prosthetics; Association of Black Cardiologists.

ABCA *See* American Black Chiropractors Association.

ABCC *See* American Board of Clinical Chemistry.

ABCP *See* American Board of Cardiovascular Perfusion.

ABCRETT *See* American Board of Certified and Registered Encephalographic Technicians and Technologists.

ABCRS *See* American Board of Colon and Rectal Surgery.

ABCT *See* American Board of Chelation Therapy.

ABD *See* American Board of Dermatology.

abdomen The part of the body that lies between the thorax and the pelvis and encloses the stomach, intestines, liver, spleen, and pancreas. *Synonyms:* belly; stomach.

abdominal Pertaining to the abdomen. *See also* abdomen.

abdominal hysterectomy *See* hysterectomy.

abdominal surgery Surgery of the abdominal viscera. *See also* surgery; viscera.

Abdominal Surgery, American Board of *See* American Board of Abdominal Surgery.

Abdominal Surgery, American Society of *See* American Society of Abdominal Surgery.

abdominal thrust *See* Heimlich maneuver.

ABDPH *See* American Board of Dental Public Health.

ABE *See* American Board of Endodontics.

ABEA *See* American Broncho-Esophagological Association.

ABEM *See* American Board of Emergency Medicine; American Board of Environmental Medicine.

ABEPC *See* American Board of Examiners in Pastoral Counseling.

ABEPSGP *See* American Board of Examiners of Psychodrama, Sociometry, and Group Psychotherapy.

ABFP *See* American Board of Family Practice; American Board of Forensic Psychiatry.

ABG *See* arterial blood gas.

ABHES *See* Accrediting Bureau of Health Education Schools.

ABHHA *See* American Baptist Homes and Hospitals Association.

ABHP *See* American Board of Health Physics.

ABHS *See* American Board of Hand Surgery.

ABIH *See* American Board of Industrial Hygiene.

ability The skill to perform something, as in the ability of a hospital to provide cardiovascular services of high quality. *See also* capability; skill.

ABIM *See* American Board of Internal Medicine.

ABIMS *See* American Board of Industrial Medicine and Surgery.

ABJS *See* Association of Bone and Joint Surgeons.

ABMG *See* American Board of Medical Genetics.

ABMLAMS *See* American Board of Medical-Legal Analysis in Medicine and Surgery.

ABMP *See* American Board of Medical Psychotherapists; Associated Bodywork and Massage Professionals.

ABMR *See* Academy of Behavioral Medicine Research.

ABMS *See* American Board of Medical Specialties.

ABMT *See* American Board of Medical Toxicology.

ABN *See* American Board of Nutrition.

ABNF *See* Association of Black Nursing Faculty in Higher Education.

ABNM *See* American Board of Neurological Microsurgery; American Board of Nuclear Medicine.

ABNN *See* American Board of Neuroscience Nursing.

ABNOLS *See* American Board of Neurological/Orthopaedic Laser Surgery.

ABNOMS *See* American Board of Neurological and Orthopaedic Medicine and Surgery.

abnormal Any departure from the normal, whether above normal or below normal. *See also* abnormal psychology; subnormal.

abnormal psychology The branch of psychology dealing with behavior disorders and disturbed individuals. Researchers in abnormal psychology, for example, may investigate the causes of violent or self-destructive behavior or the effectiveness of procedures used in treating an emotional disturbance. *See also* abnormal; psychology.

ABNS *See* American Board of Neurological Surgery.

ABO *See* American Board of Ophthalmology; American Board of Opticianry; American Board of Orthodontics; American Board of Otolaryngology.

ABO blood groups *See* blood groups.

ABOG *See* American Board of Obstetrics and Gynecology.

ABOHN *See* American Board for Occupational

Health Nurses.

ABOMS *See* American Board of Oral and Maxillofacial Surgery.

ABOP *See* American Board of Oral Pathology.

aborticide *See* abortifacient.

abortient *See* abortifacient.

abortifacient A substance or device that causes abortion. *Synonyms*: abortient; aborticide. *See also* abortion; induced abortion; RU-486.

abortion Termination of pregnancy with expulsion of the fetus. Abortion may be accidental or induced. *See also* complete abortion; habitual abortion; induced abortion; inevitable abortion; missed abortion; septic abortion; spontaneous abortion; therapeutic abortion; threatened abortion.

abortion, complete *See* complete abortion.

Abortion Federation, National *See* National Abortion Federation.

abortion, habitual *See* habitual abortion.

abortion, incomplete *See* complete abortion.

abortion, induced *See* induced abortion.

abortion, inevitable *See* inevitable abortion.

abortion, missed *See* missed abortion.

abortion, septic *See* septic abortion.

abortion, spontaneous *See* spontaneous abortion.

abortion, therapeutic *See* therapeutic abortion.

abortion, threatened *See* threatened abortion.

abortus A fetus weighing less than 500 grams (17 ounces) or being less than 20 weeks gestational age at the time of expulsion from the uterus, having no chance of survival outside the uterus. *Compare* premature birth. *See also* abortion; missed abortion.

ABOS *See* American Board of Orthopaedic Surgery.

ABO system *See* blood groups.

ABP *See* American Board of Pathology; American Board of Pediatrics; American Board of Pedodontics; American Board of Periodontology; American Board of Prosthodontics; Association for Birth Psychology.

ABPANC *See* American Board of Post Anesthesia Nursing Certification.

ABPD *See* American Board of Pediatric Dentistry.

ABPDC *See* American Board of Professional Disability Consultants.

ABPH *See* American Board of Psychological Hypnosis.

ABPLA *See* American Board of Professional Liability Attorneys.

ABPM *See* American Board of Preventive Medicine.

ABPMR *See* American Board of Physical Medicine and Rehabilitation.

ABPN *See* American Board of Psychiatry and Neurology.

ABPO *See* American Board of Podiatric Orthopedics.

ABPP *See* American Board of Professional Psychology.

ABPS *See* American Board of Plastic Surgery; American Board of Podiatric Surgery.

ABPsi *See* Association of Black Psychologists.

ABQAURP *See* American Board of Quality Assurance and Utilization Review Physicians.

ABR *See* American Board of Radiology.

ABRA *See* American Blood Resources Association.

abrasion A scrape. *See also* bruise; laceration; wound.

ABRET *See* American Board of Registration of Electroencephalographic and Evoked Potentials Technologists.

abruptio placenta A complication of pregnancy consisting of premature detachment of the placenta associated with severe hemorrhage and shock. It is an important cause of maternal death and stillbirth (fetal death). *See also* hemorrhage; maternal death; placenta previa; pregnancy; shock; stillbirth.

ABS *See* American Board of Surgery.

abscess A collection of pus, usually confined within a capsule, that forms a cavity within inflamed tissue. *See also* boil; felon; nidus; pus.

ABSS *See* American Board of Spinal Surgery.

abstinence The act or practice of refraining from indulging in something, such as alcoholic beverages or food. *See also* social detoxification.

abstract A statement summarizing the important points of a text or a case. *See also* case abstract; medical record abstraction; summary.

abstract, case *See* case abstract.

abstracter *See* medical record abstracter.

abstracting *See* medical record abstraction.

abstraction *See* medical record abstraction.

Abstracts of Clinical Care Guidelines A bimonthly publication of the Joint Commission on Accreditation of Healthcare Organizations that provides abstracts of clinical practice guidelines from selected articles published in clinical journals and government and professional society publications. *See also* Joint Commission on Accreditation of Healthcare Organizations; practice guideline.

ABT *See* American Board of Toxicology.

ABTA *See* American Board of Trial Advocates.

ABTM *See* American Board of Tropical Medicine.

ABTS *See* American Board of Thoracic Surgery.

ABTSA *See* Association for the Behavioral Treatment of Sexual Abusers.

ABU *See* American Board of Urology.

ABUAHP *See* American Board of Urologic Allied Health Professionals.

abuse Improper use or treatment, as in abuse of health services or alcohol. Abuse, in general, carries with it some sense of harm, such as child abuse, drug abuse, or fraud and abuse. *See also* abuse of process; child abuse; drug abuse; fraud and abuse; substance abuse.

abuse, chemical *See* substance abuse.

abuse, child *See* child abuse.

abuse, drug *See* drug abuse.

abuse, fraud and *See* fraud and abuse.

Abuse Listening and Mediation, Child *See* Child Abuse Listening and Mediation.

Abuse and Mental Health Services Administration, Substance *See also* Substance Abuse and Mental Health Services Administration.

abuse of process Improper use or perversion of the criminal or civil process for a purpose other than that which is intended by law. *See also* abuse; law; process.

Abuse Services, Special Constituency Section for Psychiatric and Substance *See* Special Constituency Section for Psychiatric and Substance Abuse Services.

abuse, substance *See* substance abuse.

ac Abbreviation for Latin phrase *ante cibum*, meaning "before meals."

ACA *See* American Chiropractic Association; American College of Angiology; American College of Apothecaries; American Consumers Association; American Council on Alcoholism; American Counseling Association.

ACACN *See* American Council of Applied Clinical Nutrition.

academic **1.** Pertaining to a school, especially a school of higher learning, such as a college or university; for example, an academic medical center. *See also* academic medical center. **2.** Pertaining to studies that are liberal or classical rather than technical or vocational.

academic detailing The practice of sending representatives, such as physicians or pharmacists, to physicians' offices to address physicians personally about practice guidelines. This is one approach being used by the Agency for Health Care Policy and Research to improve the probability that physicians will use sets of practice guidelines that have been developed and disseminated. Academic detailing is similar to methods used by pharmaceutical companies when promoting a drug. *See also* academic; detail person.

Academic Emergency Medicine, Society for *See* Society for Academic Emergency Medicine.

academic health center *See* academic medical center.

Academic Health Centers, Association of *See* Association of Academic Health Centers.

Academic Health Sciences Library Directors, Association of *See* Association of Academic Health Sciences Library Directors.

academic medical center A medical system typically consisting of a university hospital and medical school, often with other associated teaching hospitals, research organizations and their laboratories, outpatient clinics, libraries, and administrative facilities. *Synonym*: academic health center. *See also* academic; academic medicine; medical center.

academic medicine The part of medicine concerned with teaching, research, and medical practice, residing largely in universities and other institutions of higher learning. Those engaged in academic medicine may have university titles (professor, associate professor, assistant professor) and are often full-time university employees. *See also* academic; academic medical center; medicine; professor.

Academic Physiatrists, Association of *See* Association of Academic Physiatrists.

Academic Standards Association, Straight Chiropractic *See* Straight Chiropractic Academic Standards Association.

Academic Surgery, Association for *See* Association for Academic Surgery.

Academie Orthopaedic Society (AOS) A national organization founded in 1971 composed of 315 chairpersons and faculty members of orthopedic departments and divisions of medical schools, directors of orthopedic residency programs, and fellowship directors. It provides a forum for discussion of administrative and departmental issues concerning undergraduate and graduate orthopedic education in medical schools. It coordinates and plans activities requiring cooperation between orthopedic departments and residencies. *See also* orthopaedic/orthopedic surgery; residency.

Academy of Ambulatory Foot Surgery (AAFS) A national organization founded in 1972 composed of 1,500 podiatric physicians who advocate performing foot surgery in their offices or on an outpatient basis, thereby keeping patients ambulatory and able to function normally, and lowering the patients' medical costs. *See also* ambulatory health care; podiatric medicine.

Academy of Behavioral Medicine Research (ABMR) A national organization founded in 1979 composed of 275 individuals who are actively involved more than one aspect of biobehavioral science research, and who have been published in refereed journals relevant to the field. It seeks to foster the integration of research in biomedical and behavioral science. *See also* behavioral medicine; research.

Academy for Catholic Healthcare Leadership (ACHCL) A national organization founded in 1984 composed of 220 health care professionals interested in promoting professional and personal development of individuals working in Catholic health care organizations. It educates members about the theology, mission, and philosophy of Catholic health care, and encourages members to participate in continuing professional and spiritual education programs. It plans to confer certification upon members who have demonstrated a thorough understanding of Catholic theology as it applies to health care issues. *See also* leadership.

Academy of Certified Social Workers (ACSW) A national organization founded in 1982 by the National Association of Social Workers to certify social workers meeting its requirements. Requirements for certification include a master's or a doctorate degree in social work from a school accredited by the Council on Social Work Education; two years of full-time, paid social work experience with social work supervision in an agency or organizational setting; and successful completion of the ACSW examination. Social workers certified by the ACSW are called registered social workers. *See also* registered social worker; social worker.

Academy of Dental Materials (ADM) A national organization founded in 1940 composed of 300 licensed dentists, members of academic institutions, industrial employees, and others interested in dental

materials, such as plastics. Formerly (1983) American Academy of Plastics Research in Dentistry. *See also* dentistry.

Academy of Dentistry for the Handicapped (ADH) A national organization founded in 1950 composed of dentists, dental hygienists, dental assistants, and allied health professionals specializing in improving the oral health of persons with special dental needs. *See also* dentistry; handicapped person.

Academy of Dispensing Audiologists (ADA) A national organization founded in 1977 composed of 525 individuals with graduate degrees in audiology who dispense hearing aids as part of a rehabilitative practice. It fosters and supports professional dispensing of hearing aids by qualified audiologists and encourages audiology training programs to include pertinent aspects of hearing aid dispensing in their curriculums. *See also* audiology; hearing aid.

Academy of General Dentistry (AGD) A national organization founded in 1952 composed of 33,000 dentists engaged in the general practice of dentistry. It promotes the continuing education and professional development of general practitioners in dentistry. *See also* dentist, generalist.

Academy of Hazard Control Management (AHCM) A national organization founded in 1981 composed of 1,500 certified hazard control managers in occupational, environmental, and other aspects of safety and health. It promotes the professional development and exchange of information within the field of hazard control. *See also* hazardous waste.

Academy for Health Services Marketing (AHSM) A national organization founded in 1980 composed of 3,800 marketing professionals in the health care field, and vice presidents and directors of hospitals, health maintenance organizations, nursing homes, and other health care organizations who are interested in the marketing of health services. It sponsors continuing education for and professional development of its members. *See also* marketing.

Academy for Implants and Transplants (AIT) A national organization founded in 1972 composed of 268 dentists assisting generalist dentists in the field of implants and transplants. *See also* implant dentistry.

Academy of Operative Dentistry (AOD) A national organization founded in 1972 composed of 900 dentists and persons in allied industries interested in quality education in operative dentistry. *See also* dentistry.

Academy of Oral Diagnosis, Radiology, and Medicine (AODRM) A national organization founded in 1985 composed of 780 members that serves as a coordinating organization representing the American Academy of Oral Medicine and the Organization of Teachers of Oral Diagnosis. It seeks to establish oral diagnosis, radiology, and medicine as recognized specialties in dentistry. *See also* dentistry; oral pathology; radiology.

Academy of Orthomolecular Medicine *See* American Association of Orthomolecular Medicine.

Academy of Osteopathic Directors of Medical Education (AODME) A national organization founded in 1965 composed of 190 medical directors and directors of medical education of osteopathic hospitals or colleges. Its purposes include improving curriculum, supervision, and marketing and comanaging clerk, intern, and residency programs. *See also* osteopathic medicine.

Academy of Pharmaceutical Research and Science (APRS) A part of the American Pharmaceutical Association founded in 1965 composed of 3,800 pharmaceutical scientists from industry and academia. It sponsors national meetings to provide a forum for presentation and discussion of original laboratory research and controversial topics. It provides consultation and advice to pharmacists on scientific matters as they relate to policy, congressional committees on bills of interest to pharmaceutical scientists, and governmental agencies. *See also* American Pharmaceutical Association.

Academy of Pharmacy Practice and Management (APPM) A national organization founded in 1965 composed of 18,500 pharmacists concerned with rendering professional services directly to the public. *See also* pharmacist.

Academy of Psychosomatic Medicine (APM) A national organization founded in 1952 composed of 1,000 health professionals interested in the practice of medicine relating to the interaction of mind, body, and environment. *See also* psychosomatic medicine.

Academy of Rehabilitative Audiology (ARA) A national organization founded in 1966 composed of 300 individuals who hold graduate degrees in audiology, language or speech pathology, education of the deaf, or allied fields, and who have at least 2 years of postdegree involvement in rehabilitative or educational programs for the hearing impaired. *See* *also* audiology; hearing impaired.

Academy for Sports Dentistry (ASD) A national organization founded in 1983 composed of 300 dentists, physicians, athletic trainers, and others interested in the study and prevention of dental injuries incurred during sports participation. *See also* dentistry; sports medicine.

ACAI *See* American College of Allergy and Immunology.

ACAM *See* American College of Advancement in Medicine.

ACAP *See* American Council on Alcohol Problems.

ACATA *See* American College of Addiction Treatment Administrators.

ACC *See* American College of Cardiology; Association of Chiropractic Colleges.

ACCA *See* American Clinical and Climatological Association; American College of Cardiovascular Administrators.

ACCC *See* Association of Community Cancer Centers.

ACCE *See* American College for Continuing Education.

acceptability In health care, an overall assessment of care made by an individual or group. It is usually based on many dimensions of care including, but not limited to, its cost, appropriateness, availability, and effectiveness. *See also* appropriateness; availability; effectiveness.

acceptable alternative A common and legitimate reason for failure of an organization or a practitioner to conform to practice guideline recommendations; for example, a physician recommends a vaginal delivery after a previous cesarean section and a patient refuses. Acceptable alternatives are specified explicitly when writing review criteria. They may have been stated explicitly in a practice guideline or they may have been implied. *See also* practice guideline.

acceptable quality level (AQL) The level at which quality is "good enough." The idea that quality is "good enough" has been challenged by those persons who believe that quality never is good enough, but must be constantly improved. *Compare* continuous quality improvement. *See also* level; quality.

access, direct *See* random access.

accessibility In health care, a performance dimension addressing the degree to which an individual or a defined population can approach, enter, and make use of needed health services. *See also* availability.

Accessible Nursing Education and Licensure,

Federation for *See* Federation for Accessible Nursing Education and Licensure.

Access Management, National Association of Healthcare *See* National Association of Healthcare Access Management.

access, open *See* open access.

access, random *See* random access.

access, sequential *See* sequential access.

access time In computer science, the time lag between a request for information stored in a computer and its delivery to the user. *See also* time.

ACCH *See* Association for the Care of Children's Health.

accident An unexpected and usually undesirable incident that occurs because of chance. *See also* adverse patient occurrence; chance; incident.

ACCME *See* Accreditation Council for Continuing Medical Education.

ACCMS *See* American Center for Chinese Medical Sciences.

ACCO *See* American College of Chiropractic Orthopedists.

accomplish To succeed in doing, as in to accomplish an objective. *See also* execute; perform.

account A detailed statement of the mutual demands in the nature of debit and credit between parties, arising out of contracts or some fiduciary relation. *See also* accounts payable; accounts receivable; fiduciary; flexible spending account; national account.

accountability The obligation to disclose periodically, in adequate detail and consistent form, to all directly and indirectly responsible or properly interested parties, the purposes, principles, procedures, relationships, results, incomes, and expenditures involved in any activity, enterprise, or assignment so that they can be evaluated by the interested parties. *See also* administrative accountability; responsibility.

accountability, administrative *See* administrative accountability.

accountant An individual who works in the field of accounting and is skilled in keeping books or accounts; in designing and controlling systems of account; and in giving tax advice and preparing tax returns. *See also* certified public accountant.

accountant, certified public *See* certified public accountant.

account, flexible spending *See* flexible spending account.

account, individual health care *See* individual health care account.

account, individual retirement *See* individual retirement account.

accounting A system that provides quantitative information about the finances of a person or business entity. *See also* accounting error; accounting period; accounting records; accounting software; accounting system; auditor; bookkeeping; cost accounting; financial accounting.

accounting, cost *See* cost accounting.

accounting error Inaccurate measurement or representation of an accounting-related item not caused by intentional fraud. An error may be due to negligence or may result from the misapplication of generally accepted accounting principles. Errors may take the form of dollar discrepancies or may be compliance errors in using accounting policies and procedures. *See also* accounting; error.

accounting, financial *See* financial accounting.

Accounting Foundation, Financial *See* Financial Accounting Foundation.

Accounting Office, US General *See* US General Accounting Office.

accounting period The period covered by an income statement, such as January 1 through December 31 of a year; often a quarter, 6 months, or a year. *See also* accounting.

accounting records All documents and books used in the preparation of financial statements, including general ledgers, subsidiary ledgers, sales slips, and invoices. *See also* accounting; record.

accounting software Programs used to maintain books of account on computers. The software can be used to record transactions, maintain account balances, and prepare financial statements and reports. Many different accounting software packages exist that are designed to meet the needs of individual clients. *See also* accounting; computer software.

Accounting Standards Board, Financial *See* Financial Accounting Standards Board.

accounting system The mechanism within an organization that generates its financial information. *See also* accounting; system.

Accounting and Systems Association, Insurance *See* Insurance Accounting and Systems Association.

account manager, patient *See* patient account manager.

account, national *See* national account.

accounts payable (AP or A/P) Debts currently owed by an enterprise, such as a hospital, that arise in the normal course of business dealings and have not been replaced by a note payable of a debtor, as in bills for hospital supplies received but not yet paid. *Compare* accounts receivable. *See also* account.

accounts receivable (AR or A/R) Debts currently owed to an enterprise, such as a hospital, that arise in the normal course of business dealings and are not supported by negotiable paper. A list of such debts represents unsettled claims and transactions for services provided and goods furnished. *Compare* accounts payable. *See also* account.

ACCP *See* American College of Chest Physicians; American College of Clinical Pharmacology; American College of Clinical Pharmacy.

accredit To give official authorization or status, as to accredit a residency program or a hospital. *See also* accreditation; accredited.

accreditation A formal process by which an authorized body assesses and recognizes an organization, a program, a group, or an individual as complying with requirements, such as standards or criteria. For example, accreditation by the Joint Commission on Accreditation of Healthcare Organizations is a determination that an eligible health care organization complies with applicable standards. *See also* accreditation appeal; accreditation cycle; accreditation decision; accreditation decision processing; accreditation history; accredited; certification; Joint Commission on Accreditation of Healthcare Organizations; reaccreditation.

Accreditation of Alcoholism and Drug Abuse Counselor Credentialing Bodies, National Commission on *See* National Commission on Accreditation of Alcoholism and Drug Abuse Counselor Credentialing Bodies.

Accreditation of Ambulatory Plastic Surgery Facilities, American Association for *See* American Association for Accreditation of Ambulatory Plastic Surgery Facilities.

Accreditation, American Federation of Medical *See* American Federation of Medical Accreditation.

accreditation appeal A process through which an organization that has been denied accreditation may exercise its right to a hearing. For example, a hospital that has been denied accreditation by the Joint Commission on Accreditation of Healthcare Organizations may exercise a right to a hearing by an appeals hearing panel, followed by a review of the panel's report and recommendation by the governing body (Board of Commissioners) appeal review committee. *See also* accreditation; Board of Commissioners; Joint Commission on Accreditation of Healthcare Organizations.

Accreditation Association for Ambulatory Health Care (AAAHC) An accrediting body founded in 1979 that operates a voluntary, peer-based accreditation and consulting program for ambulatory health care organizations as a means of assisting them in efficiently providing a high level of care for patients. *See also* accreditation; ambulatory health care.

Accreditation and Certification, National Association for the Advancement of Psychoanalysis and the American Boards for *See* National Association for the Advancement of Psychoanalysis and the American Boards for Accreditation and Certification.

accreditation with commendation The highest accreditation decision awarded by the Joint Commission on Accreditation of Healthcare Organizations to a health care organization that has demonstrated exemplary performance. *See also* accreditation decision; commendation; Joint Commission on Accreditation of Healthcare Organizations.

Accreditation, Commission on Opticianry *See* Commission on Opticianry Accreditation.

Accreditation Commission for Schools and Colleges of Acupuncture and Oriental Medicine, National *See* National Accreditation Commission for Schools and Colleges of Acupuncture and Oriental Medicine.

Accreditation Commission, Utilization Review *See* Utilization Review Accreditation Commission.

Accreditation Committee The committee of the governing body (Board of Commissioners) of the Joint Commission on Accreditation of Healthcare Organizations responsible for oversight of the accreditation decision process. *See also* accreditation; accreditation decision processing; audit committee; Board of Commissioners; Joint Commission on Accreditation of Healthcare Organizations.

Accreditation, Committee on Allied Health Education and *See* Committee on Allied Health Education and Accreditation.

accreditation, conditional *See* conditional accreditation.

Accreditation Council for Continuing Medical Education (ACCME) An accrediting body founded in 1981 for sponsors of continuing medical education for physicians. Sponsoring participants are: American Board of Medical Specialties, American Hospital Association, Association for Hospital Medical Education, Federation of State Medical Boards of the United States, American Medical Association, Council of Medical Specialty Societies, and Association of American Medical Colleges. Formerly Liaison Committee on Continuing Medical Education. *See also* accreditation; continuing medical education.

Accreditation Council for Environmental Health Science and Protection, National *See* National Accreditation Council for Environmental Health Science and Protection.

Accreditation Council for Graduate Medical Education (ACGME) A council responsible for the accreditation of residency training programs, operating through 24 Residency Review Committees (RRCs). The RRCs process the actual accreditation of residency programs, but the ACGME approves standards and deals with appeals and other administrative issues. *See also* accreditation; *Directory of Residency Training Programs;* graduate medical education; Residency Review Committee.

Accreditation Council on Services for People with Developmental Disabilities (ACDD) A national organization founded in 1969 that develops, reviews, and revises standards for services provided to people with disabilities, assesses agency compliance with standards on request, and awards accreditation to agencies found to be in compliance with the council's standards. *See also* accreditation; developmental disability.

accreditation cycle A period at the conclusion of which an entity's accreditation will expire unless another survey is performed. For example, the accreditation cycle of the Joint Commission on Accreditation of Healthcare Organizations is a three-year term at the conclusion of which accreditation expires unless a full survey is performed. *See also* accreditation; accreditation survey; cycle; Joint Commission on Accreditation of Healthcare Organizations.

accreditation decision A conclusion reached by an accrediting body regarding an entity's accreditation status. For example, an accreditation decision is reached by the Joint Commission on Accreditation of Healthcare Organizations regarding a health care organization's accreditation status after evaluation of the results of an on-site survey, recommendations

of the surveyors, and any other relevant information, such as documentation of compliance with standards, documentation of plans to correct deficiencies, or evidence of recent improvements. The decision may be accreditation with commendation, accreditation, conditional accreditation, provisional accreditation, or not accredited. *See also* accreditation; accreditation with commendation; conditional accreditation; Joint Commission on Accreditation of Healthcare Organizations; not accredited; provisional accreditation.

accreditation decision aggregation The process by which a group of individual scores of compliance with standards developed by the Joint Commission on Accreditation of Healthcare Organizations determines a grid element score. Related standards are aggregated in groups. When a predetermined number of standards in a group is deficient, a type I recommendation is generated. Some standards are not grouped with others and, when deficient, in and of themselves can generate a type I recommendation. *See also* accreditation decision; accreditation decision aggregation rules; aggregation; Joint Commission on Accreditation of Healthcare Organizations; standard; type I recommendation.

accreditation decision aggregation rules The specific rules used to incorporate all survey findings made by surveyors of the Joint Commission on Accreditation of Healthcare Organizations into a number of grid element scores on an accreditation decision grid. The format of the rules is commonly referred to as the algorithm or the aggregation algorithm. The aggregation rules are listed alphabetically by grid element name. Aggregation rules are reviewed and approved by the Accreditation Committee of the Board of Commissioners. *See also* Accreditation Committee; accreditation decision; accreditation decision aggregation; aggregation; Board of Commissioners; Joint Commission on Accreditation of Healthcare Organizations.

accreditation decision grid A single-page display of performance areas that summarizes the standards of the Joint Commission on Accreditation of Healthcare Organizations for a given type of health care organization. An accreditation decision grid for a hospital, for example, summarizes the standards in the *Accreditation Manual for Hospitals*. The grid format allows for the presentation of a simplified, numerical overview of an organization's performance in each performance area. A *grid element* is a performance area, such as education and communication, or continuum of care, that receives a discrete score on the accreditation decision grid. A *grid element score* is a number representing the aggregated scores of individual standards in a performance area. A *grid score* (also referred to as the summary grid score) is the number that indicates a health care organization's overall accreditation performance. The score is calculated from the grid element scores. *See also* accreditation decision; Joint Commission on Accreditation of Healthcare Organizations; performance area.

accreditation decision processing The interrelated series of steps governing the analysis of survey findings and written progress reports, and the development of accreditation decisions and reports for health care organizations surveyed by the Joint Commission on Accreditation of Healthcare Organizations. *See also* accreditation; Accreditation Committee; accreditation decision; Joint Commission on Accreditation of Healthcare Organizations; written progress report.

accreditation decision report *See* survey report.

accreditation decision rules Statements that determine the accreditation decision developed by the Joint Commission on Accreditation of Healthcare Organizations based on grid element scores. The rules also determine the scope (which and how many elements require monitoring) and type (focused surveys and/or written progress reports) of follow-up monitoring required for compliance deficiencies. *See also* accreditation; accreditation decision; accreditation decision aggregation rules; focused survey; Joint Commission on Accreditation of Healthcare Organizations; written progress report.

accreditation, dental hygiene *See* dental hygiene accreditation.

accreditation, dental laboratory technology *See* dental laboratory technology accreditation.

accreditation duration A period of time during which an entity, such as a health care organization, is accredited by an accrediting body. For example, the accreditation duration of a hospital accredited by the Joint Commission on Accreditation of Healthcare Organizations is three years. To maintain accreditation by the Joint Commission for a three-year period, satisfactory resolution of any identified issues is required.

See also accreditation; duration; Joint Commission on Accreditation of Healthcare Organizations.

Accreditation of Healthcare Organizations, Joint Commission on *See* Joint Commission on Accreditation of Healthcare Organizations.

accreditation history An account of past accreditation decisions for an entity, such as a health care organization. The accreditation history of health care organizations that have applied for accreditation by the Joint Commission on Accreditation of Healthcare Organizations may be publicly disclosed on request. *See also* accreditation; accreditation decision; history; Joint Commission on Accreditation of Healthcare Organizations.

Accreditation of Laboratory Animal Care, American Association for *See* American Association for Accreditation of Laboratory Animal Care.

Accreditation Manual for Ambulatory Health Care (AMAHC) A publication of the Joint Commission on Accreditation of Healthcare Organizations consisting of policies and procedures relating to ambulatory health care organization accreditation surveys, current ambulatory health care standards, and scoring guidelines used to determine levels of compliance with the standards. The manual is designed for use in ambulatory health care organizations' self-assessment, and the standards are the basis for the survey report forms used by surveyors during on-site surveys. The *AMAHC* is published biannually. *See also* accreditation; Ambulatory Care Accreditation Program; ambulatory health care; Joint Commission on Accreditation of Healthcare Organizations; scoring guideline; standard.

Accreditation Manual for Health Care Networks (AMHCN) A publication of the Joint Commission on Accreditation of Healthcare Organizations consisting of policies and procedures relating to health care network accreditation surveys, current health care network standards, and scoring guidelines used to determine levels of compliance with the standards. The publication is designed for use in health care networks' self-assessment, and the standards are the basis for the survey report forms used by surveyors during on-site surveys. *See also* accreditation; Health Care Network Accreditation Program; Joint Commission on Accreditation of Healthcare Organizations; network; scoring guideline; standard.

Accreditation Manual for Home Care (AMHC)
A publication of the Joint Commission on Accreditation of Healthcare Organizations consisting of policies and procedures relating to home care accreditation surveys, current home care standards, and scoring guidelines used to determine levels of compliance with the standards. The manual is designed for use in home care organizations' self-assessment, and the standards are the basis for the survey report forms used by surveyors during on-site surveys. The *AMHC* is published biannually. *See also* accreditation; Home Care Accreditation Program; home health care; Joint Commission on Accreditation of Healthcare Organizations; scoring guideline; standard.

Accreditation Manual for Hospitals (AMH) A publication of the Joint Commission on Accreditation of Healthcare Organizations consisting of policies and procedures relating to hospital accreditation surveys, current hospital standards, and scoring guidelines used to determine levels of compliance with the standards. The manual is designed for use in hospitals' self-assessment, and the standards are the basis for the survey report forms used by surveyors during on-site surveys. The *AMH* is published annually. *See also* accreditation; Hospital Accreditation Program; Joint Commission on Accreditation of Healthcare Organizations; scoring guideline; standard.

Accreditation Manual for Long Term Care (AMLTC) A publication of the Joint Commission on Accreditation of Healthcare Organizations consisting of policies and procedures relating to long term care accreditation surveys, current long term care standards, and scoring guidelines used to determine levels of compliance with the standards. The manual is designed for use in long term care organizations' self-assessment, and the standards are the basis for the survey report forms used by surveyors during on-site surveys. The *AMLTC* is published biannually. *See also* accreditation; Joint Commission on Accreditation of Healthcare Organizations; long term care; Long Term Care Accreditation Program; scoring guideline; standard.

Accreditation Manual for Mental Health, Chemical Dependency, and Mental Retardation/ Developmental Disabilities Services (MHM) A publication of the Joint Commission on Accreditation of Healthcare Organizations consisting of policies and procedures relating to mental health care organization accreditation surveys, current mental health care standards, and scoring guidelines used to determine levels of compliance with the standards. The manual is designed for use in mental health organizations' self-assessment, and the standards are the basis for the survey report forms used by surveyors during on-site surveys. Formerly titled *Consolidated Standards Manual*. The *MHM* is published biannually. *See also* accreditation; Joint Commission on Accreditation of Healthcare Organizations; Mental Health Care Accreditation Program; mental health services; scoring guideline; standard.

Accreditation Manual for Pathology and Clinical Laboratory Services (LSM) A publication of the Joint Commission on Accreditation of Healthcare Organizations consisting of current pathology and clinical laboratory accreditation services standards. The manual is designed for use in pathology and clinical laboratories' self-assessment, and the standards are the basis for the survey report forms used by surveyors during on-site surveys. The *LSM* is published biannually. *See also* accreditation; Clinical Laboratory Improvement Amendments of 1988 (CLIA-88); Joint Commission on Accreditation of Healthcare Organizations; pathology and clinical laboratory services.

accreditation manuals *See* standards manuals.

Accreditation of Nurse Anesthesia Educational Programs/Schools, Council on *See* Council on Accreditation of Nurse Anesthesia Educational Programs/Schools.

Accreditation in Occupational Hearing Conservation, Council for *See* Council for Accreditation in Occupational Hearing Conservation.

Accreditation Program, Ambulatory Care *See* Ambulatory Care Accreditation Program.

Accreditation Program, Community Health *See* Community Health Accreditation Program.

Accreditation Program, Health Care Network *See* Health Care Network Accreditation Program.

Accreditation Program, Home Care *See* Home Care Accreditation Program.

Accreditation Program, Hospital *See* Hospital Accreditation Program.

Accreditation Program, Long Term Care *See* Long Term Care Accreditation Program.

Accreditation Program, Mental Health *See* Mental Health Care Accreditation Program.

accreditation, provisional *See* provisional accreditation.

accreditation, re- *See* reaccreditation.

Accreditation of Rehabilitation Facilities, Commission on *See* Commission on Accreditation of Rehabilitation Facilities.

Accreditation Review Committee on Education for Physician Assistants (ARC-PA) A national accrediting review body founded in 1971 for physician assistant education. It makes recommendations to the Committee on Allied Health Education and Accreditation. Formerly (1972) Joint Review Committee on Educational Programs for the Assistant to the Primary Care Physician; (1982) Joint Review Committee on Educational Programs for Physician's Assistants; (1987) Joint Review on Educational Programs for Physician Assistants; (1989) Accreditation Committee on Education for Physicians Assistants. *See also* Committee on Allied Health Education; physician assistant.

Accreditation Review Committee for Educational Programs in Surgical Technology (ARC-ST) A national body founded in 1974 that reviews accreditation applications of surgical technology programs in hospitals, community colleges, technical schools, and universities and makes recommendations to the American Medical Association's Committee on Allied Health Education and Accreditation. Formerly (1987) Joint Review Committee on Education for the Surgical Technologist. *See also* surgical technologist.

Accreditation of Services for Families and Children, Council on *See* Council on Accreditation of Services for Families and Children.

accreditation standards manuals *See* standards manuals.

accreditation survey An evaluation conducted to assess an entity's level of performance with requirements, such as standards, and to make determinations regarding its accreditation status. For example, an accreditation survey by the Joint Commission on Accreditation of Healthcare Organizations consists of an on-site evaluation of a health care organization to assess its level of compliance with applicable standards and to make determinations regarding its accreditation status. The survey includes evaluation of documentation of compliance; verbal information regarding the implementation of standards, or examples of their implementation, that will enable a determination of compliance to be made; and on-site observations by surveyors. The survey also provides the opportunity for education and consultation to health care organizations regarding standards compliance. *See also* accreditation; Joint Commission on Accreditation of Healthcare Organizations; survey; survey report form; surveyor.

accreditation survey report *See* survey report.

accredited Formally recognized by an accrediting body as meeting its standards for accreditation, as in an accredited hospital, accredited residency program, or accredited record technician. *See also* accreditation; not accredited; unaccredited.

accredited, not *See* not accredited.

accredited, un- *See* unaccredited.

accredited record technician (ART) A medical record technician (MRT) who has passed a credential examination and has met other requirements of the American Health Information Management Association. *See also* American Health Information Management Association; medical record technician.

Accrediting Agency for Clinical Laboratory Sciences, National *See* National Accrediting Agency for Clinical Laboratory Sciences.

Accrediting Bureau of Health Education Schools (ABHES) An independent accrediting body of the American Medical Technologists, founded in 1964, that accredits health education institutions and schools conducting medical laboratory technician and medical assistant education programs. Schools apply voluntarily for accreditation and, once accredited, must report to the bureau annually and be reexamined at least every six years. It currently has accredited 29 programs for medical laboratory technicians, 168 programs for medical assistants, and 118 institutions of allied health. *See also* American Medical Technologists; medical laboratory technician (associate degree); medical laboratory technician (certificate).

Accrediting Commission on Education for Health Services Administration (ACEHSA) An accrediting body founded in 1968 that accredits 60 master's degree programs in health services administration, health planning, and health policy. *See also* health administration; health services; Master of Health Administration.

ACCRYO *See* American College of Cryosurgery.

accurate **1.** Conforming exactly to fact (errorless), or deviating only slightly or within acceptable limits from a standard, as in an accurate measurement. **2.** Capable of providing a correct reading or measurement, as in an accurate scale. *Compare* inaccurate. *See* *also* accuracy of a measurement; data accuracy; measurement; standard.

accuracy, data *See* data accuracy.

accuracy of a measurement The degree to which a measurement, or an estimate based on measurements, represents the true value of the attribute that is being measured. A measurement may be accurate but not express detail (that is, it may lack a degree of precision). For instance, a temperature of 98.6° F may be accurate but not precise if a newer measuring instrument measures the temperature as 98.63432° F. Measurements should have acceptable degrees of accuracy *and* precision. *See also* accurate; data accuracy; measurement; precision.

accused *See* defendant.

ACD *See* American College of Dentists.

ACDD *See* Accreditation Council on Services for People with Developmental Disabilities.

ACDE *See* American Council for Drug Education.

ACE *See* American College of Epidemiology; Association for Continuing Education.

ACEHSA *See* Accrediting Commission on Education for Health Services Administration.

ACEP *See* American College of Emergency Physicians.

ACFO *See* American College of Foot Orthopedists.

ACFS *See* American College of Foot Surgeons.

ACG *See* American College of Gastroenterology.

ACGIH *See* American Conference of Governmental Industrial Hygienists.

ACGME *See* Accreditation Council for Graduate Medical Education.

ACGPOMS *See* American College of General Practitioners in Osteopathic Medicine and Surgery.

ACHA *See* American College Health Association.

ACHCA *See* American College of Health Care Administrators.

ACHCL *See* Academy for Catholic Healthcare Leadership.

ACHCR *See* American Council for Health Care Reform.

ache A dull, constant, prolonged pain, as in stomachache or aches and pains. *See also* pain.

ACHE *See* American College of Healthcare Executives; American Council of Hypnotist Examiners.

AChemS *See* Association for Chemoreception Sciences.

achievable standard, optimum *See* optimum achievable standard.

achievement **1.** The act of accomplishing or finishing, especially accomplishing or finishing successfully by means of exertion, skill, practice, or perseverance. **2.** Something accomplished successfully.

ACHSA *See* American Correctional Health Services Association.

acid-fast bacilli (AFB) isolation *See* tuberculosis isolation.

ACLA *See* American Clinical Laboratory Association.

ACLAM *See* American College of Laboratory Animal Medicine.

ACLM *See* American College of Legal Medicine.

ACLS *See* advanced cardiac life support.

ACM *See* American College of Medicine; Association for Computing Machinery.

ACMGA *See* American College of Medical Group Administrators.

ACMHA *See* American College of Mental Health Administration.

ACMMSCO *See* American College of Mohs Micrographic Surgery and Cutaneous Oncology.

ACN *See* American College of Neuropsychiatrists; American College of Nutrition.

ACNM *See* American College of Nuclear Medicine; American College of Nurse-Midwives.

ACNP *See* American College of Neuropsychopharmacology; American College of Nuclear Physicians.

ACOEM *See* American College of Occupational and Environmental Medicine.

ACOEP *See* American College of Osteopathic Emergency Physicians.

ACOG *See* American College of Obstetricians and Gynecologists.

ACOI *See* American College of Osteopathic Internists.

ACOMS *See* American College of Oral and Maxillofacial Surgeons.

ACOOG *See* American College of Osteopathic Obstetricians and Gynecologists.

ACOP *See* American College of Osteopathic Pediatricians.

ACORE *See* Advisory Council for Orthopedic Resident Education.

ACOS *See* American College of Osteopathic Surgeons.

acoustic coupler A device that hooks a telephone handset into a computer to allow computer communication over telephone lines through the use of a modem. *See also* modem.

ACP *See* American College of Physicians; American

College of Podopediatrics; American College of Prosthodontists; American College of Psychiatrists; Associates of Clinical Pharmacology; Association for Child Psychoanalysis.

ACPA *See* American Cleft Palate-Craniofacial Association; American College of Psychoanalysts.

ACPE *See* American College of Physician Executives; American Council on Pharmaceutical Education; Association for Clinical Pastoral Education.

ACPM *See* American College of Preventive Medicine.

ACPOC *See* Association of Children's Prosthetic-Orthotic Clinics.

ACPR *See* American College of Podiatric Radiologists.

acquired immunization *See* active immunization.

acquired immunodeficiency syndrome (AIDS) A terminal disease caused by the human immunodeficiency virus (HIV) that destroys cell-mediated immunity leading to AIDS-defining diseases, such as opportunistic infections (for example, *Pneumocystis carinii* pneumonia), neoplasms (such as Kaposi's sarcoma), and neurologic disease (such as meningoencephalitis caused by *Toxoplasma gondii*). The interval from HIV infection to development of AIDS averages four to five years, but not all infected people develop (AIDS). AIDS was first recognized in the United States in the summer of 1981. By 1984 the HIV was identified as the etiologic agent of AIDS and tests for the HIV antibody as well as for the virus itself became available. *Synonym*: full-blown AIDS. *See also* HIV; HIV infection; immunodeficiency; infectious diseases; opportunistic infection; syndrome.

ACR *See* American College of Radiology; American College of Rheumatology.

ACRM *See* American Congress of Rehabilitation Medicine.

acronym A word formed from the initial letters of a name, such as DOS for disk operating system, or by combining the initial letters or parts of a series of words, such as e-mail for electronic mail. *See also* abbreviation; initialism.

ACRRT *See* American Chiropractic Registry of Radiologic Technologists.

ACS *See* American Cancer Society; American College of Surgeons; American Cryonics Society.

ACS/DSC *See* American Celiac Society/Dietary Support Coalition.

ACSH *See* American Council on Science and Health.

ACSM *See* American College of Sports Medicine.

ACSW *See* Academy of Certified Social Workers.

act **1.** A thing done, as in an act of kindness. *See also* action. **2.** A decisional product, such as a statute, delivered by a legislative or a judicial body, for example, dental practice act. *See also* dental practice act; medical practice act; nurse practice act.

ACT *See* Alliance for Cannabis Therapeutics; American College Testing; American College of Toxicology; Association of Cytogenetic Technologists.

act, dental practice *See* dental practice act.

ACTG *See* AIDS Clinical Trials Group.

action **1.** The doing of an act or a collection of acts, as in the action of the play took place in three acts. *See also* action organization; affirmative action; political action committee. **2.** A lawsuit; the legal demand for one's rights asserted in a court. If something is "actionable," it provides legal ground for a complaint in court. *See also* action in personam; action in rem; case; complaint; lawsuit; venue.

action, affirmative *See* affirmative action.

action, cause of *See* cause of action.

action committee, political *See* political action committee.

action organization A nonprofit organization that devotes considerable effort to seeking to influence legislation, or participates in political campaigns to aid or oppose candidates for public office. *See also* organization; political action committee.

action in personam A lawsuit against a person on the basis of personal liability. *See also* action; lawsuit; liability.

action in rem A lawsuit to determine title to property. *See also* action; lawsuit.

Activation Networks, Wellness and Health *See* Wellness and Health Activation Networks.

active birth Childbirth during which the mother is encouraged to be as active as possible, mainly by moving around freely and assuming any position that feels comfortable or decreases discomfort. *See also* birth.

active euthanasia A direct medical intervention to end the life of a person suffering from the advanced stages of an incurable illness. *Synonym*: mercy killing. *Compare* passive euthanasia. *See also* euthanasia; intervention.

active immunization Stimulation of the body's immune system to confer protection against disease. Protection may be acquired by administration of a living modified agent (as in yellow fever), a suspension of killed organisms (as in whooping cough), or an inactivated toxin (as in tetanus toxoid). *Synonym*: acquired immunization. *Compare* passive immunization. *See also* diphtheria; immunization; tetanus; toxin; toxoid; vaccinate; vaccine.

active listening A counseling technique in which a counselor listens to both the facts and the feelings of the speaker. The listening is active because the counselor has the specific responsibilities of showing interest, of not passing judgment, and of helping the speaker to work through issues. Basic components of active listening include: not condoning, condemning, agreeing, or disagreeing; using reflective phrases, such as "in other words" or "sounds like"; using reflective rather than accusative "you" messages; asking expansion-type questions; using reflective body language, such as eye contact; and being genuine. *See also* listen.

activities director *See* recreational therapist.

activities of daily life *See* activities of daily living.

activities of daily living (ADL) The activities usually performed for oneself in the course of a normal day, such as eating, dressing, washing, combing hair, brushing teeth, and taking care of bodily functions. An ADL checklist is often used by providers to assess a patient prior to hospital discharge. If any activities cannot be adequately performed, arrangements are made with an outside agency, such as a visiting nurse service, or with family members to provide the necessary assistance. *See also* intermediate care; personal care; physical therapy; physical therapy assistant.

activities, risk management *See* risk management activities.

activity A defined process or pursuit in which one or more persons partakes. *See also* activity professional; process.

activity professional A specialist who develops and conducts activity programs for elderly and handicapped persons. *See also* activity; disability; handicap; professional.

Activity Professionals, National Association of *See* National Association of Activity Professionals.

ACTL *See* American College of Trial Lawyers.

act, medical practice *See* medical practice act.

act, nurse practice *See* nurse practice act.

actual charge The dollar amount a physician, hospital, or other provider actually bills a patient for a particular health service, such as a procedure. *See also* charge.

actuarial analysis Application of probability and statistical methods to calculate the risk of occurrence of events, such as illness, hospitalization, disability, or death, for a given population. A common use of actuarial analysis is the calculation of insurance premiums and, for the insurer, the necessary reserves. *See also* actuarial science; actuary; insurance; probability.

actuarial science The mathematics of insurance, including probabilities. It is used in increasing the probability that risks are carefully evaluated, that adequate premiums are charged for risks underwritten, and that adequate provision is made for future payment of benefits. *See also* actuarial analysis; actuary.

Actuaries, American Academy of *See* American Academy of Actuaries.

Actuaries, Conference of Consulting *See* Conference of Consulting Actuaries.

Actuaries, Society of *See* Society of Actuaries.

actuary A statistician who computes insurance and pension rates and premiums on the basis of experience tables, such as life expectancy and mortality tables. *See also* actuarial analysis; actuarial science; life expectancy; statistician.

acuity Acuteness, as in an acute illness that has a rapid onset and follows a short but severe course. *See also* acute; level of acuity; visual acuity.

acuity level *See* level of acuity.

acuity, visual *See* visual acuity.

acupressure A therapy in which symptoms are relieved by applying pressure with the thumbs or fingers to specific pressure points on the body. *Synonyms*: shiatsu (in Japan); G-Jo (in China). *See also* acupuncture.

Acupressure, Jin Shin Do Foundation for Bodymind *See* Jin Shin Do Foundation for Bodymind Acupressure.

acupuncture A technique originating in China for relieving pain or inducing regional anesthesia, in which thin needles are inserted into the body at specific points. *See also* acupressure.

Acupuncture Association, American *See* American Acupuncture Association.

Acupuncture and Oriental Medicine, American Association for *See* American Association for Acupuncture and Oriental Medicine.

Acupuncture and Oriental Medicine, National

Accreditation Commission for Schools and Colleges of *See* National Accreditation Commission for Schools and Colleges of Acupuncture and Oriental Medicine.

Acupuncture Research Institute (ARI) An organization founded in 1972 composed of 750 medical doctors, osteopathic physicians, homeopaths, dentists, acupuncturists, physical therapists, nurses, and other health professionals interested in investigating the validity and American application of acupuncture. It provides basic study courses in the theory and methods of acupuncture leading to licensure as a primary care physician in acupuncture by the California Board of Medical Quality Assurance and Acupuncture Examining Committee. *See also* acupuncture; licensure.

Acupuncture Schools and Colleges, National Council of *See* National Council of Acupuncture Schools and Colleges.

Acupuncturists, National Commission for the Certification of *See* National Commission for the Certification of Acupuncturists.

ACURP *See* American College of Medical Quality.

acute Having a rapid onset and following a short but severe course, as in acute disease. *Compare* chronic; subacute. *See also* acuity.

acute bronchitis Bronchitis characterized by a productive cough and fever. *Compare* chronic bronchitis. *See also* acute; bronchitis; sputum.

acute care Short-term health care; for example, for less than 30 days. *Compare* chronic care. *See also* acute; care.

acute care hospital A hospital that cares primarily for patients with acute diseases or conditions and whose average length of stay is less than 30 days. *Compare* long term care facility. *See also* acute care; hospital; short-term hospital.

acute disease A disease that begins over minutes, hours, or days that may be readily treated and cured once diagnosed but may progress despite treatment and become chronic or even cause death. An acute episode of a chronic disease, such as pneumonia in a patient with chronic obstructive pulmonary disease or sickle cell crisis in a patient with sickle cell disease, is often managed as an acute disease. *Compare* chronic disease. *See also* acute; disease.

acute myocardial infarction (AMI) Death of tissue in the heart muscle that results from insufficient blood supply to the heart, sometimes leading to cardiac arrest. *Synonyms:* coronary; heart attack; MI; myocardial infarction. *See also* atherosclerosis; heart; infarction; ischemia; myocardium; thrombosis.

Acute Physiology and Chronic Health Evaluation (APACHE) A system that classifies patients as to severity of illness using physiological values, age, and certain aspects of chronic health status. This information is used to predict the risk of dying of patients cared for in an intensive care unit. This severity measure is not dependent on the disease. *See also* severity adjustment; severity of illness.

ADA *See* Academy of Dispensing Audiologists; American Dental Association; American Dermatological Association; American Diabetes Association; American Dietetic Association.

ADAA *See* American Dental Assistants Association.

adapt To make suitable to or fit for a specific use or situation, as in adapting to rapid change. *See also* adaptation.

adaptation The process of becoming more suited to prevailing conditions, as in genetic adaptation. *See also* adapt.

ADARA *See* American Deafness and Rehabilitation Center.

ADC *See* Aid to Families with Dependent Children.

ad damnum The clause in a legal complaint (the document that initiates a lawsuit) that contains a statement of the plaintiff's money loss or the damages he or she claims. Such a clause informs an adversary of the maximum amount of the claim asserted without being proof of actual injury or of liability. *See also* lawsuit.

addiction A behavioral pattern of substance use characterized by an overwhelming involvement with the use and securing of the substance. *See also* alcoholism; alcoholism and other drug dependence; controlled substances; Controlled Substances Act of 1970; dependence; glue sniffing; morphinism; nicotine; physical dependence; withdrawal symptoms.

addiction medicine The branch of medicine dealing with addiction. *See also* addiction; addictionologist.

Addiction Medicine, American Society of *See* American Society of Addiction Medicine.

addictionologist An individual, usually a physician, who specializes in the study and treatment of addiction. *See also* addiction.

addiction psychiatrist A psychiatrist who subspecializes in addiction psychiatry. *See* addiction psychiatry.

addiction psychiatry The subspecialty of psychiatry dealing with the understanding of addictive disorders and the special and emotional problems related to addiction and substance abuse. *See also* addiction; health plan; psychiatry; substance abuse.

Addiction Research and Education, National Association for Perinatal *See* National Association for Perinatal Addiction Research and Education.

Addictions, American Academy of Psychiatrists in Alcoholism and *See* American Academy of Psychiatrists in Alcoholism and Addictions.

Addictions, National Nurses Society on *See* National Nurses Society on Addictions.

Addiction Treatment Administrators, American College of *See* American College of Addiction Treatment Administrators.

Addiction Treatment Providers, National Association of *See* National Association of Addiction Treatment Providers.

addictive A substance or practice that may result in psychological and/or physical dependence on the substance or the practice by most individuals exposed to it. *See also* addiction; addictive personality; addictive substance.

Addictive Behaviors, Society of Psychologists in *See* Society of Psychologists in Addictive Behaviors.

addictive drug *See* addictive substance.

addictive personality A personality marked by traits of compulsive and habitual use of a substance or practice. *See also* addiction; personality.

addictive substance Any substance, natural or synthetic, that causes periodic or chronic intoxication through repeated consumption by most individuals exposed to it. *Synonym*: addictive drug. *See also* addictive; drug.

additional drug benefit list A list of a limited number of prescription medications, as designated by a health plan, commonly prescribed by physicians for long-term patient use. The list is subject to periodic review and modification by the health plan. *Synonym*: drug maintenance list. *See also* drug.

additive A substance, such as a flavoring agent, preservative, or vitamin, added to another substance during manufacture to improve its color, flavor, or preservability. *Synonym*: food additive. *See also* direct food additives; indirect food additives; preservative; sulfites.

additive, food *See* additive.

additives, direct food *See* direct food additives.

additives, indirect food *See* indirect food additives.

ADDS *See* alternative dental delivery system; American Diopter and Decibel Society.

ADEC *See* Association for Death Education and Counseling.

adenoma A benign growth deriving from glandular tissue. *See also* gland; lipoma; myoma; neurinoma.

adequacy of coverage Sufficiency of insurance protection to repay the insured in the event of loss. *See also* coverage; insurance; insured; underinsured.

adequate Equal to what is required; satisfactory; suitable to a case or an occasion. For example, the coverage was adequate for the patient's needs. *Compare* inadequate. *See also* sufficient.

ADH *See* Academy of Dentistry for the Handicapped.

ADHA *See* American Dental Hygienists' Association.

ad hoc Latin phrase meaning "for this purpose"; for example, an ad hoc committee is one formed for a particular purpose, usually limited in duration until the purpose is achieved. *See also* ad hoc committee.

ad hoc committee A committee formed to accomplish certain tasks and then disband. *Compare* standing committee. *See also* ad hoc; committee.

adipose tissue Connective tissue in which fat-containing cells predominate. *Synonyms*: fat; fatty tissue. *See also* connective tissue; lipoma; liposuction surgery.

adiposity *See* obesity.

adjacent value, lower On a schematic box plot the smallest observation that is greater than or equal to the first quartile minus 1.5 times the interquartile range. *See also* adjacent value, upper; box plot; quantile; schematic box plot.

adjacent value, upper On a schematic box plot, the largest observation that is less than or equal to the third quartile plus 1.5 times the interquartile range. *See also* adjacent value, lower; box plot; quantile; schematic box plot.

adjective law Rules of legal practice that set forth methods of enforcing rights created by substantive law. For example, service of process (communication of court papers to the defendant) is a matter of adjective law. *See also* law; rights.

adjudicate **1.** To hear and settle a case by judicial procedure. **2.** The act of determining the eligibility of health services reported on a health insurance claim for payment under a policy's benefit definitions, limitations, and exclusions. Adjudication may result in full payment, partial payment, denial of payment, or a combination of these for the services reported on a given claim. **3.** The complete processing of one or more claims by an insurance company. Most insurance companies divide the claims process into the steps of claims receipt and screening to review for completeness, claimant eligibility determination, provider eligibility determination, reimbursement determination, utilization review, quality assurance, payment, and records management. *See also* claim; claims review.

adjust   To free from differences or discrepancies; to bring to proper relations, as in risk adjusting performance or quality data. *See also* adjustment; risk adjustment; severity adjustment.

adjusted autopsy rate   The number of autopsies performed on patients over a specified period in relation to the total number of inpatient and outpatient deaths, less those bodies unavailable for autopsy. *Synonym*: net autopsy rate. *See also* autopsy; autopsy rate.

adjusted daily census   The average number of patients (inpatients plus an equivalent figure for outpatients) receiving care each day during a reporting period. *See also* average daily census; census; hospital.

adjustment   A procedure for correcting differences or discrepancies in the composition of two or more populations. Adjustment is frequently employed so that valid comparisons can be made between populations. For example, adjustment for age must occur to make valid comparisons between the mortality data of a nursing home and the mortality data of a freestanding ambulatory surgical center. Adjustments used in a specific procedure are sometimes called standardization. *See also* administrative adjustment; area wage adjustment; risk adjustment; severity adjustment; standardization.

adjustment, administrative   *See* administrative adjustment.

adjustment, area wage   *See* area wage adjustment.

adjustment, contractual   *See* contractual adjustment.

adjustment, cost-of-living   *See* cost-of-living adjustment.

adjustment, risk   *See* risk adjustment.

adjustment, severity   *See* severity adjustment.

adjuvant therapy, systemic   *See* systemic adjuvant therapy.

ADL   *See* activities of daily living.

ad lib   Abbreviation for Latin phrase *ad libitum*, meaning "at pleasure," used to refer to the use of

medication as required by a patient.

ad litem   Latin phrase meaning "for purposes of the suit" being prosecuted, as in guardian ad litem. *See also* guardian ad litem; lawsuit.

ADM   *See* Academy of Dental Materials.

administer   To manage, direct, or conduct, as in administering drugs or planning, directing, budgeting, and implementing to achieve organizational objectives. *See also* administration.

administration   The guidance of an undertaking toward the achievement of its purpose, as in drug administration or hospital administration. Administration and management are often used synonymously, although they have been distinguished by applying administration to public activities and management to private, or by describing one as concerned with the making of broad policy and the other as concerned with the execution of that policy once formulated. *See also* drug administration; management; management and administration; medication administration; public administration.

Administration, Accrediting Commission on Education for Health Services   *See* Accrediting Commission on Education for Health Services Administration.

Administration, American Academy of Ambulatory Nursing   *See* American Academy of Ambulatory Nursing Administration.

Administration, American Academy of Dental Practice   *See* American Academy of Dental Practice Administration.

Administration, American Academy of Podiatric   *See* American Academy of Podiatric Administration.

Administration, American College of Mental Health   *See* American College of Mental Health Administration.

Administration, American Society for Healthcare Human Resources   *See* American Society for Healthcare Human Resources Administration.

Administration, Center for Research in Ambulatory Health Care   *See* Center for Research in Ambulatory Health Care Administration.

administration, drug   *See* drug administration.

Administration in Long Term Care, National Association of Directors of Nursing   *See* National Association of Directors of Nursing Administration in Long Term Care.

administration, management and   *See* management and administration.

administration, medication *See* medication administration.

administration, nursing home *See* nursing home administration.

administration, public *See* public administration.

Administration, Social Security *See* Social Security Administration.

administrative Pertaining to administration. *See also* administration.

administrative accountability The concept that administrators are held answerable for general notions of democracy and morality as well as for specific management responsibilities. *See also* accountability; administration; morality.

administrative adjustment In health care, bookkeeping adjustment to reflect services provided but not billed to patients because costs of billing and collection would exceed charges, or to reflect partial adjustment of charges in special circumstances. *See also* adjustment; administrative.

administrative agency A governmental body charged with administering or implementing particular legislation, often including regulation of a profession or industry. Examples are workers' compensation commissions, state boards of medical examiners, and the Federal Trade Commission. *Synonym*: public agency. *See also* administrative law; agency; regulatory agency.

administrative board *See* governing body.

administrative dietitian A registered dietitian who plans and provides for the nutritional care of groups through the management of foodservice systems. *See also* dietitian; foodservice; registered dietitian.

administrative engineer In hospitals, an engineer who has overall administrative responsibility for planning, managing, and maintaining the hospital's physical environment, equipment, and systems. *Synonyms*: chief engineer; plant engineer; director of buildings and grounds; facility manager; vice president of buildings and grounds; vice president of facilities. *See also* administrative; engineer; engineering.

administrative law A body of law created by administrative agencies in the form of rules, regulations, orders, and decisions to carry out the regulatory powers and duties of such agencies. *See also* administrative agency; law.

administrative process The procedures used by administrative agencies to make decisions, such as the procedure a hospital must follow to obtain a certificate of need from an administrative agency or the means of summoning witnesses before such agencies. *See also* administrative agency; certificate of need; process.

administrative resident A student in or graduate of a program in hospital or health care administration who participates in a practical training experience in a health care organization. *See also* administrative; resident.

administrator An executive responsible for carrying out policies established by the organization in which he or she is employed. Administrators are employed in a broad range of health care organizations including hospitals (hospital administrator), group practice clinics, large medical centers, local planning agencies, insurance plans, and governmental programs. When an administrator has authority over an entire hospital or other type of health care organization, the individual is usually the chief executive officer of that organization. *See also* assistant administrator; chief executive officer; health administration; medical administrator; public health administrator; registered record administrator; rehabilitation administrator.

administrator, assistant *See* assistant administrator.

administrator, hospital *See* administrator.

administrator, long term care *See* long term care administrator.

administrator, medical *See* medical administrator.

administrator, nursing home *See* nursing home administrator.

administrator, public health *See* public health administrator.

administrator, registered record *See* registered record administrator.

administrator, rehabilitation *See* rehabilitation administrator.

Administrators, American Academy of Medical *See* American Academy of Medical Administrators.

Administrators, American Association of Psychiatric *See* American Association of Psychiatric Administrators.

Administrators, American College of Addiction Treatment *See* American College of Addiction Treatment Administrators.

Administrators, American College of Cardiovascular *See* American College of Cardiovascular Administrators.

Administrators, American College of Health Care
See American College of Health Care Administrators.

Administrators, American College of Medical Group *See* American College of Medical Group Administrators.

Administrators, American Healthcare Radiology *See* American Healthcare Radiology Administrators.

Administrators, American Society for Hospital Food Service *See* American Society for Hospital Food Service Administrators.

Administrators, American Society of Ophthalmic *See* American Society of Ophthalmic Administrators.

Administrators, Association of Medical Rehabilitation *See* Association of Medical Rehabilitation Administrators.

Administrators, Association of Mental Health *See* Association of Mental Health Administrators.

Administrators Association, National Renal *See* National Renal Administrators Association.

Administrators, Association of Otolaryngology *See* Association of Otolaryngology Administrators.

Administrators, Association of State Drinking Water *See* Association of State Drinking Water Administrators.

Administrators of Health Occupations Education, National Association of Supervisors and *See* National Association of Supervisors and Administrators of Health Occupations Education.

Administrators, National Association of Boards of Examiners for Nursing Home *See* National Association of Boards of Examiners for Nursing Home Administrators.

Administrators, National Association of County Health Facility *See* National Association of County Health Facility Administrators.

Administrators, National Association of Public Child Welfare *See* National Association of Public Child Welfare Administrators.

Administrators, National Conference of Local Environmental Health *See* National Conference of Local Environmental Health Administrators.

Administrators Serving the Deaf, Conference of Educational *See* Conference of Educational Administrators Serving the Deaf.

administrator, social welfare *See* social welfare administrator.

Administrators, Society for Radiation Oncology *See* Society for Radiation Oncology Administrators.

Administrators of Vocational Rehabilitation, Council of State *See* Council of State Administrators of Vocational Rehabilitation.

administrator, third-party claims *See* third-party claims administrator.

admissible evidence In law, evidence (such as a medical record entry) that is relevant, not protected by specific laws (such as privileged information), and properly authenticated, and therefore is allowed to be presented to a judge or jury to prove a legal case. *See also* authenticate; discoverable; evidence; privileged communication.

admission In health care, the formal acceptance by a hospital or other health care organization of a patient who is to receive health services. *See also* clinic outpatient admission; elective admission; emergency admission; emergency department admission; inpatient admission; newborn admission; preadmission process for admission; readmission; referred outpatient admission; transfer admission; urgent admission.

admission certification *See* admissions review.

admission, clinic outpatient *See* clinic outpatient admission.

admission, elective *See* elective admission.

admission, emergency *See* emergency admission.

admission, emergency department *See* emergency department admission.

admission, inpatient *See* inpatient admission.

admission, newborn *See* newborn admission.

admission pattern monitoring The monitoring of the distribution of kinds of patients admitted to a health care organization. *See also* admission; monitor; pattern.

admission, preadmission process for *See* preadmission process for admission.

admission, re- *See* readmission.

admission, referred outpatient *See* referred outpatient admission.

admission source The point from which a patient enters a health care organization; for example, physician referral, clinic referral, health maintenance organization referral, transfer from a hospital, transfer from a skilled nursing facility, transfer from another health care facility, emergency department, or court/law enforcement admission source. *See also* admission; source.

admissions review Review of the medical necessity and appropriateness of a patient's admission to a hospital or other health care organization, conducted before, at, or shortly after admission. Admission or preadmission review, previously a requirement characteristic of some Blue Cross Plans for their participating hospitals, was performed in large part to verify the patient's eligibility for services, open the patient's claim record, and establish an expected diagnosis and length of stay. Health maintenance organizations and other prepaid plans now use admission review as a cost-containment and resources-management strategy. Only patients requiring a specific type and level of care are admitted to a health care organization, and lengths of stay appropriate for the patient's admitting diagnosis are usually assigned. *Synonyms*: admission certification; preadmission certification; preadmission review. *See also* admission; prior authorization.

admissions office *See* admitting department.

admission, transfer *See* transfer admission.

admission, urgent *See* urgent admission.

admitting department The organizational unit providing for the processing of patient admissions, discharges, and transfers and for most procedures to be carried out in the event of a patient's death. *Synonyms*: admissions office; admitting office. *See also* admission; department; discharge; discharge by transfer.

admitting diagnosis The diagnosis provided on admission, explaining the reason for admission of a patient. *See also* admission; diagnosis.

admitting function The interrelated series of organizational processes concerned with admission of patients to health care organizations. *See also* admission; function; important function.

admitting office *See* admitting department.

admitting officer An individual who specializes in arranging for admission and discharge of patients and directs the activities of the admitting department. *Synonyms*: admitting manager; hospital admitting manager; registrar. *See also* admitting department; officer.

admitting manager *See* admitting officer.

Admitting Managers, National Association of Hospital *See* National Association of Healthcare Access Management.

admitting physician The physician responsible for admission of a patient to a hospital or other inpatient health care organization. *See also* admitting privileges; physician.

admitting privileges Authorization granted by a health care organization's governing body to a prac-

titioner to admit patients to a health care organization, such as a hospital. Such individuals may practice only within the scope of their clinical privileges also granted by the governing body. *See also* admitting physician; clinical privileges; governing body.

adolescence The period of transition from childhood to adulthood, beginning with the onset of puberty to about the age of twenty years or the age of majority. *See also* adolescent medicine; age of majority; identity crisis; puberty.

Adolescence, Center for Early *See* Center for Early Adolescence.

Adolescent Development, Carnegie Council on *See* Carnegie Council on Adolescent Development.

adolescent medicine The branch of medicine and subspecialty of pediatrics and internal medicine dealing with the care and treatment of adolescents. *See also* adolescence; internal medicine; medicine; pediatrics.

Adolescent Medicine, Society for *See* Society for Adolescent Medicine.

Adolescent Pregnancy and Parenting, National Organization of *See* National Organization of Adolescent Pregnancy and Parenting.

adolescent psychiatry *See* child and adolescent psychiatry.

Adolescent Psychiatry, American Academy of Child and *See* American Academy of Child and Adolescent Psychiatry.

Adolescent Psychiatry, American Society for *See* American Society for Adolescent Psychiatry.

Adolescent Psychiatry, Society of Professors of Child and *See* Society of Professors of Child and Adolescent Psychiatry.

adopt 1. To take into one's family through legal means and raise as one's own child. **2.** To vote to accept. **3.** To take and follow by choice or assent.

ADS *See* alternative delivery system.

ADSA *See* American Dental Society of Anesthesiology.

ADT Abbreviation for Admissions, Discharges, Transfers; commonly used in hospitals to describe a daily census activity report. *See also* average daily census; census; inpatient census.

ADTA *See* American Dance Therapy Association; American Dental Trade Association.

adult One who has reached or passed the age of majority established by law, generally 18 years. *See also* child; infant.

Adult Chronic Patients, The Information Exchange

on Young   *See* The Information Exchange on Young Adult Chronic Patients.

adult basic life support   *See* basic cardiac life support.

adult day care (daycare)   Health, recreation, and social services offered to adults during daytime hours, generally Monday through Friday. These services can include health monitoring, occupational therapy, recreational therapy, personal care, meals, and transportation. *See also* adult; day care center; occupational therapy; personal care; recreational therapy; transportation.

Adult Daycare, National Institute on   *See* National Institute on Adult Daycare.

Adult Development and Aging, Association for   *See* Association for Adult Development and Aging.

adult inpatient   An inpatient who is over a certain age as determined by a hospital or other health care organization. *See also* hospital; inpatient; pediatric inpatient.

adult inpatient bed   A bed that is regularly maintained for adult inpatients who are receiving continuing organizational services. *See also* adult inpatient; bed.

adult inpatient bed count   *See* bed count.

adult-onset diabetes   *See* type II diabetes mellitus.

adult protection   *See* protection for adults.

adult protection services   *See* protection for adults.

adult respiratory distress syndrome (ARDS)   A critical illness in which an acute illness, such as hypoxia or brain injury, precipitates a severe reaction in the lungs, where fluid accumulates a few days after the initiating illness. ARDS usually necessitates the need for mechanical ventilation. *See also* lung; mechanical ventilation; respirator; respiratory distress syndrome; syndrome.

ad valorum tax   *See* value-added tax.

advance directives   Instructions or orders issued either orally or in writing to give directions about future medical care or to designate another person(s) to make medical decisions if the patient should lose the capacity to make decisions. Advance directives include living wills, durable power of attorney for health care, or similar documents portraying a patient's preferences. *See also* durable power of attorney for health care; living will; Patient Self-Determination Act.

advanced cardiac life support (ACLS)   A set of national clinical protocols, standards, guidelines, and performance criteria, developed and defined by the American Heart Association, pertaining to the initial assessment and management of the emergency cardiac care patient. The ACLS phase of emergency cardiac care consists of basic life support; the use of adjunctive equipment and special techniques for establishing and maintaining effective ventilation and circulation; electrocardiographic monitoring and arrhythmia recognition; the establishment and maintenance of intravenous access; the employment of therapies (including drug and electrical therapies) for emergency treatment of patients with cardiac and/or respiratory arrests and for stabilization in the post-arrest phase; and the treatment of patients with suspected or overt acute myocardial infarction. Qualified health professionals may be trained and certified in ACLS techniques and principles. *Synonym*: advanced life support (ALS). *See also* advanced pediatric life support; advanced trauma life support; ALS unit; American Heart Association; basic cardiac life support; basic trauma life support; golden hour; mobile intensive care unit.

advanced life support (ALS)   *See* advanced cardiac life support.

advanced pediatric life support (APLS)   A set of national clinical protocols, standards, guidelines, and performance criteria relating to pediatric cardiorespiratory support, traumatic emergencies, environmental emergencies, neonatal emergencies, and emergencies with altered levels of consciousness, developed and defined by the American Academy of Pediatrics and the American College of Emergency Medicine for health care providers who care for children in emergency settings. Qualified health professionals may be trained and certified in APLS techniques and principles. *See also* advanced cardiac life support; advanced trauma life support; American Academy of Pediatrics; American College of Emergency Medicine; basic cardiac life support; basic trauma life support.

advanced practice nurse   A nurse who has had advanced education and has met clinical practice requirements beyond the two to four years of higher education required for all registered nurses. Advanced practice nurses include nurse practitioners, nurse-midwives, clinical nurse specialists, and nurse anesthetists. *See also* clinical nurse specialist; nurse anesthetist; nurse-midwife; nurse practitioner; registered nurse.

Advanced Research in Asian Science and

Medicine, Institute for *See* Institute for Advanced Research in Asian Science and Medicine.

advanced trauma life support (ATLS) A set of national clinical standards and performance criteria, developed and defined by the American College of Surgeons Committee on Trauma, pertaining to initial assessment and management of the trauma patient. Physicians and other qualified health professionals may be trained and certified in ATLS techniques using a combined educational format of lecture presentation and associated skill technique demonstration and practicum. The approach to initial care of trauma patients was developed in 1978 in response to the desire expressed by Nebraska physicians who wanted to improve the quality of care and health outcomes of severely injured patients. *See also* advanced cardiac life support; advanced pediatric life support; American College of Surgeons; basic cardiac life support; basic trauma life support; mobile intensive care unit; traumatology.

Advance Ethical Hypnosis, Association to *See* Association to Advance Ethical Hypnosis.

Advancement of Ambulatory Care, Society for the *See* Society for the Advancement of Ambulatory Care.

Advancement of Anesthesia in Dentistry, American Society for *See* American Society for Advancement of Anesthesia in Dentistry.

Advancement of Automotive Medicine, Association for the *See* Association for the Advancement of Automotive Medicine.

Advancement of Behavior Therapy, Association for *See* Association for Advancement of Behavior Therapy.

Advancement of Blind and Retarded, Association for *See* Association for Advancement of Blind and Retarded.

Advancement of Health Education, Association for the *See* Association for the Advancement of Health Education.

Advancement of Human Behavior, Institute for the *See* Institute for the Advancement of Human Behavior.

Advancement of Management, Society for *See* Society for Advancement of Management.

Advancement of Medical Instrumentation, Association for the *See* Association for the Advancement of Medical Instrumentation.

Advancement in Medicine, American College of *See* American College of Advancement in Medicine.

Advancement of Psychiatry, Group for the *See* Group for the Advancement of Psychiatry.

Advancement of Psychoanalysis and the American Boards for Accreditation and Certification, National Association for the *See* National Association for the Advancement of Psychoanalysis and the American Boards for Accreditation and Certification.

Advancement of Psychology, Association for *See* Association for Advancement of Psychology.

Advancement of Psychotherapy, Association for the *See* Association for the Advancement of Psychotherapy.

Advancement of Science, American Association for the *See* American Association for the Advancement of Science.

Adventist Dietetic Association, Seventh-Day *See* Seventh-Day Adventist Dietetic Association.

Adventist A member of any of several Christian denominations that believe Jesus's Second Coming and the end of the world are near. *See also* Seventh-Day Adventist.

Adventist, Seventh-Day *See* Seventh-Day Adventist.

adverse Contrary to one's interest or welfare; harmful, unfavorable, or undesirable, as in an adverse patient health outcome. *See also* adverse event; adverse patient occurrence; adverse selection; drug adverse reaction.

adverse drug reaction *See* drug adverse reaction.

adverse event An untoward, undesirable, and usually unanticipated event, such as death of an inpatient, an employee, or a visitor in a health care organization. Incidents such as patient falls or improper administration of medications are also considered adverse events even if there is no permanent effect on the patient. *See also* adverse; adverse patient occurrence; drug adverse reaction; event; incident reporting; occurrence screen.

adverse patient occurrence (APO) An untoward patient care event which, under optimal conditions, is not a natural consequence of the patient's disease or treatment. Examples include falls, burns, drug reactions, surgical and anesthesia mishaps, misdiagnoses, and unexpected disabilities and deaths. All APOs, from the patient who falls but is uninjured to the patient who dies from an anesthesia error, are events that *are not* desirable outcomes of optimal medical and organizational management. An APO is not the same as a PCE (potential compensable event) or negligence. *See also* accident; adverse; incident; negligence; occurrence; potentially compensable event.

adverse selection In health insurance, the disproportionate insurance of risks (individuals) who are poorer or more prone to suffer loss or make claims than the average risk (individual). Adverse selection may result from the tendency for poorer risks or less desirable insureds, such as chronically sick people, to seek or continue insurance to a greater extent than do better risks, such as healthy people, or from the tendency for the insured to take advantage of favorable options in insurance contracts. *Compare* skimming. *See also* adverse; health insurance; risk; selection.

advertise To announce, inform, or make known by any means whatsoever, as in hospital advertising. *See also* comparative advertising; competitive advertising; deceptive advertising; false advertising; image advertising; informative advertising; least-effort principle; target audience.

advertising, comparative *See* comparative advertising.

advertising, competitive *See* competitive advertising.

advertising, deceptive *See* deceptive advertising.

advertising, false *See* false advertising.

advertising, image *See* image advertising.

advertising, informative *See* informative advertising.

advice Opinion about what could or should be done about a situation or problem. *Synonym:* counsel. *See also* adviser; counselor; opinion.

adviser An individual who counsels or gives advice, as in the president's health care advisers. *See also* advice; counselor; facilitator; medical adviser.

adviser, medical *See* medical adviser.

Advisers, Council of Economic *See* Council of Economic Advisers.

Advisors for the Health Professions, National Association of *See* National Association of Advisors for the Health Professions.

Advisory Council for Health Care Policy, Research, and Evaluation, National *See* National Advisory Council for Health Care Policy, Research, and Evaluation.

Advisory Council for Orthopedic Resident Education (ACORE) A national organization founded in 1975 that fosters and develops medical orthopedic resident education. It provides consultation and supportive services to aid in the improvement of existing orthopedic residency programs and in the organization of new programs. None of the council's activities are directly or indirectly related to the act of accreditation or certification of orthopedic residency programs. *See also* accreditation; certification; orthopaedic/orthopedic surgery; residency.

advocacy The act of pleading or arguing in favor of something, such as a cause, an idea, or a policy. *See also* lobbying.

Advocacy, National Board of Trial *See* National Board of Trial Advocacy.

Advocacy, National Institute for Trial *See* National Institute for Trial Advocacy.

Advocates, American Board of Trial *See* American Board of Trial Advocates.

AEA *See* American Electrology Association.

AEEGS *See* American Electroencephalographic Society.

AEEP *See* Association of Environmental Engineering Professors.

aerobic Requiring oxygen; for example, aerobic exercises increase the efficiency with which the body takes in and uses oxygen. *Compare* anaerobic. *See also* aerobics.

aerobics A system of physical conditioning designed to enhance circulatory and respiratory efficiency. It involves vigorous, sustained exercise, such as jogging, stepping, swimming, or cycling, which improves the body's utilization of oxygen. *See also* aerobic; exercise; fitness; workout.

Aerobics Research, Institute for *See* Institute for Aerobics Research.

Aeromedical Transport Association, Professional *See* Professional Aeromedical Transport Association.

Aerospace Medical Association (AsMA) A national organization founded in 1929 composed of 4,200 medical and scientific personnel engaged in clinical, operational, and research activities in aviation, space, and environmental medicine. *See also* space medicine.

AES *See* American Endodontic Society; American Epidemiological Society; American Epilepsy Society; American Equilibration Society.

Aesculapius The mythical god or deified hero of healing; also known as Asclepios. The staff of Aesculapius is the official symbol of the medical profession. *See also* asclepion; caduceus; heal; Hippocratic oath; Hygeia; Panacea; staff of Aesculapius.

Aesculapius, staff of   *See* staff of Aesculapius.

Aesthetic Plastic Surgery, American Society for *See* American Society for Aesthetic Plastic Surgery.

AFA   *See* American Fitness Association; American Fracture Association.

AFAR   *See* American Federation for Aging Research.

AFB   *See* Association for Fitness in Business.

AFB isolation   *See* tuberculosis isolation.

AFCR   *See* American Federation for Clinical Research.

AFDC   *See* Aid to Families with Dependent Children.

AFDO   *See* Association of Food and Drug Officials.

Affairs Professionals Society, Regulatory *See* Regulatory Affairs Professionals Society.

affairs, public   *See* public affairs.

affect   **1.** The outward manifestation of emotion, feeling, or mood. *See also* affective; affective disorder; emotion; mood. **2.** To have an influence on or effect a change in, as in affecting the outcome.

affective   In psychology, influenced by or resulting from emotions, mood, or feeling, as in an affective disorder. *See also* affect; affective disorder; psychology.

affective disorder   A disorder of mood, feeling, or emotion. *See also* affective; major affective disorder; seasonal affective disorder.

affective disorder, major   *See* major affective disorder.

affective disorder, seasonal   *See* seasonal affective disorder.

affidavit   A voluntary statement of facts, or a voluntary declaration in writing of facts, that a person swears to be true before an official authorized to administer an oath. *See also* oath.

affiliated   A condition of being in close connection, allied, associated, or attached as a member or branch. An association of affiliated organizations, such as hospitals, often affords an economic advantage in large-scale purchasing. *See also* affiliated hospital; affiliation.

Affiliated/Associated Drug Stores   *See* Chain Drug Marketing Associates.

affiliated hospital   A hospital that is associated in some degree with another institution or program; for example, a medical school, shared services organization, multihospital system, or religious organization. *See also* affiliated; affiliation; hospital.

affiliation   A form of joint venture or cooperation in which competitors or others coordinate and integrate their activities without completely merging or consolidating. *See also* affiliated hospital; joint venture.

affinity diagram   An approach to organizing facts, opinions, and issues into natural groups by listing on cards inputs from knowledgeable people and then rearranging the cards until useful groups are identified. A display of the groups of cards that express related ideas is the affinity diagram.   *See also* diagram.

affirmative action   Steps taken to correct conditions resulting from past discrimination or from violations of a law, particularly with respect to employment. Any organization that contracts with the federal government for more than $10,000 in any one year must comply with laws that prohibit discrimination based on race and sex, discrimination against handicapped individuals, and discrimination against disabled veterans. *See also* action.

affirmative defense   A response to allegations in a complaint that constitutes a defense even if the allegations being pressed are true. In effect, an affirmative defense avoids all or part of the liability by presenting new evidence to avoid judgment, rather than by denying the facts alleged in the complaint. Common examples include the statute of limitations and the contributory negligence of the opposing party. *See also* complaint; statute of limitations.

AFHHA   *See* American Federation of Home Health Agencies.

AFIP   *See* Armed Forces Institute of Pathology.

AFMA   *See* American Federation of Medical Accreditation.

AFMH   *See* Association for Faculty in the Medical Humanities.

AFOS   *See* Armed Forces Optometric Society.

African-American Natural Foods Association (AANFA)   A national organization founded in 1990 composed of natural and health food retailers, health practitioners, manufacturers, and distributors concerned with increasing awareness of natural foods and the nutritional industry in minority communities. *See also* minority; natural food.

AFROC   *See* Association of Freestanding Radiation Oncology Centers.

AFS   *See* alternative financing system; American Fertility Society.

AFTA   *See* American Family Therapy Association.

after care (aftercare)   Postdischarge services designed to help a patient maintain and improve on the gains made during treatment; for example, a support group or counseling for chemically dependent or mentally ill persons following formal treatment. *See also* care.

AG   *See* Association for Gnotobiotics.

AGA   *See* American Gastroenterological Association; American Genetic Association.

against medical advice (AMA)   A type of discharge disposition that is patient-initiated and that is contrary to the advice of a treating physician; for example, a patient leaving an emergency department against medical advice. *Synonyms*: AMA; discharge against medical advice; elopement; non-return; patient dropout; run away; signing out AMA. *See also* discharge; disposition.

AGD   *See* Academy of General Dentistry.

age   The length of time a person has lived. *See also* age of consent; age of majority; automatic retirement age; chronological age; deferred retirement age; developmental age; aged person; early retirement age; functional age; legal age; mental age; middle age.

age, automatic retirement   *See* automatic retirement age.

age, chronological   *See* chronological age.

age of consent   **1.** Age at which persons may marry without parental approval. *See also* age. **2.** Age at which an individual is legally capable of agreeing to sexual intercourse; below the age of consent, it is considered statutory rape if sexual intercourse occurs. *See also* consent; sexual intercourse; statutory rape.

age, deferred retirement   *See* deferred retirement age.

age, developmental   *See* developmental age.

aged person   A person who is advanced in years; refers to his or her chronological, not mental age. *Synonym*: elderly.

age, early retirement   *See* early retirement age.

age, functional   *See* functional age.

age, legal   *See* legal age.

age of majority   The age when an individual is considered legally capable of being responsible for all his or her actions, such as entering into contracts, and becomes legally entitled to the rights generally held by citizens, such as voting. In most states, the age of majority was traditionally 21 years but is now generally 18 years, due at least in part to the enactment in 1972 of the 26th Amendment of the US Constitution, allowing 18-year-olds to vote in federal elections. The legal age for the consumption and

purchase of alcoholic beverages is generally 21 years, prompted by state compliance with federal highway funding requirements. *Synonym*: legal majority. *See also* age; emancipated minor; mature minor; minor.

age, mental   *See* mental age.

age, middle   *See* middle age.

Agencies on Aging, National Association of Area   *See* National Association of Area Agencies on Aging.

Agencies, American Federation of Home Health   *See* American Federation of Home Health Agencies.

Agencies, Association of Health Facility Survey   *See* Association of Health Facility Survey Agencies.

agency   **1.** A relationship between two parties, by agreement or otherwise, in which one (the agent) may act on behalf of the other (the principal) and bind the principal by words and actions. *See also* apparent agency. **2.** A private or public organization set up to perform services, such as a home health agency or a collection agency. *See also* administrative agency.

agency, administrative   *See* administrative agency.

agency, apparent   *See* apparent agency.

agency, collection   *See* collection agency.

Agency for Health Care Policy and Research (AHCPR)   An administrative agency created by federal legislation (Omnibus Budget Reconciliation Act of 1989) to enhance the quality, appropriateness, and effectiveness of health care services and access to such services through the establishment of a broad base of scientific research and through the promotion of improvements in clinical practice and in the organization, financing, and delivery of health care services. The AHCPR's mission incorporates that of the previous National Center for Health Services Research and Health Care Technology Assessment. Components of AHCPR include the Medical Treatment Effectiveness Program (MEDTEP), Center for Medical Effectiveness Research, Office of the Forum for Quality and Effectiveness in Health Care, Office of Science and Data Development, Center for Research Dissemination and Liaison, Center for General Health Services Extramural Research, Center for General Health Services Intramural Research, Office of Health Technology Assessment, and National Advisory Council for Health Care Policy, Research, and Evaluation. *See also* Physician Payment Reform.

agency, home health   *See* home health agency.

agency nurse　*See* pool nurse.

agency, organ procurement　*See* organ procurement agency.

agency, private health　*See* voluntary health agency.

agency, public　*See* administrative agency.

agency, regulatory　*See* regulatory agency.

agency, state health facility licensing　*See* state health facility licensing agency.

agency, state health planning and development　*See* state health planning and development agency.

agency, voluntary health　*See* voluntary health agency.

agenda　An order of business; a sequential listing of items or initiatives to be addressed during a meeting or over a defined time interval. *See also* Agenda for Change; hidden agenda; meeting; parliamentary procedure.

Agenda for Change　The research and development initiatives of the Joint Commission on Accreditation of Healthcare Organizations designed to make continuous improvement in patient outcomes and organizational performance the central and explicit objective of Joint Commission accreditation activities. It was initiated in 1987 and encompasses a recasting of Joint Commission standards to emphasize performance of important functions, improvements in survey and decision-making processes, and creation of a national accreditation reference data system based on well-tested indicators of organization performance. *See also* Joint Commission on Accreditation of Healthcare Organizations.

agenda, hidden　*See* hidden agenda.

age, normal retirement　*See* normal retirement age.

agent　**1.** A chemical or biological substance or an organism capable of producing an effect. *See also* therapeutic agent. **2.** In law, a party authorized to act on behalf of another (the principal) and to give the other an account of such actions. *See also* agency. **3.** An instrument or means by which something is done, often used to describe a person working within an organization. *See also* change agent.

agent, change　*See* change agent.

agent, therapeutic　*See* therapeutic agent.

age, retirement　*See* retirement age.

aggravated sexual abuse　*See* rape.

aggregate　Pertaining to an entire number or quantity of something; the total amount or complete whole. For example, aggregate survey data include the collection of data collected from all surveyed health care organizations during a specified time interval. *See also* aggregate data indicator; aggregate survey data.

aggregate data indicator　A performance measure based on collection and aggregation of data about many events or phenomena. The events or phenomena may be desirable or undesirable and the data may be reported as a continuous variable or a discrete variable. The two major types of aggregate data indicators are rate-based indicators (also called discrete variable indicators) and continuous variable indicators. *Compare* sentinel event indicator. *See also* aggregate; continuous variable indicator; indicator; performance measure; rate-based indicator.

aggregate survey data　Information on key performance areas and standards collected from surveyed health care organizations and combined to produce a database that contains accumulated information concerning the standards compliance performance of the organizations during a specific time interval. *See also* aggregate; data; performance area; survey.

aggregation　The process or act of gathering into a mass, sum, or whole, as in accreditation decision aggregation rules. *See also* accreditation decision aggregation; accreditation decision aggregation rules; aggregate survey data.

aggregation, accreditation decision　*See* accreditation decision aggregation.

aggregation algorithm　*See* accreditation decision aggregation rules.

aggregation rules　*See* accreditation decision aggregation rules.

AGH　*See* American Guild of Hypnotherapists.

aging　The process of growing old or maturing. *See also* geriatric medicine; gerontology.

Aging, American Association of Homes for the　*See* American Association of Homes for the Aging.

Aging, American Society on　*See* American Society on Aging.

Aging, Association for Adult Development and　*See* Association for Adult Development and Aging.

Aging, Center for the Study of　*See* Center for the Study of Aging.

Aging and Long Term Care Services, Special Constituency Section for　*See* Special Constituency Section for Aging and Long Term Care Services.

Aging, National Association of Area Agencies on　*See* National Association of Area Agencies on Aging.

Aging, National Association of State Units on *See* National Association of State Units on Aging.

Aging, National Center on Rural *See* National Center on Rural Aging.

Aging, National Council on the *See* National Council on the Aging.

Aging Organizations, Leadership Council of *See* Leadership Council of Aging Organizations.

Aging Research, Alliance for *See* Alliance for Aging Research.

Aging Research, American Federation for *See* American Federation for Aging Research.

Aging Services Programs, National Association of Nutrition and *See* National Association of Nutrition and Aging Services Programs.

aging, state unit on *See* state unit on aging.

AGLBIC *See* Association for Gay, Lesbian, and Bisexual Issues in Counseling.

AGLP *See* Association of Gay and Lesbian Psychiatrists.

agoraphobia Irrational fear of open space. *See also* phobia.

AGOS *See* American Gynecological and Obstetrical Society.

AGPA *See* American Group Practice Association; American Group Psychotherapy Association.

agreement **1.** Harmony of opinion or accord, as in complete agreement about the need for surgery. **2.** An arrangement between parties regarding a method of action, as in a transfer agreement. *See also* collective bargaining agreement; transfer agreement.

agreement, collective bargaining *See* collective bargaining agreement.

agreement, transfer *See* transfer agreement.

AGS *See* American Geriatrics Society.

AGSG *See* Alliance of Genetic Support Groups.

AHA *See* American Healing Association; American Heart Association; American Hospital Association; American Hypnosis Association; American Hypnotists' Association.

AHA Guide to the Health Care Field A directory of hospitals, multihospital systems, health-related organizations, and American Hospital Association (AHA) members published annually by the AHA. It includes selected data on hospitals, such as number of beds, payroll, personnel, admissions, and coded classification of facilities. *See also* American Hospital Association.

AHA Hospital Statistics An annual publication of the American Hospital Association containing agge-

grate data compiled from the American Hospital Association's annual survey of hospitals. *See also* *AHA Guide to the Health Care Field*; American Hospital Association.

AHC *See* Association of Academic Health Centers; Association for the History of Chiropractic.

AHCA *See* American Health Care Association.

AHCM *See* Academy of Hazard Control Management.

AHCPR *See* Agency for Health Care Policy and Research.

AHD *See* American Health Decisions.

AHFSA *See* Association of Health Facility Survey Agencies.

AHHAP *See* Association of Halfway House Alcoholism Programs of North America.

AHIA *See* Association of Healthcare Internal Auditors.

AHIMA *See* American Health Information Management Association.

AHLC *See* American Hair Loss Council.

AHMA *See* American Holistic Medical Association.

AHME *See* Association of Hospital Medical Education.

AHNA *See* American Holistic Nurses Association.

AHP *See* Association for Healthcare Philanthropy; Association for Humanistic Psychology.

AHPA *See* American Health Planning Association; Arthritis Health Professions Association.

AHRA *See* American Healthcare Radiology Administrators.

AHSM *See* Academy for Health Services Marketing.

AHSR *See* Association for Health Services Research.

AHTA *See* American Horticultural Therapy Association.

AI *See* artificial intelligence.

AIBS *See* American Institute of Biological Sciences.

AICCP *See* Association of the Institute for Certification of Computer Professionals.

AICPA *See* American Institute of Certified Public Accountants.

AID *See* artificial insemination-donor.

Aid to the Blind A federal government categorical assistance program that includes financial assistance to states to help them provide medical aid to the blind. *See also* blindness.

aide An assistant (for example, a home health aide, nurse's aide, or psychiatric aide) with less training than the person (such as a registered nurse or physician assistant) being assisted. Aides in health care may perform tasks, such as changing clothes, diapers, and beds; assisting patients to perform exercises or personal hygiene tasks; and supporting communication or social interaction. Specific credentials and education are typically not required for this work. *See also* case aide; home health aide; nursing assistant; psychiatric aide; rehabilitation counselor aide; sanitarian aide; social service aide; speech and hearing therapy aide.

aide, case *See* case aide.

aide, home health *See* home health aide.

aide, home health care *See* home health aide.

aid, electronic hearing *See* hearing aid.

aide, nurse *See* nursing assistant.

aide, nurse's *See* nursing assistant.

aide, nursing *See* nursing assistant.

aide program, health *See* health aide program.

aide, psychiatric *See* psychiatric aide.

aide, rehabilitation counselor *See* rehabilitation counselor aide.

aide, sanitarian *See* sanitarian aide.

aide, social service *See* social service aide.

aide, speech and hearing therapy *See* speech and hearing therapy aide.

Aid to Families with Dependent Children (ADC or AFDC) A federally financed program that provides welfare for single parents who cannot otherwise take adequate care of their children.

aid, hearing *See* hearing aid.

aid, pharmaceutical *See* pharmaceutical necessity.

AIDS *See* acquired immunodeficiency syndrome.

AIDS Care, Association of Nurses in *See* Association of Nurses in AIDS Care.

AIDS Clearinghouse, CDC National *See* CDC National AIDS Clearinghouse.

AIDS Clinical Trials Group (ACTG) A federal government-administered program of the National Institutes of Health AIDS researchers. It coordinates testing of experimental drugs used in AIDS treatment and seeks to enroll HIV-infected individuals in experimental AIDS treatment programs. *See also* acquired immunodeficiency syndrome; clinical trial.

AIDS Coalition, Pediatric *See* Pediatric AIDS Coalition.

AIDS Council, National Minority *See* National Minority AIDS Council.

AIDS, Haitian Coalition on *See* Haitian Coalition on AIDS.

AIDS, National Leadership Coalition on *See* National Leadership Coalition on AIDS.

AIDS Policy, Americans for a Sound *See* Americans for a Sound AIDS Policy.

AIDS Program, HIV/ *See* HIV/AIDS Program.

AIDS-related complex (ARC) A complex in which many symptoms and signs of AIDS are present in an individual but no opportunistic infection or cancer is identified, except for HIV infection. ARC is usually a wasting syndrome that may include weight loss, fever, fatigue, lymph node enlargement, and diarrhea. *See also* acquired immunodeficiency syndrome; HIV infection.

AIDS virus *See* HIV.

AIH *See* American Institute of Homeopathy; artificial insemination-husband.

AIHA *See* American Industrial Hygiene Association.

AIHC *See* American Industrial Health Council.

AIHCA *See* American Indian Health Care Association.

AIHP *See* American Institute of the History of Pharmacy.

ailment Indisposition of the body or mind; a slight illness. *See also* illness.

AIM *See* American Institute of Management; Association for Information Management; Automatic Identification Manufacturers.

AIN *See* American Institute of Nutrition.

AIOB *See* American Institute of Oral Biology.

AIR *See* American Institutes for Research in the Behavioral Sciences.

airborne infection A transmission mechanism of an infectious agent by particles, dust, or droplet nuclei suspended in the air. *See also* infection; transmission.

aircraft, fixed-wing *See* ambulance.

Air Force Flight Surgeons, Society of United States *See* Society of United States Air Force Flight Surgeons.

Air Force Physicians, Society of *See* Society of Air Force Physicians.

AirLifeLine (ALL) A national organization founded in 1979 composed of 350 pilots who donate their time, skills, fuel, and aircraft to fly medical missions. It provides immediate transport for medical cargo, such as blood, platelets, corneas, and human organs for transplantation, or for needy patients who require specialized treatment at medical facilities far from their homes. *See also* ambulance.

Airlift, Mercy Medical *See* Mercy Medical Airlift.

Air Medical Services, Association of *See* Association of Air Medical Services.

Air National Guard Health Technicians, National Association of *See* National Association of Air National Guard Health Technicians.

airway **1.** A route for passage of atmospheric air into and out of the lungs, formed by the oral and nasal cavities, the pharynx, larynx, trachea, and bronchi. *See also* cricothyreotomy; cricothyrotomy; lung; trachea; tracheotomy. **2.** A tubular device for securing an unobstructed passageway to the lungs to ventilate the lungs, administer anesthesia, prevent aspiration of secretions, and/or prevent entrance of foreign material, such as stomach contents, from spilling into the lungs. *See also* endotracheal tube; intubation; mechanical airway; trachea.

airway, mechanical *See* mechanical airway.

AIS *See* abbreviated injury scale; American Institute of Stress.

AIT *See* Academy for Implants and Transplants.

AIUM *See* American Institute of Ultrasound in Medicine.

AJCC *See* American Joint Committee on Cancer.

AKA *See* American Kinesiotherapy Association.

ALA *See* American Longevity Association; American Lung Association.

albumin The major protein in blood plasma (approximately 60% of the total), which is responsible for much of the plasma colloidal osmotic pressure. It functions as a transport protein carrying large organic anions, such as fatty acids, bilirubin, and many drugs. It is made in the liver. Low levels of albumin occur in protein malnutrition, active inflammation, and serious liver and kidney disease. *See also* blood plasma.

alcohol An intoxicating liquor containing ethanol. *See also* alcoholism; ethanol; intoxication; potomania.

alcohol concentration, blood *See* blood alcohol concentration.

Alcohol and Drug Abuse Directors, National Association of State *See* National Association of State Alcohol and Drug Abuse Directors.

Alcohol, Drug Abuse, and Mental Health Administration *See* Substance Abuse and Mental Health Services Administration.

Alcohol and Drugs, National Episcopal Coalition on *See* National Episcopal Coalition on Alcohol and Drugs.

alcoholic An individual who drinks alcoholic substances habitually and excessively or who suffers from alcoholism. *See also* alcoholism; potomania.

Alcoholics Anonymous World Services (AA) An international organization founded in 1935 to provide supportive rehabilitation for persons with alcoholism. Local chapters are voluntarily staffed by persons formerly affected by alcoholism who have achieved abstinence through application of the organization's philosophy, principles, and methods. AA maintains that members can solve their common problems and help others achieve sobriety through a twelve-step program that includes sharing their experience, strength, and hope with each other. AA is self-supported through members' contributions and is not allied with any sect, denomination, political organization, or institution. It does not endorse or oppose any cause. *See also* abstinence; alcoholism.

alcoholism **1.** The compulsive consumption of and psychophysiological dependence on alcoholic beverages. **2.** A chronic, progressive pathological condition affecting multiple systems, especially the nervous and digestive systems. It is caused by the excessive and habitual consumption of alcohol. *See also* alcohol; alcoholism and other drug dependence; ethanol; intoxication; potomania.

Alcoholism and Addictions, American Academy of Psychiatrists in *See* American Academy of Psychiatrists in Alcoholism and Addictions.

Alcoholism, American Council on *See* American Council on Alcoholism.

Alcoholism Council, National Black *See* National Black Alcoholism Council.

Alcoholism and Drug Abuse Counselor Credentialing Bodies, National Commission on Accreditation of *See* National Commission on Accreditation of Alcoholism and Drug Abuse Counselor Credentialing Bodies.

Alcoholism and Drug Abuse Counselors, National Association of *See* National Association of Alcoholism and Drug Abuse Counselors.

Alcoholism and Drug Dependence, National Council on *See* National Council on Alcoholism and Drug Dependence.

alcoholism and other drug dependence A chronic disease characterized by a pathological pattern of alcohol and/or other drug use that causes serious impairment in social and/or occupational functioning. *See also* addiction; alcoholism; drug; psychotropic drug.

Alcoholism and Other Drug Abuse, National Certification Reciprocity Consortium/ *See* National Certification Reciprocity Consortium/Alcoholism and Other Drug Abuse.

Alcoholism Programs of North America, Association of Halfway House *See* Association of Halfway House Alcoholism Programs of North America.

Alcoholism Professionals, National Association of Lesbian/Gay *See* National Association of Lesbian/Gay Alcoholism Professionals.

alcoholism rehabilitation center A facility with an organized professional and trained staff that provides rehabilitative services to alcoholic patients. *See also* alcoholism; rehabilitation; rehabilitation center.

Alcoholism and Related Drug Problems, National Catholic Council on *See* National Catholic Council on Alcoholism and Related Drug Problems.

Alcoholism, Research Society on *See* Research Society on Alcoholism.

alcoholism treatment service An organizational unit or service for the diagnosis and treatment of alcoholism that does not offer rehabilitation services. *See also* alcoholism; service; treatment.

Alcohol Nursing Association, Drug and *See* Drug and Alcohol Nursing Association.

Alcohol Problems, American Council on *See* American Council on Alcohol Problems.

aleatory contract A contract with effects and results that depend on an uncertain event; for example, life and fire insurance are aleatory contracts. *See also* contract.

algorithm An ordered sequence of steps or instructions, with each step or instruction depending on the outcome of the previous one, that is used to tell how to solve a particular problem. An algorithm is specified exactly, so there can be no doubt about what to do next, and it has a finite number of steps. *Compare* heuristic. *See also* aggregation algorithm; clinical algorithm; computer algorithm; decision tree; flowchart.

algorithm, aggregation *See* accreditation decision aggregation rules.

algorithm, clinical *See* clinical algorithm.

algorithm, computer *See* computer algorithm.

alien FMG Abbreviation for alien foreign medical graduate. *See* foreign medical graduate.

alien foreign medical graduate *See* foreign medical graduate.

alimentary tract The mucous membrane-lined tube of the digestive system through which food passes, in which digestion takes place, and from which wastes are eliminated. It extends from the mouth to the anus and includes the pharynx, esophagus, stomach, and intestine. *Synonyms*: digestive tract; gastrointestinal tract. *See also* alimentation; digestion; esophagus; gastroenterology; intestine; rectum; stomach; tract.

Alimentary Tract, Society for Surgery of the *See* Society for Surgery of the Alimentary Tract.

alimentation The act or process of giving or receiving nourishment. *See also* alimentary tract; food; nutrition.

ALL *See* AirLifeLine.

allegation **1.** A statement asserting something without proof, as in an allegation of wrongdoing. **2.** The position of a party to a lawsuit, stated in the pleadings. *See also* alleged; lawsuit; pleadings.

alleged Represented as being as described, but not proved, as in an alleged wrongdoing. *See also* allegation.

allergist A physician who specializes in the diagnosis and treatment of allergic and immunologic conditions. *See* allergy and immunology; immunology.

Allergists, American Association of Certified *See* American Association of Certified Allergists.

allergy A state of hypersensitivity induced by exposure to a particular antigen (allergen) resulting in harmful immunologic reactions on subsequent exposures. The term is usually used to refer to hypersensitivity to an environmental antigen (atopic allergy or contact dermatitis) or to drug allergy. *See also* allergy and immunology; desensitization; drug allergy; hay fever; pollen; sneezing.

Allergy, American Academy of Otolaryngic *See* American Academy of Otolaryngic Allergy.

allergy, drug *See* drug allergy.

allergy and immunology The branch of medicine and medical specialty dealing with the evaluation, physical and laboratory diagnosis, and management of disorders potentially involving the immune system. Examples of such conditions include asthma; anaphylaxis; rhinitis; eczema; urticaria; adverse reactions to drugs, foods, and insect stings; immune deficiency diseases (both acquired and congenital); defects in host defense; and problems related to autoimmune disease, organ transplantation, or malignancies of the immune system. *See also* allergy; anaphylaxis; asthma; immunology; transplantation.

Allergy and Immunology, American Academy of *See* American Academy of Allergy and Immunology.

Allergy and Immunology, American Board of *See* American Board of Allergy and Immunology.

Allergy and Immunology, American College of *See* American College of Allergy and Immunology.

Allergy and Immunology, American Osteopathic College of *See* American Osteopathic College of Allergy and Immunology.

Allergy and Immunology, Joint Council of *See* Joint Council of Allergy and Immunology.

Allergy Society, Pan American *See* Pan American Allergy Society.

Alliance for Aging Research (AAR) A nonmembership organization founded in 1986 composed of gerontologists and other medical professionals, executives, and members of Congress concerned with increasing private and public research into aging. *See also* aging; gerontology.

Alliance for Alternatives in Healthcare (AAH) A national organization founded in 1983 composed of 1,000 holistic physicians, corporations, and other individuals seeking to enhance public recognition of holistic, homeopathic, naturopathic, chiropractic, and acupuncture treatments. *See also* acupuncture; chiropractic; holistic health; holistic medicine; homeopathy; naturopathy.

alliance area According to the proposed Health Security Act (1993), an area served by a regional alliance. *See also* Health Security Act; regional alliance.

Alliance for Cannabis Therapeutics (ACT) A national organization founded in 1980 composed of medical professionals, policymakers, and lay persons who support the medical use of cannabis (marijuana) in treating the side effects of chemotherapy experienced by some cancer patients, and in aiding glaucoma, AIDS, and multiple sclerosis patients. It works to end federal prohibition of cannabis in medicine and to construct a medically meaningful, ethically correct and compassionate system of regulation which permits the seriously ill to legally obtain cannabis. *See also* cannabis; drug side effect; therapeutics.

alliance, corporate *See* corporate alliance.

alliance eligible individual, corporate *See* corporate alliance eligible individual.

alliance eligible individual, regional *See* regional alliance eligible individual.

alliance employer, corporate *See* corporate alliance employer.

alliance employer, regional *See* regional alliance employer.

Alliance to End Childhood Lead Poisoning A nonmembership public interest organization founded in 1990 concerned with the elimination of childhood lead poisoning. It seeks to raise awareness of and change preconceptions about the causes and widespread occurrence of childhood lead poisoning. *See also* lead; poison; saturnism.

Alliance of Genetic Support Groups (AGSG) A national organization founded in 1985 composed of 334 voluntary genetic organizations and professional and other individuals interested in promoting the health and well-being of individuals and families affected by genetic disorders. It fosters a partnership among consumers and professionals to enhance education and service for, and represent the needs of, individuals affected by genetic disorders. *See also* genetic disease; genetics.

alliance, health *See* health alliance.

alliance, health care *See* health alliance.

alliance, health insurance purchasing *See* health alliance.

alliance health plan, corporate *See* corporate alliance health plan.

alliance health plan, regional *See* regional alliance health plan.

alliance, large-employer *See* large-employer alliance.

Alliance for the Prudent Use of Antibiotics (APUA) A national organization founded in 1981 composed of 600 physicians, scientists, medical and public health personnel, and other individuals supporting prudent use of antibiotics. It believes that extensive use of antibiotics leads to development of resistant strains of pathogenic and common, nonpathogenic bacteria with resistance traits transferable from one bacterium to others. These resistant strains are no longer susceptible to antibiotics and therefore can undermine treatment of infectious bacterial diseases. The APUA defines good use of antibiotics, informs and educates the public about the dangers of misusing and overusing antibiotics and other antimicrobial agents, and provides data to individuals and organizations interested in preventing antibiotic misuse and overuse. *See also* antibiotic; bacteria; infectious diseases; plasmid; prudence.

alliance, purchasing *See* health alliance.

alliance, regional　*See* regional alliance.

alliance, regional health　*See* regional alliance.

alliance, regional purchasing　*See* regional alliance.

Allied, American Urological Association　*See* American Urological Association Allied.

Allied Health Education and Accreditation, Committee on　*See* Committee on Allied Health Education and Accreditation.

allied health personnel　*See* allied health professional.

Allied Health Personnel in Ophthalmology, Joint Commission on　*See* Joint Commission on Allied Health Personnel in Ophthalmology.

allied health profession　*See* paraprofession.

allied health professional　A health professional qualified by training and frequently by licensure to assist, facilitate, or complement the work of physicians, dentists, podiatrists, nurses, pharmacists, and other specialists in the health care system. For example, a specialist in blood bank technology and a emergency medical technician (EMT) are allied health professionals. *Synonyms*: allied health personnel; allied health specialist; paramedical personnel; paraprofessionals. *See also* health professional; licensure; paraprofession.

Allied Health Professionals, American Board of Urologic　*See* American Board of Urologic Allied Health Professionals.

Allied Health Professions, American Society of　*See* American Society of Allied Health Professions.

allied health specialist　*See* allied health professional.

allocation　Assignment or allotment, as in allocation of hospital resources or cost allocation. *See also* cost allocation; resource allocation.

allocation, cost　*See* cost allocation.

allocation of resources　*See* resource allocation.

allograft　A transplant of an organ or tissues between non-identical individuals of the same species, formerly termed homograft. Most organ transplants today, such as kidney and liver transplants, are allografts. *Synonyms*: allogeneic graft; homograft. *See also* organ; transplant.

allopathic medicine　*See* allopathy.

allopathic physician　A physician who practices allopathic medicine and views his or her role as an active interventionist who should attempt to counteract the effect of a disease by using surgical or medical treatments to produce effects opposite those

of the disease. Most American physicians with a Doctor of Medicine (MD) degree practice allopathic medicine. *See also* allopathy; intervention; physician.

allopathy　A system of medicine based on the theory that successful therapy, either medical or surgical, depends on actively creating a condition antagonistic to or incompatible with the condition to be treated. For example, drugs, such as antibiotics, are given to combat diseases caused by the microorganisms to which the antibiotics are antagonistic. *Compare* homeopathy; naprapathy; naturopathy; osteopathic medicine. *See also* allopathic physician; health intervention; intervention.

alloplastic　Pertaining to an inert foreign body used for implantation into tissue. *See also* implant; implantation; plastic surgery.

allowable cost　A cost incurred by a health care provider during the course of providing services that is recognized as payable by a third-party payer. *See also* cost; third-party payer.

all-payer system　A system in which prices for health services and payment methods are the same, regardless of who is paying. For instance, in an all-payer system, the government, a private insurer, a big company, an individual, or any other payer, pays the same rates, usually set by a government agency, for specific health services. The uniform fee bars health care providers from shifting costs from one payer to another (for example, those more able to pay). *See also* cost shifting; payer; single-payer system.

ALMI　*See* American Leprosy Missions.

alopecia　Loss of hair from the head or other normally hair-bearing areas. *See also* dermatology.

ALOS　*See* average length of stay.

alpha error　*See* type I error.

Alpha Omega Alpha (AOA)　An honor society founded in 1902 composed of 70,000 men and women in medicine at graduate and postgraduate levels. It sponsors professorships, offers student research fellowships, and sponsors the "Leaders in American Medicine" videotape series. *See also* physician.

ALPNA　*See* American Licensed Practical Nurses Association.

ALROS　*See* American Laryngological, Rhinological and Otological Society.

ALS　Abbreviation for advanced life support. *See* advanced cardiac life support.

ALS unit　An emergency ground vehicle (ambulance) usually staffed by two emergency medical technician-paramedics and stocked with intravenous fluids, cardiac monitor, defibrillation equipment, certain medications, and system-approved telecommunication. *See also* advanced cardiac life support; defibrillation; emergency medical technician-paramedic; ambulance; mobile intensive care unit.

alteration A change or a difference, as in fraudulent alteration of a medical record.

alternative Offering a different approach from the conventional or established one, as in an alternative delivery system. *See also* alternative delivery system; alternative dental delivery system; alternative financing system; alternative hypothesis; alternative level of care; alternative medicine; alternative reproduction; choice; option.

alternative delivery system (ADS) Any system that delivers health care on a basis other than fee-for-service by integrating financing issues with patient care issues. *See also* alternative; alternative dental delivery system; fee for service; fee-for-service plan.

alternative dental delivery system (ADDS) A dental care delivery and financing approach distinguishable from payment of fees and charges to independent and unselected dental providers. *See also* alternative delivery system.

alternative financing system (AFS) A structured health care financing mode that is distinguishable from the traditional fee-for-service approach. Capitation through a health maintenance organization (HMO), for example, is an alternative financing system to fee for service. *See also* alternative delivery system; fee for service.

Alternative Health Care Policy, National Council on *See* National Council on Alternative Health Care Policy.

alternative hypothesis In statistical testing, the hypothesis accepted if a sample contains sufficient evidence to reject the null hypothesis. In most cases, the alternative hypothesis is the expected conclusion, that is, why the test was completed in the first place. *See also* alternative; hypothesis; null hypothesis; statistics.

alternative level of care Care provided to patients who are no longer in the acute phase of care, but who require restorative services. *See also* alternative; level of care.

Alternative Medical Association (AMA) A nation-

al organization founded in 1978 to prepare and distribute two six-year, home-study degree programs in herbal medicine and holistic nutrition. *See also* alternative medicine; holistic medicine; medical association.

alternative medicine Systems of therapeutics that differ from orthodox medical care. *See also* acupuncture; acupressure; allopathy; herbalism; holistic medicine; homeopathy; naprapathy; naturopathy; osteopathic medicine.

alternative reproduction Technologies, such as artificial insemination, that promote conception and pregnancy. *See also* artificial reproduction; conception; noncoital reproduction; pregnancy.

Alternatives in Healthcare, Alliance for *See* Alliance for Alternatives in Healthcare.

altitude sickness *See* mountain sickness.

altruism The act of generosity and unselfishness in which a duty is not involved. The donation of blood or a kidney is an example of altruism, not duty. *See also* duty; supererogation.

Alzheimer's disease The most common cause of dementia, marked by progressive loss of mental capacity over a period of years resulting from degeneration of brain cells. Named after Alois Alzheimer (1864-1915), a German neurologist. *See also* dementia; disease.

AMA *See* against medical advice; Alternative Medical Association; American Management Association; American Medical Association.

AMAA *See* American Medical Athletic Association.

AMAHC *See Accreditation Manual for Ambulatory Health Care.*

amalgam Any alloy of mercury. Amalgams are widely used in dental fillings. *See also* dentistry; filling.

ambulance An emergency vehicle used for transporting patients to a health care facility after injury or illness. Types of ambulances used in the United States include ground (surface) ambulance, rotor-wing (helicopter), and fixed-wing aircraft (airplane). *See also* ALS unit; BLS unit; emergency medical services system; emergency medical technician; emergency medical technician-paramedic; emergency services; medevac; medicar; mobile intensive care unit.

Ambulance Association, American *See* American Ambulance Association.

ambulance attendant *See* emergency medical technician; emergency medical technician-paramedic.

ambulance chaser **1.** A person who solicits negligence cases for an attorney for a fee or in consideration of a percentage of the recovery. *See also* attorney. **2.** An attorney who, on hearing of a personal injury that may have been caused by the negligence or wrongful act of another, at once seeks out the injured person with a view to securing authority to bring action on behalf of the injured. *See also* ambulance; lawyer.

ambulatory Walking or capable of walking about. *Synonym*: ambulant. *See also* ambulatory health care; ambulatory surgery; ambulatory surgical facility; ambulatory visit group.

ambulatory care *See* ambulatory health care.

Ambulatory Care Accreditation Program The survey and accreditation program of the Joint Commission on Accreditation of Healthcare Organizations for eligible ambulatory health care organizations, including the following types: ambulatory care clinics; ambulatory surgery centers; college or university health centers; group practices; armed services ambulatory health care organizations; cardiac catheterization centers; Native American health service centers; primary care centers; and urgent/emergency care centers. *See also Accreditation Manual for Ambulatory Health Care*; ambulatory health care; Joint Commission on Accreditation of Healthcare Organizations; program.

ambulatory care center *See* freestanding ambulatory care center.

ambulatory care center, hospital-based *See* hospital-based ambulatory care center.

Ambulatory Care, Division of *See* Division of Ambulatory Care.

Ambulatory Care, National Association for *See* National Association for Ambulatory Care.

Ambulatory Care, Society for the Advancement of *See* Society for the Advancement of Ambulatory Care.

Ambulatory Foot Surgery, Academy of *See* Academy of Ambulatory Foot Surgery.

ambulatory health care All types of health services provided to patients who are not confined to an institutional bed as inpatients during the time services are rendered. Ambulatory care services are provided in many settings ranging from freestanding ambulatory surgical facilities to cardiac catheterization centers. *See also* ambulatory; ambulatory

surgery; mobile health unit; outpatient care.

Ambulatory Health Care, Accreditation Association for *See* Accreditation Association for Ambulatory Health Care.

Ambulatory Health Care, Accreditation Manual for *See* Accreditation Manual for Ambulatory Health Care.

Ambulatory Health Care Accreditation Program *See* Ambulatory Care Accreditation Program.

Ambulatory Health Care Administration, Center for Research in *See* Center for Research in Ambulatory Health Care Administration.

Ambulatory Nursing Administration, American Academy of *See* American Academy of Ambulatory Nursing Administration.

ambulatory inpatient An inpatient who is able to walk about and does not require confinement to a bed. *See also* ambulatory health care; inpatient.

Ambulatory Pediatric Association (APA) A national organization founded in 1960 composed of 1,200 health care providers interested in the care of children in ambulatory care facilities, such as outpatient departments in private university and other teaching hospitals and those engaged in public health work or private practice. *See also* ambulatory health care; pediatrics.

Ambulatory Plastic Surgery Facilities, American Association for Accreditation of *See* American Association for Accreditation of Ambulatory Plastic Surgery Facilities.

ambulatory surgery Surgical services provided for patients who are admitted and discharged on the day of surgery. Examples of ambulatory surgery procedures include arthroscopy and hernia repair. *Synonyms*: in-and-out surgery; outpatient surgery; same-day surgery. *See also* ambulatory health care; ambulatory surgical facility; freestanding ambulatory surgical facility; surgery.

Ambulatory Surgery Association, Federated *See* Federated Ambulatory Surgery Association.

ambulatory surgery center *See* ambulatory surgical facility.

ambulatory surgical facility A freestanding or a hospital-based facility, with an organized professional staff, that provides surgical services to patients who do not require an inpatient bed. *Synonyms*: ambulatory surgery center; surgical center; surgicenter. *See also* freestanding ambulatory surgical facility.

ambulatory surgical facility, freestanding *See* freestanding ambulatory surgical facility.

ambulatory visit group (AVG) A counterpart of the diagnosis-related group (DRG) classification but designed for use in ambulatory care settings, rather than hospital settings. *See also* ambulatory; diagnosis-related groups.

AMCHP *See* Association of Maternal and Child Health Programs.

AMCPA *See* American Managed Care Pharmacy Association.

AMCRA *See* American Managed Care and Review Association.

AMDA *See* American Medical Directors Association.

AMDM *See* Association of Microbiological Diagnostic Manufacturers.

AMEEGA *See* American Medical Electroencephalographic Association.

amenorrhea Abnormal suppression or absence of menstruation. *See also* menstruation; pregnancy; pseudocyesis.

American Academy of Actuaries (AAA) A national organization founded in 1965 composed of 10,000 actuaries. It promulgates standards and facilitates interrelations between actuaries and government bodies. *See also* actuarial science; actuary; standard.

American Academy of Allergy *See* American Academy of Allergy and Immunology.

American Academy of Allergy and Immunology (AAAI) A national organization founded in 1943 composed of 4,200 physicians specializing in allergy and immunology. Formerly (1982) American Academy of Allergy. *See also* allergy and immunology.

American Academy of Ambulatory Nursing Administration (AAANA) A national organization founded in 1978 composed of 1,000 nurses with administrative/management responsibilities in ambulatory care. *See also* administration; ambulatory health care; nursing.

American Academy for Cerebral Palsy and Developmental Medicine (AACPDM) A national organization founded in 1947 composed of 1,800 physicians, researchers, and health professionals interested in the diagnosis, care, treatment, and research of cerebral palsy and developmental disabilities and with acceptance of the challenges caused by these conditions. Associate members are occupational, physical, and speech therapists. *See also* cerebral palsy; developmental disability.

American Academy of Child Psychiatry *See* American Academy of Child and Adolescent Psychiatry.

American Academy of Child and Adolescent Psychiatry (AACAP) A national organization founded in 1953 composed of 5,000 physicians who have completed five years of residency in child and adolescent psychiatry. It seeks to stimulate and advance medical contributions to the knowledge and treatment of psychiatric illnesses of children and adolescents. Formerly (1986) American Academy of Child Psychiatry. *See also* child and adolescent psychiatry; residency.

American Academy of Clinical Psychiatrists (AACP) A national organization founded in 1975 composed of 600 practicing board-prepared or board-certified psychiatrists who promote the scientific practice of psychiatric medicine. *See also* psychiatry.

American Academy of Clinical Toxicology (AACT) A national organization founded in 1968 composed of 400 physicians, veterinarians, pharmacists, research scientists, and analytical chemists interested in clinical toxicology. *See also* medical toxicology.

American Academy of Compensation Medicine *See* American Society of Legal and Industrial Medicine.

American Academy of Cosmetic Surgery (AACS) A national organization founded in 1985 composed of 1,250 licensed cosmetic surgeons. It seeks to encourage high-quality cosmetic medical and dental care and provides continuing education for cosmetic surgeons. It operates the American Board of Cosmetic Surgery. *See also* continuing education; cosmetic surgery; plastic surgery.

American Academy of Crisis Interveners (AACI) A national organization founded in 1977 composed of 200 professionals from the fields of mental health, law enforcement, education, religion, and medicine whose work causes them to deal with behavioral and psychological crises and emergencies. It sponsors training institutes and workshops and provides instructors in all areas of crisis intervention. *See also* crisis; intervention.

American Academy of Crown and Bridge Prosthodontics *See* American Academy of Fixed Prosthodontics.

American Academy of Dental Electrosurgery (AADE) A national organization founded in 1963 composed of 200 dentists who are qualified by special training to use electrosurgery therapeutically and research scientists who investigate the behavior of the therapeutic electrosurgical high-frequency currents and their effects on oral structures. It promotes the introduction of instruction in dental electrosurgery at the undergraduate basic science and clinical levels and the improvement of electronic circuitry and clinical techniques. *See also* dentistry; electrotherapy.

American Academy of Dental Group Practice (AADGP) A national organization founded in 1973 composed of 1,600 dentists and dental group practices interested in practice management and treatment in group practice settings. *See also* dentistry; group practice.

American Academy of Dental Practice Administration (AADPA) A national organization founded in 1958 composed of 250 dentists interested in efficient administration of dental practice. *See also* administration; dentistry.

American Academy of Dental Radiology *See* American Academy of Oral and Maxillofacial Radiology.

American Academy of Dermatology (AAD) A national organization founded in 1938 composed of 8,800 physicians specializing in skin diseases. It conducts educational programs and provides placement services. *See also* dermatology.

American Academy of Disability Evaluating Physicians (AADEP) A national organization founded in 1987 composed of 500 physicians interested in performance of disability evaluations. *See also* disability; physician.

American Academy of Environmental Engineers (AAEE) A national organization founded in 1955 composed of 2,600 environmentally-oriented registered engineers certified by examination as diplomates of the academy. It recognizes the following areas of specialization: air pollution control, hazardous waste management, industrial hygiene, radiation protection, solid waste management, water supply, and wastewater. *See also* engineer; environmental health; hazardous waste.

American Academy of Environmental Medicine (AAEM) A national organization founded in 1965 composed of 450 physicians, engineers, and others interested in the clinical aspect of environmental medicine. *See also* environmental health.

American Academy of Facial Plastic and Reconstructive Surgery (AAFPRS) A national organization founded in 1964 composed of 3,200 physicians specializing in facial plastic surgery. *See also* plastic surgery.

American Academy of Family Physicians (AAFP) A national organization founded in 1947 composed of approximately 60,000 family physicians who provide continuing comprehensive care to patients. It sponsors continuing medical education, bestows awards, and maintains placement services. *See also* family physician; family practice.

American Academy of Family Physicians, Fellow of *See* Fellow of the American Academy of Family Physicians.

American Academy of Federal Civil Service Physicians *See* Federal Physicians Association.

American Academy of Fixed Prosthodontics (AACBP) A national organization founded in 1952 composed of 485 dentists. It provides a two-day professional continuing education course in the specialty of fixed prosthodontics. Formerly (1991) American Academy of Crown and Bridge Prosthodontics. *See also* bridge; continuing education; crown; prosthodontics.

American Academy of Forensic Psychology (AAFP) A national organization founded in 1980 composed of individuals who have met requirements, including passing an examination, set by the American Board of Professional Psychology. *See also* American Board of Professional Psychology; forensic sciences; psychology.

American Academy of Forensic Sciences (AAFS) A national organization founded in 1948 composed of 3,500 criminalists, scientists, members of the bench and bar, pathologists, biologists, psychiatrists, examiners of questioned documents, toxicologists, odontologists, anthropologists, and engineers interested in improving the practice and elevating the standards of forensic sciences. *See also* forensic sciences.

American Academy of Gnathologic Orthopedics (AAGO) A national organization founded in 1970 composed of 400 dentists dealing with the prevention or correction of malocclusion and bony malformation of the jaw and face. *See also* dentistry; gnathic.

American Academy of Gold Foil Operators (AAGFO) A national organization founded in 1950 composed of 400 dentists who perform restorative procedures using gold foil and the rubber dam. It formulates and applies new ideas for research on gold foil and the rubber dam and encourages members of the dental profession and research institutions to study gold foil and rubber dam procedures. *See also* dentistry.

American Academy of Head, Facial and Neck Pain and TMJ Orthopedics A national organization founded in 1985 composed of 200 dentists who treat head, facial, and neck pain. It functions as a referral service for patients suffering from head, facial, and neck pain. *See also* dentistry; temporomandibular joint syndrome.

American Academy of the History of Dentistry (AAHD) A national organization founded in 1951 composed of 600 individuals seeking to stimulate interest, study, and research in the history of dentistry and promote the teaching of dental history. *See also* dentistry; history.

American Academy of Hospital Attorneys (AAHA) A national organization founded in 1968 composed of 2,700 attorneys who represent or are employees of hospitals or other health care organizations. Formerly (1984) American Society of Hospital Attorneys. *See also* hospital attorney.

American Academy of Husband-Coached Childbirth (AAHCC) A for-profit organization founded in 1970 composed of 1,200 individuals. It trains instructors in the Bradley method of natural childbirth. *See also* natural childbirth.

American Academy of Implant Dentistry (AAID) A national organization founded in 1952 composed of 2,300 dentists interested in furthering scientific research and development in the field of implantology. *See also* implant dentistry; prosthodontics.

American Academy of Implant Prosthodontics (AAIP) A national organization founded in 1980 composed of 300 experts in implant dentistry. It encourages continuing education, advancement, and research in implant dentistry and promotes the surgical insertion of dental transplants and the design and insertion of prosthodontic devices to replace missing teeth. *See also* continuing education; implant dentistry; prosthodontics.

American Academy of Industrial Hygiene (AAIH) A national organization founded in 1960 composed of 3,500 certified industrial hygiene professionals. It monitors the professional aspects of industrial hygienists who have passed board examinations and have become certified members. *See also* certification; environmental health; industrial hygienist.

American Academy of Insurance Medicine (AAIM)

A national organization founded in 1889 composed of 800 medical directors of life insurance companies. Formerly (1992) Association of Life Insurance Medical Directors of America. *See also* life insurance; medical director.

American Academy of Legal and Industrial Medicine *See* American Society of Legal and Industrial Medicine.

American Academy of Maxillofacial Prosthetics (AAMP) A national organization founded in 1953 composed of 148 dentists specializing in maxillofacial prosthetics. *See also* maxillofacial; prosthetics.

American Academy of Medical Administrators (AAMA) A national organization founded in 1957 composed of 2,000 individuals involved in medical administration at the executive or middle-management levels. It promotes educational courses for training people in medical administration, conducts research, maintains biographical archives of members, and offers placement services. *See also* medical administrator.

American Academy of Medical Directors *See* American College of Physician Executives.

American Academy of Medical Preventics *See* American College of Advancement in Medicine.

American Academy of Medical-Legal Analysis (AAMLA) A national organization founded in 1981 composed of 500 physicians and attorneys certified as diplomates of the American Board for Medical-Legal Analysis in Medicine and Surgery and other individuals interested in the field. *See also* American Board for Medical-Legal Analysis in Medicine and Surgery; forensic medicine.

American Academy on Mental Retardation (AAMR) A national organization founded in 1960 composed of 250 scientists actively engaged in research in any discipline relating to mental retardation. *See also* mental retardation.

American Academy of Microbiology (AAM) A national organization founded in 1955 composed of 1,000 microbiologists constituting the professional arm of the American Society for Microbiology. *See also* American Society for Microbiology; microbiology.

American Academy of Natural Family Planning (AANFP) A national organization founded in 1982 composed of 300 individuals who participate in natural family planning instruction. It seeks to improve the quality of natural family planning services by establishing specific certification and accreditation requirements for teachers and educational programs. *See also* accreditation; certification; family planning; natural family planning.

American Academy of Neurological and Orthopaedic Surgeons (AANaOS) A national organization founded in 1977 composed of 1,100 neurological and orthopaedic surgeons, neurologists, physiatrists, and professionals in allied medical or surgical specialities. It maintains the American Board of Neurological and Orthopaedic Medicine and Surgery and the American Board for Medical-Legal Analysis in Medicine and Surgery. *See also* American Board for Medical-Legal Analysis in Medicine and Surgery; American Board of Neurological and Orthopaedic Medicine and Surgery; neurological surgeon; orthopaedic surgeon.

American Academy of Neurological Surgery A national organization founded in 1938 composed of 168 leaders in the field of neurological surgery who are interested in neurosurgical education. *See also* neurological surgery.

American Academy of Neurology (AAN) A national organization founded in 1948 composed of 11,000 physicians specializing in nerve and nervous system diseases. *See also* neurology.

American Academy of Nurse Practitioners (AANP) A national organization founded in 1985 composed of 3,600 groups and individuals promoting high standards of health care delivered by nurse practitioners. It acts as a forum to enhance the identity and continuity of nurse practitioners and addresses national and state legislative issues that affect members. *See also* nurse practitioner.

American Academy of Nursing (AAN) A national organization founded in 1973 composed of 800 members and sponsored by the American Nurses Association. The purposes of the AAN include advancing new concepts in nursing and health care and addressing issues and problems confronting nursing and health. Members of the AAN are Fellows of the American Academy of Nursing. *See also* American Nurses Association; Fellow of the American Academy of Nursing; fellow; nurse; registered nurse.

American Academy of Nursing, Fellow of the *See* Fellow of the American Academy of Nursing.

American Academy of Ophthalmology (AAO) A national organization founded in 1896 composed of 17,000 ophthalmologists interested in high-quality eye care and continuing education. It operates the American Academy of Ophthalmology Government Affairs Office which serves as a liaison between the AAO and the federal government; monitors pending legislation affecting ophthalmology; and prepares statements and testimonies to be presented to congressional committees and regulatory agencies. *See also* continuing education; ophthalmology.

American Academy of Optometry (AAO) A national organization founded in 1921 composed of 3,850 optometrists, educators, and scientists interested in clinical practice standards, optometric education, and experimental research in visual problems. It conducts postgraduate education for optometrists and physicians and confers diplomate status in five fields of optometric practice. *See also* optometry.

American Academy of Oral and Maxillofacial Radiology (AAOMR) A national organization founded in 1949 composed of 500 dentists who teach or specialize in oral radiology. It serves as the authoritative body on radiation hygiene and hazards for the American Dental Association. Formerly (1991) American Academy of Dental Radiology. *See also* oral and maxillofacial surgery; radiology.

American Academy of Oral Medicine (AAOM) A national organization founded in 1946 composed of 800 dental educators, specialists, general dentists, and physicians interested in the study of diseases of the mouth. *See also* oral pathology.

American Academy of Oral Pathology (AAOP) A national organization founded in 1946 composed of 800 oral pathologists who study and treat diseases of the mouth and oral cavity. *See also* dental specialties; oral pathology.

American Academy of Orthodontics for the General Practitioner (AAOGP) A national organization founded in 1959 composed of 250 licensed dentists. The AAOGP provides dentists in general practice with an organization through which they can augment their basic knowledge and training in orthodontics. *See also* dentist, generalist; orthodontics.

American Academy of Orthopaedic Surgeons (AAOS) A national organization founded in 1933 composed of 15,100 orthopedic surgeons certified by the American Board of Orthopedic Surgery. *See also* American Orthopaedic Foot and Ankle Society; Fellow of the American Academy of Orthopaedic Surgeons; orthopaedic/orthopedic surgery.

American Academy of Orthopaedic Surgeons,

Fellow of the   See Fellow of the American Academy of Orthopaedic Surgeons.

American Academy of Orthotists and Prosthetists (AAOP)   A national organization founded in 1970 composed of 1,700 certified professional practitioners in orthotics and prosthetics. See also orthotist/prosthetist.

American Academy of Osteopathy (AAO)   A national organization founded in 1937 composed of 3,500 osteopathic physicians. It seeks to develop and teach the science and art of osteopathic manipulative therapy and encourage greater proficiency in the use of osteopathic structural diagnostic and therapeutic procedures. See also Cranial Academy; osteopathic medicine.

American Academy of Otolaryngic Allergy (AAOA)   A national organization founded in 1941 composed of 1,900 otolaryngologists who are interested in the treatment of otolaryngic allergy. See also allergy; otolaryngology.

American Academy of Otolaryngology - Head and Neck Surgery (AAO-HNS)   A national organization founded in 1982 composed of 9,000 physicians specializing in otolaryngology and head and neck surgery. See also Fellow of the American Academy of Otolaryngology - Head and Neck Surgery; otolaryngology.

American Academy of Otolaryngology - Head and Neck Surgery, Fellow of the   See Fellow of the American Academy of Otolaryngology - Head and Neck Surgery.

American Academy of Pediatric Dentistry (AAPD)   A national organization founded in 1947 composed of 3,100 teachers and researchers in pediatric dentistry and dentists whose practice is limited to children. Formerly (1984) American Academy of Pedodontics. See also dental specialties; pediatric dentistry.

American Academy of Pediatrics (AAP) A national organization founded in 1930 composed of 40,000 pediatricians and pediatric subspecialists. It maintains 42 committees, councils, and task forces including Accident and Poison Prevention; Early Childhood, Adoption, and Dependent Care; and Infectious Diseases. It sponsors the Pediatric Review and Education Program, a self-assessment, continuing education program for practicing pediatricians. See also advanced pediatric life support; continuing education; Fellow of the American Academy of Pedi-

atrics; pediatrics.

American Academy of Pediatrics, Fellow of the   See Fellow of the American Academy of Pediatrics.

American Academy of Pedodontics   See American Academy of Pediatric Dentistry.

American Academy of Periodontology (AAP)   A national organization founded in 1914 composed of 6,007 dentists specializing in the treatment of supporting and surrounding tissues of the teeth and their diseases. See also dental specialties; gingiva; gingivitis; periodontics.

American Academy of Physical Medicine and Rehabilitation (AAPMR)   A national organization founded in 1938 composed of 3,200 diplomates of the American Board of Physical Medicine and Rehabilitation. See also American Board of Physical Medicine and Rehabilitation; physical medicine and rehabilitation.

American Academy of Physician Assistants (AAPA)   A national organization founded in 1968 composed of 13,000 physician assistants, who have graduated from an American Medical Association accredited program and/or are certified by the National Commission on Certification of Physician Assistants, and individuals who are enrolled in an accredited physician assistant educational program. See also allied health professional; certification; physician assistant.

American Academy of Podiatric Administration (AAPA)   A national organization founded in 1961 composed of 200 doctors of podiatric medicine interested in practice administration. It works to standardize office management procedures to create more efficient podiatry practices and develops formalized procedures for obtaining and training podiatry office assistants. See also administration; podiatric medicine.

American Academy of Podiatric Sports Medicine (AAPSM)   A national organization founded in 1970 composed of 800 podiatrists, physicians, and athletic trainers interested in promoting professional participation and research in sports medicine. See also athletic trainer; physician; podiatric medicine; sports medicine.

American Academy of Psychiatrists in Alcoholism and Addictions (aaPaa)   A national organization founded in 1985 composed of 1,000 psychiatrists and psychiatric residents interested in substance abuse. See also addiction psychiatry; alcoholism;

alcoholism and other drug dependence; psychiatry; resident.

American Academy of Psychiatry and the Law (AAPL) A national organization founded in 1969 composed of 1,350 psychiatrists who are members of the American Psychiatric Association or the American Academy of Child and Adolescent Psychiatry and who are interested in areas where psychiatry and the law overlap. *See also* forensic medicine; medical law; psychiatry.

American Academy of Psychoanalysis (AAP) A national organization founded in 1956 composed of 825 psychoanalysts who are fellows of the academy; associates are psychiatrists, scientists, or educators. It seeks to develop communication among psychoanalysts and persons in other disciplines in science and the humanities. *See also* psychoanalysis.

American Academy of Psychotherapists (AAP) A national organization founded in 1955 composed of 725 psychologists, psychiatrists, clergy, and social workers engaged in the practice of psychotherapy. It provides a meeting ground for psychotherapists of differing backgrounds and orientations and facilitates cross-discipline thinking, planning, and research in psychotherapy. *See also* psychotherapist; psychotherapy.

American Academy of Restorative Dentistry (AARD) A national organization founded in 1928 composed of 285 dentists practicing restorative dentistry and educators interested in dentistry as it applies to treatment of the natural teeth to restore and maintain a healthy functioning mouth as part of a healthy body. *See also* dentistry.

American Academy of Sanitarians (AAS) A national organization founded in 1966 composed of 400 registered sanitarians who possess at least a master's degree in public health, environmental health sciences, or environmental management. Its purpose is to certify sanitarians. *See also* certification; industrial hygienist; public health; sanitarian.

American Academy of Somnology (AAS) A national organization founded in 1986 composed of clinicians, researchers, and students interested in promoting the field of somnology. *See also* somnology.

American Academy of Spinal Surgeons (AASS) A national organization founded in 1982 composed of 600 physicians specializing in spinal surgery. It promotes scientific and educational advancement in the field. *See also* spinal cord; surgeon.

American Academy of Sports Physicians (AASP) A national organization founded in 1979 composed of 150 physicians engaged in the practice of sports medicine who have made contributions in research, academics, or related fields. Its objectives are to educate and inform physicians whose practices comprise mainly sports medicine and to register and recognize physicians who have expertise in sports medicine. *See also* physician; sports medicine.

American Academy of Thermology (AAT) A national organization founded in 1968 composed of 400 physicians, physicists, and technicians interested in the field of thermography. Its objectives are to disseminate knowledge concerning the application of thermography to various medical specialties and to promote technical advancement in the field. Its committees are Breast Thermography; Cerebrovascular Thermography; Neuromusculoskeletal Thermography; and Peripheral Vascular Thermography. Formerly (1983) American Thermographic Society. *See also* thermography.

American Academy of Tropical Medicine (AATM) A national organization founded in 1984 composed of physicians and allied health professionals interested in tropical medicine. *See also* allied health professional; physician; tropical medicine.

American Acupuncture Association (AAA) A national organization founded in 1972 composed of 400 physicians, nurses, acupuncturists, physical therapists, and herbologists promoting acceptance of acupuncture as a viable medical method. It works to legalize acupuncture at the state level. *See also* acupuncture.

American Aerobics Association *See* American Fitness Association.

American Ambulance Association (AAA) A national organization founded in 1977 composed of 640 private suppliers of ambulance services. *See also* ambulance.

American Apitherapy Society (AAS) A national organization founded in 1978 composed of 300 beekeepers, physicians, scientists, and others interested in apitherapy, the therapeutic use of honey bee products. It encourages investigation of hive products in order to provide a scientific foundation for their curative properties and use in human medicine. It seeks to prove the effectiveness of bee venom in treating inflammatory diseases, such as arthritis and rheumatisms. Formerly (1989) North American

ApioTherapy Society.

American Art Therapy Association (AATA) A national organization founded in 1969 composed of 3,600 art therapists, students and individuals in related fields interested in the progressive development of therapeutic uses of art. It has established professional criteria for training art therapists. *See also* art therapy.

American Assembly for Men in Nursing (AAMN) A national organization founded in 1971 composed of registered nurses interested in helping eliminate prejudice in nursing, drawing men to the nursing profession, and promoting the principles and practices of positive health care. It acts as a clearinghouse for information on men in nursing. Formerly (1982) National Male Nurse Association. *See also* clearinghouse; nursing; registered nurse.

American Association for Accreditation of Ambulatory Plastic Surgery Facilities (AAAAPSF) An accrediting body founded in 1981 to maintain high standards through adherence to a voluntary program of inspection and accreditation of ambulatory plastic surgery facilities. There are 400 members. *See also* accreditation; ambulatory health care; ambulatory surgical facility; plastic surgery.

American Association for Accreditation of Laboratory Animal Care (AAALAC) A national organization founded in 1965 composed of 31 national education, health, and research organizations professionally interested in the care, study, and use of laboratory animals in research, breeding, teaching, and testing programs. It operates an accreditation program for laboratory animal care whereby organizations are site-visited, peer-reviewed, and evaluated. *See also* accreditation; animal care technologist; animal experimentation; antivivisectionist; vivisection.

American Association for Acupuncture and Oriental Medicine (AAAOM) A national organization founded in 1981 composed of 1,000 professional acupuncturists and other individuals interested in acupuncture and oriental medicine. *See also* acupuncture.

American Association for the Advancement of Science (AAAS) The largest general scientific organization founded in 1848 composed of 135,000 individuals and 296 scientific societies, professional organizations, and state and city academies representing all fields of science. Its objectives are to further the work of scientists and to improve the effectiveness of science in the promotion of human welfare. *See also* science.

American Association of Anatomists (AAA) A national organization founded in 1888 composed of 2,661 anatomists and scientists in related fields. *See also* anatomy.

American Association for Artificial Intelligence (AAAI) A national organization founded in 1979 composed of 13,000 artificial intelligence researchers, students, libraries, and corporations interested in uniting researchers and developers of artificial intelligence in order to provide an element of cohesion in the field. Its areas of interest include interpretation of visual data, robotics, expert systems, natural language processing, knowledge representation, and artificial intelligence programming technologies. *See also* artificial intelligence; natural language processing; robotics.

American Association for Automotive Medicine *See* Association for the Advancement of Automotive Medicine.

American Association of Ayurvedic Medicine (WMAFPH) A national organization founded in 1978 composed of physicians interested in developing within themselves the highest ideal of the perfect physician. It assists physicians in encouraging patients to use transcendental meditation programs to prevent disease and improve health, improving doctor-patient relationships, and bringing perfect health to society. Also known as United States Association of Physicians. Formerly (1986) American Association of Physicians Practicing the Transcendental Meditation Program; (1990) World Medical Association for Perfect Health. *See also* ayurvedic medicine; transcendental meditation.

American Association of Behavioral Therapists (BT) A national organization founded in 1987 composed of 955 professionals from many fields, including mental health counseling, biofeedback therapy, hypnotherapy, and medicine, who share a common interest in the use of the behavioral sciences. *See also* behavioral medicine; behavioral science; behavior therapy.

American Association of Bioanalysts (AAB) A national organization founded in 1956 composed of 1,000 directors, owners, managers, and supervisors of bioanalytical clinical laboratories interested in clinical laboratory procedures and testing. It sponsors a Proficiency Testing Service open to individuals engaged in the clinical laboratory field. *See also* American Board of Bioanalysis; clinical laboratory.

American Association of Blood Banks (AABB) A national organization founded in 1947 composed of 10,000 community and hospital blood banks and transfusion services, physicians, nurses, technologists, administrators, and others interested in blood banking and transfusion medicine. Its purpose is to make whole blood or its components available through blood banks, operate a clearinghouse for exchange of blood and blood credits, and encourage development of blood banks. It conducts educational programs for blood bank personnel, trains and certifies blood bank technologists, maintains a rare donor file and Reference Laboratory System, and sponsors workshops. It sets standards, and inspects and accredits blood banks through a nationwide program. *See also* accreditation; bank; blood bank; blood banking; blood banking specialist; certification; clearinghouse; donor; specialist in blood bank technology.

American Association for Cancer Education (AACE) A national organization founded in 1966 composed of 550 physicians, dentists, nurses, health educators, social workers, and occupational therapists interested in cancer education. It provides a forum for improvement of cancer education that focuses on prevention, early detection, treatment, and rehabilitation. Its committees include Basic Science; Dental; Education Evaluation; Medical; Nursing; and Radiation. *See also* cancer; education.

American Association for Cancer Research (AACR) A national organization founded in 1907 composed of 7,000 research workers for presentation and discussion of new and significant observations and problems in cancer. *See also* cancer; research.

American Association of Cardiovascular and Pulmonary Rehabilitation (AACVPR) A national organization founded in 1985 composed of 2,000 allied health professionals involved in the field of cardiovascular and pulmonary rehabilitation. It fosters the improvement of clinical practice in the area. *See also* allied health professional; cardiovascular; pulmonary; rehabilitation.

American Association of Certified Allergists (AACA) A national organization founded in 1968 composed of 510 physicians specializing in allergy and clinical immunology. Its objectives include improving expertise in allergy treatment and pro-

moting improved standards for the practice and teaching of allergy. *See also* allergy and immunology.

American Association of Certified Allied Health Personnel in Ophthalmology *See* Association of Technical Personnel in Ophthalmology.

American Association of Certified Orthoptists (AACO) A national organization founded in 1940 composed of 400 orthoptists certified by the American Orthoptic Council, after completing a minimum of 24 months training, to treat defects in binocular function. *See also* orthoptics; orthoptist.

American Association of Chairmen of Departments of Psychiatry (AACDP) A national organization founded in 1967 composed of 136 chairpersons of departments of psychiatry in colleges of medicine. Its purposes include promoting medical education, research, and patient care, particularly as these concern psychiatry. *See also* chairperson; psychiatry.

American Association of Children's Residential Centers (AACRC) A national organization founded in 1956 composed of 325 multidisciplinary mental health professionals involved in treatment services for emotionally disturbed children. *See also* mental health professional; residential care; residential care facility.

American Association for Clinical Chemistry (AACC) A national organization founded in 1948 composed of 10,000 clinical laboratory scientists and others engaged in the practice of clinical chemistry in independent laboratories, hospitals, and allied institutions. *See also* chemical pathology; chemistry technologist; laboratory.

American Association of Clinical Urologists (AACU) A national organization founded in 1969 composed of 1,700 clinical urologists who are members of the American Urological Association or its sections and the American Medical Association. *See also* American Medical Association; American Urological Association; urology.

American Association of Colleges of Nursing (AACN) A national organization founded in 1969 composed of 414 institutions offering baccalaureate and/or graduate degrees in nursing. *See also* baccalaureate degree program; nursing; registered nurse.

American Association of Colleges of Osteopathic Medicine (AACOM) A national organization founded in 1898 composed of 15 osteopathic medical colleges. It operates a centralized application service, monitors and works with the US Congress and government agencies in the planning of health care programs, and gathers statistics on osteopathic medical students, faculty, and diplomates. *See also* osteopathic medicine.

American Association of Colleges of Pharmacy (AACP) A national organization founded in 1900 composed of corporations, individuals, and 2,000 colleges of pharmacy programs accredited by the American Council on Pharmaceutical Education. *See also* American Council on Pharmaceutical Education; pharmacy.

American Association of Colleges of Podiatric Medicine (AACPM) A national organization founded in 1932 composed of administrators, faculty, practitioners, students, and other individuals associated with podiatric medical education. It provides vocational material for secondary schools and colleges and conducts public affairs activities and legislative advocacy. *See also* podiatric medicine.

American Association of Community Psychiatrists (AACP) A national organization founded in 1984 composed of 350 psychiatrists practicing in community mental health centers or similar programs that provide care to populations of the mentally ill regardless of their ability to pay. *See also* community mental health center; psychiatry.

American Association for Continuity of Care (AACC) A national organization founded in 1982 composed of 700 health professionals involved in discharge planning, social work, hospital administration, home health care, long term care, home health agencies, and continuity of care. *See also* continuity of care; discharge planning; home health agency; home health care; long term care; social work.

American Association of Correctional Psychologists *See* American Association for Correctional Psychology.

American Association for Correctional Psychology (AACP) A national organization founded in 1953 composed of 400 practitioners, academicians, and researchers interested in community and institutional programs for juvenile and adult offenders and their victims. Formerly (1983) American Association of Correctional Psychologists. *See also* psychology.

American Association for Counseling and Development *See* American Counseling Association.

American Association of Critical-Care Nurses (AACN) A national organization founded in 1969 composed of 72,000 registered nurses specializing in critical care that provides certification, education and training, standards, and other services to its members. *See also* certification; certified critical care nurse; critical care medicine; critical care nurse.

American Association of Dental Consultants (AADC) A national organization founded in 1977 composed of 275 dental insurance consultants and others interested in dental insurance plans from administrative and design perspectives. It operates a certification program. *See also* certification; consultant; dental insurance.

American Association of Dental Editors (AADE) A national organization founded in 1931 composed of 325 dental editors seeking to promote and advance dental journalism. *See also* journalism.

American Association of Dental Examiners (AADE) A national organization founded in 1883 composed of 850 present and past members of state dental examining boards and board administrators. It assists member agencies with problems relating to state dental board examinations and licensure and enforcement of the state dental practice act. *See also* dental practice act; dentistry; specialty board examination.

American Association for Dental Research (AADR) A national organization founded in 1972 composed of 5,000 dentists, researchers, dental schools, and dental products-manufacturing companies interested in promoting better dental health and research activities. *See also* dentistry; research.

American Association of Dental Schools (AADS) A national organization founded in 1923 composed of 3,600 individuals interested in dental education; schools of dentistry, graduate dentistry, and dental auxiliary education in the United States, Canada, and Puerto Rico; and affiliated institutions of the federal government. It promotes better teaching and education in dentistry and dental research. *See also* dental school; dentistry.

American Association of Diabetes Educators (AADE) A national organization founded in 1974 composed of 7,000 nurses, dietitians, social workers, physicians, pharmacists, podiatrists, and others involved in teaching diabetes management to diabetics. *See also* diabetes mellitus.

American Association of Directors of Psychiatric

Residency Training (AADPRT) A national organization founded in 1973 composed of 428 directors of psychiatric residency training programs. *See also* psychiatry; residency.

American Association of Electrodiagnostic Medicine (AAEM) A national organization founded in 1953 composed of 2,700 practicing physicians who are active in electromyography and electrodiagnosis and who have made contributions to this field. Its objective is to increase knowledge of electromyography and electrodiagnostic medicine and to improve patient care. Formerly (1990) American Association of Electromyography and Electrodiagnosis. *See also* electrodiagnosis; electromyography.

American Association of Electromyography and Electrodiagnosis *See* American Association of Electrodiagnostic Medicine.

American Association of Endodontists (AAE) A national organization founded in 1943 composed of 4,000 dentists engaged in clinical practice, teaching, and research in endodontics. *See also* dental specialties; endodontics.

American Association of Entrepreneurial Dentists (AAED) A national organization founded in 1983 composed of dentists and other dental professionals involved in research, industry, manufacturing, marketing, publication, and other entrepreneurial activities. Its activities include informing the public, dentists, educators, and manufacturing companies of new and beneficial techniques, products, and services; coordinating the review of specifications for dental materials and products by regulatory agencies; evaluating and representing new ideas and products to manufacturing companies at convention trade expositions; and providing lists of foreign dental dealers and buyers. *See also* dentistry; entrepreneur.

American Association of Eye and Ear Hospitals (AAEEH) A national organization composed of the chief executive officers and administrators of 14 eye and ear specialty hospitals interested in fair economic treatment for their hospitals and sharing business functions, such as purchasing, planning, and information and data collection. *See also* chief executive officer; hospital; ophthalmology; otolaryngology.

American Association of First Responders *See* National Association of First Responders.

American Association for Fitness in Business *See* Association for Fitness in Business.

American Association of Functional Orthodontics

(AAFO) A national organization founded in 1981 composed of 1,800 dentists involved in the use of functional appliances for orthodontic malocclusions and temporomandibular joint dysfunctions. Its purpose is to facilitate exchange of information and case reports on current development in this type of treatment. Previously (1985) American Association of Functional Orthodontists. *See also* orthodontic appliance; orthodontics; temporomandibular joint.

American Association of Functional Orthodontists *See* American Association of Functional Orthodontics.

American Association of Genito-Urinary Surgeons (AAGUS) A national organization founded in 1886 composed of 180 physicians specializing in genito-urinary surgery. *See also* urology.

American Association for Geriatric Psychiatry (AAGP) A national organization founded in 1978 composed of 1,468 psychiatrists interested in promoting better mental health care for the elderly. *See also* geriatric psychiatry.

American Association of Gynecological Laparoscopists (AAGL) A national organization founded in 1972 composed of 5,200 physicians who specialize in obstetrics and gynecology and who are interested in gynecological endoscopic procedures. *See also* endoscopy; gynecology; laparoscopy.

American Association for Hand Surgery (AAHS) A national organization founded in 1970 composed of 960 plastic, orthopaedic, and general surgeons and other individuals having a specific interest in hand surgery. *See also* hand surgery.

American Association of Healthcare Consultants (AAHC) A national organization founded in 1949 composed of 250 individuals exclusively devoted to hospital and health care consultation including the provision of consulting services in strategic planning and marketing, organization and management, human resource management, and other areas. Formerly (1984) American Association of Hospital Consultants. *See also* consultant; health care consultant.

American Association for the History of Medicine (AAHM) A national organization founded in 1925 composed of 1,300 physicians and other individuals with professional or vocational interest in the history of medicine. It promotes research, study, interest, and writing in the history of medicine, including public health, dentistry, pharmacy, nursing, medical social work, and allied sciences and professions. *See* *also* history; medicine.

American Association for the History of Nursing (AAHN) A national organization founded in 1980 composed of 375 individuals interested in promoting the history of nursing. It conducts research and educational programs. *See also* history; nursing.

American Association of Homeopathic Pharmacists (AAHP) A national organization founded in 1922 composed of 20 manufacturing pharmacists of homeopathic preparations and associate members (distributors). The organization works for the preservation and promotion of the use of homeotherapeutics. *See also* homeopathy; pharmacist.

American Association of Homes for the Aging (AAHA) A national organization founded in 1961 composed of 4,000 voluntary nonprofit and governmental nursing homes, housing, and health-related facilities and services for the elderly; state associations; and interested persons. It provides a unified means of identifying and solving problems in order to protect and advance the interests of the elderly persons served. *See also* aging.

American Association of Hospital Consultants *See* American Association of Healthcare Consultants.

American Association of Hospital Dentists (AAHD) A national organization founded in 1960 composed of 900 directors and staff members of dental departments in hospitals. *See also* dentist; hospital.

American Association of Hospital Podiatrists (AAHP) A national organization founded in 1950 composed of 800 podiatrists affiliated with hospitals. *See also* hospital; podiatrist.

American Association of Immunologists (AAI) A national organization founded in 1913 composed of 5,500 scientists engaged in immunological research in virology, bacteriology, biochemistry, and related areas. *See also* immunology.

American Association of Industrial Management (AAIM) A national organization founded in 1899 composed of 180 companies in diverse fields ranging from manufacturing to banks to hospitals. *See also* industrial; management.

American Association of Industrial Nurses *See* American Association of Occupational Health Nurses.

American Association of Industrial Social Workers (AAISW) A national organization founded in 1982 composed of industrial social work practitioners, professors, and students interested in educating the public about the profession and promoting an understanding of industrial social work and employee assistance programs. It grants the qualification of registered industrial social worker. *See also* industrial social worker.

American Association for Laboratory Animal Science (AALAS) A national organization founded in 1949 composed of 4,500 persons and institutions professionally interested in the production, use, care, and study of laboratory animals. It serves as clearinghouse for the collection and exchange of information on all phases of laboratory animal care and management and on the care, use, and procurement of laboratory animals used in biomedical research. It conducts examinations and certification through its animal technician certification program. *See also* animal care technologist; animal experimentation; antivivisectionist; certification; vivisection.

American Association of Legal Nurse Consultants (AALNC) A national organization founded in 1989 composed of 710 registered nurses providing medical consultation to the legal profession. *See also* registered nurse.

American Association for Marriage and Family Therapy (AAMFT) A national organization founded in 1942 composed of 18,000 marriage and family therapists. It has 50 accredited training centers throughout the United States. *See also* counselor; marital counseling.

American Association of Medical Assistants (AAMA) A national organization founded in 1956 composed of 13,000 assistants, receptionists, secretaries, bookkeepers, nurses, and laboratory personnel employed in the offices of physicians and other medical facilities. It conducts a certification program, the passage of which entitles the individual to certification as a certified medical assistant (CMA). It also conducts accreditation of one-year and two-year programs in medical assisting in conjunction with the Committee on Allied Health Education and Accreditation. *See also* allied health professional; certified medical assistant; medical assistant.

American Association of Medical Milk Commissions (AAMMC) A national organization founded in 1907 composed of 35 physician members of local Medical Milk Commissions, including sanitarians and bacteriologists who supervise production of certified milk (milk from dairies conforming to official standards of sanitation). *See also* sanitarian.

American Association of Medical Society Executives (AAMSE) A national organization founded in 1946 composed of 1,000 executives of national, state, regional, or county medical and specialty societies. *See also* executive; medical society; specialty societies.

American Association for Medical Systems and Informatics *See* American Medical Informatics Association.

American Association for Medical Transcription (AAMT) A national organization founded in 1978 composed of 9,000 medical transcriptionists, their supervisors, teachers and students of medical transcription, owners and managers of medical transcription services, and other interested health personnel. *See also* transcription.

American Association of Medico-Legal Consultants (AAMC) A national medical malpractice screening panel founded in 1972 composed of 1,200 physicians and physician-attorneys. The organization performs medical malpractice screening, peer review, medical and hospital risk management, and medical audits. It holds seminars for physicians and attorneys in the field of medical-legal problems. *See also* consultant; medical malpractice; peer review; risk management.

American Association of Mental Deficiency *See* American Association on Mental Retardation.

American Association of Mental Health Professionals in Corrections (AAMHPC) A national organization founded in 1940 composed of 2,000 psychiatrists, psychologists, social workers, nurses, and other mental health professionals working in correctional settings and interested in improving the treatment, rehabilitation, and care of persons with mental illness, mental retardation, and emotional disturbances. *See also* mental health professional; mental illness; mental retardation.

American Association on Mental Retardation (AAMR) A national organization founded in 1876 composed of 9,500 physicians, educators, administrators, social workers, psychologists, psychiatrists, students, and others interested in the general welfare of persons with mental retardation and the study of the cause, treatment, and prevention of mental retardation. Formerly (1987) American Association on Mental Deficiency. *See also* mental retardation.

American Association for Music Therapy (AAMT) A national organization founded in 1971 composed of 650 certified music therapists, students, and colleges and universities offering music therapy programs. *See also* music therapy.

American Association of Naturopathic Physicians (AANP) A national organization founded in 1985 composed of 225 naturopathic physicians. *See also* naturopath; naturopathy.

American Association of Nephrology Nurses and Technicians *See* American Nephrology Nurses' Association.

American Association of Neurological Surgeons (AANS) A national organization founded in 1931 composed of 3,470 neurological surgeons interested in promoting excellence in neurological surgery and its related sciences. *See also* neurological surgery.

American Association of Neuropathologists (AANP) A national organization founded in 1924 composed of 660 physicians specializing in neuropathology. *See also* neuropathology.

American Association of Neuroscience Nurses (AANN) A national organization founded in 1968 composed of 3,400 registered nurses engaged in or primarily interested in neurosurgical or neurological nursing. *See also* neurology; neurological surgery; registered nurse.

American Association of Neurosurgical Nurses *See* American Association of Neuroscience Nurses.

American Association of Nurse Anesthetists (AANA) A national organization founded in 1931 composed of 24,500 active registered nurses who have successfully completed an accredited program in nurse anesthesia and passed a national examination for certification. *See also* certification; certified registered nurse anesthetist; nurse anesthetist.

American Association of Nurse Attorneys, The *See* The American Association of Nurse Attorneys.

American Association of Nursing Homes *See* American Health Care Association.

American Association of Nutritional Consultants (AANC) A national organization founded in 1948 composed of 5,000 nutritional consultants. *See also* nutrition; consultant.

American Association of Occupational Health Nurses (AAOHN) A national organization founded in 1988 composed of 11,500 registered nurses employed by business and industry, nurse educators, nurse editors, nurse writers, and others interested in occupational health nursing. *See also* occupational health nurse.

American Association of Office Nurses (AAON) A national organization founded in 1988 composed of 2,200 nurses working primarily in physicians' offices. *See also* office nurse.

American Association of Oral and Maxillofacial Surgeons (AAOMS) A national organization founded in 1918 composed of 5,870 dentists specializing in disease diagnosis and surgical and adjunctive treatment of diseases, injuries, and defects of the oral and maxillofacial region. *See also* dental specialties; oral and maxillofacial surgery.

American Association of Orthodontists (AAO) A national organization founded in 1901 composed of 11,000 orthodontists. It seeks to advance the art and science of orthodontics through continuing education, encouragement of research, provision of information to the public, and cooperation with other health groups. *See also* continuing education; dental specialties; orthodontics.

American Association of Orthomolecular Medicine (AAOM) A national organization founded in 1971 composed of 310 psychiatrists, biochemists, researchers, nutritional scientists, biologists, and other scientists interested in nutrition altered metabolic states, defects in brain chemistry, molecular biology, genetics, research in brain enzymes, and treatment based upon altering molecular levels and concentrations of essential substances for optimum functioning. Formerly (1987) Academy of Orthomolecular Medicine. *See also* orthomolecular medicine therapy.

American Association of Orthopedic Medicine (AAOrthMed) A national organization founded in 1982 composed of 300 physicians and allied health professionals interested in the advancement of knowledge, diagnosis, and nonsurgical treatment of musculoskeletal and related disorders. *See also* orthopaedic/orthopedic surgery.

American Association of Osteopathic Examiners (AAOE) A national organization founded in 1935 composed of private physicians and state medical boards working for adequate osteopathic representation on all physician-licensing boards. It conducts examinations and offers certification of osteopathic physicians. *See also* certification; licensure; osteopathic medicine.

American Association of Osteopathic Specialists (AAOS) A national organization founded in 1952 composed of 400 osteopathic physicians interested in improving the practice of the specialty disciplines. It maintains continuing education programs: American Academy of Osteopathic Anesthesiologists; American Academy of Osteopathic Family Practitioners; American Academy of Osteopathic Internists; American Academy of Osteopathic Neurologists and Psychiatrists; American Academy of Osteopathic Obstetricians and Gynecologists; American Academy of Osteopathic Radiologists; American Academy of Osteopathic Orthopedic Surgeons. It provides certification programs in 26 different areas of specialization. Formerly (1984) American Academy of Osteopathic Surgeons. *See also* certification; continuing education; osteopathic medicine.

American Association for Parapsychology (AAP) A national organization founded in 1971 interested in encouraging interest in parapsychology, bridging the gap between academic parapsychology and experimental extrasensory perception participation among laymen, stimulating interest in scientific research, and encouraging public involvement in future research. It offers a course in parapsychology including basic theories, principles, and histories of phenomena involving telepathy, clairvoyance, hypnosis, sensory awareness, and social and transpersonal psychology. Formerly (1986) American Parapsychological Research Association. *See also* clairvoyance; hypnosis; parapsychology; telepathy.

American Association for Partial Hospitalization (AAPH) A national organization founded in 1965 composed of 775 individuals interested in the development and improvement of partial hospitalization within the continuum of psychiatric treatment. *See also* partial hospitalization.

American Association of Pastoral Counselors (AAPC) A national organization founded in 1963 composed of 3,100 clergy and other religious professionals of all faiths with special training in counseling. It works to set standards and establish criteria for the operation of church-related counseling programs; provide certification for religious professionals engaged in specialized ministries of counseling; and approve church-related counseling centers. *See also* certification; counselor; pastoral.

American Association of Pathologists (AAP) A national organization founded in 1976, composed of 2,000 experimental research pathologists who have made significant contributions to the knowledge of disease. *See also* pathology.

American Association of Pathologists' Assistants (AAPA) A national organization founded in 1972 composed of 300 pathologists' assistants and individuals qualified by academic and practical training to provide service in anatomic pathology under the direction of a qualified pathologist who is responsible for the performance of the assistant. *See also* pathologist's assistant.

American Association for Pediatric Ophthalmology and Strabismus A national organization founded in 1974 composed of 500 ophthalmologists who limit their practice largely to children. *See also* ophthalmology; strabismus.

American Association of Pharmaceutical Scientists (AAPS) A national organization founded in 1986 composed of 5,200 pharmaceutical scientists interested in exchanging scientific information and forming public policies to regulate pharmaceutical sciences and related issues of public concern. *See also* pharmaceutical.

American Association of Physicians for Human Rights (AAPHR) A national organization founded in 1979 composed of 450 physicians and medical students seeking elimination of discrimination on the basis of sexual orientation in the health professions and promoting unprejudiced medical care for gay and lesbian patients. It maintains a referral and support program for HIV-infected physicians. *See also* gay; HIV infection; human rights; lesbianism; physician.

American Association of Physicists in Medicine (AAPM) A national organization founded in 1958 composed of 3,100 persons and organizations engaged in application of physics to medicine and biology in medical research. *See also* medical physics; physics; radiological physics.

American Association of Plastic Surgeons (AAPS) A national organization founded in 1921 composed of 425 plastic surgeons. *See also* plastic surgery.

American Association of Podiatric Physicians and Surgeons (AAPPS) A national organization founded in 1979 composed of 1,500 podiatrists. It provides training and certification for podiatry and podiatric surgery and offers accreditation to agencies providing podiatric services and podiatric peer review. *See also* accreditation; certification; peer review; podiatric medicine.

American Association of Poison Control Centers (AAPCC) A national organization founded in 1958 composed of 1,000 individuals and organizations engaged in the operation of poison control centers. It aids in the procurement of information on the ingredients and potential acute toxicity of substances that may cause poisonings and on the management of such poisonings. It has established standards for poison information and control centers. *See also* medical toxicology; poison; poison control center.

American Association of Preferred Provider Organizations (AAPPO) A national organization founded in 1983 composed of 800 health care executives, health care consultants, corporations, and preferred provider organizations who are interested in the development and promotion of preferred provider organizations. It provides educational and legislative support to organizations and individuals involved with the development of preferred provider organizations, and conducts educational seminars, consulting services, and accreditation services for preferred provider organizations. *See also* preferred provider organization.

American Association of Professional Hypnotherapists (AAPH) A national organization founded in 1980 composed of 1,550 hypnotherapists, marriage and family therapists, psychologists, clinical social workers, physicians, pastoral counselors, and others trained in hypnosis therapy. It promotes public awareness of hypnosis as applied to personal motivation and improvement, habit control, mental health services, and assistance in the healing process. *See also* hypnosis; hypnotherapy.

American Association of Professional Standards Review Organizations *See* American Medical Peer Review Association.

American Association for Protecting Children (AAPC) A national organization founded in 1877 composed of 2,000 individuals and agencies seeking to protect children from neglect and abuse. It works for effective and responsive community child-protective services and provides comprehensive in-service training for professionals, including social workers, physicians, teachers, and law enforcement personnel. It offers evaluation and technical assistance to community and state child-protective programs. *See also* child abuse.

American Association of Psychiatric Administrators (AAPA) A national organization founded in

1960 composed of 300 psychiatrists who occupy the position of chief administrative or clinical officer of a public or private neuropsychiatric hospital or clinic. *See also* administrator; clinic; hospital; psychiatry.

American Association of Psychiatric Services for Children (AAPSC) A national organization founded in 1948 composed of 165 members interested in the prevention and treatment of mental and emotional disorders of the young. It acts as an information clearinghouse and provides accreditation services. *See also* child and adolescent psychiatry; psychiatry.

American Association of Psychiatrists *See* American Association of Psychiatrists from India.

American Association of Psychiatrists from India (AAP) A national organization composed of 400 psychiatrists and other mental health professionals of Asian-Indian descent in the United States. It seeks to further the education and training of members and to enhance their interest in the mental health field. Formerly (1990) American Association of Psychiatrists. *See also* psychiatry.

American Association of Public Health Dentistry (AAPHD) A national organization founded in 1937 composed of 650 dentists, dental hygienists, health educators, and other persons actively engaged in dental public health. *See also* public health dentistry.

American Association of Public Health Physicians (AAPHP) A national organization founded in 1954 composed of 200 physicians actively engaged in public health. *See also* public health physician - administrative; public health physician - clinical.

American Association for Public Opinion Research (AAPOR) A national organization founded in 1947 composed of 1,450 individuals interested in the methods and applications of public opinion and social research. *See also* public opinion; public opinion poll.

American Association of Railway Surgeons (AARS) A national organization founded in 1888 composed of 500 physicians engaged in professional work with railroad personnel. *See also* surgeon.

American Association for Rehabilitation Therapy (AART) A national organization founded in 1950 composed of 400 medical rehabilitation therapists and specialists and others interested in vocational rehabilitation of the mentally and physically disabled. *See also* rehabilitation.

American Association of Religious Therapists

(AART) A national organization founded in 1958 composed of 417 psychiatrists, psychologists, social workers, and clergymen promoting religious views in psychotherapy. *See also* psychotherapy; religion; religious.

American Association for Respiratory Care (AARC) A national organization founded in 1947 composed of 30,000 respiratory care technicians and therapists employed by hospitals, group practices, educational institutions, and municipal organizations. Formerly (1986) American Association for Respiratory Therapy. *See also* respiratory therapist; respiratory therapy technician.

American Association for Respiratory Therapy *See* American Association for Respiratory Care.

American Association of Retired Persons (AARP) A national organization founded in 1958 composed of 32,000,000 working or retired persons 50 years of age or older. It seeks to improve every aspect of living for older people and has targeted health care as an area of immediate concern. It is active in health legislation, health care financing, access, and quality issues. *See also* retirement; retirement age; retirement center.

American Association of Senior Physicians (AASP) A national organization founded in 1975 composed of 5,000 retired and nonretired physicians and their spouses who are 50 years of age or older. It is with furthering the rights and benefits of senior physicians. It holds retirement seminars. *See also* physician; retirement.

American Association of Sex Educators, Counselors and Therapists (AASECT) A national organization founded in 1967 composed of 2,600 professionals interested in sex education, counseling, and therapy. It assists, among other activities, educational, religious, clinical, and social agencies in developing human relations and sex curricula. *See also* counselor; education; sex; sex therapy.

American Association for Social Psychiatry (AASP) A national organization founded in 1971 composed of 500 professionals and trainees devoted to the study, prevention, and treatment of mental illness, behavioral disorders, and human vicissitudes. *See also* social psychiatry.

American Association of Spinal Cord Injury Nurses (AASCIN) A national organization founded in 1983 composed of 1,600 nurses who care for patients with spinal cord injuries, nurses interested in the field of spinal cord injury, and persons who have provided extraordinary service to improve the quality of life for spinal cord injury patients. *See also* nurse; paraplegia; quadriplegia; spinal cord.

American Association of Spinal Cord Injury Psychologists and Social Workers A national organization founded in 1986 composed of 500 psychologists and social workers who treat patients with spinal cord injuries. It promotes improvement of psychological care of spinal cord injury patients and focuses on topics, such as sexuality and alcohol and drug dependence among spinal cord injury patients. *See also* paraplegia; psychologist; quadriplegia; social worker; spinal cord.

American Association of State Social Work Boards (AASSWB) A national organization founded in 1979 composed of 47 state boards and authorities empowered to regulate the practice of social work within their own jurisdictions. It seeks to protect the recipient of social work service and promote confidence in and accountability of the social work profession by establishing national regulatory standards for the practice of professional social work. *See also* social work.

American Association for the Study of Headache (AASH) A national organization founded in 1959 composed of 950 physicians, dentists, and scientists interested in the study of headaches. *See also* headache.

American Association for the Study of Liver Diseases (AASLD) A national organization founded in 1950 composed of 1,300 physicians interested in exchanging scientific information about liver disease and liver research. *See also* gastroenterology; hepatologist.

American Association of Suicidology (AAS) A national organization founded in 1967 composed of 1,400 psychologists, psychiatrists, social workers, nurses, health educators, physicians, directors of suicide prevention centers, clergy, and others sharing a common interest in the advancement of studies of suicide prevention and life-threatening behavior. *See also* suicidology.

American Association of Surgeon Assistants (AASA) A national organization founded in 1973 composed of 500 surgeon assistants, surgical physician assistants, students, physicians, surgeons, and allied health professionals. Formerly (1990) American Association of Surgeon's Assistants. *See also* sur-

geon assistant.

American Association for the Surgery of Trauma (AAST) A national organization founded in 1938 composed of 800 surgeons interested in the cultivation and improvement of the science and art of the surgery of trauma and allied sciences. *See also* trauma; traumatology.

American Association of Testifying Physicians (AATP) A national organization founded in 1948 composed of 2,553 physicians and insurance companies interested in training doctors to effectively testify in court. *See also* physician; testify; testimony.

American Association of Therapeutic Humor (AATH) A national organization founded in 1987 composed of 500 health care providers, clergy, and educators promoting the use of humor as a therapeutic technique. *See also* humor; laughter; therapeutic.

American Association for Thoracic Surgery (AATS) A national organization founded in 1917 composed of 900 specialists in surgery of the chest region, including cardiovascular surgeons. *See also* thoracic surgery.

American Association of Tissue Banks (AATB) A national organization founded in 1976 composed of 800 tissue banks that encourages the development of regional tissue banks and the establishment of guidelines and standards for the retrieval, preservation, distribution, and use of tissues for transplantation. *See also* bank; tissue; tissue bank; transplantation.

American Association of University Affiliated Programs for the Developmentally Disabled *See* American Association of University Affiliated Programs for Persons with Developmental Disabilities.

American Association of University Affiliated Programs for Persons with Developmental Disabilities (AAUAP) A national organization founded in 1968 composed of 52 university-based or affiliated clinical service and interdisciplinary training centers for graduate students and others interested in the field of mental retardation and other developmental disabilities. It provides coordination of federal funding for programs and technical assistance to Congress. Formerly (1983) American Association of University Affiliated Programs for the Developmentally Disabled. *See also* developmental disability; disability; mental retardation.

American Association of Women Dentists

(AAWD) A national organization founded in 1921 composed of 2,000 women dentists and dental students. *See also* dentist.

American Association for Women Radiologists (AAWR) A national organization founded in 1980 composed of 1,600 women physicians involved in diagnostic or therapeutic radiology, nuclear medicine, or radiologic physics. It facilitates exchange of knowledge and information as it relates to women in radiology, encourages publication of materials on radiology and medicine by members, supports women who are training in the field, and encourages women radiologists to participate in radiological societies. *See also* nuclear medicine; radiologic physics; radiology.

American Association for World Health (AAWH) A national organization founded in 1951 composed of 1,200 organizations and individuals interested in strengthening US commitment to world health. It supports programs of the World Health Organization and the Pan American Health Organization. Also known as US Committee for the World Health Organization. *See also* Pan American Health Organization; World Health Organization.

American Association for Vital Records and Public Health Statistics *See* Association for Vital Records and Health Statistics.

American Athletic Trainers Association and Certification Board (AATA) A national organization founded in 1978 to qualify and certify active athletic trainers; to establish minimum competence standards for individuals participating in the prevention and care of athletic injuries; and to inform the public of the importance of having competent leadership in the area of athletic training. *See also* allied health professional; athletic trainer; certification.

American Audiology Society *See* American Auditory Society.

American Auditory Society (AAS) A national organization founded in 1976 composed of 2,688 audiologists, otolaryngologists, scientists, hearing aid industry professionals, educators of hearing impaired people, and individuals involved in industries serving hearing impaired people, including the amplification system industry. Formerly (1982) American Audiology Society. *See also* audiology; otolaryngology.

American Baptist Homes and Hospitals Association (ABHHA) A national organization founded in 1935 composed of 99 nursing homes and hospitals, retirement facilities, and children's homes and special services. It provides special programs and educational events for member institutions. *See also* hospital; nursing home; retirement center.

American Bar Association (ABA) A national organization founded in 1878 composed of 360,000 attorneys in good standing of the bar of any state. It conducts research and educational projects and activities to encourage professional improvement, provides public services, improves the administration of civil and criminal justice, and increases the availability of legal services to the public. *See also* attorney; bar; lawyer; Model Rules of Professional Conduct.

American Bar Association Center for Professional Responsibility (ABACPR) A nonmembership organization that supports the work of committees of the American Bar Association involved in the design and implementation of policy in the fields of legal ethics, professional discipline and regulation, professionalism, unauthorized practice of law, and client security funds. It maintains liaison with courts, disciplinary agencies, and advisory committees in each state. *See also* American Bar Association; bar.

American Black Chiropractors Association (ABCA) A national organization founded in 1980 composed of individuals who have earned a recognized doctorate degree in chiropractic and students who are enrolled in a chiropractic college. Its objectives include educating the public, health care organizations, and health care providers about chiropractic and promoting black chiropractic practitioners in the community. Formerly (1981) Association of Black Chiropractors. *See also* chiropractic.

American Blood Commission (ABC) An organization founded in 1975 composed of 32 national organizations representing medical professionals, health agencies, insurance carriers, patients, and donors who promote the development of a publicly stated national blood policy. It proposes a system under which the existing major organizations in the field would work together under the policy direction of a commission representing many national organizations interested in services. *See also* blood; donor.

American Blood Resources Association (ABRA) A national organization founded in 1972 composed of 100 operators of blood plasma centers. It represents the interests of plasma collection centers, promotes plasma as an important part of the blood industry, and has developed a code of ethics. *See also* blood plasma; donor.

American Board of Abdominal Surgery (ABAS) A national board founded in 1865 that certifies as diplomates specialists in abdominal surgery. It establishes minimum educational and training standards for the specialty and determines whether candidates have received adequate preparation as defined by the board. It provides comprehensive oral and written examinations to determine the ability and fitness of candidates. *See also* abdomen; abdominal surgery; board; certification; diplomate.

American Board of Allergy and Immunology (ABAI) A joint medical specialty board of the American Board of Internal Medicine and the American Board of Pediatrics founded in 1972 composed of internists and pediatricians with special competency in treating problems of allergy and immunology. It establishes qualifications and examines physician candidates for certification as specialists in allergy and immunology. *See also* allergy and immunology; American Board of Internal Medicine; American Board of Pediatrics; board; certification; medical specialty boards.

American Board of Anesthesiology (ABA) A national medical specialty board founded in 1938 that seeks to improve standards of the practice of anesthesiology and to establish criteria of fitness for the designation of a specialist in the field. It advises the Accreditation Council for Graduate Medical Education of the American Medical Association concerning training of individuals seeking certification; arranges and conducts examinations to determine the competence of physicians who apply; and issues certificates to individuals meeting the required standards. *See also* anesthesiology; board; certification; medical specialty boards.

American Board of Bioanalysis (ABB) A national board founded in 1968 consisting of scientists, educators, and recognized authorities in the clinical laboratory field. It certifies individuals as bioanalyst laboratory directors, bioanalytic laboratory managers, and laboratory supervisors. It accredits continuing education programs. *See also* American Association of Bioanalysts; board; certification; clinical laboratory.

American Board of Bionic Rehabilitative Psychology (ABBRP) An organization founded in 1983 composed of 475 physicians specializing in bionic rehabilitative psychology. *See also* bionic; bionics; board; psychology; rehabilitation.

American Board of Cardiovascular Perfusion (ABCP) A national board founded in 1975 composed of 1,800 certified clinical perfusionists. The organization seeks to protect the public through the establishment and maintenance of standards in the field. It establishes qualifications for examination and recertification and administers annual board examinations. *See also* board; cardiovascular; certification; perfusionist; recertification.

American Board for Certification in Orthotics and Prosthetics (ABC) A national board founded in 1948 that establishes qualifications, conducts examinations, and certifies individuals (3,400 members) and facilities (600 facilities) whom the board finds qualified to practice orthotics and prosthetics. *See also* board; certification; orthotist/prosthetist; specialty boards.

American Board of Certified and Registered Encephalographic Technicians and Technologists (ABCRETT) An organization founded in 1980 composed of 1,200 certified encephalography (EEG) technologists that conducts educational and certification programs for EEG technologists. *See also* board; certified; electroencephalographic technician/technologist; electroencephalography; technician; technologist.

American Board of Chelation Therapy (ABCT) A national board founded in 1982 and sponsored by the American Holistic Medical Association and the American College of Advancement in Medicine to define and establish qualifications required of licensed physicians for certification in the field of chelation therapy. *See also* American College of Advancement in Medicine; American Holistic Medical Association; board; certification; chelation therapy.

American Board of Clinical Chemistry (ABCC) A national board founded in 1950 that works to establish and enhance the standards of competence for the practice of clinical chemistry, including toxicological chemistry, and to certify qualified specialists. It conducts examinations annually for certification in clinical chemistry and clinical toxicology. It is sponsored by the American Association for Clinical Chemistry, American Chemical Society, American

Institute of Chemists, American Society for Biochemistry and Molecular Biology, and other organizations. *See also* board; certification; clinical chemistry; toxicology.

American Board of Colon and Rectal Surgery (ABCRS) A national medical specialty board established in 1934 to investigate qualifications, administer examinations, and provide certification as diplomates for physicians specializing in colon and rectal surgery. Formerly American Board of Proctology. *See also* board; certification; colon and rectal surgery; diplomate; medical specialty boards.

American Board of Dental Public Health (ABDPH) A national dental board founded in 1950 to investigate the qualifications of, administer examinations to, and certify as diplomates dentists specializing in dental public health. *See also* board; certification; dental specialties; diplomate; public health dentistry; specialty boards.

American Board of Dermatology (ABD) A national medical specialty board founded in 1932 composed of 12 directors. It seeks to ensure provision of competent care for patients with cutaneous diseases by establishing requirements of postdoctoral training and creating and conducting annual comprehensive examinations to determine the competence of physicians who meet the requirements for examination by the board. It issues certificates to those who satisfactorily complete the examination. *See also* board; certification; dermatology; medical specialty boards.

American Board of Emergency Medicine (ABEM) A national medical specialty board founded in 1976 that designs and administers an annual two-part examination (written and oral) to evaluate physicians seeking certification as specialists in emergency medicine. Recertification is required every ten years. *See also* board; certification; emergency medicine; medical specialty boards; recertification.

American Board of Endodontics (ABE) A national board that certifies dentists who have successfully completed study and training in an advanced endodontics education program accredited by the Commission on Dental Accreditation of the American Dental Association and who have successfully completed the examinations administered by the board. There are approximately 650 diplomates. *See also* board; certification; dental specialties; diplomate; endodontics; specialty boards.

American Board of Environmental Medicine (ABEM) A national board founded in 1988 that examines, evaluates, and certifies physicians, training programs, and hospital units; environmental control and biodetoxification units; and rehabilitation centers. *See also* board; certification; detoxification; environmental health; physician.

American Board of Examiners of Pastoral Counseling (ABEPC) An national interdenominational board founded in 1921 providing certification in pastoral counseling to individuals, centers, and institutions. It conducts certification testing in chaplaincy and pastoral counseling and annual reviews. *See also* board; certification; chaplain; counsel; pastoral.

American Board of Examiners of Psychodrama, Sociometry, and Group Psychotherapy (ABEPS-GP) A national organization founded in 1975 that certifies professionals in the field of group psychotherapy, psychodrama, and sociometry. *See also* board; certification; psychodrama; psychotherapy; sociometry.

American Board of Family Practice (ABFP) A national medical specialty board of physicians certified in family practice. *See also* board; certification; family physician; family practice; medical specialty boards.

American Board of Forensic Psychiatry (ABFP) A national board founded in 1976 composed of 227 persons in the medical profession certified in forensic psychiatry. It establishes and revises, as necessary, standards for individuals who wish to practice forensic psychiatry and certifies applicants who comply with the board's requirements. It seeks to provide the judicial system with a uniform system of identifying qualified specialists in forensic psychiatry. *See also* board; certification; forensic psychiatry.

American Board of Hand Surgery (ABHS) A national board composed of 500 hand surgeons interested in advancing scientific knowledge and providing educational opportunities in the field of hand surgery. *See also* board; hand surgeon; hand surgery.

American Board of Health Physics (ABHP) A national board founded in 1960 that promotes the health physics profession by establishing standards and procedures for certification and conducting certification examinations. *See also* board; certification; health physics; standard.

American Board of Industrial Hygiene (ABIH) A national board founded in 1960 that certifies industrial hygienists. *See also* board; certification; hygiene; industrial hygienist.

American Board of Industrial Medicine and Surgery (ABIMS) A national board founded in 1984 composed of 300 physicians specializing in industrial medicine and surgery interested in promoting scientific advancement and providing educational courses in the field. *See also* board; industrial health services.

American Board of Internal Medicine (ABIM) A national medical specialty board founded in 1936 to determine the qualifications of, administer examinations to, and certify as specialists in internal medicine those physicians meeting its standards of clinical competence. Board members are elected from certified leaders in internal medicine. The board has certified approximately 91,000 internists and 43,000 subspecialist diplomates and issued 8,600 recertification certificates. *See also* board; certification; diplomate; internal medicine; medical specialty boards; recertification.

American Board of Medical Genetics (ABMG) A national medical specialty board founded in 1979 composed of 1,640 individuals who have passed the board's examination. The board certifies individuals for the delivery of medical genetics services and accredits medical geneticist training programs. *See also* board; certification; medical genetics; medical specialty boards.

American Board of Medical-Legal Analysis in Medicine and Surgery (ABMLAMS) A national board founded in 1981 composed of 400 physicians and attorneys who are candidates for certification in the field of medical-legal analysis, which deals with forensic and jurisprudential aspects of medicine and surgery. It is maintained by the American Academy of Neurological and Orthopaedic Surgeons. *See also* American Academy of Neurological and Orthopaedic Surgeons; board; certification; forensic medicine.

American Board of Medical Psychotherapists (ABMP) A national board founded in 1982 composed of 2,349 psychiatrists, psychologists, social workers, and psychiatric nurses interested in psychotherapy. It offers certification review and continuing education programs. *See also* board; certification; continuing education; psychotherapy.

American Board of Medical Specialties (ABMS) A national organization founded in 1970 composed of primary medical specialty boards and joint boards; organizations with related interests are associate members. It acts for approved medical specialty boards as a group. Medical specialty boards of the ABMS currently include allergy and immunology, anesthesiology, colon and rectal surgery, dermatology, emergency medicine, family practice, internal medicine, medical genetics, neurological surgery, nuclear medicine, obstetrics and gynecology, ophthalmology, orthopaedic surgery, otolaryngology, pathology, pediatrics, physical medicine and rehabilitation, plastic surgery, preventive medicine, psychiatry and neurology, radiology, surgery, thoracic surgery, and urology. *See also* allergy and immunology; anesthesiology; board; colon and rectal surgery; dermatology; emergency medicine; family practice; internal medicine; medical genetics; medical specialties; medical specialty boards; neurological surgery; nuclear medicine; obstetrics and gynecology; ophthalmology; orthopaedic surgery; otolaryngology; pathology; pediatrics; physical medicine and rehabilitation; plastic surgery; preventive medicine; psychiatry and neurology; radiology; surgery; thoracic surgery; urology.

American Board of Medical Toxicology (ABMT) A national board founded in 1968 that evaluates and certifies physicians in medical toxicology. *See also* board; certification; medical toxicology; physician; specialty boards.

American Board of Neurological Microsurgery (ABNM) A national board composed of 175 neurological microsurgery specialists. It promotes scientific advancement and provides educational courses in neurological microsurgery. *See also* board; continuing medical education; microsurgery; neurological surgery.

American Board of Neurological/Orthopaedic Laser Surgery (ABNOLS) A national board composed of 150 laser surgeons interested in advancing scientific knowledge and education in the field. *See also* board; laser; surgery.

American Board of Neurological and Orthopaedic Medicine and Surgery (ABNOMS) A national board founded in 1977 composed of 500 individuals proficient in neurological and orthopaedic medicine and surgery who have previous board certification and proper preceptorship and have made significant contributions to the field of neurological and orthopaedic medicine and surgery. *See also* board; certification; neurological surgery; orthopaedic/orthopedic surgery; surgery.

American Board of Neurological Surgery (ABNS) A national medical specialty board founded in 1940 composed of 3,761 diplomates that investigates qualifications of, administers examinations to, and certifies as diplomates physicians specializing in neurological surgery. *See also* board; certification; diplomate; medical specialty boards; neurological surgery.

American Board of Neuroscience Nursing (ABNN) A national board founded in 1978 composed of 765 registered nurses who have passed a written examination demonstrating achievement in neuroscience nursing. Formerly (1984) American Association of Neurosurgical Nurses. *See also* board; neuroscience; nursing; registered nurse; specialty boards.

American Board of Nuclear Medicine (ABNM) A national medical specialty board founded in 1971 sponsored by the American Boards of Internal Medicine, Pathology, and Radiology and the Society of Nuclear Medicine. It certifies as diplomates physicians specializing in nuclear medicine. *See also* American Board of Internal Medicine; American Board of Pathology; American Board of Radiology; board; certification; diplomate; medical specialty boards; nuclear medicine; Society of Nuclear Medicine.

American Board of Nutrition (ABN) A national board founded in 1948 composed of physicians qualified to treat nutritional and metabolic disorders and doctoral recipients working on problems of human nutrition and nutrient requirements. It establishes standards for qualification of persons as specialists in the field of human nutrition, holds examinations, and certifies as diplomates those who meet its qualifications. *See also* board; certification; diplomate; nutrition; physician; standard.

American Board of Obstetrics and Gynecology (ABOG) A national medical specialty board founded in 1927 to establish qualifications, conduct examinations, and certify as diplomates those physicians qualified to specialize in obstetrics and gynecology. *See also* board; certification; diplomate; medical specialty boards; obstetrics and gynecology.

American Board for Occupational Health Nurses (ABOHN) A national board founded in 1972 that establishes standards and confers initial and ongo-

ing certification in occupational health nursing. *See also* board; certification; occupational health nurse; recertification; standard.

American Board of Ophthalmology (ABO) A national medical specialty board founded in 1916 to determine the adequacy of training, the professional preparation, and ophthalmic knowledge of ophthalmologists who wish to be certified. It certifies as diplomates physicians specializing in ophthalmology. *See also* board; certification; diplomate; medical specialty boards; ophthalmology.

American Board of Opticianry (ABO) A national board founded in 1947 that provides uniform standards for certifying dispensing opticians by administering the National Opticianry Competency Examination and by issuing certified optician certificates to those passing the examination. *See also* board; certification; opticianry.

American Board of Oral and Maxillofacial Surgery (ABOMS) A national dental board that certifies as diplomates dentists specializing in oral and maxillofacial surgery. *See also* board; certification; dental specialties; diplomate; oral and maxillofacial surgery; specialty boards.

American Board of Oral Pathology (ABOP) A national board founded in 1948 that arranges, conducts, and controls examinations to determine the competence of applicants wishing to be certified in oral pathology. There are 260 diplomates of the organization. *See also* board; certification; diplomate; oral pathology.

American Board of Orthodontics (ABO) A national board founded in 1929 that investigates the qualifications of, administers examinations to, and certifies as diplomates dentists specializing in orthodontics. There currently are 1,695 diplomates. *See also* board; certification; dental specialties; diplomate; orthodontics; specialty boards.

American Board of Orthodontics, College of Diplomates of the *See* College of Diplomates of the American Board of Orthodontics.

American Board of Orthopedic Surgery (ABOS) A national medical specialty board founded in 1934 to establish qualifications, conduct annual examinations, and certify as diplomates those physicians qualified to practice orthopedic surgery. *See also* board; certification; diplomate; medical specialty boards; orthopaedic/orthopedic surgery.

American Board of Otolaryngology (ABO) A

national medical specialty board founded in 1924 that holds examinations and certifies as diplomates qualified physicians specializing in otolaryngology. *See also* board; certification; diplomate; medical specialty boards; otolaryngology.

American Board of Pathology (ABP) A national medical specialty board founded in 1936 that maintains a registry of certified pathologists, participates in the evaluation and review of graduate medical school pathology programs, and examines and certifies as specialists in pathology doctors of medicine or osteopathic medicine who have had three to five years postgraduate training in laboratory medicine and pathology. *See also* board; certification; medical specialty boards; pathology; registry.

American Board of Pediatric Dentistry (ABPD) A national board founded in 1940 composed of approximately 800 diplomates whose purpose is to investigate the qualifications of, administer examinations to, and certify as diplomates dentists specializing in the care of children. Formerly (1986) the American Board of Pedodontics. *See also* board; certification; diplomate; pediatric dentistry; specialty boards.

American Board of Pediatrics (ABP) A national medical specialty board founded in 1933 composed of 40,000 diplomates that establishes qualifications, conducts examinations, and certifies as diplomates physicians qualified as specialists in pediatrics. *See also* board; certification; diplomate; medical specialty boards; pediatrics.

American Board of Pedodontics (ABP) *See* American Board of Pediatric Dentistry.

American Board of Periodontology (ABP) A national board founded in 1939 that conducts examinations to determine the qualifications and competence of dentists who voluntarily apply for certification as diplomates in the field of periodontology (periodontics). *See also* board; certification; diplomate; periodontics; specialty boards.

American Board of Physical Medicine and Rehabilitation (ABPMR) A national medical specialty board founded in 1947 composed of 3,800 certified physicians. The board establishes qualifications, conducts examinations, and certifies physicians qualified to specialize in physical medicine and rehabilitation. *See also* board; certification; medical specialty boards; physical medicine and rehabilitation.

American Board of Plastic Surgery (ABPS) A national medical specialty board founded in 1937 to investigate the qualifications of, administer examinations to, and certify as diplomates physicians specializing in plastic surgery. *See also* board; certification; diplomate; medical specialty boards; plastic surgery.

American Board of Podiatric Orthopedics (ABPO) A national board founded in 1975 composed of 617 podiatrists who have taken a competency examination prepared by the board. It offers a certifying examination in foot orthopedics for podiatrists. *See also* board; certification; podiatric orthopedics.

American Board of Podiatric Surgery (ABPS) A national board founded in 1975 for the purpose of certifying the competence of legally licensed podiatrists. To date, there are approximately 3,000 board-certified podiatric surgeons. *See also* board; certification; podiatric surgery; specialty boards.

American Board of Post Anesthesia Nursing Certification (ABPANC) A national board founded in 1985 that administers examinations to individuals wishing to attain post-anesthesia nursing certification. *See also* anesthesia; board; certification; nursing.

American Board of Preventive Medicine (ABPM) A national medical specialty board founded in 1948 that determines eligibility requirements, administers examinations, and certifies physicians in the specialized fields of public health, aerospace medicine, occupational medicine, and preventive medicine. There are approximately 5,600 diplomates. *See also* board; certification; diplomate; medical specialty boards; preventive medicine.

American Board of Professional Disability Consultants (ABPDC) A for-profit board founded in 1988 composed of 350 physicians, psychologists, counselors, and attorneys. It identifies and awards diplomate standing to specialists in disability and personal injury. *See also* board; consultant; diplomate; disability; personal injury.

American Board of Professional Liability Attorneys (ABPLA) A national board founded in 1972 composed of 300 liability-litigation attorneys who have satisfied requirements of litigation experience and who have passed the National Board of Trial Advocacy written examination for civil litigation specialists and the oral ABPLA examination. Its objectives include promoting and improving ethical and technical standards of advocacy and litigation practice in product and professional liability litigation and establishing basic standards for training, qualification, and recognition of specialists. *See also* advocacy; attorney; board; National Board of Trial Advocacy; product liability; professional liability.

American Board of Professional Psychology (ABPP) A national board founded in 1947 composed of 3,750 members who have successfully passed oral examinations administered in eight specialties: clinical psychology, industrial and organizational psychology, forensic psychology, counseling psychology, clinical neuropsychology, family psychology, health psychology, and school psychology. Candidates must have five years of qualifying experience in psychological practice. *See also* board; certification; psychology.

American Board of Prosthodontics (ABP) A national dental board that certifies as diplomates dentists specializing in fixed, removable, and maxillofacial prosthodontics. *See also* board; certification; diplomate; prosthodontics; specialty boards.

American Board of Psychiatry and Neurology (ABPN) A national medical specialty board founded in 1934 that determines eligibility requirements, administers examinations, and certifies physicians with specialized training in psychiatry, neurology, child neurology, child adolescent psychiatry, clinical neurophysiology, and geriatric psychiatry. There are 37,000 diplomates. *See also* board; certification; diplomate; medical specialty boards; neurology; psychiatry.

American Board of Psychological Hypnosis (ABPH) A national board founded in 1959 that awards specialty diplomas to psychologists meeting requirements in experimental and clinical hypnosis. Its purpose is to raise the standards of individuals conducting research in hypnosis and using it in clinical practice by requiring specialized training and experience as evidenced by advanced credentials in psychology, published research, written and oral examinations, and recommendations of colleagues. *See also* board; hypnosis.

American Board of Quality Assurance and Utilization Review Physicians (ABQAURP) A national board founded in 1977 composed of 5,000 physicians and coordinators involved in quality assurance and utilization review. It certifies as diplomates physicians and other qualified individuals specializing in quality assurance and utilization review. *See*

also board; certification; diplomate; quality assurance; utilization review.

American Board of Radiology (ABR) A national medical specialty board founded in 1934 that establishes qualifications, conducts examinations, and certifies physicians in the specialty of radiology and physicists in radiological physics and related branches (sciences dealing with x-rays or rays from radioactive substances for medical use). *See also* board; certification; medical specialty boards; radiology.

American Board of Registration of Electroencephalographic and Evoked Potentials Technologists (ABRET) A national board founded in 1961 that determines the competency of electroencephalography technologists through administration of written and oral examinations. *See also* board; electroencephalographic technician/technologist; electroencephalography; evoked potentials.

American Boards for Accreditation and Certification, National Association for the Advancement of Psychoanalysis and the *See* National Association for the Advancement of Psychoanalysis and the American Boards for Accreditation and Certification.

American Board of Spinal Surgery (ABSS) A national board composed of 250 spinal surgeons seeking to advance knowledge and provide education in the field of spinal surgery. *See also* board; physician; spinal cord; surgery.

American Board of Surgery (ABS) A national medical specialty board founded in 1937 that certifies as diplomates physicians specializing in surgery. It also certifies Special Qualifications in pediatric surgery and general vascular surgery and Added Qualifications in general vascular surgery, surgical critical care, and hand surgery. It currently offers recertification in general surgery and pediatric surgery. *See also* American Pediatric Surgical Association; board; certification; diplomate; general surgery; medical specialty boards; pediatric surgery; recertification; vascular surgery.

American Board of Thoracic Surgery (ABTS) A national medical specialty board founded in 1948 that investigates the qualifications of, administers examinations to, and certifies physicians specializing in thoracic surgery. *See also* board; certification; thorax; medical specialty boards; thoracic surgery.

American Board of Toxicology (ABT) A national board founded in 1979 that conducts a certification program in toxicology and administers annual certification and recertification examinations. There are 1,200 diplomates. *See also* board; certification; diplomate; recertification; toxicology.

American Board of Trial Advocates (ABTA) A national board founded in 1958 composed of 3,210 civil trial plaintiff and defense attorneys and judges. It seeks to preserve the jury system. *See also* attorney; board; jury; trial.

American Board of Tropical Medicine (ABTM) A national board founded in 1980 that investigates the qualifications and determines the competency of candidates applying for membership and provides continuing medical education to specialists in tropical medicine. *See also* board; certification; continuing medical education; tropical medicine.

American Board of Urologic Allied Health Professionals (ABUAHP) A national board founded in 1972 that conducts an annual certification examination for urological professionals. Its parent organization is American Urological Association Allied. *See also* allied health professional; American Urological Association Allied; board; certification; urology.

American Board of Urology (ABU) A national medical specialty board founded in 1935 that conducts examinations and certifies physicians in the specialty of urology. *See also* board; certification; medical specialty boards; urology.

American Boards for Accreditation and Certification, National Association for the Advancement of Psychoanalysis and the *See* National Association for the Advancement of Psychoanalysis and the American Boards for Accreditation and Certification.

American Broncho-Esophagological Association (ABEA) A national organization founded in 1917 composed of 300 otolaryngologists, chest specialists, thoracic surgeons, and gastroenterologists engaged in the practice of broncho-esophagology (diseases and injuries of the respiratory system and upper digestive tract). *See also* gastroenterology; otolaryngology; thoracic surgery.

American Burn Association (ABA) A national organization founded in 1967 composed of 3,500 physicians, nurses, physical therapists, occupational therapists, dietitians, biomedical engineers, social workers, and researchers interested in the care of burn patients. *See also* burn; burn unit.

American Cancer Society (ACS) A national organization founded in 1913 composed of 2,500,000 volunteers supporting education and research in cancer

prevention, diagnosis, detection, and treatment. *See also* cancer.

American Cardiology Technologists Association *See* National Society for Cardiovascular/Pulmonary Technology.

American Celiac Society *See* American Celiac Society/Dietary Support Coalition.

American Celiac Society/Dietary Support Coalition (ACS/DSC) A national organization founded in 1970 composed of 4,000 physicians who diagnose and care for individuals with gluten-sensitive intestinal disease, dietitians, nutritionists, agencies that serve individuals with gluten-sensitive intestinal disease, and other individuals interested in a gluten-free diet. It provides information on how to follow a gluten-free diet, assists members in locating specialty foods that are gluten-free, and encourages retailers to make gluten-free products available. Formerly (1990) American Celiac Society. *See also* celiac disease; gluten; nutrition.

American Center for Chinese Medical Sciences (ACCMS) A national organization founded in 1974 composed of 200 medical and scientific professionals from the US and China working to develop medical contacts, share experiences, and promote the exchange of scientific information between American and China. It sponsors meetings and tours to China, promotes joint research, and conducts lectures. Formerly (1980) American Center for Chinese Medicine.

American Center for Chinese Medicine *See* American Center for Chinese Medical Sciences.

American Chinese Medical Society *See* Chinese American Medical Society.

American Chiropractic Association (ACA) A national organization founded in 1930 composed of 20,000 chiropractors. Specialized councils include Chiropractic Orthopedics, Diagnosis and Internal Disorders, Diagnostic Imaging, Mental Health, Neurology, Nutrition, Physiological Therapeutics, Sports Injuries and Physical Fitness, and Technical. *See also* chiropractic; chiropractor.

American Chiropractic Board of Radiology *See* Council on Diagnostic Imaging.

American Chiropractic Board of Thermography *See* Council on Diagnostic Imaging.

American Chiropractic Registry of Radiologic Technologists (ACRRT) A national organization founded in 1982 composed of 2,000 chiropractic assistants and radiologic technologists employed in chiropractic offices. It serves as a certifying agency for individuals in the field and maintains a registry of certified chiropractic radiologic technologists. *See also* certification; chiropractic; registry.

American Cleft Palate-Craniofacial Association (ACPA) A national organization founded in 1943 composed of 2,500 physicians, dentists, speech pathologists, audiologists, psychologists, nurses and other individuals engaged in the care of individuals with cleft lip and palate and associated craniofacial deformities. Formerly (1988) American Cleft Palate Association. *See also* cleft palate.

American Clinical and Climatological Association (ACCA) A national organization founded in 1884 composed of 375 internists interested in the clinical study of diseases associated with various climates. *See also* climatology; internal medicine.

American Clinical Laboratory Association (ACLA) A national organization founded in 1971 composed of corporations, partnerships, and individuals owning or controlling one or more independent clinical laboratory facilities operating for a profit and licensed under the Clinical Laboratories Improvement Act of 1967 or the Clinical Laboratories Improvement Amendment of 1988 or accredited by the Medicare program. Its purposes include elimination of inequalities in the standards applied to different segments of the clinical laboratory market and the discouragement of the enactment of restrictive legislative or regulatory policies. *See also* clinical laboratory; Clinical Laboratory Improvement Act of 1967 (CLIA '67); Clinical Laboratory Improvement Amendments of 1988 (CLIA '88); Medicare; standard.

American College of Addiction Treatment Administrators (ACATA) A national organization founded in 1984 composed of 300 administrators of addiction treatment facilities interested in educational and professional standards in the field of addiction treatment administration. *See also* addiction; administrator.

American College of Advancement in Medicine (ACAM) A national organization founded in 1973 composed of 450 physicians interested in promoting preventive medicine throughout the world. It conducts research programs in the fields of chelation therapy, nutritional medicine, and other preventive modalities. Formerly (1987) American Academy of Medical Preventics. *See also* chelation therapy; holistic medicine; preventive medicine.

American College of Allergy and Immunology (ACAI) A national organization founded in 1987 composed of 3,400 practicing allergists, educators, researchers, and clinical immunologists interested in encouraging the study, improving the practice, and advancing the cause of clinical immunology and allergy. Formed by merger of American College of Allergists (founded 1942) and American Association for Clinical Immunology and Allergy (founded 1964). *See also* allergy and immunology.

American College of Angiology (ACA) A national organization founded in 1954 composed of 2,500 physicians and basic scientists in health care industries interested in the advancement of the study and research of vascular diseases. *See also* angiology; Fellow of the American College of Angiology.

American College of Angiology, Fellow of the *See* American College of Angiology.

American College of Apothecaries (ACA) A national organization founded in 1940 composed of 1,000 pharmacists who own and operate prescription pharmacies, including hospital pharmacists, pharmacy students, and faculty of colleges of pharmacy. Its primary objective is the translation, transformation, and dissemination of knowledge, research data, and recent developments in the pharmaceutical industry and public health. It sponsors the Community Pharmacy Residency Program and offers continuing education courses. *See also* apothecary; continuing education; pharmacy.

American College of Cardiology (ACC) A national organization founded in 1949 composed of 18,000 physicians and scientists specializing in cardiology and cardiovascular diseases. It operates Heart House Learning Center and maintains numerous committees. *See also* cardiology; Fellow of the American College of Cardiology.

American College of Cardiology, Fellow of the *See* Fellow of the American College of Cardiology.

American College of Cardiovascular Administrators (ACCA) A chapter of the American Academy of Medical Administrators, founded in 1986 and composed of 750 upper-level and middle-level managers in the cardiovascular health care field. It represents members with the medical industry and provides credentialing of cardiology administrators. *See also* administrator; American Academy of Medical Administrators; cardiovascular.

American College of Chemosurgery *See* American College of Mohs Micrographic Surgery and Cutaneous Oncology.

American College of Chest Physicians (ACCP) A national organization founded in 1935 composed of 15,000 physicians and surgeons specializing in diseases of the chest (diseases of the heart and lungs). It promotes undergraduate and postgraduate medical education and research in the field. *See also* Fellow of the American College of Chest Physicians.

American College of Chest Physicians, Fellow of the *See* Fellow of the American College of Chest Physicians.

American College of Chiropractic Orthopedists (ACCO) A national organization founded in 1964 composed of 755 certified and noncertified chiropractic orthopedists and students enrolled in a postgraduate chiropractic orthopedic program. *See also* certification; chiropractic.

American College of Clinical Pharmacology (ACCP) A national organization founded in 1969 composed of 875 individuals who have earned the degree of Doctor of Medicine or a doctorate in any one of the biomedical sciences and individuals who have had at least three years of training or the equivalent in basic science, internal medicine, or an allied field. It promotes the science of clinical pharmacology including excellence in the investigational and clinical testing of drugs. *See also* internal medicine; pharmacology.

American College of Clinical Pharmacy (ACCP) A national organization founded in 1979 composed of 1,600 clinical pharmacists dedicated to promoting the rational use of drugs in society and advancing the practice of clinical pharmacy and interdisciplinary health care. *See also* drug; pharmacy.

American College for Continuing Education (ACCE) A national organization founded in 1968 that promotes programs for continuing education in podiatry. Formerly (1983) American College of Foot Specialists. *See also* continuing education; podiatric medicine.

American College of Cryosurgery (ACCRYO) A national organization founded in 1977 composed of 336 physicians, general surgeons, scientists, and other individuals involved in the clinical application of cryosurgery. It serves, among other activities, as a national faculty to educate members and teach at university training centers. *See also* cryosurgery.

American College of Dentists (ACD) A national

organization founded in 1920 composed of 5,700 dentists and other individuals interested in advancing the standards of the profession of dentistry. *See also* dentistry; Fellow of the American College of Dentists; standard.

American College of Dentists, Fellow of the *See* Fellow of the American College of Dentists.

American College of Emergency Physicians (ACEP) A national organization founded in 1968 composed of 14,800 physicians who devote a significant portion of their professional time to emergency medicine. It aims to provide a unifying direction of purpose in the field of the emergency medicine. *See also* advanced pediatric life support; emergency medicine; emergency physician; Fellow of the American College of Emergency Physicians.

American College of Emergency Physicians, Fellow of the *See* Fellow of the American College of Emergency Physicians.

American College of Epidemiology (ACE) A national organization founded in 1979 composed of 850 medical professionals involved in the field of epidemiology. It promotes education in the practice of epidemiology and maintains professional standards in the field. *See also* epidemiology; standard.

American College of Foot Orthopedists (ACFO) A national organization founded in 1949 composed of 675 podiatrists sanctioned as specialists to practice foot orthopedics. *See also* podiatric medicine.

American College of Foot Specialists *See* American College for Continuing Education.

American College of Foot Surgeons (ACFS) A national organization founded in 1940 composed of 3,000 podiatric surgeons interested in promoting and disseminating information on podiatric surgery among the public, podiatric surgeons, and other health professionals. *See also* Fellow of the American College of Foot Surgeons; podiatric medicine.

American College of Foot Surgeons, Fellow of the *See* Fellow of the American College of Foot Surgeons.

American College of Gastroenterology (ACG) A national organization founded in 1932 composed of 4,000 physicians and surgeons specializing in diseases and disorders of the gastrointestinal tract and accessory organs of digestion, including disorders due to nutrition. *See also* disease; gastroenterology; nutrition.

American College of General Practice *See* American College of Medicine.

American College of General Practitioners in Osteopathic Medicine and Surgery (ACGPOMS) A national organization founded in 1950 composed of 9,000 osteopathic physicians in general practice. It aims to advance the standards of general practice through increasing educational opportunities and establishing a department of general practice in hospitals. It awards the degree of Fellow for outstanding contributions in education to the college. *See also* osteopathic medicine; standard.

American College Health Association (ACHA) A national organization founded in 1920 composed of 3,000 institutions and individuals interested in promoting health for students and all other members of the college community.

American College of Health Care Administrators (ACHCA) A national organization founded in 1962 composed of 6,700 persons engaged in the administration of long term care institutions, in medical administration, or in activities designed to improve the quality of nursing home administration. It certifies members' competence in nursing home and long term care administration. Formerly American College of Nursing Home Administrators. *See also* administrator; certification; long term care; nursing home administrator.

American College of Healthcare Executives (ACHE) A national organization founded in 1933 composed of 23,000 hospital and health service administrators. It works to keep members abreast of current and future trends, issues, and developments; shape productive and effective organizational strategies and professional performance; increase the visibility and recognition of the health care management profession; and maintain professional standards. It maintains numerous committees and task forces, conducts research programs, and compiles statistics. Formerly (1985) American College of Hospital Administrators. *See also* administrator; executive; Fellow of the American College of Healthcare Executives.

American College of Healthcare Executives, Fellow of the *See* Fellow of the American College of Healthcare Executives.

American College of Hospital Administrators *See* American College of Healthcare Executives.

American College of Laboratory Animal Medicine (ACLAM) A national organization founded in 1957 composed of 360 veterinarians specializing in laboratory animal medicine. It establishes standards of training and experience for qualification of specialists in the field, administers examinations, and certifies eligible specialists. It sponsors symposia on infectious and metabolic diseases of laboratory animals and conducts education for diplomates on topics including quality assurance, biohazards, and animal production. *See also* animal care technologist; animal experimentation; antivivisectionist; certification; diplomate; vivisection.

American College of Legal Medicine (ACLM) A national organization founded in 1955 composed of 1,053 individuals who hold degrees in medicine and law. It promotes and advances the field of legal medicine or medical jurisprudence and arranges for meetings with medical, legal, and professional groups and legislative, judicial, and enforcement bodies interested in any province where law and medicine are contiguous. It also makes available postgraduate training in legal medicine and/or medical jurisprudence. *See also* health law; hospital law; jurisprudence.

American College of Medical Group Administrators (ACMGA) A national certification organization founded in 1956 composed of 1,200 members drawn from the Medical Group Management Association. It encourages medical group practice administrators to improve and maintain their proficiency and to establish a program with uniform standards of admission, advancement, and certification in order to achieve the highest possible standards in the profession of medical group practice administration. *See also* certification; Fellow of the American College of Medical Group Administrators; group practice; Medical Group Management Association; standard.

American College of Medical Group Administrators, Fellow of the *See* Fellow of the American College of Medical Group Administrators.

American College of Medical Quality (ACURP) A national organization founded in 1973 composed of physicians, affiliates, and institutions seeking to set standards of competence in the field of quality assurance and utilization review. It conducts educational seminars and workshops in quality assurance and utilization review and compiles statistics on numbers of physicians and allied health personnel working in quality assurance and utilization review.

See also allied health professional; physician; quality assurance; utilization review.

American College of Medicine (ACM) A national organization founded in 1981 that promotes the specific needs of general practitioners and provides continuing medical education programs for maintaining competence in the practice of medicine. Formerly (1984) American College of General Practice. *See also* continuing medical education; general practice.

American College of Mental Health Administration (ACMHA) A national organization founded in 1980 composed of 250 mental health clinicians and administrators. *See also* administration; mental health professional.

American College of Mohs Micrographic Surgery and Cutaneous Oncology (ACMMSCO) A national organization founded in 1967 composed of 260 physicians, including dermatologists, surgeons, plastic surgeons, and other specialists, who have had a minimum of one year of training in chemosurgery at an approved institution. It provides accreditation of physicians who have become proficient in the method and strives to facilitate education and the exchange of ideas. Formerly (1987) American College of Chemosurgery. *See also* accreditation; chemosurgery; dermatologist; plastic surgeon; surgeon.

American College of Neuropsychiatrists (ACN) A national organization founded in 1937 composed of 420 psychiatrists, neurologists, and other individuals interested in study and research in neurology and psychiatry in the osteopathic profession. *See also* osteopathic medicine; psychiatry.

American College of Neuropsychopharmacology (ACNP) A national organization founded in 1961 composed of 606 investigators whose work is related to neuropsycho-pharmacology. It promotes the scientific study and application of neuropsychopharmacology and conducts study groups and plenary sessions. *See also* neuropharmacology; pharmacology.

American College of Nuclear Medicine (ACNM) A national organization founded in 1972 composed of 500 physicians and medical scientists in nuclear medicine interested in advancing the science of nuclear medicine, studying the socioeconomic aspects of the practice of nuclear medicine, and encouraging improved and continuing education for practitioners in the field. *See also* continuing edu-

cation; nuclear medicine.

American College of Nuclear Physicians (ACNP) A national organization founded in 1974 composed of 1,200 nuclear medicine physicians, scientists, and corporations interested in fostering high standards of nuclear medicine service and promoting the continuing competence of practitioners of nuclear medicine. Problem-solving areas include unnecessary and costly regulations and restrictions; public fear, lack of understanding, and misinformation; complex state and federal legislation; transportation difficulties involving nuclear medicine supplies; and previous lack of cohesive efforts in addressing such problems. *See also* nuclear medicine; nuclear medicine physician.

American College of Nurse-Midwives (ACNM) A national organization founded in 1955 composed of 3,000 registered nurses certified to extend their practice into providing gynecological services and care of mothers and babies throughout the maternity cycle. Members have completed an ACNM-accredited program of study and clinical experience in midwifery and passed a national certification examination. *See also* certification; certified nurse-midwife; nurse-midwife; registered nurse.

American College of Nursing Home Administrators *See* American College of Health Care Administrators.

American College of Nutrition (ACN) A national organization founded in 1959 composed of 1,010 physicians, research scientists, nutritionists, dietitians, allied health personnel, and postbaccalaureate students and trainees in these fields. It provides education on clinical and experimental developments in the field of nutrition and provides continuing education of physicians and other scientists on nutritional subjects. *See also* continuing education; nutrition.

American College of Obstetricians and Gynecologists (ACOG) A national organization founded in 1951 composed of 31,000 physicians specializing in childbirth and the diseases of women. It sponsors continuing professional development programs. *See also* Fellow of the American College of Obstetricians and Gynecologists; obstetrician-gynecologist.

American College of Obstetricians and Gynecologists, Fellow of the *See* Fellow of the American College of Obstetricians and Gynecologists.

American College of Occupational and Environmental Medicine (ACOEM) A national organization founded in 1988 composed of 5,200 physicians specializing in occupational and environmental medicine. Formerly (1992) American College of Occupational Medicine. *See also* environmental health; occupational medicine; physician.

American College of Occupational Medicine *See* American College of Occupational and Environmental Medicine.

American College of Oral and Maxillofacial Surgeons (ACOMS) A national organization founded in 1975 composed of 1,350 diplomates of the American Board of Oral and Maxillofacial Surgery who practice oral and maxillofacial surgery. *See also* American Board of Oral and Maxillofacial Surgery; diplomate; oral and maxillofacial surgery.

American College of Osteopathic Emergency Physicians (ACOEP) A national organization founded in 1975 composed of 420 osteopathic emergency physicians. It provides and evaluates postdoctoral and continuing education for osteopathic emergency physicians; encourages and implements the training of emergency physicians; and promotes the coordination of community emergency care facilities and personnel. It maintains the American Osteopathic Board of Emergency Medicine; sponsors the Emergency Medicine Continuing Medical Education Program for Accreditation; and serves as the evaluating body for Osteopathic Emergency Medicine Residency Programs. *See also* continuing medical education; emergency medicine; osteopathic medicine; residency.

American College of Osteopathic Hospital Administrators *See* College of Osteopathic Healthcare Executives.

American College of Osteopathic Internists (ACOI) A national organization founded in 1943 composed of 1,300 osteopathic physicians who limit their practice to internal medicine and various subspecialties and who intend, through postdoctoral education, to qualify as certified specialists in the field. *See also* certification; internal medicine; osteopathic medicine.

American College of Osteopathic Obstetricians and Gynecologists (ACOOG) A national organization founded in 1934 composed of 538 osteopathic physicians and surgeons specializing in obstetrics and gynecology. It conducts educational programs and reviews osteopathic obstetric and gynecologic residency training programs. *See also* obstetrics and gynecology; osteopathic medicine.

American College of Osteopathic Pediatricians (ACOP) A national organization founded in 1940 composed of 350 osteopathic physicians who have received or are receiving advanced training in pediatrics and who are specializing in pediatric practice. *See also* osteopathic medicine; pediatrics.

American College of Osteopathic Surgeons (ACOS) A national organization founded in 1927 composed of 1,300 osteopathic physicians specializing in surgery and surgical specialties, including general surgery, neurological surgery, orthopedic surgery, plastic surgery, thoracic-cardiovascular surgery, and urological surgery. *See also* osteopathic medicine; surgery.

American College of Physician Executives (ACPE) A national organization founded in 1978 composed of 6,000 physicians whose primary professional responsibility is the management of health care organizations. The ACPE, among other activities, certifies physician executives as diplomates. Absorbed (1989) American Academy of Medical Directors (founded 1975). *See also* certification; diplomate; executive; Fellow of the American College of Physician Executives; physician executive.

American College of Physician Executives, Fellow of the *See* Fellow of the American College of Physician Executives.

American College of Physicians (ACP) A national organization founded in 1915 composed of 70,000 physicians specializing in internal medicine and closely related specialties, such as dermatology, neurology, psychiatry, cardiology, gastroenterology, and public health. It sponsors annual postgraduate courses for practicing physicians. *See also* continuing medical education; Fellow of the American College of Physicians; internal medicine.

American College of Physicians, Fellow of the *See* Fellow of the American College of Physicians.

American College of Podiatric Radiologists (ACPR) A national organization founded in 1944 composed of 80 podiatrists interested in the use and interpretation of x-rays in treating ailments of the lower extremities. It sponsors postgraduate seminars on podiatric radiology and supports research. *See also* podiatric medicine; radiology.

American College of Podopediatrics (ACP) A national organization founded in 1977 composed of 200 podiatric physicians and surgeons, general physicians and surgeons, psychologists, and physical therapists interested in children's foot health. *See also* podiatric medicine; podopediatrics.

American College of Preventive Medicine (ACPM) A national organization founded in 1954 composed of 2,000 physicians specializing in preventive medicine, public health, occupational medicine, or aerospace medicine. It sponsors special education programs. *See also* Fellow of the American College of Preventive Medicine; preventive medicine.

American College of Preventive Medicine, Fellow of the *See* Fellow of the American College of Preventive Medicine.

American College of Prosthodontists (ACP) A national organization founded in 1970 composed of approximately 2,100 dentists specializing in prosthetics who are either board certified, board prepared, or under training in an approved graduate or residency program. *See also* board certified; board prepared; prosthodontics.

American College of Psychiatrists (ACP) A national organization founded in 1963 composed of 800 individuals who have made a significant contribution to psychiatry. *See also* psychiatry.

American College of Psychoanalysts (ACPA) A national organization founded in 1969 composed of 200 physician psychoanalysts. Its goal is to contribute to the development of psychoanalysis. *See also* physician; psychoanalysis.

American College of Radiology (ACR) A national organization founded in 1923 composed of 20,000 physicians and radiologic physicists who specialize in the use of x-ray, ultrasound, nuclear medicine magnetic resonance, and other imaging modalities for the diagnosis of disease and the treatment and management of cancer. *See also* Fellow of the American College of Radiology; radiology.

American College of Radiology, Fellow of the *See* Fellow of the American College of Radiology.

American College of Rheumatology (ACR) A national organization founded in 1934 composed of 4,700 physicians, scientists, and academicians with a common interest in patients with joint and connective tissue diseases. Formerly (1989) American Rheumatism Association. *See also* connective tissue; joint; rheumatology.

American College of Sports Medicine (ACSM) A national organization founded in 1954 composed of 12,500 physicians and other individuals interested in the benefits and effects of exercise and the treatment

and prevention of injuries incurred in sports, exercise, and fitness activities. *See also* exercise; Fellow of the American College of Sports Medicine; fitness; sports medicine.

American College of Sports Medicine, Fellow of the *See* Fellow of the American College of Sports Medicine.

American College of Surgeons (ACS) A national organization founded in 1913 composed of 51,000 surgeons organized primarily to improve the quality of care for surgical patients by elevating standards of surgical education and practice. It conducts, among other activities, nationwide programs to improve emergency medical services and hospital cancer programs. *See also* advanced trauma life support; cancer; emergency medical services system; Fellow of the American College of Surgeons; general surgery; tumor registry.

American College of Surgeons, Fellow of the *See* Fellow of the American College of Surgeons.

American College Testing (ACT) An organization founded in 1959 that administers tests, including the Medical College Admission Test. *See also* Medical College Admission Test; standardized test.

American College of Toxicology (ACT) A national organization founded in 1977 composed of 900 individuals interested in toxicology and related disciplines, such as analytical chemistry, biology, pathology, teratology, and immunology. *See also* biology; chemistry; immunology; pathology; teratology; toxicology.

American College of Trial Lawyers (ACTL) A national honorary organization founded in 1950 composed of 4,200 practicing trial lawyers, former trial lawyers now holding elective or appointed posts, and judges of courts of record. *See also* lawyer; trial; trial court.

American Conference of Governmental Industrial Hygienists (ACGIH) A national organization founded in 1938 composed of 3,800 individuals employed by official governmental units who are responsible for full-time programs of industrial hygiene, educators, and other individuals conducting research in industrial hygiene. *See also* industrial hygiene; industrial hygienist.

American Congress of Rehabilitation Medicine (ACRM) A national organization founded in 1921 composed of 3,300 physicians and allied health specialists active in and contributing to advancement in the field of rehabilitation medicine. *See also* allied health professional; physical medicine and rehabilitation; physician.

American Consumers Association (ACA) A national organization founded in 1984 that provides information on consumer services and goods, including product quality, cost, safety, and effectiveness. It promotes exchange of information beneficial to the health and welfare of the American consumer. *See also* consumer; consumerism.

American Correctional Health Services Association (ACHSA) A national organization founded in 1975 composed of 1,600 health care providers interested in improving the quality of correctional health services. Its aims are to provide acceptable health services to incarcerated persons. It conducts conferences on correctional health care management, nursing, mental health, juvenile corrections, and dentistry.

American Corrective Therapy Association *See* American Kinesiotherapy Association.

American Council on Alcoholism (ACA) A national organization founded in 1953 composed of 14,000 local, state, regional, and national groups and individuals working to end alcohol abuse and alcoholism. *See also* alcoholism.

American Council on Alcohol Problems (ACAP) A national federation founded in 1895 composed of 37 state affiliates, 22 denominational judicatories, and 2,000 associate members seeking long-range solutions to the problems posed by alcohol. *See also* alcoholism.

American Council of Applied Clinical Nutrition (ACACN) A national organization founded in 1974 composed of 500 clinical nutrition specialists. It offers structured academic courses and certification. *See also* certification; nutrition.

American Council on Chiropractic Physiotherapy *See* Council on Chiropractic Physiological Therapeutics.

American Council for Drug Education (ACDE) A national organization founded in 1977 composed of 1,500 doctors, mental health counselors, teachers, clergymen, school librarians, parent groups, industry leaders, and individuals interested in disseminating information and research on marijuana, cocaine, and other psychoactive drugs. *See also* drug abuse; education.

American Council for Health Care Reform (ACHCR) A national organization founded in 1980 composed of 15,000 members organized to eliminate what the council terms as unnecessary and costly federal and state health care regulations and laws, such as certificate of public need restrictions that limit public choice in the selection of health care providers. It supports reform of the National Health Planning Act. It testifies before congressional and state legislative committees and coordinates grassroots support for free market approaches to health care delivery. *See also* certificate of need; National Health Planning and Resources Development Act of 1974.

American Council of Hypnotist Examiners (ACHE) A national organization founded in 1980 composed of 7,400 individuals certified in the field of hypnotherapy. The organization educates, examines, and awards certification in the field of hypnotherapy. *See also* certification; hypnosis; hypnotherapy.

American Council on Pharmaceutical Education (ACPE) A national accrediting body for professional programs of colleges and schools of pharmacy and approval of providers of continuing pharmaceutical education. *See also* accreditation; pharmaceutical; pharmacy.

American Council on Science and Health (ACSH) A national organization founded in 1978 composed of 200 individuals who provide consumers with scientifically balanced evaluations of food, chemicals, the environment, and human health. Council personnel participate in government regulatory proceedings, congressional hearings, radio and television programs, and public debates and other forums and write for professional and scientific journals, popular magazines, and newspaper columns. *See also* consumer.

American Counseling Association (ACA) A national organization founded in 1952 composed of 58,000 counseling and human development professionals in elementary and secondary schools, higher education, community agencies and organizations, rehabilitation programs, government, industry, business, and private practice. Formerly (1992) American Association for Counseling and Development. *See also* counsel; counseling.

American Cryonics Society (ACS) A national organization founded in 1969 composed of 204 individuals interested in life extension through cryonics. It promotes education and provides information about cryonic suspension, suspended animation, and low-temperature medicine. It enables individuals to arrange for their own cryonic suspension. It conducts programs to freeze tissue samples from endangered species for possible future cloning. Formerly (1985) Bay Area Cryonics Society. *See also* cryonics.

American Dance Therapy Association (ADTA) A national organization founded in 1966 composed of 1,000 individuals professionally practicing dance therapy, students interested in becoming dance therapists, university departments with dance therapy programs, and individuals in related therapeutic fields. Its purpose is to establish and maintain high standards of professional education and competence in dance therapy. *See also* dance therapy; standard.

American Deafness and Rehabilitation Association (ADARA) A national organization founded in 1966 composed of 1,000 psychiatrists, mental health counselors, teachers, students, researchers, rehabilitation facility personnel, interpreters, speech therapists, social workers, physicians, and other individuals who serve persons with hearing and/or visual impairments. *See also* deafness; hearing impaired; physician; rehabilitation; social worker; speech therapist.

American Dental Assistants Association (ADAA) A national organization founded in 1923 composed of 15,000 individuals employed as dental assistants in dental offices, clinics, hospitals, or institutions; instructors of dental assistants; and dental students. *See also* dental assistant.

American Dental Association (ADA) A national organization founded in 1859 composed of 140,000 dentists. It encourages the improvement of the dental health of the public and promotes the art and science of dentistry in matters of legislation and regulations. It inspects and accredits dental schools and schools for dental hygienists, assistants, and laboratory technicians. It operates a library of 50,000 volumes. *See also* accreditation; dental assistant; dental hygienist; dental laboratory technician; dental laboratory technology accreditation; dental school; dentistry.

American Dental Hygienists' Association (ADHA) A national organization founded in 1923 composed of 30,000 licensed dental hygienists possessing a degree or certificate in dental hygiene granted by an accredited school of dental hygiene. It maintains an accrediting service through the American Dental Association's Commission on Dental Accreditation. *See also* accreditation; dental hygienist.

American Dental Society of Anesthesiology (ADSA) A national organization founded in 1953 composed of 3,200 dentists and physicians interested in encouraging study and progress in dental anesthesiology. *See also* anesthesiology; dentistry.

American Dental Trade Association (ADTA) A national organization founded in 1882 composed of 200 manufacturers and distributors of dental instruments, supplies, and equipment, and dental laboratories. Membership represents 400 dental supply houses and 90% of the total volume of sales in the dental industry. *See also* dentistry.

American Dermatological Association (ADA) A national organization founded in 1876 composed of 350 physicians specializing in dermatology. It promotes teaching, practice, and research in dermatology. *See also* dermatology; physician.

American Diabetes Association (ADA) A national organization founded in 1940 composed of 280,000 health professionals and laypersons interested in diabetes mellitus. It promotes the free exchange of information about diabetes mellitus by educating the public in the early recognition of the disease, the importance of medical supervision in its treatment, and the development of educational methods designed for people with diabetes. *See also* diabetes mellitus.

American Dietetic Association (ADA) A national organization founded in 1917 composed of 60,000 dietetic professionals and registered dietitians in hospitals, colleges, universities, school food services, day care centers, research, business, and industry, and dietetic technicians who meet ADA requirements. It sets and approves standards of education and practice. *See also* dietetic technician; dietitian.

American Diopter and Decibel Society (ADDS) A national organization founded in 1960 composed of 200 physicians specializing in ophthalmology, otolaryngology, rhinology, or allied sciences. It devotes any available income in excess of cost of operation or other resources to research and educational projects. *See also* decibel; diopter; ophthalmology; otolaryngology; physician; rhinology.

American Electroencephalographic Society (AEEGS) A national organization founded in 1946 composed of 1,320 electroencephalographers and neurophysiologists. *See also* electroencephalography; neurophysiology.

American Electrology Association (AEA) A national organization founded in 1958 composed of 1,800 electrologists interested in promoting uniform legislative standards throughout the states, coordinating efforts of affiliated associations in dealing with problems of national scope, and granting accreditation. Formerly (1986) American Electrolysis Association. *See also* accreditation; electrology; electrolysis.

American Electrolysis Association *See* American Electrology Association.

American Endodontic Society (AES) A national organization founded in 1969 composed of 10,000 dentists that promotes and provides educational and scientific information on simplified root canal therapy for the generalist dentist. *See also* endodontics.

American Epidemiological Society (AES) A national organization founded in 1927 composed of 300 individuals from diverse disciplines with a common interest in the study of diseases or conditions in human populations. *See also* epidemiology.

American Epilepsy Society (AES) A national organization founded in 1946 composed of 1,550 physicians and researchers engaged in practice and research in epilepsy or closely related fields, such as electroencephalography. It fosters treatment of epilepsy in its biological, clinical, and social phases and promotes better care and treatment of persons subject to convulsions (seizures). *See also* convulsion; electroencephalography; epilepsy.

American Equilibration Society (AES) A national organization founded in 1955 composed of 1,500 dentists, orthodontists, oral surgeons, and physicians interested in study and proficiency in the diagnosis and treatment of occlusive and temporomandibular joint disorders. *See also* dentist; oral and maxillofacial surgeon; orthodontist; physician; temporomandibular joint syndrome.

American Family Therapy Association (AFTA) A national organization founded in 1977 composed of 900 family therapy teachers, researchers, and practitioners working to advance theory and therapy that views the family as a unit. *See also* family; therapy.

American Federation for Aging Research (AFAR) An organization founded in 1979 composed of physicians, scientists, and other individuals involved or interested in research in aging and associated diseases. Its purpose is to stimulate and fund research on aging. *See also* aging; physician; research.

American Federation for Clinical Research (AFCR) A national organization founded in 1940 composed of 12,500 clinical scientists under age 43 years interested in original research in clinical and laboratory medicine. *See also* research.

American Federation of Home Health Agencies (AFHHA) A national organization founded in 1980 composed of 325 agencies providing therapeutic services, such as nursing, speech therapy, and physical therapy, in the home. It promotes home health by influencing public policy. *See also* home health agency; nursing; physical therapy; speech therapy.

American Federation of Medical Accreditation (AFMA) A national organization founded in 1979 composed of 60 scientific organizations and medical associations that have primary certifying boards. It accredits medical and scientific organizations and continuing medical education for member organizations. *See also* accreditation; board; certification; continuing medical education.

American Fertility Society (AFS) A national organization founded in 1944 composed of 10,000 gynecologists, obstetricians, urologists, reproductive endocrinologists, veterinarians, research workers, and other individuals interested in reproductive health in humans and animals. It seeks to extend knowledge of all aspects of fertility and problems of infertility and mammalian reproduction. *See also* fertility; infertility; reproduction.

American Fitness Association (AFA) A national organization founded in 1981 composed of 3,000 individuals interested in conducting research and educational activities in the field of aerobic exercise and disseminating information on research findings, such as the effects of stress on muscles, joints, and tendons. It monitors the aerobics industry; tests exercise products, such as shoes, mats, and weights; and conducts surveys on injury rates. This organization is unrelated to another group of the same name (see next entry). Formerly (1990) American Aerobics Association. *See also* aerobics; fitness; physical fitness program; wellness.

American Fitness Association (AFA) A national organization founded in 1986 composed of 5,000 physicians, psychologists, exercise physiologists, and other health and fitness professionals interested in promoting involvement and education in health and fitness. It attempts to influence legislative action and sponsors seminars, sports clinics, and competitions. This organization is unrelated to another group of the same name (see previous entry). *See also* fitness; physical fitness program.

American Fracture Association (AFA) A national

organization founded in 1938 composed of 500 orthopaedic, general, industrial, plastic, traumatic, and dental surgeons and physicians interested in the care and treatment of fractures. It seeks to further and create interest in the study of the various accepted types of bone fracture therapy. *See also* bone; fracture.

American Gastroenterological Association (AGA) A national organization founded in 1897 composed of 6,400 physicians of internal medicine certified in gastroenterology and radiologists, pathologists, surgeons, and physiologists with an interest and competency in gastroenterology. *See also* certified; gastroenterology; general surgery; internal medicine; pathology; physiology; radiology.

American Genetic Association (AGA) A national organization founded in 1903 composed of 1,500 biologists, geneticists, and other individuals engaged in basic and applied research in genetics. It seeks to improve human welfare and plant and animal stocks. *See also* genetic; genetics.

American Geriatrics Society (AGS) A national organization founded in 1942 composed of 6,011 physicians and other health professionals interested in problems of the elderly. It promotes the study of geriatrics and stresses the importance of medical research in the field of aging. *See also* geriatric medicine.

American Group Practice Association (AGPA) A national organization founded in 1949 composed of 300 private group practice medical and dental clinics representing more than 21,000 physicians. It fosters accreditation of medical clinics and compiles statistics. *See also* accreditation; group practice; physician.

American Group Psychotherapy Association (AGPA) A national organization founded in 1942 to provide a forum for the exchange of ideas among approximately 3,500 psychiatrists, psychologists, psychiatric nurses, social workers, and other mental health professionals in group psychotherapy practice meeting membership requirements. *See also* group therapy; mental health professional; psychotherapy.

American Guild of Hypnotherapists (AGH) A national organization founded in 1975 composed of 1,106 hypnotherapists and professional hypnotists, and mental health, medical, dental, and chiropractic professionals who use hypnosis in their practices. *See also* hypnotherapy.

American Gynecological and Obstetrical Society (AGOS) A national organization founded in 1981 composed of 300 physicians interested in cultivating and promoting knowledge of obstetrics and gynecology. Formed by merger of American Gynecological Society (founded 1876) and American Association of Obstetricians and Gynecologists (founded in 1888 and formerly American Association of Obstetricians, Gynecologists, and Abdominal Surgeons). *See also* obstetrics and gynecology; physician.

American Hair Loss Council (AHLC) A national organization founded in 1985 composed of 320 dermatologists, plastic surgeons, cosmetologists, barbers, and other individuals interested in nonbiased information regarding treatments for hair loss in men and women. *See also* alopecia.

American Healing Association (AHA) A national organization founded in 1975 composed of practitioners, counselors, and other individuals interested in psychic, spiritual, and faith healing and counseling. *See also* alternative medicine; heal.

American Health Care Association (AHCA) A national organization founded in 1949 composed of 9,800 long term care facilities. It promotes standards for professionals in long-term health care delivery and quality care for patients and residents in a safe environment. It focuses on issues of availability, quality, affordability, and fair payment. It maintains liaison with governmental agencies, Congress, and professional associations. Absorbed (1984) National Council of Health Centers (formerly National Council of Health Care Services). Formed by merger of American Association of Nursing Homes and National Association of Registered Nursing Homes. *See also* long term care facility.

American Healthcare Institute *See* Association AMHS Institute.

American Healthcare Radiology Administrators (AHRA) A national organization founded in 1973 composed of 3,100 radiology managers interested in improving management of radiology departments in hospitals and other health care organizations and providing liaisons between related organizations, such as radiology, health care and management groups, and government agencies. Formerly (1986) American Hospital Radiology Administrators. *See also* administrator; hospital; manager; radiology.

American Health Decisions (AHD) A confederation founded in 1989 of 21 state health programs. It assists in establishing public education programs about health care and policy and promotes personal autonomy on ethical issues, such as a patient's decision to refuse or accept treatment. *See also* autonomy; decision; health; patient's right of autonomy.

American Health Information Management Association (AHIMA) A national organization founded in 1928 composed of 31,000 registered record administrators and accredited record technicians with expertise in health information management, biostatistics, classification systems, and systems analysis. It conducts annual qualification examinations to certify medical record personnel as registered record administrators (RRA) and accredited record technicians (ART). Formerly (1991) American Medical Record Association. *See also* accreditation; accredited record technician; certification; certified coding specialist; medical record; medical record administrator; medical record technician; registered record administrator.

American Health Planning Association (AHPA) A national organization founded in 1970 composed of state and local development agencies, health planning agencies, university health science centers, insurance and industry organizations, and affiliated organizations and individuals. The organization conducts research, disseminates information, and performs clearinghouse functions and activities in health planning tasks and concepts. *See also* health planning.

American Health Security Act *See* Health Security Act.

American Heart Association (AHA) A national organization founded in 1924 composed of 200,000 physicians, scientists, and laypersons. Its activities include support of research, education, and community service programs with the objective of reducing premature death and disability from cardiovascular diseases and stroke (cerebrovascular accident). It is financed entirely by voluntary contributions of the public, principally during the Heart Campaign held each year in February. *See also* acute myocardial infarction; advanced cardiac life support; cardiology; cerebrovascular accident.

American Heart Association, Council on Arteriosclerosis of the *See* Council on Arteriosclerosis of the American Heart Association.

American Holistic Medical Association (AHMA) A national organization founded in 1978 composed of 400 medical doctors, osteopathic physicians, and students who are interested in furthering the prac-

tice of holistic health care. *See also* holistic health; holistic medicine; osteopathic physician; physician.

American Holistic Nurses Association (AHNA) A national organization founded in 1981 composed of 1,900 registered, licensed practical, vocational, and student nurses promoting education for nurses and the public on the concept of holistic health care. *See also* holistic health; holistic medicine; licensed practical nurse; licensed vocational nurse; nurse; registered nurse.

American Horticultural Therapy Association (AHTA) A national organization founded in 1973 composed of 691 professional horticultural therapists, rehabilitation specialists, institutions, and commercial organizations interested in the development of horticulture and related activities as a therapeutic and rehabilitative medium. Horticultural therapy is considered particularly useful in the fields of geriatrics and developmental disabilities. Formerly (1987) National Council for Therapy and Rehabilitation Through Horticulture. *See also* developmental disability; geriatric medicine; horticulture; therapy.

American Hospital Radiology Administrators *See* American Healthcare Radiology Administrators.

American Hospital Association (AHA) A national organization founded in 1898 composed of 54,500 individuals and health care organizations including hospitals, health care systems, and preacute and postacute health care delivery organizations. It carries out research and education projects in areas, such as health care administration, hospital economics, and community relations; represents hospitals in national legislation; offers programs for institutional effectiveness review, technology assessment, and hospital administrative services; collects and analyzes data; and maintains a 44,000 volume health care administration library and biographical archive. The AHA publishes *Hospital Statistics* and *Guide to the Health Care Field* annually, and *Hospitals and Health Networks* monthly. *See also AHA Hospital Statistics; AHA Guide to the Health Care Field*; hospital; *Hospitals and Health Networks; Master Facility Inventory of Hospitals and Institutions*.

American Hospital Association, American Society for Healthcare Education and Training of the *See* American Society for Healthcare Education and Training of the American Hospital Association.

American Hospital Association, American Society

for Healthcare Environmental Services of the
See American Society for Healthcare Environmental Services of the American Hospital Association.

American Hospital Association, National Society of Patient Representation and Consumer Affairs of the *See* National Society of Patient Representation and Consumer Affairs of the American Hospital Association.

American Hospital Association, Society for Healthcare Planning and Marketing of the *See* Society for Healthcare Planning and Marketing of the American Hospital Association.

American Hospital Radiology Administrators *See* American Healthcare Radiology Administrators.

American Hypnosis Association (AHA) A national organization founded in 1972 composed of 500 professionals and paraprofessionals in hypnotherapy. It maintains a rental library of 50 videotapes and acts as a resource center for members. *See also* hypnosis.

American Hypnotists' Association (AHA) A national organization founded in 1959 composed of 401 holders of the following degrees: doctorate degree in psychology, DDS (Doctor of Dental Surgery), MD (Doctor of Medicine); DC (Doctor of Chiropractic), ND (Doctor of Naturopathy), DO (Doctor of Osteopathy), or doctorate degree in public health. It promotes scientific research in ethical hypnosis and related sociology and maintains records of all known types or methods of inducing hypnosis. It disseminates information on ethical hypnosis to professional medical and dental societies and conducts a training program. *See also* ethical; hypnosis.

American Indian *See* Native American.

American Indian Health Care Association (AIHCA) A national organization founded in 1975 composed of Native American Indian health programs. It provides training, technical assistance, health care delivery management, research, and evaluation for Indian health programs and organizations. *See also* Native American.

American Industrial Health Council (AIHC) A national organization founded in 1977 composed of 60 industrial and commercial firms and trade associations working to advocate and promote the implementation of scientific methods to identify potential industrial carcinogens (cancer-inducing substances) and other health hazards, such as mutagens (agents that induce mutation) and teratogens (agents that cause developmental malformations). It seeks to develop a basis for the review, risk assessment, and regulation of substances that may pose significant chronic health risks. *See also* carcinogen; mutagen; occupational medicine; teratogen.

American Industrial Hygiene Association (AIHA) A national organization founded in 1939 composed of 9,500 industrial hygienists. It promotes the study and control of environmental factors affecting the health of workers. It accredits laboratories and maintains 35 technical committees. *See also* accreditation; environmental health; industrial hygienist; occupational medicine.

American Institute of Biological Sciences (AIBS) A national organization founded in 1947 composed of 7,200 biological associations and laboratories whose members have an interest in the life sciences. It promotes effectiveness of effort among persons engaged in biological research, education, and application of biological sciences, including medicine and agriculture. It conducts symposium series and maintains an educational consultant panel. *See also* biology.

American Institute of Certified Public Accountants (AICPA) A national organization founded in 1887 composed of 280,000 accountants certified by the states and territories. Its responsibilities include establishing auditing and reporting standards; influencing the development of financial accounting standards underlying the presentation of US corporate financial statements; and preparing and grading the national Uniform Certified Public Accountant Examination for the state licensing bodies. *See also* certified; certified public accountant.

American Institute of the History of Pharmacy (AIHP) A national organization founded in 1941 composed of 1,200 pharmacists, firms, and organizations interested in historical and social aspects of the pharmaceutical field. *See also* history; pharmacy.

American Institute of Homeopathy (AIH) A national organization founded in 1844 composed of 160 physicians and dentists practicing homeotherapeutics according to the three natural laws of cure proposed by Samuel CF Hahnemann. *See also* homeopathy.

American Institute of Life Threatening Illness and Loss, (Division of Foundation of Thanatology) (FT) A national organization founded in 1967 composed of 400 health, theology, psychology, and social science professionals devoted to scientific and humanistic inquiries into death, loss, grief, and bereavement. It promotes improved psychosocial and medical care for critically ill and dying patients, and assistance for their families. It stimulates and coordinates professional, educational, and research programs interested in mortality and the management of grief. Formerly (1991) Foundation of Thanatology. *See also* thanatology.

American Institute of Management (AIM) A national research and educational organization founded in 1948 composed of 1,500 executives interested in management efficiency and methods of appraising management performance. It conducts professional development correspondence courses for members and management audits. *See also* executive; management.

American Institute of Nutrition (AIN) A national organization founded in 1928 composed of 2,770 nutrition research scientists from universities, government, and industry. American Society for Clinical Nutrition is a division. *See also* American Society for Clinical Nutrition; nutrition.

American Institute of Oral Biology (AIOB) A national organization founded in 1943 composed of dental and medical health professionals interested in continuing education in the field of oral biology. *See also* dentistry; oral pathology.

American Institute of Stress (AIS) A national organization founded in 1979 composed of physicians, health professionals, scholars, and other individuals from varied disciplines interested in the personal and social consequences of stress. It compiles research data on topics, such as relationships between emotional factors and cardiovascular disease; stress and the immune system with specific emphasis on cancer; and stress reduction programs for industry. It seeks a definition of health that recognizes the need for harmony between the individual and the physical and social environments as well as the effects of positive emotions, such as creativity, faith, and humor on health. *See also* stress.

American Institute of Ultrasound in Medicine (AIUM) A national organization founded in 1951 composed of 10,000 physicians, engineers, scientists, sonographers, and other professionals using diagnostic medical ultrasound. It promotes the application of ultrasound in clinical medicine and in research; studies its effects on tissue; and recommends standards for its use. *See also* ultrasound imaging.

American Institutes for Research in the Behavioral Sciences (AIR) A nonmembership organization founded in 1946 composed of 240 individuals who conduct programs of research and development on socially relevant problems in the behavioral sciences. It seeks to establish general principles to enhance the scientific understanding of a broad range of human behaviors. It is supported by contracts and grants from industry. *See also* behavioral science.

American In-Vitro Allergy/Immunology Society A national organization founded in 1988 composed of physicians, scientists, and other professionals who study or use in-vitro technology in the diagnosis and treatment of allergic and immunologic disorders. It promotes the appropriate use of in-vitro procedures in allergy and immunology. It offers services in third-party payer negotiation and in-vitro testing standardization. *See also* allergy and immunology; in vitro.

American Joint Committee on Cancer (AJCC) An organization founded in 1959 composed of 40 surgeons, physicians, radiologists, pathologists, American Cancer Society representatives, and National Cancer Institute representatives. The AJCC formulates and publishes systems of classification and staging of cancer and reports of end results for the purpose of selecting the most effective treatment, determining prognosis, and continuing evaluation of cancer control measures. It promotes the use of developed systems of classification of cancer and evaluates systems of recording and reporting data. Formerly (1981) American Joint Committee for Cancer Staging and End Results Reporting. *See also* American Joint Committee on Cancer pathologic stage classification system; cancer.

American Joint Committee on Cancer (AJCC) pathologic stage classification system A method of describing the extent of cancer based on the pathologic examination of a resected specimen. The pathologic stages are AJCC stages I through V; pT is the pathologic assessment of the primary tumor; pN is the pathologic assessment of the regional lymph nodes. *See also* American Joint Committee on Cancer; cancer; pathology; resect; staging.

American Joint Committee for Cancer Staging

and End Results Reporting *See* American Joint Committee on Cancer.

American Journal of Nursing The monthly journal of the American Nurses Association containing articles of general and specialized clinical interest to nurses. It is the principal resource about the nursing profession in the United States. *See also* American Nurses Association; journal; nursing; registered nurse.

American Kinesiotherapy Association (AKA) A national organization founded in 1946 composed of 1,000 kinesiotherapists, exercise therapists, and other individuals interested in physical and mental rehabilitation. Formerly (1987) American Corrective Therapy Association. *See also* kinesiology.

American Laryngological, Rhinological and Otological Society (ALROS) A national organization founded in 1895 composed of 750 medical specialists dealing with the ear, nose, and throat. Also known as Triological Society. *See also* otolaryngology; physician; rhinology.

American Leprosy Missions (ALMI) A nonmembership organization founded in 1906 providing medical, rehabilitative, and social care for individuals with leprosy in 30 countries. Its activities include conducting specialized training for medical workers and providing personnel and resources to conduct training programs at National Hansen's Disease Center in Carville, Louisiana. *See also* leprosy.

American Licensed Practical Nurses Association (ALPNA) A national organization founded in 1984 composed of 6,400 licensed practical nurses. It lobbies and maintains relations with the government on issues and legislation that may have an impact on licensed practical nurses and conducts continuing education classes. *See also* continuing education; licensed practical nurse.

American Longevity Association (ALA) An organization founded in 1980 composed of scientists and laypersons interested in the acceleration of research programs that study the mechanisms of aging, arteriosclerosis, heart attack, stroke, use of artificial hearts, cryopreservation of organs, and other areas relevant to longevity. *See also* aging; longevity.

American Lung Association (ALA) A national organization founded in 1904 composed of 9,500 physicians, nurses, and laymen interested in the prevention and control of lung disease. It works with other organizations in planning and conducting programs in community services; public, professional and patient education; and research. It maintains the American Thoracic Society as its medical section. It is financed by the annual Christmas Seal Campaign and other fundraising activities. *See also* American Thoracic Society; Congress of Lung Association Staff; lung.

American Managed Care Pharmacy Association (AMCPA) A national organization founded in 1975 composed of 11 preferred provider organizations that specialize in maintenance drug therapy in managed care environments and make available home-delivery pharmacy services. It promotes managed care prescription services as suppliers of medicine to home-delivery pharmacy services and seeks to assist health plan officers and consumers in obtaining maximum value from prescription services. Formerly (1989) National Association of Mail Service Pharmacies. *See also* managed care; pharmacy.

American Managed Care and Review Association (AMCRA) A national organization founded in 1971 composed of 500 medical organizations from the managed health care industry representing over 250,000 practicing physicians and 25 million individuals with health insurance. It seeks to provide better medical care at a reasonable cost and to render the most appropriate and economical setting for its delivery. Formerly (1989) American Medical Care and Review Association. *See also* health insurance; managed care.

American Management Association (AMA) A national organization founded in 1923 composed of 70,000 managers in industry, commerce, and government; charitable and noncommercial organizations; university teachers of management; and administrators. *See also* management.

American Massage Therapy Association (AMTA) A national organization founded in 1943 composed of 12,000 massage therapists or technicians. It provides referrals to area therapists and certified schools, accredits massage training programs, and offers a national certification program for massage therapists. *See also* accreditation; massage.

American Medical Association (AMA) A national membership organization founded in 1847 composed of 271,000 physicians and county medical societies. It disseminates scientific information to members and the public, informs members of medical health legislation on state and national levels, and represents the profession before Congress and governmental agencies. It cooperates in setting standards for medical schools, hospitals, residency programs, and continuing medical education courses. The AMA is governed by a board of trustees and a house of delegates representing various state and local medical associations and government agencies, such as the Public Health Service and medical departments of the uniformed services. It offers numerous publications, including the *Journal of the American Medical Association (JAMA)*. *See also Journal of the American Medical Association*; medical association; physician.

American Medical Association, Council on Medical Education of the *See* Council on Medical Education of the American Medical Association.

American Medical Athletic Association (AMAA) A national organization founded in 1969 composed of 5,000 persons in the medical or allied fields interested in fostering endurance sports among physicians in the United States so that they, in turn, will encourage endurance sports among their patients. One of its committees reviews jogging deaths. Also known as American Medical Joggers Association. *See also* fitness; sports medicine.

American Medical Care and Review Association *See* American Managed Care and Review Association.

American Medical Directors Association (AMDA) A national organization founded in 1975 composed of 1,400 physicians providing care in long term care organizations, such as nursing homes and other geriatric facilities. *See also* geriatric medicine; long term care; medical director.

American Medical Electroencephalographic Association (AMEEGA) A national organization founded in 1946 composed of 850 individuals interested in clinical electroencephalography. *See also* electroencephalography.

American Medical Informatics Association (AMIA) A national organization founded in 1981 composed of 850 medical personnel, physicians, physical scientists, engineers, data processors, researchers, educators, hospital administrators, nurses, medical record administrators, and computer professionals interested in applying advanced systems and information technologies to scientific, literary, and educational activities. Formerly (1990) American Association for Medical Systems and Informatics. *See also* informatics; medical informatics.

American Medical Joggers Association *See* American Medical Athletic Association.

American Medical Peer Review Association (AMPRA) A national organization founded in 1973 composed of 1,400 institutions and individuals interested in developing communications programs for physicians, institutions, and other individuals interested in peer review organizations. It conducts on-site assistance programs to increase physicians' involvement and leadership in peer review organizations (PROs), improve practice patterns through review, and understand and use PRO data to improve service delivery. Formerly (1982) American Association of Professional Standards Review Organizations. *See also* peer review; peer review organization.

American Medical Political Action Committee (AMPAC) A national committee composed of 68,000 physicians, their spouses, and other persons interested in political action and participation in public affairs. *See also* political action committee.

American Medical Publishers' Association (AMPA) A national organization founded in 1961 composed of 50 US medical publishing companies interested in exchanging information among members; improving the creation, distribution, and sale of medical books and journals; and facilitating communication with medical organizations, schools, and the medical community.

American Medical Record Association *See* American Health Information Management Association.

American Medical Society on Alcoholism and Other Drug Dependencies *See* American Society of Addiction Medicine.

American Medical Technologists (AMT) A national professional registry founded in 1939 composed of 22,150 medical laboratory technologists, technicians, medical assistants, and dental assistants. *See also* dental assistant; medical assistant; medical laboratory technician; medical technologist; registry.

American Medical Technologists, Registered Medical Assistants of *See* Registered Medical Assistants of American Medical Technologists.

American Medical Women's Association (AMWA) A national organization founded in 1915 composed of 11,000 women holding a Doctor of Medicine (MD) or a Doctor of Osteopathy (DO) degree from approved medical colleges, and women interns, residents, and medical students. It seeks to find solutions to problems common to women studying or practicing medicine, such as career advancement and the integration of professional and family responsibilities. *See also* physician.

American Medical Writers Association (AMWA) A national organization founded in 1940 composed of 3,400 medical writers, editors, audiovisualists, public relations and pharmaceutical personnel, and publishers interested in communication in medicine and allied sciences. *See also* communication; language; public relations; writer.

American Mental Health Counselors Association (AMHCA) A national association founded in 1976 composed of 12,000 professional counselors employed in mental health services. *See also* counselor.

American Microscopical Society (AMS) A national organization founded in 1878 composed of 697 microscopical biologists and microscopists interested in fostering biological research that uses the microscope. *See also* microscope.

American Motility Society (AMS) A national organization founded in 1980 composed of 220 professionals interested in the study of gastrointestinal motility. It promotes research on topics, such as the esophagus and clinical disorders of esophageal and gastric emptying. *See also* alimentary tract; esophagus; gastroenterology; gastroesophageal reflux; gastrointestinal; reflux esophagitis; stomach.

American Naprapathic Association (ANA) A national organization founded in 1909 composed of 300 naprapathic physicians. It promotes and publishes the principles of natural healing and seeks to further legislation and recognition of the naprapathic system of treatment. *See also* naprapathy.

American National Standards Institute (ANSI) A national organization founded in 1918 composed of 1,250 industrial firms, trade associations, technical societies, labor organizations, consumer organizations, and government agencies. It serves as a clearinghouse for nationally coordinated voluntary standards for fields ranging from information technology to building construction. It gives status as American National Standards to standards developed by agreement from all groups interested in such areas as: definitions, terminology, symbols, and abbreviations; materials, performance characteristics, procedures, and methods of rating; methods of testing and analysis; size, weight, and volume; practice,

safety, health, and building construction. It provides information on foreign standards and represents US interests in international standardization work. *See also* clearinghouse; standard.

American Natural Hygiene Society (ANHS) A national public health organization founded in 1948 composed of 6,500 individuals interested in promoting health maintenance through natural means, such as natural foods, fresh air, pure water, sunshine, fasting, exercise, and rest. It emphasizes a lifestyle that encourages people to maximize their health by living in harmony with their physiological needs. *See also* exercise; hygiene; public health.

American Nephrology Nurses' Association (ANNA) A national organization founded in 1966 composed of 6,500 registered nurses, physicians, dietitians, social workers, and technicians interested in care of patients with kidney disorders. Formerly (1984) American Association of Nephrology Nurses and Technicians. *See also* dietitian; kidney; nephrology; nursing; physician; registered nurse; social worker.

American Neurological Association (ANA) A national organization founded in 1875 composed of 960 physicians and scientists interested in the form, functioning, and disorders of the nervous system. *See also* neurology.

American Neurotology Society (ANS) A national organization founded in 1965 composed of 315 physicians and audiologists interested in the diagnosis and treatment of hearing and balance disorders. It promotes education and research in the field of neurotology. *See also* audiology; otology/neurotology; physician.

American Nurses Association (ANA) A national organization founded in 1896 representing 200,000 registered nurses. The ANA is made up of 53 state groups and 860 local groups. It sponsors American Nurses Foundation (for research), American Academy of Nursing, Center for Ethics and Human Rights, International Nursing Center, and American Nurses Credentialing Center. Publications include the *American Journal of Nursing*. *See also* American Academy of Nursing; *American Journal of Nursing*; registered nurse.

American Nursing Assistant's Association (ANAA) A national organization founded in 1982 composed of 210 certified nursing assistants and nurses' aides. *See also* certified; nursing assistant.

American Nutritionists Association (ANA) A national organization founded in 1986 composed of 250 nutritionists holding graduate degrees from accredited universities interested in representing nutritionists before federal and state policymakers. *See also* nutrition; nutritionist.

American Occupational Therapy Association (AOTA) A national organization founded in 1917 composed of 45,000 registered occupational therapists and certified occupational therapy assistants who provide services to people whose lives have been disrupted by physical injury or illness, developmental problems, the aging process, or social or psychological difficulties. *See also* certified; Fellow of the American Occupational Therapy Association; occupational therapist; occupational therapy; occupational therapy assistant.

American Occupational Therapy Association, Fellow of the *See* Fellow of the American Occupational Therapy Association.

American Occupational Therapy Certification Board (AOTCB) A national board that administers a certification program for occupational therapists and occupational therapy assistants. It also operates disciplinary mechanisms. *See also* board; certification; occupational therapy.

American Ophthalmological Society (AOS) A national honorary organization founded in 1864 composed of 225 physicians specializing in the functions and treatment of the eye. *See also* ophthalmology; physician.

American Optometric Association (AOA) A national organization founded in 1898 composed of 29,000 optometrists, students of optometry, and paraoptometric assistants and technicians. Its purposes include improving the quality, availability, and accessibility of eye and vision care; representing the optometric profession; helping members conduct their practices; and promoting high standards of patient care. It monitors and promotes legislation concerning the scope of optometric practice, alternate health care delivery systems, health care cost containment, Medicare, and other issues relevant to eye/vision care. *See also* optometry.

American Organization of Nurse Executives (AONE) A national organization founded in 1967 composed of 5,500 registered nurses active in the field of nursing service administration and nurses responsible for the management of nursing depart-

ments in health care organizations. *See also* executive; nurse executive; nurse manager; registered nurse.

American Oriental Bodywork Therapy Association (AOBTA) A national organization founded in 1984 composed of 650 professional oriental bodyworkers and teachers. It identifies qualified practitioners and serves as a legal entity representing members when dealing with the government, especially in establishing professional status. It sets teaching standards for all styles of oriental bodywork, including acupressure, five-element shiatsu, macrobiotic shiatsu, nippon, and zen. *See also* acupressure; massage.

American Orthodontic Society (AOS) A national organization founded in 1974 composed of 1,900 general and pediatric dentists. The organization's objectives include making orthodontic information readily available to ethical dentists and monitoring third-party services and government programs. It offers courses in orthodontic techniques. *See also* dentist, generalist; orthodontics.

American Orthopaedic Association (AOA) A national organization founded in 1887 composed of 300 bone and joint surgeons interested in furthering knowledge in the diagnosis and treatment of crippling diseases. *See also* bone; joint; orthopaedic/orthopedic surgery.

American Orthopaedic Foot and Ankle Society (AOFAS) A national organization founded in 1969 composed of 550 members of American Academy of Orthopaedic Surgeons interested in research on education in and care of the foot and ankle. It sponsors continuing medical education courses. Formerly (1983) American Orthopedic Foot Society. *See also* American Academy of Orthopaedic Surgeons; continuing medical education; orthopaedic/orthopedic surgery.

American Orthopaedic Society for Sports Medicine (AOSSM) A national organization founded in 1972 composed of 1,000 orthopaedic surgeons working in the field of sports medicine. *See also* orthopaedic/orthopedic surgery; sports medicine.

American Orthopedic Foot Society *See* American Orthopaedic Foot and Ankle Society.

American Orthopsychiatric Association (ORTHO) A national organization founded in 1923 composed of 10,000 psychiatrists, psychologists, social workers, educators, psychiatric nurses, lawyers, and other individuals in related fields, including anthropology, sociology, and economics. *See also* orthopsychiatry.

American Orthoptic Council (AOC) A national board composed of 19 ophthalmologists and orthoptists that administers the national board examination required for certification. *See also* board; certification; ophthalmologist; orthoptist.

American Orthotic and Prosthetic Association (AOPA) A national organization founded in 1917 composed of 1,250 firms that manufacture and fit artificial limbs, braces, and cosmetic replacements, such as fingers and ears. *See also* orthotics; prosthetics.

American Osteopathic Academy of Orthopedics (AOAO) A national organization founded in 1941 composed of 326 osteopathic orthopedic surgeons. *See also* orthopaedic/orthopedic surgery; osteopathic medicine.

American Osteopathic Academy of Sclerotherapy (AOAS) A national organization founded in 1954 composed of 125 osteopathic physicians interested in sclerotherapy. The academy defines sclerotherapy as the stimulation of the formation of fibrous connective tissues by the body, in a specific location, by the application of a sclerosing agent, typically the injection of certain medications known as sclerosants. Primary studies involve the treatment of unstable joints, venous abnormalities, and tendonbone points of hyperirritability. *See also* osteopathic medicine.

American Osteopathic Academy of Sports Medicine (AOASM) A national organization founded in 1975 composed of 1,300 members of the American Osteopathic Association and other individuals interested in standards development, education, and research in the field of sports medicine. *See also* osteopathic medicine; sports medicine.

American Osteopathic Association (AOA) A national organization founded in 1897 composed of approximately 22,000 osteopathic physicians, surgeons, and graduates of approved colleges of osteopathic medicine. The AOA inspects and accredits colleges and hospitals; conducts a specialty certification program; sponsors a national examining board satisfactory to state licensing agencies; maintains a mandatory program of continuing medical education for members; and conducts other activities. *See also* accreditation; board; continuing medical education; licensure; osteopathic medicine.

American Osteopathic Association, Bureau of

Professional Education of the *See* Bureau of Professional Education of the American Osteopathic Association.

American Osteopathic Board of Emergency Medicine (AOBEM) A national board founded in 1980 whose purpose is to administer examinations and certify osteopathic physicians in the specialty of emergency medicine. It sets eligibility standards for osteopathic emergency physicians and offers annual certification examinations in emergency medicine. *See also* board; certification; emergency medicine; osteopathic medicine; standard.

American Osteopathic Board of General Practice (AOBGP) A national board founded in 1972 that prepares and administers a certification examination for osteopathic physicians. *See also* board; certification; general practice; osteopathic medicine.

American Osteopathic Board of Pediatrics (AOBP) A national board that prepares and administers a certification examination for osteopathic pediatricians. Standards are formulated by the American Osteopathic Association, and certification is conducted by annual examination. *See also* certification; osteopathic medicine; pediatrics.

American Osteopathic College of Allergy and Immunology (AOCAI) A national organization founded in 1974 composed of 75 osteopathic physicians interested in allergies and immunology. It works to improve education in the field. *See also* allergy; allergy and immunology; osteopathic medicine.

American Osteopathic College of Anesthesiologists (AOCA) A national organization founded in 1952 composed of 500 members of the American Osteopathic Association who are engaged in the practice of anesthesiology. *See also* anesthesiology; osteopathic medicine.

American Osteopathic College of Dermatology (AOCD) A national organization founded in 1955 composed of 130 members of the osteopathic profession certified or involved in dermatology. It conducts specialized education programs. *See also* certified; dermatology; osteopathic medicine.

American Osteopathic College of Pathologists (AOCP) A national organization founded in 1954 composed of 180 osteopathic physicians who have completed residency training programs in pathology and clinical pathology; candidate members are in residency training in pathology. It establishes guidelines for training programs in pathology and clinical pathology for osteopathic physicians and maintains standards in residency training programs. *See also* osteopathic medicine; pathology; residency.

American Osteopathic College of Preventive Medicine (AOCPM) A national organization founded in 1982 composed of 160 osteopathic physicians interested in aerospace medicine, occupational/environmental medicine, or public health preventive medicine. *See also* occupational medicine; osteopathic medicine; preventive medicine; public health.

American Osteopathic College of Proctology (AOCPr) A national organization composed of 155 osteopathic physicians specializing in treatment of diseases of the anus, rectum, and colon. *See also* colon and rectal surgery; osteopathic medicine.

American Osteopathic College of Radiology (AOCR) A national organization founded in 1940 composed of 600 certified radiologists, residents-in-training and other osteopathic physicians involved in radiology. *See also* certified; osteopathic medicine; radiology.

American Osteopathic College of Rehabilitation Medicine (AOCRM) A national organization founded in 1954 composed of 125 osteopathic physicians interested in physical and rehabilitation medicine as a specialty. Active members are certified in the specialty by the American Osteopathic Board of Rehabilitation Medicine of the American Osteopathic Association. *See also* certified; osteopathic medicine; physical medicine and rehabilitation.

American Osteopathic Hospital Association (AOHA) A national organization founded in 1934 composed of 100 osteopathic hospitals. It holds educational institutes on health care management, conducts research programs, and compiles statistics, among other activities. *See also* hospital; osteopathic medicine.

American Otological Society (AOS) A national organization founded in 1868 composed of 220 otologists and contributors to the advancement of disorders of the ear and temporal bone. *See also* otology/neurotology.

American Pain Society (APS) A national organization founded in 1977 composed of 1,827 physicians, dentists, psychologists, nurses, and other health professionals interested in the study of pain. It promotes control, management, and understanding of pain through scientific meetings and research

activities. It develops standards for training and ethical management of pain patients. *See also* pain.

American Pancreatic Association (APA) A national organization founded in 1970 composed of 325 individuals interested in clinical and basic research related to diseases of the pancreas. It provides a forum for presentation of scientific research related to the pancreas. *See also* pancreas.

American Paraplegia Society (APS) A national organization founded in 1954 composed of 300 physicians and researchers in the spinal cord injury field interested in advancing and fostering improved health care of spinal cord injury patients and developing and promoting education and research in the neuroscience fields. *See also* paralysis; paraplegia; spinal cord.

American Parapsychological Research Association *See* American Association for Parapsychology.

American Pathology Foundation (APF) A national organization founded in 1959 composed of 500 board-certified pathologists interested in promoting the practice of pathology in private laboratories, exchanging information that will improve anatomic and clinical pathology, and attending seminars on direct billing and management. *See also* board certified; pathology.

American Pediatric Society (APS) A national organization founded in 1888 composed of 1,039 physician educators and researchers interested in the study of children and their diseases, prevention of illness, and promotion of health in childhood. *See also* pediatrics; physician.

American Pediatric Surgical Association (APSA) A national organization founded in 1970 composed of 488 pediatric surgeons certified by the American Board of Surgery for competence in dealing with surgical problems of infancy and childhood. *See also* American Board of Surgery; pediatric surgery.

American Pharmaceutical Association (APhA) A national organization founded in 1852 composed of 40,000 pharmacists, educators, students, researchers, editors and publishers of pharmaceutical literature, pharmaceutical chemists and scientists, food and drug officials, hospital pharmacists, and pharmacists in government service. It works to ensure the quality of drug products, represents the interests of the profession before governmental bodies, and interprets and disseminates information on developments in health care. It maintains a headquarters building in Washington, DC, called the American Institute of Pharmacy. *See also* pharmaceutical; pharmacy.

American Pharmacy The monthly journal of the American Pharmaceutical Association. *See also* American Pharmaceutical Association; journal.

American Physical Therapy Association (APTA) A national organization founded in 1921 composed of 51,000 physical therapists, physical therapy assistants, and students. It acts as an accrediting body for educational programs in physical therapy and is responsible for establishing standards, among other activities. *See also* accreditation; Orthopaedic Section, American Physical Therapy Association; physical therapy; Private Practice Section/American Physical Therapy Association; standard.

American Physical Therapy Association, Orthopaedic Section, *See* Orthopaedic Section, American Physical Therapy Association.

American Physical Therapy Association, Private Practice Section/ *See* Private Practice Section/American Physical Therapy Association.

American Physician Art Association (APAA) A national organization founded in 1936 composed of 350 physicians interested in art. It stimulates physician artists to produce works of art in the fields of painting, sculpture, photography, graphic arts, design, and creative crafts and is currently establishing a central photographic archive of members' artworks. *See also* art therapy; physician.

American Physicians, Association of *See* Association of American Physicians.

American Physicians Association of Computer Medicine (APACM) A national organization founded in 1984 composed of 350 physicians, interns, and medical students interested in the use of computers in patient care, education, and research. It is developing a database of programs and a certifying board of computer medicine. *See also* computer; database; medical computer science; medical informatics; physician.

American Physicians and Dentists, Union of *See* Union of American Physicians and Dentists.

American Physicians Fellowship for Medicine in Israel (APF) A national organization founded in 1950 composed of 8,500 American physicians whose goals are to foster and aid medical progress in Israel. It secures fellowships for selected Israeli physicians; arranges lectureships in Israel by prominent Ameri-

can physicians; sends financial aid, medical supplies, and books; and helps maintain the Jerusalem Academy of Medicine, the Home for Retired Physicians in Haifa, Israel, and the Institute of Medical History. *See also* fellowship; physician.

American Physicians Poetry Association (APPA) A national organization founded in 1976 composed of 150 physicians who support the principle that sensitivity in the practice of medicine can be maintained and developed through poetry. It provides a forum of communication for physician-poets, and assists members in publishing and reading poetry. *See also* physician; poetry therapy; sensitivity.

American Physicians and Surgeons, Association of *See* Association of American Physicians and Surgeons.

American Physiological Society (APS) A national organization founded in 1887 composed of 6,600 physiologists interested in all aspects of physiology ranging from animal experimentation to public affairs to cardiovascular, renal, and respiratory physiology. *See also* physiology.

American Podiatric Circulatory Society (APCS) A national organization founded in 1979 composed of 675 podiatrists interested in information on the suffuse osmotic chemisorb asphyxiation (SOCA) therapy devised by Dr Tereno for treatment of geriatric patients suffering from arterial blockage in their limbs. SOCA therapy uses vitamins to enrich the blood and enlarge subcutaneous capillaries and lymph vessels, thus creating an alternate circulatory network that bypasses blocked arteries. SOCA therapy is an alternative to major surgery and/or amputation in geriatric patients with poor circulation in their limbs. *See also* circulatory system; podiatric medicine; vitamin.

American Podiatric Medical Association (APMA) A national organization founded in 1912 composed of 9,200 podiatrists. Its list of committees includes Appeals and Control, Hospitals, Podiatric Therapeutics, Podiatry Political Action, and Public Health and Preventive Podiatric Medicine. Formerly (1984) American Podiatry Association. *See also* podiatric medicine.

American Podiatry Association *See* American Podiatric Medical Association.

American Productivity Center *See* American Productivity and Quality Center.

American Productivity Management Association
See Quality and Productivity Management Association.

American Productivity and Quality Center (APQC)
A national organization founded in 1977 composed of 300 major corporations, foundations, and individuals interested in improving productivity and the quality of work life in the United States. It works with businesses, unions, academic institutions, and government agencies to find ways to improve productivity and quality. Formerly (1988) American Productivity Center. *See also* productivity; quality.

American Professional Practice Association (APPA) A national organization founded in 1959 composed of 70,000 physicians and dentists that provides economic benefits and services, such as unsecured loan plans; equipment, furniture, and automobile leasing; estate planning services; group insurance; and leisure and personal service programs. *See also* dentist; physician; practice.

American Prosthodontic Society (APS) A national organization founded in 1927 composed of 1,300 dentists interested in prosthodontics. *See also* prosthodontics.

American Protestant Health Association (APHA) A national organization founded in 1920 composed of 120 Protestant health and welfare institutions. Formerly (1984) American Protestant Hospital Association.

American Protestant Hospital Association *See* American Protestant Health Association.

American Psychiatric Association (APA) A national organization founded in 1844 composed of 37,000 psychiatrists interested in the study of the nature, treatment, and prevention of mental disorders. It assists in formulating programs to meet mental health needs, compiles and disseminates facts and figures about psychiatry, and furthers psychiatric education and research. *See also* Fellow of the American Psychiatric Association; psychiatry.

American Psychiatric Association, Fellow of the *See* Fellow of the American Psychiatric Association.

American Psychiatric Nurses Association (APNA) A national organization founded in 1987 composed of 2,800 psychiatric nurses interested in improving patient care by fostering clinical research and encouraging community involvement. *See also* psychiatric nursing.

American Psychoanalytic Association (APsaA) A national organization founded in 1911 composed of 3,025 psychoanalysts who have graduated from or are currently attending an accredited institute and who are interested in establishing and maintaining standards for the training of psychoanalysts and for the practice of psychoanalysis. It fosters the integration of psychoanalysis with other branches of medicine and encourages research. *See also* accredited; psychoanalysis; standard.

American Psychological Association (APA) A national organization founded in 1892 composed of 70,000 psychologists. It works to advance psychology as a science, profession, and means of promoting human welfare. It maintains 46 divisions and publishes numerous journals. *See also* Fellow of the American Psychological Association; psychology.

American Psychological Association, Fellow of the *See* Fellow of the American Psychological Association.

American Psychological Association, Division of Psychotherapy of the *See* Division of Psychotherapy of the American Psychological Association.

American Psychology - Law Society (AP-LS) A division of the American Psychological Association founded in 1968 composed of 1,700 psychologists and other individuals interested in promoting exchanges between the disciplines of psychology and law; for example, promoting the education of lawyers at all levels regarding psychology and of psychologists at all levels regarding the law and promoting the effective use of psychologists in the legal process. *See also* American Psychological Association; jurisprudence; psychology.

American Psychopathological Association (APPA) A national organization founded in 1912 composed of 500 physicians and scientists interested in the field of psychopathology and investigating scientific problems of abnormal psychology. These include the study of phenomena arising from abnormal mental processes, organic pathological conditions directly connected with abnormal mental processes, means that may remove or modify social or individual factors operating in the production of mental diseases, and the relationship between psychopathological and social or cultural problems. *See also* abnormal psychology; psychopath.

American Psychosomatic Society (APS) A national organization founded in 1943 composed of 750 specialists from all medical disciplines, social scientists, and psychologists interested in scientific research and clinical practice in the field of psychosomatic medicine. *See also* psychosomatic medicine.

American Public Health Association (APHA) A national organization founded in 1872 composed of 31,500 physicians, nurses, educators, nutritionists, dentists, other health specialists, and members of the public interested in public health issues. It seeks to protect and promote personal, mental, and environmental health. It promulgates standards, establishes uniform practices and procedures, develops the etiology of communicable diseases, and explores medical care programs and their relationship to public health. *See also* communicable disease; Fellow of the American Public Health Association; public health; standard.

American Public Health Association, Fellow of the *See* Fellow of the American Public Health Association.

American Public Health Association, New Professionals Section of the *See* New Professionals Section of the American Public Health Association.

American Public Welfare Association (APWA) A national organization founded in 1930 composed of 5,000 public welfare agencies, their professional staff members, and other individuals and organizations interested in public welfare. *See also* public welfare.

American Radiological Nurses Association (ARNA) A national organization founded in 1981 composed of 650 radiological nurses interested in sharing professional experiences and concerns. It conducts educational programs. *See also* nurse; radiology.

American Radium Society (ARS) A national organization founded in 1916 composed of 850 medical specialists and allied scientists interested in cancer treatment. *See also* cancer; radium.

American Red Cross *See* American Red Cross National Headquarters.

American Red Cross National Headquarters (ARC) A humanitarian organization led by volunteers that provides relief to victims of disasters and helps people prevent, prepare for, and respond to emergencies. Founded by Clara Barton with a group of friends on May 21, 1881 as the American Association of the Red Cross, it was granted a charter by the US Congress in 1900 as the American Red Cross, responsible for providing services to members of the US Armed Forces and relief to disaster victims at home and abroad. The American Red Cross provides social work services in Department of Defense hospitals. Today, the Red Cross has 25,394 staff members, 2,763 chapters, and a budget of over one billion dollars. It maintains 56 regional blood centers and collects, processes, and distributes half the nation's blood supply. *See also* blood; blood bank; blood banking; Red Cross.

American Registry of Clinical Radiography Technologists (ARCRT) A national organization founded in 1955 for radiologic technologists who meet membership requirements, including successfully completing a registry examination. *See also* radiographer; registry; technologist.

American Registry of Diagnostic Medical Sonographers (ARDMS) A national organization founded in 1975 that develops and administers examinations in diagnostic medical sonography and vascular technology and registers successful candidates. There are currently 11,000 members. *See also* diagnostic medical sonographer; registry.

American Registry of Medical Assistants (ARMA) A national organization founded in 1950 composed of 4,000 medical assistants who have completed an accredited medical assistant training course or who have trained with a physician. *See also* accredited; medical assistant; registry.

American Registry of Pathology (ARP) A national organization founded in 1976 composed of national medical professional societies engaging in cooperative enterprises in medical research and education with the Armed Forces Institute of Pathology. It functions as a fiscal agent in the management of research grants and monies derived from tuition fees and contributions and serves as a link between the military and civilian medical, dental, and veterinary communities for the mutual benefit of military and civilian medicine. *See also* Armed Forces Institute of Pathology; pathology; registry.

American Registry of Radiologic Technologists (ARRT) A national organization founded in 1922 that has certified 180,000 radiographers, nuclear medicine technologists, and radiation therapy technologists. The board is governed by trustees appointed by the American College of Radiology and the American Society of Radiologic Technologists. *See also* American College of Radiology; American Society of Radiologic Technologists; certification; nuclear medicine technologist; radiation therapy technologist; radiographer; registry; specialty boards.

American Rehabilitation Counseling Association (ARCA) A division founded in 1958 of the American Association for Counseling and Development composed of 3,000 rehabilitation counselors and professionals interested in improving the rehabilitation counseling profession and its services to individuals with disabilities. *See also* American Association for Counseling and Development; counseling; rehabilitation.

American Rheumatism Association   *See* American College of Rheumatology.

American Rhinologic Society (ARS)   A national organization founded in 1954 composed of 550 physicians who are diplomates of the American Board of Otolaryngology, the American Board of Plastic Surgery, and other boards and who have additional training and interest in the study of medical and surgical rhinology. *See also* American Board of Otolaryngology; American Board of Plastic Surgery; board; diplomate; rhinology.

American Roentgen Ray Society (ARRS)   A national organization founded in 1900 composed of 6,150 specialists in diagnostic and/or therapeutic radiology. *See also* radiology; x-ray.

American Rural Health Association   *See* National Rural Health Association.

American School Health Association (ASHA)   A national organization founded in 1927 composed of 4,000 school physicians, school nurses, dentists, nutritionists, health educators, dental hygienists, and public health workers interested in the development and advancement of school health programs. *See also* dental hygienist; dentist; nutritionist; physician; public health; school nurse; school psychologist.

Americans with Disabilities Act of 1990   Legislation enacted to provide a clear and comprehensive national mandate for the elimination of discrimination against individuals with disabilities; to provide clear, strong, consistent, enforceable standards addressing discrimination against individuals with disabilities; and to ensure that the federal government plans a central role in enforcing the standards established in the act. *See also* disability.

American Sleep Disorders Association (ASDA) A national organization founded in 1975 composed of 1,700 sleep disorders centers and individuals interested in providing full diagnostic and treatment services for patients with all types of sleep disorders. It fosters educational activities at medical schools and in continuing medical education programs and conducts site visits to ensure minimum standards at

member centers. It trains and evaluates the competence of individuals who care for patients with sleep disorders. *See also* polysomnographic technology; sleep; sleep apnea; somnology.

American Small and Rural Hospital Association *See* National Rural Health Association.

American Social Health Association (ASHA)   A national voluntary health organization founded in 1912 interested in the prevention, control, and eventual elimination of the consequences of sexually-transmitted diseases as a social health problem. It operates Herpes Resource Center, a national program for sufferers of incurable genital herpes. *See also* herpes simplex; sexually-transmitted disease.

American Society of Abdominal Surgery (ASAS) A national organization founded in 1959 composed of 9,300 physicians specializing in abdominal surgery. It sponsors an extensive program of surgical education including study courses, postgraduate programs, lectures, and demonstrations. *See also* abdomen; abdominal surgery.

American Society of Addiction Medicine (ASAM) A national organization founded in 1954 composed of 3,500 physicians with special interest and experience in the field of alcoholism and other drug dependencies. Formerly (1989) American Medical Society on Alcoholism and Other Drug Dependencies. *See also* addiction medicine; alcoholism and other drug dependence.

American Society for Adolescent Psychiatry (ASAP)   A national organization founded in 1967 composed of 1,500 psychiatrists interested in the behavior of adolescents. It provides for the exchange of psychiatric knowledge and encourages the development of adequate standards and training facilities for treatment of adolescents. *See also* adolescence; child and adolescent psychiatry; psychiatry; standard.

American Society for Advancement of Anesthesia in Dentistry (ASAAD)   A national organization founded in 1929 composed of 400 dentists and physicians interested in dental anesthesia. It studies new anesthetics and chemicals and researches pain control methods. It sponsors continuing education seminars, symposia, and scientific sessions. *See also* anesthesia; continuing education; dentistry; pain.

American Society for Aesthetic Plastic Surgery (ASAPS)   A national organization founded in 1967 composed of 942 board-certified plastic surgeons.

See also plastic surgery.

American Society on Aging (ASA) A national organization founded in 1954 composed of 8,000 health care and social service professionals, educators, researchers, administrators, businesspersons, students, and senior citizens. It offers 25 continuing education programs for professionals in aging-related fields. *See also* aging; continuing education; geriatric medicine; gerontology.

American Society of Allied Health Professions (ASAHP) A national organization founded in 1967 composed of 750 national allied health professional membership organizations, clinical service programs, academic institutions, and other institutions whose interests include the advancement of allied health education, research, and service delivery. *See also* allied health professional.

American Society of Anesthesiologists (ASA) A national organization founded in 1905 composed of 28,000 physicians specializing or interested in anesthesiology. It seeks to develop and further the specialty of anesthesiology for the general elevation of the standards of medical practice. *See also* American Society of Anesthesiologists - Physical Status classification system; anesthesiology; physician; standard.

American Society of Anesthesiologists - Physical Status (ASA-PS class) classification system A system of classifying patients into categories based on the presence and severity of disease: ASA-P1, a normal healthy patient; P2, a patient with mild systemic disease; P3, a patient with severe systemic disease; P4, a patient with severe systemic disease that is a constant threat to life; P5, a dying patient who is not expected to survive; P6, a declared brain-dead patient whose organs are being removed for donor purposes. An emergency patient in one of the classes above whose procedure is performed on an emergency basis is designated with an "E" following the classification, for example, P2E. *See also* American Society of Anesthesiologists; anesthesiology; classification system.

American Society for Apheresis (ASFA) A national organization founded in 1981 composed of 500 physicians, nurses, technologists, and other individuals active in the field of apheresis. It assists in forming standards and regulations in the field of apheresis and promotes training and research in apheresis therapy for patients. *See also* apheresis.

American Society for Artificial Internal Organs

(ASAIO) A national organization founded in 1955 composed of 1,700 individuals seeking to increase knowledge about artificial internal organs and their utilization. *See also* artificial; organ.

American Society of Bariatric Physicians (ASBP) A national organization founded in 1950 composed of 700 physicians with an interest in the study and treatment of obesity and associated conditions. *See also* bariatrics; obesity; physician.

American Society for Biochemistry and Molecular Biology (ASBMB) A national organization founded in 1906 composed of 8,500 biochemists and molecular biologists who have conducted and published original investigations in biological chemistry and/or molecular biology. Formerly (1987) American Society of Biological Chemists. *See also* biochemistry; molecular biology.

American Society of Biological Chemists *See* American Society for Biochemistry and Molecular Biology.

American Society for Bone and Mineral Research (ASBMR) A national organization founded in 1977 composed of 1,850 physicians, dentists, veterinarians, and other doctors interested in research in bone and mineral diseases. It has established guidelines to aid in preventing osteoporosis. *See also* bone; osteoporosis.

American Society of Cataract and Refractive Surgery (ASCRS) A national organization founded in 1974 composed of 4,500 ophthalmologists interested in surgery of the anterior segment of the eye, including intraocular lens implant surgery and refractive corneal surgery. *See also* cataract; lens; ophthalmology.

American Society for Cell Biology (ASCB) A national organization founded in 1960 composed of 7,100 scientists with educational or research experience in cell biology or an allied field. *See also* biology; cell.

American Society of Childbirth Educators (ASCE) A national organization founded in 1972 that provides for the exchange and dissemination of information relating to prepared childbirth as a shared family experience. It disseminates information to qualified professionals regarding standards and techniques relevant to prepared childbirth. *See also* labor; standard.

American Society for Clinical Evoked Potentials (ASCEP) A national organization founded in 1981 composed of 410 physicians in physical medicine and rehabilitation, neurology, neurosurgery, ophthalmology, and anesthesiology interested in studying the central nervous system's transmissions and to teach electrodiagnostic reading of evoked potentials. *See also* central nervous system; electroneurodiagnostic technologist; evoked potentials; physician.

American Society of Clinical Genetics and Dysmorphology *See* Birth Defect and Clinical Genetic Society.

American Society of Clinical Hypnosis (ASCH) A national organization founded in 1957 composed of 4,000 physicians, dentists, and psychologists with doctoral degrees interested in the field of hypnosis. It sets standards of training and conducts teaching sessions at basic and advanced levels. *See also* hypnosis; hypnotherapy.

American Society for Clinical Investigation (ASCI) A national organization founded in 1909 composed of 2,300 physicians who have accomplished meritorious original investigations in the clinical or allied sciences of medicine. Active members are physicians under age 48 years; emeritus members are those over age 48 years. *See also* investigation; physician.

American Society for Clinical Nutrition (ASCN) A national organization founded in 1959 composed of 1,200 physicians and scientists actively engaged in clinical nutrition research. It is a division of the American Institute of Nutrition. *See also* American Institute of Nutrition; nutrition.

American Society of Clinical Oncology (ASCO) A national organization founded in 1964 composed of 8,700 physicians and paramedical personnel who have a predominant interest in the diagnosis and care of patients with cancer. *See also* oncology; paramedical personnel; physician.

American Society of Clinical Pathologists (ASCP) A national organization founded in 1922 composed of 45,000 clinical pathologists, clinical scientists, chemists, microbiologists, medical technologists, and other individuals interested in clinical pathology. It promotes a wider application of pathology and laboratory medicine to the diagnosis and treatment of disease, conducts a program for the examination and certification of medical laboratory personnel, and conducts educational programs. *See also* certification; continuing education; pathology.

American Society for Clinical Pharmacology and Therapeutics (ASCPT) A national organization founded in 1900 composed of 2,025 physician members interested in the promotion and advancement of the science of human pharmacology and therapeutics. It provides a continuing medical education program for practicing physicians. *See also* clinical pharmacology; continuing medical education; pharmacology; physician; therapeutics.

American Society of Clinic Radiologists (ASCR) A national organization founded in 1977 composed of 20 organizations of radiologists representing major multispecialty clinics. Its purpose is to maintain and improve the quality and efficiency of radiologic care by convening radiologists to share information about educational, operational, technical, political, and socioeconomic aspects of radiologic practice. *See also* clinic; radiology.

American Society of Colon and Rectal Surgeons (ASCRS) A national organization founded in 1899 composed of 1,500 surgeons specializing in the diagnosis and treatment of diseases of the colon, rectum, and anus. *See also* colon and rectal surgery.

American Society for Colposcopy and Cervical Pathology (ASCCP) A division founded in 1964 of the American College of Obstetricians and Gynecologists composed of 2,000 obstetricians, gynecologists, and other individuals interested in the accurate and ethical application of colposcopy. *See also* American College of Obstetricians and Gynecologists; colposcopy.

American Society of Consultant Pharmacists (ASCP) A national professional membership organization founded in 1969 composed of 4,600 registered pharmacists and educators who are interested in pharmaceutical procedures within nursing homes and related health facilities. *See also* consultant; nursing home; long term care facility; pharmacist.

American Society of Contemporary Medicine and Surgery (ASCMS) A national organization founded in 1968 composed of 8,000 medical and surgical specialists interested in the dissemination of medical information and continuing medical education by means of conferences, seminars, and print and audiovisual media. It offers continuing education programs at its regular scientific assemblies. *See also* continuing medical education.

American Society of Contemporary Ophthalmology (ASCO) A national organization founded in 1966 composed of 6,000 ophthalmologists interested in the advancement of clinical research and the availability of continuing education in ophthalmology. *See also* continuing medical education; ophthalmology.

American Society for Cybernetics (ASC) A national organization founded in 1964 composed of 250 persons with professional standing or interest in the field of cybernetics. It fosters projects in theoretical and applied cybernetics by means of multidisciplinary scientific research programs and encourages education in cybernetics in schools and universities. *See also* cybernetics; medical cybernetics.

American Society of Cytology (ASC) A national organization founded in 1951 composed of 3,600 cytologists, pathologists, clinicians, researchers, and cytotechnologists interested in making the cytological method of early cancer detection universally available to the public. *See also* cancer; cytology; cytopathology; cytotechnologist; pathology.

American Society for Cytotechnology (ASCT) A national organization founded in 1979 composed of 1,400 cytotechnologists, physicians, and other individuals in the field of cytopathology. *See also* cytopathology; cytotechnologist; physician.

American Society of Dentistry for Children (ASDC) A national organization founded in 1927 composed of 10,000 general practitioners and specialists interested in dentistry for children. It conducts specialized education and research programs and provides placement service for graduates in dentistry. *See also* pediatric dentistry.

American Society for Dermatologic Surgery (ASDS) A national organization founded in 1970 composed of 2,157 physicians specializing in dermatologic surgery. *See also* dermatology; surgery.

American Society of Dermatopathology (ASD) A national organization founded in 1962 composed of 880 dermatopathologists and other individuals interested in dermatopathology. *See also* dermatopathology.

American Society of Directors of Volunteer Services (ASDVS) A national organization founded in 1968 composed of 1,700 persons who are employed or recognized by the administration of a health care organization as having major or continuing responsibility for managing and coordinating its volunteer services program and who are eligible for personal membership in the American Hospital Association. Its purposes include developing the knowledge and increasing the competence of indi-

vidual members and providing a means of communication for directors of volunteer services and health care organizations. *See also* American Hospital Association; director; volunteer; volunteer services.

American Society of Echocardiography (ASE) A national organization founded in 1976 composed of 4,000 physicians and technicians specializing in ultrasound heart imaging and diagnosis. *See also* diagnostic medical sonographer; echocardiography; physician; ultrasound imaging.

American Society of Electroneurodiagnostic Technologists (ASET) A national organization founded in 1959 composed of persons engaged in clinical electroencephalographic (EEG) technology, with some individuals performing both clinical and research EEG and related neurodiagnostic procedures, such as evoked potential responses and polysomnography. *See also* electroneurodiagnostic technologist; evoked potentials.

American Society of Extra-Corporeal Technology (AmSECT) A national organization founded in 1964 composed of 3,000 perfusionists, technologists, physicians, nurses, and other individuals interested in the practice of extracorporeal technology (involving heart-lung machines). *See also* heart-lung machine; nurse; perfusionist; physician.

American Society of Forensic Odontology (ASFO) A national organizations composed of 450 individuals interested in the field of forensic dentistry. *See also* forensic dentistry; odontology.

American Society for Gastrointestinal Endoscopy (ASGE) A national organization founded in 1941 composed of 5,000 gastroenterologists, internists, and surgeons who perform gastroscopic, esophagoscopic, coloscopic, and perineoscopic examinations. It aims to further the knowledge of digestive diseases by endoscopic methods. *See also* endoscopy; gastroenterology; general surgery; internal medicine.

American Society for Geriatric Dentistry (ASGD) A national organization founded in 1965 composed of 450 dentists, dental hygienists, and dental students interested in oral health care for older adults in all health care settings (acute care, ambulatory care, home care, and long term care). It promotes continuing education of the practitioner of geriatric dentistry; nursing home administrators and personnel; and dental hygienists, nurses, and students. *See also* continuing education; dental geriatrics; dentistry;

geriatric medicine.

American Society of Group Psychotherapy and Psychodrama (ASGPP) A national organization founded in 1942 composed of 800 social workers, psychologists, psychiatrists, clergy members, nurses, and other individuals interested in group psychotherapy, psychodrama, and sociometry. *See also* art therapy; dance therapy; drama therapy; manual arts therapy; music therapy; poetry therapy; recreational therapy; sociometry.

American Society of Hand Therapists (ASHT) A national organization founded in 1977 composed of 532 registered and licensed occupational and physical therapists specializing in hand therapy and hand rehabilitation. *See also* occupational therapist; physical therapist.

American Society of Handicapped Physicians (ASHP) A national organization founded in 1981 composed of 1,200 handicapped physicians and other individuals interested in the problems faced by handicapped physicians. It acts as a forum to address the needs of physically disabled physicians and works against discrimination of the handicapped. *See also* handicapped person; physician.

American Society for Head and Neck Surgery (ASHNS) A national organization founded in 1959 composed of 600 otolaryngologists and other individuals of the American College of Surgeons whose primary interest is head and neck surgery. *See also* American College of Surgeons; otolaryngologist - head and neck surgeon.

American Society for Healthcare Central Service Personnel (ASHCSP) A national organization founded in 1967 composed of 1,700 individuals interested in central services in health care organizations. Formerly (1987) American Society for Hospital Central Service Personnel. *See also* central service department.

American Society for Healthcare Education and Training of the American Hospital Association (ASHET) A national organization founded in 1970 composed of 1,500 education personnel and trainers from hospitals and other health care organizations involved in staff development and patient and community education. Its purposes include demonstrating the value of comprehensive education as a management strategy and promoting continuing education among all health care personnel. *See also* American Hospital Association; continuing education.

American Society for Healthcare Environmental Services of the American Hospital Association (ASHES) An organization of the American Hospital Association founded in 1986 composed of 1,200 managers and directors of hospital environmental services, laundry and linen services, housekeeping departments, and long term care units. *See also* American Hospital Association; environmental services.

American Society for Healthcare Human Resources Administration (ASHHRA) A national organization founded in 1964 composed of 2,550 individuals interested in providing effective and continuous leadership in the field of health care human resources administration. *See also* human resources; human resources management; leadership.

American Society for Health Care Marketing and Public Relations (ASHCMPR) A national organization founded in 1964 composed of 3,000 persons in hospitals, hospital councils or associations, hospital-related schools, and health care organizations who are responsible for marketing and public relations. Formerly (1984) American Society for Hospital Public Relations; (1990) American Society for Hospital Marketing and Public Relations. *See also* marketing; public relations.

American Society for Healthcare Risk Management (ASHRM) A national organization founded in 1980 composed of 2,500 employees actively involved in the risk management functions of hospitals or other health care providers. It promotes professional development of hospital risk managers and addresses risk management issues affecting the health care industry. Formerly (1986) called American Society for Hospital Risk Management. *See also* risk management; risk management activities; risk manager.

American Society of Hematology (ASH) A national organization founded in 1957 composed of 4,600 hematologists and other individuals holding doctorate degrees with an interest in the field. It promotes exchange of information and ideas related to blood and blood-forming tissues and investigation of hematologic problems. *See also* hematology.

American Society for Histocompatibility and Immunogenetics (ASHI) A national organization founded in 1968 composed of 1,000 scientists, physicians, and technologists involved in research and clinical activities related to histocompatibility testing. It conducts proficiency testing and educational programs. *See also* histocompatibility; immuno-genetics.

American Society of Hospital Attorneys *See* American Academy of Hospital Attorneys.

American Society of Hospital-Based Emergency Air Medical Services *See* Association of Air Medical Services.

American Society for Hospital Central Service Personnel *See* American Society for Healthcare Central Service Personnel.

American Society for Hospital Engineering of the AHA (ASHE) An organization of the American Hospital Association (AHA) founded in 1962 composed of 5,000 hospital engineers, facilities managers, directors of buildings and grounds, assistant administrators, directors of maintenance, directors of clinical engineering, design and construction professionals, and safety officers. It works to promote better patient care by encouraging and assisting members to develop their knowledge and increase their competence in the field of facilities management. *See also* administrative engineer; American Hospital Association; engineer.

American Society for Hospital Food Service Administrators (ASHFSA) A national organization founded in 1967 composed of 1,800 directors and assistant directors of food service departments in health care organizations who are eligible for personal membership in the American Hospital Association. It promotes improved administration of food-service departments through continuing education and development of management skills. *See also* American Hospital Association; continuing education; foodservice department.

American Society for Hospital Marketing and Public Relations *See* American Society for Health Care Marketing and Public Relations.

American Society for Hospital Materials Management (ASHMM) A national organization founded in 1962 composed of 2,000 individuals active in the fields of purchasing, inventory and distribution, and materials management as performed in hospitals, related patient care institutions, or government and voluntary health care organizations. *See also* materials management department; purchasing department.

American Society of Hospital Pharmacists (ASHP) A national organization founded in 1942 composed of 23,000 pharmacists employed by hos-

pitals and other types of health care organizations. It provides personnel placement service for members and sponsors a professional and personal liability program. It conducts educational and exhibit programs. *See also* hospital; pharmacist.

American Society for Hospital Public Relations *See* American Society for Health Care Marketing and Public Relations.

American Society for Hospital Risk Management *See* American Society for Healthcare Risk Management.

American Society of Human Genetics (ASHG) A national organization founded in 1948 composed of 4,200 physicians, researchers, genetic counselors, and other individuals interested in human genetics. *See also* genetic counselor; genetics; human genetics; physician.

American Society of Hypertension (ASH) A national organization founded in 1985 composed of 4,000 medical professionals, paraprofessionals, and postgraduate students interested in hypertension and related cardiovascular diseases. *See also* hypertension.

American Society for Information Science (ASIS) A national organization founded in 1937 composed of 4,000 information specialists, scientists, administrators, and other individuals interested in the use, organization, storage, retrieval, evaluation, and dissemination of recorded specialized information. Members are engaged in activities and specialties including classification and coding systems, automatic and associative indexing, machine translation of languages, and copyright issues. *See also* classification system; information; information science.

American Society of Internal Medicine (ASIM) A national organization founded in 1956 composed of 25,000 physicians specializing in internal medicine. It focuses on the delivery and financing of medical care in areas including access to care, appropriate reform of the American health care system, issues affecting the elderly, health insurance and reimbursement, managed care, and documentation of physician performance. *See also* internal medicine; physician.

American Society for Laser Medicine and Surgery (ASLMS) A national organization founded in 1980 composed of 1,728 physicians, physicists, nurses, dentists, podiatrists, technicians, and commercial representatives interested in the medical applications of lasers. *See also* laser.

American Society of Law and Medicine (ASLM)
A national organization founded in 1972 composed of 4,500 physicians, attorneys, health care management executives, nurses, insurance company personnel, members of the judiciary, and other individuals interested in medicolegal relations and health law. It provides opportunities for continuing education through publications, conferences, and information clearinghouse services. *See also* health law.

American Society of Legal and Industrial Medicine (AALIM) A national organization founded in 1946 composed of 200 physicians who meet qualifications established by the academy and are interested in compensation medicine. It seeks to advance the study of industrial medicine and workers' disability compensation. Formerly (1985) American Academy of Compensation Medicine; (1991) American Academy of Legal and Industrial Medicine. *See also* workers' compensation.

American Society of Lipo-Suction Surgery (ASLSS) A national organization founded in 1982 composed of 650 surgeons specializing in dermatology, general surgery, gynecology, otolaryngology, plastic and reconstructive surgery, and cosmetics surgery who are interested in the art and methods of liposuction surgery. *See also* liposuction surgery.

American Society of Maxillofacial Surgeons (ASMS) A national organization founded in 1947 composed of 385 physicians and dentists who have at least five years of recognized graduate training and experience in maxillofacial surgery. It seeks to stimulate and advance knowledge of the science and art of maxillofacial surgery and improve and elevate the standard of practice. *See also* oral and maxillofacial surgery; standard of care.

American Society for Medical Technology (ASMT)
A national organization founded in 1932 composed of 20,000 medical laboratory personnel who have an associate or a baccalaureate degree and clinical training and specialists who hold at least a master's degree in one of the major fields of medical technology, such as bacteriology, mycology, or biochemistry. *See also* bacteriology; biochemistry; medical laboratory technician; medical technology; mycology.

American Society for Microbiology (ASM) A national organization founded in 1899 composed of 38,000 microbiologists. It maintains numerous committees, 22 divisions, placement services, and biographical archives. *See also* microbiology.

American Society of Nephrology (ASN) A national organization founded in 1966 composed of 4,300 nephrologists interested in education and improving the quality of patient care. *See also* internal medicine; kidney; nephrology; physician.

American Society of Neuroimaging (ASN) A national organization founded in 1977 composed of 600 neurologists, neurosurgeons, neuroradiologists, and scientists interested in the development of computerized axial tomography, magnetic resonance imaging, and other neurodiagnostic techniques for clinical service, teaching, and research. *See also* computerized axial tomography; magnetic resonance imaging; neuroradiology; radiology.

American Society of Neuroradiology (ASNR) A national organization founded in 1962 composed of 1,900 radiologists who spend at least half their time practicing neuroradiology. *See also* neuroradiology; radiology.

American Society of Ophthalmic Administrators (ASOA) A division of the American Society of Cataract and Refractive Surgery founded in 1986 composed of 1,500 persons involved with the administration of an ophthalmic office or clinic. *See also* administrator; American Society of Cataract and Refractive Surgery; ophthalmology; optometry.

American Society of Ophthalmic Registered Nurses (ASORN) A national organization founded in 1976 composed of 1,800 registered nurses specializing in the field of ophthalmology. It facilitates continuing education of its members and represents members' interests before governmental agencies, hospitals, industries, research organizations, technical societies, universities, and other professional associations. *See also* continuing education; ophthalmology; registered nurse.

American Society of Outpatient Surgeons (ASOS)
A national organization founded in 1978 composed of 400 anesthesiologists and surgeons in various specialties who practice surgery in an office-based setting. It seeks to provide improved surgical care at lower costs. It is affiliated with the Accreditation Association for Ambulatory Health Care. *See also* Accreditation Association for Ambulatory Health Care; ambulatory surgery; anesthesiology; surgeon.

American Society of Parasitologists (ASP) A national organization founded in 1924 composed of 1,500 persons interested in improving the teaching and promoting the study of parasites. Its committees include nomenclature and terminology and techniques in clinical laboratory medicine. *See also* parasite; parasitology.

American Society for Parenteral and Enteral Nutrition (ASPEN) A national organization founded in 1975 composed of 7,200 physicians, dietitians, nurses, pharmacists, and other health specialists interested in nutritional support for patients during hospitalization and rehabilitation. *See also* enteral and parenteral nutrition and infusion therapy services; nutrition; total parenteral nutrition.

American Society of Pediatric Hematology/Oncology (ASPHO) A national organization founded in 1981 composed of 850 physicians who have served residencies in pediatrics and fellowships in pediatric hematology-oncology; specialists in allied disciplines including surgery, pathology, radiology, pedodontics, and psychiatry; physicians trained in hematology or oncology of adults who are interested in the treatment of blood diseases and cancer in children; and individuals holding doctoral degrees who are involved in research relevant to the field. Affiliated members include nurses and physician assistants working with children with cancer, sickle cell disease, thalassemia, hemophilia, and other hematological disorders, and psychologists, social workers, and research scientists. *See also* cancer; hematology; hemophilia; pediatric hematology-oncology; sickle cell anemia.

American Society for Pediatric Neurosurgery (ASPN) A national organization founded in 1978 composed of 50 pediatric neurosurgeons. It represents the interests of pediatric neurosurgery as they relate to government, the public, universities, and professional societies; supports basic and clinical research in pediatric neurosurgery; and provides leadership in undergraduate, graduate, and continuing education in pediatric neurosurgery. *See also* neurological surgery; pediatrics.

American Society for Personnel Administration *See* Society for Human Resource Management.

American Society of Pharmacognosy (ASP) A national organization founded in 1959 composed of 900 pharmacognosists and other persons interested in the plant sciences and natural products. *See also* pharmacognosy.

American Society for Pharmacology and Experimental Therapeutics (ASPET) A national organization founded in 1908 composed of 4,200 investiga-

tors in pharmacology and toxicology. Its committees cover topics, such as substance abuse and public information, and its divisions include Clinical Pharmacology, Drug Metabolism, and Neuropharmacology. *See also* pharmacology; therapeutics; toxicology.

American Society for Pharmacy Law (ASPL) A national organization founded in 1974 composed of 800 pharmacists, lawyers, and students. Its purposes are to further legal knowledge, communicate accurate legal information to pharmacists, and foster knowledge and education pertaining to the rights and duties of pharmacists. *See also* law; pharmacist; pharmacy.

American Society of Plastic and Reconstructive Surgeons (ASPRS) A national organization founded in 1931 composed of 4,000 plastic surgeons interested in promoting care for plastic surgery patients through research, service, and education. It sponsors patient education programs, holds clinical symposia, and acts as a liaison between members and government and medical education. It offers a toll-free patient referral service providing names of certified plastic surgeons and information on procedural brochures. *See also* certified; plastic surgery.

American Society of Plastic and Reconstructive Surgical Nurses (ASPRSN) A national organization founded in 1975 composed of 1,200 registered nurses, licensed practical nurses, and licensed vocational nurses working with plastic surgeons or interested in plastic and reconstructive nursing. Its objectives include enhancing leadership qualities of nurses in the field of plastic surgery and increasing the skills, knowledge, and understanding of personnel in plastic surgery nursing through continuing education. It is affiliated with the American Society of Plastic and Reconstructive Surgeons. *See also* continuing education; licensed practical nurse; licensed vocational nurse; plastic surgery; registered nurse; surgical nurse.

American Society of Podiatric Assistants *See* American Society of Podiatric Medical Assistants.

American Society of Podiatric Dermatology (ASPD) A national organization founded in 1914 composed of 267 doctors of podiatric medicine with expertise in foot dermatology and candidates for the Doctor of Podiatric Medicine (DPM) degree in colleges of podiatric medicine who are interested in the field of podiatric dermatology. *See also* dermatology; podiatric medicine.

American Society of Podiatric Medical Assistants

(ASPMA) A national organization founded in 1964 composed of 1,100 podiatric assistants interested in educational seminars. It administers certification examinations. Formerly (1985) American Society of Podiatric Assistants. *See also* certification; medical assistant; podiatric assistant; podiatric medicine.

American Society of Podiatric Medicine (ASPM) A national organization founded in 1944 composed of 110 podiatrists interested in research in podiatry, postgraduate courses, and scientific programs at annual meetings. *See also* podiatric medicine.

American Society of Post Anesthesia Nurses (ASPAN) A national organization founded in 1980 composed of 6,600 postanesthesia nurses interested in upgrading standards of postanesthesia patient care and the professional growth of licensed nurses involved in the care of patients in the immediate postanesthesia period. *See also* nurse; postoperative care; recovery room.

American Society of Preventive Oncology (ASPO) A national organization founded in 1977 composed of 300 professionals in clinical, educational, or research disciplines interested in the area of cancer prevention. It promotes exchange of information, including environmental exposures and life-styles, and works to implement programs for the prevention and early detection of cancer. *See also* oncology; preventive medicine.

American Society for Psychical Research (ASPR) A national organization founded in 1885 composed of 2,000 members interested in telepathy, vision and apparition, dowsing, precognition, psychokinesis (mind over matter), automatic writing and other forms of automatism, psychometry, psychic healing, dreams, clairvoyance, clairaudience, and predictions and the physical phenomena of mediumship (such as materialization, telekinesis, rapping, and other sounds) and other unclassified parapsychological phenomena. *See also* parapsychology.

American Society of Psychoanalytic Physicians (ASPP) A national organization founded in 1985 composed of 300 psychiatrists, psychoanalysts, and other individuals interested in fostering a wider understanding and utilization of psychoanalytic concepts and providing an opportunity to study psychoanalytic theory from all schools of thought. It offers lectures on therapy that combine a psychoanalytic orientation with other disciplines. *See also* physician; psychoanalysis.

American Society of Psychopathology of Expression (ASPE) A national organization founded in 1964 composed of 137 physicians, psychologists, art therapists, artists, social workers, criminologists, writers, and other individuals interested in the problems of expression and the artistic activities connected with psychiatric, sociological, and psychological research. It disseminates information about research and clinical applications in the field of psychopathology of expression. *See also* abnormal psychology; express; psychopath.

American Society for Psychoprophylaxis in Obstetrics (ASPO/LAMAZE) A national organization founded in 1960 composed of 5,000 physicians, nurses, nurse-midwives, certified teachers of the psychoprophylactic (Lamaze) method of childbirth, and other individuals interested in Lamaze childbirth preparation and family-centered maternity care. It disseminates information about the theory and practical application of psychoprophylaxis in obstetrics, administers teacher training courses, and certifies qualified Lamaze teachers. It sponsors prenatal classes in the Lamaze method for expectant parents. *See also* certification; obstetrics; prophylaxis.

American Society for Quality Control (ASQC) A national organization founded in 1946 composed of 68,500 professionals interested in the advancement of quality. It offers courses in quality engineering, reliability engineering, managing for quality, management of quality costs, quality audit-development and administration, management of the inspection function, probability and statistics for engineers and scientists, and product liability and prevention. *See also* quality control.

American Society of Radiologic Technologists (ASRT) A national organization founded in 1920 composed of 16,000 diagnostic radiography, radiation therapy, ultrasound, and nuclear medicine technologists interested in advancing the science of radiologic technology and establishing and maintaining high standards of education and training in the field. *See also* diagnostic medical sonographer; nuclear medicine technologist; radiation therapy technologist; radiographer.

American Society of Regional Anesthesia (ASRA) A national organization founded in 1974 composed of 6,000 physicians and researchers involved with the study and clinical use of regional anesthesia. *See also* anesthesia; regional anesthesia.

American Society of Retired Dentists (ASRD) A national organization founded in 1981 composed of 1,600 retired and active dentists interested in maintaining financial security and continued social, cultural, and professional activity. It provides members with opportunities to serve their communities, information on continuing education programs, and assistance in maintaining good physical and mental health. It offers retirement and preretirement programs. *See also* continuing education; dentist; retirement.

American Society of Safety Engineers (ASSE) A national organization founded in 1911 composed of 26,000 safety engineers, safety directors, and other individuals interested in accident prevention and safety programs. *See also* accident; engineer; safety management.

American Society of Sanitary Engineering (ASSE) A national organization founded in 1906 composed of 2,700 plumbing officials, sanitary engineers, plumbers, plumbing contractors, building officials, architects, engineers, designing engineers, physicians, and other persons interested in health. *See also* engineering; sanitary engineer.

American Society for Stereotactic and Functional Neurosurgery (ASSFN) A national organization founded in 1968 composed of 200 neurosurgeons practicing stereotactic surgery and interested in promoting communication in the field. *See also* neurological surgery; stereotactic surgery.

American Society for the Study of Orthodontics (ASSO) A national organization founded in 1945 composed of members of the American Dental Association or other societies, with special interest in orthodontics but not limited to those who practice in the field. Its purposes include encouraging and assisting the diffusion of orthodontic knowledge to all dentists who include orthodontics as an integral part of their health service or limit their practice to orthodontics. It conducts clinical study groups throughout the United States. *See also* American Dental Association; dentistry; orthodontics.

American Society for Surgery of the Hand (ASSH) A national organization founded in 1946 composed of 1,037 surgeons specializing in surgery of the hand. It promotes research and worthwhile contributions to the field of hand surgery. *See also* hand surgery.

American Society for Testing and Materials *See* ASTM.

American Society of Therapeutic Radiologists *See* American Society for Therapeutic Radiology and Oncology.

American Society for Therapeutic Radiology and Oncology (ASTRO) A national organization founded in 1955 composed of 3,116 physicians who limit their practice to radiation therapy. Formerly (1983) American Society of Therapeutic Radiologists. *See also* radiation oncology; radiation therapy; radiology.

American Society of Transplant Surgeons (ASTS) A national organization founded in 1975 composed of 444 surgeons specializing in transplantation. It promotes education and research and participates in developing programs that will benefit organ recipients. Its committees deal with topics, such as heart transplantation and ethics. *See also* ethics; surgeon; transplant; transplantation.

American Society of Tropical Medicine and Hygiene (ASTMH) A national organization founded in 1952 composed of 2,300 physicians and scientists interested in tropical medicine and hygiene, including the areas of arborvirology, entomology, medicine, nursing, and parasitology. *See also* tropical medicine.

Americans for a Sound AIDS Policy (ASAP) A national advisory group founded in 1987 composed of physicians, public health professionals, legislators, and businessmen assisting in the formulation of a workable public policy on AIDS that will be understood and accepted by the public. It advocates early diagnosis and promotes reducing transmission of the virus through public health intervention strategies, such as confidential and voluntary partner notification. *See also* acquired immunodeficiency syndrome; public policy.

American Speech-Language-Hearing Association (ASHA) A national organization founded in 1925 composed of 60,000 speech-language pathologists and audiologists. It acts as an accrediting body for college and university graduate school programs, clinics, and hospital programs and as a certifying body for professionals providing speech, language, and hearing therapy to the public. *See also* accreditation; audiologist; certification; speech pathologist; speech therapist.

American Spinal Injury Association (ASIA) A national organization founded in 1973 composed of 400 physicians who have been trained in the care of spinal paralytic patients and who are either actively engaged in the field and acknowledged to be competent by their peers or who have made a significant contribution to the advancement of the basic sciences or one of the clinical fields of practice relating to treatment of the spine. *See also* paraplegia; quadriplegia; spinal cord.

American Standard Code for Information Interchange (ASCII) A common code for the computer representation of letters, numbers, and function symbols used for data communications. The code employs eight computer bits in various combinations to handle all 128 standard characters. *See also* computer; bit.

American Statistical Association (ASA) A national organization founded in 1839 composed of 15,000 persons interested in the theory, methodology, and application of statistics to all fields of human endeavor. Sections include Biometrics, Biopharmaceutical, and Quality and Productivity. *See also* biometrics; productivity; quality; statistics.

American Surgical Association (ASA) A national organization founded in 1880 composed of 990 interested in promoting the science and art of surgery. *See also* surgery.

American Surgical Trade Association *See* Health Industry Distributors Association.

American Therapeutic Recreation Association (ATRA) A national organization founded in 1984 composed of 2,000 therapeutic recreation professionals and students who use sports, handicrafts, and other recreational activities to improve the physical, mental, and emotional functions of persons with illnesses or disabling conditions in hospitals, mental rehabilitation centers, physical rehabilitation centers, senior citizen treatment centers, and public health facilities. *See also* recreational therapy.

American Thermographic Society *See* American Academy of Thermology.

American Thoracic Society (ATS) The medical section of the American Lung Association founded in 1905 composed of 10,000 specialists in pulmonary diseases, physicians in the public health field interested in tuberculosis control, thoracic surgeons, and research workers in lung disease. It acts as adviser in scientific matters. *See also* American Lung Association; thoracic surgery.

American Thyroid Association (ATA) A national

organization founded in 1923 composed of 650 internists, surgeons, pathologists, radiologists, and research workers interested in the thyroid gland and its diseases. *See also* thyroid gland.

American Tort Reform Association (ATRA) A national organization founded in 1986 composed of 400 professional groups, businesses, and business and trade associations interested in remedying the current liability insurance "crisis" by developing, promoting, and coordinating the US tort law system. *See also* tort.

American Transplant Association (ATA) A nonmembership organization founded in 1985 that acts as an informational referral network for transplant patients and offers support for financial expenses and emergency transportation. It provides public education on organ and tissue donation awareness. *See also* organ procurement; transplantation.

American Trauma Society (ATS) A national organization founded in 1968 composed of 2,500 physicians, nurses, emergency medical services personnel, other health professionals, institutions, and corporations. It seeks to prevent trauma situations, improve trauma care through professional and paraprofessional education, and educate the public through campaigns and dissemination of information. *See also* trauma; traumatology.

American Type Culture Collection (ATCC) A private, nonmembership organization founded in 1925 with 210 staff seeking to collect, propagate, preserve, and distribute authentic cultures of microorganisms and genetic materials for reference purposes for use in educational, research, and other scientific and industrial activities. It conducts research in cryobiology, microbial systematics, and karyology. It maintains a depository for cultures involved in patent application and for confidential safekeeping of proprietary cultures. It aids in processing and packaging of biohazardous materials, identifies cultures, and conducts workshops on topics relating to microbiology, cell culture, biotechnology, and management of culture collections. *See also* cell; culture; culture medium; karyology; microorganism; tissue; tissue culture.

American Urological Association (AUA) A national organization founded in 1902 composed of 6,100 physicians specializing in urology. *See also* American Association of Clinical Urologists; physician; urology.

American Urological Association Allied (AUAA) A national organization founded in 1972 composed of 1,700 registered and licensed practical nurses, technicians, physician assistants, persons working in urology-related industries, and secretarial employees in urology offices. It supersedes the Urological Nurses Association. *See also* licensed practical nurse; physician assistant; registered nurse; urology.

American Venereal Disease Association (AVDA) A national organization founded in 1934 composed of 1,150 professionals and laypersons interested in clinical and laboratory research in the diagnosis, medical and social pathology, treatment, and public health control of venereal diseases. Its primary interest is reduction of the prevalence of sexually-transmitted diseases. *See also* sexually-transmitted disease; venereology.

AMERSA *See* Association of Medical Education and Research in Substance Abuse.

AMH *See Accreditation Manual for Hospitals.*

AMHA *See* Association of Mental Health Administrators.

AMHC *See Accreditation Manual for Home Care.*

AMHC *See* Association of Mental Health Clergy.

AMHCA *See* American Mental Health Counselors Association.

AMHCN *See Accreditation Manual for Health Care Networks.*

AMHE *See* Association of Haitian Physicians Abroad.

AMHPS *See* Association of Minority Health Professions Schools.

AMI *See* acute myocardial infarction; Association of Medical Illustrators.

AMIA *See* American Medical Informatics Association.

aminoglycoside Any of a group of bacterial antibiotics (for example, amikacin, gentamicin, streptomycin) derived from various species of *Streptomyces* or produced synthetically. Serious adverse effects of aminoglycosides include nephrotoxicity (toxic to kidneys) and ototoxicity (toxic to ears and hearing). *See also* antibacterial; antibiotic.

AMLTC *See Accreditation Manual for Long Term Care.*

amniocentesis A prenatal obstetric procedure in which amniotic fluid containing fetal amniocytes is removed through a needle inserted through the abdominal wall into the uterus of a pregnant woman. The amniotic fluid is used for laboratory analysis. The procedure is usually performed between the sixteenth and twentieth weeks of gestation as an aid in the diagnosis of fetal abnormalities, such as chromosomal abnormalities, neural tube defects, and Tay-Sachs disease and to assess fetal maturity later in pregnancy. *See also* amniotic fluid; Down syndrome; obstetrics; pregnancy.

amniotic fluid The liquid surrounding the fetus throughout pregnancy. *See also* amniocentesis; amnioscopy.

amnioscopy Direct observation of the fetus and the color and amount of the amniotic fluid by means of an endoscope inserted through the vagina and the uterine cervix. *See also* amniocentesis.

AMP *See* Association for Media Psychology.

AMPA *See* American Medical Publishers' Association.

AMPAC *See* American Medical Political Action Committee.

amphetamines Drugs that stimulate the central nervous system, often used as decongestant inhalants, to combat fatigue, and to suppress appetite. They are also used illegally for their euphoric effects. *See also* controlled substances; drug; euphoria; stimulant.

AMPRA *See* American Medical Peer Review Association.

AMRA *See* Association of Medical Rehabilitation Administrators.

AMS *See* American Microscopical Society; American Motility Society.

AmSECT *See* American Society of Extra-Corporeal Technology.

AMSPDC *See* Association of Medical School Pediatric Department Chairmen.

AMSUS *See* Association of Military Surgeons of the United States.

AMT *See* American Medical Technologists.

AMTA *See* American Massage Therapy Association.

amulet A charm worn about the person as a preventive measure against disease, mischief, or witchcraft. *Synonym:* talisman. *See also* amuletic medicine.

amuletic medicine A therapy believed to exert its effect by occult means. *See also* amulet; medicine.

AMWA *See* American Medical Women's Association; American Medical Writers' Association.

amygdalin *See* laetrile.

ANA *See* American Naprapathic Association; American Neurological Association; American Nurses' Association; American Nutritionists Association.

ANAA *See* American Nursing Assistant's Association.

anabolic steroids Synthetic derivatives of testosterone, the male sex hormone that helps the human body build muscle and synthesize proteins. Anabolic steroids may be prescribed for certain anemias and leukemias and for lessening the pain or severity of breast cancer in women. They are taken illegally by some individuals to enhance muscle size and strength. Adverse effects of anabolic steroids in these individuals include increased irritability, restlessness, feelings of violence, and impotence. Anabolic steroids are classified as a schedule III controlled substance. *See also* controlled substances; schedule III substances; sex hormone; steroid; testosterone.

anabolism The constructive phase of metabolism in which smaller molecules, such as amino acids, are converted to large molecules, such as proteins. *Compare* catabolism. *See also* metabolism.

ANAC *See* Association of Nurses in AIDS Care.

anaerobic Without oxygen, as in anaerobic bacteria which thrive in the absence of oxygen. *Compare* aerobic.

analgesia Insensibility to pain. *See also* analgesic; pain.

analgesic An agent that removes or diminishes sensibility to pain. *See also* pain.

anal intercourse *See* sodomy.

analog computer A computer most frequently used in scientific, mathematical, and aerospace applications, in which numerical data are represented by measurable physical variables, such as voltages or rotations. *Compare* digital computer. *See also* computer.

analog data Data that are represented by an infinite number of variable measurable quantities along a continuum. An example of analog data is the infinite number of measurements of body temperature that occur along a continuum, such as 98.600° F, 98.601° F, 98.602° F, and so forth. Digital data, by contrast, are data expressed in discrete numbers (for example, 0 to 9 in the decimal system or 1 and 0 in the binary system), especially by a computer. *See also* analog-to-digital conversion; data; digit; digital data.

analog-to-digital conversion A process or device by which analog data are translated into digital form. *See also* analog data; digital data.

analysis The separation of an intellectual whole into its constituent parts for individual study. *See also* actuarial analysis; cost-benefit analysis; cost-effectiveness analysis; market analysis; medical-legal analysis; multivariate analysis; profile analysis; qualitative analysis; quantitative analysis.

analysis, actuarial *See* actuarial analysis.

Analysis, American Academy of Medical-Legal *See* American Academy of Medical-Legal Analysis.

Analysis, Association for Behavior *See* Association for Behavior Analysis.

analysis, cost-benefit *See* cost-benefit analysis.

analysis, cost-effectiveness *See* cost-effectiveness analysis.

analysis of data *See* data analysis.

analysis, factor *See* factor analysis.

analysis, force-field *See* force-field analysis.

analysis, market *See* market analysis.

analysis, medical-legal *See* medical-legal analysis.

Analysis in Medicine and Surgery, American Academy of Medical-Legal *See* American Academy of Medical-Legal Analysis in Medicine and Surgery.

analysis, meta- *See* meta-analysis.

analysis, multiple regression *See* regression analysis.

analysis, multivariate *See* multivariate analysis.

analysis, narco- *See* narcoanalysis.

analysis, Pareto *See* Pareto analysis.

analysis, policy *See* policy analysis.

analysis, practice pattern *See* practice pattern analysis.

analysis, process capability *See* process capability analysis.

analysis, profile *See* profile analysis.

analysis, qualitative *See* qualitative analysis.

analysis, quantitative *See* quantitative analysis.

analysis, regression *See* regression analysis.

analysis, risk *See* risk analysis.

analysis, risk-benefit *See* risk-benefit analysis.

analysis, systems *See* systems analysis.

analysis unit, special *See* special analysis unit.

analyst, health record *See* medical record analyst.

analyst, medical record *See* medical record analyst.

analyst, policy *See* policy analyst.

analyst, systems *See* systems analyst.

analytic study, cohort *See* cohort analytic study.

anaphylactic shock *See* anaphylaxis.

anaphylaxis An immediate and exaggerated hypersensitivity reaction to a previously encountered outside antigen, such as penicillin. *See also* allergy; antigen; shock.

anaplasia Reversion of cells to an immature or a

less differentiated form, as occurs in most malignant tumors. *See also* anaplastic; cancer.

anaplastic Characterized by cells that have become less differentiated. *See also* anaplasia.

anatomical Pertaining to anatomy, as in an anatomical gift. *See also* anatomical gift; anatomical pathologist; anatomy.

anatomical gift Testamentary donation of a vital organ(s) generally for the purpose of medical research or transplantation. Most states have adopted the Uniform Anatomical Gift Act of 1969, which authorizes the gift of all or part of a human body after death for specified purposes. *See also* organ procurement; Uniform Anatomical Gift Act of 1969.

anatomical pathologist A specialist in the gross and microscopic study of organs and tissues removed for biopsy or during postmortem examinations (autopsies). *See also* anatomy; autopsy; gross anatomy; microscopic anatomy; pathology.

anatomist A specialist in anatomy. *See also* anatomy; morbid anatomist.

anatomist, morbid *See* morbid anatomist.

Anatomists, American Association of *See* American Association of Anatomists.

anatomy The science of the shape and structure of organisms and their parts. *See also* gross anatomy; microscopic anatomy; morphology; nervous system; neuroanatomy.

anatomy, gross *See* gross anatomy.

anatomy, macroscopic *See* gross anatomy.

anatomy, microscopic *See* microscopic anatomy.

anatomy, neuro- *See* neuroanatomy.

ancillary Supporting, as in ancillary hospital services. *See also* ancillary charge; ancillary services.

ancillary charge **1.** The dollar amount associated with additional service performed prior to and/or secondary to a procedure, such as pathology, radiology, and anesthesia services. *See also* anesthesiology; pathology; radiology. **2.** A charge in addition to a copayment that a member of a health plan is required to pay to a participating pharmacy for a prescription that, through the request of the member or participating prescriber, has been dispensed in nonconformance with the health plan's maximum allowable cost list. *See also* allowable cost; charge; copayment; health plan; prescription.

ancillary services Hospital or other health care organization services other than room and board and professional services. Examples of ancillary services are diagnostic imaging, pharmacy, laboratory, and therapy services not separately itemized. *See also* ancillary charge; environmental services; pharmacy; radiology; support services.

ANDA *See* abbreviated new-drug application.

androgen A steroid hormone, such as testoterone, that controls the development and maintenance of masculine characteristics. *See also* andropause; hormone; sex hormone; testis; testosterone.

andropause A change of life for men frequently expressed as a career change, divorce, or reordering of one's life. It is associated with a decline in androgen levels that occurs in many men during their late forties or early fifties. *Compare* menopause. *See also* androgen; climacteric.

anecdotal Based on descriptions of unmatched individual cases rather than on controlled studies, as in a curious conclusion based on anecdotal cases rather than on data from controlled studies. *See also* anecdote; control experiment; control group.

anecdote A short account of an interesting incident. *See also* anecdotal.

anemia A deficiency in the number or volume of red blood cells or hemoglobin. Anemia may result from decreased red cell production (for example, iron-deficiency anemia), increased red cell destruction (for example, hemolytic anemia), or blood loss (for example, a ruptured abdominal aortic aneurysm or traumatic hemorrhage from a wound). *See also* hemorrhage; iron-deficiency anemia; sickle cell anemia.

anemia, iron-deficiency *See* iron-deficiency anemia.

anemia, sickle cell *See* sickle cell anemia.

anesthesia Loss of feeling or sensation, especially loss of the sensation of pain. In medicine, anesthesia is induced to permit performance of surgery or other painful procedures. *See also* epidural anesthesia; general anesthesia; local anesthesia; pain; regional anesthesia.

Anesthesia, American Society of Regional *See* American Society of Regional Anesthesia.

Anesthesia and Critical Care, Society of Neurosurgical *See* Society of Neurosurgical Anesthesia and Critical Care.

Anesthesia in Dentistry, American Society for Advancement of *See* American Society for Advancement of Anesthesia in Dentistry.

Anesthesia Educational Programs/Schools, Council on Accreditation of Nurse *See* Council on Accreditation of Nurse Anesthesia Educational

Programs/Schools.

anesthesia, epidural *See* epidural anesthesia.

anesthesia, general *See* general anesthesia.

anesthesia, local *See* local anesthesia.

Anesthesia Nurses, American Society of Post *See* American Society of Post Anesthesia Nurses.

Anesthesia Nursing Certification, American Board of Post *See* American Board of Post Anesthesia Nursing Certification.

anesthesia patients, classification of *See* American Society of Anesthesiologists - Physical Status classification system.

Anesthesia and Perinatology, Society for Obstetric *See* Society for Obstetric Anesthesia and Perinatology.

anesthesia, regional *See* regional anesthesia.

anesthesia, spinal *See* regional anesthesia.

anesthesiologist A physician specializing in anesthesiology. *See also* anesthesiology.

Anesthesiologists, American Osteopathic College of *See* American Osteopathic College of Anesthesiologists.

Anesthesiologists, American Society of *See* American Society of Anesthesiologists.

anesthesiologist's assistant (AA) An allied health professional who functions under the direction of an anesthesiologist and assists him or her in tasks ranging from collecting preoperative data to insertion of intravenous and arterial catheters and special catheters for central venous pressure monitoring to performing airway management and drug administration for induction and maintenance of anesthesia. Anesthesiologist's assistants are one type of allied health professional for which the Committee on Allied Health Education and Accreditation has accredited education programs. *See also* accredited; airway; allied health professional; anesthesia; anesthesiology.

Anesthesiologists, Association of University *See* Association of University Anesthesiologists.

Anesthesiologists - Physical Status classification system, American Society of *See* American Society of Anesthesiologists - Physical Status classification system.

Anesthesiologists, Society of Cardiovascular *See* Society of Cardiovascular Anesthesiologists.

anesthesiology The branch of medicine and medical specialty dealing with providing pain relief and maintenance, or restoration, of a stable condition during and immediately following an operation or

an obstetric or a diagnostic procedure. Two subspecialties of anesthesiology are critical care medicine and pain management. *See also* anesthesia; critical care medicine; pain management; physician.

Anesthesiology, American Board of *See* American Board of Anesthesiology.

Anesthesiology, American Dental Society of *See* American Dental Society of Anesthesiology.

anesthetic A drug or agent that is used to abolish or decrease the sensation of pain or feeling. *See also* general anesthetic; inhalation anesthetic; intravenous anesthetic; local anesthetic; nitrous oxide; pain; topical anesthetic.

anesthetic, general *See* general anesthetic.

anesthetic, inhalation *See* inhalation anesthetic.

anesthetic, intravenous *See* intravenous anesthetic.

anesthetic, local *See* local anesthetic.

anesthetic, topical *See* topical anesthetic.

anesthetist A physician, anesthesiologist's assistant, registered nurse, dentist, or other qualified individual who administers anesthetics to patients. *See also* anesthesiologist; anesthesiologist's assistant; nurse anesthetist; physician.

anesthetist, nurse *See* nurse anesthetist.

Anesthetists, American Association of Nurse *See* American Association of Nurse Anesthetists.

Anesthetists, Council on Certification of Nurse *See* Council on Certification of Nurse Anesthetists.

angel dust *See* PCP.

Angel Planes, The *See* The Angel Planes.

angina Severe pain.

angina pectoris Severe chest pain that occurs when the oxygen flow to the heart muscle is insufficient, usually the result of narrowing of the coronary arteries. *See also* angina; atherosclerosis; ischemia.

angiography A procedure in which substances opaque to radiation are injected into blood vessels so that diagnostic x-rays of those blood vessels may be made; for example, coronary (artery) angiography. *Synonym:* arteriography. *See also* arteriogram; cardiovascular medicine; coronary angiography; radiology.

Angiography and Interventions, Society for Cardiac *See* Society for Cardiac Angiography and Interventions.

angiology The branch of medicine dealing with the blood vessels of the body. *See also* American College of Angiology; blood vessel.

Angiology, American College of *See* American College of Angiology.

angioplasty A procedure for eliminating areas of narrowing or blockages in blood vessels, as in coronary artery angioplasty. *See also* cardiovascular medicine; laser angioplasty; percutaneous transluminal angioplasty; percutaneous transluminal coronary angioplasty; radiology.

angioplasty, balloon *See* percutaneous transluminal angioplasty.

angioplasty, laser *See* laser angioplasty.

angioplasty, percutaneous transluminal *See* percutaneous transluminal angioplasty.

angioplasty, percutaneous transluminal coronary *See* percutaneous transluminal coronary angioplasty.

ANHS *See* American Natural Hygiene Society.

anima Inner self. *Compare* persona.

Animal Care, American Association for Accreditation of Laboratory *See* American Association for Accreditation of Laboratory Animal Care.

animal care technologist An individual who cares for animals used in laboratory experiments, biological tests, and medical research. *See also* animal experimentation; technologist.

animal experimentation Conduct of experiments on animals to advance medicine and science by finding cures for diseases or new methods of treatment. *See also* antivivisectionist; experiment; vivisection.

Animal Management Association, Laboratory *See* Laboratory Animal Management Association.

Animal Medicine, American College of Laboratory *See* American College of Laboratory Animal Medicine.

Animal Resources, Institute of Laboratory *See* Institute of Laboratory Animal Resources.

Animal Science, American Association for Laboratory *See* American Association for Laboratory Animal Science.

Ankle Society, American Orthopaedic Foot and *See* American Orthopaedic Foot and Ankle Society.

ANNA *See* American Nephrology Nurses' Association.

anorexia nervosa An eating disorder, most common in adolescent and young women, characterized by preoccupation with body image, fear of obesity, self-induced starvation, and excessive exercising. Anorexia refers to a loss of appetite, compared to bulimia, which refers to an insatiable appetite. *Compare* bulimia nervosa. *See also* adolescence; eating disorder.

ANS *See* American Neurotology Society.

ANSI *See* American National Standards Institute.

answer **1.** A reply. **2.** A correct solution to a prob-

lem. **3.** A document filed with a court that contains the response of a defendant to the allegation set out in a plaintiff's complaint. *See also* allegation; complaint; plaintiff; pleadings.

antacid Any substance administered to counteract gastric acidity, relieve symptoms associated with gastroesophageal reflux, gastritis, and peptic ulcer, and promote healing of peptic ulcer. *See also* gastroesophageal reflux; milk of magnesia; peptic ulcer.

antenatal *See* prenatal.

anterior At or toward the front of a part, organ, or structure; for example, anterior fontanelle in a newborn. *Compare* posterior.

anthracosis *See* black lung disease.

anthropology The study of the origin, behavior, and physical, social, and cultural development of human beings. *See also* anthropophobia; social science.

Anthropology, Society for Medical *See* Society for Medical Anthropology.

anthropophobia Irrational fear of human society. *See also* antrhopology; phobia.

antibacterial Counteracting bacteria through killing (bacteriocidal) or inhibiting (bacteriostatic) their growth or replication, as in soap or penicillin. *See also* aminoglycoside; antibiotic; bacteria; bacteriocidal; bacteriostatic; cephalosporin; penicillin.

antibiotic Any drug, such as penicillin or streptomycin, containing any quantity of any chemical substance produced by a microorganism, which has the capacity to inhibit the growth of or destroy bacteria and other microorganisms (or a chemically synthesized equivalent of such a substance). Antibiotics are used in the prevention and treatment of infectious diseases. *See also* aminoglycoside; bacteria; cephalosporin; infectious diseases; microorganism; penicillin.

Antibiotics, Alliance for the Prudent Use of *See* Alliance for the Prudent Use of Antibiotics.

antibodies Immunoglobulins produced by lymphoid tissues in response to bacteria, viruses, or other antigenic substances. Antibodies are specific for antigens and work by attaching to invading organisms or foreign substances to help defend the body. *See also* antibody positive; antigen; immunoglobulin; immunology.

antibody positive Having had a positive result in a blood test, especially for the AIDS virus. *See also* acquired immunodeficiency syndrome; antibodies.

anti-choice Opposed to the principle of allowing a

woman to choose for herself whether or not to have an abortion; a derogatory synonym for pro-life. *See also* abortion; pro-life.

anticoagulant A substance that inhibits blood coagulation, used therapeutically in conditions where there is undesirable or excessive clotting (for example, pulmonary embolism) or in circumstances where there is an increased risk of such clotting (for example, during certain surgical operations, such as insertion of a prosthetic heart valve). The agent usually employed is either heparin, which is short-lived and must be administered by injection, or one of the oral anticoagulants, such as warfarin sodium, which inhibit the hepatic synthesis of the vitamin-K-dependent factors. *See also* anticoagulant therapy; heparin; thrombolysis; warfarin.

anticoagulant therapy Treatment of patients with substances, such as streptokinase, warfarin, or heparin, that prevent blood from clotting. *See also* anticoagulant; heparin; streptokinase; thrombolytic therapy; warfarin.

anticoagulation *See* anticoagulant therapy.

anticonvulsant A drug that counteracts convulsions (seizures), as in dilantin and phenobarbital are two common anticonvulsants. *See also* convulsion; epilepsy.

antidiarrheal Counteracting diarrhea, as in an antidiarrheal medication. *See also* diarrhea; dysentery; schedule V substances; traveler's diarrhea.

antidepressant A medication that is used in the treatment of depressive disorders, such as monoamine oxidase inhibitors, tricyclics, and tetracyclics. *See also* depression.

antidote A remedy for counteracting a poison. *See also* poison; poison control center.

antidumping law *See* patient dumping.

antiduplication clause *See* coordination of benefits.

antiemetic Counteracting nausea and vomiting, as in an antiemetic medication.

Anti-Fraud Association, National Health Care *See* National Health Care Anti-Fraud Association.

antigen A foreign substance capable, under certain conditions, of inducing a specific immune response and of reacting with the products of that response. *See also* anaphylaxis; antibodies; histocompatibility antigen; immunoassay.

antigen, histocompatibility *See* histocompatibility antigen.

antihemophilic factor *See* factor VIII.

antihistamine Counteracting the effect of histamine, which plays an important role in allergies. *See also* allergy.

antihypertensive Counteracting high blood pressure. *See also* blood pressure; hypertension.

antipruritic Counteracting itchiness. *See also* itch.

antipsychotic *See* neuroleptic.

antisepsis Destruction of pathogenic microorganisms to prevent infection. *See also* disinfect; infection; microorganism.

antiseptics Agents that inhibit the growth of (though they may not destroy) microorganisms, such as bacteria and viruses. Numerous chemicals possess this ability including ethanol and potassium permanganate solution. Antiseptics are used to prepare the skin before operations and in any other situation when surgical cleanliness is desirable. *See also* antisepsis.

antisocial personality disorder *See* psychopath.

antisubstitution laws State laws that require pharmacists to dispense a drug precisely as written in a prescription issued by a physician, dentist, or other authorized health professional. The effect is to prohibit pharmacists from substituting a different brand name of the drug or a generic equivalent of the drug that is prescribed, even in instances when the substitute drug is acknowledged to be therapeutically equivalent to the drug prescribed and perhaps less expensive. *See also* law; dentist; pharmacist; physician; prescription; substitution.

antitrust injury Injury resulting directly from a lessening of competition, not merely from harm to an individual competitor. *See also* antitrust laws; injury; legal injury.

antitrust laws Federal and state statutes to protect trade and commerce from unlawful restraints, price discriminations, price fixing, and monopolies, and aimed at promoting free competition in the market place. Any agreement or cooperative effort or intent by two or more entities that affects or restrains, or is likely to affect or restrain their competitors, is illegal under these statutes. In health care, antitrust claims often concern arrangements between physicians (such as radiologists, anesthesiologists, pathologists, and sometimes cardiologists and emergency physicians) involved in exclusive service contracts with their hospitals. Plaintiffs, such as a physician or physician group excluded from the hospital as a result of the contract, have alleged that these contracts violate the Sherman Antitrust Act. The principle federal antitrust acts are: Sherman Antitrust Act (1890); Clayton Act (1914); Federal Trade Commission Act (1914); Robinson-Patman Act (1936). *See also* Clayton Act; monopoly; per se violation; restraint of trade; rule of reason; Sherman Antitrust Act.

antitussive Counteracting coughing, as in antitussive medication. *See also* cough; expectorant; schedule V substances.

antivivisectionist Individuals who are opposed to experiments on living animals. *Compare* vivisection. *See also* animal experimentation.

anxiety An unpleasant state of uneasiness or apprehension, as in having an expectation but not the certainty of something happening or something that is going to imminently happen. Anxiety is sometimes manifested as a sense of fear, poorly understood by the subject, which arises without justifiable cause. *See also* globus hystericus; identity crisis; worry.

Anxiety Disorders, Council on *See* Council on Anxiety Disorders.

AOA *See* Alpha Omega Alpha; American Optometric Association; American Orthopaedic Association; American Osteopathic Association; Association of Otolaryngology Administrators.

AOAO *See* American Osteopathic Academy of Orthopedics.

AOAS *See* American Osteopathic Academy of Sclerotherapy.

AOASM *See* American Osteopathic Academy of Sports Medicine.

AOBEM *See* American Osteopathic Board of Emergency Medicine.

AOBGP *See* American Osteopathic Board of General Practice.

AOBP *See* American Osteopathic Board of Pediatrics.

AOBTA *See* American Oriental Bodywork Therapy Association.

AOC *See* American Orthoptic Council.

AOCA *See* American Osteopathic College of Anesthesiologists.

AOCAI *See* American Osteopathic College of Allergy and Immunology.

AOCD *See* American Osteopathic College of Dermatology.

AOCP *See* American Osteopathic College of Pathologists.

AOCPM *See* American Osteopathic College of Preventive Medicine.

AOCPr *See* American Osteopathic College of Proctology.

AOCR *See* American Osteopathic College of Radiology.

AOCRM *See* American Osteopathic College of Rehabilitation Medicine.

AOD *See* Academy of Operative Dentistry.

AODME *See* Academy of Osteopathic Directors of Medical Education.

AODRM *See* Academy of Oral Diagnosis, Radiology, and Medicine.

AOE *See* Association of Optometric Educators.

AOFAS *See* American Orthopedic Foot and Ankle Society.

AOHA *See* American Osteopathic Hospital Association.

AONE *See* American Organization of Nurse Executives.

AOPA *See* American Orthotic and Prosthetic Association.

AORN *See* Association of Operating Room Nurses.

AOS *See* Academie Orthopaedic Society; American Ophthalmological Society; American Orthodontic Society; American Otological Society.

AOSED *See* Association of Osteopathic State Executive Directors.

AOSSM *See* American Orthopaedic Society for Sports Medicine.

AOTA *See* American Occupational Therapy Association.

AOTCB *See* American Occupational Therapy Certification Board.

AP or A/P *See* accounts payable.

APA *See* Ambulatory Pediatric Association; American Pancreatic Society; American Psychiatric Association; American Psychological Association.

APAA *See* American Physician Art Association.

APACHE *See* Acute Physiology and Chronic Health Evaluation.

APACM *See* American Physicians Association of Computer Medicine.

APACVS *See* Association of Physician's Assistants in Cardio-Vascular Surgery.

APAP *See* Association of Physician Assistant Programs.

APBP *See* Association of Professional Baseball Physicians.

APC *See* Association of Pathology Chairmen.

APCS *See* American Podiatric Circulatory Society.

APDIM *See* Association of Program Directors in

Internal Medicine.

aperient *See* laxative.

APF *See* American Pathology Foundation; American Physicians Fellowship for Medicine in Israel.

APFC *See* Association of Physical Fitness Centers.

Apgar scale A method of quantifying the condition of a newborn infant, developed by Dr Virginia Apgar (1909-1974), an anesthesiologist. The Apgar score is usually determined at one minute, and again at five minutes, after birth and is the sum of points, to a maximum of 10, gained on assessment of heart rate, respiratory effort, muscle tone, reflex irritability, and color. A score of 0 to 3 represents severe distress, a score of 4 to 7 indicates moderate distress, and a score of 7 to 10 indicates an absence of difficulty in adjusting to extrauterine life. The five-minute score is normally higher than the one-minute score. *See also* neonate; scale; score.

APGO *See* Association of Professors of Gynecology and Obstetrics.

APHA *See* American Protestant Health Association; American Public Health Association.

APhA *See* American Pharmaceutical Association.

aphasia Partial or total loss of the faculty or power to articulate ideas or comprehend spoken or written language, resulting from damage to the cerebral cortex caused by injury or disease. *See also* cerebrovascular accident; language; motor aphasia; sensory aphasia.

aphasia, expressive *See* motor aphasia.

aphasic, motor *See* motor aphasia.

aphasia, receptive *See* sensory aphasia.

aphasia, sensory *See* sensory aphasia.

apheresis A procedure in which blood is drawn from a donor and separated into its components, some of which are retained, such as plasma or platelets, and the remainder returned by transfusion to the donor. *Synonym*: hemapheresis. *See also* blood donor; blood plasma; blood transfusion; platelet.

Apheresis, American Society for *See* American Society for Apheresis.

aphrodisiac A substance that induces sexual arousal.

aphthous stomatitis A recurring condition of unknown etiology characterized by the eruption of painful ulcers (canker sores) on the mucous membranes of the mouth and lips. *See also* canker sore.

APIC *See* Association for Practitioners in Infection Control.

Apitherapy Society, American *See* American Apitherapy Society.

AP-LS *See* American Psychology - Law Society.

APLS *See* advanced pediatric life support; Association for Politics and the Life Sciences.

APM *See* Academy of Psychosomatic Medicine; Association of Professors of Medicine; Association for Psychoanalytic Medicine.

APMA *See* American Podiatric Medical Association.

APNA *See* American Psychiatric Nurses Association.

apnea Temporary absence or cessation of breathing, as in sleep apnea. *See also* sleep apnea.

Apnea Professionals, National Association of *See* National Association of Apnea Professionals.

apnea, sleep *See* sleep apnea.

APO *See* adverse patient occurrence.

APON *See* Association of Pediatric Oncology Nurses.

APOSW *See* Association of Pediatric Oncology Social Workers.

apothecary Pharmacist who owns and operates a prescription pharmacy. *See also* druggist; pharmacist; pharmacy.

Apothecaries, American College of *See* American College of Apothecaries.

APP *See* Association of Pakistani Physicians.

APPA *See* American Physicians Poetry Association; American Professional Practice Association; American Psychopathological Association; Association of Philippine Physicians in America.

apparent agency An agency relationship created not by agreement, but rather, due to circumstances created by parties that indicate that an agency existed. Observers would assume that one party was acting as agent for another. For example, an emergency physician has, under certain circumstances, been held to be the apparent agent of a hospital even though he or she was not, in fact, employed by the hospital. *See also* agency.

appeal, accreditation *See* accreditation appeal.

appellant **1.** A party that takes an appeal from one court or jurisdiction to a different one. **2.** A party that appeals the decision of a lower court and brings it to a court of higher jurisdiction.

appellate court A court to which a judgment reached in a trial court is appealed. An appellate court is responsible for determining whether the trial court made an error of law in deciding the case. Appellate courts are frequently divided into intermediate appellate courts to which a party may always appeal and a supreme appellate court, which has discretion over which cases it chooses to hear. *See also* court; trial court.

appellee The party in a case against whom an appeal is lodged. Another name for the appellee is the respondent, that is, the party that does not want the appeal to successfully overturn the lower court ruling. *See also* appellate court.

appendicitis Inflammation of the appendix that, if undiagnosed and untreated, can lead rapidly to perforation and generalized peritonitis. *See also* appendectomy; McBurney's point; peritonitis.

appendectomy The surgical removal of the appendix through a incision in the right lower quadrant of the abdomen. *See also* appendicitis; McBurney's point.

APPIC *See* Association of Psychology Postdoctoral and Internship Centers.

appliance A device or apparatus for performing or facilitating the performance of a particular function, as in an orthodontic appliance. *See also* orthodontic appliance; orthosis.

appliance, dental *See* orthodontic appliance.

appliance, orthodontic *See* orthodontic appliance.

applicable Pertinent, related to, or appropriate, as in applicable standards.

application, abbreviated new drug *See* abbreviated new drug application.

application, computer *See* computer application.

application, new drug *See* new drug application.

Applied Clinical Nutrition, American Council of *See* American Council of Applied Clinical Nutrition.

Applied Psychoanalysis, Association for *See* Association for Applied Psychoanalysis.

Applied Psychophysiology and Biofeedback, Association for *See* Association for Applied Psychophysiology and Biofeedback.

APPM *See* Academy of Pharmacy Practice and Management.

apportionment of damages The allocation of an award determined by verdict among those entitled to receive its benefit or against those obligated to pay. *See also* apportionment of fault; award; damages; verdict.

apportionment of fault The allocation of responsibility for damages among those whose acts contributed to the injuries or loss. For example, a plaintiff may be partially responsible for his or her own injury or loss and may be apportioned a percentage of fault that may reduce or bar his or her recovery. Additionally, when multiple defendants have contributed to an injury or loss, they may each be assigned a percentage of fault. Depending on the rules of that jurisdiction, such an apportionment may form the basis for determining the amount of the total verdict for which each party is responsible. *See also* apportionment of damages; damages; plaintiff.

appraisal cost The cost incurred while conducting inspections, tests, and other planned evaluations used to determine whether products or services meet their requirements. Appraisal cost includes, for example, prototype inspections and testing, supplier surveillance, and packaging inspection. *See also* cost; cost of quality; failure cost; inspection; prevention cost.

appropriate Suitable for a particular person, condition, occasion, or place, as in an appropriate therapy for the disease. *Compare* inappropriate. *See also* appropriateness.

appropriateness In health care, a performance dimension addressing the degree to which the care/intervention provided is relevant to a patient's clinical needs, given the current state of knowledge. *See also* acceptability; appropriate; care; dimensions of performance; intervention.

appropriate self-insured health plan According to the Health Security Act introduced to Congress, a group health plan that is a self-insured health plan. *See also* group health plan; health plan; Health Security Act; state-certified health plan.

appropriation A legislative act authorizing the expenditure of a designated amount of public funds for a specific purpose. *See also* backdoor authority.

Appropriations, Committee on *See* Committee on Appropriations.

approved Sanctioned by an appropriate authority. *See also* appropriate; sanction.

APQC *See* American Productivity and Quality Center.

a priori Latin phrase meaning "from cause to effect, from what goes before"; refers to the process of deducing facts that must necessarily follow from a general principle or admitted truth. *See also* deduce; deductive reasoning.

APRS *See* Academy of Pharmaceutical Research and Science.

APS *See* American Pain Society; American Paraplegia Society; American Pediatric Society; American Physiological Society; American Prosthodontic Society; American Psychosomatic Society.

APSA *See* American Pediatric Surgical Association.

APsaA *See* American Psychoanalytic Association.

APSS *See* Association of Professional Sleep Societies.

APT *See* Association of Polysomnographic Technologists; Association for Psychological Type.

APTA *See* American Physical Therapy Association.

APUA *See* Alliance for the Prudent Use of Antibiotics.

APWA *See* American Public Welfare Association.

AQL *See* acceptable quality level.

AQP *See* Association for Quality and Participation.

AR or A/R *See* accounts receivable.

ARA *See* Academy of Rehabilitative Audiology; Association of Retired Americans.

arbiter One appointed by a court to decide a controversy according to law or equity, although the decision maker is not a judicial officer. Unlike an arbitrator, an arbiter needs the court's confirmation of the decision for it to be final. *See also* arbitrator.

arbitrate To judge or decide. *See also* arbitration.

arbitration The process of dispute resolution in which a neutral third party (arbitrator) renders a decision after a hearing at which both parties have an opportunity to be heard. Arbitration is one arrangement for taking and abiding by the judgment of selected persons in some disputed matter, instead of carrying it to established tribunals of justice and is intended to avoid the formalities, delay, expense, and vexation of ordinary litigation. *See also* arbitration panel; arbitrator; binding arbitration; mediation; negotiation.

arbitration, binding *See* binding arbitration.

arbitration, compulsory *See* binding arbitration.

arbitration panel A group chosen by the parties to a dispute to hear a case and make a final, binding decision concerning the dispute. *See also* arbitration; panel.

arbitrator An impartial person chosen to settle an issue between parties engaged in a dispute. He or she may be chosen by the parties to a dispute or appointed by a court to hear the parties' claims and render a decision. *Compare* arbiter. *See also* arbitration.

ARC *See* AIDS-related complex; American Red Cross National Headquarters.

ARCA *See* American Rehabilitation Counseling Association.

ARC-PA *See* Accreditation Review Committee on Education for Physician Assistants.

ARCRT *See* American Registry of Clinical Radiogra-

phy Technologists.

ARC-ST *See* Accreditation Review Committee for Educational Programs in Surgical Technology.

ARDMS *See* American Registry of Diagnostic Medical Sonographers.

ARDS *See* adult respiratory distress syndrome.

Area Agencies on Aging, National Association of *See* National Association of Area Agencies on Aging.

area, alliance *See* alliance area.

area, catchment *See* catchment area.

area coverage, out-of- *See* out-of-area coverage.

area, health service *See* health service area.

area, medically underserved *See* medically underserved area.

area, metropolitan statistical *See* metropolitan statistical area.

area network, local *See* local area network.

area network, wide *See* wide area network.

area, performance *See* performance area.

area, physician shortage *See* physician shortage area.

area, scarcity *See* scarcity area.

area, service *See* catchment area.

area wage adjustment The differences in diagnosis-related groups (DRGs) payment rates that reflect variations in area hospital wage levels, based on Bureau of Labor Statistics data. *See also* adjustment; diagnosis-related groups; wage.

ARHP *See* Association of Reproductive Health Professionals.

ARI *See* Acupuncture Research Institute.

arithmetically In mathematics, the rate of change in which a constant is added to each number in the series. For example, an arithmetical progression beginning with 6 and with a constant of 2 would be: 6, 8, 10, 12, 14. *Compare* exponentially; geometrically. *See also* linear; logarithmic.

arithmetic mean *See* mean.

ARMA *See* American Registry of Medical Assistants.

Armed Forces Institute of Pathology (AFIP) A national organization founded in 1862 and chartered by the US Department of Defense. The AFIP maintains a consultation service for the diagnosis of pathologic material; conducts experimental, statistical, and morphological research in pathology; provides instruction in advanced pathology and related subjects; prepares, procures, and duplicates teaching aids; operates the AFIP Repository and Research Services; and maintains the National Museum of

Health and Medicine of the AFIP and a Medical Illustration Service for the collection, preparation, duplication, reference, and filing of medical illustrative material. *See also* pathology.

Armed Forces Optometric Society (AFOS) A national organization founded in 1970 composed of 600 uniformed service optometrists, optometry students, and former military optometrists interested in advancing and improving the vision care of service personnel, their dependents, and others under the care of optometry officers in the uniformed services. *See also* optometry.

Armed Forces, Society of Medical Consultants to the *See* Society of Medical Consultants to the Armed Forces.

Armed Services, Committee on *See* Committee on Armed Services.

ARMT *See* American Registry of Medical Assistants.

Army Nurse Corps Association, Retired *See* Retired Army Nurse Corps Association.

ARN *See* Association of Rehabilitation Nurses.

ARNA *See* American Radiological Nurses Association.

ARNMD *See* Association for Research in Nervous and Mental Disease.

ARP *See* American Registry of Pathology.

arrangement A structure or combination of things organized in a particular way or for a specific purpose, as in multihospital arrangement for providing health care services. *See also* tying arrangement.

arrangement, tying *See* tying arrangement.

arrest, cardiac *See* cardiac arrest.

arrhythmia An irregularity of heart rhythm, as in atrial fibrillation or ventricular tachycardia. *Synonym*: dysrhythmia. *See also* artificial cardiac pacemaker; bradycardia; cardiac arrest; cardiovascular medicine; defibrillation; emergency medicine; fibrillation; rhythm; tachycardia; ventricular fibrillation.

ARRS *See* American Roentgen Ray Society.

ARRT *See* American Registry of Radiologic Technologists.

ARS *See* American Radium Society; American Rhinologic Society.

ART *See* accredited record technician.

Art Association, American Physician *See* American Physician Art Association.

arterial blood gas (ABG) A diagnostic laboratory test used to determine the amount of important gases, such as oxygen and carbon dioxide, in the blood. *See also* artery; blood gas determination.

arterial blood pressure Blood pressure measured within the arteries of the body usually with a specially designed intra-arterial catheter. *See also* artery; blood pressure.

arteriogram An x-ray image of an artery after injection of a radiopaque medium, as in performing angiography to obtain an arteriogram of the coronary arteries. *See also* angiography.

arteriography *See* angiography.

arteriosclerosis A condition in which the wall of the arteries harden; this may cause insufficient blood circulation to the area supplied by the artery or arteries, as in coronary arteriosclerosis. *Synonym*: arteriosclerosis obliterans. *See also* atherosclerosis.

Arteriosclerosis of the American Heart Association, Council on *See* Council on Arteriosclerosis of the American Heart Association.

arteriosclerosis obliterans *See* arteriosclerosis.

artery A vessel through which blood passes away from the heart to the various parts of the body. *See also* arterial blood gas; arterial blood pressure; blood vessel; vein.

arthralgia Pain affecting the joints. *Compare* myalgia. *See also* arthritis; joint; pain.

arthritis Painful inflammation of a joint or joints, a characteristic of over 100 disorders, such as rheumatoid arthritis and osteoarthritis. *See also* arthralgia; inflammation; joint; osteoarthritis; rheumatism.

Arthritis Health Professions Association (AHPA) A national organization founded in 1965 composed of 2,000 nurses, occupational and physical therapists, social workers, psychologists, vocational counselors, physicians, pharmacists, and other health professions interested in the practice, education, and research of rheumatic disease. *See also* arthritis; rheumatology.

Arthritis and Musculoskeletal and Skin Diseases Information Clearinghouse, National *See* National Arthritis and Musculoskeletal and Skin Diseases Information Clearinghouse.

arthritis, osteo- *See* osteoarthritis.

arthroscope A thin instrument for examining the interior of a joint, such as the knee joint, and for carrying out diagnostic and therapeutic procedures within the joint. *See also* arthroscopy; orthopaedic/orthopedic surgery.

arthroscopy Examination of the interior of a joint with an arthroscope, which is inserted into a joint. The surgeon can either look directly into the arthroscope or observe on a screen the view projected by the arthroscope. The surgeon can diagnose a condition using only a small incision for insertion of the arthroscope and can use a tool with the arthroscope to perform certain surgical procedures within viewing range of the scope. *See also* arthroscope; joint; orthopaedic/orthopedic surgery.

Arthroscopy Association of North America (AANA) An organization founded in 1982 composed of 900 orthopedic surgeons interested in advancing arthroscopy. *See also* arthroscopy; orthopaedic/orthopedic surgery.

articles of incorporation *See* articles of organization.

articles of organization The creating document for an organization, such as the articles of incorporation for a corporation or a constitution for an unincorporated entity. Bylaws are not articles of organization. *See also* bylaws; governing instrument; organization.

artificial Made by human beings; produced rather than natural, as in artificial insemination. *Compare* natural. *See also* artificial cardiac pacemaker; artificial insemination; artificial intelligence; artificial respiration; artificial selection.

artificial cardiac pacemaker A device designed to stimulate, by electrical impulses, contraction of the heart muscle at a certain rate. It is employed in heart block or in the absence of normal function of the heart's sinoatrial node. It may be connected from the outside, as with a temporary transvenous or transthoracic pacemaker, or implanted within the subcutaneous tissues of the body. *See also* arrhythmia; demand pacemaker; fixed-rate pacemaker; natural cardiac pacemaker; pacemaker.

artificial insemination The introduction of semen from a man into a woman's genital tract by artificial means. *See also* artificial insemination - donor; artificial insemination - husband; artificial reproduction; insemination; noncoital reproduction; semen.

artificial insemination - donor (AID) A technique of fertilization in which sperm from an anonymous donor is injected (inseminated) into the vagina of a consenting woman (recipient). This technique may be indicated when the husband is sterile or has a genetic disorder. *Compare* artificial insemination - husband. *See also* fertility; noncoital reproduction.

artificial insemination - husband (AIH) A technique of fertilization in which a husband's sperm is injected into his wife's vagina, cervix or uterus in order to improve fertility. *Compare* artificial insemi-

nation - donor. *See also* fertility; infertility; noncoital reproduction.

artificial intelligence (AI) 1. A discipline in which an attempt is made to approximate the human thinking process through use of computers. **2.** A computer programming methodology whereby masses of data or knowledge can be used to resolve problems. *See also* computer; expert system; intelligence.

Artificial Intelligence, American Association for *See* American Association for Artificial Intelligence.

Artificial Internal Organs, American Society for *See* American Society for Artificial Internal Organs.

artificial pacemaker *See* artificial cardiac pacemaker.

artificial reproduction *See* noncoital reproduction.

artificial respiration A procedure used to restore or maintain respiration in a person who has stopped breathing. The method uses mechanical or manual means to force air into and out of the lungs in a rhythmic manner. *See also* cardiopulmonary resuscitation; mechanical ventilation; respiration; respirator.

artificial selection The interference by humans in the selection of the genotypes to produce succeeding generations of humans. *Compare* natural selection. *See also* genotype; selection.

Arts Therapy Associations, National Coalition of *See* National Coalition of Arts Therapy Associations.

art therapist An individual who specializes in art therapy. *See also* art therapy.

art therapy The use of art to achieve the therapeutic goals of symptom relief, emotional integration, and recovery from or adjustment to illness or disability. *See also* dance therapy; drama therapy; manual arts therapy; music therapy; poetry therapy; recreational therapy.

Art Therapy Association, American *See* American Art Therapy Association.

ARVO *See* Association for Research in Vision and Ophthalmology.

ASA *See* American Society on Aging; American Society of Anesthesiologists; American Statistical Association; American Surgical Association.

ASAAD *See* American Society for Advancement of Anesthesia in Dentistry.

ASAHP *See* American Society of Allied Health Professions.

ASAIO *See* American Society for Artificial Internal Organs.

ASAM *See* American Society of Addiction Medicine.

ASAP *See* American Society for Adolescent Psychiatry; Americans for a Sound AIDS Policy.

ASAPS *See* American Society for Aesthetic Plastic Surgery.

ASA-PS class *See* American Society of Anesthesiologists-Physical Status classification system.

ASAS *See* American Society of Abdominal Surgery.

ASBMB *See* American Society for Biochemistry and Molecular Biology.

ASBMR *See* American Society for Bone and Mineral Research.

ASBP *See* American Society of Bariatric Physicians.

ASC *See* American Society for Cybernetics; American Society of Cytology.

ASCB *See* American Society for Cell Biology.

ASCCP *See* American Society for Colposcopy and Cervical Pathology.

ASCE *See* American Society of Childbirth Educators.

ASCEP *See* American Society for Clinical Evoked Potentials.

ASCH *See* American Society of Clinical Hypnosis.

ASCI *See* American Society for Clinical Investigation.

ASCII *See* American Standard Code for Information Interchange.

asclepion An early Greek temple of healing. Greek temple medicine flourished during the time of Hippocrates (late fifth century) but was largely independent of his school. *See also* Aesculapius; Hippocrates of Cos.

ASCMS *See* American Society of Contemporary Medicine and Surgery.

ASCN *See* American Society for Clinical Nutrition.

ASCO *See* American Society of Clinical Oncology; American Society of Contemporary Ophthalmology; Association of Schools and Colleges of Optometry.

ascorbic acid *See* vitamin C.

ASCP *See* American Society of Clinical Pathologists; American Society of Consultant Pharmacists.

ASCPT *See* American Society for Clinical Pharmacology and Therapeutics.

ASCR *See* American Society of Clinic Radiologists.

ASCRS *See* American Society of Cataract and Refractive Surgery; American Society of Colon and Rectal Surgeons.

ASCT *See* American Society for Cytotechnology.

ASD *See* Academy for Sports Dentistry; American Society of Dermatopathology; Association for the Study of Dreams.

ASDA *See* American Sleep Disorders Association.

ASDC *See* American Society of Dentistry for Children.

ASDS *See* American Society for Dermatologic Surgery.

ASDVS *See* American Society of Directors of Volunteer Services.

ASDWA *See* Association of State Drinking Water Administrators.

ASE *See* American Society of Echocardiography; Association for Surgical Education.

aseptic Free from infection or septic material. *See also* sterile.

ASET *See* American Society of Electroneurodiagnostic Technologists.

ASFA *See* American Society for Apheresis.

ASFO *See* American Society of Forensic Odontology.

ASGD *See* American Society for Geriatric Dentistry.

ASGE *See* American Society for Gastrointestinal Endoscopy.

ASGPP *See* American Society of Group Psychotherapy and Psychodrama.

ASH *See* American Society of Hematology; American Society of Hypertension.

ASHA *See* American School Health Association; American Social Health Association; American Speech-Language-Hearing Association.

ASHCMPR *See* American Society for Health Care Marketing and Public Relations.

ASHCSP *See* American Society for Healthcare Central Service Personnel.

ASHE *See* American Society for Hospital Engineering of the AHA.

ASHES *See* American Society for Healthcare Environmental Services of the American Hospital Association.

ASHET *See* American Society for Healthcare Education and Training of the American Hospital Association.

ASHFSA *See* American Society for Hospital Food Service Administrators.

ASHG *See* American Society of Human Genetics.

ASHHRA *See* American Society for Healthcare Human Resources Administration.

ASHI *See* American Society for Histocompatibility and Immunogenetics.

ASHMM *See* American Society for Hospital Materials Management.

ASHMPR *See* American Society for Hospital Marketing and Public Relations.

ASHNS *See* American Society for Head and Neck Surgery.

ASHP *See* American Society of Handicapped Physicians; American Society of Hospital Pharmacists.

ASHRM *See* American Society for Healthcare Risk Management.

ASHT *See* American Society of Hand Therapists.

ASIA *See* American Spinal Injury Association.

Asian American Psychological Association (AAPA) A national organization founded in 1972 composed of 260 psychologists and graduate students in psychology interested in advancing the welfare of Asian-Americans and other individuals through the use and development of psychology. It assists in and encourages research and services that affect Asian-Americans. *See also* psychology.

Asian Science and Medicine, Institute for Advanced Research in *See* Institute for Advanced Research in Asian Science and Medicine.

ASIM *See* American Society of Internal Medicine.

ASIS *See* American Society for Information Science.

ASLM *See* American Society of Law and Medicine.

ASLMS *See* American Society for Laser Medicine and Surgery.

ASLSS *See* American Society of Lipo-Suction Surgery.

ASM *See* American Society for Microbiology; Association for Systems Management.

AsMA *See* Aerospace Medical Association.

ASMS *See* American Society of Maxillofacial Surgeons.

ASMT *See* American Society for Medical Technology.

ASN *See* American Society of Nephrology; American Society of Neuroimaging.

ASNR *See* American Society of Neuroradiology.

ASOA *See* American Society of Ophthalmic Administrators.

ASORN *See* American Society of Ophthalmic Registered Nurses.

ASOS *See* American Society of Outpatient Surgeons.

ASP *See* American Society of Parasitologists; American Society of Pharmacognosy.

ASPAN *See* American Society of Post Anesthesia Nurses.

ASPD *See* American Society of Podiatric Dermatology.

ASPE *See* American Society of Psychopathology of Expression.

aspects of care, important *See* important aspects of care.

ASPEN *See* American Society for Parenteral and Enteral Nutrition.

ASPET *See* American Society for Pharmacology and Experimental Therapeutics.

ASPH *See* Association of Schools of Public Health.

ASPHO *See* American Society of Pediatric Hematology/Oncology.

aspirate **1.** To treat by aspiration. **2.** The material or substance obtained by the process of aspirating. *See also* aspirating needle; aspiration; aspiration biopsy.

aspirating needle A long, hollow needle for removing fluid from a cavity. *See also* aspiration; hypodermic needle; needle; syringe.

aspiration **1.** The removal of fluids or other substances from a cavity by the application of suction. **2.** The process of inhaling, as in aspiration pneumonia.

aspiration biopsy A biopsy in which tissue is obtained by the application of suction through a needle attached to a syringe. *See also* aspiration; biopsy; syringe.

ASPL *See* American Society for Pharmacy Law.

ASPM *See* American Society of Podiatric Medicine.

ASPMA *See* American Society of Podiatric Medical Assistants.

ASPN *See* American Society for Pediatric Neurosurgery.

ASPO *See* American Society of Preventive Oncology.

ASPO/LAMAZE *See* American Society for Psychoprophylaxis in Obstetrics.

ASPP *See* American Society of Psychoanalytic Physicians.

ASPR *See* American Society for Psychical Research.

ASPRS *See* American Society of Plastic and Reconstructive Surgeons.

ASPRSN *See* American Society of Plastic and Reconstructive Surgical Nurses.

ASQC *See* American Society for Quality Control.

ASRA *See* American Society of Regional Anesthesia.

ASRD *See* American Society of Retired Dentists.

ASRT *See* American Society of Radiologic Technologists.

Assault, National Coalition Against Sexual *See* National Coalition Against Sexual Assault.

Assault Prevention Center, National *See* National Assault Prevention Center.

assault, sexual *See* sexual assault.

assay **1.** The quantitative or qualitative evaluation of a substance. **2.** The results of such an evaluation. *See also* bioassay; immunoassay; ligand assay; radioimmunoassay.

assay, bio- *See* bioassay.

assay, immuno- *See* immunoassay.

assay, ligand *See* ligand assay.

assay, radioimmuno- *See* radioimmunoassay.

AS-SCORE index Severity-of-illness classification system based on five factors: age of patient, systems involved in illness, stage of disease, complications, and patient's response to therapy. *See also* classification system; index; severity of illness.

ASSE *See* American Society of Safety Engineers; American Society of Sanitary Engineering.

Assembly of Hospital Schools of Nursing *See* Institute for Hospital Clinical Nursing Education.

assessment **1.** The process of determining the value, significance, or extent of something, as in data assessment (the process of determining the significance of data) or quality assessment (the process of determining the extent to which quality is present). *See also* audiological assessment; needs assessment; outcome assessment; patient assessment; performance assessment; process assessment; quality assessment; risk assessment; technology assessment; vocational assessment. **2.** The value, significance, or extent of a thing assessed, as in a high tax assessment.

assessment, audiological *See* audiological assessment.

Assessment, Commission on Office Laboratory *See* Commission on Office Laboratory Assessment.

Assessment Commission, Prospective Payment *See* Prospective Payment Assessment Commission.

Assessment in Counseling, Association for *See* Association for Assessment in Counseling.

Assessment, National Center for Health Services Research and Health Care Technology *See* National Center for Health Services Research and Health Care Technology Assessment.

assessment, needs *See* needs assessment.

Assessment, Office of Health Technology *See* Office of Health Technology Assessment.

assessment, outcome *See* outcome assessment.

assessment, patient *See* patient assessment.

assessment, performance *See* performance assessment.

assessment, process *See* process assessment.

Assessment Program, Diagnostic and Therapeutic Technology *See* Diagnostic and Therapeutic Technology Assessment Program.

assessment, quality *See* quality assessment.

assessment, reliability *See* reliability testing.

assessment, risk *See* risk assessment.

Assessment, Society for Personality *See* Society for Personality Assessment.

assessment, technology *See* technology assessment.

assessment, vocational *See* vocational assessment.

asset Anything owned that has monetary value.

See also capital asset; current asset; fixed asset; liquid asset.

asset, capital *See* capital asset.

asset, current *See* current asset.

asset, fixed *See* fixed asset.

asset, liquid *See* liquid asset.

ASSFN *See* American Society for Stereotactic and Functional Neurosurgery.

ASSH *See* American Society for Surgery of the Hand.

assignable cause *See* special cause.

assignable cause variation *See* special cause variation.

assignment **1.** An agreement in which a patient assigns to a health care provider the right to reserve payment from a third-party payer for the service the patient has received. *See also* third-party payer. **2.** The acceptance by a physician of Medicare payment as full payment for services rendered. *Synonym*: assignment of benefits. *See also* Medicare.

assignment of benefits *See* assignment.

assistance, public *See* public assistance.

assistant administrator An individual holding an upper-level line management position who is responsible for certain discrete segments, units, or functions within a hospital or other health care organization. This person usually reports directly to the hospital administrator or an associate administrator. *See also* administrator; line management.

assistant, anesthesiologist's *See* anesthesiologist's assistant.

assistant, dental *See* dental assistant.

assistant, dietetic *See* dietetic assistant.

assistant, medical *See* medical assistant.

assistant, nursing *See* nursing assistant.

assistant, occupational therapy *See* occupational therapy assistant.

assistant, ophthalmic *See* ophthalmic medical technician; ophthalmic medical technologist.

assistant, pathologist's *See* pathologist's assistant.

assistant, pharmacy *See* pharmacy assistant.

assistant, physical therapy *See* physical therapy assistant.

assistant, physician *See* physician assistant.

assistant, physician's *See* physician assistant.

assistant, podiatric *See* podiatric assistant.

Assistants, Accreditation Review Committee on Education for Physician *See* Accreditation Review Committee on Education for Physician Assistants.

Assistants, American Academy of Physician *See* American Academy of Physician Assistants.

Assistants, American Association of Medical *See* American Association of Medical Assistants.

Assistants of American Medical Technologists, Registered Medical *See* Registered Medical Assistants of American Medical Technologists.

Assistants, American Registry of Medical *See* American Registry of Medical Assistants.

Assistants, American Society of Podiatric Medical *See* American Society of Podiatric Medical Assistants.

Assistants Association, American Dental *See* American Dental Assistants Association.

Assistants Association, National Dental *See* National Dental Assistants Association.

Assistants in Cardio-Vascular Surgery, Association of Physician's *See* Association of Physician's Assistants in Cardio-Vascular Surgery.

Assistants, National Association of Childbirth *See* National Association of Childbirth Assistants.

Assistants, National Association of Dental *See* National Association of Dental Assistants.

Assistants, National Commission on Certification of Physician *See* National Commission on Certification of Physician Assistants.

assistant, social work *See* social work assistant.

assistant, surgeon *See* surgeon assistant.

assistant and technician, optometric *See* optometric assistant and technician.

Assisted Reproductive Technology, Society for *See* Society for Assisted Reproductive Technology.

ASSO *See* American Society for the Study of Orthodontics.

Associacion Medica Pan Americana *See* Pan American Medical Association.

associate A person united with another or others in an act, an enterprise, or a business; a partner or colleague. This term replaces "subordinate" and "employee" in the continuous quality improvement and total quality management paradigms. *See also* continuous quality improvement; employee; subordinate; total quality management.

Associated Bodywork and Massage Professionals (ABMP) A national organization founded in 1986 composed of 6,500 professional massage therapists and bodyworkers; polarity, movement, and sports massage therapists; Shiatsu and Trager practitioners, reflexologists, orthobionomists, and infant massage instructors; and massage therapy schools.

It promotes massage therapy and bodywork and encourages ethical therapy practices. Formerly (1990) Associated Professional Massage Therapists and Bodyworkers. *See also* acupressure; massage.

Associated Professional Massage Therapists and Bodyworkers See Associated Bodywork and Massage Professionals.

associate degree In nursing and other health profession education, the degree conferred on an individual who successfully graduates from an educational unit in a junior college, community college, college, or university that offers an accredited two-year program in professional nursing and other health professional areas. An associate degree in nursing or an equivalent degree is granted on successful completion of the program. *Compare* baccalaureate degree program. *See also* accredited; degree; diploma school; nurse; university.

Associate Degree Nursing, National Organization for *See* National Organization for Associate Degree Nursing.

Associated Information Managers *See* Association for Information Management.

associate hospital *See* medical control.

Associates of Clinical Pharmacology (ACP) A national organization founded in 1977 composed of 3,000 individuals engaged in clinical pharmacology and other related research professions, including research associates, nurses, pharmacists, pharmacologists, physicians, and regulatory professionals. It provides continuing education credits to pharmacy and nursing professionals through the American Council on Pharmaceutical Education and the American Nurses Association. *See also* American Council on Pharmaceutical Education; American Nurses Association; clinical pharmacology; continuing education; nurse; pharmacology; pharmacy.

association **1.** A group of people or organizations joined together for a particular purpose. *See also* medical association. **2.** In statistics, the statistical dependence between two or more events, characteristics, or other variables. An association is present if the probability of occurrence of an event or characteristic, or the quantity of a variable, depends upon the occurrence of one or more other events, the presence of one or more other characteristics, or the quantity of one or more other variables. The association between two variables is described as positive when the occurrence of higher values of a variable is associated with the occurrence of higher values of another variable. In a negative association, the occurrence of higher values of one variable is associated with lower values of the other variable. An association may be fortuitous or may be produced by various other circumstances; the presence of an association does not, therefore, necessarily imply a causal relationship. *See also* correlation.

Association of Academic Health Centers (AHC) A national organization founded in 1969 composed of 104 chief executive officers of university-based health centers in the United States. It is interdisciplinary and focuses primarily on total health personnel education. *See also* academic medical center; chief medical officer; university.

Association of Academic Health Sciences Library Directors (AAHSLD) A national organization founded in 1978 composed of 126 academic medical and allied health science school libraries, represented by their directors. *See also* health sciences library.

Association of Academic Physiatrists (AAP) A national organization founded in 1967 composed of 880 academic physicians practicing physical medicine and rehabilitation and certified by the American Board of Physical Medicine and Rehabilitation. *See also* American Board of Physical Medicine and Rehabilitation; physiatrist; physical medicine and rehabilitation.

Association for Academic Surgery (AAS) A national organization founded in 1966 composed of 2,400 surgeons with backgrounds in all surgical specialties in academic surgical centers at chief resident level or above. Its objectives include encouraging new surgeons to pursue careers in academic surgery and supporting them in establishing themselves as investigators and educators by providing a forum. *See also* academic medical center; surgery.

Association for Adult Development and Aging (AADA) A division of the American Association for Counseling and Development founded in 1952 composed of 1,969 individuals holding a master's degree or its equivalent in adult counseling or a related field. It seeks to improve the competence and skills of members, promote the development of guidelines for professional preparation of counselors, and provide leadership and information to families, legislators, community service agencies, counselors, and other service providers or professionals related to adult development and aging. *See*

also American Association for Counseling and Development; counseling.

Association to Advance Ethical Hypnosis (AAEH) A national organization founded in 1955 composed of 1,500 practitioners of all the healing arts, educators, police officers, attorneys, and lay technicians interested in establishing a code of ethics in the practice of hypnosis, exposing and discouraging malpractice and the use and granting of nonacademic titles and degrees, and opposing the restriction of hypnosis to members of special professional groups. It conducts a three-phase examination (written, oral, and practical) and certifies members as hypno-technicians. *See also* certification; ethical; hypnosis.

Association for the Advancement of Automotive Medicine (AAAM) A national organization founded in 1957 composed of 650 physicians and other professionals interested in motor vehicle safety, design, and road engineering. It works to reduce the number of injuries and fatalities on the nation's highways by encouraging research on the effects of diseases, disabilities, and environmental factors on driver capabilities. It supports laws and regulations to upgrade the standards for licensing drivers and the use of appropriate protective devices. Formerly (1987) American Association for Automotive Medicine.

Association for Advancement of Behavior Therapy (AABT) A national organization founded in 1966 composed of 4,100 psychologists, psychiatrists, social workers, dentists, nurses, physiotherapists, and other professionals interested in the field of behavior modification, with special emphasis on clinical applications. *See also* behavior modification.

Association for Advancement of Blind and Retarded (AABR) An organization founded in 1955 composed of community groups and individuals interested in multihandicapped blind and adults with severe mental retardation. It operates ten group residences providing intermediate care facilities for blind and retarded adults; two-day to six-day treatment centers for blind, multihandicapped, and severely retarded adults; and a summer camp for blind and multihandicapped people. It provides information and referral services. *See also* blindness; handicap; mental retardation.

Association for the Advancement of Health Education (AAHE) A national organization founded in 1937 composed of 11,000 professionals who have responsibility for health education in schools, colleges, communities, hospitals and clinics, and industries. It advances health education through program activities and federal legislation and encourages close working relationships between all health education and health service organizations. *See also* health education.

Association for the Advancement of Medical Instrumentation (AAMI) A national organization founded in 1965 composed of 5,500 clinical engineers, biomedical equipment technologists, hospital administrators, physicians, consultants, engineers, and manufacturers of medical devices interested in the advancement of health care through effective application and management of health care technology. *See also* bioinstrumentation; technology.

Association for Advancement of Psychology (AAP) A national organization founded in 1974 composed of 6,000 members of the American Psychological Association or other national psychological associations, students of psychology, and organizations with a primarily psychological focus. *See also* psychology.

Association for the Advancement of Psychotherapy (AAP) A national organization founded in 1939 composed of 400 physicians who are psychiatrists or in psychiatric training. It creates a forum where all concepts of psychotherapeutic thought can be aired for the advancement of psychotherapy in practice, research, and training. *See also* physician; psychiatry; psychotherapy.

Association of Air Medical Services (AAMS) A national organization founded in 1980 composed of 300 air medical transport providers and manufacturers and distributors of air medical transport equipment. It seeks to develop standards for aircraft configuration, minimum professional and educational requirements for personnel on board, operations, and communications equipment. Formerly (1988) American Society of Hospital-Based Emergency Air Medical Services. *See also* ambulance; medical services.

Association of American Cancer Institutes (AACI) A national organization founded in 1959 composed of 78 directors of cancer centers. It informs members of important legislative and program developments in the field and promotes discussion among cancer center leadership throughout the world. *See also* cancer.

Association of American Indian Physicians (AAIP) A national organization founded in 1971 composed of 152 physicians (medical doctors or doctors of osteopathy) of American Indian descent. It encourages American Indians to enter the health professions; establishes contracts with government agencies to provide consultation and other expert opinion regarding health care of American Indians and Alaskan Natives; and receives contracts and grant monies and other forms of assistance from these sources. *See also* Native American; physician.

Association of American Medical Colleges (AAMC) A national organization founded in 1876 composed of 2,200 medical schools, graduate affiliate medical colleges, academic societies, teaching hospitals, and individuals interested in the advancement of medical education, biomedical research, and health care. It provides a centralized application service and offers management education programs for medical school deans, teaching hospital directors, department chairs, and service chiefs of affiliated hospitals. It develops and administers the Medical College Admissions Test (MCAT). *See also* Council of Teaching Hospitals; Medical College Admissions Test; medical education; medical school.

Association of American Physicians (AAP) A national organization founded in 1886 composed of 1,200 medical school faculty and clinical investigators. *See also* faculty; medical school; physician.

Association of American Physicians and Surgeons (AAPS) A national organization founded in 1943 composed of 5,000 physicians interested in the socioeconomic and legal aspects of medical practice, such as medical economics, public relations, and legislation. It conducts an Expert Witness Program and makes available legal consultation services. *See also* expert witness; physician; surgeon.

Association AMHS Institute A national organization founded in 1984 composed of 40 nonprofit multihospital systems. It sponsors educational programs for corporate officers and trustees of multihospital systems and monitors, investigates, and develops policy positions on developments in the field. Formerly (1988) American Healthcare Institute. *See also* multihospital system.

Association for Applied Poetry (AAP) A national organization founded in 1984 composed of 2,000 poets, teachers, therapists, social workers, creative artists, and librarians interested in the application of poetry and creative writing to human services, healing, self-awareness, and self-actualization. *See also* poetry therapy.

Association for Applied Psychoanalysis (AAP) A national organization founded in 1952 composed of 300 practicing and research psychoanalysts who have undergone at least 300 hours of personal psychoanalysis. It seeks to facilitate and promote training and research in applied psychoanalysis. *See also* psychoanalysis.

Association for Applied Psychophysiology and Biofeedback (AAPB) A national organization founded in 1969 composed of 2,100 persons interested in the interrelationship of external feedback systems, states of consciousness, and the physiological mechanisms involved. Formerly (1988) Biofeedback Society of America. *See also* biofeedback.

Association for Assessment in Counseling (AAC) A national organization founded in 1965 and composed of 1,684 persons who plan, administer, and conduct testing programs, provide test scoring services, interpret and use test results, and develop evaluation instruments. It supports increasing competency in assessment, testing, measurement, and evaluation of professional counselors. Formerly (1992) Association for Measurement and Evaluation in Counseling and Development. *See also* counseling; measurement.

Association for Automated Reasoning (AAR) A national organization founded in 1984 composed of 400 scientists interested in promoting research in the field of automated reasoning programs for computer systems. *See also* reasoning.

Association of Aviation Psychologists (AAP) A national organization founded in 1964 composed of 350 behavioral scientists who are employed or interested in the field of aviation psychology or related fields dealing with human factors in aviation. It includes psychologists, engineers, physiologists, education specialists, sociologists, and statisticians employed by the federal government, universities, commercial airlines, industry, and the armed forces. It promotes aviation psychology and related aerospace and environmental disciplines through information exchange, meetings, stimulation of educational and research interest, and application of psychologic principles and research to problems in aviation. *See also* psychology.

Association for Behavior Analysis (ABA) A national organization founded in 1974 composed of 2,000 professionals, such as psychologists interested

in the applied, experimental, and theoretical analysis of behavior. It conducts workshops and seminars in 16 areas including, for example, behavioral pharmacology and toxicology and developmental disabilities. *See also* analysis; behavior.

Association for the Behavioral Treatment of Sexual Abusers (ABTSA) A national organization founded in 1985 composed of 250 professionals working with sex offenders or victims of sexual assault. It provides training to professionals on the treatment of sex offenders and offers instruction in the operation of penile plethysmography, a device used to determine and record variations in the size of the penis due to the amount of blood present in it. Formerly (1986) Association for the Behavioral Treatment of Sexual Aggression. *See also* behavior therapy; sexual assault.

Association for the Behavioral Treatment of Sexual Aggression *See* Association for the Behavioral Treatment of Sexual Abusers.

Association for Birth Psychology (ABP) A national organization founded in 1978 composed of 352 obstetricians, pediatricians, midwives, nurses, psychotherapists, psychologists, counselors, social workers, sociologists, and other individuals interested in birth psychology, a developing discipline interested in the experience of birth and the correlation between the birth process and personality development. *See also* birth; psychology.

Association of Black Cardiologists (ABC) A national organization founded in 1974 composed of 350 physicians and other health professionals interested in lowering mortality and morbidity resulting from cardiovascular diseases. *See also* cardiologist; cardiovascular medicine.

Association of Black Chiropractors *See* American Black Chiropractors Association.

Association of Black Nursing Faculty in Higher Education (ABNF) A national organization founded in 1987 composed of 127 black nursing faculty teaching in baccalaureate and higher degree programs accredited by the National League for Nursing. It works to promote health-related issues and educational concerns of interest to the black community and the ABNF. It assists members in professional development; develops and sponsors continuing education activities; fosters networking and guidance in employment and recruitment activities; and promotes health-related issues of legislation, government programs, and community activities. *See also* faculty; National League for Nursing; nursing.

Association of Black Psychologists (ABPsi) A national organization founded in 1968 composed of 1,250 psychologists and other persons interested in enhancing the psychological well-being of black people in America; defining mental health in consonance with newly established psychological concepts and standards; and developing policies for local, state, and national decision making that have impact on the mental health of the black community. *See also* psychology.

Association of Bone and Joint Surgeons (ABJS) A national organization founded in 1947 composed of 185 orthopedic surgeons interested in clinical aspects of orthopedics and in training leaders in the specialty. *See also* bone; joint; orthopaedic/orthopedic surgery.

Association for the Care of Children's Health (ACCH) A national organization founded in 1965 composed of 4,300 child life specialists, nurses, pediatricians, parents, child psychiatrists, psychologists, and social workers who are interested in the emotional, psychological, or social needs of children in pediatric health care settings, such as hospitals. *See also* child life specialist.

Association for Chemoreception Sciences (AChemS) A national organization founded in 1979 composed of 649 research scientists, experimental psychologists, and industrial researchers interested in studying chemoreception (the physiological reception of chemical stimuli) by the senses of taste and smell. It conducts research on the differences in human and animal perception of chemical stimuli in taste and smell. *See also* chemistry; sense.

Association for Child Psychoanalysis (ACP) A national organization founded in 1965 composed of 500 child psychoanalysts interested in discussion and dissemination of information in their field. *See also* psychoanalysis.

Association of Children's Prosthetic-Orthotic Clinics (ACPOC) A national organization founded in 1980 composed of 450 prosthetic-orthotic clinics for children. It promotes the exchange of information concerning children's prosthetic-orthotic devices. *See also* orthotics; prosthetics.

Association of Chiropractic Colleges (ACC) A national organization founded in 1977 composed of 18 presidents of chiropractic colleges that are members of the Council on Chiropractic Education. *See also* chiropractic.

Association for Clinical Pastoral Education (ACPE) A national organization founded in 1967 composed of 3,600 certified clinical pastoral education supervisors, theological schools and seminaries, and denominational agencies. It accredits institutions, agencies, and parishes that offer clinical pastoral education to theological students, ordained clergy, members of religious orders, and laypeople. It certifies ministers as supervisors of clinical pastoral education. Clinical pastoral education programs are offered as part of theological degree and graduate degree programs, as continuing education for the ministry, as training for chaplaincy and pastoral counseling, and as training for certification as supervisor of clinical pastoral education. *See also* certification; clinical pastoral counselor.

Association of Clinical Scientists A national organization founded in 1949 composed of 700 physicians and scientists working in various fields of laboratory medicine. It promotes education and research in clinical science by practical methods, maintains and improves the accuracy of measurements in clinical laboratories, and promotes uniformity in clinical laboratory procedures. *See also* clinical laboratory.

Association of Community Cancer Centers (ACCC) An organization founded in 1974 composed of 715 institutions and individuals involved in the provision of community cancer care. It seeks to improve communication among providers of community cancer care and encourages clinical research using the community as a setting. *See also* cancer; community.

Association for Computing Machinery (ACM) A national organization founded in 1947 composed of 75,000 computer scientists, engineers, physical scientists, business system specialists, analysts, and social scientists interested in computing and data processing. It seeks to advance information processing including the study, design, development, construction, and application of modern technology and computing techniques. *See also* computer; data processing.

Association for Continuing Education (ACE) A national organization founded in 1982 composed of 2,000 physicians, dentists, and allied health professionals pursuing continuing education credit in their fields. It conducts a weekly educational program. *See also* continuing education; continuing medical education.

Association of Cytogenetic Technologists (ACT) A national organization founded in 1975 composed of 1,500 persons interested in the field of cytogenetics. It offers a certification program for technologists, compiles statistics, and maintains placement services. *See also* cytogenetics; technologist.

Association for Death Education and Counseling (ADEC) A national organization founded in 1976 composed of 900 individuals and institutions interested in responsible and effective death education and counseling. Its goals include upgrading the quality of death education and patient care in hospitals, residential care facilities, and other organizations. It formulates and enforces codes of ethics and certifies death educators and counselors. Formerly (1986) Forum for Death Education and Counseling. *See also* thanatology.

Association of Environmental Engineering Professors (AEEP) A national organization founded in 1963 composed of 500 college and university professors in the fields of environmental engineering; air, land, and water resources; pollution control; environmental health engineering; and related programs. It studies graduate curricula, entrance requirements, enrollment, and physical facilities at universities to establish criteria and improve education in environmental engineering. *See also* engineering; environmental health; pollution; professor.

Association Executives, National Council of State Pharmaceutical *See* National Council of State Pharmaceutical Association Executives.

Association for Faculty in the Medical Humanities (AFMH) A national organization founded in 1983 composed of 350 faculty in the humanities at medical schools. It promotes teaching and research in the humanities in the context of medical education and closer links among scholars in the humanities who work in medical education. *See also* faculty; humanities.

Association for Fitness in Business (AFB) A national organization founded in 1974 composed of 3,500 health and fitness professionals employed by major companies to conduct fitness programs for employees; interested persons in personnel and sales to fitness facilities; health educators and other health professionals; and students interested in the field. It recommends adherence to American College of Sports Medicine qualifications and professional standards for fitness directors and stimulates active research in and serves as a clearinghouse on employee health and fitness. It sponsors seminars and an educational committee that studies effectiveness of preparation, training programs, and certification. Formerly (1983) American Association of Fitness Directors in Business and Industry. *See also* business; fitness.

Association of Food and Drug Officials (AFDO) A national organization founded in 1897 composed of 500 officials who enforce federal, state, district, county, and municipal laws and regulations relating to food, drugs, cosmetics, and consumer product safety. It seeks to prevent fraud in production, manufacture, distribution, and sale of these items. It promotes uniform laws and administrative procedure and disseminates information concerning law enforcement. *See also* consumer; drug; food; safety.

Association of Freestanding Radiation Oncology Centers (AFROC) A national organization founded in 1986 composed of 300 freestanding radiation oncology center employees, radiologists, oncologists, physicists, radiation therapists, and laboratory clinicians. *See also* radiation oncology.

Association of Gay and Lesbian Psychiatrists (AGLP) A national organization founded in 1975 composed of 450 gay, lesbian, and bisexual members of the American Psychiatric Association, and other psychiatrists. It provides support for gay and lesbian psychiatrists, furthers the understanding of members, colleagues, and the public on matters relating to homosexuality, and promotes improved mental health services for gays and lesbians. *See also* American Psychiatric Association; gay; lesbianism; psychiatry.

Association for Gay, Lesbian, and Bisexual Issues in Counseling (AGLBIC) A national organization founded in 1974 composed of 210 counselors and personnel and guidance workers interested in lesbian and gay issues. Formerly (1988) Association for Gay and Lesbian Issues in Counseling. *See also* bisexuality; gay; lesbianism.

Association for Gnotobiotics (AG) A national organization composed of 415 gnotobiologists, veterinarians, doctors, and animal-husbandry personnel interested in gnotobiotics. It provides researchers with information about raising animals in a germ-free and controlled environment so that the animals may be used for research, especially for studies on cancer and infectious disease. It is working to develop a certification program and to establish acceptable nomenclature in the field. *See also* gnotobiotics.

Association of Haitian Physicians Abroad (AMHE) An organization founded in 1972 composed of 900 Haitian doctors. Its purpose is to unite Haitian doctors abroad and to organize professional activities among them. It provides charitable assistance to the Haitian community. Formerly (1986) Haitian Medical Association Abroad. *See also* physician.

Association of Halfway House Alcoholism Programs of North America (AHHAP) An organization founded in 1966 composed of 300 halfway house corporations, staff, board members, and individuals closely related to the halfway house movement. It is a charitable organization dedicated to educating and serving halfway house programs through technical assistance, consultant services, workshops, and related services. *See also* alcoholism; halfway house.

Association of Healthcare Internal Auditors (AHIA) A national organization founded in 1981 composed of 900 health care internal auditors promoting cost containment and increased productivity in health care organizations through internal auditing. Formerly (1989) Healthcare Internal Audit Group. *See also* auditor.

Association for Healthcare Philanthropy (AHP) A national organization founded in 1967 composed of 2,500 persons employed by health care organizations in the field of health care resource development and fundraising; hospital administrators and trustees; and hospitals. *See also* fundraising; philanthropy.

Association of Health Facility Licensure and Certification Directors *See* Association of Health Facility Survey Agencies.

Association of Health Facility Survey Agencies (AHFSA) A national organization founded in 1968 composed of 51 directors of state or territorial health facility licensure and certification programs; staff members of a state or territorial health facility licensure and certification agency; and employees of the federal Health Care Financing Administration (HCFA). Its purposes are to exchange information between members and the Association of State and Territorial Health Officials (ASTHO); constitute a reservoir of expertise to aid in the guidance of

ASTHO; improve the quality of health facility licensure and certification programs; and provide a forum for state and territorial issues at the national level. It has a representative on an ASTHO standing committee and provides liaisons with the federal Department of Health and Human Services and the HCFA. Formerly (1991) Association of Health Facility Licensure and Certification Directors. *See also* Association of State and Territorial Health Officials; certification; health facility; licensure.

Association for Health Services Research (AHSR) A national organization founded in 1981 composed of 1,500 individuals and organizations interested in health services research. Its objectives include fostering productive cooperation among researchers, public and private funding agencies, health professionals, policymakers, and the public; representing the views of members in the development and implementation of national legislative and administrative policies concerning health services research; and educating the public concerning the need for and contribution of health services research in improving health care in the United States. *See also* health services research.

Association for the History of Chiropractic (AHC) A national organization founded in 1980 composed of 700 chiropractors, students, educators, and writers; chiropractic colleges; and other organizations interested in researching and recording the history of the chiropractic profession. *See also* chiropractic; history.

Association for Hospital Medical Education (AHME) A national organization founded in 1954 composed of 700 physician directors of medical education in hospitals and clinics and other health profession educators. It conducts educational programs and workshops for members and other individuals in the area of graduate and continuing medical education. *See also* continuing medical education; graduate medical education; hospital; medical education director.

Association for Humanistic Psychology (AHP) A national organization founded in 1962 composed of 3,500 psychologists, social workers, clergy, educators, psychiatrists, and laypeople interested in the development of human sciences in ways that recognize distinctive human qualities and working toward fulfilling the innate capacities of people. *See also* psychology.

Association for Information Management (AIM)
A national organization founded in 1978 composed of 1,000 information managers and chief information officers in corporations, government agencies, and nonprofit organizations. It serves the management and career needs of information executives and managers and promotes information management as a management function. Formerly (1990) Associated Information Managers. *See also* information system; management information system.

Association of the Institute for Certification of Computer Professionals (AICCP) An organization founded in 1982 composed of 45,000 computer professionals who have passed the examination given semiannually by the Institute for Certification of Computer Professionals and who have been awarded the certified data processors certificate, certified computer programmer certificate, and certified systems professionals certificate. It encourages professionalism, certification, and adherence to standards by promoting the certification examinations. *See also* certification; computer; Institute for Certification of Computer Professionals; standard.

Association of Life Insurance Medical Directors of America *See* American Academy of Insurance Medicine.

Association of Maternal and Child Health Programs (AMCHP) A national organization founded in 1944 composed of 300 individuals responsible for or involved in the administration of state and territorial maternal and child health care programs and programs for children with special health care needs. It seeks to inform public and private sector decision makers of the health care needs of mothers and children; develop and recommend maternal and child health policies and programs; and develop coalitions with other organizations. *See also* maternal and child health services.

Association for Measurement and Evaluation in Counseling and Development *See* Association for Assessment in Counseling.

Association for Media Psychology (AMP) A division of the American Psychological Association founded in 1982 composed of 520 psychologists, psychiatrists, social workers, psychiatric nurses, and members of the communications media. It seeks to publicize scientific psychology and promote research on the influence of the media on attitude, behavior, and well-being. It encourages innovative

use of the media in the prevention of physical and mental disorders and assists mental health professionals in developing program ideas and ways of effectively communicating to the public through the media. *See also* media; psychology.

association, medical *See* medical association.

Association of Medical Education and Research in Substance Abuse (AMERSA) A national organization founded in 1976 composed of 500 medical school faculty members and other persons interested in general medical education who are involved with providing information on alcohol and other drug-related topics to medical professionals and students. *See also* faculty; medical education; medical school; substance abuse.

Association of Medical Illustrators (AMI) A national organization founded in 1945 composed of 900 medical illustrators interested in promoting the study and advancement of medical illustration. *See also* medical illustrator.

Association of Medical Rehabilitation Directors and Coordinators *See* Association of Medical Rehabilitation Administrators.

Association of Medical Rehabilitation Administrators (AMRA) A national organization founded in 1953 composed of 250 individuals engaged in administering medical rehabilitation programs for federal, state, and nongovernmental hospitals and centers; physicians specializing in rehabilitation medicine; and rehabilitation educators. It maintains the American Board for Certification of Medical Rehabilitation Administrators. Formerly (1989) Association of Medical Rehabilitation Directors and Coordinators. *See also* administrator; rehabilitation.

Association of Medical School Pediatric Department Chairmen (AMSPDC) A national organization founded in 1961 composed of 147 chairs of the department of pediatrics of each accredited medical school in the United States and Canada. It fosters education and research in the field of child health and human development. *See also* accredited; department chair; medical school; pediatrics.

Association of Mental Health Administrators (AMHA) A national organization founded in 1959 composed of 1,500 administrators of services for persons with the emotional disturbances, mental illness, mentally retardation, developmental disabilities, and problems of alcohol and substance abuse. *See also* administrator; alcoholism and other drug dependence; developmental disability; mental illness; mental retardation.

Association of Mental Health Clergy (AMHC) A national organization founded in 1948 composed of 550 clergy of all faiths (including pastors, priests, sisters, and rabbis) who minister to the religious needs of the mentally and emotionally troubled. It establishes standards for clergy in psychiatric and mental health facilities. *See also* chaplain; clergy.

Association of Microbiological Diagnostic Manufacturers (AMDM) A national organization founded in 1976 composed of 75 medical device manufacturers, distributors, and users. It informs members of regulatory policies and government legislation affecting the microbiological diagnostic equipment manufacturing industry. *See also* medical device; microbiology.

Association of Military Surgeons of the United States (AMSUS) A national organization founded in 1891 composed of 15,000 physicians, dentists, veterinarians, pharmacists, nurses, dietitians, physiotherapists, and other persons of commissioned rank or equivalent in the Army, Navy, Air Force, Public Health Service, Veterans Administration, Medical Reserve, and National Guard. The organization is interested in the advancement of federal medicine and allied medical sciences in the federal medical services. *See also* surgeon.

Association of Minority Health Professions Schools (AMHPS) An organization founded in 1978 composed of 8 predominantly black health professional schools seeking to increase the number of minorities in health professions; improve the health of blacks in the United States; and increase the federal resources available to minority schools and students. *See also* health professionals; minority.

Association of Nurses in AIDS Care (ANAC) A national organization founded in 1987 composed of 800 nurses and other health care professionals involved in caring for people who are HIV-infected or have AIDS. It functions as a network and provides leadership and educational services for members. *See also* acquired immunodeficiency syndrome; HIV infection; nurse.

Association of Operating Room Nurses (AORN) A national organization founded in 1949 composed of 45,000 registered nurses engaged in perioperative nursing on supervisory, teaching, or staff levels. It studies existing practices and new developments in operating room nursing and education and sponsors national and regional institutes and scholarships. *See also* operating room nurse; registered nurse.

Association of Optometric Educators (AOE) A national organization founded in 1972 composed of 100 teachers in schools and colleges of optometry who are interested in enhancing the professional and academic status and conditions of services of optometric educators and in promoting communication among members. The AOE is concerned with faculty welfare, faculty-administration relations, faculty-student relations, and faculty-professional relations. *See also* faculty; optometry.

Association of Osteopathic State Executive Directors (AOSED) A national organization founded in 1918 composed of 112 executives of divisional and affiliated societies of the American Osteopathic Association. *See also* American Osteopathic Association; osteopathic medicine.

Association of Otolaryngology Administrators (AOA) A national organization founded in 1983 composed of 360 persons employed in a managerial capacity for private or academic group medical practices specializing in otolaryngology. It provides a forum for interaction and exchange of information among otolaryngological managers and presents educational programs. *See also* administrator; otolaryngology.

Association of Pakistani Physicians (APP) A national organization founded in 1976 composed of 1,200 physicians and dentists who are native to Pakistan but now live and practice in North America. It assists Pakistani physicians newly arrived in North America in orientation and adjustment and arranges for donation of medical literature and medical supplies to Pakistan. It offers scientific programs for which continuing medical education credits are awarded. *See also* continuing medical education; physician.

Association for Past Life Research and Therapy *See* Last Word: Therapies, Inc.

Association of Pathology Chairmen (APC) A national organization founded in 1967 composed of 138 chairs of medical school departments of pathology. It acts as a communications center for exchange of information and for workshops on innovations for teaching and resident training, department administration, and relationships with governmental and other nonuniversity agencies. *See also* department chair; medical school; pathology.

Association of Pediatric Oncology Nurses (APON) A national organization founded in 1973 composed of 1,000 nurses caring for children with cancer. It encourages updating of literature, development of standards, and improved communication among nurses caring for children with cancer. *See also* cancer; pediatric hematology-oncology; nurse.

Association of Pediatric Oncology Social Workers (APOSW) A national organization founded in 1977 composed of 170 social workers involved with pediatric cancer patients in medical settings. Its activities include advancing the practice of pediatric oncology social work and formulating and recording local and federal legislation relating to pediatric oncology. *See also* pediatric hematology-oncology; social worker.

Association of Philippine Physicians in America (APPA) A national organization founded in 1972 composed of 3,000 individuals from the Philippines who are licensed to practice medicine in the United States. It renders free medical care to indigent persons, establishes a continuing medical education program for physicians, provides aid for education of physicians, and supports medical research. Formerly (1986) Association of Philippine Practicing Physicians in America. *See also* continuing medical education; physician.

Association of Phillipine Practicing Physicians in America *See* Association of Philippine Physicians in America.

Association of Physical Fitness Centers (APFC) A national organization founded in 1975 composed of 115 owners and operators of 500 physical fitness centers, defined as businesses or organizations promoting physical fitness by stressing exercise, training, recreational, and athletic activities; associate members are suppliers of physical fitness centers. It informs the public of the role of the full-service physical fitness center industry and its relation to health and fitness. It promotes a code of ethical practices for the industry and monitors and acts on state legislative activities. *See also* fitness; physical fitness program.

Association of Physician Assistant Programs (APAP) An organization founded in 1972 composed of educational institutions with training programs for assistants to primary care and surgical

physicians. It assists in the development and organization of educational curricula for physician assistant programs and contributes to defining the roles of physician assistants in the field of medicine. It sponsors the Annual Survey of Physician Assistant Educational Programs in the United States. *See also* physician assistant.

Association of Physician's Assistants in Cardio-Vascular Surgery (APACVS) A national organization founded in 1981 composed of 675 physician assistants who work with cardiovascular surgeons. Its objective is to assist in defining the role of physician assistants in the field of cardiovascular surgery through educational forums. It offers a placement service and compiles statistics. *See also* physician assistant; thoracic surgery.

Association of Planned Parenthood Professionals *See* Association of Reproductive Health Professionals.

Association for Politics and the Life Sciences (APLS) A national organization founded in 1980 composed of 450 individuals and libraries interested in the interaction of human biology and public policy. It emphasizes study of behavioral biology as it relates to political science and the legal and public policy implications of advances in biotechnology and biomedical technology. *See also* biotechnology; politics; technology.

Association of Polysomnographic Technologists (APT) A national organization founded in 1978 composed of 750 individuals who practice polysomnography in research or clinical settings. *See also* polysomnographic technology; sleep apnea; somnology.

Association for Practitioners in Infection Control (APIC) A national organization founded in 1972 composed of 9,000 physicians, nurses, epidemiologists, microbiologists, medical technicians, pharmacists, and sanitarians interested in infection control. It promotes quality research and standardization of practices and procedures, develops communications among members, and assesses and influences legislation related to the field. *See also* infection control; practitioner.

Association of Professional Baseball Physicians (APBP) A national organization founded in 1970 composed of 36 physicians and surgeons of the professional baseball teams in the United States. It aims to provide the best possible medical care to all players and associated personnel. It conducts drug abuse seminars on topics, such as amphetamine, steroid, and cocaine use by athletes. *See also* drug abuse; physician; sports medicine.

Association of Professional Sleep Societies (APSS) A national organization founded in 1985 composed of the Sleep Research Society, American Sleep Disorders Association, and Association of Polysomnographic Technologists. It works to facilitate sleep research and development of sleep disorders medicine by encouraging cooperation and exchange of information among its members. *See also* American Sleep Disorders Association; Association of Polysomnographic Technologists; polysomnographic technology; sleep; sleep apnea; Sleep Research Society; somnology.

Association of Professors of Gynecology and Obstetrics (APGO) A national organization founded in 1962 composed of 146 departments of obstetrics and gynecology in approved medical schools in the United States and Canada. Its purposes include improving the study of gynecology and obstetrics and providing a means of exchanging information relating to the programs of study, teaching methods, and research activities of such departments. *See also* gynecology; obstetrics.

Association of Professors of Medicine (APM) A national organization founded in 1954 composed of 125 heads of departments of medicine (internal medicine) in US medical schools. It conducts educational programs. *See also* internal medicine; medical school; professor.

Association of Program Directors in Internal Medicine (APDIM) A national organization founded in 1977 composed of 940 physicians in internal medicine, including departmental chairs and directors of internal medicine, directors of residency-training programs, associate program directors, medical education directors, and chiefs of medical services. It advances medical education through assisting accredited hospital internal medicine residency training programs in the United States and Puerto Rico. It conducts annual courses for chief residents and program directors. *See also* chief resident; internal medicine; residency.

Association for Psychoanalytic Medicine (APM) A national organization founded in 1945 composed of 241 physicians who are psychoanalysts. It provides a forum on psychoanalytic developments for its membership and the community and conducts postgraduate seminars. *See also* psychoanalysis.

Association for Psychological Type (APT) A national organization founded in 1979 composed of 3,500 individuals interested in organizational development, religious communities, management, education, and counseling, and who are interested in psychological type, the Myers-Briggs Type Indicator, and the works of Carl G. Jung, the Swiss psychologist and founder of analytical psychology. *See also* psychology.

Association of Psychology Internship Centers *See* Association of Psychology Postdoctoral and Internship Centers.

Association of Psychology Postdoctoral and Internship Centers (APPIC) A national organization founded in 1968 composed of 525 Veterans Administration hospitals, medical centers, state hospitals, university counseling centers, and other facilities that provide internship and postdoctoral programs in professional psychology. It serves as a clearinghouse to provide college students with internship placement assistance at member facilities. Formerly (1991) Association of Psychology Internship Centers. *See also* psychology.

Association for the Psychophysiological Study of Sleep *See* Sleep Research Society.

Association for Quality and Participation (AQP) A national organization founded in 1977 composed of 8,000 quality managers, manufacturing executives, professionals in personnel relations, organization presidents, and employee involvement professionals, such as training directors, facilitators, and coordinators. *See also* quality control.

Association of Rehabilitation Nurses (ARN) A national organization founded in 1974 composed of 7,500 registered nurses interested in or actively engaged in the practice of rehabilitation nursing. Its committees involve members in issues of organizational, local, and national importance and provide an avenue to effect change. *See also* rehabilitation; rehabilitation nurse.

Association of Reproductive Health Professionals (ARHP) A national organization founded in 1963 composed of 600 physicians, scientists, educators, and reproductive health professionals interested in educating the public and health professionals on matters pertaining to reproductive health, including sexuality, contraception, prevention of sexually transmitted disease, family planning, and abortion. It supports the right of women to decide to sustain or terminate their pregnancies. Formerly (1987) Association of Planned Parenthood Professionals. *See also* contraception; family planning; health professional; reproduction; sexually transmitted diseases.

Association for Research in Nervous and Mental Disease (ARNMD) A national organization founded in 1920 composed of 950 individuals engaged in the practice or research of neurology, neurosurgery, or psychiatry who are members of neurologic or psychiatric societies. *See also* neurological surgery; neurology; psychiatry.

Association for Research in Vision and Ophthalmology (ARVO) A national organization founded in 1928 composed of 6,000 researchers in the field of blinding eye diseases. *See also* ophthalmology; vision.

Association of Retired Americans (ARA) A national organization founded in 1973 composed of 55,000 senior Americans interested in group benefits. Its purpose is to offer a program of high-quality, low-cost benefits and services to members, such as discounts on prescriptions, eyeglasses, and hearing aids, and insurance benefits including emergency air medical transportation. It assists governmental bodies and agencies with the development of programs and legislation that benefit and promote the well-being of retired Americans. *See also* retirement.

Association of Schools and Colleges of Optometry (ASCO) A national organization founded in 1941 composed of 17 colleges of optometry in the United States and two in Canada. It encourages optometric education and fosters optometric and visual research. *See also* optometry.

Association of Schools of Public Health (ASPH) A national organization founded in 1941 composed of 24 accredited graduate schools of public health interested in the advancement of academic public health programs. *See also* accredited; public health.

Association of State Drinking Water Administrators (ASDWA) A national organization founded in 1984 composed of 57 managers of state and territorial drinking water programs and state regulatory personnel. It works to meet the communication and coordination needs of state drinking water program managers and facilitates the exchange of information and experience among state drinking water agencies. It acts as a collective voice for the protection of public health through assurance of high-quality drinking water. It oversees the implementa-

tion of the Safe Drinking Water Act. It acts as a liaison with Congress and the Environmental Protection Agency. *See also* administrator; Environmental Protection Agency; public health.

Association of State and Territorial Dental Directors (ASTDD) A national organization composed of 53 directors of state and territorial dental programs. It provides a forum for consideration of dental health administrative problems. *See also* dentistry.

Association of State and Territorial Directors of Nursing (ASTDN) A national organization composed of 54 directors of nursing in the states and territories. It serves as a channel for sharing methods and disseminates information to increase the effectiveness of public health nursing services. *See also* nursing; public health nurse.

Association of State and Territorial Directors of Public Health Education (ASTDPHE) A national organization founded in 1946 composed of 76 directors of public health education in state and territorial departments of health and Native American health service areas. It develops, among other activities, practice guidelines and supports collection and dissemination of data and information relevant to public health education. Its parent organization is the Association of State and Territorial Health Officials. Formerly (1989) Conference of State and Territorial Directors of Public Health Education. *See also* public health.

Association of State and Territorial Health Officials (ASTHO) A national organization founded in 1942 composed of 55 executive officers of state and territorial health departments. It represents state and territorial health officers on matters of federal health, legislation, and policies and aids public or private agencies dealing with human health, especially in interstate and federal relationships. *See also* public health.

Association for the Study of Dreams (ASD) A national organization founded in 1984 composed of 600 medical professionals, sociologists, counselors, educators, researchers, and other individuals whose disciplines are related to the study of dreams and dreaming. It provides an interdisciplinary forum for the promotion and public dissemination of information regarding research into the physiological and therapeutic aspects of dreams and their interpretation. *See also* dream; sleep.

Association for Surgical Education (ASE) A

national organization founded in 1980 composed of 350 surgeons and individuals involved in undergraduate surgical education interested in developing and disseminating information on motivation, techniques, research, and applications for presenting curricula in undergraduate surgical education. *See also* surgery.

Association of Surgical Technologists (AST) A national organization founded in 1969 composed of 11,500 individuals who have received education and training to work in specifically delineated areas of patient care in the operating room. Emphasis is placed on preparing members to take the National Certifying Examination and to participate actively in a continuing education program. *See also* surgical technologist.

Association for Systems Management (ASM) A national organization founded in 1947 composed of 7,000 executives and specialists in management information systems serving business, commerce, education, government, and the military. It offers seminars, conferences, and courses in all phases of information systems and management. *See also* management information system.

Association of Teachers of Maternal and Child Health (ATMCH) A national organization founded in 1968 composed of 200 faculty and graduate students in maternal and child health. It promotes the teaching and research of maternal and child health programs in public health schools and professional schools in the United States and participates in the development and support of policy initiatives related to the field. *See also* maternal and child health programs/services.

Association of Teachers of Preventive Medicine (ATPM) A national organization founded in 1942 composed of 700 teachers in medical schools, research, and other phases of preventive medicine and public health. *See also* preventive medicine.

Association of Technical Personnel in Ophthalmology (ATPO) A national organization founded in 1969 composed of 1,000 certified and noncertified allied health personnel in ophthalmology. Formerly (1989) American Association of Certified Allied Health Personnel in Ophthalmology. *See also* ophthalmology.

Association of Tongue Depressors (ATD) A national organization founded in 1978 composed of 28 health care companies, researchers, and manufac-

turers of wooden tongue depressors. Its objective is to strive for safe, sturdy, sterile sticks. Its monthly publication is *Wooden Stick*. *See also* tongue depressor.

Association of Trial Lawyers of America (ATLA) A national organization founded in 1946 composed of 65,000 lawyers, judges, law professors, and students engaged in civil plaintiff or criminal defense advocacy. It objectives include advancing jurisprudence and the law as a profession and advancing the cause of persons seeking redress for damages against person or property. *See also* jurisprudence; lawyer; trial; trial court.

Association of University Anesthesiologists (AUA) A national organization founded in 1953 composed of 600 academic anesthesiologists from medical school faculties. It encourages members to pursue original investigations in the clinic and the laboratory and develops methods of teaching anesthesiology. Formerly (1990) Association of University Anesthetists. *See also* anesthesiology; medical school; university.

Association of University Anesthetists *See* Association of University Anesthesiologists.

Association of University Environmental Health/Sciences Centers (AUEHSC) A national organization founded in 1980 composed of 14 university-based environmental health science centers supported by the National Institute of Environmental Health Sciences. It serves as a forum for exchange of information. *See also* environmental health; university.

Association of University Professors of Ophthalmology (AUPO) A national organization founded in 1966 composed of 190 heads of departments or divisions of ophthalmology in accredited medical schools in the United States, and directors of ophthalmology residency programs in institutions not connected to medical schools. It operates the Ophthalmology Matching Program and a faculty placement service. *See also* accredited; medical school; ophthalmology; professor; university.

Association of University Programs in Health Administration (AUPHA) A national organization founded in 1948 composed of 1,200 universities offering graduate and undergraduate study in health services and hospital administration. Its purposes include improving the quality of education in health services administration. *See also* health administration; university.

Association of University Programs in Occupa-

tional Health and Safety (AUPOHS) A national organization founded in 1977 composed of 14 universities offering graduate training and continuing education for occupational health safety professionals. It provides a forum for the exchange of information among members on graduate training in occupational medicine, occupational health nursing, industrial hygiene, and industrial safety engineering. It works in conjunction with the National Institute for Occupational Safety and Health to facilitate the operation of training programs. *See also* National Institute for Occupational Safety and Health; occupational health and safety; occupational medicine; university.

Association of University Radiologists (AUR) A national organization founded in 1953 composed of 1,600 physicians and scientists who have been appointed to a university faculty. It provides a forum for university-based radiologists to present and discuss results of research, teaching, and administrative issues. *See also* faculty; radiology; university.

Association for Vital Records and Health Statistics (AVRHS) A national organization founded in 1933 composed of 220 officials of state and local health agencies responsible for registration, tabulation, and analysis of births, deaths, fetal deaths, marriages, divorces, and other health statistics. Formerly (1980) American Association for Vital Records and Public Health Statistics. *See also* vital records; vital statistics.

Association for Voluntary Sterilization *See* Association for Voluntary Surgical Contraception.

Association for Voluntary Surgical Contraception (AVSC) A national organization founded in 1943 that disseminates information on voluntary surgical contraception, promotes safer, simpler techniques in surgical contraception, and fosters, stimulates, and supports voluntary surgical contraception activities in various types of health programs throughout the world by providing local medical groups with training equipment and technical assistance. Formerly (1985) Association for Voluntary Sterilization. *See also* contraceptive sterilization; sterilization.

Association for Women in Psychology (AWP) A national organization founded in 1969 composed of 1,500 members interested in ending the role that the association feels psychology has had in perpetuating unscientific and unquestioned assumptions about the "natures" of women and men, and

encouraging unbiased psychological research on sex and gender in order to establish facts and expose myths. *See also* gender; myth; psychology; sex.

Association of Women's Health, Obstetric, and Neonatal Nurses (AWHONN) A national organization founded in 1969 composed of 24,000 registered nurses and allied health workers with an interest in obstetric, gynecologic, and neonatal nursing. It sponsors educational meetings and stimulates interest in obstetric, gynecologic, and neonatal nursing. Formerly (1993) NAACOG: The Organization for Obstetric, Gynecologic, and Neonatal Nurses. *See also* neonate; obstetrics and gynecology; registered nurse.

assumption The act of taking for granted, as in accepting as true without proof. *See also* judgment; opinion; principle; tenet; theorem.

assumption of risk In torts, an affirmative defense used by a defendant to a negligence suit claiming that the plaintiff had knowledge of a condition or situation obviously dangerous to himself or herself and yet voluntarily exposed himself or herself to the hazard created by the defendant, thereby relieving him or her of legal responsibility for any resulting injury. When a plaintiff knowingly and voluntarily exposes himself or herself to a risk of harm, he or she is said to "assume the risk." *See also* assumption; risk; tort.

assurance The act or action of making certain and putting beyond doubt, as in performing "quality assurance" activities to reduce the risk of poor quality care. Assurance is often a declaration intended to inspire belief and full confidence. *See also* quality assurance; quality assurance professional; quality assurance program.

Assurance, National Committee for Quality *See* National Committee for Quality Assurance.

Assurance, National Organization for Competency *See* National Organization for Competency Assurance.

assurance professional, quality *See* quality assurance professional.

assurance program, quality *See* quality assurance program.

assurance, quality *See* quality assurance.

AST *See* Association of Surgical Technologists.

ASTDD *See* Association of State and Territorial Dental Directors.

ASTDN *See* Association of State and Territorial Directors of Nursing.

ASTDPHE *See* Association of State and Territorial Directors of Public Health Education.

asthma A clinical syndrome characterized by increased responsiveness of the tracheobronchial tree to a variety of stimuli. The primary physiological manifestation of this hyperresponsivness is a variable airway obstruction. These changes are reversible either spontaneously or as a result of therapy. *See also* bronchospasm; chronic obstructive pulmonary disease; emergency medicine; peak flow meter; pediatrics; pulmonary medicine; spirometer.

ASTHO *See* Association of State and Territorial Health Officials.

ASTM A national organization founded in 1898 composed of 33,000 engineers, scientists, managers, professionals, academicians, consumers, and skilled technicians holding membership as individuals in or representatives of business firms, government agencies, education institutions, and laboratories. It establishes test standards for materials, products, systems, and services and has 133 technical committees (each having 5 to 50 subcommittees). New committees are organized periodically to keep pace with technological advances. It has developed more than 9,000 standard test methods, specifications, classifications, definitions, and recommended practices now in use. Also known as American Society for Testing and Materials. *See also* standard; testing.

ASTMH *See* American Society of Tropical Medicine and Hygiene.

ASTRO *See* American Society for Therapeutic Radiology and Oncology.

ASTS *See* American Society of Transplant Surgeons.

asymptomatic HIV infection Infection characterized by a positive test for the human immunodeficiency virus (HIV) but lacking symptoms or signs of illness. *See also* HIV infection.

ATA *See* American Thyroid Association; American Transplant Association.

ataxia An abnormal condition involving impaired ability to coordinate movement, resulting from lesions in the spinal cord or cerebellum. *See also* central nervous system; cerebellum; spinal cord.

ATCC *See* American Type Culture Collection.

ATD *See* Association of Tongue Depressors.

atherosclerosis A form of arteriosclerosis in which, in addition to a hardening of the walls of the arteries, fatty deposits build up on the inner arterial walls and interfere with blood flow. *See also* acute myocardial infarction; angina pectoris; arteriosclerosis; cardiovascular medicine; cholesterol; infarction; ischemia; morbid obesity; plaque.

Athletic Association, American Medical *See* American Medical Athletic Association.

athletic trainer An allied health professional who, with the consultation and supervision of attending and/or consulting physicians, provides a variety of services, including injury prevention, recognition, immediate care, treatment, and rehabilitation after athletic trauma. Athletic trainers typically provide their services in one or more of the following settings: secondary schools, colleges and universities, professional athletic organizations, and private or hospital-based clinics. Athletic trainers are one type of allied health professional for which the Committee on Allied Health Education and Accreditation has accredited education programs. *See also* allied health professional; Committee on Allied Health Education and Accreditation; sports medicine; train.

Athletic Trainers Association and Certification Board, American *See* American Athletic Trainers Association and Certification Board.

Athletic Trainers Association, National *See* National Athletic Trainers Association.

ATLA *See* Association of Trial Lawyers of America.

ATLS *See* advanced trauma life support.

ATMCH *See* Association of Teachers of Maternal and Child Health.

ATPM *See* Association of Teachers of Preventive Medicine.

ATPO *See* Association of Technical Personnel in Ophthalmology.

ATRA *See* American Therapeutic Recreation Association; American Tort Reform Association.

at risk The state of being subject to some uncertain event that can cause loss or difficulty; for example, a person who smokes cigarettes is at risk of developing lung cancer or an insurance company is at risk of incurring a financial loss by agreeing to provide or pay for more services than are paid for through premiums or per capita payments. *See also* risk.

ATS *See* American Thoracic Society; American Trauma Society.

attack, transient ischemic *See* transient ischemic attack.

attempted vaginal birth after cesarean section *See* vaginal birth after cesarean section.

attempt to monopolize Conduct short of actual

monopolization that is prohibited by Section 2 of the Sherman Antitrust Act. There are two elements to an attempt to monopolize claim: specific intent to destroy competition or build monopoly, and a dangerous probability that the attempt will be successful in the relevant market. *See also* monopoly; Sherman Antitrust Act.

attempt, suicide   *See* suicide attempt.

attending physician   A member of a health care organization's medical staff who is legally responsible for the care and treatment provided a given patient. *See also* medical staff; physician.

attention-deficit disorder   A syndrome affecting certain children and adolescents and, rarely, adults (ten times more frequently in boys than girls) with learning and behavior disabilities. Its characteristics include varying degrees of impairment in perception; conceptualization; language, memory, and motor skills; excessive motor activity; inattentiveness; impulsiveness; impatience; poor tolerance for frustration; and distractibility. *Synonym*: attention-deficient hyperactivity disorder. *See also* disorder; hyperactivity; learning disability; syndrome.

attestation   The act of witnessing a document in writing; bearing witness.

Attitudinal Healing, Center for   *See* Center for Attitudinal Healing.

attorney   An individual who is usually, but not necessarily, a lawyer empowered to act for another, as in plaintiff's attorney. Such an individual is also called an attorney-at-law and an attorney-in-fact. *See also* attorney general; Juris Doctor; jurisprudence; lawyer; power of attorney.

attorney-at-law   *See* attorney.

attorney-client privilege   The legally established policy that communication is confidential between an attorney and a client in the course of the professional relationship and that it cannot be disclosed without the consent of the client. It may be oral or written statements or may be actions and gestures. Its purpose is to encourage full and frank communication between attorneys and their clients and thereby promote broader public interest in the observance of law and administration of justice. *See also* attorney; client; physician-patient privilege; privileged communication.

attorney-in-fact   *See* attorney.

attorney general   The chief law officer of the federal government or of each state government. *See also* attorney.

attorney, power of   *See* power of attorney.

attorney, prosecuting   *See* prosecuting attorney.

Attorneys, American Academy of Hospital   *See* American Academy of Hospital Attorneys.

Attorneys, American Association of Nurse   *See* The American Association of Nurse Attorneys.

Attorneys, American Board of Professional Liability   *See* American Board of Professional Liability Attorneys.

Attorneys, National Association of Black Women   *See* National Association of Black Women Attorneys.

Attorneys, The American Association of Nurse   *See* The American Association of Nurse Attorneys.

attributable cause variation   *See* special-cause variation; variation.

attribute   A quality or characteristic inherent in or ascribed to someone or something; for example, length is a quantifiable attribute of a ruler, and efficiency and/or effectiveness of a specified process is a quantifiable attribute of a health care practitioner's or a health care organization's performance. *See also* attribute data; variable.

attribute data   Data that arise from the classification of items into categories; from counts of the number of items in a given category or the proportion in a given category; and from counts of the number of occurrences per unit. For instance, data indicating a hospital's compliance *or* noncompliance with a standard would be attribute data. *Compare* variables data. *See also* attribute; data.

AUA   *See* American Urological Association; Association of University Anesthesiologists.

AUAA   *See* American Urological Association Allied.

audience, target   *See* target audience.

audiological assessment   A process that uses audiological tests for delineating the site of auditory dysfunction, including such tests as pure tone air-conduction thresholds, speech reception thresholds, speech discrimination measurements, and impedance measurements. *See also* assessment; audiologist.

audiologist   An individual qualified by education and authorized by law (where applicable) to evaluate and treat patients with impaired hearing, including the fitting and dispensing of hearing aids. *See also* audiology; hearing aid; hearing impaired; speech pathology.

Audiologists, Academy of Dispensing   *See* Academy of Dispensing Audiologists.

audiology   The study of hearing, especially hearing defects and their treatment. *See also* audiologist.

Audiology, Academy of Rehabilitative   *See* Academy of Rehabilitative Audiology.

Audiology, Council on Professional Standards in Speech-Language Pathology and   *See* Council on Professional Standards in Speech-Language Pathology and Audiology.

audiometer   An instrument for measuring hearing activity for pure tones of normally audible frequencies. *Synonym:* sonometer. *See also* audiology.

audiometrician   An individual who administers hearing tests prescribed by audiologists and physicians to patients for diagnostic and evaluative purposes. *See also* audiologist; audiometric screening; industrial audiometric technician.

audiometric screening   A process that may include such tests as pure tone air-conduction thresholds, pure tone air-conduction suprathreshold screenings, impedance measurements, or observations of reactions to auditory stimuli. *See also* audiometrician; screening.

audiometric technician, industrial   *See* industrial audiometric technician.

audit   A systematic inspection of records or accounts to verify their accuracy and completeness. *See also* dental audit; financial audit; independent audit; internal audit; medical audit; nursing audit; patient care audit; process quality audit; product quality audit; quality audit; quality system audit.

audit committee   A committee of the governing body of a corporation responsible for overseeing auditing activities, such as nominating independent auditors and discussing their work with them. For example, the audit and oversight committee of the Joint Commission on Accreditation of Healthcare Organization is a five-member subcommittee of the Accreditation Committee of the Board of Commissioners. The audit and oversight committee audits staff's application of the aggregation and decision rules when processing accreditation reports that are not presented to the accreditation committee for review and final decision determination. The audit and oversight committee also reviews and recommends approval of decision grids, aggregation rules, and decision rules to the Accreditation Committee and presents all recommendations for modifications to the decision grids, aggregation rules, and decision rules to the accreditation committee for final

approval. *See also* Accreditation Committee; audit; auditor; Joint Commission on Accreditation of Healthcare Organizations.

audit, dental   *See* dental audit.

audit, financial   *See* financial audit.

audit, independent   *See* independent audit.

audit, internal   *See* internal audit.

audit, medical   *See* medical audit.

audit, nursing   *See* nursing audit.

auditor   **1.** One who checks the accuracy, fairness, and general acceptability of accounting records and statements and then attests to them; for example, a certified public accountant. *See also* accounting; certified public accountant. **2.** A public officer charged by law with the duty of examining and verifying the expenditure of public fund, or an accountant who performs a similar function for private parties. *See also* audit.

Auditors, Association of Healthcare Internal   *See* Association of Healthcare Internal Auditors.

Auditory Society, American   *See* American Auditory Society.

auditory substitutional device   *See* hearing aid.

audit, patient care   *See* patient care audit.

audit, process quality   *See* process quality audit.

audit, product quality   *See* product quality audit.

audit, quality   *See* quality audit.

audit, quality system   *See* quality system audit.

AUEHSC   *See* Association of University Environmental Health/Sciences Centers.

AUPHA   *See* Association of University Programs in Health Administration.

AUPO   *See* Association of University Professors of Ophthalmology.

AUPOHS   *See* Association of University Programs in Occupational Health and Safety.

AUR   *See* Association of University Radiologists.

auscultation   In physical diagnosis, the act of hearing to obtain physical signs, such as cardiac murmurs, pericardial rubs and knocks, or a noise over an arteriovenous fistula. A stethoscope is an instrument often used in auscultating the human body. *See also* physical examination; rales; stethoscope.

authenticate   To confirm the accuracy of an entry in a medical record and that the person who says he or she wrote the entry, did write it. *See also* authentication; authorship.

authentication   A process of confirming authorship of an entry in a medical record, for example, by verifying a written signature, identifiable initials, computer key, or other methods. *See also* admissible evidence; authenticate; authorship; forgery.

authoritarianism Seeking weakness in others, then setting out to control and manipulate; favoring absolute obedience to authority, as opposed to individual freedom. *See also* authority.

authority **1.** An accepted source of expert information or advice, as in a recognized authority on risk management. *See also* expert. **2.** The power to enforce laws, exact obedience, or judge, as in authority to make a final decision. *See also* authoritarianism; backdoor authority; borrowing authority; contract authority; entitlement authority; staff authority.

authority, backdoor *See* backdoor authority.

authority, borrowing *See* backdoor authority.

authority, contract *See* backdoor authority.

authority, entitlement *See* entitlement authority.

authority, staff *See* staff authority.

authorization, prior *See* prior authorization.

authorize To empower or to give a right or authority to act, as in a patient authorizing release of his or her patient care information. *See also* authority.

authorship Source or origin, as in authorship of an entry made in a patient's medical record. *See also* authorship determination.

authorship determination A process of identifying a health professional responsible for a health care entry (for example, in a medical record), as by his or her written signature, biometric identifier, or computer key. *See also* authentication; authorship; determination.

autism A developmental disability characterized by abnormal introversion and egocentricity. *See also* developmental disability.

autoclave Equipment that sterilizes (for example, surgical instruments) through steam under pressure. *See also* sterile; sterilization.

autologous Relating to self; originating within an organism, as in an autologous blood transfusion. *See also* autologous blood transfusion.

autologous blood transfusion A transfusion of an individual using his or her own blood, which usually was drawn previously and stored for later use, typically in elective surgery. *See also* autotransfusion; blood transfusion; elective surgery.

Automated Reasoning, Association for *See* Association for Automated Reasoning.

automated speech technology *See* voice input/output technology.

automatic data processing *See* electronic data processing.

automatic fire-extinguishing system A sprinkler or other fire-extinguishing system that is activated by the presence of heat. *See also* system.

Automatic Identification Manufacturers (AIM) A national organization founded in 1972 composed of 165 suppliers of automatic identification equipment and systems, such as bar code, magnetic stripe, radio frequency, machine vision, voice technology, optical character recognition, and systems integration technologies. *See also* automated speech technology; bar code; machine readable; optical character recognition; scanner; voice input/output technology.

automatic retirement age The age at which retirement is automatically effective, as decided by an organization's policy. *See also* retirement age.

automation The reduction of human work by fully or partially replacing it with machine work. *See also* mechanization; mechatronics.

autonomy The condition of having one's life under one's control and making decisions or plans and acting on them. Autonomy also dictates the duty of individuals not to interfere either intentionally or negligently in another person's making of decisions or plans or acting on them. Autonomy forms the ethical basis for patient's right of autonomy, which includes, among other rights, the right to informed consent, the right to refuse treatment, and the right to die. *See also* informed consent; patient's right of autonomy; rights.

autonomy, patient's right of *See* patient's right of autonomy.

autopsy Dissection of a dead body, including the internal organs and structures, to determine the cause of death or the nature of pathological changes. An autopsy is normally required by statute for deaths by violent, unexplained, or unnatural means. *Synonyms*: necropsy; postmortem. *See also* hospital autopsy; morgue; pathologist; prosector.

autopsy data Data derived from autopsied deaths for the study of the natural history of disease, trends in frequency of disease, and other topics. Autopsies are done on nonrandomly selected persons in the population and findings are not necessarily generalizable to a given population. *See also* autopsy; autopsy rate; data.

autopsy, hospital *See* hospital autopsy.

autopsy rate The number of autopsies performed on patients over a given period in relation to the total number of inpatient and outpatient deaths. *Synonym*: gross autopsy rate. *See also* adjusted autopsy rate; autopsy; rate.

autopsy rate, adjusted *See* adjusted autopsy rate.

autopsy rate, gross *See* autopsy rate.

autopsy rate, net *See* adjusted autopsy rate.

autotransfusion Reinfusion of blood or blood products derived from a patient's own circulation. *See also* autologous blood transfusion; intraoperative autotransfusion; MAST; postoperative autotransfusion.

autotransfusion, intraoperative *See* intraoperative autotransfusion.

autotransfusion, postoperative *See* postoperative autotransfusion.

auxilian A member of a health care organization's (such as a hospital or medical society) auxiliary. *See also* auxiliary.

auxiliary A self-governing membership organization founded by individuals from the community to assist a hospital or other health care organization in promoting the health and welfare of the community; for example, a hospital auxiliary or medical society auxiliary. *See also* volunteer.

availability In health care, a performance dimension addressing the degree to which the care/intervention is performed when required by a patient. It is a measure of the supply of health resources and services relative to the needs or demands of an individual or a community. Health care is available when it can be obtained from appropriate personnel at the time and place it is needed. Availability is a function of the distribution of appropriate resources and services and the willingness of the provider to render services to particular patients in need. *See also* acceptability; accessibility; dimensions of performance.

availability, bio- *See* bioavailability.

AVDA *See* American Venereal Disease Association.

average *See* mean; measures of central tendency; median; mode.

average cost The total cost of producing a good or service divided by the number of units produced. *See also* cost.

average daily census The average number of inpatients, excluding newborns, receiving care each day in a health care organization during a reporting period. *See also* ADT; census.

average length of stay (ALOS) Average stay counted by days of all or a class of inpatients discharged over a given period, calculated by dividing the number of inpatient days by the number of discharges. *See also* length of stay.

AVG *See* ambulatory visit group.

Aviation Medical Association, Civil *See* Civil Aviation Medical Association.

Aviation Psychologists, Association of *See* Association of Aviation Psychologists.

AVRHS *See* Association for Vital Records and Health Statistics.

AVSC *See* Association for Voluntary Surgical Contraception.

award **1.** To grant or concede as due, as in awarding a plaintiff. *See also* apportionment of damages. **2.** The decision or determination rendered by arbitrators or commissioners, or other private or extrajudicial deciders, upon a controversy submitted to them.

AWHONN *See* Association of Women's Health, Obstetric, and Neonatal Nurses.

awkward zone In a Pareto analysis, those factors that are not clearly in the "vital few" or the "useful many." *See also* Pareto chart; Pareto principle.

AWP *See* Association for Women in Psychology.

axis One of the dimensions of a graph. A two-dimension graph has two axes, the horizontal, or x, axis, and the vertical, or y, axis. Mathematically there may be more than two axes, and graphs are sometimes drawn with a third dimension. The human mind cannot comprehend more than three dimensions in visual space. *See also* graph; x-axis; y-axis.

axis, x- *See* x-axis.

axis, y- *See* y-axis.

ayurvedic medicine The traditional Hindu science of medicine. *See also* transcendental meditation; yoga.

Ayurvedic Medicine, American Association of *See* American Association of Ayurvedic Medicine.

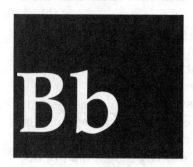

Bb

babies, blue *See* blue babies.

baby An infant or very young child. *See also* neonate; newborn.

baby boomer *See* boomer.

baby buster *See* buster.

baby, sick *See* sick baby.

baby, test-tube *See* test-tube baby.

baccalaureate *See* bachelor's degree.

baccalaureate degree program In nursing education, a program educating registered nurses and other health professionals in a four-year college or university, at the end of which a bachelor's degree is awarded. Classroom and laboratory teaching is provided by the college, typically through its nursing or other professional school, and clinical teaching by the college's own or an affiliated hospital. *Compare* associate degree; degree program; diploma school. *See also* bachelor's degree; degree; registered nurse.

bachelor's degree An academic degree conferred by a college or university upon those persons who complete the undergraduate curriculum, as in a bachelor's degree in science (BS or BSc), the arts (BA), nursing (BSN), social work (BSW), or pharmacy (PharB). *Synonym:* baccalaureate. *See also* degree; degree nurse; doctorate; master's degree; university.

backdoor authority Legislative authority for the obligation of funds outside the normal appropriation process. The most common forms of backdoor authority are borrowing authority (authority to spend debt receipts) and contract authority. Entitlement authority is sometimes considered to be a form of backdoor authority, since the enactment of the basic benefit legislation may effectively mandate the subsequent enactment of an appropriation to pay for the statutory benefits. The Environmental Protection Agency's construction grant program and the Social Security Administration's trust funds are two more examples of programs with backdoor authority. *Synonym:* backdoor spending. *See also* appropriation; authority; entitlement authority; Environmental Protection Agency; Social Security Administration.

backdoor spending *See* backdoor authority.

back order A request for an item for sale or inventory that is not available immediately. *See also* order.

back-up hospital A hospital that provides specialized services and inpatient care for patients receiving services in ambulatory care centers, such as a freestanding ambulatory care center or a freestanding ambulatory surgical facility, should the patients require these services, especially on an emergency basis. *See also* freestanding ambulatory care center; freestanding ambulatory surgical facility; hospital; hospital-based ambulatory care center.

bacteremia The presence of bacteria in the blood. *Synonym:* blood poisoning. *See also* blood culture; sepsis; septicemia.

bacteria Unicellular microorganisms that commonly multiply by cell division and are typically contained within cell walls. They may be aerobic or anaerobic, motile or nonmotile, and may be free-living, saprophytic, parasitic, or even pathogenic, the last causing disease in animals, including humans. *See also* aerobic; anaerobic; antibacterial; bacteriocidal; bacteriostatic; campylobacter; cholera; germ; gonorrhea; Gram's stain; microorganism; pneumococcus; strain; tetanus.

bacteria, gram-negative *See* Gram's stain.

bacteria, gram-positive *See* Gram's stain.

bacteriocidal Destroying bacteria, as in a bacteriocidal antibiotic. *See also* antibacterial; antibiotic; bacteria; bacteriostatic.

bacteriologist A physician, medical technologist, or other person who specializes in the study of bacteria and the diagnosis of bacterial diseases. *See also* bacteria; bacteriology; microbiology.

bacteriology The study of bacteria, especially in relation to medicine and agriculture. Bacteriology is part of the more general science of microorganisms known as microbiology. *See also* bacteria; clinical diagnostic bacteriology; clinical laboratory; medical bacteriology; microbiology; Petri dish; public health bacteriology.

bacteriology, clinical diagnostic *See* clinical diagnostic bacteriology.

bacteriology, medical *See* medical bacteriology.

bacteriology, public health *See* public health bacteriology.

bacteriostatic Inhibiting the growth or multiplication of bacteria, as in a bacteriostatic soap. *See also* antibacterial; antibiotic; bacteria; bacteriocidal.

bacterium Singular of bacteria. *See also* bacteria.

bad apples *See* continuous quality improvement.

bad debt A debt that is uncollectible. A health care provider, such as a hospital or physician, may absorb the cost of bad debt by increasing charges for other patients, especially for private patients and patients with commercial health insurance. *See also* commercial health insurance; cost shifting; debt; private patient.

BaE *See* barium enema.

balance **1.** A state of equilibrium characterized by the cancellation of all forces by equal opposing forces. **2.** In accounting, the difference between debits and credits of an account. *See also* account; balance billing; balance sheet.

balance billing The practice of physicians, dentists, and other independent practitioners to seek payment from the patient of that portion of a patient's bill not covered by the government or other third-party payers. *See also* balance; billing.

balanced budget A budget in which receipts are equal to outlays. *See also* budget.

balance sheet A statement of a business or an institution that lists the assets, debts, and owners' investment as of a specified date. *See also* asset; balance; debt; financial statement.

Baldridge Award *See* Malcolm Baldridge National Quality Award.

ballistics The scientific study of the motion of projectiles in flight, as in wound ballistics, which involves the study of the speed and direction of missiles (such as bullets and other projectiles) in relation to the injuries they produce.

balloon angioplasty *See* percutaneous transluminal angioplasty.

balloon, trial *See* trial balloon.

bandage **1.** A strip or roll of gauze or other material for wrapping or binding a part of the body. **2.** To cover a part of the body by wrapping with a strip of gauze or other material.

Bangladesh Medical Association of North America (BMA) A national organization founded in 1982 composed of 200 physicians from Bangladesh or physicians who have graduated from a medical college in Bangladesh. It assists medical students and physicians in obtaining specialized medical training and postgraduate job placement in North America. *See also* medical association.

bank **1.** A business establishment in which money is kept for saving or commercial purposes or is invested, supplied for loans, or exchanged. *See also* bank credit. **2.** In medicine, a stored supply of human material or tissues for future use, as in blood, bone, eye, human-milk, skin, or sperm banks. *See also* blood bank; cryobank; organ bank; ova banking; sperm banking; tissue bank.

Bank Association of America, Eye *See* Eye Bank Association of America.

bank, blood *See* blood bank.

bank, commercial blood *See* commercial blood bank.

bank, community blood *See* community blood bank.

bank credit A written promise by a bank that an organization or person may borrow up to a specified amount. *See also* bank.

bank, cryo- *See* cryobank.

banking, blood *See* blood banking.

banking, ova *See* ova banking.

banking, sperm *See* sperm banking.

banking, zygote *See* zygote banking.

Bank, Living *See* The Living Bank.

Bank, National Practitioner Data *See* National Practitioner Data Bank.

bank, organ *See* organ bank.

bankrupt **1.** A legal state of insolvency in which all assets of an individual or an organization are put in the hands of a court-supervised trustee who proportionately pays debts to creditors. *See also* asset.

2. Complete lack of a specified resource or quality, as in an individual who is morally bankrupt.

Banks, American Association of Blood *See* American Association of Blood Banks.

Banks, American Association of Tissue *See* American Association of Tissue Banks.

Bank for Sight Restoration, Eye- *See* Eye-Bank for Sight Restoration.

Bank, The Living *See* The Living Bank.

bank, tissue *See* tissue bank.

BAPHR *See* Bay Area Physicians for Human Rights.

Baptist Homes and Hospitals Association, American *See* American Baptist Homes and Hospitals Association.

Baptist Hospital Association (BHA) A national organization founded in 1975 composed of four Baptist or Baptist-oriented hospitals. It assists member hospitals in their growth, development, and accreditation by exchange of information, ideas, and experiences. *See also* hospital.

bar **1.** In law, attorneys considered as a group, as in the American Bar Association. *See also* attorney; lawyer. **2.** The profession of law. *See also* law.

Bar Association, American *See* American Bar Association.

Bar Association, Federal *See* Federal Bar Association.

Bar Association, Hispanic National *See* Hispanic National Bar Association.

Bar Association, National *See* National Bar Association.

bar chart *See* bar graph.

bar code Computer-readable product labels used in electronic inventory maintenance, invoicing, and pricing; for example, bar coding is used to identify many materials coming into, or generated within, hospitals, such as laboratory specimens, medical records, and x-rays. *See also* Health Industry Business Communications Council.

bargain The process between two or more parties of determining obligations that each party promises to carry out, as in when something is bought, sold, exchanged, or agreed upon.

bar graph A pictorial display of sets of rectangles, each rectangle being identified with a particular classification of data and the height of the rectangle representing a data value for that classification. *See also* graph; grouped bar graph; histogram; stacked bar graph.

bar graph, grouped *See* grouped bar graph.

bar graph, stacked *See* stacked bar graph.

barbiturate A class of sedative-hypnotic agents, classified into long-acting, intermediate-acting, short-acting, and ultrashort-acting groups. The ultrashort-acting barbiturates, such as thiopental, are often used as intravenous anesthetics. The long-acting barbiturate phenobarbital is used as an anticonvulsant in the treatment of epilepsy. The benzodiazepines have replaced the barbiturates for most uses. Some barbiturates have a high potential for abuse and are, therefore, schedule II controlled substances. *See also* benzodiazepines; controlled substances; depressants; intravenous anesthetic; schedule II substances.

Bariatric Physicians, American Society of *See* American Society of Bariatric Physicians.

bariatrics The branch of medicine dealing with the causes, prevention, and treatment of obesity. *See also* obesity.

barium A metallic element whose compounds are poisonous and not used in modern medicine. Barium sulphate, however, is a white insoluble powder that in suspension provides a contrast medium for radiography of the digestive tract. *See also* barium enema; radiology.

barium enema (BaE, BE) A suspension of barium sulphate administered as a enema and retained in the intestines during x-ray examination. The column of radiopaque barium may reveal the presence of filling defects or deformities of the intestine produced by cancer or other abnormalities. *Synonym*: contrast enema. *See also* barium; contrast medium; enema; GI series; intestine; radiology; radiopaque.

Baromedical Nurses Association (BNA) A national organization founded in 1985 composed of 160 registered nurses practicing baromedicine (hyperbaric medicine), involved in research relating to baromedical nursing, completing basic orientation in baromedicine, or contributing to literature on baromedicine or baromedical nursing. It defines, develops, and promotes the standards of baromedical nursing. *See also* hyperbaric medicine; registered nurse; standard.

baromedicine *See* hyperbaric medicine.

barrier Something that separates, holds apart, or obstructs, as in inability to perform sign language acting as a barrier to communication between a hearing-impaired patient and practitioner.

barrister An English lawyer who is specially trained and appears exclusively as a trial lawyer in higher courts. He is retained by a solicitor, not directly by the client. There is no equivalent term in the United States. *See also* lawyer; solicitor.

basal metabolic rate (BMR) The minimum rate of energy expenditure required by the body under resting (basal) conditions in order to maintain essential functions, such as circulation, respiration, and thermogenesis. *See also* metabolism; rate; respiration; thermogenesis.

Baseball Physicians, Association of Professional *See* Association of Professional Baseball Physicians.

base capitation The stipulated dollar amount to cover the cost of health services, less mental health/substance abuse services, pharmacy, and administrative charges. *See also* capitation.

base, knowledge *See* knowledge base.

baseline An observation or value that represents the current background level of a measurable quantity, as in baseline mammography or a baseline rate (expressed as number of procedures per patient per pregnancy) for performance of ultrasonography during pregnancy. The baseline rate is used for comparison with values representing responses to experimental intervention or an environmental stimulus, usually implying that the baseline and response values refer to the same individual or system.

Baseline An on-line statistical-reporting system and service provided by the Commission on Professional and Hospital Activities. This computer-based service provides demographic data on a local, state, regional, or national basis and includes a marketing module that provides a subscribing hospital with information on the hospitals in the region, population demographic data by zip code and census track, and health care utilization statistics, including average charges for hospital services. *See also* Commission on Professional and Hospital Activities.

base pay *See* base salary.

base period The amount of time that an employee must work before becoming eligible for certain employment benefits. *See also* benefits; employee.

base salary Earnings before the addition of overtime, bonuses, or premium pay. *Synonym*: base pay. *See also* salary.

base year, hospital *See* hospital base year.

base year Medicare costs A hospital's costs for the base year from which computations are made in the Medicare payment formula. The base year is, by definition, always several years behind the present. *See also* Forms 1007 and 1008; hospital base year; Medicare.

BASIC *See* Beginners' All-purpose Symbolic Instruction Code.

basic benefits package *See* basic health services.

basic cardiac life support (BCLS) The phase of emergency cardiac care that either prevents circulatory or respiratory arrest or insufficiency through prompt recognition and intervention or externally supports the circulation and ventilation of a victim of cardiac or respiratory arrest through cardiopulmonary resuscitation (CPR). Health professionals and the public may be trained and certified in basic life support techniques and principles. *See also* advanced cardiac life support; BLS unit; cardiopulmonary resuscitation; certification; emergency medical technician.

basic health coverage *See* basic health services.

basic health services A minimum set of health services that should be generally and uniformly available in order to provide adequate health protection of the population from disease or to meet some other criteria or standards. For example, basic health services might include physician visits, drugs, hospital expenses, dental services, and mental health care. There is much debate on what set of services constitutes an appropriate minimum of basic health services and how to ensure availability of the services. *Compare* optional services. *See also* availability; comprehensive benefit package; health services.

basic trauma life support (BTLS) A training course developed in 1982 for emergency medical technicians to improve the prehospital management of trauma patients. Modern trauma training teaches rapid primary assessment, extrication, packaging, and immediate transport of the critical trauma patient. *See also* advanced trauma life support; emergency medical technician-paramedic; golden hour; load and go; trauma.

bassinet A hospital bed regularly maintained for infants newly born in a hospital. *Synonym*: newborn bed. *See also* bed; hospital.

batch processing The manual or computerized grouping and processing of similar data in a single operational sequence, as in batch processing of health insurance claims. *See also* data.

bath A conductive or convective medium, such as water, vapor, sand, or mud, with which the body is cleansed or in which the body is wholly or partly immersed for therapeutic or cleansing purposes. *See also* paraffin bath; sitz bath; sponge bath.

bath, paraffin *See* paraffin bath.

bath, sitz *See* sitz bath.

bath, sponge *See* sponge bath.

battered child syndrome Unexplained or inappropriately explained physical trauma and other manifestations of severe, repeated physical abuse of children, usually by a parent. *See also* child abuse; syndrome.

battery **1.** Any set, series, or grouping of similar things, as in a battery of blood tests. **2.** A nonconsensual touching; the unlawful application of force to another person. For example, a battery occurs when, in the absence of an emergency or other legally justifiable reason, a patient is treated without consent. *See also* consent; informed consent.

baud In computer science, the number of signals sent and received per second; a measure of the flow speed of computer data over telecommunications lines. *See also* computer.

bay, sick *See* sick bay.

Bay Area Cryonics Society *See* American Cryonics Society.

Bay Area Physicians for Human Rights (BAPHR) An organization founded in 1977 composed of 350 graduates of and students in approved schools of medicine and osteopathic medicine, dentistry, and podiatry interested in improving the quality of medical care for gay and lesbian patients and educating the public about health care needs of the homosexual. It maintains liaison with public officials about gay and lesbian health concerns and offers support to gay and lesbian physicians through social functions and consciousness-raising groups. *See also* gay; human rights; homosexuality; lesbianism.

BC *See* Blue Cross; board certified.

BCAC *See* Breast Cancer Advisory Center.

BCBSA *See* Blue Cross and Blue Shield Association.

BC/BS plan *See* Blue Cross/Blue Shield plan.

B cell *See* lymphocyte.

BCHCM *See* Board of Certified Hazard Control Management.

BCLS *See* basic cardiac life support.

B complex *See* vitamin B complex.

BCP *See* Board of Certification in Pedorthics.

BCSP *See* Board of Certified Safety Professionals.

BDCGS *See* Birth Defect and Clinical Genetic Society.

BE *See* barium enema.

beam radiation A type of radiation therapy in which treatment is given with x-ray, cobalt linear accelerator, neutron beam, betatron, or spray radiation, regardless of the source of the radiation. *See also* radiation; radiation therapy.

beat A throb or pulsation, as of the heart (heartbeat) or of an artery. *Synonym:* pulse.

bed **1.** A supporting structure (such as a piece of furniture for reclining and sleeping). *See also* water bed. **2.** An accommodation for a single person at a hospital or other type of health care organization. Beds are often used as a measure of organizational capacity and size. Licenses and certificates-of-need may be granted for specific numbers or types of beds. *See also* adult inpatient bed; constructed beds; day bed; hospital bed; incubator bed; isolation bed; licensed beds; night bed; outpatient bed; pediatric inpatient bed; regularly maintained beds; resident bed; specialty bed; swing bed; temporary bed.

bed, adult inpatient *See* adult inpatient bed.

bed conversion The conversion of a bed allocated for one type of care to a bed allocated for another type of care, as in converting an acute-care bed to a long term care bed. *See also* swing bed.

bed count The total number of beds regularly maintained by a health care organization for inpatients. Adult inpatient bed count, pediatric inpatient bed count, and newborn bed count are the total number of beds regularly maintained for adult inpatients, pediatric patients, and newborn patients, respectively. *Synonym:* bed size. *See also* occupancy.

bed, day *See* day bed.

bed, hospital *See* hospital bed.

bed, incubator *See* incubator bed.

bed, isolation *See* isolation bed.

bed, night *See* night bed.

bed, outpatient *See* outpatient bed.

bed pan A vessel for receiving the urinary and fecal discharges of a patient confined to bed.

bed, pediatric inpatient *See* pediatric inpatient bed.

bed, resident *See* resident bed.

beds, constructed *See* constructed beds.

bed, sick *See* sick bed.

bedside Literally, at the side of a patient's bed, or in a patient's presence, as in bedside diagnosis. *See also* bedside diagnosis; chairside; sick bed.

bedside diagnosis Making a determination of a patient's disease or condition by taking a medical history and performing physical examination in the patient's presence and yielding immediate conclusions. *Synonym*: office diagnosis. *See also* diagnosis; medical history; physical examination.

bed size *See* bed count.

beds, licensed *See* licensed beds.

bed sore *See* pressure sore.

bed, specialty *See* specialty bed.

beds, regularly maintained *See* regularly maintained beds.

bed, swing *See* swing bed.

bed, temporary *See* temporary bed.

bed turnover rate The average number of times over a given period that there is a change of occupant of a bed regularly maintained by a health care organization. *See also* bed; rate.

bed, water *See* water bed.

before-after trial In research, a clinical trial in which therapeutic alternatives are investigated in individuals of one period and under one treatment and then are compared with individuals at a subsequent time, treated in a different fashion. If the disorder being treated is not fatal and the "before" treatment is not curative, the same individuals may be studied in the before and after periods, strengthening the design through increased group comparability for the two periods. *See also* clinical trial; crossover trial; trial.

Beginners' All-purpose Symbolic Instruction Code (BASIC) A widely used, introductory, symbolic programming language for computer applications, often employed with remote or time-sharing computer centers. *See also* computer.

behavior The manner in which one acts; the actions or reactions of persons or things in response to external or internal stimuli. *See also* behavioral epidemic; behavioral medicine; behavioral norms; behavioral science; behavior modification; behavior therapy; organizational behavior; reinforcement.

Behavioral Disorders, Council for Children with *See* Council for Children with Behavioral Disorders.

behavioral epidemic A widespread occurrence originating in behavioral patterns as opposed to invading microorganisms or physical agents. Examples include the dancing manias of the Middle Ages, episodes of mass fainting or convulsions, crowd panic, or waves of fashion or enthusiasm. The communicable nature of the behavior is dependent not only on person-to-person transmission of the behavioral pattern but also on group reinforcements (as with tobacco, alcohol, or drug use). Behavioral epidemics may be difficult to differentiate from, or may complicate, outbreaks of organic disease, for example, due to contamination of the environment by a toxic substance. *See also* behavior; epidemic; tarantism.

behavioral medicine The application of behavior therapy techniques, such as biofeedback, relaxation training, and hypnosis, to the prevention and treatment of medical and psychosomatic disorders and to the treatment of undesirable behaviors, such as overeating and substance abuse. *See also* behavior therapy; biofeedback; hypnosis; psychosomatic illness; substance abuse.

Behavioral Medicine Research, Academy of *See* Academy of Behavioral Medicine Research.

Behavioral Medicine, Society of *See* Society of Behavioral Medicine.

Behavioral Neuropsychology Special Interest Group (BNSIG) A national organization founded in 1978 composed of 250 neuropsychologists involved in behavior therapy. It conducts research on implications for behavior therapy or neuropsychology. It is a special interest group of the Association for the Advancement of Behavior Therapy. *See also* Association for the Advancement of Behavior Therapy; psychology.

behavioral norms Socially enforced requirements and expectations about basic responsibilities and behaviors of individuals in groups of all sizes and complexity. A *pivotal norm* is one to which adherence is a requirement of continued membership in the group. A *peripheral norm* is considered desirable, but adherence to it is not essential to continued membership in the organization. *See also* behavior; norm.

Behavioral Pediatrics, Society for *See* Society for Behavioral Pediatrics.

Behavioral Pharmacology Society (BPS) A national organization founded in 1957 composed of 200 professional psychologists and pharmacologists interested in behavioral pharmacology and psychopharmacology or the connection between drugs and behavior. *See also* behavioral medicine; pharmacology.

Behavioral, Psychological and Cognitive Sciences, Federation of *See* Federation of Behavioral, Psychological and Cognitive Sciences.

behavioral science A scientific discipline, such as sociology, anthropology, or psychology, in which the actions and reactions of human beings and animals are studied through observational and experimental methods. *See also* behavior; science.

Behavioral Sciences, American Institutes for Research in the *See* American Institutes for Research in the Behavioral Sciences.

Behavioral Therapists, American Association of *See* American Association of Behavioral Therapists.

Behavioral Treatment of Sexual Abusers, Association for the *See* Association for the Behavioral Treatment of Sexual Abusers.

Behavior Analysis, Association for *See* Association for Behavior Analysis.

Behavior Genetics Association (BGA) A national organization founded in 1971 composed of individuals engaged in teaching or research in some area of behavior genetics. Its objectives include encouraging and aiding the education and training of research workers in the field of behavior genetics and the aiding in public dissemination and interpretation of information concerning the interrelationship of genetics and behavior and its implications for health, human development, and education. *See also* behavior; human genetics.

behavior, health *See* health behavior.

Behavior, Institute for the Advancement of Human *See* Institute for the Advancement of Human Behavior.

behavior modification The use of basic learning techniques, such as conditioning, biofeedback, reinforcement, or aversion therapy, to manage and improve human behavior. *See also* behavior; behavioral medicine; biofeedback; operant conditioning; sex therapy.

behavior, organizational *See* organizational behavior.

Behavior Resources, Institutes for *See* Institutes for Behavior Resources.

Behaviors, Society of Psychologists in Addictive *See* Society of Psychologists in Addictive Behaviors.

behavior therapy A form of psychotherapy that uses basic learning techniques to modify maladaptive behavior patterns by substituting new responses to given stimuli for undesirable ones. *See also* behavioral medicine; operant conditioning; psy-

chotherapy.

Behavior Therapy, Association for Advancement of *See* Association for Advancement of Behavior Therapy.

belief Mental acceptance of something as true, especially a tenet or a body of tenets accepted by a group. *See also* myth; taboo; tenet.

belief model, health *See* health belief model.

bell-shaped curve *See* normal distribution.

belly *See* abdomen.

BEMI *See* Bio-Electro-Magnetics Institute.

BEMS *See* Bioelectromagnetics Society.

benchmark **1.** A point of reference or standard by which something can be measured, compared, or judged, as in benchmarks of performance. *See also* compare; measure. **2.** A standard unit for the basis of comparison, that is, a universal unit that is identified with sufficient detail so that other similar classifications can be compared as being above, below, or comparable to the benchmark. *See also* benchmarking; gold standard; standard; yardstick.

benchmarking A process of measuring another organization's product or service according to specified standards in order to compare it with and improve one's own product or service. *Internal benchmarking* occurs within the same organization. *External benchmarking* occurs outside of the organization with another organization that produces the same product or provides the same service. *Functional benchmarking* refers to benchmarking a similar function or process, such as scheduling, in another industry. *See also* benchmark; measure; standard.

benchmarking, external *See* benchmarking.

benchmarking, functional *See* benchmarking.

benchmarking, internal *See* benchmarking.

beneficence The state or quality of being charitable or producing favorable effects. For example, beneficence towards patients can be defined as preventing harm to them, benefiting them, and, if harm is unavoidable, to make certain the harm is substantially outweighed by the benefit. *See also* benefit; duty; implied consent; paternalism.

beneficial occupancy permit A permit issued by building departments of municipalities or states allowing owners to take possession of a building at the completion of construction. Issuance of the permit generally signifies that the building meets applicable law and regulation. *See also* permit.

beneficiary A person who is eligible to receive, or is

receiving, benefits from an insurance policy or other health care financing program, such as Medicare or a health maintenance organization. *See also* benefits; insurance; insured; voucher system.

benefit Something that promotes or enhances well-being, as in fringe benefit. *See also* benefit-cost ratio; benefits; hospice benefit; marginal benefit; net social benefit; perquisite; risk benefit analysis.

benefit analysis, risk- *See* risk-benefit analysis.

benefit-cost ratio The ratio of net present value of measurable benefits to costs. Calculation of a benefit-cost ratio is used, for example, to determine the economic feasibility of success of a program. *See also* benefit; cost; ratio.

benefit, fringe *See* perquisite.

benefit, hospice *See* hospice benefit.

benefit, marginal *See* marginal benefit.

benefit, net social *See* net social benefit.

benefit package, comprehensive *See* comprehensive benefit package.

benefit plan, employee health *See* employee health benefit plan.

benefit plan, incentive *See* incentive benefit plan.

benefit program, employee *See* employee benefit program.

benefits In insurance, the money, care, or other services to which an individual is entitled by virtue of insurance. In health care insurance, there are two major kinds of benefits: indemnity benefits and service benefits. *See also* comprehensive benefit package; coordination of benefits; duplication of benefits; extended benefits; hospital benefits; indemnity benefits; maternity benefits; service benefits.

benefits, coordination of *See* coordination of benefits.

benefits, duplication of *See* duplication of benefits.

benefits, explanation of *See* explanation of benefits.

Benefits, Explanation of Medicare *See* Explanation of Medicare Benefits.

benefits, extended *See* extended benefits.

benefits, hospital *See* hospital benefits.

benefits, indemnity *See* indemnity benefits.

benefits, maternity *See* maternity benefits.

benefits, service *See* service benefits.

benevolence A moral value characterized by a person behaving toward other persons in a kindly way that is not menacing or harmful. *See also* morals.

benign Favorable for recovery as in a benign tumor or benign prostatic hypertrophy; not malignant, recurrent, or progressive. *Compare* malignant. *See*

also benign prostatic hypertrophy.

benign prostatic hypertrophy (BPH) A benign tumor of the prostate gland, which originates from the prostate tissue surrounding the urethra. Symptoms are related to mechanical obstruction, including diminished forcefulness and projection of the urinary stream, nocturia, hematuria, infection, and acute retention of urine. *See also* hematuria; nocturia; prostate.

benzodiazepine Any of a group of tranquilizers, including diazepam (*Valium*), having a common molecular structure and similar pharmacological activities, such as antianxiety, muscle-relaxing, sedative, and hypnotic effects. *See also* controlled substances; schedule IV substances.

Bernoulli distribution *See* binomial distribution.

best-before date A date marked on a food package to show the latest time by which the contents can be used without risk of deterioration. *See also* open date; pack date.

best interest In health care, regard for one's own benefit or advantage, or regard for the welfare of a patient, as in surrogate decision making when factors, such as the quality of life and the extent of life sustained, are taken into consideration in the patient's best interest.

beta error *See* type II error.

BGA *See* Behavior Genetics Association.

BHA *See* Baptist Hospital Association.

BHI *See* Bureau of Health Insurance.

bias **1.** A preference or inclination that inhibits impartial judgment. *See also* slant. **2.** In any measurement process, systematic errors in data or deviation from the truth, resulting from the methods, tools, or environment of the data collection and processing. There are many kinds of bias including, but not limited to, interviewer bias, measurement bias, observer bias, bias in the presentation of data, bias in publication, recall bias, reporting bias, response bias, sampling bias, and selection bias. Three strategies of eliminating conscious and unconscious bias in both subjects (subject bias) and investigators (observer bias) include the single-blind technique, double-blind technique, triple-blind technique, and use of a placebo. Bias is distinguished from random error. *See also* double-blind technique; placebo; placebo effect; random error; selection bias; single-blind technique; triple-blind study.

bid Abbreviation for Latin phrase *bis in di'e*, meaning "twice a day."

bilateral Having two sides, or pertaining to both sides, as in bilateral scalp hematomas. *Compare* medial; lateral; unilateral.

bile A viscous, dark yellow, alkaline secretion of the liver in humans used in the digestion of fats and the absorption of the fat-soluble vitamins A, D, and K. The major constituents of bile are cholesterol, bile salts, bile pigments, other waste products, and electrolytes. The bile is secreted into the duodenum via the common bile duct after storage between meals in the gallbladder, in which it is concentrated by reabsorption of water. *See also* gallbladder; gastroenterology; vitamin A; vitamin D; vitamin K.

biliary tract surgery Surgery involving the bile-conveying structures: the duodenum, gallbladder, and liver. *See also* bile; duodenum; gallbladder; liver; surgery.

bilirubin Bile pigment that can cause jaundice when normal bile excretion from the liver to the intestine is blocked. *See also* jaundice; kernicterus; liver.

bill **1.** An order drawn by a person or an organization on another person or organization to pay a certain sum of money, as in a health care provider sending a bill to a patient or a third-party payer for services provided. *See also* invoice. **2.** A document or notice containing a formal statement of a matter, as in a bill of patient rights. *See also* bill of patient rights.

billing The process of formally notifying recipients of services or goods of an amount of money due. *Synonym:* invoicing. *See also* balance billing; bill; billing cycle; invoice; third-party billing.

billing, balance *See* balance billing.

billing cycle The interval between periodic billings for goods sold or services rendered, normally one month, or a system whereby bills or statements are mailed at periodic intervals in the course of a month in order to distribute the clerical workload evenly. *See also* billing; cycle.

Billing System, National Uniform *See* National Uniform Billing System.

billing, third-party *See* third-party billing.

bill of patient rights A statement of ethical and legal principles adopted by a health care organization to regulate its operational policies and procedures, operations staff, professional staff, and volunteers in a manner that recognizes and obligates the organization to protect and promote the human dignity and rights of patients. *See also* a bill; patient rights.

bimanual Performed with both hands, as in a bimanual pelvic examination. *See also* pelvic examination.

bimodal distribution A distribution with two regions of high frequency separated by a region of low frequency of observations; a two-peak distribution. *See also* distribution.

binding Obligatory, as used in statute; for example, binding arbitration. *See also* binding arbitration.

binding arbitration Arbitration in which the parties agree to be bound by the determination of the arbitrator. *Synonym:* compulsory arbitration. *See also* arbitrator; arbitration; binding.

binomial distribution A probability distribution associated with two mutually exclusive outcomes, for example, death and survival. The binomial distribution is used to model prevalence rates and cumulative incidence rates. *Synonym:* Bernouilli distribution. *See also* distribution; probability distribution.

Bioanalysis, American Board of *See* American Board of Bioanalysis.

Bioanalysts, American Association of *See* American Association of Bioanalysts.

bioassay The measurement of the strength or concentration of a drug or other biologically active substance by comparing its effect on an organism, organ, or tissue with that of a standard preparation. *Synonym:* biological assay. *See also* assay; pregnancy test.

bioavailability In pharmacology, the relative amount of, and rate at which, a medication dose reaches the systemic circulation in a therapeutically active form after administration. *See also* bioequivalence; pharmacology.

biochemist An individual who specializes in the study of the chemistry of living organisms and life processes for clinical or research purposes. *Synonyms:* biological chemist; physiological chemist. *See also* biochemistry.

biochemistry The study in living organisms of chemical substances and vital processes including metabolism, biological oxidation and bioenergetics, enzymes, proteins, nucleic acids, and protein biosynthesis. *See also* chemistry; enzyme; metabolism.

Biochemistry and Molecular Biology, American Society for *See* American Society for Biochemistry and Molecular Biology.

Bioelectrical Repair and Growth Society (BRAGS) A national organization founded in 1980 composed of 300 medical professionals, engineers, biological and physical scientists, and representatives of industry interested in furthering research, communication, cooperation, and education in the study and clinical applications of the effects of electricity and magnetism in growth, repair, and regeneration of human cells and tissues.

Bio-Electro-Magnetics Institute (BEMI) A national organization founded in 1986 composed of 450 medical professionals, alternative health practitioners, and other individuals interested in the study of the relationship between living organisms and electromagnetic fields and radiation. It promotes the fields of energy field medicine and bioenergetics.

Bioelectromagnetics Society (BEMS) A national organization founded in 1978 composed of 700 scientists, engineers, and other individuals who conduct research in or are interested in the interaction of electromagnetic energy and acoustic energy with biological systems.

bioengineer An individual who applies engineering principles to the fields of biology and medicine, as in the development of aids or replacements for defective or missing body organs and the development of instrumentation for diagnosis, treatment, and monitoring of physiological conditions. *Synonyms*: biomedical engineer; medical engineer. *See also* engineer; engineering.

bioengineering The application of engineering principles to the fields of biology and medicine, as in the development of replacements for defective or missing body organs, or genetic engineering. *Synonym*: biomedical engineering. *See also* bioengineer.

bioequivalence In pharmacology, the degree to which two formulations of the same drug have equal bioavailability. *See also* bioavailability; chemical equivalence; pharmaceutical equivalence; pharmacology.

bioethics The study of the ethical and moral implications of new biological discoveries and biomedical advances, as in the fields of genetic engineering and drug research. *See also* biomedical ethics; ethics.

biofeedback A technique of providing an individual with information regarding one or more physiological variables, such as heart rate, blood pressure, or skin temperature, in an attempt to gain some voluntary control over that function. It may be used clinically to treat certain conditions, such as hypertension and migraine headache. *See also* behavioral

medicine; behavior modification.

Biofeedback, Association for Applied Psychophysiology and *See* Association for Applied Psychophysiology and Biofeedback.

Biofeedback Society of America *See* Association for Applied Psychophysiology and Biofeedback.

biohazard A biological agent, such as an infectious microorganism, or a condition that constitutes a threat to human beings, especially in biological research or experimentation. *See also* hazard.

bioinstrumentation Instruments, such as a thermometer, for the measurement, recording, and transmission of physiological information, such as body temperature. *See also* biosensor; clinical thermometer; instrument; thermometer.

biologic *See* biological.

biological Any virus, therapeutic serum, toxin, antitoxin, or analogous product of plant or animal origin used in the prevention, diagnosis, or treatment of disease. Biologicals, including vaccines and blood plasma products, are regulated by the Bureau of Biologics, a division of the Food and Drug Administration. They differ from drugs in that biologicals are usually derived from living microorganisms and cannot be synthesized or readily standardized by chemical or physical means. They tend to be chemically less stable than drugs, their safety cannot be as easily assured, and they are never as chemically pure as drugs. *Synonyms*: biologic; biological product. *Compare* drug; medication.

biological assay *See* bioassay.

biological chemist *See* biochemist.

biological clock An innate mechanism in living organisms that controls the periodicity or rhythm of various physiological functions or activities. *See also* clock.

biological half-life The rate of removal of a substance, such as a drug, by biological processes, such as excretion or metabolism. *See also* half-life.

Biological Photographic Association (BPA) A national organization founded in 1931 composed of 1,200 photographers, technicians, doctors, scientists, educators, and other individuals interested in photography in the health sciences and related fields. It seeks to advance the techniques of biophotography and biomedical communications through meetings, seminars, and workshops. It has established a Board of Registry to offer qualifying examinations for registered biological photographers.

biological response modifier therapy (BRM) A generic term that covers all chemical or biological agents that alter the immune system or change the host's response (defense mechanism) to a cancer, as in allogenic cells, bone marrow transplant, and interferon. *See also* immune system.

Biological Sciences, American Institute of *See* American Institute of Biological Sciences.

Biological Stain Commission (BSC) A national organization founded in 1922 composed of scientists in biology, medicine, and related fields working for the establishment of standards for the identification, purity, performance, and labeling of the more important biological stains, in order to improve their reliability as tools in biological research. It conducts a program of stain certification, in cooperation with manufacturers and distributors. *See also* Gram's stain; stain.

biological warfare The use of disease-producing microorganisms, toxic biological products, or organic biocides to cause death or injury to humans, animals, or plants.

biological waste *See* hazardous waste.

biology The scientific study of life and of living organisms, including their structure, function, growth, origin, evolution, and distribution. The two main branches of biology are botany and zoology. Further subdivisions include cytology, histology, morphology, physiology, embryology, ecology, genetics, and microbiology. Related subjects are biochemistry, biophysics, and biometrics. *See also* biochemistry; biometrics; biophysics; botany; cryobiology; embryology; genetics; histology; molecular biology; morphology; physiology; radiobiology; reproduction; sociobiology; teratology.

Biology, American Academy of Micro- *See* American Academy of Microbiology.

Biology, American Institute of Oral *See* American Institute of Oral Biology.

Biology, American Society for Cell *See* American Society for Cell Biology.

Biology, American Society for Micro- *See* American Society for Microbiology.

biology, chrono- *See* chronobiology.

Biology Council, Human *See* Human Biology Council.

biology, cryo- *See* cryobiology.

Biology and Medicine, Society for Experimental *See* Society for Experimental Biology and Medicine.

biology, molecular *See* molecular biology.

biology, radio- *See* radiobiology.

Biology (A Reticuloendothelial Society), Society for Leukocyte *See* Society for Leukocyte Biology (A Reticuloendothelial Society).

Biology, Society for Cryo- *See* Society for Cryobiology.

Biology, Society for Developmental *See* Society for Developmental Biology.

Biology, Society of Ethno- *See* Society of Ethnobiology.

Biology Society, IEEE Engineering in Medicine and *See* IEEE Engineering in Medicine and Biology Society.

Biology, Society for the Study of Social *See* Society for the Study of Social Biology.

biology, socio- *See* sociobiology.

Biomaterials, Society for *See* Society for Biomaterials.

biomechanics The study of the mechanics of a living body, especially of the forces exerted by muscles and gravity on the skeletal structure. *See also* bionic.

biomedical Pertaining to the application of the natural sciences, such as biology, biochemistry, and biophysics, to the study of medicine. *See also* biochemistry; biology; biomedicine; biophysics.

Biomedical Communications Associations, Council for *See* Council for Biomedical Communications Associations.

Biomedical Computing, Special Interest Group on *See* Special Interest Group on Biomedical Computing.

biomedical engineer *See* bioengineer.

biomedical engineering *See* bioengineering.

biomedical engineering department *See* clinical engineering department.

Biomedical Engineering Society (BMES) A national organization founded in 1968 composed of 1,600 engineers, physicians, managers, and university professors representing all fields of biomedical engineering. *See also* bioengineer.

Biomedical Equipment Technicians, Society of *See* Society of Biomedical Equipment Technicians.

biomedical ethics A branch of ethics dealing with the practice of medicine and biomedical research. *See also* bioethics; biomedical; ethics.

Biomedical Marketing Association (BMA) A national organization composed of 700 diagnostic marketers in the biomedical field. It conducts research and educational seminars, presents awards, and compiles statistics. *See also* biomedical; marketing.

Biomedical Research, National Association for *See* National Association for Biomedical Research.

biomedicine **1.** The field of medical science dealing with the ability of human beings to tolerate environmental stresses and variations, as in space travel. **2.** The application of the principles of the natural sciences, especially biology and physiology, to clinical medicine.

biometrics The science of the application of statistical methods to the analysis of biological data; the quantitative measurement of biological facts, especially with respect to variation. *Synonym*: biometry. *See also* statistics.

Biometric Society (IBS) A national organization founded in 1947 composed of 6,800 biologists, statisticians, and other individuals interested in applying statistical techniques to biological research data. *See also* biometrics.

bionic Having anatomical structures or physiological processes that are replaced or enhanced by electronic or mechanical components. *See also* biomechanics; bionics.

Bionic Rehabilitative Psychology, American Board of *See* American Board of Bionic Rehabilitative Psychology.

bionics The application of biological principles to the study and design of engineering systems, especially electronic systems. *See also* bionic.

biophysics The branch of biology that applies the laws of physics to the explanation of biological phenomena. *See also* biology; physics.

biopsy The removal and examination, usually microscopic, of tissue from a living body, performed to establish precise diagnosis. Abbreviated bx. *Synonym*: tissue sample. *See also* aspiration biopsy; needle biopsy.

biopsy, aspiration *See* aspiration biopsy.

biopsy, needle *See* needle biopsy.

biosensor A device that detects, records, and transmits information regarding a physiological change or process. *See also* bioinstrumentation.

Biosocial Research, Huxley Institute for *See* Huxley Institute for Biosocial Research.

biostatistician An individual specializing in the application of mathematics and statistics to health care research, planning, and services. *Synonym*: health statistician. *See also* biostatistics; statistics.

biostatistics Application of statistics to the analysis of biological and medical problems. *See also* biostatistician; statistics.

biotechnology The branch of technology concerned with the use of living organisms (usually microorganisms) in industrial, medical, and other scientific processes. Applications include the production of certain drugs, synthetic hormones, and bulk foodstuffs as well as the bioconversion of organic waste and the use of genetically altered bacteria in the cleanup of oil spills. *See also* recombinant DNA; technology.

biotelemetry The monitoring, recording, and measuring of a living organism's basic physiological functions, such as heart rate, muscle activity, and body temperature, by the use of telemetry techniques. *See also* telemetry.

bipolar disorder *See* manic-depressive illness.

bipolar illness *See* manic-depressive illness.

birth The emergence and separation of offspring from the body of the mother. *See also* active birth; delivery; extramural birth; labor; live birth; natural childbirth; posthumous birth; premature birth; wrongful birth.

birth, active *See* active birth.

birth after cesarean section, vaginal *See* vaginal birth after cesarean section.

birth certificate A legal document recording details of a live birth, usually comprising name, date, place, identity of parents, and sometimes additional information, such as birth weight. It provides the basis for vital statistics of birth and birthrates in a political or administrative jurisdiction and for the denominator for infant mortality and certain other vital rates. *Compare* death certificate. *See also* certificate; vital statistics.

birth control Artificial measures taken to prevent conception, especially by planned use of contraceptive techniques. *See also* conception; contraception; family planning.

birth control pill *See* oral contraceptive.

Birth Defect and Clinical Genetic Society (BDCGS) A national organization founded in 1980 composed of 275 physicians and dentists whose practices involve caring for children with birth defects or providing genetic counseling. Its goals are to educate health professionals, governmental agencies, insurance, providers, and the public on the significance of genetic and dysmorphological research. Formerly

(1985) American Society of Clinical Genetics and Dysmorphology. *See also* clinical genetics; deformity.

birth, extramural   *See* extramural birth.

birthing center   A freestanding or hospital-based facility that provides prenatal, childbirth, and post-natal care, often incorporating family-centered maternity care concepts and practices. It is typically designed to provide a comfortable, homelike setting during childbirth and is generally less restrictive than a hospital in its regulations, as in permitting midwifery or allowing family members or friends to attend the delivery. *Synonym*: childbirth center. *See also* birth; birthing room.

birthing room   An area of a hospital or outpatient medical facility equipped for labor, delivery, and recovery and designed as a natural, homelike environment. *Compare* labor room. *See also* birthing center.

birth, live   *See* live birth.

birth mark   Visible congenital marks on the skin.

birth mother   Biological mother. *See also* noncoital reproduction.

birth, posthumous   *See* posthumous birth.

birth, premature   *See* premature birth.

Birth Psychology, Association for   *See* Association for Birth Psychology.

birth rate   A summary rate based on the number of live births in a population over a given period, usually a year; for example, the number of live births per 1,000 persons per year. *See also* birth; live birth; rate.

birth trauma   An injury to the infant received in or due to the process of being born, as in brachial plexus injury. *See also* injury.

birth weight   Infant's weight recorded at the time of birth. Certain variants of birth weight are precisely defined. Low birth weight, for example, is below 2500 grams; very low birth weight is below 1500 grams; ultralow birth weight is below 1000 grams. Large for gestational age is birth weight above the 90th percentile; average weight for gestational age is birth weight between 10th and 90th percentiles; and small for gestational age is a birth weight below 10th percentile. *See also* low birth weight; weight.

birth weight, low   *See* low birth weight.

birth, wrongful   *See* wrongful birth.

Bisexual Issues in Counseling, Association for Gay, Lesbian, and   *See* Association for Gay, Lesbian, and Bisexual Issues in Counseling.

bisexuality   **1.** Sexual attraction to persons of both sexes; exhibition of both homosexual and heterosexual behavior. **2.** True hermaphroditism (having gonads of both sexes in the same individual). *See also* heterosexuality; homosexuality; transsexuality.

Bisexual People in Medicine, Lesbian, Gay and   *See* Lesbian, Gay and Bisexual People in Medicine.

bit   In computer science, a single character of a language having just two characters, as either of the binary digits 0 or 1. It is the smallest unit of information that can be stored by a computer. A byte, by contrast, is a group of adjacent bits and the most common byte contains eight bits. A byte represents a single character or the amount of information that a computer can handle with a single instruction. Examples of bytes include a letter, space, numeral, or punctuation mark. *See also* byte; contrast resolution; field; megabit; parity.

bite, sound   *See* sound bite.

bit, mega-   *See* megabit.

Black Alcoholism Council, National   *See* National Black Alcoholism Council.

black box method   A method of reasoning or studying a problem in which the methods or procedures are not described, explained, or even understood. Nothing is stated or inferred about the method; discussion and conclusions relate solely to the empirical relationships observed. *See also* method; reasoning.

Black Cardiologists, Association of   *See* Association of Black Cardiologists.

Black Chiropractors Association, American   *See* American Black Chiropractors Association.

Black Lawyers, National Conference of   *See* National Conference of Black Lawyers.

black lung disease   Common name for anthracosis (a form of pneumoconiosis), a chronic lung disease caused by inhaling coal dust and found among coal miners. It is named after the black appearance of lung tissue among affected individuals. Certain medical benefits for victims of the disease are available under Title IV of the Federal Coal Mine Health and Safety Act of 1969. *See also* disease; pneumoconiosis.

Black Lung and Respiratory Disease Clinics, National Coalition of   *See* National Coalition of Black Lung and Respiratory Disease Clinics.

Black Nurses Association, National   *See* National Black Nurses Association.

Black Nursing Faculty in Higher Education, Association of   *See* Association of Black Nursing

Faculty in Higher Education.

blackout *See* syncope.

Black Psychiatrists of America (BPA) A national organization founded in 1968 composed of 550 black psychiatrists united to promote black behavioral science and foster high-quality psychiatric care for blacks and minority group members. *See also* minority; psychiatry.

Black Psychologists, Association of *See* Association of Black Psychologists.

Blacks in the Health Professions, National Center for the Advancement of *See* National Center for the Advancement of Blacks in the Health Professions.

Black Social Workers, National Association of *See* National Association of Black Social Workers.

Black Women Attorneys, National Association of *See* National Association of Black Women Attorneys.

Black Women's Health Project, National *See* National Black Women's Health Project.

blind Sightless. *See also* blindness.

Blind, Aid to the *See* Aid to the Blind.

blinded Unaware, as in clinicians or patients being blinded to the treatments that patients are receiving or observers being blinded to each other's assessments, making their observations uninfluenced by one another. *Synonym*: masked. *See also* blinded study.

blinded study A study in which observer(s) and/or subjects are kept ignorant of the group to which the subjects are assigned, as in an experiment. *See also* blinded; double-blind technique; single-blind technique; triple-blind study.

blindness Lack of sightedness, from whatever cause. *See also* ophthalmology; talking books.

Blind and Retarded, Association for Advancement of *See* Association for Advancement of Blind and Retarded.

blip A temporary movement in statistics (usually in an unexpected or unwelcome direction); hence any kind of temporary problem or hold-up. *See also* statistics.

blister A localized epidermal swelling containing clear fluid. *See also* epidermis; skin.

block, nerve *See* nerve block.

blood The fluid tissue present in the circulatory system of humans consisting of plasma, blood cells, and platelets that is circulated by the heart through the vertebrate vascular system carrying oxygen and nutrients to and waste materials away from all body tissues. *See also* blood bank; blood cell; blood compo-

nents; blood transfusion; blood typing; hemorrhage.

blood alcohol concentration The concentration of alcohol in the blood, expressed as the weight of alcohol in a fixed volume of blood and used as a measure of the degree of intoxication in an individual. The concentration depends on body weight, the quantity and the rate of alcohol ingestion, and the rates of alcohol absorption and metabolism. *See also* alcohol; breathalyzer test.

blood bank **1.** A store of donated blood for use in blood transfusion. **2.** A division of a health care organization responsible for collecting, processing, storing, and distributing blood to be used for transfusion by the same or other individuals. *See also* bank; blood banking; commercial blood bank; community blood bank; hospital blood bank.

blood bank, commercial *See* commercial blood bank.

blood bank, community *See* community blood bank.

blood bank, hospital *See* hospital blood bank.

blood banking The branch of medicine and medical specialty dealing with the maintenance of an adequate blood supply, blood donor and patient-recipient safety, and appropriate utilization of blood components. Blood banking specifically involves pretransfusion compatibility testing, highly specialized testing procedures for antibodies, and the preparation and safe use of specially prepared blood components, including red blood cells, white blood cells, platelets, and plasma constituents. *See also* antibodies; blood; blood bank; pathology.

blood banking specialist A pathologist who subspecializes in blood banking. A blood bank technologist, by contrast, is called a "specialist in blood bank technology." *See also* blood banking; pathology; specialist in blood bank technology.

Blood Banks, American Association of *See* American Association of Blood Banks.

blood bank technologist *See* specialist in blood bank technology.

blood bank technology, specialist in *See* specialist in blood bank technology.

blood/body fluid precautions A category of patient isolation that involves prevention of direct or indirect contact with infected blood or body fluids. A private room is indicated if the patient's hygiene is poor. Masks are not indicated, but gowns should be used if soiling of clothing with blood or body fluids is likely. Gloves should be used for touching blood or body fluids. *See also* isolation.

blood cell A formed element of the blood including red blood cells (erythrocytes), white blood cells (leukocytes), and platelets (thrombocytes). Together they normally constitute about 50% of the total volume of the blood. *See also* lymphocyte; platelet; red blood cell; white blood cell.

blood cell, red *See* red blood cell.

blood cell, white *See* white blood cell.

Blood Centers, Council of Community *See* Council of Community Blood Centers.

blood clot A semisolid, gelatinous mass of coagulated blood that consists of red blood cells, white blood cells, and platelets entrapped in a fibrin network. *See also* fibrin; platelet; red blood cell; streptokinase; thrombolysis; thrombosis; thrombus; urokinase; white blood cell.

Blood Club, National Rare *See* National Rare Blood Club.

blood coagulation *See* coagulation.

Blood Commission, American *See* American Blood Commission.

blood components The various parts of human blood, including, for example, red blood cells, white blood cells, platelets, and plasma. *See also* blood plasma; lymphocyte; platelet; red blood cell; white blood cell.

blood count The number of red blood cells, white blood cells, and platelets in a definite volume of blood. *Synonym*: complete blood count. *See also* hematocrit; hemocytometer.

blood count, complete *See* blood count.

blood culture A culture of microorganisms from specimens of blood to determine the presence and nature of bacteremia. *See also* bacteremia; blood; culture.

blood derivative A pooled blood product, such as albumin, gamma globulin, or Rh immune globulin, which usually carries a significantly lower risk of complications with use than blood or blood components.

blood distribution Issue, exchange, or sale by a blood bank of processed whole blood or blood components and derivatives. *See also* blood bank.

blood donor Volunteers who provide blood for blood transfusion. *See also* apheresis; donor; professional blood donor; replacement blood donor; voluntary blood donor.

blood donor, professional *See* professional blood donor.

blood donor, replacement *See* replacement blood donor.

blood donor, voluntary *See* voluntary blood donor.

blood gas determination An analysis of the pH and the concentration and pressure of oxygen, carbon dioxide, and hydrogen ions in the blood. It is used to assess acid-base balance and ventilatory status in a wide range of conditions, including cardiac failure, respiratory failure, and diabetic ketoacidosis. A blood gas determination may be performed on arterial or venous blood. *Synonym*: ABG; arterial blood gas. *See also* arterial blood gas; diabetic ketoacidosis.

blood glucose The concentration of glucose in the blood, measured in milligrams of glucose per deciliter of blood. *Synonym*: blood sugar. *See also* diabetes mellitus; glucose; hyperglycemia; hypoglycemia.

blood groups The classification of blood on the presence or absence of genetically determined antigens on the surface of the red blood cell. There are many grouping systems, including ABO, Duffy, Kell, and Rh. Their importance derives from their clinical significance in transfusion therapy, organ transplantation, disputed paternity cases, maternal-fetal compatibility, and genetic studies. ABO blood groups, the most important system for classifying blood, is identified by the presence or absence of two different antigens, A or B. The four blood types in this grouping are A, B, AB, and O; they are determined by and named for the A and B antigens. Type AB indicates the presence of both antigens; type O, the absence of both. *See also* blood transfusion; paternity test; Rh factor.

blood letting The therapeutic removal of a quantity of blood (phlebotomy). Once a panacea for many ills, it is now restricted to a small number of specific conditions, such as polycythemia. *Compare* blood transfusion. *See also* phlebotomy.

blood, occult *See* occult blood.

blood, outdated *See* outdated blood.

blood plasma Pale gray or gray-yellow fluid part of the blood that contains specific proteins for clotting the blood and in which blood cells and platelets are normally suspended. *See also* American Blood Resources Association; blood cell; platelet.

blood poisoning *See* bacteremia; septicemia.

blood pressure (BP) The pressure exerted by the blood against blood vessel walls, especially arteries, as it circulates. Systolic pressure reflects the maximum force (with the heart muscle contracted) and diastolic pressure reflects the minimum force (with the heart muscle relaxed). *See also* hypertension; hypotension; sphygmomanometer; vital signs.

blood processing Serological testing, grouping, and typing of whole blood for direct use and preparation of blood components and derivatives.

blood repository A facility for storage and distribution of whole blood and its components by arrangement with a blood bank. *See also* blood bank.

Blood Resources Association, American *See* American Blood Resources Association.

blood serum The clear liquid that separates from the blood when it is allowed to clot completely. It is therefore blood plasma from which clotting agents (fibrinogen) have been removed in the process of clotting. *See also* blood; blood plasma; serodiagnosis; serology.

Blood, Society for the Study of *See* Society for the Study of Blood.

blood sugar *See* blood glucose.

blood test An examination of a sample of blood to determine its chemical, physical, or serologic characteristics. *See also* blood; test.

blood transfusion The administration of blood, blood components, and/or blood products to replace blood lost through disease, trauma, or surgery. *Compare* blood letting; phlebotomy. *See also* autologous blood transfusion; autotransfusion; blood groups; hemophilia; Jehovah's Witness; major crossmatching; minor crossmatching; overtransfusion; packed cells; transfusion reaction.

blood transfusion, autologous *See* autologous blood transfusion.

blood transfusion services Organizational services relating to transfusing and infusing patients with blood, blood components, and/or blood products. *See also* blood transfusion.

blood typing Identification of genetically determined antigens on the surface of the red blood cell, used to determine a person's blood group. Typically a blood bank procedure, blood typing is the first step in testing donor's and recipient's blood to be used in blood transfusion and is followed by crossmatching. *See also* blood groups; crossmatching; transfusion reaction.

blood usage review A function that entails measuring, assessing, and improving performance relating to blood usage in health care organizations. *See also* blood; usage.

blood vessel A tube that carries blood, including arteries, arterioles, capillaries, veins, and venules. *See also* angiology; artery; capillary; vascular; vascular surgery; vein.

blood, whole *See* whole blood.

BLS Abbreviation for basic life support. *See* basic cardiac life support.

BLS unit An emergency ground vehicle usually staffed with 2 emergency medical technicians or an emergency medical technician and an emergency medical technician-paramedic capable of providing basic cardiac life support to patients in the prehospital phase of emergency care. A BLS unit is not stocked with intravenous fluids, cardiac monitor, defibrillation equipment, or certain medications. *Compare* ALS unit; mobile intensive care unit. *See also* ambulance; basic cardiac life support; emergency medical technician; emergency medical technician-paramedic.

blue babies Infants born with cyanotic congenital heart disease that causes their skin and mucous membranes to appear bluish. *See also* baby; cyanosis.

Blue Cross and Blue Shield Association (BCBSA) A national federation founded in 1982 composed of nonprofit health care prepayment insurance plans, developed and sponsored by hospitals and physicians, called Blue Cross (BC) and Blue Shield (BS) plans, respectively. These plans contract with hospitals and other health care providers to make payment for health care services to their subscribers. One important impetus for creation of the national association was to facilitate BC and BS plans entering into national contracts with large corporations having plants or offices in the areas of several autonomous BC and BS plans, each with differing policies and benefits. *See also* Blue Cross plan; Blue Shield plan; national account; not-for-profit carrier.

Blue Cross/Blue Shield (BC/BS) plan A nonprofit health care prepayment insurance plan originating with hospitals (Blue Cross) and physicians (Blue Shield). In many locales, the Blue Cross and Blue Shield plans have joined. Blue Cross and Blue Shield plans in the United States are linked by a national association known as the Blue Cross and Blue Shield Association (BCBSA). Most subscribers enroll at their place of employment in group plans. *See also* Blue Cross and Blue Shield Association; national account; not-for-profit carrier.

Blue Cross (BC) plan A nonprofit, tax-exempt hospital care prepayment insurance plan originally developed and sponsored by hospitals. A BC plan must be a nonprofit community service organization that has a governing body with a membership including a majority of public representatives. Many BC plans have linked with physician-sponsored Blue Shield (BS) plans. There are approximately 77 autonomous Blue Cross plans in the United States. When BC and BS plans are linked in a locale, they may be referred to as Blue Cross/Blue Shield (BC/BS) plans. *See also* Blue Cross/Blue Shield plan; Blue Shield plan; home plan; national account; not-for-profit carrier.

Blue Shield (BS) plan A nonprofit, tax-exempt physician care prepayment insurance plan originally developed and sponsored by physicians in 1939. Many BS plans have linked with hospital-sponsored Blue Cross (BC) plans. There are approximately 77 autonomous plans of each type in the United States typically governed by state statutes. When BS and BC plans are joined in a locale they may be referred to as Blue Cross/Blue Shield (BCBS) plans. *See also* Blue Cross/Blue Shield plan; Blue Cross plan; national account; not-for-profit carrier.

blunt trauma Trauma due to nonpenetrating force that may occur as a result of, for example, a crushing injury, a motor vehicle accident, a fall, or an assault with a blunt weapon. *See also* penetrating trauma; trauma.

BMA *See* Bangladesh Medical Association of North America; Biomedical Marketing Association.

BMES *See* Biomedical Engineering Society.

BMR *See* basal metabolic rate.

BNA *See* Baromedical Nurses Association; Bureau of National Affairs.

BNDD *See* Bureau of Narcotics and Dangerous Drugs.

BNDD number An outmoded term for the registration number assigned by the US Drug Enforcement Administration (DEA) to a physician, hospital, pharmacy, or other qualified "business activity." The BNDD number is now called the DEA registration number and authorizes the recipient to prescribe or dispense controlled substances. *See also* controlled substances; DEA number; number.

BNSIG *See* Behavioral Neuropsychology Special Interest Group.

board An organized body of administrators or investigators, as in a board of trustees. *See also* administrator; governing body.

board certification A method of formally identifying a physician or other health professional who has completed a specified amount of training and a certain set of requirements and passed an examination required by a specialty board. For example, 23 medical specialty boards currently grant certification to physicians when all requirements have been met. *See also* certification; specialty boards.

Board of Certification in Pedorthics (BCP) A national organization founded in 1958 composed of 400 pedorthists. It sponsors a mandatory certification program and seeks to maintain high standards of practice in pedorthics and facilitate continuing education of members. *See also* certification; pedorthics.

board certified (BC) Refers to a physician or other health professional who has passed an examination given by a specialty board and been certified by that board as a specialist in the subject matter. The examination can be taken when the professional meets requirements set by the specialty board for board eligibility. *Compare* board prepared. *See also* board certification; certification; medical specialist; specialist.

Board of Certified Hazard Control Management (BCHCM) An organization founded in 1976 composed of 2,000 safety managers interested in the establishment of professional standards and refinement in the industry. It evaluates and certifies individuals involved primarily in the administration of safety and health programs. Its levels of certification are senior and master, with master being the highest attainable status indicating that the individual possesses the skill and knowledge necessary to manage comprehensive safety and health programs. It establishes curricula in conjunction with colleges, universities, and other training institutions to better prepare hazard control managers for their duties. *See also* certified; hazard; safety management.

board-certified physician A physician who has been certified by a specialty board as a specialist, as in board-certified dermatologist or board-certified thoracic surgeon. *See also* board certification; physician; specialist.

Board of Certified Safety Professionals (BCSP) A national board founded in 1969 that grants the designation of certified safety professional (CSP) to safety engineers, industrial hygienists, safety managers, fire protection engineers, and other persons who have passed the two written examinations administered by the board and who have met other established criteria. Over 10,000 individuals have been certified as CSPs. *See also* certification; industrial hygienist.

board of commissioners *See* governing body.

Board of Commissioners The governing body of the Joint Commission on Accreditation of Healthcare Organizations. *See also* governing body; Joint Commission on Accreditation of Healthcare Organizations.

board of directors *See* governing body.

board eligible *See* board prepared.

board examination, national *See* national board examination.

board examination, specialty *See* specialty board examination.

board of health A public body with oversight and governing responsibility for a local public health department and its community health programs. Members of a board of health usually are appointed by an elected official or governing body, such as a mayor or county commission. *See also* public health.

board of governors *See* governing body.

board and lodging *See* residential community-based care.

board of medical examiners, state *See* state board of medical examiners.

Board of Medical Specialties, American *See* American Board of Medical Specialties.

board, mother *See* mother board.

Board of Nephrology Examiners - Nursing and Technology (BONENT) A national organization founded in 1974 composed of 3,000 registered nurses, licensed practical nurses, licensed vocational nurses, and dialysis technicians that provides nephrology nursing and technology certification examinations. *See also* certification; dialysis technician; licensed practical nurse; licensed vocation nurse; nephrology; registered nurse.

board prepared Refers to a physician or other health professional who is prepared for specialty board examination (including those who may have failed the examination if they remain eligible). Each of the specialty boards has requirements that must be met before the examination for specialty board certification can be taken. These include, for instance, graduation from an approved school, training experience of specified type and length, and specified time in practice or on the job. *Synonym*: board eligible. *Compare* board certified. *See also* certification; eligible.

Boards, American Association of State Social Work *See* American Association of State Social Work Boards.

Boards of Examiners for Nursing Home Administrators, National Association of *See* National Association of Boards of Examiners for Nursing Home Administrators.

boards, medical specialty *See* medical specialty boards.

boards, national *See* national board examination.

Boards of Pharmacy, National Association of *See* National Association of Boards of Pharmacy.

board, sounding *See* sounding board.

boards, specialty *See* specialty boards.

boards, state *See* state boards.

boards, state medical *See* state medical boards.

board of trustees *See* governing body.

body language *See* nonverbal communication.

body louse A surface parasite (*Pediculosis*) of humans that flourishes under conditions of overcrowding and poor hygiene. It causes skin irritation and local reaction, and is an important vector of relapsing fever and some forms of typhus. *See also* head louse; parasite; pediculosis.

Bodymind Acupressure, Jin Shin Do Foundation for *See* Jin Shin Do Foundation for Bodymind Acupressure.

body snatching The illegal procurement of dead bodies, as for anatomical dissection, especially robbing a grave of a recently buried corpse.

Bodywork and Massage Professionals, Associated *See* Associated Bodywork and Massage Professionals.

Bodywork Therapy Association, American Oriental *See* American Oriental Bodywork Therapy Association.

boil An acute staphylococcal abscess of the skin and subcutaneous tissues. *Synonym*: furuncle. *See also* abscess; felon; infection.

boilerplate A term for paragraphs, sections, and exhibits used in documents, such as contracts, written in similar language to convey uniform information that is not central to the unique content of the document.

bomb, logic *See* logic bomb.

bond A certificate of debt issued by a government or corporation guaranteeing payment of the original investment plus interest by a specified future date. *See also* bond rating.

bond rating A method of evaluating the possibility of default by a bond issuer, such as a government body or a corporation. Standard & Poor's and Moody's Investors Service, for example, analyze the financial strength of each bond's issuer; their rating ranges from AAA (highly unlikely to default) to D (in default). *See also* bond; rating.

bone The dense, calcified, porous connective tissue forming the major portion of the skeleton. *See also* bone marrow; long bone; orthopaedic/orthopedic surgery; osteomyelitis; osteoporosis; osteotripsy; rheumatology; skeleton; tendon.

Bone and Joint Surgeons, Association of *See* Association of Bone and Joint Surgeons.

bone, long *See* long bone.

bone marrow The soft, fatty, vascular tissue that fills most bone cavities and is the source of red blood cells and many white blood cells. *See also* bone marrow transplant; long bone; red blood cell; white blood cell.

bone marrow transplant A technique used to enhance or restore a person's immune response or supply of blood cells or to replace diseased or destroyed bone marrow, as by radiation, with normally functioning bone marrow. Bone marrow is removed from a donor's pelvic bone and administered intravenously to a patient. *See also* bone marrow; National Marrow Donor Program; transplant.

Bone and Mineral Research, American Society for *See* American Society for Bone and Mineral Research.

BONENT *See* Board of Nephrology Examiners - Nursing and Technology.

bonus, recruitment *See* recruitment bonus.

book **1.** A set of written, printed, or blank pages fastened along one side and encased between protective covers. **2.** A written or printed work. *See also* talking books.

bookkeeping A component of accounting consisting of the collection, compilation, and retention of an organization's financial information in an organized

fashion. It precedes the preparation of financial statements. *See also* accounting; book.

books, talking *See* talking books.

boomer Short for baby boomer: a person born as a result of the baby boom, a sharp increase in the birth rate that occurred in the United States at the end of World War II and lasted until the mid-1960s. *Compare* buster.

boot To start up a computer. Boot (earlier, bootstrap) derives from the idea that the computer has to "pull itself up by its bootstraps," that is, to load into memory a small program that enables it to load larger programs. *See also* computer; operating system.

borderline In psychiatry, on the borderline between neurosis and psychosis, as in borderline psychosis. *See also* neurosis; psychiatry; psychosis.

borrowed servant An employee of one person or organization who is temporarily employed by another. For example, a nurse employed by a hospital may be temporarily employed by a surgeon to work with his or her surgical team. In such instances, the temporary employer may be responsible for the actions of the nurse (the borrowed servant). *See also* captain of the ship doctrine; charitable immunity; master and servant; respondent superior.

borrowing authority *See* backdoor authority.

boss An employer, supervisor, or other person who makes decisions or exercises authority. This word is sometimes replaced with "leader" or "team leader" in the continuous quality improvement and total quality management paradigms. *See also* authority; leader.

botany The scientific study of plants. *See also* biology.

bottom line Net profit or loss. It is often used as an expression when seeking the result or main point without asking for the reasons, as in "What is the bottom line?"

botulism An often fatal form of food poisoning caused by an endotoxin produced by the bacillus *Clostridium botulinum*. These bacteria grow in anaerobic (without oxygen) conditions of low acidity, such as in improperly canned vegetables and fruits. *See also* endotoxin; food poisoning.

bougie A slender, flexible, hollow or solid, cylindrical instrument for introduction into the urethra or other tubular organ, usually to measure, dilate, or medicate constricted passages. *See also* instrument; surgery; urology.

boundary A border or limit. For example, in

process improvement, a boundary is the beginning or end point in the portion of a process from a supplier to a customer that will help focus the process improvement effort. *See also* limit; process improvement.

bowel *See* intestine.

box Enclosure of the space between the third and first quartile values on a basic box plot. *See also* box plot.

box plot A five-number summary of a set of data. A box encloses the space between the first and third quartiles. The median is indicated by a line dividing the box. The highest and lowest values are shown as the ends of lines extending from the box. *See also* median; quantile; schematic box plot.

box plot, schematic *See* schematic box plot.

boycott Concerted action by two or more competing persons or distinct business entities to prevent another competitor from having access to a particular service, product, facility, or markets resulting in an anticompetitive effect. *Synonym*: concerted refusals to deal. *See also* antitrust laws.

BP *See* blood pressure.

BPA *See* Biological Photographic Association; Black Psychiatrists of America.

BPEAOA *See* Bureau of Professional Education of the American Osteopathic Association.

BPH *See* benign prostatic hypertrophy.

BPS *See* Behavioral Pharmacology Society.

BR *See* Business Roundtable.

brace An orthopedic or orthodontic appliance for supporting or correcting the alignment of bony structures or the teeth. *See also* orthodontic appliance; orthosis.

bradycardia An abnormal slowing of the heartbeat, such as to a rate of 60 beats per minute or less. *Compare* tachycardia. *See also* arrhythmia.

BRAGS *See* Bioelectrical Repair and Growth Society.

brain The part of the central nervous system that occupies most of the skull. The two cerebral hemispheres occupy the anterior and middle fossae of the skull, while the cerebellum and brainstem occupy the posterior fossa. Around all parts of the brain are three meninges: the pia mater, arachnoid mater, and dura mater. *See also* brainstem; central nervous system; cerebellum; cerebrum; hypothalamus; meninges; skull.

brain, computer *See* central processing unit.

brain death A clinical state marked by the absence of neurologic function. Declaration of brain death is based on the clinical criteria of irreversible brainstem damage and the inability of an individual to maintain functions vital to life, such as heart beat, respiration, and blood pressure, without external mechanical support or medication. The exact criteria vary among institutions. Tests used to confirm the clinical impression of brain death include an isoelectric electroencephalogram (EEG) documented at six-hour intervals, no flow in the cerebral angiogram, and a brain scan without isotope uptake. Brain death differs from a persistent vegetative state. *See also* brain; brainstem; death; vegetative state.

brain scan A radiological examination of the brain by means of computerized axial tomographic scanning or following the intravenous injection of radioisotopes. *See also* computerized axial tomography; radioisotopes; scan.

brainstem The part of the brain connecting the cerebral hemispheres with the spinal cord, comprising, from top to bottom, the midbrain, the pons, and the medulla oblongata. *See also* brain.

brainstorming A process used to elicit a large number of ideas from a group of people who are encouraged to use their collective thinking power to generate ideas and unrestrained thoughts in a relatively short period of time.

brainwashing 1. Intensive, forcible indoctrination aimed at destroying a person's basic convictions and attitudes and replacing them with an alternative set of fixed beliefs. 2. The application of a concentrated means of persuasion, such as an advertising campaign or repeated suggestion, in order to develop a specific belief or motivation. *See also* belief; persuasion.

bran The nonabsorbable residue (husk) of wheat, barley, oats, or other grains. *See also* fiber.

brand name A name used to identify a commercial product or service, which may or may not be registered as a trademark; for example, *Mandol* is the name given to the drug product cefamandol by its manufacturer. Drugs are primarily advertised to practitioners by brand name. *Synonym*: trade name. *Compare* chemical name; established name; generic name. *See also* antisubstitution laws; trademark.

breach of duty A failure to perform a duty owed to another human being or to society; a failure to exercise that care which a reasonable person would exercise under similar circumstances. *See also* duty.

breakdown, nervous *See* nervous breakdown.

breast *See* mammary gland.

Breast Cancer Advisory Center (BCAC) A non-membership organization founded in 1975 that makes referrals and disseminates information about breast cancer.

Breast Cancer Organizations, National Alliance of *See* National Alliance of Breast Cancer Organizations.

Breast Disease, Society for the Study of *See* Society for the Study of Breast Disease.

breastfeed *See* nurse.

breathalyzer test A chemical test of a person's breath to determine whether he or she is intoxicated, usually when he or she is suspected of drunken driving. The test is normally administered by a police officer trained in the use of the equipment. The equipment must be calibrated on a regular basis. A person operating a motor vehicle is usually presumed to have consented to taking the test, and refusal to take the test may result in the automatic loss of one's driver's license. The results of the test are admissible as evidence in court. *See also* blood alcohol concentration; test.

breathing The drawing into and expulsion from the lungs of air or other gaseous mixtures. *See also* Kussmaul breathing; respiration; ventilation.

breathing, Kussmaul *See* Kussmaul breathing.

breech The back end of anything, often used to describe the rear of the barrel of a rifle or cannon. In health care, a breech delivery occurs when the breech (rear end) of the infant appears first. *See also* breech delivery.

breech delivery A delivery of an infant when the buttocks of the infant are presented in labor (breech presentation). *See also* breech; delivery.

bridge In dentistry, a fixed or removable replacement for one or several but not all of the natural teeth, usually anchored at each end to a natural tooth. *See also* dentistry; prosthodontics.

brittle diabetes *See* type I diabetes mellitus.

BRM *See* biological response modifier therapy.

brokered partnership A legal relationship between health care providers and purchasers of health care in a self-regulating organization that acts as a broker by matching providers and employers through negotiating price, use, and health services from a competitive position, with both buyers and sellers participating in the decision making. *See also* partnership.

bronchitis An acute or a chronic inflammation of the mucous membranes of the tracheobronchial tree. *See also* acute bronchitis; chronic bronchitis; pulmonary medicine; sputum.

bronchitis, acute *See* acute bronchitis.

bronchitis, chronic *See* chronic bronchitis.

Broncho-Esophagological Association, American *See* American Broncho-Esophagological Association.

bronchoscope An endoscope for visualization of the tracheobronchial tree of the lungs. The tube contains fibers that carry light down the tube and project an enlarged image up the tube to the viewer. Two types of bronchoscope are the rigid, tubular metal bronchoscope and the narrower, flexible fiberoptic bronchoscope. *See also* bronchoscopy; endoscope; lung.

bronchoscopy The process of visualizing the tracheobronchial tree using a bronchoscope. Bronchoscopy enables the practitioner to examine the bronchi, obtain a specimen for biopsy or culture, or remove a foreign body from the respiratory tract. Fiberoptic bronchoscopy is performed with a fiberoptic bronchoscope. *See also* bronchoscope; pulmonary medicine; thoracic surgery.

bronchospasm An abnormal contraction of the smooth muscle of the bronchi, resulting in an acute narrowing and obstruction of the respiratory airway. Cough and wheezing may be indicative of bronchospasm, which is a chief characteristic of asthma and bronchitis. *See also* asthma; bronchitis.

brown lung The common name for byssinosis, a chronic lung disease among textile workers, caused by the inhalation of cotton dust. *See also* pneumoconiosis; pulmonary medicine.

bruise A patchy blue discoloration of the skin following injury. *Synonyms*: black-and-blue mark; contusion. *See also* abrasion; hematoma; laceration; wound.

BS *See* Blue Shield.

BSC *See* Biological Stain Commission.

BSN Abbreviation for Bachelor of Science in Nursing. *See* bachelor's degree; registered nurse.

BSW Abbreviation for Bachelor of Social Work. *See* bachelor's degree; social worker.

BT *See* American Association of Behavioral Therapists.

BTLS *See* basic trauma life support.

bubo A swelling in the groin or the armpits due to

enlarged lymph nodes. *See also* lymph node.

budget An itemized summary of estimated or intended expenditures for a given period along with proposals for financing them. A systematic plan for the expenditure of a usually fixed resource, such as money or time, during a given period. *See also* balanced budget; global budget.

budget, balanced *See* balanced budget.

Budget, Committee on the *See* Committee on the Budget.

budget, congressional *See* congressional budget.

budget, global *See* global budget.

budgeting, top-down global *See* top-down global budgeting.

budget neutrality Limitation imposed on an overall budget to ensure that it will neither increase nor decrease the total amount of the previous budget. *See also* budget.

Budget Office, Congressional *See* Congressional Budget Office.

Budget, Office of Management and *See* Office of Management and Budget.

budget, president's *See* president's budget.

budget reconciliation Federal government budgeting process in which Congress changes programs and laws so that program costs match the amount Congress wants to spend. *See also* budget.

budget, tax expenditure *See* tax expenditure budget.

bug **1.** A disease-producing microorganism, as in a flu bug. **2.** An illness or disease produced by a disease-producing microorganism, as in "got the bug." **3.** A defect or difficulty, as in a system or design. **4.** In computer science, an error in a computer program's design that produces incorrect results.

building codes Standards or regulations for construction that are developed to provide a built environment that is safe for patient care. *See* American National Standards Institute; *Life Safety Code®*.

Building Codes and Standards, National Conference of States on *See* National Conference of States on Building Codes and Standards.

building, medical office *See* medical office building.

building, scenario *See* scenario building.

building, team *See* team building.

bulimia nervosa An eating disorder characterized by alternating episodes of gorging and then purging, usually by vomiting or abusing laxatives. It occurs predominantly in females, with onset usually in adolescence or early adulthood. There is an awareness that the binges are abnormal; a fear of not being able to stop eating voluntarily; and self-deprecation and depressed mood following the binges. Bulimia differs from anorexia nervosa, in which bulimic episodes may occur, but there usually is no extreme weight loss in bulimia. *Compare* anorexia nervosa. *See also* adolescence; laxative; vomit.

bulletin board In computer science, a center of computer information that can be accessed or added to and modified by authorized personal computer terminals, used generally by people who have common areas of interest and wish to exchange information and ideas on those subjects. *See also* computer.

bunion An enlarged and deformed knuckle joint of the great toe with overlying bursitis. *See also* joint; orthopaedic/orthopedic surgery; podiatric medicine.

burden of proof The responsibility in a legal proceeding of presenting sufficient evidence to prove a matter. *See also* evidence; proof.

bureau A department, agency, or office, as in the Federal Bureau of Investigation. *See also* bureaucracy; bureaucrat.

bureaucracy Administration of a government chiefly through bureaus or departments staffed with nonelected officials. *See also* bureaucrat; Parkinson's Law.

bureaucrat An official of a bureaucracy who may be rigidly devoted to the details of administrative procedure. *See also* bureaucracy.

bureaucratese A style of language characterized by jargon and euphemism that is used especially by bureaucrats. *See also* bureaucrat; euphemism; jargon; legalese; officialese.

Bureau of Health Care Delivery and Assistance *See* Health Resources and Services Administration.

Bureau of Health Education Schools, Accrediting *See* Accrediting Bureau of Health Education Schools.

Bureau of Health Insurance (BHI) The former name of one of the organizational elements that formed the basis for the Health Care Financing Administration when it was an agency within the Social Security Administration. *See also* Health Care Financing Administration; Social Security Administration.

Bureau of Health Professions *See* Health Resources and Services Administration.

Bureau of Narcotics and Dangerous Drugs (BNDD) The federal agency replaced by the Drug Enforcement Agency (DEA). *See also* Drug

Enforcement Agency.

Bureau of National Affairs (BNA) The largest employer of information specialists in the nation's capital whose function is to report, analyze, and explain the activities of the federal government and the courts to those persons who are directly affected by them. BNA is generally recognized as a leading source of information services. *See also* information.

Bureau of Professional Education of the American Osteopathic Association (BPEAOA) A group composed of chairpersons of component committees of the bureau, representatives of the American Association of Colleges of Osteopathic Medicine, and public representatives. It approves policy regarding new and/or different intern and residency training programs in approved osteopathic hospitals. It serves as an accrediting agency for colleges of osteopathic medicine and all other types of postdoctoral osteopathic education. Final approval of postdoctoral training activities rests with the American Osteopathic Association Board of Trustees. *See also* accreditation; American Osteopathic Association; osteopathic medicine.

Bureau of Resources Development *See* Health Resources and Services Administration.

Bureaus of America, Medical-Dental-Hospital *See* Medical-Dental-Hospital Bureaus of America.

burn A skin lesion caused by injury from fire, heat, radiation, electricity, or a caustic agent. *See also* burn unit.

Burn Association, American *See* American Burn Association.

Burn Information Exchange, National *See* National Burn Information Exchange.

Burn Medicine, National Institute for *See* National Institute for Burn Medicine.

burnout Physical or emotional exhaustion, especially as a result of long-term stress, as in physician burnout. *See also* worn-out.

burn unit An intensive (special) care unit for treatment of inpatients with severe burns. Severely burned patients may include those with the following injuries: second-degree burns of more than 25% total body surface area for adults or 20% total body surface area for children; third-degree burns of more than 10% total body surface area; any severe burns of the hands, face, eyes, ears, or feet; and all inhalation injuries, electrical burns, complicated burn injuries involving fractures and other major trau-

mas. *See also* special care unit; unit.

burp To expel gas from the stomach. *See also* flatus; gas.

business **1.** The occupation, work, or trade in which a person is engaged. **2.** Commercial, industrial, or professional dealings. **3.** A commercial enterprise or establishment. *See also* business health care coalition; business office; business office manager; small business; trade.

Business, Association for Fitness in *See* Association for Fitness in Business.

Business Association, National Nurses in *See* National Nurses in Business Association.

Business Administration, Master of *See* Master of Business Administration.

Business Communications Council, Health Industry *See* Health Industry Business Communications Council.

Business Consultants, Institute of Certified Professional *See* Institute of Certified Professional Business Consultants.

Business Consultants, Society of Professional *See* Society of Professional Business Consultants.

business health care coalition A voluntary organization of employers formed to monitor and communicate information on a wide range of health care issues affecting employees of the individual companies. The coalitions consist largely of employers who purchase group health insurance coverage and become members of coalitions to improve their capacity to plan and manage health care benefits and expenditures. *See also* business; coalition; health care coalition.

Business Management Association, Radiology *See* Radiology Business Management Association.

business office In health care organizations, the unit that conducts routine financial operations, including the preparation and mailing of patient bills, filing of insurance claims, collecting of past-due bills, preparing and maintaining of financial records and budgets, and preparing of payrolls and financial reports. *See also* business; business office manager.

business office manager The individual who supervises and coordinates the operations of a health care organization's business office, including the supervision of office functions, such as bookkeeping, clerical services, filing, recordkeeping, preparing reports, and word processing. *See also* business; business office; manager; office manager.

Business Roundtable (BR)   A group founded in 1972 composed of 200 major US corporations represented by their chief executive officers. It an influential lobbying force representing the views of American business. Its members examine public issues that affect the economy and develop positions that seek to reflect sound economic and social principles. Its 12 task forces conduct extensive research, often drawing on the staffs of member companies for talent and expertise. The Business Roundtable began informally in 1969 as Construction Users Anti-Inflation Roundtable and combined with the Labor Law Study Committee and other business groups in 1972.

buster   Short for baby buster: a person born in the generation after the baby boom, at a time when the birth rate fell dramatically in most Western countries. *Compare* boomer.

buy *See* purchase.

buyer principle, prudent   *See* prudent buyer principle.

buyer's market   A market condition characterized by low prices and a supply of commodities exceeding demand. *Compare* seller's market. *See also* market.

buzzword   A slang word or phrase used by an in-group, sometimes having imprecise meaning but sounding impressive to outsiders. If, however, the meaning is sufficiently clear, and enough people use a buzzword, it can become widely used, as in "bottom line." *See also* catchword; euphemism; jargon.

Bx   Abbreviation for biopsy. *See* biopsy.

bylaws   In health care, the rules, regulations, or laws adopted by a health care organization or components thereof (such as the medical staff) for the reg-

ulation of its own actions. In corporate law, bylaws are self-imposed rules that constitute an agreement or contract between a corporation and its members to conduct the corporate business in a particular way. *See also* governing body bylaws; governing instrument; medical staff bylaws.

bylaws, governing body *See* governing body bylaws.

bylaws, medical staff   *See* medical staff bylaws.

bypass   **1.** In medicine, a permanent alternative pathway for a blood vessel, especially near the heart or brain, created by transplanting a vessel from elsewhere in the body or inserting an artificial one. **2.** An operation by which this is achieved or an artificial device is inserted. For example, a coronary artery bypass is a procedure in which a section of saphenous vein (from the leg) is grafted between the aorta and a coronary artery distal to an obstructive lesion in the latter. *See also* coronary artery bypass graft procedure.

bypass graft procedure, coronary *See* coronary artery bypass graft procedure.

byssinosis   *See* brown lung.

byte   A grouping of eight bits processed by an computer as a unit; bytes are the building blocks for characters in computer language. A computer with eight-bit bytes can distinguish 2 to the 8th power, or 256 different characters. The size of a computer's memory is measured in kilobytes, where 1 kilobyte (K) equals 1,024 bytes. *See also* bit; gigabyte; megabyte.

byte, giga-   *See* gigabyte.

byte, mega-   *See* megabyte.

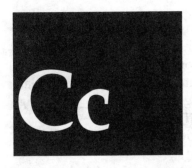

Cc

C Abbreviation for Celsius degree; centigrade. *See* Celsius scale; centigrade.

CA *See* cancer; Consumer Alert; Cranial Academy.

CAAHA *See* Council on Arteriosclerosis of the American Heart Association.

CABG procedure *See* coronary artery bypass graft procedure.

cachexia A wasting of the body, often occurring in people with tumors of the liver, pancreas, and digestive tract, and widespread malignancies. Cachexia appears to be related to the body's release of tumor necrosis factor, also called cachectin. *See also* hunger; starvation.

CAD *See* computer-aided design; coronary artery disease; Council on Anxiety Disorders.

cadaver The body of a deceased person. The term is generally applied to a human body preserved for anatomical dissection and study. *See also* autopsy; corpse; dissect.

caduceus The wand with two snakes winding around it, carried by Hermes (or Mercury), the messenger of the gods. It is used as a medical symbol and as the emblem of the US Army Medical Corps. The official symbol of the medical profession is the staff of Aesculapius. *See also* Aesculapius; staff of Aesculapius; symbol.

caffeine A central nervous system stimulant that belongs to a group of drugs called methylxanthines, found in more than 60 species of plants, including coffee, tea, and cocoa plants. *See also* caffeinism; stimulant; theobromine; theophylline.

caffeinism A condition manifested by insomnia, restlessness, excitement, tachycardia, tremors, and diuresis, resulting from ingestion of excessive amounts of caffeine. *See also* caffeine; stimulant.

CAH *See* Center for Attitudinal Healing.

CAHEA *See* Committee on Allied Health Education and Accreditation.

CAI *See* computer-aided instruction.

CAIR *See* Child Abuse Institute of Research.

calcitonin A hormone secreted by the thyroid gland that blocks the action of the hormone parathormone and thus prevents the release of calcium from bone; used in the treatment of osteoporosis to prevent bone resorption. *See also* calcium; hormone; osteoporosis; thyroid gland.

calcium The most plentiful mineral in the human body, making up parts of the bones, teeth, soft tissues, and body fluids. It is required for effective nerve and muscle function, for blood clotting (coagulation), and to activate enzymes necessary for the conversion of food to energy. Calcium is found in milk and milk products, green leafy vegetables, sardines, oysters, citrus fruits, and dried peas and beans. *See also* calcitonin; coagulation; osteoporosis; rickets.

calendar year A continuous period beginning January 1 and ending December 31. *Compare* fiscal year.

calibration The process or act of determining the accuracy of an instrument, usually by measurement of its variation from a standard, to ascertain necessary correction factors. *See also* measure; measurement; instrument; standard; variation.

California Medical Insurance Feasibility Study A study (1976) sponsored by the California Medical Association and the California Hospital Association in which researchers used occurrence criteria to review over 20,000 patient charts from 23 hospitals to identify the presence of adverse events that might result in litigation for malpractice compensation. These events were termed "potentially compensable events" (PCEs). The study determined that 17% of

PCEs involved negligence that would justify a verdict for the patient if the claim were brought to litigation. *See also* occurrence criteria; occurrence screening; potentially compensable events.

CALM *See* Child Abuse Listening and Mediation.

calorie The gram or small calorie is the amount of heat required to raise one gram of water one degree Celsius at atmospheric pressure. A large calorie (also called great calorie, kilocalorie, kilogram calorie) is the quantity of heat equal to 1,000 small calories. A unit equal to the large calorie is often used to denote the heat expenditure of an organism and the fuel or energy value of food, as in the hot fudge sundae is 3,000 (large) calories. *See also* empty calories.

calorie, low *See* low calorie.

calories, empty *See* empty calories.

CAMA *See* Civil Aviation Medical Association.

campylobacter A bacterium occurring in unpasteurized dairy produce and other everyday foods; it is capable of causing food poisoning in humans. *See also* bacteria; food poisoning.

CAMS *See* Chinese American Medical Society.

cancer (CA) Any malignant neoplasm or tumor, the natural course of which is fatal. Cancer cells, unlike benign tumor cells, are characterized by proliferation, invasion, and metastasis. *See also* anaplasia; carcinoma; chemotherapy; malignancy; metastasis; tumor.

Cancer Advisory Center, Breast *See* Breast Cancer Advisory Center.

Cancer, American Joint Committee on *See* American Joint Committee on Cancer.

Cancer Centers, Association of Community *See* Association of Community Cancer Centers.

Cancer Council, United *See* United Cancer Council.

Cancer Education, American Association for *See* American Association for Cancer Education.

Cancer Information Service (CIS) An organization founded in 1975 and funded by the National Cancer Institute composed of trained counselors who provide information about cancer causes, prevention, detection, diagnosis, rehabilitation, and research. *See also* cancer; counselor.

Cancer Institute, National *See* National Institutes of Health.

Cancer Institutes, Association of American *See* Association of American Cancer Institutes.

cancerophobia A morbid fear of cancer; an unwarranted belief by an individual that he or she is suffering from cancer. *See also* cancer; phobia.

Cancer Organizations, National Alliance of Breast *See* National Alliance of Breast Cancer Organizations.

cancer registry *See* tumor registry.

Cancer Research, American Association for *See* American Association for Cancer Research.

Cancer Research, National Coalition for *See* National Coalition for Cancer Research.

Cancer Society, American *See* American Cancer Society.

Candida A yeastlike fungus, commonly part of the normal flora of the skin, mouth, intestinal tract, and vagina, but that can cause many infections, including candidiasis, onychomycosis, vaginitis, and thrush. *Candida albicans* is the usual pathogen. *See also* candidiasis.

candidiasis Infection with the fungus *Candida*, typically a superficial infection of the moist cutaneous areas of the body, such as the vaginal area (vaginitis) or the oral cavity and esophagus (thrush). *Synonym:* moniliasis. *See also Candida;* opportunistic infection; thrush; vaginitis.

candy striper A volunteer in a health care organization who performs specified support tasks as a means of helping the ill, handicapped, and elderly, or exploring health careers. *See also* volunteer.

cane A stick used as an aid in walking or carried as an accessory. *See also* crutch; walker; wheelchair.

canker sore An ulcer, chiefly of the mouth or lips, characteristic of aphthous stomatitis. *See also* aphthous stomatitis; sore.

cannabis Products of the hemp plants *Cannabis indica* and *Cannabis sativa* which contain the active ingredient tetrhydrocannabinol and compounds closely related to it. Normally smoked, this drug is essentially an intoxicant and has no psychoactive effect or hallucinogenic effect. While it currently has no general medicinal use in the United States, it has been recognized as a treatment for glaucoma and as an antiemetic in some cancer patients afflicted with nausea and vomiting associated with chemotherapy. *Synonyms:* bhang; ganja; grass; hashish; marijuana; pot; reefer; tea; weed. *See also* antiemetic; controlled substances; Schedule I substances.

Cannabis Therapeutics, Alliance for *See* Alliance for Cannabis Therapeutics.

cannibalism The consumption of the flesh of one's own species.

CAO   Chief administrative officer. *See* chief executive officer.

CAOHC   *See* Council for Accreditation in Occupational Hearing Conservation.

CAP   *See* College of American Pathologists.

cap   An upper limit or ceiling, as in a statutorily-imposed limit on recovery of noneconomic damages in tort actions. *See also* pain and suffering.

capability   A talent or ability that has potential for development or use, as in measuring a hospital's actual performance as opposed to its capability to perform well. *See also* ability; process capability.

capability, process   *See* process capability.

capacity   The ability to perform or produce; the innate potential for accomplishment. *See also* optimum capacity; resource capacity.

capacity, optimum   *See* optimum capacity.

capacity, resource   *See* resource capacity.

CAPD   Continuous ambulatory peritoneal dialysis. *See* peritoneal dialysis.

capillary   The smallest blood vessels in the circulatory system, which connect arterioles and venules, forming a network in nearly all parts of the body. The walls of capillaries act as semipermeable membranes, allowing the free exchange of respiratory gases, fluids, nutrients, and waste products between the blood and the tissue spaces, but normally retaining the blood cells and the larger molecules, such as proteins. *See also* blood vessel; vitamin P.

capital   All the money and other property of a corporation or other enterprise used in the production of goods and/or services, for example, a hospital's buildings, beds, and equipment used in the provision of health care services. Capital goods are permanent and durable goods, as opposed to supplies, which are usually disposable goods. *See also* capital asset; capital expenditure; capital improvement; risk capital.

capital asset   Property with a relatively long life, such as buildings or equipment, that is not held for sale in the regular course of business. For tax purposes, capital assets are property, the sale or exchange of which gives rise to capital gain or loss rather than ordinary income or a deduction. *See also* asset; capital; capital depreciation; capital gains tax.

capital cost   The cost of investing in the development of new facilities, services, or equipment, excluding operational costs. *See also* capital; cost.

capital depreciation   The decline in value of capital assets over time with use. *See also* capital asset.

capital expenditure   The cost of an acquisition, such as facilities and equipment, or repair to property, which has a useful life extending substantially beyond the taxable year. Such costs are not deductible for income tax purposes; they may be subject to depreciation or depletion. *See also* capital; capital expenditure review.

capital expenditure review   Prospective review by a designated state regulatory agency of the need to expend capital on specific organizational proposals. *See also* capital expenditure.

capital factor, uniform   *See* uniform capital factor.

capital financing   Organizational funding for facilities and equipment that become part of the capital assets of the organization. *See also* capital; capital asset.

capital gains or losses   Gains or losses realized from the sale or exchange of capital assets, calculated as the difference between the amount realized on the sale or exchange and the taxpayer's investment in the asset. *See also* capital asset; capital gains tax.

capital gains tax   A tax on profits realized from the sale of stocks, property, or capital assets. *See also* capital asset; tax.

capital improvement   A modification, addition, restoration, or other improvement that increases the usefulness, productivity, or serviceable life of an existing building, structure, or major item of equipment, and that increases the recorded worth of the item or entity. *See also* capital; improvement.

capital intensive   Requiring a large amount of equipment or machinery relative to the quantity of labor or land required for production or manufacture of items or services. *See also* capital.

capital investment   Money paid out for acquisition of a capital asset, or something for permanent use of value in a business or home. *See also* capital asset; investment.

capitalism   An economic system in which private ownership of property exists, the income from property or capital accrues to the individuals or organizations that accumulated it and own it, individuals and organizations are relatively free to compete with other individuals and organizations for their own economic gain, and the profit motive is basic to economic life. *See also* profit; socialism.

capital, risk   *See* risk capital.

capita, per   *See* per capita.

capitation A method of payment for health services in which a health care provider is paid a fixed, per capita amount for each person served without regard to the actual number or nature of services provided to each person. Under this system, a managed care plan, such as a health maintenance organization, pays a physician or a hospital a fixed amount to care for a patient over a given time; health care providers do not receive extra money even if the costs of care exceed the fixed amount. *See also* base capitation; capitation grant; health care provider; health services; per capita.

capitation, base *See* base capitation.

capitation grant A method of federal support for health professional schools, such as medical schools, in which an eligible school receives a fixed capitation payment, called a capitation grant, from the federal government for each student enrolled. *See also* capitation; grant.

cap, legal *See* legal cap.

CAPS *See* Christian Association for Psychological Studies.

captain of the ship doctrine In health care, the principle that the person in charge of a group, such as a surgeon in charge of a surgical team, is responsible and liable for the actions of every member under his or her supervision, such as all of the members of a surgical team. Under the "borrowed servant" doctrine, hospital employees making up a surgical team are considered "borrowed" from the hospital by the surgeon and if any of those individuals were negligent, the surgeon would be liable as their "employer." These two theories developed because of the doctrine of charitable immunity, which protected many hospitals from liability for the negligence of their employees. Charitable immunity is now abolished or limited in all jurisdictions, and it is no longer necessary to hold physicians liable for hospital employees' negligence because the hospital can be sued directly. The trend is to abolish these doctrines and to impose liability on the party who has actual control over the employee who performed negligently. *See also* borrowed servant; charitable immunity; doctrine; master and servant; *respondeat superior*.

captive insurance company An insurance company formed to insure the risks of its owner(s), such as a hospital(s) or physicians. *See also* insurance company; risk.

capture, data *See* data capture.

carbohydrates Organic molecules, composed primarily of carbon, hydrogen, and oxygen atoms, that provide energy for the central nervous system and muscles. Carbohydrates are divided into three groups: monosaccharides, disaccharides, and polysaccharides. *See also* ketoacidosis; ketogenic diet; ketone; ketosis.

carbon dioxide monitoring, transcutaneous oxygen/ *See* transcutaneous oxygen/carbon dioxide monitoring.

carbon monoxide (CO) A colorless, odorless, highly poisonous gas, formed by the incomplete combustion of carbon or a carbonaceous material, such as gasoline. *See also* gas; poison.

carcass A nonhuman dead body. *See also* corpse.

carcinoembryonic antigen (CEA) An antigen existing in small amounts in adult tissue. An elevated amount is suggestive of cancers of the colon, pancreas, stomach, lung, and breast, although CEA levels may also be elevated in patients with alcoholic cirrhosis, pancreatitis, and inflammatory bowel disease, and in patients who smoke. The primary use of CEA is monitoring response to treatment of colorectal cancer. *See also* cancer.

carcinogen Any cancer-producing substance. *See also* cancer.

carcinoma A malignant new growth made up of epithelial cells tending to infiltrate the surrounding tissues and give rise to metastases. *See also* cancer; malignancy; metastasis.

card, electronic-striped *See* electronic-striped card.

card, health *See* health card.

card in health care, smart *See* smart card in health care.

cardiac Pertaining to the heart.

Cardiac Angiography and Interventions, Society for *See* Society for Cardiac Angiography and Interventions.

cardiac arrest Sudden cessation of cardiac function with disappearance of arterial blood pressure, connoting either ventricular fibrillation or ventricular standstill (asystole). *See also* arrhthymia; respiratory arrest; ventricular fibrillation.

cardiac care nurse A registered nurse who is qualified by advanced training in cardiac care to provide care to cardiac patients, typically in a hospital cardiac care unit. *See also* cardiac care unit; registered nurse.

cardiac care unit (CCU) An intensive (special) care unit for treatment and continuous monitoring of inpatients with cardiac disorders. *Synonyms:* cardiac intensive care unit (CICU); cardiovascular care unit (CCU); coronary intensive care unit (CICU); coronary care unit (CCU). *See also* special care unit.

cardiac catheterization An invasive procedure consisting of the passage of a radiopaque catheter into a peripheral vein (or an artery when the left side of the heart is being catheterized) followed by its advancement under fluoroscopic control until the tip lies in one of the chambers of the heart. Though the technique was first performed in 1929, it has only been fully exploited during the past 30 years in the diagnosis of heart disease and the performance of hemodynamic studies. *See also* cardiac catheterization laboratory; catheter; catheterization; invasive procedure; radiopaque.

cardiac catheterization laboratory A laboratory that provides special diagnostic procedures, such as cardiac catheterization, necessary for the care of patients with cardiac conditions. *See also* cardiac catheterization; laboratory.

cardiac decompensation The failure of the heart at a stage of disease in which available compensatory mechanisms (for example, myocardial hypertrophy) are no longer able to overcome the extra work load imposed (for example, by a stenotic aortic valve). Symptoms therefore arise (for example, shortness of breath, exercise intolerance). *See also* cardiac arrest; decompensation.

cardiac electrophysiology, clinical *See* clinical cardiac electrophysiology.

cardiac pacemaker *See* pacemaker.

cardiac rehabilitation program Restorative services used after open heart surgery, angioplasty, and acute myocardial infarction and for patients identified as being at high risk for undesirable cardiovascular events. Through such programs, patients are reconditioned from a state of cardiac injury or high risk to resume activities of daily living (ADL) at an optimal level. Programs often include counseling, education, and exercise. *See also* activities of daily living; acute myocardial infarction; angioplasty; exercise; open heart surgery; rehabilitation program.

cardinal number A number used to compare quantity or frequency, as in how many or how often; for example, three (3), sixty-four (64), twenty-two (22). *Compare* ordinal number. *See also* number.

Card Industry Association, Smart *See* Smart Card Industry Association.

cardiogram *See* electrocardiogram.

Cardiography, American Society of Echo- *See* American Society of Echocardiography.

cardiologist An internist who subspecializes in cardiovascular medicine. *See also* cardiovascular medicine; internist.

cardiologist, pediatric *See* pediatric cardiologist.

Cardiologists, Association of Black *See* Association of Black Cardiologists.

cardiology *See* cardiovascular medicine.

Cardiology, American College of *See* American College of Cardiology.

cardiology, pediatric *See* pediatric cardiology.

cardiology service The unit in a health care organization providing diagnosis and treatment of patients with cardiovascular disorders. *See also* cardiovascular medicine; service.

cardiomyopathy A general diagnostic term designating primary myocardial disease, such as postpartum cardiomyopathy or congestive cardiomyopathy, often of obscure or unknown etiology.

cardiopulmonary resuscitation (CPR) The administration of artificial heart and lung action in the event of cardiac and/or respiratory arrest. The two major components of cardiopulmonary resuscitation are artificial ventilation and closed-chest cardiac massage. *Compare* slow code. *See also* artificial respiration; basic cardiac life support; cardiac arrest; code blue; crash cart; mouth-to-mouth resuscitation; resuscitation.

cardiothoracic *See* thoracic.

cardiothoracic surgeon *See* thoracic surgeon.

cardiothoracic surgery *See* thoracic surgery.

cardiovascular (CV) Pertaining to the heart and blood vessels. *See also* cardiovascular medicine; vascular.

Cardiovascular Administrators, American College of *See* American College of Cardiovascular Administrators.

Cardiovascular Anesthesiologists, Society of *See* Society of Cardiovascular Anesthesiologists.

Cardiovascular Credentialing International (CCI/NBCVT) A national organization founded in 1988 composed of cardiovascular and cardiopulmonary technicians involved in the allied health professions. It conducts testing of allied health professionals throughout the United States and Canada and provides study guides and reliability and validity testing. Formed by merger of National Board of Cardiovascular Technology and Cardiovascular Credentialing International. Formerly (1984) National Board for Cardiopulmonary Credentialing; and (1986) National Board of Cardiovascular and Pulmonary Credentialing; (1991) Cardiovascular Credentialing International/National Board of Cardiovascular Technology. *See also* allied health professional; cardiovascular technologist.

Cardiovascular and Interventional Radiology, Society of *See* Society of Cardiovascular and Interventional Radiology.

cardiovascular medicine The branch of medicine and subspecialty of internal medicine dealing with diseases of the heart and blood vessels and management of complex cardiac conditions, such as heart attacks and life-threatening abnormal heart rhythms. *Synonym*: cardiology. *See also* acute myocardial infarction; angioplasty; arrhythmia; blood vessel; clinical cardiac electrophysiology; heart; internal medicine; stress test.

Cardiovascular Perfusion, American Board of *See* American Board of Cardiovascular Perfusion.

cardiovascular perfusionist *See* perfusionist.

Cardiovascular and Pulmonary Rehabilitation, American Association of *See* American Association of Cardiovascular and Pulmonary Rehabilitation.

cardiovascular surgeon *See* thoracic surgeon.

cardiovascular surgery *See* thoracic surgery.

Cardio-Vascular Surgery, Association of Physician's Assistants in *See* Association of Physician's Assistants in Cardio-Vascular Surgery.

cardiovascular technologist An allied health professional who performs diagnostic examinations at the request or direction of a physician in one or more of the following three areas: invasive cardiology, noninvasive cardiology, and noninvasive peripheral vascular study. Cardiovascular technologists are one type of allied health professional for which the Committee on Allied Health Education and Accreditation has accredited education programs. *See also* allied health professional; technologist; technology.

Cardiovascular Technology/National Society for Pulmonary Technology, National Society for *See* National Society for Cardiovascular Technology/National Society for Pulmonary Technology.

cardioversion The restoration or attempt at restoration of a normal rhythm of the heart by electrical shock or administration of certain medications. *See also* arrhythmia; defibrillation; ventricular fibrillation.

carditis Inflammation of the heart, as in rheumatic carditis or streptococcal carditis. *See also* heart; inflammation.

card, optical-stripe *See* optical-stripe card.

card, report *See* report card.

card, single magnetic-striped *See* single magnetic-striped card.

card, smart *See* smart card.

Card Systems, National Medic- *See* National Medic-Card Systems.

care Provision of accommodations, comfort, and attentive treatment to an individual, also implying responsibility for safety. *See also* caring; respect and caring.

care, acute *See* acute care.

care, adult day *See* adult day care.

care, after *See* after care.

care, alternative level of *See* alternative level of care.

care, ambulatory *See* ambulatory health care.

care, ambulatory health *See* ambulatory health care.

care, aspects of *See* important aspects of care.

care center, primary *See* primary care center.

care, charity *See* charity care.

Care of Children's Health, Association for the *See* Association for the Care of Children's Health.

care, chronic *See* chronic care.

care, comfort *See* palliative care.

care, community health *See* community health care.

care, comprehensive health *See* comprehensive health care.

care, continuing *See* continuing care.

care, continuity of *See* continuity of care.

care, corporatization of health *See* corporatization of health care.

care, custodial *See* custodial care.

care, domiciliary *See* domiciliary care.

care, due *See* due care.

care, durable power of attorney for health *See* durable power of attorney for health care.

care, elder *See* elder care.

care, emergency *See* emergency care.

care, evaluation of *See* evaluation of care.

care, extended *See* extended care.

care, extraordinary *See* extraordinary care.

care facility, extended *See* extended care facility.

care facility, intermediate *See* intermediate care facility.

care facility, residential *See* residential care facility.

care facility, skilled nursing *See* skilled nursing facility.

care, foundation for dental *See* foundation for dental care.

care, health *See* health care.

care, home *See* home health care.

care, home health *See* home health care.

care, hospice *See* hospice care.

care hospital, acute *See* acute care hospital.

care hospital, tertiary *See* tertiary care hospital.

care, important aspects of *See* important aspects of care.

care, inpatient *See* inpatient care.

care, intensive *See* intensive care.

care, intensive home health *See* intensive home health care.

care, intermediate *See* intermediate care.

care, intermediate home health *See* intermediate home health care.

care, intermittent *See* intermittent care.

care, interpersonal aspects of *See* interpersonal aspects of care.

care, level of *See* level of care.

care, life *See* life care.

care, life support *See* life support care.

care, long term *See* long term care.

care, maintenance home health *See* maintenance home health care.

care, managed *See* managed care.

care, managed health *See* managed care.

care, medical *See* medical care.

care medicine, critical *See* critical care medicine.

care nurse, critical *See* critical care nurse.

care nurse, intensive *See* intensive care nurse.

care, nursing *See* nursing care.

care, ordinary *See* ordinary care.

care organization, health *See* health care organization.

care, outcome of *See* patient health outcome.

care, outpatient *See* outpatient care.

care, palliative *See* palliative care.

care path *See* critical pathway.

care, patient-centered *See* patient centered care.

care, pattern of *See* pattern of care.

care, personal *See* personal care.

care physician, critical *See* critical care physician.

care physician, primary *See* primary care physician.

care plan A formal plan of activities to be conducted by personnel of a health care organization on behalf of a patient and to be used to evaluate that patient's needs and progress. *Synonyms*: patient care plan; patient treatment plan. *See also* interdisciplinary patient care plan; nursing care plan.

care plan, interdisciplinary patient *See* interdisciplinary patient care plan.

care plan, nursing *See* nursing care plan.

care plan, patient *See* care plan.

care, postoperative *See* postoperative care.

care, postpartum *See* postpartum care.

care, postsurgical *See* postsurgical care.

care, preoperative *See* preoperative care.

care, primary *See* primary care.

care program, home *See* home care program.

care, progressive patient *See* progressive patient care.

care provider, primary *See* primary care provider.

care, psychiatric *See* psychiatric care.

care, quality of *See* quality of care.

care, referred *See* referred care.

care, residential *See* residential care.

care, residential community-based *See* residential community-based care.

care, respite *See* respite care.

care, secondary *See* secondary care.

care, skilled nursing *See* skilled nursing care.

care, specialized *See* secondary care.

care, standard of *See* standard of care.

care, subacute *See* subacute care.

care, support *See* support care.

care, surgical critical *See* surgical critical care.

care, terminal *See* terminal care.

care, tertiary *See* tertiary care.

care, uncompensated *See* uncompensated care.

care unit, inpatient *See* inpatient care unit.

care unit, intensive *See* intensive care unit.

care unit, intermediate *See* intermediate care unit.

CARF *See* Commission on Accreditation of Rehabilitation Facilities.

caries Molecular decay of the teeth and bone. *Synonyms*: cavity; dental caries. *See also* dentistry.

caring Committed, compassionate, as in nursing and social work as caring professions. *See also* care; respect and caring.

Carnegie Council on Adolescent Development (CCAD) A program founded in 1986 of the

Carnegie Corporation of New York in which researchers, physicians, psychologists, religious leaders, elected officials, school administrators, and parents conduct research on adolescent development focusing on the prevention of health-damaging and compromising behavior. It seeks to interest the public in the development of preventive measures to combat adolescent youth crimes, teenage pregnancy, drug and alcohol abuse, and teenage suicide. *See also* adolescence; adolescent medicine.

carotid Relating to the principal artery of the neck, as in carotid endarterectomy. *See also* artery; blood vessel; carotid endarterectomy.

carotid endarterectomy A procedure in which the thickened, atheromatous inner layer of the carotid artery is excised. *See also* carotid; endarterectomy.

carrier 1. An individual who harbors the specific organisms of a disease without manifesting symptoms and is capable of transmitting the infection. Examples of diseases that produce carriers are acquired immunodeficiency syndrome (AIDS), hepatitis, and typhoid fever. *See also* vector. **2.** An insurance company (a commercial health insurer, a government agency, an insurance plan, a service plan, or a prepaid plan) that underwrites or administers programs that pay for insured health services. Under Medicare, Part B, a carrier is an agency or organization that is retained via a contract to administer various functions, including the payment of claims. *See also* not-for-profit carrier; third-party payer.

carrier, not-for-profit *See* not-for-profit carrier.

cart A wheeled vehicle for moving patients or equipment and supplies within a hospital or other type of health care organization. *See also* crash cart; gurney; litter.

cart, crash *See* crash cart.

cascade iatrogenesis A sequence of two or more serious undesirable occurrences resulting from a diagnostic, prophylactic, or therapeutic intervention; an error of omission involving a reasonable clinical standard; or an accidental injury occurring in a health care setting. *See also* iatrogenesis; iatrogenic.

case 1. An instance of something, or occurrence. **2.** In medicine, a particular instance of disease, such as a case of leukemia, or a person in a population or study group identified as having a particular disease or condition of interest. *See also* case abstract; case-based review; case-control study; case mix. **3.** In law,

an action or a suit or just grounds for an action. *See also* action.

case abstract A group of data elements summarizing information in a medical record and used for billing, performance review and research. *See also* abstract; case; data element; medical record.

case aide A paraprofessional who works on aspects of cases or provides services to less complex cases under the close and regular supervision of a caseworker. Qualifications for case aides vary including a high school degree, related experience, an associate's degree, or a bachelor's degree. *See also* aide; caseworker; paraprofession; social worker.

case-based review An approach to quality-of-care evaluation based on review of individual medical records by health professionals who make judgments as to whether the care delivered was of acceptable quality. *See also* case; judgment; medical record.

case comparison study *See* case-control study.

case conference *See* morbidity and mortality conference.

case-control study An inquiry in which groups of individuals are selected because they do (the cases) or do not (the controls) have the disease whose cause and other attributes are being studied; the groups are then compared with respect to their past, existing, or future characteristics judged likely to be relevant to the disease to see which of the characteristics differ and how, in the cases as compared to the controls. For example, persons with hepatic cancer (cases) are compared with persons without hepatic cancer (controls) and history of hepatitis B is determined for the two groups. A case-control study is a type of retrospective study. *Synonyms:* case-comparison study; case-referent study. *See also* case; control group; retrospective study.

case finding The identification of instances of a particular disease or condition through screening of asymptomatic people or surveillance of defined populations. *See also* case; screening.

case history The collected data concerning an individual, his or her family, and environment, including his or her medical history and any other information that may be useful in analyzing and diagnosing his or her condition for instructional purposes. *See also* case; history.

case, index *See* index case.

case law The aggregate of reported decisions in

cases on a particular legal subject. *See also* case; law.

case mix The relative frequency of patients classified into categories by disease, procedure, method of payment, and other characteristics. *See also* case-mix index; diagnosis-related group; patient mix.

case-mix index In prospective payment systems, the comparison of a hospital's cost for its case mix to the national or regional average hospital cost for a similar case mix. *See also* case mix; index; prospective payment system.

case-mix management information system (CMMIS) A computerized data system in which data elements from case abstracts and patient bills are analyzed for costs and charges by diagnosis-related groups (DRGs) in relation to hospital and physician fees for those DRGs. *See also* case mix; diagnosis-related groups; management information system.

case-mix severity Level of severity of illness or disability within a particular case-mix grouping. *See also* case mix; case severity; severity of illness.

case-mortality rate The proportion of cases of a specified disease or condition that are fatal within a specified time. *See also* case; mortality rate.

case, prima facie *See* prima facie case.

case-referent study *See* case-control study.

case review, surgical *See* surgical case review.

case series In research, a series of patients with a defined disorder, as in series of patients with false aneurysms of the femoral artery. The term usually describes a study reporting on a consecutive collection of patients treated in a similar manner, without a concurrent control group. For example, a surgeon might describe the characteristics of and outcomes for 30 consecutive patients with a femoral artery false aneurysm who received a revascularization procedure. *See also* case; consecutive sample; series.

case severity A measure of the intensity or gravity of a patient's illness for a specified condition or diagnosis; also, the average severity of illnesses for all patients of a health care organization during a given period. Case severity is often indirectly measured by the average length of stay, implying that "sicker" patients require longer periods of hospitalization. The direct measurement of case severity has become increasingly important with the use of diagnosis-related groups (DRGs) to determine hospital reimbursements by Medicare and other third-party payers. Case severity is viewed by many as a needed

modifier to DRG-based reimbursement. *See also* diagnosis-related groups; severity of illness.

casework Social work devoted to the needs of individual clients or cases. *See also* caseworker; casework supervisor; social work.

caseworker A social worker or other qualified individual who performs casework. *See also* child welfare caseworker; social service caseworker; family counselor.

caseworker, child welfare *See* child welfare caseworker.

caseworker, family *See* family counselor.

caseworker, social service *See* social service caseworker.

casework supervisor An individual, usually with a master's degree in social work, who supervises social service agency staff, volunteers, and students of schools of social work. A casework supervisor may assign caseloads and related duties, evaluate staff performance, and recommend needed actions. *See also* caseworker; social worker; supervisor.

case, worst- *See* worst-case.

cast A rigid dressing, usually made of gauze and plaster of Paris, used to immobilize part of the body. *Synonym:* plaster cast. *See also* plaster of Paris; spica; splint.

casual sex Sexual activity between people who are not regular or established sexual partners. *See also* safe sex; sex.

casualty Any injury or persons injured by an accident, an act of terrorism, a police action, or an act of war.

CAT *See* computerized axial tomography.

catabolism The destructive phase of metabolism in which larger molecules, such as glycogen, are converted to smaller molecules, such as pyruvic acid. *Compare* anabolism. *See also* metabolism.

Catalogue of Federal Domestic Assistance *See* federal assistance programs.

catamenia *See* menses.

cataract An opacity, partial or complete, of one or both eyes, on or in the lens or capsule, especially an opacity impairing vision or causing blindness. *See also* ophthalmology.

Cataract and Refractive Surgery, American Society of *See* American Society of Cataract and Refractive Surgery.

catastrophic illness An illness that is usually considered to be life-threatening or with the threat of serious residual disability and that involves or results in substantial, often ruinous, medical expense. *See also* catastrophic insurance; illness.

catastrophic insurance Insurance intended to protect against the cost of a catastrophic illness, with "catastrophic" defined as greater than a predetermined cost. *See also* catastrophic illness; health insurance; insurance.

catchment area A region from which the patients of a health care organization are drawn. It may be defined on the basis of population distribution, natural geographic boundaries, transportation accessibility, and other factors. *Synonym:* service area. *See also* health service area; Medicare locality; patient origin study.

catchword A well-known, catchy acronym, word, or phrase, as in TQM, quality improvement, or managed competition. *See also* buzzword; euphemism; jargon.

Catecholamine Club (CC) A national organization founded in 1969 composed of 350 neuroscience researchers interested in catecholamines. *See also* catecholamines.

catecholamines Neurotransmitters (transmitters of signals in the nervous system) and hormones that include norepinephrine, epinephrine, and dopamine. All three compounds function in brain chemistry. Norepinephrine and dopamine act as agents that transfer nerve impulses; epinephrine mainly initiates physiological and metabolic responses in stress situations. The function of these compounds are significant in the study of the biochemistry of the brain and nervous system and of nervous system and brain disorders. *See also* biochemistry; neuroscience.

categorical program A medical residency program that includes a first postgraduate year (PGY-1-year) in its specialty. *See also* PGY-1; residency.

categorically needy Individuals who are members of certain categories or groups eligible to receive public assistance and who are economically needy (for example, the aged, blind, disabled, or a member of a family with children under age 18 or 21 years, if in school). These individuals generally are receiving cash assistance under the Aid to Families with Dependent Children (AFDC) or Supplemental Security Income programs. States must cover all recipients of AFDC payments under Medicaid. The categorically needy must meet state income and

resource requirements. *See also* Aid to Families with Dependent Children; Medicaid; supplemental security income.

category A specifically defined division in a system of classification; a class. *See also* stratification category.

category, stratification *See* stratification category.

cathartic *See* laxative.

Catherine T. MacArthur Foundation, The John D. and *See* The John D. and Catherine T. MacArthur Foundation.

catheter A hollow, flexible, surgical instrument for withdrawing fluids from or introducing fluids into a cavity of the body. For example, a urinary catheter is introduced into the bladder through the urethra for the withdrawal of urine, and a central venous catheter is introduced via a large vein into the superior vena cava or right atrium for the purposes of measurement or introducing fluids. *See also* catheterization; central line; central venous pressure; instrument; umbilical line.

catheterization The process of passing a catheter into a cavity of the body. For example, urinary catheterization is the process of passing a small catheter through the urethra into the bladder. *See also* cardiac catheterization.

catheterization, cardiac *See* cardiac catheterization.

catheter, Swan-Ganz *See* Swan-Ganz catheter.

cathexis Concentration of emotional energy on an object, a person, or an idea.

cathode ray tube (CRT) Electronic display tube used to portray data on a terminal screen and found in computer applications as well as in certain clinical imaging equipment. It consists of a vacuum tube in which a hot cathode emits electrons that are accelerated as a beam through a relatively high-voltage anode, further focused or deflected electrostatically or electromagnetically, and allowed to fall on a phosphorescent screen. *See also* oscilloscope; terminal.

Catholic Council on Alcoholism and Related Drug Problems, National *See* National Catholic Council on Alcoholism and Related Drug Problems.

Catholic Health Association of the United States (CHA) A national organization founded in 1915 composed of 1,200 Catholic hospitals, health care facilities, religious orders, health care systems, and extended care facilities.

Catholic Healthcare Leadership, Academy for *See* Academy for Catholic Healthcare Leadership.

Catholic Hospital Association *See* Catholic Health

Association of the United States.

Catholic Medical Mission Board (CMMB) An organization founded in 1928 that provides medical supplies and lay personnel to assist the staffs of Catholic medical institutions in all areas of the world. Its purpose is to send cost-free medicines overseas to improve the care given charitably to the destitute sick.

Catholic Pharmacists Guild of the United States, National See National Catholic Pharmacists Guild of the United States.

Catholic Physicians Guilds, National Federation of See National Federation of Catholic Physicians Guilds.

CAT scan An image produced by a CAT scanner. *Synonym*: CT scan. *See also* computerized axial tomography; EMI scan.

CAT scanner A device that produces cross-sectional images of an internal body structure using computerized axial tomography. *Synonym*: CT scanner. *See also* computerized axial tomography; scanner.

caudal Relating to the tail or hind parts; posterior. *Compare* cephalic.

causality See causation.

causation The relating of causes to the effects they produce. For instance, in epidemiology, causation of disease means that certain factors (predisposing, enabling, precipitating, and/or reinforcing factors) relate to disease occurrence. In law, the tort of negligence requires that a duty was breached and that the breached duty *caused* damage to the plaintiff. *Synonym*: causality. *See also* cause; multiple causation.

causation, multiple See multiple causation.

cause That which brings about any condition or produces any effect. Cause is that which effects a result. *See also* causation; common cause; direct cause; immediate cause; intervening cause; necessary cause; proximate cause; root cause; superseding cause.

cause of action A set of facts or legal circumstances adequate to claim judicial attention. *See also* action; cause; release.

cause, common See common cause.

cause, direct See direct cause.

cause-and-effect diagram A pictorial display drawn to represent the relationship between some "effect" and all the possible "causes" influencing it. *Synonyms*: cause-effect diagram; fishbone diagram (because of its appearance); Ishikawa diagram (after

the individual, Kaoru Ishikawa, who first developed and applied the tool). *See also* cause; diagram.

cause-effect diagram See cause-and-effect diagram.

cause, immediate See immediate cause.

cause, intervening See intervening cause.

cause, necessary See necessary cause.

cause, proximate See proximate cause.

cause, remote See remote cause.

cause, root See root cause.

causes of death See death certificate.

cause, special See special cause.

cause, sufficient See cause.

cause, superseding See superseding cause.

cause, supervening See intervening cause.

cause variation, common See common cause variation.

cause variation, special See special cause variation.

cautery The application of a caustic substance, a hot instrument, an electric current, or other agent to destroy abnormal tissue by searing, burning, or scarring.

cavity **1.** A hollow place or space, or a potential space, within the body or in one of its organs, as in the chest cavity or the peritoneal cavity. *See also* peritoneal cavity. **2.** *See* caries.

cavity, peritoneal See peritoneal cavity.

CBC Abbreviation for complete blood count. *See* blood count.

CBMT See Certification Board for Music Therapists.

CBO See Congressional Budget Office.

CC See Catecholamine Club; Credentialing Commission.

CCA See Conference of Consulting Actuaries.

CCAD See Carnegie Council on Adolescent Development.

CCBC See Council of Community Blood Centers.

CCBD See Council for Children with Behavioral Disorders.

CCC See Council on Clinical Classifications.

CCE See Council on Chiropractic Education.

CCI/NBCVT See Cardiovascular Credentialing International.

CCMS See Congress of County Medical Societies.

CCNA See Council on Certification of Nurse Anesthetists.

CCNCC See Commission on Clinical Nomenclatures, Coding, and Classification.

CCO See Council on Chiropractic Orthopedics.

CCOC See Council on Clinical Optometric Care.

CCPT See Council on Chiropractic Physiological Therapeutics.

CCRN *See* certified critical care nurse.

CCS *See* certified coding specialist.

CCU Abbreviation for cardiac care unit; cardiovascular care unit; coronary care unit; or critical care unit. *See also* cardiac care unit; special care unit.

CCU nurse *See* critical care nurse.

CD *See* compact disk.

CDABO *See* College of Diplomates of the American Board of Orthodontics.

CDC *See* Centers for Disease Control and Prevention.

CDC National AIDS Clearinghouse (NAC) A service of the Centers for Disease Control and Prevention that collects, analyzes, and disseminates information on acquired immunodeficiency syndrome (AIDS), primarily for health professionals, educators, social service workers, attorneys, employers and human resource professionals, state HIV/AIDS programs, community organizations, and service associations. Formerly (1991) National AIDS Information Clearinghouse; (1993) National AIDS Clearinghouse. *See also* acquired immunodeficiency syndrome; Centers for Disease Control and Prevention; clearinghouse.

CDER *See* Center for Death Education and Research.

CDF *See* Children's Defense Fund.

CDHCF *See* Consultant Dietitians in Health Care Facilities.

CDI *See* Clearinghouse on Disability Information.

CDL *See* National Board for Certification of Dental Laboratories.

CDM *See* Center for Dance Medicine.

CDMA *See* Chain Drug Marketing Associates.

CD-ROM disc *See* CD-ROM disk.

CD-ROM disk In computer science, a compact disk that functions as a read-only memory. A CD-ROM disk holds a database that is usually updated monthly or quarterly. CD-ROM drives and disks are relatively expensive, but they replace the cost of modem and telecommunications charges and they may be shared with multiple computers. On-line is an alternative method of accessing a database. *Synonyms*: CD-ROM; CD-ROM disc. *See also* modem; on-line; read-only memory.

CDS *See* Christian Dental Society; Christian Doctors Sodality.

CEA *See* carcinoembryonic antigen; Center for Early Adolescence.

CEASD *See* Conference of Educational Administrators Serving the Deaf.

cease dependency on mass inspection One of Deming's Fourteen Points emphasizing the need to improve processes and to emphasize prevention of mistakes, rather than spending considerable resources on mass inspection that separates defective products, which are either thrown out or reworked, from acceptable products. *See also* Deming's Fourteen Points; Deming, W. Edwards; inspection; quality inspection.

CEC *See* Cryogenic Engineering Conference.

CEE *See* Council on Electrolysis Education.

celiac disease A chronic nutritional disturbance, usually of young children, caused by the inability to metabolize gluten, which results in malnutrition, a distended abdomen, muscle wasting, and the passage of stools having a high fat content. The disorder can be controlled by a special diet that emphasizes the elimination of all foods containing gluten. *See also* disease; gluten; malabsorption.

Celiac Society/Dietary Support Coalition, American *See* American Celiac Society/Dietary Support Coalition.

celioscope *See* laparoscope.

cell A minute protoplasmic mass that makes up organized tissue, consisting of a nucleus surrounded by cytoplasm that contains the various organelles and is enclosed in the cell or plasma membrane. A cell is the fundamental structural and functional unit of living organisms. *See also* cell kinetics; collagen; protoplasm; sickle cell.

cell anemia, sickle *See* sickle cell anemia.

Cell Biology, American Society for *See* American Society for Cell Biology.

cell crisis, sickle *See* sickle cell crisis.

Cell Disease, National Association for Sickle *See* National Association for Sickle Cell Disease.

cell disease, sickle *See* sickle cell anemia.

cell kinetics The study of the rates and mechanisms by which cells undergo a divisional cycle. *See also* cell; kinetics.

cell-mediated immune response An immune response mediated by T lymphocytes (T cells) chiefly against viral and fungal invasion and transplanted tissue. *See also* immune response; lymphocyte.

cell, sickle *See* sickle cell.

cells, packed *See* packed cells.

cell trait, sickle *See* sickle cell trait.

cellulitis An acute suppurative inflammation of the

deep subcutaneous tissues and sometimes muscle, which may be associated with abscess formation. It is usually caused by infection of an operative or traumatic wound or burn. The most common bacteria causing cellulitis are group A streptococci and *Staphylococcus aureus. See also* bacteria; inflammation; infection.

Celsius scale   A temperature scale on which zero degrees is officially 273.15 kelvins and 100 degrees is 373.15 kelvins. The degree Celsius is commonly called the degree centigrade with O degrees centigrade at the freezing point of fresh water and 100 degrees centigrade at the boiling point of fresh water at normal atmospheric pressure of 760 mm. The Celsius scale was developed by the Swedish astronomer, Anders Celsius (1701-1744). The Celsius scale is an example of an interval scale. *See also* centigrade scale; Fahrenheit scale; interval scale; scale; temperature; thermometer.

census   An official, usually periodic enumeration of a population, such as the number of individuals (for example, patients) in an area or building (for example, a hospital) at a given time. *See also* adjusted daily census; average daily census; inpatient census; occupancy.

census, adjusted daily   *See* adjusted daily census.

census, average daily   *See* average daily census.

census, inpatient   *See* inpatient census.

Center for Attitudinal Healing (CAH)   A nonsectarian organization founded in 1975 to supplement traditional health care by offering free services in attitudinal healing for children and adults with life-threatening illnesses or other crises. The concept of attitudinal healing is based on the belief that it is possible to choose peace rather than conflict and love rather than fear; the center defines health as inner peace and healing as the process of letting go of fear. *See also* heal.

Center for Dance Medicine (CDM)   An organization founded in 1978 to educate dancers about their bodies and preventive medicine in order to help them avoid injuries. It conducts workshops and seminars. *See also* preventive medicine.

Center for Death Education and Research (CDER)   A national organization founded in 1969 interested in bringing recent and relevant ideas, information, and insights concerning death to the public. It sponsors research into grief and bereavement and studies of attitudes and responses to death and dying. *See also* mourn; thanatology.

Center for Devices and Radiologic Health   *See* Food and Drug Administration.

Center for Drugs and Biologics   *See* Food and Drug Administration.

Center for Early Adolescence (CEA)   An organization founded in 1978 that provides training, technical assistance, and information services to agencies and individuals, such as teachers, social service personnel, physicians, and clergy, who work with youth aged 10 to 15 years. *See also* adolescence.

Center for Environmental Health   *See* Centers for Disease Control and Prevention.

Center for Food Safety and Applied Nutrition   *See* Food and Drug Administration.

Center for General Health Services Extramural Research and the Center for General Health Services Intramural Research   Components of the Agency for Health Care Policy and Research that fund projects within and outside the agency, including the use of large databases for policy research on costs, utilization, access, and long term care. *See also* access; Agency for Health Care Policy and Research; long term care.

Center for Hazardous Materials Research (CHMR)   A nonmembership organization founded in 1985 that conducts applied research programs on the use and disposal of hazardous materials and wastes. It develops and implements policy on the economic, environmental, institutional, public health, public policy, and technological issues presented by hazardous materials and wastes. It offers many services, such as technical assistance to industry and government in the areas of pollution prevention, recycling, and waste minimization and management; technical services to communities relating to hazardous waste site cleanup; and educational and training programs in health and safety, emergency response, and hazardous materials handling. *See also* hazardous materials; hazardous waste.

Center for Health Promotion and Education   *See* Centers for Disease Control and Prevention.

Center for Humane Options in Childbirth Experiences (CHOICE)   A national organization founded in 1977 composed of 1,200 medical professionals, paraprofessionals, and other individuals who teach and encourage parents, parents-to-be groups, and other persons working in family-oriented hospital birth centers and out-of-hospital situations. It trains and certifies attendants to attend or coach births and acts as a consumer advocate for hospital births. *See also* childbirth center.

Center for Infectious Diseases *See* Centers for Disease Control and Prevention.

center line The line on a graph representing the average (for example, the mean or median) value of the items being plotted. *See also* graph; mean; median.

Center for Medical Consumers and Health Care Information (CMC) A national organization founded in 1976 that encourages individuals to make a critical evaluation of all information received from health professionals, to use medical services more selectively, and to understand the limitations of modern medicine. It promotes awareness that life-style choices, such as smoking, exercise habits, and nutritional practices, have more effect on health than access to medical care. *See also* consumer; evaluation; health professional; information.

Center for Medical Effectiveness Research A component of the Agency for Health Care Policy and Research that focuses on patient outcomes and alternative strategies for prevention, treatment, and management of medical conditions, including possible overuse or underuse of services and issues of accessibility. *See also* Agency for Health Care Policy and Research.

Center for Mental Health Services *See* Substance Abuse and Mental Health Services Administration.

Center for Prevention Services *See* Centers for Disease Control and Prevention.

Center for Professional Development and Training *See* Centers for Disease Control and Prevention.

Center for Research in Ambulatory Health Care Administration (CRAHCA) A nonmembership organization founded in 1973 that assists in upgrading the quality of medical care through innovative education programs and research on management systems, cost, and productivity. It works with administrators of medical group practices in the United States, Canada, Mexico, and Europe. *See also* administrator; ambulatory health care; group practice.

Center for Research Dissemination and Liaison A component of the Agency for Health Care Policy and Research that will identify mechanisms for compiling or cataloguing research findings and applying them in various practice settings. *See also* Agency for Health Care Policy and Research.

Center for the Rights of the Terminally Ill (CRTI) A national organization founded in 1986 composed of physicians, nurses, attorneys, pro-life organizations, and disability rights groups seeking to secure for the elderly, the handicapped, and the sick and dying the right to competent, compassionate, and ethical health care. It opposes euthanasia, assisted suicide, and abortion. It opposes "living will" legislation as unnecessary and dangerous. It promotes a federal conscience clause law that would allow health professionals to decline to perform any act of omission or commission that would cause or hasten the death of a patient. *See also* abortion; disability; euthanasia; living will; pro-life; terminal illness.

Center for Science in the Public Interest (CSPI) A national organization founded in 1971 composed of 250,000 scientists, nutrition educators, journalists, and lawyers interested in effects of science and technology on society. Its past work has centered primarily on food safety and nutrition problems at the national level. It monitors current research and federal agencies that oversee food safety, trade, and nutrition. It has initiated legal actions to ban unsafe and poorly tested food additives and has petitioned federal agencies for better food labeling and action against deceptive food advertising, especially advertising directed at children. *See also* public interest.

Centers for Disease Control and Prevention (CDC) An agency of the US Department of Health and Human Services, with headquarters in Atlanta, concerned with all phases of control of communicable, vector-borne, and other occupational diseases. The CDC's responsibilities include epidemiology, surveillance, detection, laboratory science, ecologic investigations, training, and disease control methods for an increasing variety of health issues. The CDC's four centers and one institute are: the Center for Environmental Health, the Center for Health Promotion and Education, the Center for Infectious Diseases, the Center for Prevention Services, and the National Institute for Occupational Safety and Health. The CDC was formerly called Communicable Disease Center (1946) and Center for Disease Control (1970). *See also* epidemiology; occupational disease; surveillance.

centers of excellence Tertiary care facilities that have established a reputation for quality in one or more areas. Their reputation tends to draw patients from extended geographical areas, thereby achieving economies of scale. *See also* catchment area;

economies of scale; tertiary care center; tertiary care hospital.

Center for Social Gerontology, The   *See* The Center for Social Gerontology.

Center for the Study of Aging (CSA)   A nonmembership organization founded in 1957 composed of behavioral scientists, educators, gerontologists, physicians, and other health professionals interested in education, research, and training, and providing leadership in the field of health and fitness for older people. Its services include programs for volunteers and professionals in aging, gerontology, geriatrics, wellness, fitness, and health, and consultant services, including adult day care, nutrition, nursing homes, and retirement. *See also* adult day care; aging; fitness; geriatric medicine; gerontology; wellness.

Center for the Study of Pharmacy and Therapeutics for the Elderly (CSPTE)   An organization founded in 1978 that conducts research in pharmacotherapeutic and pharmacodynamic geriatrics and gerontology. *See also* geriatric medicine; gerontology; pharmacy; therapeutics.

Center for Substance Abuse Prevention   *See* Substance Abuse and Mental Health Services Administration.

Center for Substance Abuse Treatment   *See* Substance Abuse and Mental Health Services Administration.

Center for the Well-Being of Health Professionals (CWBHP)   A national society founded in 1979 composed of 800 health and other professional associations interested in promoting the well-being of health professionals and their families through preventive education on manifestations of disabilities, increased awareness about the stresses inherent in the system of providing health services, and efforts to improve and maintain effectiveness. It conducts research and supports efforts to study the incidence and causes of professional impairment, with prevention as a goal. *See also* health maintenance.

centigrade   Having 100 gradations (steps or degrees). *See also* Celsius scale; centigrade scale.

centigrade scale   A scale in which the interval between two fixed points is divided into 100 equal units. *See also* Celsius scale; centigrade; scale; thermometer.

centile   *See* quantile.

central line   A catheter inserted into a major blood vessel, typically through the subclavian vein or internal jugular vein. *See also* catheter; umbilical line.

central nervous system (CNS)   The portion of the human nervous system consisting of the brain and spinal cord. *See also* brain; cerebellum; cerebrum; hypothalamus; meninges; nervous system; spinal cord.

Central Neuropsychiatric Association (CNPA)   An organization founded in 1922 composed of 250 neurologists, neurosurgeons, and psychiatrists interested in promoting neuropsychiatry and related fields through presentations on theoretical and chemical topics. It fosters friendly interaction and sociability among neurologists, psychiatrists, and neurosurgeons. *See also* neurological surgery; neurology; neuropsychiatry; psychiatry.

central processing   In health care, the receiving, decontaminating, cleaning, preparing, disinfecting, and sterilizing of reusable items. Central processing is the function of the central service unit of a hospital or other type of health care organization. *See also* central service department.

central processing unit   The hardware and program instructions that control the interpretation and execution of all other instructions to a computer. *Synonym:* computer brain. *See also* computer; unit.

central service (CS) department   The department that provides sterilization, storage, and distribution of sterile equipment and supplies. *Synonyms:* central processing department; central processing unit; central supply. *See also* central processing; sterilization.

Central Service Personnel, American Society for Healthcare   *See* American Society for Healthcare Central Service Personnel.

Central Society for Clinical Research (CSCR)   A national organization founded in 1928 composed of 1,294 individuals who have accomplished a meritorious original investigation in the clinical or allied sciences of medicine and who enjoy unimpeachable moral standing in the profession. *See also* research.

central supply   *See* central service department.

central tendency, measures of   *See* measures of central tendency.

central venous pressure (CVP)   Blood pressure measured within the main veins of the body, usually with a specially designed catheter called a central venous pressure catheter. *See also* catheter.

CEO   *See* chief executive officer.

CEPH   *See* Council on Education for Public Health.

cephalagia   *See* headache.

cephalhematoma A subperiosteal hemorrhage (bruise) limited to the surface of one cranial (skull) bone, usually a benign condition seen frequently in newborns as a result of bone (birth) trauma. *Synonym*: cephalohematoma. *See also* birth trauma.

cephalic Relating to the head. *Compare* caudal.

cephalohematoma *See* cephalhematoma.

cephalosporin A broad-spectrum antibiotic closely related to penicillin and originally derived from the fungus *Cephalosporium*. Cephalosporins are commonly referred to as first-generation, second-generation, or third-generation cephalosporins. *See also* antibacterial; antibiotic.

cerebellum The part of the brain largely responsible for posture, balance, and muscle movement, located in the human at the base of the brain in back. It is connected to the cerebrum. *See also* ataxia; brain; brainstem; cerebrum; central nervous system.

cerebral death *See* vegetative state.

cerebral palsy A disorder usually caused by damage to the motor areas of the brain occurring at or before birth and marked by muscular impairment, such as poor coordination. *See also* brain; developmental disability; palsy.

Cerebral Palsy Associations, United *See* United Cerebral Palsy Associations.

Cerebral Palsy and Developmental Medicine, American Academy for *See* American Academy for Cerebral Palsy and Developmental Medicine.

cerebrospinal fluid (CSF) Fluid that surrounds the brain and spinal cord. It is typically withdrawn during a lumbar puncture procedure to determine whether meningitis is present. *See also* lumbar puncture; meningitis.

cerebrospinal meningitis *See* meningitis.

cerebrovascular accident (CVA) An abnormal condition of the blood vessels of the brain characterized by occlusion by an embolus or cerebrovascular hemorrhage, resulting in decreased blood supply to the brain tissues normally supplied by the damaged blood vessel. The sequelae of a CVA depend on the location of the occlusion or bleeding and the extent of the area of decreased blood supply. Manifestations include paralysis, weakness, speech defect, or death. *Synonym*: stroke. *See also* accident; aphasia; ischemia; multi-infarct dementia; thrombosis; transient ischemic attack.

cerebrum The large, rounded structure that makes up most of the brain; it controls and integrates motor, sensory, and higher mental functions, such as thought, reason, emotion, and memory. *See also* brain; brainstem; central nervous system; cerebellum.

certificate A formal declaration that can be used to document a fact, such as a birth certificate or a certificate of insurance. *See also* birth certificate; certificate of compliance; certificate of insurance; certificate of need; death certificate; diploma.

certificate, birth *See* birth certificate.

certificate of compliance A document signed by an authorized party affirming that the supplier of a service or product has met the requirements of the relevant specifications, contract, or regulation. *Synonyms*: certificate of conformance; certificate of conformity. *See also* certificate; compliance.

certificate of conformance *See* certificate of compliance.

certificate of conformity *See* certificate of compliance.

certificate, death *See* death certificate.

certificate, fetal death *See* fetal death certificate.

certificate of insurance (COI) A certificate issued by an insurance company to verify that an individual (such as a physician) or an institution is insured for a certain type of risk during a specific period. *See also* certificate; insurance.

certificate of necessity *See* certificate of need.

certificate of need (CON) A certificate issued by a governmental body, such as a state health planning and development agency, to an individual or a health care organization proposing to construct or modify a facility, incur a major capital expenditure, or offer a new or different health service. When a certificate is required (for instance, for all proposals involving more than a minimum capital investment or that change bed capacity), it is a condition of licensure of the organization or service and is intended to control expansion of health care organizations and services in the public interest by preventing excessive or duplicate development of organizations and services. *See also* administrative process; certificate; licensure; public interest; state health planning and development agency.

certification The procedure and action by which a duly authorized body evaluates and recognizes (certifies) an individual, institution, or educational program as meeting predetermined requirements, such as standards. Certification is essentially synonymous with accreditation, except that certification is often, but not always, applied to individuals (such as certifying a medical specialist), whereas accreditation is applied to institutions or programs (such as accrediting a hospital or a residency program). Certification programs are generally nongovernmental and do not exclude the uncertified from practice as do licensure programs. While licensure is meant to establish the minimum competence required to protect the public health, safety, and welfare, certification enables the public to identify those practitioners who have met a standard of training and experience set above the level required for licensure. *Synonym*: occupational certification. *See also* accreditation; board certified; licensure; qualify; recertification; uncertified.

Certification of Acupuncturists, National Commission for the *See* National Commission for the Certification of Acupuncturists.

Certification Agency for Medical Lab Personnel, National *See* National Certification Agency for Medical Lab Personnel.

Certification, American Board of Post Anesthesia Nursing *See* American Board of Post Anesthesia Nursing Certification.

certification, board *See* board certification.

Certification Board, American Athletic Trainers Association and *See* American Athletic Trainers Association and Certification Board.

Certification Board, American Occupational Therapy *See* American Occupational Therapy Certification Board.

Certification Board for Music Therapists (CBMT) A national board founded in 1982 that certifies and recertifies (every five years) professional music therapists. There are 4,000 board-certified professional music therapists. *See also* board; certification; music therapy; recertification.

Certification Board, Nuclear Medicine Technology *See* Nuclear Medicine Technology Certification Board.

Certification Board of Pediatric Nurse Practitioners and Nurses, National *See* National Certification Board of Pediatric Nurse Practitioners and Nurses.

Certification of Computer Professionals, Association of the Institute for *See* Association of the Institute for Certification of Computer Professionals.

Certification of Computer Professionals, Institute for *See* Institute for Certification of Computer Professionals.

Certification of Dental Laboratories, National

Board for *See* National Board for Certification of Dental Laboratories.

Certification in Dental Technology, National Board for *See* National Board for Certification in Dental Technology.

certification examination A test given by a certifying body, such as a medical specialty board, for the purpose of determining whether an individual, such as a physician, meets the requirements for the certification sought, such as pediatrics. *See also* certification; examination.

certification by HCFA A statement by the Health Care Financing Administration (HCFA) that a hospital meets HCFA's conditions of participation. Certification by HCFA is required for Medicare and Medicaid reimbursement. *See also* certification; deemed status; Health Care Financing Administration.

Certification Institute, Human Resource *See* Human Resource Certification Institute.

certification, labor *See* labor certification.

certification by a medical specialty board. *See* board certification.

Certification, National Association for the Advancement of Psychoanalysis and the American Boards for Accreditation and *See* National Association for the Advancement of Psychoanalysis and the American Boards for Accreditation and Certification.

Certification, National Commission for Electrologist *See* National Commission for Electrologist Certification.

Certification, National Council for Therapeutic Recreation *See* National Council for Therapeutic Recreation Certification.

certification, occupational *See* occupational certification.

Certification of Orthopaedic Technologists, National Board for *See* National Board for Certification of Orthopaedic Technologists.

Certification in Orthotics and Prosthetics, American Board for *See* American Board for Certification in Orthotics and Prosthetics.

Certification in Pedorthics, Board of *See* Board of Certification in Pedorthics.

Certification of Physician Assistants, National Commission on *See* National Commission on Certification of Physician Assistants.

certification, re- *See* recertification.

Certification Reciprocity Consortium/Alcoholism

and Other Drug Abuse *See* National Certification Reciprocity Consortium/Alcoholism and Other Drug Abuse.

certified Formally approved and recognized by a certifying body, as in a certified hospital or certified counselor. *Compare* uncertified. *See also* accreditation; board certified; certification; licensure.

Certified Allergists, American Association of *See* American Association of Certified Allergists.

certified, board *See* board certified.

certified coding specialist (CCS) A health information management professional certified by the American Health Information Management Association, who assigns and sequences codes to classify diagnoses and procedures for use in medical research, reimbursement, and health care planning. *See also* American Health Information Management Association; certification; certified; medical record abstractor; medical record coder.

certified computer programmer A computer programmer certified by the Institute for Certification of Computer Professionals. *See also* certification; certified; computer programmer; Institute for Certification of Computer Professionals.

certified counselor A counselor who assists persons with aging, vocational development, adolescent, family, and marital concerns and who has been certified by the National Board for Certified Counselors. *See also* certification; certified; counselor; National Board for Certified Counselors.

Certified Counselors, National Board for *See* National Board for Certified Counselors.

certified critical care nurse (CCRN) A registered nurse who is certified by the American Association of Critical-Care Nurses. *See also* American Association of Critical-Care Nurses; certification; certified; critical care nurse.

certified data processor A data processor who is certified by the Institute for Certification of Computer Professionals. *See also* certified; data processing; data processing department; Institute for Certification of Computer Professionals.

Certified Hazard Control Management, Board of *See* Board of Certified Hazard Control Management.

certified health plan, state- *See* state-certified health plan.

certified hospital A hospital recognized by the US Department of Health and Human Services as meeting its standards for participation as a provider in the Medicare program. *See also* certification; certified; hospital; Medicare.

certified medical assistant (CMA) A medical assistant who is certified by the American Association of Medical Assistants. *See also* American Association of Medical Assistants; certification; certified; medical assistant.

certified medical representative An individual who is certified by the Certified Medical Representatives Institute. *See also* certification; certified; Certified Medical Representatives Institute.

Certified Medical Representatives Institute (CMRI) An institute founded in 1966 devoted to pharmaceutical education. It administers a program to provide pharmaceutical representatives with scientific information to help them communicate with physicians and pharmacists. The program consists of three years of home study with examinations each trimester. Upon successful completion, participants are awarded the designation of certified medical representative. *See also* certification; detail person.

certified nurse A registered nurse who has obtained a credential of certification in a nursing specialty. About 40 percent of the certified nurses in the United States have their credentials from the American Nurses Association, which examines and certifies in many clinical and administrative areas of nursing ranging from adult nurse practitioner to school nurse. *See also* American Nurses Association; certification; certified; nurse; nurse practitioner; registered nurse.

certified nurse-midwife (CNM) A registered nurse specializing in management of maternal and perinatal care in normal pregnancy, labor, and childbirth, who is certified by the American College of Nurse-Midwives. *See also* American College of Nurse-Midwives; certification; certified; nurse-midwife.

Certified Orthoptists, American Association of *See* American Association of Certified Orthoptists.

certified patient account manager (CPAM) A patient account manager who has satisfied certification requirements established by the American Guild of Patient Account Managers. *See also* certified; patient account manager.

certified professional bureau executive (CPBE) A professional bureau executive who has met the requirements for certification of the Medical-Dental-Hospital Bureaus of America. *See also* certification; certified; Medical-Dental-Hospital Bureaus of

America.

Certified Professional Business Consultants, Institute of *See* Institute of Certified Professional Business Consultants.

certified professional in quality assurance (CPQA) A quality assurance professional who has met the requirements for certification by the National Association of Quality Assurance Professionals. *See also* certification; certified; National Association of Quality Assurance Professionals; quality assurance professional.

certified public accountant (CPA) An accountant who has satisfied the statutory and administrative requirements of his or her jurisdiction to be registered or licensed as a public accountant. *See also* accountant; auditor; certification; certified.

Certified and Registered Encephalographic Technicians and Technologists, American Board of *See* American Board of Certified and Registered Encephalographic Technicians and Technologists.

certified registered nurse anesthetist (CRNA) A licensed registered nurse who has met the certification requirements of the Council on Certification of Nurse Anesthetists and is qualified by education and experience to administer anesthesia. *See also* certification; certified; Council on Certification of Nurse Anesthetists; nurse anesthetist.

certified safety professional (CSP) A safety engineer, industrial hygienist, safety manager, fire protection engineer, or other persons who have met the certification requirements of the Board of Certified Safety Professionals. *See also* Board of Certified Safety Professionals; certification; certified; industrial hygienist.

Certified Social Workers, Academy of *See* Academy of Certified Social Workers.

certified systems professional A systems professional certified by the Institute for Certification of Computer Professionals. *See also* certification; certified; Institute for Certification of Computer Professionals.

certified, un- *See* uncertified.

Certifying Board of the American Dental Assistants Association *See* Dental Assisting National Board.

certiorari, writ of *See* writ of certiorari.

cerumen Earwax.

Cervical Pathology, American Society for Colposcopy and *See* American Society for Col-

poscopy and Cervical Pathology.

cesarean delivery *See* cesarean section.

Cesarean Prevention Movement (CPM) A national organization founded in 1982 composed of 2,000 individuals interested in the increasing rate of cesarean births. Its objectives include promoting vaginal births, offering encouragement, information, and support for women wanting vaginal births after cesareans (VBAC), and assisting in organizing and informing new parents and cesarean parents on preventing future cesareans by opposing unnecessary medical interventions during the birth process and by working to make hospital routines more responsive to women in labor. It offers teacher training and course materials and sponsors a childbirth education certification program. *See also* birth; certification; cesarean section; labor.

cesarean section (CS) Delivery of a fetus through incisions in the abdominal wall (laparotomy) and the uterine wall (hysterotomy). This definition does not include removal of the fetus from the abdominal cavity in case of rupture of the uterus or abdominal pregnancy. *Synonyms*: abdominal delivery; cesarean delivery. *See also* primary cesarean section; section; vaginal birth after cesarean section.

cesarean section, primary *See* primary cesarean section.

cesarean section, vaginal birth after *See* vaginal birth after cesarean section.

CFCM *See* Committee for Freedom of Choice in Medicine.

CFD *See* Choice in Dying - The National Council for the Right to Die.

CFH *See* Council on Family Health.

CFMA *See* Council for Medical Affairs.

CFO *See* chief financial officer.

CGFNS *See* Commission on Graduates of Foreign Nursing Schools.

CHA *See* Catholic Health Association of the United States.

Chain Drug Marketing Associates (CDMA) A national organization founded in 1988 composed of 72 drug store chains located in the United States, Puerto Rico, and Canada. It represents members in the market for merchandise. Formerly (1992) Affiliated/Associated Drug Stores. *See also* drugstore; marketing; pharmacy.

Chain Drug Stores, National Association of *See* National Association of Chain Drug Stores.

chair A nonsexist way of saying "chairman or chairwoman"; a chairperson. *See also* chairperson; department chair; gender neutral.

chairman, department *See* department chair (of a clinical service).

chairman of service *See* chief of service; department chair.

Chairmen, Association of Medical School Pediatric Department *See* Association of Medical School Pediatric Department Chairmen.

Chairmen, Association of Pathology *See* Association of Pathology Chairmen.

Chairmen of Departments of Psychiatry, American Association of *See* American Association of Chairmen of Departments of Psychiatry.

chairperson The presiding officer of an organization, department, committee, task force, or meeting. "Chairperson" or "chair" increasingly is replacing the term "chairman." *See also* chair; person.

chairside The dentistry equivalent of bedside in medicine. *See also* dentistry.

Champlin Foundations, The *See* The Champlin Foundations.

CHAMPUS *See* Civilian Health and Medical Program of the Uniformed Services.

CHAMPVA *See* Civilian Health and Medical Program of the Veterans Administration.

chance The unknown and unpredictable element in events that seems to have no assignable (special) cause. *See also* accident; probable error; random error; special cause; stochastic.

chance of cure, lost *See* lost chance of cure.

chance of survival, lost *See* lost chance of survival.

change To cause to be different. *Compare* inertia. *See also* change agent; stability.

change agent An individual whose efforts facilitate change in a group or organization. *See also* agent; change.

change, sex *See* sex change.

CHAP *See* Community Health Accreditation Program.

chaplain A member of the clergy or a layperson who performs religious functions and who may provide pastoral counseling to patients, their families, and organizational staff in institutional settings, such as a hospital. *See also* chaplaincy service; clinical pastoral counselor.

chaplaincy service A service ministering religious activities and providing pastoral counseling to patients, their families, and staff of a health care organization. *Synonyms*: pastoral care; pastoral counseling department. *See also* chaplain; clinical pastoral counselor.

Chaplains, College of *See* College of Chaplains.

characteristic, key quality *See* key quality characteristic.

characteristics, quality *See* quality characteristics.

charge **1.** The dollar amount assigned to a unit of service, such as a physician visit or a day in a hospital special care unit, charged by a physician, hospital, or other health care provider. The dollar amount charged for services may not reflect actual costs of providing the services. Further, the methods by which charges are related to cost vary substantially from service to service and institution to institution. Different third-party payers may require use of different methods of determining either charges or costs. Charges for one service provided by an organization are often used to subsidize the costs of other services. Charges to one type or group of patients may also be used to subsidize the costs of providing services to other groups of patients. *Compare* cost. *See also* actual charge; ancillary charge; covered charge; customary, prevailing, and reasonable charge; daily service charge; fixed charge; prevailing charge; reasonable charge; risk charge. **2.** A statement of purpose given to a group convened to accomplish stated objectives, as in the task force listened to its charge. **3.** To impose a duty, responsibility, or obligation on, as in charging the task force with carrying out the project. **4.** To accuse, as in charged with medical malpractice. **5.** An accusation, as in an unsubstantiated charge.

charge, actual *See* actual charge.

charge, ancillary *See* ancillary charge.

charge, covered *See* covered charge.

charge, customary, prevailing, and reasonable *See* customary, prevailing, and reasonable charge.

charge, daily service *See* daily service charge.

charge, fixed *See* fixed charge.

charge nurse A registered nurse or other qualified individual who directs and supervises the provision of nursing care in a nursing unit for a given period of time, as in one shift. *See also* nurse; registered nurse; unit manager.

charge, prevailing *See* prevailing charge.

charge, reasonable *See* reasonable charge.

charge, risk *See* risk charge.

charge, take- *See* take-charge.

charge, usual, customary, and reasonable *See* usual, customary, and reasonable charge.

charitable **1.** Generous in giving help or money to the needy, as in a charitable hospital. **2.** Mild or tolerant in judging other persons.

Charitable Foundation, G. Harold and Leila Y. Mathers *See* G. Harold and Leila Y. Mathers Charitable Foundation.

charitable hospital A hospital whose revenues are generated in whole or in substantial part from charitable donations and that specializes in inpatient services for the indigent. Many children's hospitals are charitable hospitals. *See also* children's hospital.

charitable immunity A now largely discarded doctrine under which charitable enterprises, such as a hospital, were held blameless for their negligent actions. *See also* charity; immunity.

charitable organization A public charity or a private foundation that is generally eligible to receive tax-deductible charitable contributions. A substantial number of hospitals belong to one or the other category. The theory behind tax exemption for charitable organizations is that in their absence, the government would need to provide services with public funds. *Synonym*: charitable institution. *See also* foundation; organization; philanthropy.

Charitable Trust, Lucille P. Markey *See* Lucille P. Markey Charitable Trust.

Charitable Trusts, The Pew *See* The Pew Charitable Trusts.

charity A gift or an activity that benefits an indefinite number of persons by the provision of religion, education, or relief from disease, by assisting people to establish themselves in life or by erecting or maintaining public works. The essence of charity is that it is for the public at large, rather than for specific individuals. Charity, in contrast to philanthropy, usually does not expect some form of improvement in return for donation of services or money. *Compare* philanthropy. *See also* care; charity allowance; charity care.

charity allowance A reduced charge for health care services for indigent or medically indigent patients. *See also* charity; charity care; medically indigent.

charity care Free or reduced-fee care provided to patients with financial constraints. *See also* charity; charity allowance.

charlatan One who pretends to more knowledge or

skill than he or she possesses. *See also* knowledge; mountebank; quack; skill.

chart **1.** A pictorial device, such as a pie chart or bar graph, used to illustrate relationships. *See also* graph. **2.** A diagram that exhibits a relationship, often functional, between two sets of numbers as a set of points having coordinates determined by the relationship. *See also* control chart; run chart. **3.** A patient's medical record. *See also* medical record.

chart, control *See* control chart.

charter statement In quality improvement, a list of the duties and responsibilities of a quality improvement project team. *See also* quality improvement team.

charting, open *See* open charting.

chart, organizational *See* organizational chart.

chart, Pareto *See* Pareto chart.

chart, pie *See* pie chart.

chart, run *See* run chart.

chauvinism Prejudiced belief in the superiority of one's own gender, group, or kind, as in male chauvinism. *See also* male chauvinism.

chauvinism, male *See* male chauvinism.

CHC *See* Coalitions for Health Care; community health center.

checklist A list of actions or items to be reviewed during a process; the actions or items are "checked off" as they are completed or identified. *See also* process.

check sheet A data collection form that helps to summarize data based on sample observations and begin to identify patterns. A check sheet is used to answer the question, "How often are certain events happening?" It starts the process of translating "opinions" into "facts." The completed form displays the data in a simple graphic summary. *Synonym*: checksheet. *See also* Pareto chart.

chelation therapy The use of metal binding and bioinorganic agents given to patients intravenously in cases of blood poisoning to "pick up" and remove calcium, lead, or other toxic heavy metals and restore cellular homeostasis. Because of lack of controlled studies for conditions other than calcinosis, digitalis toxicity, and excessive body storage of heavy metals, chelation therapy is not considered standard medical procedure. *See also* calcium; digitalis; lead.

Chelation Therapy, American Board of *See* American Board of Chelation Therapy.

chemical **1.** Pertaining to chemistry. *See also* chemistry. **2.** Pertaining to the action of chemicals, as in chemical equivalence. *See also* chemical equivalence. **3.** A drug, particularly an illegal drug, as in chemical dependency. *See also* chemical dependency.

chemical abuse *See* substance abuse.

Chemical and Allied Trades Association, Drug, *See* Drug, Chemical and Allied Trades Association.

chemical dependency A physical and psychological habituation to drugs or alcohol. *See also* chemical dependency services.

Chemical Dependency Nurses, National Consortium of *See* National Consortium of Chemical Dependency Nurses.

chemical dependency services Services of a health care organization including diagnosis and treatment of alcohol-dependent and/or drug-dependent patients. *See also* alcohol and other drug dependence; chemical dependency.

chemical equivalence The degree to which drug products contain identical amounts of the same active ingredients in the same dosage forms, meet existing physiochemical standards in official compendia, and are chemically indistinguishable. *See also* bioequivalence; pharmaceutical equivalence.

chemical name The description of the chemical structure of a drug, based on the rules of standard chemical nomenclature. *Compare* brand name; established name; generic name. *See also* name.

chemical pathologist A pathologist who specializes in chemical pathology. *See* chemical pathology; pathologist.

chemical pathology The branch of medicine and subspecialty of pathology dealing with the application of biochemical data to the detection, confirmation, or monitoring of disease. *See also* pathology.

Chemical Society, Histo- *See* Histochemical Society.

chemistry The science dealing with the elements and atomic relations of matter and the various compounds of the elements. *See also* biochemistry; clinical chemistry; forensic chemistry; histochemistry; neurochemistry; physical science; radiochemistry.

Chemistry, American Association for Clinical *See* American Association for Clinical Chemistry.

Chemistry, American Board of Clinical *See* American Board of Clinical Chemistry.

chemistry, bio- *See* biochemistry.

chemistry, clinical *See* clinical chemistry.

chemistry, forensic *See* forensic chemistry.

chemistry, geo- *See* geochemistry.

chemistry, histo- *See* histochemistry.

Chemistry, National Registry in Clinical *See* National Registry in Clinical Chemistry.

chemistry, neuro- *See* neurochemistry.

chemistry, radio- *See* radiochemistry.

chemistry technologist A medical technologist who performs chemical analyses of body fluids and discharges. *See also* medical technologist.

chemoprophylaxis The administration of any chemical, drug, or food supplement to prevent or control the further development of a disease or condition. *Synonym*: chemoprevention. *See also* prophylaxis.

Chemoreception Sciences, Association for *See* Association for Chemoreception Sciences.

chemosurgery A surgical technique in which skin cancer is microscopically excised. *See also* American College of Mohs Micrographic Surgery and Cutaneous Oncology; cancer; skin.

chemotherapy The administration of any chemical or drug to treat a disease or condition to limit its further progress, as in cancer chemotherapy. *Synonym*: drug therapy. *See also* antibiotic.

chest *See* thorax.

Chest Physicians, American College of *See* American College of Chest Physicians.

chest surgeon *See* thoracic surgeon.

chest surgery *See* thoracic surgery.

Chexchange Network (CN) A national organization founded in 1980 composed of 555 continuing health education directors and health seminar coordinators. It teaches marketing techniques to health professionals and develops strategies for health seminars and conferences. *See also* continuing education.

CHF *See* Coalition for Health Funding; congestive heart failure.

chickenpox A contagious disease affecting mainly children and caused by the varicella-zoster virus. It is characterized by vesicular rash that appears in crops over a few days after an incubation period of two to three weeks. The rash is chiefly on the trunk and face and is accompanied by fever. Encephalitis is a rare complication. *Synonym*: varicella. *See also* communicable disease; herpes zoster; infectious diseases; pox.

chief of clinical affairs *See* medical director.

chief, department *See* department chair (of a clinical service).

chief engineer A hospital or other health care organization engineer who directs and administers the organization's equipment, buildings, and grounds maintenance and repair programs. *Synonym*: maintenance engineer. *See also* administrative engineer; engineering.

chief executive officer (CEO) The individual appointed by a governing body to act on its behalf in the overall management of an organization. *Synonyms*: administrator; chief administrative officer; director; executive director; executive vice-president; president; vice-president. *See also* executive; governing body; superintendent.

chief executive officer exit conference A meeting involving surveyor(s), chief executive officer, chairperson of the governing body, nurse executive, president or chief of the medical staff, and, if applicable, the chief operating officer, which is held at the conclusion of an on-site accreditation survey by the Joint Commission on Accreditation of Healthcare Organizations. The purpose of the meeting is the presentation by the surveyor(s) of any findings of significant standards compliance problems and the potential impact of this performance, when accreditation is an issue, on the accreditation decision. The conference also offers an opportunity for participants to clarify issues prior to the conclusion of the survey. *Synonym*: leadership exit conference. *See also* Accreditation Committee; accreditation survey; Joint Commission on Accreditation of Healthcare Organizations; leadership interview.

chief financial officer (CFO) The individual responsible for management of an organization's overall financial plans and policies and the administration of accounting practices. The job typically includes directing the treasury, budgeting, auditing, and tax accounting and purchasing real estate. Specific responsibilities typically include developing and coordinating all necessary and appropriate accounting and statistical data with and for all the departments. *See also* controller.

chief information officer (CIO) The individual in charge of the information systems function of an organization. *Synonym*: information systems director. *See also* information; information system; management information system.

chief of medical affairs *See* medical director.

chief of nursing The individual responsible for the management of all nursing services in a health care organization. *Synonyms*: director of nursing; vice president for/of nursing services. *See also* nurse executive.

chief operating officer (COO) The individual responsible for the management of day-to-day and internal operations of an organization. In many organizations the COO is the second highest management officer and, in the absence of the chief executive officer, is responsible for administration. *Synonyms*: associate administrator; executive vice-president; senior vice-president.

chief resident A resident who has completed minimum training required in a specialty and assumes a leadership role in the supervision, design, and management of a residency program. *See also* residency program; resident.

chief of service A member of an organization's medical staff who is elected or appointed to serve as the medical and administrative head of a clinical service. *See also* department chief; medical staff.

chief of staff The member of an organization's medical staff who is elected, appointed, or employed by the organization and who serves as the medical and administrative head of the medical staff. Working with the medical executive committee and the clinical departments, the chief of staff typically sees that all functions required by law, professional standards, or the Joint Commission on Accreditation of Healthcare Organizations, and the medical staff bylaws, rules, and regulations, are carried out satisfactorily. The chief of staff position varies from organization to organization. He or she may be elected or appointed; serve full time or part time; be salaried, receive a stipend, or serve voluntarily; be an employee of the organization or an independent practitioner; and serve for a set term of one to several years or be employed on a contractual basis. A hospital may have both an elected chief of staff and a hospital-salaried medical director or it may have only one or the other. If the chief of staff is elected by the medical staff, he or she generally chairs the medical executive committee, which reports to the governing board. If the chief of staff is a salaried position, the organization charter usually shows the medical director reporting to the hospital chief executive officer, with the medical executive committee chaired by the elected president of the medical staff and accountable to the governing board. *Synonyms for a salaried chief of* *staff*: chief of clinical affairs; chief of medical services; dean for clinical affairs; director of medical affairs; medical director; vice president for professional services; vice president for medical affairs. *Synonyms for an elected chief of staff*: chairman of the staff; president of the staff. *See also* Joint Commission on Accreditation of Healthcare Organizations; medical director; medical staff; president of the medical staff.

child A person between birth and 13 years of age.

CHILD *See* Children's Healthcare Is a Legal Duty.

child abuse Physical, emotional, or sexual maltreatment of children, usually by parents, relatives, or caretakers. *See also* abuse; battered child syndrome; medical neglect.

Child Abuse and Family Violence, National Council on *See* National Council on Child Abuse and Family Violence.

Child Abuse Institute of Research (CAIR) An organization founded in 1988 composed of individuals interested in improving the quality of life for children by focusing on the problems of child abuse. It promotes education and research into the cause and prevention of child abuse. *See also* child abuse.

Child Abuse Listening and Mediation (CALM) A national organization founded in 1970 that conducts a social service program to prevent and treat sexual, physical, and emotional abuse of children, and offer early intervention for stressed families. It provides emergency child care for parents under stress and conducts a program of public information and education and an in-school education program for students, parents, and teachers on prevention and recognition of child maltreatment. *See also* child abuse.

Child Abuse, National Committee for Prevention of *See* National Committee for Prevention of Child Abuse.

child and adolescent psychiatrist A psychiatrist who subspecializes in child and adolescent psychiatry. *See also* child and adolescent psychiatry.

child and adolescent psychiatry The branch and subspecialty of psychiatry dealing with the diagnosis and treatment of mental, addictive, and emotional disorders of childhood and adolescence. *See also* adolescence; play therapy; psychiatry.

Child and Adolescent Psychiatry, American Academy of *See* American Academy of Child and Adolescent Psychiatry.

Child and Adolescent Psychiatry, Society of Professors of *See* Society of Professors of Child and Adolescent Psychiatry.

child, battered *See* battered child syndrome.

childbearing The human act or process of giving birth. *See also* birth; labor.

childbearing center A center for giving birth. *See also* childbearing; Maternity Center Association; National Association of Childbearing Centers.

Childbearing Centers, National Association of *See* National Association of Childbearing Centers.

childbed fever *See* puerperal fever.

childbirth *See* labor.

Childbirth, American Academy of Husband-Coached *See* American Academy of Husband-Coached Childbirth.

Childbirth Assistants, National Association of *See* National Association of Childbirth Assistants.

childbirth center *See* birthing center.

Childbirth Educators, American Society of *See* American Society of Childbirth Educators.

Childbirth Experiences, Center for Humane Options in *See* Center for Humane Options in Childbirth Experiences.

childbirth, natural *See* natural childbirth.

child death rate The number of deaths of children aged 1 to 4 years in a given year per 1,000 children in this age group. This rate is a useful measure of the burden of preventable communicable diseases in the child population. *See also* communicable disease; disease-specific death rate; fetal death rate; hospital death rate; infant death rate; maternal mortality rate; mortality rate; neonatal death rate; rate.

Child Development, Society for Research in *See* Society for Research in Child Development.

Child Health Act A part of the federal Social Security Act that authorizes funds for maternal and infant care and care for preschool and school-age children. Dental care, crippled children's services, family planning services, and training and research funding are covered under this act. *See also* Social Security Act.

Child Health, Association of Teachers of Maternal and *See* Association of Teachers of Maternal and Child Health.

Child Health Clearinghouse, National Maternal and *See* National Maternal and Child Health Clearinghouse.

Child Health and Human Development, National Institute of　*See* National Institute of Child Health and Human Development.

Child Health, National Center for Education in Maternal and　*See* National Center for Education in Maternal and Child Health.

Child Health Programs, Association of Maternal and　*See* Association of Maternal and Child Health Programs.

child health services, maternal and　*See* maternal and child health services.

Childhood Lead Poisoning, Alliance to End　*See* Alliance to End Childhood Lead Poisoning.

Child Life Council (CLC)　A national organization founded in 1982 composed of child life personnel, patient activities specialists, and students in the field interested in the psychological well-being and optimum development of children, adolescents, and their families in health care settings. *See also* child life specialist.

child life specialist　A specialist in the field of child life who works to reduce the stress of hospitalization for children, adolescents, and their families. *See also* Child Life Council; stress.

Child Mental Health Services, National Consortium for　*See* National Consortium for Child Mental Health Services.

Child Neurology Society (CNS)　A national organization founded in 1971 composed of 900 neurologists certified by the American Board of Psychiatry and Neurology and other individuals specializing in child neurology. *See also* neurology.

Child Nutrition Coalition　*See* Child Nutrition Forum.

Child Nutrition Forum (CNF)　A national organization founded in 1981 composed of 230 organizations involved in agriculture, civil rights, education, and nutrition advocacy; and consumer and religious groups, unions, and elected officials that support effective and adequately funded federal food programs for children. Formerly (1981) Child Nutrition Coalition. *See also* nutrition.

child protection　*See* protection for children.

child protection services　*See* protection for children.

child psychiatrist　*See* child and adolescent psychiatrist.

child psychiatry　*See* child and adolescent psychiatry.

Child Psychoanalysis, Association for　*See* Association for Child Psychoanalysis.

Children, Aid to Families with Dependent　*See* Aid to Families with Dependent Children.

Children, American Association for Protecting　*See* American Association for Protecting Children.

Children, American Association of Psychiatric Services for　*See* American Association of Psychiatric Services for Children.

Children, American Society of Dentistry for　*See* American Society of Dentistry for Children.

Children with Behavioral Disorders, Council for　*See* Council for Children with Behavioral Disorders.

Children, Council on Accreditation of Services for Families and　*See* Council on Accreditation of Services for Families and Children.

Children in Hospitals (CIH)　A national organization founded in 1971 composed of 200 educators, health professionals, and parents seeking to minimize the trauma of a child's hospitalization by supporting and educating parents and medical personnel regarding the need for children to have parents present whenever possible. It encourages hospitals to adopt flexible visiting policies and to provide live-in accommodations for parents with hospitalized children.

Children, Medical Network for Missing　*See* Medical Network for Missing Children.

Children, National Association of Counsel for　*See* National Association of Counsel for Children.

Children, National Association of Homes and Services for　*See* National Association of Homes and Services for Children.

Children, National Association of Psychiatric Treatment Centers for　*See* National Association of Psychiatric Treatment Centers for Children.

Children's Health, Association for the Care of　*See* Association for the Care of Children's Health.

Children's Healthcare Is a Legal Duty (CHILD)　A national organization founded in 1983 composed of 300 physicians, lawyers, and individuals interested in promoting the legal rights of children in obtaining medical care. It opposes religion-based denial of medical care to children; child discipline through physical abuse that is sanctioned by religious beliefs; and the exemption of religious day care centers from state licensing because they are religious bodies. It collects and disseminates information regarding state laws and court cases dealing with the legal rights of children to receive medical care regardless of religious convictions.

children's hospital　A hospital devoted exclusively to the care and treatment of children. *See also* hospital.

Children's Hospitals and Related Institutions, National Association of *See* National Association of Children's Hospitals and Related Institutions.

Children, Shriners Hospitals for *See* Shriners Hospitals for Crippled Children.

Children, Society for Ear, Nose, and Throat Advances in *See* Society for Ear, Nose, and Throat Advances in Children.

Children's Prosthetic-Orthotic Clinics, Association of *See* Association of Children's Prosthetic-Orthotic Clinics.

Children's Residential Centers, American Association of *See* American Association of Children's Residential Centers.

Children and Youth With Disabilities, National Information Center for *See* National Information Center for Children and Youth With Disabilities.

Child Safety Council, National *See* National Child Safety Council.

Child Welfare Administrators, National Association of Public *See* National Association of Public Child Welfare Administrators.

child welfare caseworker A social worker qualified by education to perform many activities relating to child welfare including, but not limited to the following: investigating homes to protect children from harmful environments; arranging for adoption and foster care for children; identifying evidence of abuse or neglect; advising parents on the care of severely handicapped infants; counseling children and youth with social adjustment difficulties; arranging homemaker's services during parents' illness; starting legal action to protect neglected or abused children; helping unmarried parents; counseling couples on adoption; evaluating homes and parents for possible placement of children for adoption or foster care; and consulting with parents, teachers, counselors, and other persons to help identify problems. *See also* caseworker; social worker.

Child Welfare Institute (CWI) A nonmembership organization founded in 1984 composed of individuals interested in child welfare issues. It supports programs promoting foster parenting, minor emancipation (endowing minors with legal rights of adults), adoption, reunification of foster children with their birth parents, child abuse and neglect, and other issues. *See also* child abuse.

Child Welfare League of America (CWLA) A national organization founded in 1920 composed of 650 members working to improve care and services for abused, dependent, or neglected children, youth, and their families. It provides consultation, conducts research, conducts agency and community surveys, develops standards for services, and administers special projects. *See also* child abuse; welfare.

chill *See* rigor.

Chinese American Medical Society (CAMS) A national organization founded in 1962 composed of 500 physicians of Chinese origin residing in the United States and Canada. It seeks to advance medical knowledge and research among members, establish scholarships, and hold meetings for professional purposes. It maintains a placement service and bestows a Scientific Award annually to the member with the highest scholastic achievements. Formerly (1985) American Chinese Medical Society. *See also* medical society.

Chinese Medical Sciences, American Center for *See* American Center for Chinese Medical Sciences.

chip *See* microchip.

CHIP *See* Comprehensive Health Insurance Plan.

chiropodist *See* podiatrist.

chiropody *See* podiatric medicine.

chiropractic A system of medicine, founded in 1895 by DD Palmer, based on the principles that the nervous system largely determines the state of health and that disease results from nervous system malfunctioning. Treatment consists primarily of the adjustment or manipulation of parts of the body, especially the spinal column, and radiography is used for diagnosis only. Operations, drugs, and immunizations are usually rejected as violations of the human body. A practitioner is called a Doctor of Chiropractic (DC), chiropractor, or chiropractic physician. *See also* chiropractor; Doctor of Chiropractic.

Chiropractic Academic Standards Association, Straight *See* Straight Chiropractic Academic Standards Association.

Chiropractic Association, American *See* American Chiropractic Association.

Chiropractic, Association for the History of *See* Association for the History of Chiropractic.

Chiropractic Board of Radiology, American *See* Council on Diagnostic Imaging.

Chiropractic Board of Thermography, American *See* Council on Diagnostic Imaging.

Chiropractic Colleges, Association of *See* Association of Chiropractic Colleges.

Chiropractic Education, Council on *See* Council on Chiropractic Education.

Chiropractic Organizations, Federation of Straight *See* Federation of Straight Chiropractic Organizations.

Chiropractic Orthopedics, Council on *See* Council on Chiropractic Orthopedics.

Chiropractic Orthopedists, American College of *See* American College of Chiropractic Orthopedists.

chiropractic physician *See* chiropractor.

Chiropractic Physiological Therapeutics, Council on *See* Council on Chiropractic Physiological Therapeutics.

Chiropractic Registry of Radiologic Technologists, American *See* American Chiropractic Registry of Radiologic Technologists.

Chiropractic Research Society, Precision *See* Precision Chiropractic Research Society.

chiropractor An individual who is qualified by education and authorized by law to practice chiropractic. *Synonyms*: chiropractic physician; doctor of chiropractic. *See also* chiropractic.

Chiropractors Association, American Black *See* American Black Chiropractors Association.

chirurgeon Archaic term for a surgeon. *See* surgeon.

chirurgery Archaic term for surgery. *See* surgery.

chi-square distribution In statistics, a variable with K degrees of freedom that is distributed like the sum of the squares of K independent random variables, each of which has a normal distribution with mean zero and variance one. *See also* chi-square test; distribution.

chi-square test Any statistical test based on comparison of a test statistic to a chi-square distribution that can be used to determine whether two or more variables are related. It is best used with nominal data. *Synonym*: chi-squared test. *See also* chi-square distribution; goodness-of-fit test; nominal data; nominal scale; test.

chlamydia Any of various gram-negative, coccoid microorganisms of the genus *Chlamydia* that cause disease in humans and animals, including trachoma and sexually transmitted diseases, such as nonspecific urethritis in men and pelvic inflammatory disease in women. *See also* pelvic inflammatory disease; sexually transmitted disease.

CHMR *See* Center for Hazardous Materials Research.

CHN *See* community health network.

choice The freedom to choose from a set, as of persons or things. *Synonyms*: alternative; option; preference.

CHOICE *See* Center for Human Options in Childbirth Experiences.

Choice in Dying - The National Council for the Right to Die (CFD) A national organization founded in 1992 composed of 160,000 persons interested in education, judicial, and legislative activities relating to protecting the rights of dying patients and protecting physicians, hospitals, and other health care providers from liability threats for complying with the mandated desires of terminally ill persons wishing to die. Formed by merger of Society for the Right to Die and Concern for Dying. *See also* euthanasia; right to die; suicide.

choice, dual *See* dual choice.

Choice in Medicine, Committee for Freedom of *See* Committee for Freedom of Choice in Medicine.

cholecystectomy Removal of the gallbladder. *See also* gallbladder; laparoscopic cholecystectomy.

cholecystectomy, laparoscopic *See* laparoscopic cholecystectomy.

cholera An acute infectious disease of the small intestine caused by the bacterium *Vibrio cholerae* and characterized by profuse watery diarrhea, vomiting, muscle cramps, severe dehydration, and depletion of electrolytes. *See also* bacteria.

cholesterol A fatty substance that is a major component of all cell membranes and myelin sheaths of nerve fibers. From it our cells make adrenal and sex hormones, bile acids, and vitamin D in the skin (with the aid of sunlight). The body produces and stores cholesterol mainly in the liver. It is also found in foods from animal sources (egg yolks, meat, milk). It is essential for life in moderate amounts; harmful (associated with the pathogenesis of atherosclerosis) in excess. *See also* atherosclerosis; high-density lipoprotein; hypercholesterolemia; low-density lipoprotein; saturated fat; very-low-density lipoprotein.

CHP *See* comprehensive health planning.

CHPA *See* comprehensive health planning agencies.

CHP agencies *See* comprehensive health planning agencies.

Christian Association for Psychological Studies (CAPS) A national organization founded in 1956 composed of 2,200 psychologists, marriage and family therapists, social workers, educators, physicians, nurses, ministers, pastoral counselors, and rehabilitation workers engaged in the fields of psychology, counseling, psychiatry, pastoral counseling, and related areas. It helps members as Christians to explore the fields of psychology, pastoral counseling, and psychotherapy for a better insight into personality and interpersonal relations. *See also* psychology.

Christian Dental Society (CDS) An organization founded in 1962 composed of 300 members who encourage dentists of the American Dental Association to donate their professional services to Christian schools, clinics, and hospitals. Members also supply materials and equipment to missions. *See also* American Dental Association; dentistry.

Christian Doctors Sodality (CDS) A national organization founded in 1924 composed of 672 licensed chiropractors and physicians who are also ordained ministers, elders, or deacons. It conducts research and compiles statistics on the importance of religious faith combined with traditional health care in healing. *See also* chiropractor; physician; religion.

Christian Medical and Dental Society (CMDS) A national organization founded in 1931 composed of 8,000 physicians, dentists, and medical and dental students who share a belief in the necessity of satisfying people's spiritual as well as physical needs. It seeks to extend the reality of the Christian faith through members' daily contact and through the active support of medical missions. It sponsors Medical Group Missions, a project that sends health teams to underdeveloped countries. It also provides a health insurance program for missionaries in groups. Formerly (1988) Christian Medical Society. *See also* Medical Group Missions of the Christian Medical and Dental Society.

Christian Medical and Dental Society, Medical Group Missions of the *See* Medical Group Missions of the Christian Medical and Dental Society.

Christian Medical Society *See* Christian Medical and Dental Society.

Christian Science The religion and system of healing founded by Mary Baker Eddy in 1879, who attributed her recovery from an illness to insights she gained from reading the Scripture. The religion upholds the idea that disease and sin are caused by mental error and may be eliminated by spiritual treatment without medical intervention. This belief is protected by the principle of autonomy. If, however, a child of a Christian Scientist family is ill and these beliefs would seriously jeopardize the child's health, the parents would have limited power in decision making. The services of Christian Science sanatoria are covered under some health insurance programs including Medicare and, in some states, Medicaid. *Synonyms:* Christian Science Church; Church of Christ, Scientist; Churches of Christ Scientist.

Christmas Seal Campaign *See* American Lung Association.

chromosome A threadlike strand of DNA (deoxyribonucleic acid) and associated proteins in the nucleus of animal and plant cells that carries the genes and function in the transmission of hereditary information. *See also* cytogenetics; deoxyribonucleic acid; gene.

chromotherapy Color therapy, which involves the use of projected colors of light to treat specific health problems. *See also* Dinshah Health Society.

chronic Lasting a long time, as in chronic disease. *Compare* acute. *See also* subacute.

chronic bronchitis Bronchitis characterized by an excessive secretion of mucus in the bronchi with a productive cough for at least three consecutive months in at least two successive years. *Compare* acute bronchitis. *See also* bronchitis; chronic obstructive pulmonary disease; sputum.

chronic care Care provided to patients on a long-term basis. *Compare* acute care. *See also* care.

chronic disease A disease or illness that lasts a long time, usually developing gradually over months or years, and that is marked by frequent recurrence, as in chronic obstructive pulmonary disease. Chronic disease leaves residual disability, is caused by nonreversible pathological alteration, requires special training of the patient for rehabilitation, and/or may be expected to require a long period of supervision, observation, or care. *Synonym:* chronic illness. *Compare* acute disease. *See also* disease.

chronic disease hospital A hospital that provides medical and skilled nursing services to patients with long-term illnesses who are not in an acute phase but who require an intensity of services not available in nursing homes. *See also* chronic disease; long-term hospital.

Chronic Health Evaluation (APACHE), Acute Physiology and *See* Acute Physiology and Chronic Health Evaluation (APACHE).

chronic illness *See* chronic disease.

chronic obstructive lung disease *See* chronic obstructive pulmonary disease.

chronic obstructive pulmonary disease (COPD) A disorder characterized by abnormal tests of expiratory flow that do not change markedly over several months of observation; includes emphysema, asthma, and chronic bronchitis. *Synonym*: chronic obstructive lung disease. *See also* asthma; bronchitis; chronic bronchitis; emphysema.

Chronic Pain Outreach Association, National *See* National Chronic Pain Outreach Association.

Chronic Patients, The Information Exchange on Young Adult *See* The Information Exchange on Young Adult Chronic Patients.

chronobiology The scientific study of the effect of time on living systems. *See also* circadian; time.

chronological age The age of a person expressed as the period of time that has elapsed since birth. *Compare* developmental age; mental age. *See also* age.

CHSS *See* Cooperative Health Statistics System.

Church of Christ, Scientist *See* Christian Science.

CI *See* confidence interval.

CIC *See* Consumer Information Center.

CICU Cardiac intensive care unit; coronary intensive care unit. *See* cardiac care unit.

CIH *See* Children in Hospitals.

CIO *See* chief information officer.

CIR *See* Committee of Interns and Residents; Cosmetic Ingredient Review.

circadian Pertaining to a period of about 24 hours and applied especially to the rhythmic repetition of certain phenomena in living organisms at about the same time each day. *See also* chronobiology; circadian rhythm; jet lag.

circadian rhythm The rhythmic repetition of certain phenomena in living organisms at about the same time each day. *See also* chronobiology; circadian; jet lag.

circle, quality *See* quality circle.

circuit In electronics, a closed path followed or capable of being followed by an electric current. *See also* integrated circuit; microcircuit.

circuit, integrated *See* integrated circuit.

circuit, micro- *See* microcircuit.

circular file *See* round file.

circulating nurse A registered nurse qualified by education and training in operating room techniques who is responsible for establishing and main-taining a safe and therapeutic environment for patients during surgery. *See also* operating room nurse.

circulation Movement in a regular circle or circuit, as in the movement of the blood through the heart and blood vessels. *See also* circulatory system.

circulation technologist *See* perfusionist.

Circulatory Society, American Podiatric *See* American Podiatric Circulatory Society.

circulatory system The system of structures, consisting of the heart, blood vessels, and lymphatics, by which blood and lymph are circulated throughout the body. *See also* rheology; shock; system.

circumcision Removal of all or part of the prepuce, or foreskin, in males or the incision of the fold of skin over the clitoris in females. *See also* clitoris; penis; ritual.

Circumcision Information Center, Non- *See* Non-Circumcision Information Center.

Circumcision Information Resource Centers, National Organization of *See* National Organization of Circumcision Information Resource Centers.

circumstantial evidence In law, testimony based on deduction from facts and not on personal, first-hand knowledge or observation. *See also* deduction; direct evidence; evidence; fact.

cirrhosis of the liver A group of conditions characterized by extensive destruction of liver tissue and replacement fibrosis. There are many causes and corresponding pathology, only one of which is correlated with the prolonged excessive consumption of alcohol. *See also* liver; liver failure.

CIS *See* Cancer Information Service; Clinical Immunology Society.

CISC *See* RISC.

citizen A person owing loyalty to and entitled by birth or naturalization to the protection of a state or nation. *See also* citizenship; second-class citizen.

Citizen Health Research Group, Public *See* Public Citizen Health Research Group.

Citizen Litigation Group, Public *See* Public Citizen Litigation Group.

Citizen, Public *See* Public Citizen.

Citizens Coalition for Nursing Home Reform, National *See* National Citizens Coalition for Nursing Home Reform.

citizen, second-class *See* second-class citizen.

citizenship The status of a citizen with its attendant duties, rights, and privileges. *See also* citizen.

city hospital *See* municipal hospital.

Civil Aviation Medical Association (CAMA) A national organization founded in 1948 composed of 700 aviation medical examiners, physicians who are pilots, aviation medical educators, flight instructors, airline medical department physicians, NASA physicians, and fixed base operators interested in ascertaining the basic mental and physical requirements of civil air personnel and the proper methods for the physical assessment of air personnel engaged in civil aviation.

civil commitment A type of confinement order used in the civil context for mentally ill, incompetent, alcoholic, and drug-addicted individuals, as contrasted with the criminal commitment of a sentence. *See also* commitment.

civil court A trial court that hears disputes arising under the common law and civil statutes. *Compare* criminal court. *See also* court; trial court.

Civilian Health and Medical Program of the Uniformed Services (CHAMPUS) An entitlement health care program administered by the Department of Defense that pays for care delivered by civilian health providers to retired members and to dependents of active and retired members of the uniformed services of the United States (Army, Navy, Air Force, Marine Corps, Commissioned Corps of the Public Health Service, Coast Guard, and National Oceanic and Atmospheric Administration). The CHAMPUS hires third-party administrators (fiscal intermediaries) and pays benefit dollars directly. It does not charge premiums but requires the dependents of service personnel on active duty to share the costs of outpatient care, and retirees and their dependents to share the costs of both outpatient and inpatient care. *See also* Civilian Health and Medical Program of the Veterans Administration; entitlement.

Civilian Health and Medical Program of the Veterans Administration (CHAMPVA) An entitlement health care program administered by the Department of Defense for the Veterans Administration that pays for care delivered by civilian health providers to eligible dependents and survivors of certain veterans. It is administered through CHAMPUS and has the same cost-sharing requirements. *See also* Civilian Health and Medical Program of the Uniformed Services; Department of Veterans Affairs; entitlement.

civil law The body of law that describes the private rights and responsibilities of individuals. It involves actions (for example, in tort or contract) filed by one person against another. It does not encompass criminal law (crimes against society). *Compare* criminal law. *See also* contract; law; tort.

claim **1.** A request to an insurer by an insured person (or, on his behalf, by the provider of a service or good) for payment of benefits under an insurance policy. *See also* adjudicate; pending claim; uniform claim form. **2.** A demand for money or other property due, or believed to be due, such as a medical malpractice claim. *See also* counterclaim.

claim, counter- *See* counterclaim.

claim, cross *See* cross claim.

claim form, uniform *See* uniform claim form.

claim number, health insurance *See* health insurance claim number.

claim, pending *See* pending claim.

claims administrator, third-party *See* third-party claims administrator.

claims data **1.** Data derived from providers' claims to third-party payers. **2.** Data derived from liability claims. *See also* claim; data.

claims-incurred coverage Insurance that covers the insured, such as a physician, for any claims arising from an event that occurred or is alleged to have occurred during the policy period, regardless of when the claim is made. *See also* claim; coverage.

claims-made coverage Insurance that covers the insured (such as a physician) for any claim made, rather than any injury occurring, while the policy is in effect. Claims made after the insurance policy lapses are not covered as they are by claims-incurred coverage. *Compare* occurrence policy. *See also* claim; coverage; tail coverage.

Claims of the Paranormal, Committee for the Scientific Investigation of *See* Committee for the Scientific Investigation of Claims of the Paranormal.

claims review A retrospective review by government agencies, medical foundations, insurers, or other organizations responsible for payment to determine the financial liability of the payer, eligibility of the beneficiary and the provider, appropriateness of the service provided, amount requested under an insurance or prepayment contract, and utilization rates for specific plans. *See also* adjudicate; claim; review.

clairvoyance Extrasensory perception. *See also* perception; telepathy.

clamp A device used for gripping, compressing, joining, or fastening parts, as in an aortic clamp used to compress the aorta to stop bleeding. *See also* forceps.

CLAO *See* Contact Lens Association of Ophthalmologists.

clap *See* gonorrhea.

Clark, Foundation, The Edna McConnell *See* The Edna McConnell Clark Foundation.

CLAS *See* Clinical Ligand Assay Society; Congress of Lung Association Staff.

classification of diseases Arrangement of diseases into groups based on common characteristics and frequently given numeric labels. One widely used classification of diseases is the *International Classification of Diseases, Ninth Revision, Clinical Modification (ICD-9-CM)*. *See also* classification system; coding; disease; nosology; taxonomy.

classification system An arrangement of the elements of a subject into groups according to preestablished criteria. For example, in *International Classification of Diseases, Ninth Revision, Clinical Modification*, the diseases are arranged in chapters, sections, categories, and subcategories for tabulating events or episodes of morbidity and mortality. *See also* classification of diseases; nosology; taxonomy.

clause, recurring *See* recurring clause.

clause, severability *See* severability clause.

claustrophobia Irrational fear of enclosed or confined space. *See also* phobia.

Clayton Act A 1914 federal antitrust law enacted as a reaction to the vagueness of the Sherman Antitrust Act of 1890. The Clayton Act specifically prohibits price discrimination, tying agreements, exclusive dealing contracts, mergers, and interlocking directorates, when the effect may be to substantially lessen competition or tend to create a monopoly in any line of commerce. *See also* antitrust laws; monopoly; restraint of trade; Sherman Antitrust Act.

CLC *See* Child Life Council.

CLD *See* Council for Learning Disabilities.

Clean Air Act A federal statute passed in 1963 and amended since, to protect public health and welfare from the effects of air pollution. The act establishes national air quality standards and specific automobile emission standards to achieve these goals.

cleanliness *See* hygiene.

CLEAR *See* Council on Licensure, Enforcement and Regulation.

clearinghouse An organization or center that col-

lects, reviews, and disseminates information on topics of interest to people.

Clearinghouse on Disability Information (CDI) A national clearinghouse founded in 1973 that responds to inquiries on topics concerning federally-funded programs serving disabled persons and federal legislation affecting the disabled community. Formerly (1989) Clearinghouse on the Handicapped. *See also* clearinghouse; disability.

Clearinghouse on Family Violence Information A national organization founded in 1987 that provides information services to practitioners and researchers studying family violence prevention. *See also* clearinghouse.

Clearinghouse on the Handicapped *See* Clearinghouse on Disability Information.

cleft palate A congenital fissure in the roof of the mouth, resulting from incomplete fusion of the palate during embryonic development. It may involve only the uvula or extend through the entire palate to the lip. *See also* hare lip; otolaryngology; palate; plastic surgery.

Cleft Palate-Craniofacial Association, American *See* American Cleft Palate-Craniofacial Association.

clergy The body of people ordained for religious service. *See also* religion.

Clergy, Association of Mental Health *See* Association of Mental Health Clergy.

clerk **1.** A person who works in an office performing tasks, such as keeping records, attending to correspondence, or filing. *See also* health unit coordinator; secretary. **2.** A person who works at a sales counter or service desk, for example, in a hotel. **3.** A person who keeps records and performs the regular business of a court or legislative body. **4.** A law clerk, as for a judge. **5.** *See* clinical clerk.

clerk, clinical *See* clinical clerk.

clerk, health unit *See* health unit coordinator.

CLIA '67 *See* Clinical Laboratory Improvement Act of 1967.

CLIA '88 *See* Clinical Laboratory Improvement Amendments of 1988.

cliché A trite or overused expression or idea. *See also* buzzword; catchword; euphemism; jargon.

client An individual who has retained or consented to treatment or receipt of services from a professional. This term is usually employed by health professionals educated in the social sciences (such as psychologists and counselors), while the term "patient" is more typically used by health professionals educated in the medical sciences. *See also* patient.

client privilege, attorney- *See* attorney-client privilege.

climacteric The syndrome of endocrine, somatic, and psychic changes occurring at the termination of the reproductive period in the female, ending with menopause; it may also accompany the normal diminution of sexual activity in the male. *Synonym:* climacterium. *See also* andropause; menopause.

Climatological Association, American Clinical and *See* American Clinical and Climatological Association.

climatology The meteorological study of climates and their phenomena. *See also* meteorotropism.

climax *See* orgasm.

clinic A facility, or part of one, for diagnosis and treatment of outpatients. *See also* dental clinic; free clinic; outpatient service.

clinical Involving or based on direct observation of a patient, originally meaning at the patient's bedside, as distinguished from theoretical or basic sciences.

clinical algorithm A description of steps to be taken in patient care in specified circumstances, such as a description of the steps to be taken in the care of adult patients presenting with nontraumatic chest pain. This approach makes use of branching logic and of all pertinent data, both about the patient and from epidemiologic and other sources, to arrive at decisions that yield maximum benefit and minimum risk. *Synonym:* clinical protocol. *See also* algorithm.

clinical biochemical geneticist A medical geneticist who specializes in clinical biochemical genetics. *See also* clinical biochemical genetics; genetics; medical genetics.

clinical biochemical genetics The subspecialty of medical genetics dealing with performing and interpreting biochemical analyses relevant to the diagnosis and management of human genetic diseases. *See also* genetics; medical genetics.

clinical cardiac electrophysiology A subspecialty of cardiology involving complicated technical procedures to evaluate heart rhythms and determine appropriate treatment for them. These procedures are performed in different settings, including emergency and operating rooms, intensive care units, and clinics or laboratories. *See also* cardiology; electrophysiology.

clinical chemistry Chemistry as it relates to medicine, for example, measurement of blood serum sodi-

um or potassium levels. *See also* chemistry; clinical.

Clinical Chemistry, American Association for *See* American Association for Clinical Chemistry.

Clinical Chemistry, American Board of *See* American Board of Clinical Chemistry.

Clinical Chemistry, National Registry in *See* National Registry in Clinical Chemistry.

clinical clerk A medical or dental student who, as part of a medical or dental school's curriculum, receives clinical experience by performing supervised duties in a hospital. *See also* clinical clerkship; dental school; dental student; medical school; medical student.

clinical clerkship A period in which a medical or dental student receives clinical experience by performing supervised duties in a hospital. *See also* clinical clerk; dental school; dental student; hospital; medical school; medical student.

Clinical and Climatological Association, American *See* American Clinical and Climatological Association.

clinical criteria *See* practice guideline.

clinical cytogeneticist A medical geneticist who specializes in clinical cytogenetics. *See also* clinical cytogenetics.

clinical cytogenetics The subspecialty of medical genetics dealing with cytogenetic laboratory diagnostic and clinical interpretive services. *See also* cytogenetics; genetics; medical genetics.

clinical data Data derived from clinical examinations, as by a physician or other health professional, and tests, such as diagnostic laboratory tests, x-rays, and electrocardiograms. *See also* clinical database; data.

clinical database An organized collection of clinical data in a standardized format, relating to patients, diagnoses, treatments, prognoses, and outcomes. *See also* database.

Clinical Data Set, Uniform *See* Uniform Clinical Data Set.

clinical decision analysis The application of decision analysis in a clinical setting with the aim of applying epidemiologic and other data on probability of outcomes when alternative decisions can be made. *See also* decision analysis; decision tree.

clinical department A functional division of a health care organization devoted to a clinical area, often a specialty area, such as surgery, cardiovascular medicine, or obstetrics. *Synonym:* clinical service. *See also* department; department chair; hospital department; service.

clinical diagnosis A diagnosis made on the basis of knowledge obtained by medical history and physical examination, and usually without benefit of laboratory tests, x-rays, or other ancillary diagnostic modalities. *See also* clinical; diagnosis.

clinical diagnostic bacteriology The branch of bacteriology dealing with the collection of specimens from persons or the environment, examination for bacteria or evidence of bacterial infection, and evaluation of the results. *See also* bacteriology; clinical laboratory.

clinical dietitian A registered dietitian who assesses nutritional needs of patients, develops and implements nutritional care plans, and evaluates and reports results. *See also* dietitian; registered dietitian.

clinical engineer A professional who supports and advances patient care by applying engineering and managerial skills to health care technology. *See also* bioengineer; clinical engineering department; engineering.

clinical engineering department A department that provides management, maintenance, service, and, in some cases, design and development, for a health care organization's medical equipment and instrumentation. *Synonym*: biomedical engineering department. *See also* clinical engineer; department.

clinical evoked potential *See* evoked potentials.

Clinical Evoked Potentials, American Society for *See* American Society for Clinical Evoked Potentials.

Clinical and Experimental Hypnosis, Society for *See* Society for Clinical and Experimental Hypnosis.

clinical geneticist A medical geneticist who specializes in clinical genetics. *See* clinical genetics.

clinical genetics The branch of medical genetics dealing with health and disease in individuals and their families or the science and practice of diagnosis, prevention, and management of genetic disorders, such as inborn errors of metabolism, hemoglobinopathies, chromosome abnormalities, and neural tube defects. *See also* genetics; medical genetics.

Clinical Genetic Society, Birth Defect and *See* Birth Defect and Clinical Genetic Society.

clinical hypnosis *See* hypnosis.

Clinical Hypnosis, American Society of *See* American Society of Clinical Hypnosis.

Clinical Immunology Society (CIS) A national organization founded in 1986 composed of 800 investigators and clinicians interested in immuno-

logic diseases. It promotes research on the causes and mechanisms of immunologic diseases and improved treatment, evaluation, and prevention of diseases related to immunity. *See also* immunology.

clinical information system An information system that collects, stores, and transmits information that is used to support clinical applications (for example, pharmacy, laboratory, radiology, nursing, performance measurement). Billing systems and other financial systems would not be considered clinical information systems. *See also* hospital information system; information system; management information system.

clinical instructor, nurse *See* nurse clinical instructor.

Clinical Investigation, American Society for *See* American Society for Clinical Investigation.

clinical laboratory Any facility that examines materials from the human body for purposes of providing information for the diagnosis, prevention, or treatment of any disease or impairment of, or the assessment of, the health of human beings. Typical divisions of a clinical laboratory include hematology, cytology, bacteriology, histology, biochemistry, medical toxicology, and serology. *Synonyms*: laboratory; medical laboratory. *See also* hematology laboratory; laboratory; pathology and clinical laboratory services; special function laboratory.

Clinical Laboratory Association, American *See* American Clinical Laboratory Association.

Clinical Laboratory Improvement Act of 1967 (CLIA '67) An amendment to the Public Health Service Act requiring federal licensure of clinical laboratories operating as interstate commerce. *See also* Clinical Laboratory Improvement Amendments of 1988; Public Health Service Act.

Clinical Laboratory Improvement Amendments of 1988 (CLIA '88) Standards for laboratory personnel, quality control, and quality assurance based on the complexity of a laboratory test, set by Congress to improve the quality of clinical laboratory testing in all laboratories in the United States. These regulations, which became effective September 1, 1992, expand government oversight from 12,000 previously regulated Medicare, Medicaid, and interstate laboratories to more than 150,000 laboratories, primarily physician office laboratories. *See also* clinical laboratory; laboratory; standard.

Clinical Laboratory Management Association (CLMA) A national organization founded in 1971 composed of 5,000 individuals holding managerial or supervisory positions with clinical laboratories, persons engaged in education of these individuals, and manufacturers or distributors of equipment or services to clinical laboratories. *See also* clinical laboratory; management.

Clinical Laboratory Sciences, National Accreditation Agency for   *See* National Accrediting Agency for Clinical Laboratory Sciences.

Clinical Laboratory Services, Accreditation Manual for Pathology and   *See Accreditation Manual for Pathology and Clinical Laboratory Services.*

clinical laboratory services, pathology and   *See* pathology and clinical laboratory services.

Clinical Laboratory Standards, National Committee for   *See* National Committee for Clinical Laboratory Standards.

Clinical Ligand Assay Society (CLAS)   A national organization founded in 1976 composed of 1,000 clinical laboratory directors and doctors, hospital technologists, private laboratories, and representatives of industry interested in ligand assays. Its objectives include advancing standards of ligand assay practice as applied to physiology in the prevention, diagnosis, and treatment of disease. Formerly (1981) Clinical Radioassay Society. *See also* ligand assay.

Clinical and Medical Electrologists, Society of   *See* Society of Clinical and Medical Electrologists.

clinical medicine   The study of disease by direct examination of the living patient. *See also* medicine.

clinical molecular geneticist   A medical geneticist who specializes in clinical molecular genetics. *See also* clinical molecular genetics; medical geneticist.

clinical molecular genetics   A subspecialty of medical genetics dealing with performing and interpreting molecular analyses relevant to the diagnosis and management of human genetic diseases. *See also* genetics; medical genetics.

clinical neurophysiologist   A neurologist or a psychiatrist who subspecializes in clinical neurophysiology. *See also* clinical neurophysiology; neurology; neurophysiology.

clinical neurophysiology   The branch of medicine and subspecialty of neurology and psychiatry dealing with the diagnosis and management of central and peripheral nervous system disorders using electrophysiological techniques. *See also* neurology; neurophysiology.

Clinical Nomenclatures, Coding, and Classification, Commission on   *See* Commission on Clinical Nomenclatures, Coding, and Classification.

clinical nurse specialist (CNS)   A registered nurse who has acquired advanced knowledge, clinical skills, and competence in a specialized area of nursing and health care. These skills are made directly available through the provision of nursing care to clients and are indirectly available through guidance and planning of care with other nursing personnel. Clinical nurse specialists hold a master's degree in nursing, preferably with an emphasis in clinical nursing. *Synonym:* nurse specialist. *See also* advanced practice nurse; nurse; registered nurse.

Clinical Nursing Education, Institute for Hospital   *See* Institute for Hospital Clinical Nursing Education.

Clinical Nutrition, American Council of Applied   *See* American Council of Applied Clinical Nutrition.

Clinical Nutrition, American Society for   *See* American Society for Clinical Nutrition.

clinical oncology   *See* gynecologic oncology; medical oncology; pediatric oncology.

Clinical Oncology, American Society of   *See* American Society of Clinical Oncology.

Clinical Optometric Care, Council on   *See* Council on Clinical Optometric Care.

Clinical Orthopaedic Society (COS)   An organization founded in 1912 composed of 700 orthopedic surgeons practicing in cities of the Midwest. *See also* orthopaedic/orthopedic surgery.

clinical pastoral counselor   A minister who works with patients or clients and their families in health care settings. He or she assists patients in dealing with acute, chronic, and terminal illnesses through individual and group counseling. *See also* chaplain; counselor; pastoral.

Clinical Pastoral Education, Association for   *See* Association for Clinical Pastoral Education.

clinical path   *See* clinical pathway.

clinical pathologist   A pathologist who specializes in the study of disease-induced and physiological changes in body fluids and tissues as they pertain to treatment of disease. *See also* pathologist.

Clinical Pathologists, American Society of   *See* American Society of Clinical Pathologists.

clinical pathology   The application of laboratory methods to clinical problems. *See also* pathology.

clinical pathway   A treatment regime, agreed upon by consensus, that includes all of the elements of care, regardless of the effect on patient outcomes. It is a broader look at care and may include tests and x-rays that do not affect patient recovery. *Synonyms*: care path; clinical path. *See also* critical pathway; practice parameter.

clinical pharmacology The branch of pharmacology that deals with the actions and uses of drugs in patients. *See also* pharmacology.

Clinical Pharmacology, American College of *See* American College of Clinical Pharmacology.

Clinical Pharmacology, Associates of *See* Associates of Clinical Pharmacology.

Clinical Pharmacology and Therapeutics, American Society for *See* American Society for Clinical Pharmacology and Therapeutics.

Clinical Pharmacy, American College of *See* American College of Clinical Pharmacy.

clinical practice guideline *See* practice guideline.

clinical practice plan *See* medical practice plan.

clinical privileges Authorization granted by an appropriate authority (for example, a governing body) in a health care organization to a practitioner to provide specific patient care services in the health care organization within defined limits, based on an individual practitioner's license, education, training, experience, competence, health status, and judgment. A practitioner may have clinical privileges to diagnose and treat, but not have admitting privileges. *Synonym*: privileging. *See also* admitting privileges; delineation of clinical privileges; emergency privileges; licensed independent practitioner; temporary privileges.

clinical privileges, delineated *See* delineated clinical privileges.

clinical privileges, delineation of *See* delineation of clinical privileges.

clinical protocol *See* clinical algorithm.

Clinical Psychiatrists, American Academy of *See* American Academy of Clinical Psychiatrists.

clinical psychologist A health professional qualified by education and authorized as necessary by law to practice clinical psychology. Clinical psychologists do not treat physical causes of mental illness with drugs or other medical or surgical measures since they are not licensed to practice medicine. *See also* clinical psychology.

clinical psychology The branch of psychology in which psychological principles and methods derived from developmental and abnormal psychol-

ogy are applied to the diagnosis and treatment of mental and behavioral disorders. *See also* clinical psychologist; psychology.

Clinical Radioassay Society *See* Clinical Ligand Assay Society.

Clinical Radiography Technologists, American Registry of *See* American Registry of Clinical Radiography Technologists.

clinical record *See* medical record.

Clinical Research, American Federation for *See* American Federation for Clinical Research.

Clinical Research, Central Society for *See* Central Society for Clinical Research.

clinical resumé A component of the medical record consisting of a concise recapitulation of the reasons for hospitalization, the significant findings, the procedures performed, the treatment rendered, the condition of the patient on discharge, and any specific instructions given to the patient and/or family. *Synonym*: discharge summary. *See also* medical record.

Clinical Scientists, Association of *See* Association of Clinical Scientists.

clinical service *See* clinical department.

clinical social worker A social worker, usually with a master's degree in social work, who provides psychotherapy or counseling in all types of health delivery systems, ranging from hospitals and clinics to fee-for-service private practice settings. *See also* social worker.

clinical social worker, private practice A social worker who offers psychotherapy or counseling to individual families or groups in the private practice setting. They often counsel families of troubled adolescents and people with marital problems and may also organize group sessions for families of people with special health problems, such as cancer. *See also* social worker.

Clinical Social Work, National Federation of Societies for *See* National Federation of Societies for Clinical Social Work.

clinical thermometer A thermometer used to measure body temperature. *See also* thermometer.

clinical toxicology *See* medical toxicology.

Clinical Toxicology, American Academy of *See* American Academy of Clinical Toxicology.

clinical trial An organized inquiry that is conducted to provide a large body of data for statistically valid evaluation of a defined treatment. Patients are commonly used as research subjects in real-life settings. *Synonyms*: research trial; therapeutic trial. *See also* crossover trial; double-blind technique; nonrandomized trial; randomized trial.

Clinical Trials Group, AIDS *See* AIDS Clinical Trials Group.

Clinical Trials, Society for *See* Society for Clinical Trials.

Clinical Urologists, American Association of *See* American Association of Clinical Urologists.

clinic, dental *See* dental clinic.

clinic, free *See* free clinic.

clinician A practitioner, such as a physician, psychologist, or nurse clinician, who is involved in clinical practice or clinical studies. *Compare* laboratorian. *See also* clinical.

Clinic, Karen Horney *See* Karen Horney Clinic.

clinic manager An individual who is in charge of managing a medical or dental clinic. *See also* clinic; manager.

clinicopathologic conference A case conference at which presentation and discussion of the clinical features and diagnosis precede exposition of the pathological findings, the latter being presented usually on the basis of autopsy examination. *See also* autopsy; conference.

clinic outpatient admission The formal acceptance by a health care organization of a patient who is to receive diagnostic services or treatment in a formally organized unit of a medical or surgical specialty or subspecialty, but who is not to be lodged in the organization's inpatient unit. *See also* admission; outpatient; outpatient care.

clinic patient An outpatient who either uses the services of a hospital, which may be offered at a reduced rate, or those offered at private clinics at regular charges. *See also* clinic; patient.

Clinic Radiologists, American Society of *See* American Society of Clinic Radiologists.

Clinics, Association of Children's Prosthetic-Orthotic *See* Association of Children's Prosthetic-Orthotic Clinics.

clinic, screening *See* screening clinic.

Clinics, National Coalition of Black Lung and Respiratory Disease *See* National Coalition of Black Lung and Respiratory Disease Clinics.

Clinton health plan *See* Health Security Act.

clipping service Review and collection of media output on specific topics for organizations that typically are involved in numerous activities in multiple communities or states. Information so gathered is useful for evaluating the effectiveness of organizations' public information programs and for maintaining awareness of media exposure or responsiveness. *See also* service.

clitoris A small erectile protrusion situated in the front part of the vulva, homologous with the male penis. *See also* circumcision; genitalia; penis.

CLMA *See* Clinical Laboratory Management Association; Contact Lens Manufacturers Association.

clock An instrument for measuring time. *See also* biological clock; instrument; measurement; time.

clock, biological *See* biological clock.

clone **1.** One that closely resembles or copies another, as in appearance or function; for example, a personal computer clone. *See also* PC clone. **2.** A group of genetically identical cells descended from a single common ancestor, such as a bacterial colony whose members arose from a single original cell as a result of binary fission. **3.** A replica of a DNA sequence, such as a gene, produced by genetic engineering. *See also* deoxyribonucleic acid; genetic engineering.

clone, PC *See* PC clone.

closed access *See* closed panel group practice.

closed date A production code that manufacturers stamp on a food product to ensure quality and monitor distribution.

closed medical staff *See* closed staff.

closed panel group practice A medical or dental practice or plan whose beneficiaries are allowed to use only those specified facilities and physicians or dentists that accept the organization's plan's conditions of membership and reimbursement. Services provided in a group practice facility and prepaid by some agency are more precisely called "prepaid group practice." *Synonym*: closed access; gatekeeper model. *Compare* open panel group practice; prepaid group practice. *See also* group practice; panel.

closed staff An arrangement wherein no new applicants are accepted to a health care organization's medical staff unless a vacancy exists or is anticipated. The phrase is also applied to hospital-physician contracts in which a physician or physician group provides administrative and clinical services required for the operation of a hospital department on an exclusive basis. Other physicians are excluded from practicing that specialty in that institution for the period of the contract. *Compare* open staff. *See also* exclusive contract; medical staff; staff.

closing statement In litigation, a summation made by each client's attorney, at the end of the case, which sets forth that client's case. *See also* opening statement.

clostridial myonecrosis *See* gas gangrene.

closure, hospital *See* hospital closure.

clot *See* blood clot.

clot, blood *See* blood clot.

CLSA *See* Contact Lens Society of America.

cluster A group of the same or similar elements gathered or occurring closely together, as in a cluster of hospital standards or a cluster headache. *See also* cluster headache.

cluster headache A severe recurring headache that is associated with the release of histamine and is characterized by sudden sharp pain, watering of the eye, and runny nose on one side of the head. *See also* cluster; headache; migraine.

clyster An injection into the rectum. *Synonym*: enema.

CMA *See* certified medical assistant.

CMC *See* Center for Medical Consumers and Health Care Information.

CMDS *See* Christian Medical and Dental Society.

CME *See* continuing medical education.

CME-AMA *See* Council on Medical Education of the American Medical Association.

CMHC *See* community mental health center.

CMIS *See* Computerized Medical Imaging Society.

CMMB *See* Catholic Medical Mission Board.

CMMIS *See* case-mix management information system.

CMPDL *See* Commission on Mental and Physical Disability Law.

CMRI *See* Certified Medical Representative Institute.

CMSS *See* Council of Medical Specialty Societies.

CN *See* Chexchange Network.

CNF *See* Child Nutrition Forum.

CNHI *See* Committee for National Health Insurance.

CNHS *See* Coalition for a National Health System.

CNI *See* Community Nutrition Institute.

CNM *See* certified nurse-midwife.

CNPA *See* Central Neuropsychiatric Association.

CNRHSPP *See* Council for the National Register of Health Service Providers in Psychology.

CNS *See* central nervous system; Child Neurology Society; clinical nurse specialist.

CO *See* carbon monoxide.

COA *See* Commissioned Officers Association of the United States Public Health Service; Commission on Opticianry Accreditation; Council on Accreditation of Services for Families and Children.

coach In quality improvement, a key resource person from within an organization who supports the organization's leadership in quality and performance improvement activities. A coach is knowledgeable about quality improvement, respected, enthusiastic, eager to learn, and eager to help other persons learn. *See also* continuous quality improvement.

coagulation The process of blood clot formation. *Synonym*: blood clotting. *See also* blood clot; calcium; coagulopathy; factor VIII; hemophilia.

coagulopathy Any disorder of coagulation. *See also* coagulation; hemophilia.

coalition An alliance, especially a temporary one, of people or groups, as in a business health care coalition. *See also* business health care coalition; health care coalition.

coalition, business health care *See* business health care coalition.

Coalition for Cancer Research, National *See* National Coalition for Cancer Research.

Coalition of Digestive Disease Organizations *See* Digestive Disease National Coalition.

coalition, health care *See* health care coalition.

Coalition for Health Funding (CHF) A coalition founded in 1970 composed of 45 health and health-related organizations concerned with identifying inadequacies in existing and proposed levels of support for selective federal health programs and communicating the need for adequate funding for specific health programs to the public, the press, the administration, and Congress. *See also* coalition.

Coalition for a National Health Service *See* Coalition for a National Health System.

Coalition for a National Health System (CNHS) A coalition founded in 1977 seeking to educate people about the needs for a national health system and proposing guidelines for such a system. Formerly (1986) Coalition for a National Health Service. *See also* coalition; national health service.

Coalition for Nursing Home Reform, National Citizens *See* National Citizens Coalition for Nursing Home Reform.

Coalition on Sexuality and Disability (CSD) A coalition founded in 1978 composed of 300 members interested in promoting sexual health care services through education, training, and advocacy for people with disabilities. It seeks to educate health professionals and disabled people and promote research in the area of sexuality and disability. *See also* coalition; disability; sex.

Coalitions for Health Care (CHC) An alliance founded in 1982 composed of 170 members representing the AFL-CIO, American Hospital Association, American Medical Association, Blue Cross and Blue Shield Association, the Business Roundtable, and Health Insurance Association of American. The alliance is concerned with managing health care expenditures, with attention to private and public policies on the quality of and access to health care, by stimulating formation of community-level coalitions sharing this goal. *See also* coalition; health care coalition.

Coalition on Smoking or Health (CSH) A coalition formed in 1982 by the American Lung Association, American Heart Association, and American Cancer Society to more effectively bring tobacco use prevention and education issues to the attention of federal legislators and policymakers. It has supported an increase in cigarette excise tax; replacement of current health warnings on cigarette packages and advertisements with more specific and effective warnings concerning tobacco-use and its effects on health; a smoking ban on all domestic and international passenger airline flights and in federal buildings; restriction of US exports of tobacco products; elimination of federal support for the tobacco industry; and regulation by the Food and Drug Administration of tobacco and tobacco products. *See also* American Cancer Society; American Heart Association; American Lung Association; involuntary smoking; smoking.

COB *See* coordination of benefits.

COBOL Acronym for common business-oriented language; a computer language developed in the early 1960s by several computer manufacturers and the US Department of Defense. COBOL is often used to write programs to process business data, such as payrolls and accounts payable records. Many programs and application software systems used in health care business offices are also written in COBOL. *See also* computer software.

COBRA *See* Consolidated Omnibus Budget Reconciliation Act of 1985.

COC *See* College of Chaplains.

cocaine An addictive, toxic alkaloid, derived from the leaves of the coca plant, having narcotic and euphoric effects. Cocaine hydrochloride may be used as a local anesthetic, especially in the examination and treatment of the eye, ear, nose, and throat. The vasoconstrictive action of the drug slows bleeding and limits absorption. *See also* crack; controlled substances; schedule II substances.

codable diagnosis A diagnosis that can be placed into a classification system of symbols, as in the coding of hospital diagnoses using the *International Classification of Disease, Ninth Revision, Clinical Modification (ICD-9-CM). See also* classification system; coding; diagnosis.

code **1.** A systematic collection, compendium, or compilation of laws, rules, or regulations, as in the Criminal Code (referring to penal laws) or code of ethics. *See also* code of ethics; Code of Hammurabi. **2.** A patient whose heart has stopped beating, as in cardiac arrest. *See also* cardiopulmonary resuscitation; code blue. **3.** A system of symbols used to represent assigned meanings. **4.** To put into the form of or symbols of a code, as in coding hospital diagnoses. *See also* coder; coding.

code, bar *See* bar code.

code blue A moniker given to an individual in cardiopulmonary arrest who requires the immediate care of a designated team of health professionals who may be dispersed throughout a hospital. "Code blue" is announced over the organization's communications system to summon providers to the scene of the emergency. *Compare* cardiopulmonary resuscitation. *See also* cardiac arrest; do-not-resuscitate order; slow code.

code of ethics A statement of principles and standards concerning the conduct of those who subscribe to the code, as in a code of ethics that defines proper professional behavior and practices. Codes of ethics are distinguished from licensure laws or practice acts in that they are a form of collective self-regulation rather than of regulation by external bodies. *See also* dental practice act; ethics; Hippocratic oath; licensure; medical practice act; nurse practice act; principle; regulation; standard.

code, genetic *See* genetic code.

Code of Hammurabi Hammurabi, the founder of the first Babylonian empire, laid down a legal code circa 2,100 BC, which was discovered in Susa (in what is now western Iran) in 1902. Clauses 215-223 relate to medicine, laying down the fees appropriate to various services. The code also set penalties for an unsuccessful outcome; for example, in the case of loss of life or of an eye, the physician was to have his hands cut off if the patient was a nobleman, or to render value for value if a slave. *See also* code.

code, no *See* do-not-resuscitate order.

Code®, Life Safety *See* Life Safety Code®.

coder An individual skilled in the translation of language descriptions or text, such as diagnoses or procedures, into symbolic codes, such as numbers, derived from an established coding structure such as the *International Classification of Diseases, Ninth Revision, Clinical Modification*. *See also* code; coding; medical record coder.

coder, medical record *See* medical record coder.

codes, building *See* building codes.

code, show *See* slow code.

code, slow *See* slow code.

Codes and Standards, National Conference of States on Building *See* National Conference of States on Building Codes and Standards.

coding The process by which a number or other symbol is substituted for a more extensive item of information, such as a description of a disease entity or diagnosis. *Compare* decoding. *See also* classification of diseases; code; coder; coding system; computer-assisted coding; medical record coding; procedure-coding manual.

Coding, and Classification, Commission on Clinical Nomenclatures, *See* Commission on Clinical Nomenclatures, Coding, and Classification.

coding, computer-assisted *See* computer-assisted coding.

coding manual, procedure- *See* procedure-coding manual.

coding, medical record *See* medical record coding.

coding system A structured set of characters used to represent data items; for example, the codes 01, 02, . . ., 12 may be used to represent the months January, February, . . ., December of the data-element months of the year. *See also* coding.

Codman, Ernest Amory A surgeon (1869-1940) who practiced in Boston at the Massachusetts General Medical School in the first quarter of the twentieth century. He was an ardent and outspoken advocate of the need for surgeons and hospitals to collect performance and outcomes data and make these data available to the public. *See also* end result; physician.

COE *See* Council on Optometric Education.

coefficient A numeric factor multiplying a term in an algebraic equation, as in a correlation coefficient. *See also* coefficient of determination; coefficient of variation; confidence coefficient; correlation coefficient.

coefficient of confidence *See* confidence coefficient.

coefficient of correlation *See* correlation coefficient.

coefficient of determination A statistic that shows the amount of variability in a dependent variable explained by the regression model's independent variable(s). It is denoted by R to the second power and ranges from 0 to 1. If 0, there is no explanation of the dependent variable at all; if 1, the independent variables explain all the variability of the dependent variable. *See also* coefficient; dependent variable; independent variable.

coefficient, interobserver reliability *See* interobserver reliability coefficient.

coefficient of variation (CV) In statistics, the standard deviation divided by the mean, sometimes multiplied by 100. It is a dimensionless quantity indicating the relative variability around a mean. *See also* coefficient; mean; standard deviation; variation.

cognition The mental process or faculty of knowing, including aspects, such as awareness, perception, reasoning, and judgment. *See also* cognitive; judgment; mentation; perception.

cognitive Pertaining to cognition, as in cognitive development or cognitive dissonance. *See also* cognition; cognitive dissonance; cognitive science.

cognitive dissonance In psychology, a condition of conflict or anxiety resulting from inconsistency between one's beliefs and one's actions. *See also* cognition; cognitive.

cognitive science **1.** The study of the nature of mental tasks and the processes that permit them to be performed. **2.** A branch of artificial intelligence that seeks to simulate human reasoning and associative powers on a computer, using specialized software. *See also* artificial intelligence; cognition; cognitive; science.

Cognitive Sciences, Federation of Behavioral, Psychological and *See* Federation of Behavioral, Psychological and Cognitive Sciences.

Cognitive Science Society (CSS) A national organization founded in 1979 composed of 800 researchers in the fields of psychology, artificial intelligence, and cognitive science that promotes the dissemination of research in cognitive science and allied sciences. *See also* artificial intelligence; cognitive science.

COHE *See* College of Osteopathic Healthcare Executives.

coherent Marked by an orderly and a logical consistency of internal elements, as in speaking coherently or a coherent speech. *Compare* incoherent.

cohort In research, any defined group of persons sharing a common characteristic, such as members of the same age or the same sex, who are followed or traced over a period of time to determine the incidence of a disorder or complications of an established disorder. *See also* cohort analytic study; cohort study; inception cohort.

cohort analytic study In research, a prospective investigation of the factors that might cause a disorder in which a cohort of individuals who do not have evidence of an outcome of interest but who are exposed to the putative cause are compared with a concurrent cohort who are also free of the outcome but not exposed to the putative cause. Both cohorts are then followed to compare the incidence of the outcome under study. *See also* cohort.

cohort, inception *See* inception cohort.

cohort study In research, a longitudinal study concerning a defined subpopulation, such as adult males who died between June and August 1940 and adult males who died during the same months in 1945. *See also* cohort; longitudinal study.

COI *See* certificate of insurance.

coinsurance In a health insurance policy, a form of cost sharing in which the insured pays a set portion or percentage of the cost of each health service provided. *See also* copayment; cost sharing.

coitus *See* sexual intercourse.

coitus interruptus Sexual intercourse in which withdrawal takes place prior to male ejaculation, the intention being to avoid female insemination and conception. *See also* contraception; onanism; sexual intercourse.

COLA *See* Commission on Office Laboratory Assessment; cost-of-living adjustment.

cold A viral inflammation of the mucous membranes of the nasopharyngeal passages. No specific remedy yet exists for this common affliction. *See also* virus.

cold sore *See* herpes simplex.

colic Severe abdominal pain caused by spasm, obstruction, or distention of any of the hollow organs, such as the intestines or ureters. *See also* pain; renal colic.

colic, renal *See* renal colic.

coliform bacillus *See* Escherichia coli.

collaborate To work together, especially in a joint intellectual effort, as in researchers collaborating on a project or health professionals collaborating in the provision of health services. *See also* collaborative culture.

collaborative culture An organizational culture characterized by a shared vision, shared leadership, empowered workers, cooperation among organizational units as they work to improve processes, a high degree of openness to feedback and data, and optimization of the organizational whole versus its many parts. *See also* collaborate; culture.

collagen Connective tissue that helps hold cells together. *See also* cell.

collapse Circulatory failure, or extreme prostration from some other cause.

collateral **1.** Property, insurance, money, or other assets offered and accepted as an inducement and security against a loan or pledge of performance. **2.** Of a secondary nature; subordinate, as in collateral damage from a bombing run. **3.** Situated or running side by side; parallel, as in collateral blood flow that allows perfusion to continue when flow in main vessels is obstructed.

colleague A fellow member of a profession, association, occupation, or organization. *See also* collegial.

collection The act or process of bringing things together in a group; a gathering. *See also* data collection.

collection agency An organization that collects past-due monies for an individual or another organization. Health care providers, for instance, often employ collection agencies when their own collection attempts are unsuccessful. *See also* agency; collection; patient collection.

Collection, American Type Culture *See* American Type Culture Collection.

collection, concurrent data *See* concurrent data collection.

collection cycle The time interval between the rendering of a service or a bill and payment of the bill in full. *See also* collection; cycle.

collection, data *See* data collection.

collection, patient *See* patient collection.

collection, prospective data *See* prospective data collection.

collection rate The amount of revenue collected

divided by the amount of revenue billed (or invoiced). *See also* collection; rate.

collection, retrospective data *See* retrospective data collection.

Collections, US Federation for Culture *See* US Federation for Culture Collections.

collective bargaining Negotiation between the representatives of organized workers and representatives of their employer or employers to determine wages, hours, rules, and working conditions. *See also* collective bargaining agreement. ·

collective bargaining agreement The contract or formal agreement between organized workers and their employer resulting from the negotiation of demands. *See also* agreement; collective bargaining.

College Admission Test, Medical *See* Medical College Admission Test.

College of American Pathologists (CAP) A national organization founded in 1947 composed of 12,200 physicians practicing pathology. It fosters improvement of education, research, and medical laboratory service to physicians, hospitals, and the public. It provides placement information for members and conducts a laboratory accreditation program and laboratory proficiency testing surveys. *See also* Fellow of the College of American Pathologists; pathology.

College of American Pathologists, Fellow of the *See* Fellow of the College of American Pathologists.

College of Chaplains (COC) A national organization founded in 1946 composed of 2,200 ordained clergy or full-time nonordained ministers serving as chaplains or in a similar capacity, in any setting, who have a bachelor of arts, bachelor of divinity, or masters degree and are endorsed as chaplains by their faith group. Members who are certified chaplains hold status as Fellows of the college. Formerly (1991) College of Chaplains (of APHA). *See also* certification; chaplain; chaplaincy service.

College of Chaplains (of APHA) *See* College of Chaplains.

College of Diplomates of the American Board of Orthodontics (CDABO) A national organization composed of 1,391 diplomates of the American Board of Orthodontics who qualify by passing extra examinations. It promotes self-evaluation and ongoing professional improvement among orthodontists. *See also* American Board of Orthodontics; diplomate; orthodontics.

College Health Association, American *See* American College Health Association.

College of Optometrists in Vision Development (COVD) A national organization founded in 1970 composed of 1,400 optometrists involved in orthoptics and optometric vision therapy with emphasis on visual information processing in visually-related learning problems. Its purposes include establishing a body of practitioners who are knowledgeable in functional and developmental concepts of vision, and ensuring that the public will receive continuously improving vision care. *See also* optometry; orthoptics; vision.

College of Osteopathic Healthcare Executives (COHE) A national organization founded in 1954 composed of 150 executives of osteopathic hospitals. It sets criteria of competency in hospital administration and assists in education programs. Formerly (1986) American College of Osteopathic Hospital Administrators. *See also* executive; osteopathic medicine.

college, quality *See* quality college.

Colleges of Acupuncture and Oriental Medicine, National Accreditation Commission for Schools and *See* National Accreditation Commission for Schools and Colleges of Acupuncture and Oriental Medicine.

Colleges, Association of American Medical *See* Association of American Medical Colleges.

Colleges, Association of Chiropractic *See* Association of Chiropractic Colleges.

Colleges, National Council of Acupuncture Schools and *See* National Council of Acupuncture Schools and Colleges.

Colleges of Nursing, American Association of *See* American Association of Colleges of Nursing.

Colleges of Optometry, Association of Schools and *See* Association of Schools and Colleges of Optometry.

Colleges of Osteopathic Medicine, American Association of *See* American Association of Colleges of Osteopathic Medicine.

Colleges of Pharmacy, American Association of *See* American Association of Colleges of Pharmacy.

Colleges of Podiatric Medicine, American Association of *See* American Association of Colleges of Podiatric Medicine.

collegial Refers to an equitable relationship of power, responsibility, and authority among colleagues. *See also* colleague.

colon Part of the large intestine extending from the cecum to the rectum. The word is sometimes used as a synonym for the entire large intestine. *See also* colon and rectal surgery; intestine; rectum.

colonoscope An elongated flexible endoscope that permits visual examination of the entire colon. *Synonym*: coloscope. *See also* colon; colonoscopy; endoscope.

colonoscopy Inspection of the entire colon with a colonoscope. *Synonym*: coloscopy. *See also* colon; colonoscope.

colon and rectal surgeon A physician specializing in colon and rectal surgery. *See* colon and rectal surgery; surgeon.

Colon and Rectal Surgeons, American Society of *See* American Society of Colon and Rectal Surgeons.

colon and rectal surgery The branch of medicine and medical specialty dealing with the diagnosis and treatment of various diseases of the intestinal tract, colon, rectum, anal canal, and perianal area by medical and surgical means. Colon and rectal surgery involves management of hemorrhoids, anal fissures (painful tears in the anal lining), and abscesses and fistulae (infections located around the anus and rectum); the use of endoscopy to evaluate and treat problems, such as cancer, polyps (precancerous growths), and inflammatory conditions; and performance of abdominal surgical procedures involving inflammatory bowel diseases, such as chronic ulcerative colitis and Crohn's disease, and diverticulitis and cancer. *See also* colon; colonoscope; rectum; surgery.

Colon and Rectal Surgery, American Board of *See* American Board of Colon and Rectal Surgery.

Colon and Rectal Surgery, American Society of *See* American Society of Colon and Rectal Surgery.

colon, sigmoid *See* sigmoid colon.

coloscope *See* colonoscope.

coloscopy *See* colonoscopy.

colostomy A surgical procedure in which a pathway for fecal matter is made leading from the colon through the wall of the abdomen where the wastes are collected in a bag. *See also* colon; enterostomy; ileostomy; ostomy; stoma.

colposcope An instrument inserted into the vagina for examination of the tissues of the cervix and vagina by means of a magnifying lens. *See also* colposcopy.

colposcopy Examination of the vagina and cervix with a colposcope. *See also* colposcope.

Colposcopy and Cervical Pathology, American Society for *See* American Society for Colposcopy and Cervical Pathology.

coma **1.** A state of unconsciousness from which an individual cannot be aroused, even by powerful stimulation. *See also* consciousness. **2.** Glasgow coma score of 8 or less. *See also* Glasgow coma scale.

comfort care *See* palliative care.

COMISS *See* Commission on Pastoral Research.

command A user-generated computer instruction. *See also* computer.

commencement of coverage The date at which insurance protection begins. *See also* coverage.

commendation The act of expressing approval and praising, as in hospital that earns accreditation with commendation because of its exemplary performance in providing health care of high quality. *See also* accreditation with commendation.

commendation, accreditation with *See* accreditation with commendation.

Commerce, Committee on Energy and *See* Committee on Energy and Commerce.

Commerce, Department of *See* Department of Commerce.

commercial blood bank A blood bank whose surplus income inures to the benefit of the owner(s). *Synonym*: proprietary blood bank. *Compare* community blood bank. *See also* blood bank.

commercial health insurance Any health insurance for hospital or medical care other than that written by Blue Cross and Blue Shield, which are considered to be noncommercial because they are nonprofit organizations. *See also* health insurance.

commission **1.** The act of committing or perpetrating. *Compare* omission. **2.** A group of people officially authorized to perform specified functions or duties.

Commission on Accreditation of Rehabilitation Facilities (CARF) An organization founded in 1966 sponsored by 31 rehabilitation/habilitation organizations. It is the standard-setting and accrediting authority for rehabilitation/habilitation organizations providing services to people with disabilities. *See also* accreditation; habilitation; rehabilitation.

Commission on Clinical Nomenclatures, Coding, and Classification (CCNCC) A nonprofit organization, sponsored by various health care organizations, concerned with health care coding and nomenclature issues. It is primarily focused on developing and implementing a coding system for clinical entities. *See also* coding; nomenclature.

Commissioned Officers Association of the US Public Health Service (COA) A national organization founded in 1910 composed of 7,300 commissioned officers of the US Public Health Service, including career active duty, retired, and inactive reserve officers who are physicians, dentists, scientists, engineers, pharmacists, nurses, and other types of professional personnel. *See also* Public Health Service.

Commission on Graduates of Foreign Nursing Schools (CGFNS) A national organization founded in 1977 to help ensure safe nursing care for the American public and to protect graduates of foreign nursing schools from employment exploitation. It administers a nursing and English language proficiency examination to foreign-educated nurses who wish to practice as registered nurses in the United States. It identifies those foreign-educated nurses qualified to become registered nurses in the United States. *See also* nurse.

Commission on the Mentally Disabled *See* Commission on Mental and Physical Disability Law.

Commission on Mental and Physical Disability Law (CMPDL) A national organization founded in 1976 that gathers and disseminates information on court decisions, legislation, and administrative developments affecting people with mental and physical disabilities. Topics covered include the insanity defense, civil commitment, institutional rights, rights in the community, education of children with disabilities, discrimination against people with disabilities, and environmental barriers. Formerly (1991) Commission on the Mentally Disabled. *See also* disability.

Commission on Office Laboratory Assessment (COLA) A national organization founded in 1993 sponsored by the American Academy of Family Physicians, the American Society of Internal Medicine, the College of American Pathologists, and the American Medical Association, for the purpose of accrediting office laboratories. It has published a handbook describing the voluntary educational and accreditation program for physician office laboratories. *See also* accreditation; assessment; laboratory.

Commission on Opticianry Accreditation (COA) An accrediting agency founded in 1979 for oph-

thalmic dispensing and ophthalmic laboratory technology programs in postsecondary institutions. *See also* accreditation; optician.

Commission on Pastoral Research (COMISS) An organization founded in 1972 composed of 8 pastoral care and counseling organizations. It disseminates information on research in the field. *See also* clinical pastoral counselor; pastoral.

Commission on Professional and Hospital Activities (CPHA) A medical information center concerned with the improvement of hospital and medical care. It serves as a national repository for patient and health care data and maintains the Professional Activity Study, the basic component of a family of computerized patient-record-information systems developed to display hospital medical practices. *See also* hospital discharge abstract system; Professional Activity Study.

commitment **1.** The state of being bound emotionally or intellectually to a course of action or to another person or persons, as in the organizational leadership demonstrating its commitment to quality improvement. **2.** The proceedings directing confinement of a mentally ill or an incompetent person for treatment. Commitment proceedings may be either civil or criminal and voluntary or involuntary. Due process protections are afforded to persons involuntarily committed, for example, periodic judicial review of continued confinement. *See also* civil commitment; involuntary commitment; medical hold.

commitment, civil *See* civil commitment.

commitment, involuntary *See* involuntary commitment.

committee A group of persons to whom the consideration or determination of certain business is referred or confided, as in a hospital's quality assurance committee. *See also* Accreditation Committee; ad hoc committee; audit committee; executive committee; expert panel; financing committee; infection control committee; joint conference committee; medical staff executive committee; patient care committee; peer review committee; pharmacy and therapeutics committee; political action committee; product evaluation committee; standing committee; steering committee; task force; tissue committee; utilization review committee.

committee, accreditation *See* accreditation committee.

committee, ad hoc *See* ad hoc committee.

Committee on Allied Health Education and Accreditation (CAHEA) A committee of the

American Medical Association. Founded in 1976, it serves as an accrediting agency for 2,885 allied health programs in 28 occupational areas including the following: anesthesiologist assistant, athletic trainer, specialist in blood bank technology, cardiovascular technologist, cytotechnologist, diagnostic medical sonographer, electroneurodiagnostic technologist, emergency medical technician-paramedic, medical assistant, medical illustrator, histologic technician/technologist, medical laboratory technician (associate degree), medical laboratory technician (certificate), medical technologist, medical record administrator, medical record technician, nuclear medicine technologist, occupational therapy assistant, occupational therapist, ophthalmic medical technician/technologist, perfusionist, physician assistant, surgeon assistant, radiation therapy technologist, radiographer, respiratory therapist, respiratory therapy technician, and surgical technologist. *See also* accreditation; allied health professional.

Committee on Appropriations   A committee of the United States Senate and a committee of the House of Representatives concerned with the spending authority of legislated programs, including health. *See also* appropriation.

Committee on Armed Services   A committee of the United States Senate and a committee of the House of Representatives whose concerns include the health care programs, facilities, and human resources of the Uniformed Services. *See also* Department of Defense.

committee, audit   *See* audit committee.

Committee on the Budget   Committee of the US House of Representatives whose concerns include budgeting for health care programs and resources. *See also* budget.

Committee on Energy and Commerce   A committee of the US House of Representatives whose concerns include public health and quarantines and health and health facilities, except health care supported by payroll deductions.

Committee on Energy and Natural Resources Committee of the US Senate whose concerns include nuclear waste and insurance programs.

committee, executive   *See* executive committee.

committee, finance   *See* finance committee.

Committee on Finance   Committee of the US Senate concerned with national social security, general revenue sharing, and the health programs financed

by a specific tax or trust fund and health programs under the Social Security Act. *See also* finance; Social Security Act.

Committee for Freedom of Choice in Cancer Therapy   *See* Committee for Freedom of Choice in Medicine.

Committee for Freedom of Choice in Medicine (CFCM)   A national organization founded in 1972 composed of 30,000 members interested in freedom of choice for any therapy that shows clear evidence of efficacy and to prohibit the interference of government or any third party in the relationship between an informed patient and his or her physician. It conducts symposia on alternative therapies in order to educate the public and the medical profession about new discoveries in the treatment of degenerative diseases, and directs people with questions concerning alternative therapies to physicians in their areas. It maintains databases, conducts research, and compiles statistics on people with degenerative diseases. Formerly (1985) Committee for Freedom of Choice in Cancer Therapy. *See also* alternative medicine; choice; efficacy.

committee, infection control   *See* infection control committee.

Committee of Interns and Residents (CIR)   A national organization founded in 1957 composed of 5,000 medical and dental interns, residents, chief residents, and fellows at 50 member hospitals located in New York, New Jersey, and Washington, DC. Its purposes include representing house staff in matters pertaining to compensation, benefits, hours, working conditions, and other issues affecting their employment, education, training, and the quality of health services and patient care. *See also* fellow; intern; resident.

committee, joint conference   *See* joint conference committee.

Committee on Labor and Human Resources   A committee of the US Senate whose concerns include disabled individuals, equal employment opportunity, occupational safety and health, public health, Saint Elizabeth's Hospital, and biomedical research and development. *See also* human resources.

committee, medical staff executive   *See* medical staff executive committee.

Committee for National Health Insurance (CNHI) A national organization founded in 1969 composed of 100 citizen's organizations and individuals from health care fields, government, labor, academic, business, and economics interested in conducting research and education on the health care system in the United States, including its problems and the ways in which to bring about reform through enactment of a comprehensive national health insurance program. *See also* national health insurance.

committee, patient care   *See* patient care committee.

committee, peer review   *See* peer review committee.

committee, pharmacy and therapeutics   *See* pharmacy and therapeutics committee.

committee, political action   *See* political action committee.

committee, product evaluation   *See* product evaluation committee.

Committee for Responsible Genetics   *See* Council for Responsible Genetics.

Committee for the Scientific Investigation of Claims of the Paranormal (CSICOP)   A national organization founded in 1976 composed of 200 psychologists, philosophers, astronomers, science writers, and other individuals interested in the field of the paranormal, including unidentified flying objects, astrology, and psychic phenomena. It is concerned about biased, pseudoscientific media presentations of claims of paranormal occurrences, fearing that the ready acceptance of such claims erodes the spirit of scientific skepticism and opens the public to gullibility in other areas. Its subcommittees focus on areas, such as paranormal health claims and parapsychology. *See also* paranormal; parapsychology.

committee, standing   *See* standing committee.

committee, steering   *See* steering committee.

committee, tissue   *See* tissue committee.

committee, utilization review   *See* utilization review committee.

Committee on Veterans' Affairs   A committee of the US Senate and a committee of the House of Representatives concerned with vocational rehabilitation of veterans, readjustment of service personnel to civilian life, soldiers' and sailors' civil relief, and veterans' hospitals, medical care, and treatment of veterans among its responsibilities. *See also* veteran.

Committee on Ways and Means   Committee of the US House of Representatives concerned with revenue measures, tax-exempt foundations and charitable trusts, and national social security, except for health care and facilities programs that are supported from general revenues as opposed to payroll

deductions, among its responsibilities. Its Subcommittee on Health is concerned with health care, health delivery systems, health research, tax credit and deduction provisions of the Internal Revenue Code dealing with health insurance premiums and health care costs, and health care programs of the Social Security Act, except Medicaid. *See also* Medicaid; Social Security Act.

common business oriented language (COBOL)   *See* COBOL.

common cause   An ever-present factor that contributes to the random variation inherent in all processes. Common causes of variation are endogenous to a system and are not disturbances (they *are* the system) and can be removed or eliminated only by making basic changes in the system. *Synonyms*: endogenous cause; systemic cause. *See also* cause; common-cause variation; variation;.

common-cause variation   Variation in a process that is due to the process itself and is produced by interactions of variables of that process. Common-cause variation is inherent in all processes. *Synonyms*: endogenous cause variation; systemic cause variation. *See also* common cause; process variation; tampering; variation.

common law   Law that derives its authority from judicial decisions, as distinguished from law created by legislative enactment. *See also* law.

common sense   Innate good judgment. *See also* intuition; judgment; pragmatism.

Commonwealth Fund, The   *See* The Commonwealth Fund.

communicable disease   A disease, such as chickenpox, caused by a defined infectious agent or its toxic products that arises through transmission of that agent or its products from an infected person, animal, or reservoir to a susceptible host, either directly or indirectly through an intermediate plant or animal host, vector, or the inanimate environment. *See also* child death rate; disease; infectious diseases; notifiable disease; transmission.

communicate   To exchange thoughts, messages, or information, as by speech, signals, writing, or behavior. *See also* communication; language.

communication   The act of exchanging thoughts, messages, or information, as by speech, signals, writing, or behavior. *See also* electronic data interchange; language; mass communication; miscommunication; nonverbal communication; privileged communication.

communication, mass   *See* mass communication.

communication, mis-   *See* miscommunication.

communication, nonverbal   *See* nonverbal communication.

communication, privileged   *See* privileged communication.

Communications Association, Health Sciences *See* Health Sciences Communications Association.

Communications Associations, Council for Biomedical   *See* Council for Biomedical Communications Associations.

Communications Council, Health Industry Business *See* Health Industry Communications Council.

communications, satellite   *See* satellite communications.

communications software   *See* on-line searching.

communications, tele-   *See* telecommunications.

community   A body of individuals living in a defined area or having a common interest or organization, as in a community blood bank.

community-acquired infection   An infection that a patient acquires prior to hospitalization. *Compare* nosocomial infection. *See also* community; infection.

Community-Based Long-Term Care, National Institute on   *See* National Institute on Community-Based Long-Term Care.

community-based planning   Health services planning that emphasizes local efforts to stimulate, support, and improve health care quality in communities.

community blood bank   A blood bank that is not for profit, serving various hospitals in a community. *Compare* commercial blood bank. *See also* bank; blood bank; community.

Community Blood Centers, Council of   *See* Council of Community Blood Centers.

Community Cancer Centers, Association of   *See* Association of Community Cancer Centers.

community diagnosis   The process of appraising the health status of a community. *See also* community; diagnosis.

Community Health Accreditation Program (CHAP)   A subsidiary of the National League for Nursing that accredits home and community-based health care organizations. *See also* accreditation; home health agency; National League for Nursing.

community health care   Activities and programs intended to improve the general health status of a community. *See also* care; community.

community health center (CHC)   A health care organization established in a residential community that generally has scarce or nonexistent health services, capable of delivering health and social services. *Synonym*: neighborhood health center. *See also* community.

Community Health Centers, National Association of   *See* National Association of Community Health Centers.

community health network (CHN)   State, county, or city health system for delivering health care to the poor. *Synonym*: community network. *See also* community; network.

community health services   Diagnostic, therapeutic, and preventive health services provided for individuals in a community. This phrase does not connote any organizational structure. *See also* community; health services.

community hospital   A hospital established to meet the medical needs of the residents of the community in which the hospital is located. Generally, community hospitals are short-term, general, not-for-profit hospitals, but they may be proprietary or governmental hospitals. *See also* community; hospital.

Community Hospitals, National Council of   *See* National Council of Community Hospitals.

community living facility   *See* halfway house.

community mental health center (CMHC)   A health care organization capable of providing comprehensive, principally ambulatory, mental health services to individuals residing or employed in a defined catchment area. Patients develop skills for daily living and prevent or minimize the need for hospitalization through vocational rehabilitation, counseling, and short-term stabilization services. *See also* catchment area.

Community Mental Health Centers, National Council of   *See* National Council of Community Mental Health Centers.

community network   *See* community health network.

Community Nutrition Institute (CNI)   An organization founded in 1970 composed of citizen advocates specializing in food and nutrition issues, which include hunger, food quality and safety, nutrition research, food programs, education, and food labeling and marketing. Its major goal is to secure a food system that provides access to a diet that sustains cultural and social values and maintains human health. It develops standards for food products. *See also* citizen; community; nutrition.

community organization worker A social worker who plans, organizes, and works with community groups concerned with social problems of the community. *See also* community; social worker.

Community Psychiatrists, American Association of *See* American Association of Community Psychiatrists.

Community Psychiatry, Institute on Hospital and *See* Institute on Hospital and Community Psychiatry.

community rating A method of determining premiums for health insurance in which a premium is based on the average cost of the actual or anticipated health services used by all subscribers in a specific geographic area or industry. The premium does not vary for different groups of subscribers or with the group's claims experience, age, sex, or health status. The intent of community rating is to spread the cost of illness evenly over all subscribers to an insurance plan, rather than charging the sick more than the healthy for health insurance. *Compare* experience rating. *See also* community; premium; rating.

community relations *See* public relations.

community relations director *See* public relations director.

community residential facility A facility that provides living accommodations and guidance in daily living activities principally to persons with mental retardation. *See also* intermediate care facility; residential care facility.

community trust A trust that generally solicits funds from, is controlled by people from, and focuses its efforts on a particular community, as in a nonprofit hospital or a migrant worker health clinic. *See also* community.

comorbidity A disease or condition present at the same time as the principal disease or condition of a patient. Comorbidities may cause an increase in hospital length of stay and are used in third-party payer reimbursement methodologies for inpatient stays. *See also* length of stay; morbidity; other diagnosis; severity of illness; third-party payer.

compact disk (CD) A small optical disk on which information, such as business or scientific data or music, is encoded. The data are applied by laser impressions on the disk. The disk holds data more compactly than do electronic tapes and disks and so is especially useful for applications requiring large amounts of information. *Synonyms*: laser disk; optical disk. *See also* CD-ROM disk.

compact disk-read only memory *See* CD-ROM disk.

companies, telecommunications *See* telecommunications companies.

company A union or association of persons for carrying on a commercial or an industrial enterprise.

company, captive insurance *See* captive insurance company.

company, holding *See* holding company.

company, insurance *See* insurance company.

company, mutual insurance *See* mutual insurance company.

company, parent *See* parent company.

company, stock insurance *See* stock insurance company.

comparative Founded on and estimated by comparison. For example, comparative interpretation of performance data is the method of interpretation that seeks to arrive at the meaning of data by comparing their several parts (say, trending data of a hospital over time) and also by comparing data as a whole with other data (say, comparing two or more organizations' data) obtained in like manner and referring to the same subject (say, performance of cesarean section for failure to progress). *See also* comparative advertising; comparative psychology; compare.

comparative advertising Advertising that specifically compares the advertised service or product with another's service or product. *See also* advertise; comparative; competitive advertising; deceptive advertising; false advertising; image advertising; informative advertising.

comparative psychology The branch of psychology dealing with the differences and similarities in the behavior of animals of different species. Psychologists in this field make systematic studies of the abilities, needs, and activities of various animal species as compared with human beings. *See also* comparative; psychology.

compare To measure and/or judge with the intent of determining the degree to which two or more objects of interest being compared are similar and different and by how much. *Compare* contrast. *See also* benchmark; benchmarking; comparative.

compendium A collection of information; for example, the *United States Pharmacopeia*, the *Homeopathic Pharmacopeia of the United States*, and the *National Formulary*. *See also* Homeopathic Pharmacopeia of the United States; National Formulary; United States

Pharmacopeia.

compensable Entitled to compensation. *See also* compensable injury; compensation.

compensable injury In workers' compensation law, an injury caused by an accident arising out of and in the course of employment and for which the affected employee is entitled to receive compensation. *See also* compensation; injury; workers' compensation.

compensation **1.** Direct and indirect monetary and nonmonetary rewards given to employees on the basis of the value of the job, their personal contributions, and their performance. **2.** Payment of damages; indemnification. Usually the equivalent in money for a loss sustained. *See also* workers' compensation. **3.** The counterbalancing of any defect of structure or function. For example, in psychology, a conscious or unconscious process by which a person attempts to make up for real or imagined physical or psychological deficiencies.

compensation acts, workers' *See* workers' compensation acts.

compensation disability, unemployment *See* unemployment compensation disability.

compensation fund, patient *See* patient compensation fund.

compensation insurance, workers' *See* workers' compensation insurance.

compensation, over- *See* overcompensation.

compensation programs, workers' *See* workers' compensation programs.

compensation statutes, workers' *See* workers' compensation statutes.

compensation, workers' *See* workers' compensation.

compensation, workmens' *See* workers' compensation.

compensatory damages Damages that are awarded in court as the measure of actual loss suffered. The doctrine is designed to place the injured party in the same position he or she occupied prior to the injury and to provide nothing in addition. *See also* damages; punitive damages.

compete To strive for the position, reward, profit, or goal for which another is striving. *See also* competition.

competence **1.** Capacity equal to requirement, as in the competence of a medical or professional staff member to meet the requirements of the task assigned. *Synonym:* competency. **2.** Sufficient mental ability to understand the nature and consequence of one's actions and make a rational decision. A competent patient possesses the ability to understand and communicate information, reason and deliberate about his or her choices, and choose in the light of some goals and values. Legally, all adults are competent until proven incompetent. Competence is defined by state statute. *Compare* incompetence. *See also* decisional capacity.

competency *See* competence.

Competency Assurance, National Organization for *See* National Organization for Competency Assurance.

competition A contest by two or more rivals, as in rivalry in the marketplace. Goods and services will be bought from those who, in the view of buyers, provide "the most for the money." Competition tends to reward more efficient producers and/or suppliers and lead the economy toward efficient use of resources. *See also* compete; managed competition; perfect competition.

competition, managed *See* managed competition.

competition, perfect *See* perfect competition.

competition, pure *See* perfect competition.

competitive advertising Advertising containing very little information and used only to allow a producer to create or maintain a share of the market for that service or product. *See also* advertise; comparative advertising; deceptive advertising; false advertising; image advertising; informative advertising.

complaint **1.** An expression of pain, dissatisfaction, or resentment, as in a patient's chief complaint. *See also* patient complaint. **2.** In civil action, the first pleading of a plaintiff setting out the facts on which the claim is based. The purpose is to give notice to the adversary of the nature and basis of the claim asserted. In criminal law, the preliminary charge or accusation made by one person against another to the appropriate court or officer, usually a magistrate. Court proceedings, such as a trial, cannot be instituted until an indictment or information has been handed down against a defendant. *See also* affirmative defense; pleadings.

complaint, patient *See* patient complaint.

complete abortion An abortion in which all of the products of conception have been expelled from the uterus and identified, compared to an incomplete abortion in which the uterus is not entirely emptied of the products of conception. *See also* abortion; conceptus.

complete blood count (CBC) *See* blood count.

completed suicide An attempted suicide that results in death. *See also* suicide.

complete medical record   A medical record whose contents reflect the diagnosis, results of diagnostic tests, therapy rendered, condition and in-hospital progress of the patient, and condition of the patient at discharge; and whose contents, including any required clinical resume or final progress notes, are assembled and authenticated; in which all final diagnoses and any complications are recorded without the use of symbols or abbreviations. *See also* medical record.

compliance   **1.** To act in accordance with stated requirements, such as standards, as in compliance with a standard. *See also* compliance level; comply; conformance. **2.** In health care, a willingness to follow a prescribed course of treatment or action, as in patient compliance with a treatment regimen, or physician compliance with generally accepted medical practice.

compliance level   A measurement of the extent to which an entity acts in accordance with requirements, for example, a health care organization's level of compliance with a specified standard or group of standards. The Joint Commission on Accreditation of Healthcare Organizations assigns one of five levels of compliance to a standard or groups of standards. *Substantial compliance* means that an organization consistently meets all major provisions of a specified standard (designated by a score 1); *significant compliance* means that an organization meets most provisions of a standard (designated by a score 2); *partial compliance* means that an organization meets some provisions of the standard (designated by a score 3); *minimal compliance* means that an organization meets few provisions of the standard (designated by a score 4); *noncompliance* means that an organization fails to meet the provisions of the standard (designated by a score 5); and *not applicable* means that the standard does not apply to the organization (designated by NA). *See also* compliance; Joint Commission on Accreditation of Healthcare Organizations.

compliance, minimal   *See* compliance level.

compliance, non-   *See* compliance level.

compliance, partial   *See* compliance level.

compliance, significant   *See* compliance level.

compliance, substantial   *See* compliance level.

complication   In medicine, a detrimental patient condition that arises during the process of providing health care, regardless of the setting in which the

care is provided. For instance, perforation, hemorrhage, bacteremia, and adverse reactions to medication (particularly in the elderly) are four complications of colonoscopy and the associated anesthesia and sedation. A complication may prolong an inpatient's length of stay or lead to other undesirable outcomes. *See also* morbidity.

comply   To act in accordance with another's command, request, rule, or wish, as in patients who do not comply with a physician's prescribed course of treatment. *See also* compliance.

component   **1.** A constituent element or part of a process or system, as in the many components of an information management system or the sensory component of the nervous system. *See also* blood components; federal component. **2.** An organized site of service in a health care network for which the Joint Commission on Accreditation of Healthcare Organizations has standards (for example, hospital, ambulatory surgical center, long term care facility) or other entities with which a network contracts for specific services (for example, mental health). This is contrasted with a practitioner site, which is the office of a practitioner member of the panel of a network. *See also* Joint Commission on Accreditation of Healthcare Organizations; network.

component, federal   *See* federal component.

components, blood   *See also* blood components.

compound   A substance that consists of two or more elements in union.

comprehensive benefit package   According to the Health Security Act recently (1993) introduced to Congress, benefits consisting of hospital services, services of health professionals, emergency and ambulatory medical and surgical services, clinical preventive services, mental illness and substance abuse services, family planning services and services for pregnant women, hospice care, home health care, extended care services, ambulance services, outpatient laboratory, radiology, and diagnostic services, outpatient prescription drugs and biologicals, outpatient rehabilitation services, durable medical equipment and prosthetic and orthotic devices, vision care, dental care, health education classes, and investigational treatments. *See also* basic health services; benefits; health plan; Health Security Act.

comprehensive health care   Services that meet the total health care needs of a patient, including outpatient, inpatient, and home care. *Compare* basic health services. *See also* care; comprehensive health care delivery system.

comprehensive health care delivery system The provision of comprehensive health care services by health care providers (health care organizations and practitioners) to a defined population. *See also* comprehensive health care.

comprehensive health insurance Insurance that provides broad coverage including most medical and surgical services in both inpatient and outpatient settings. *See also* health insurance.

Comprehensive Health Insurance Plan (CHIP) A national health insurance proposal submitted to Congress in 1974 as H.R. 12684. The plan would have given all US citizens identical benefits under three separate plans that had different administrative, financing, and cost-sharing arrangements. Each plan would have covered a segment of the population according in part to income and in part to employment status. CHIP and other national health insurance proposals failed to obtain a national consensus. *See also* health insurance.

comprehensive health planning (CHP) A health planning initiative, initiated by the Comprehensive Health Planning and Public Health Services Amendments of 1966 and replaced by the National Health Planning and Resources Development Act of 1974, that was meant to encompass all factors and programs affecting the health of the American people. It was meant to be conducted by areawide and state CHP agencies that had the authority to intervene in matters of environmental and occupational health, health education, and health behaviors, as well as medical resources and services. A council guided the planning in CHP and was composed of a majority of health services consumers, not providers. Federal support for CHP was completely eliminated in 1986.

comprehensive health planning agencies (CHPA) Agencies originally established under the Comprehensive Health Planning and Public Health Services Amendment of 1966 to perform specified health care planning functions. These agencies were superseded by Health Systems Agencies, state health planning and development agencies, and statewide health coordination councils established by the Health Planning and Resources Development Act of 1974. *See also* comprehensive health planning.

comprehensive major medical insurance Insurance that includes both basic and major medical health coverage. It is characterized by a relatively small deductible sum, a coinsurance provision, and maximum benefits of $250,000 or more. *See also* catastrophic insurance.

Comprehensive Smoking Education Act of 1984 A federal law providing for research, education, and communication of information about the effects and dangers to human health presented by cigarette smoking. The law also provides for cigarette packages and advertising to carry one of four specified warnings from the Surgeon General. *See also* smoking.

compromise The trade-off of one factor of comparable value for another. In true compromise each party concedes something the other side finds acceptable.

comptroller *See* controller.

Comptroller General of the United States *See* General Accounting Office.

compulsion A persistent and irresistable impulse to perform an irrational or apparently useless action, such as handwashing or counting. These actions are engaged in for unknown or unconscious purposes. *See also* obsession; obsessive-compulsive.

compulsive, obsessive- *See* obsessive-compulsive.

compulsive personality disorder, obsessive- *See* obsessive-compulsive personality disorder.

compulsory arbitration *See* binding arbitration.

computed axial tomography *See* computerized axial tomography.

computed tomography *See* computerized axial tomography.

computer A programmable electronic device that performs high-speed mathematical or logical operations on data that are furnished to it directly or are stored in its memory. The basic components of a computer include input devices (for example, keyboard), a memory, an arithmetical and logical section (the processor), output devices (such as a printer or screen), and a control section. Computers are sometimes classified into microcomputers, minicomputers, and mainframe computers. *See also* analog computer; central processing unit; computer hardware; computer software; digital computer; joystick; mainframe computer; microchip; microcomputer; minicomputer; modem; mother board; semiconductor; window; word processor.

computer-aided design (CAD) Use of computers

and computer programs for design of products. *Synonym*: computer-assisted design. *See also* computer.

computer-aided instruction (CAI) The application of computers to educational programming. *Synonym*: computer-assisted instruction. *See also* computer.

computer-aided manufacturing A process whereby the scheduling and monitoring of the production steps and related inventory movements are controlled automatically by computer.

computer-aided software engineering A software process designed to lessen work hours spent performing tedious and time-consuming programming routines. *See also* computer; engineering.

computer algorithm An algorithm written in a language that a computer can understand. *See also* algorithm; clinical algorithm; computer.

computer, analog *See* analog computer.

computer application A program or series of programs that perform a group of work routines, such as for payroll or inventory control. *See also* computer.

computer-assisted coding A process in which a coder is assisted by a computer in the coding process, meaning that the coder uses a computer keyboard, enters the words of the diagnosis, and the computer identifies the correct code (usually a number). Interactive systems prompt the coder to enter more specific information, thereby increasing diagnostic precision in coding. *See also* coder; coding.

computer-assisted design *See* computer-aided design.

computer-assisted instruction *See* computer-aided instruction.

computer-based patient record A computerized record of all of the data and images collected over the course of a patient's health history. *See also* medical record.

Computer-Based Patient Record Institute (CPRI) A national membership organization founded in 1992 that initiates and coordinates activities to facilitate and promote the routine use of computer-based patient records throughout health care. Its activities include promoting the development and use of standards for computer-based patient record messages, communications, codes, and identifiers; encouraging creation of policies and mechanisms to protect patient and provider confidentiality and ensure data security; and demonstrating how computer-based patient record systems can lead to improvements in effective and efficient patient care. *See also* computer-based patient record; computer-based patient record system.

computer-based patient record system A record system that captures, stores, retrieves, and transmits patient-specific health care related data, including clinical, administrative, and payment data. *See also* computer; system.

computer crime Criminal activity directly related to the use of computers, specifically illegal trespass into the computer system or database of another, manipulation or theft of stored or on-line data, or sabotage of equipment and data.

computer, digital *See* digital computer.

computer hardware The tangible parts of a computer (for example, microchips, boards, wires, and transformers) and computer systems (for example, mainframe computer, all input and output attachments, all data storage devices). *Compare* computer software; firmware. *See also* computer; drive.

computerized axial tomography (CAT) The recording of internal body images at a predetermined plane by means of an emergent x-ray beam that is measured by a scintillation counter. The electronic impulses are recorded on a magnetic disk and then are processed by a minicomputer for reconstruction display of the body in cross-section on a cathode ray tube. *Synonyms*: CAT scan; computed tomography. *See also* tomography.

computerized axial tomography (CAT) scan *See* CAT scan.

computerized axial tomography (CAT) scanner *See* CAT scanner.

Computerized Medical Imaging Society (CMIS) A national organization founded in 1976 composed of 350 physicians and other medical personnel interested in computerized axial tomography and other radiological diagnostic procedures. It provides a forum for exchange of information about the medical use of computerized axial tomography in radiological diagnosis. Formerly (1983) Computerized Tomography Society; (1988) Computerized Radiology Society. *See also* computerized axial tomography.

Computerized Radiology Society *See* Computerized Medical Imaging Society.

computerized tomography (CT) *See* computerized axial tomography.

Computerized Tomography Society *See* Computerized Medical Imaging Society.

computer literacy The ability to operate a computer and to understand the language used in working with a specific system or systems. *See also* computer.

Computer Medicine, American Physicians Association of *See* American Physicians Association of Computer Medicine.

computer, micro- *See* microcomputer.

computer, mini- *See* minicomputer.

computer modeling Use of computers to simulate real-world operating environments so that the outcome of proposed changes can be estimated before they are implemented. Computer modeling is used extensively in systems analysis and systems thinking. *See also* systems analysis; systems thinking.

computer, personal *See* personal computer.

computer, pocket *See* pocket computer.

computer, portable *See* portable computer.

Computer Professionals, Association of the Institute for Certification of *See* Association of the Institute for Certification of Computer Professionals.

Computer Professionals, Institute for Certification of *See* Institute for Certification of Computer Professionals.

computer program A set of instructions for a computer to execute. A program can be written in a programming language, such as BASIC, or in an assembly language. Programs that direct a computer are called computer software. *See also* Beginners' All-purpose Symbolic Instruction Code; debug; loop; program.

computer programmer An individual who prepares instructions for computers. A programmer receives directions from a systems analyst. *See also* certified computer programmer; systems analyst.

computer programmer, certified *See* certified computer programmer.

computer science, medical *See* medical computer science.

computer screen The screen on which a computer or electronic typewriter operator sees what he or she is doing. It is similar to, but not the same as, a television screen. *See also* cathode ray tube.

computer software The programs, routines, and symbolic languages that control the functioning of the computer hardware and direct its operation. *Compare* computer hardware; firmware. *See also* system software.

computer, super- *See* supercomputer.

computer system, interactive *See* interactive computer system.

computer terminal A device with which people communicate with a computer. It typically has a keyboard and cathode ray tube (CRT) display. The terminal may be directly connected to the host computer or may use telephone lines via a modem. *See also* cathode ray tube; dumb terminal; intelligent terminal; interactive terminal; modem.

Computer Users in Speech and Hearing (CUSH) A national organization founded in 1981 composed of 1,000 professionals involved in communication sciences and communication disorders; companies that develop products for remediation and treatment of communication disorders; and individuals and family members who are experiencing communication disorders. It maintains a software lending library. *See also* computer; hearing.

computer virus A computer program designed to replicate itself by copying itself into the other programs stored in a computer. It may be benign or have a deleterious effect, such as causing a program to operate incorrectly or filling a computer's memory with unwanted codes. *See also* worm.

computer worm *See* worm.

computing *See* electronic data processing.

Computing Machinery, Association for *See* Association for Computing Machinery.

Computing, Special Interest Group on Biomedical *See* Special Interest Group on Biomedical Computing.

CON *See* certificate of need.

concept A general idea derived or inferred from specific instances or occurrences. *See also* idea. **2.** Something formed in the mind. *See also* conception; preconception.

concept, marketing *See* marketing concept.

conception **1.** Formation of a viable zygote by the union of the male sperm and the female ovum. *Compare* contraception. *See also* artificial reproduction; pregnancy; safe period. **2.** *See* concept.

conception, pre- *See* preconception.

conceptus The sum of derivatives of a fertilized ovum at any stage of development from fertilization until birth, including the embryo or fetus. *Synonym:* products of conception. *See also* live birth.

concern A matter of interest, requiring attention.

Concern for Dying *See* Choice in Dying-The National Council for the Right to Die.

concerted refusals to deal *See* boycott.

conciliation *See* mediation.

conciliator An individual who is assigned to or

assumes the responsibility for working with disputing parties until they reach a voluntary settlement. *See also* arbiter; mediation; mediator.

conclusion **1.** The result or outcome of an act or process. **2.** A judgment or decision reached after deliberation. *See also* illation.

conclusion error *See* statistical conclusion validity.

conclusion validity, statistical *See* statistical conclusion validity.

concordance A measure of the degree to which there is agreement or concord.

concur To agree. *Compare* dissent.

concurrent data collection In health care performance measurement, the process of gathering data on how a process works or is working while a patient is in active treatment. *See also* concurrent review; data collection; prospective data collection; retrospective data collection.

concurrent review **1.** In health care, evaluative activities conducted while a patient is in active treatment. **2.** Assessment activities conducted by surveyors from the Joint Commission on Accreditation of Healthcare Organizations, limited to the level of compliance at the time of survey. *See also* compliance level; Joint Commission on Accreditation of Healthcare Organizations; surveyor.

condition A state or mode of being, as in a heart condition or a comorbid condition. *See also* comorbidity; preexisting condition; state.

conditional accreditation A determination by the Joint Commission on Accreditation of Healthcare Organizations that standards compliance deficiencies exist in a health care organization. Findings of correction, which serve as the bases for further consideration of awarding full accreditation, must be demonstrated through a follow-up survey. *See also* accreditation; accreditation decision; follow-up survey; Joint Commission on Accreditation of Healthcare Organizations; special analysis unit.

conditioned reflex In psychology, a new or modified response elicited by a stimulus after conditioning. *Synonym*: conditioned response. *See also* conditioning.

conditioned response *See* conditioned reflex.

conditioned stimulus In psychology, a previously neutral stimulus that, after repeated association with an unconditioned stimulus, elicits the response affected by the unconditioned stimulus itself.

conditioning In psychology, a process of behavior modification by which a subject comes to associate a

desired behavior with a previously unrelated stimulus; discovered by Pavlov. *See also* behavior modification; conditioned reflex; Pavlov, Ivan; stimulus.

conditioning, operant *See* operant conditioning.

condition, preexisting *See* preexisting condition.

conditions of enrollment Rules that determine eligibility for health insurance enrollment. *See also* enrollment; health insurance.

conditions of participation The various conditions that a health care provider (for example, a hospital, home health agency, or skilled nursing facility) desiring to participate in a health care or insurance program (such as the Medicare program) is required to meet before participation is permitted. Investigations to determine whether health care providers meet or continue to meet conditions of participation are made by an appropriate state health agency, which is responsible for certifying that the conditions have been met and that the provider is eligible to participate. *See also* certified; Medicare; Medicare conditions of participation; participation.

conditions of participation, Medicare *See* Medicare conditions of participation.

condolence Sympathy with a person who has experienced pain, grief, or misfortune.

condom A sheathe used to cover the genitals, worn during intercourse to reduce the probability of impregnation and infection. *Synonym*: sheath. *See also* genitalia.

conduct **1.** To direct the course of, manage, or control. **2.** The way a person acts, especially from the standpoint of morality and ethics. *See also* unethical conduct.

conductivity testing Measurement of the conductive properties (capacity to conduct a current of electricity) of floors in areas where inhalation anesthetics are used. *See also* inhalation anesthetic; testing.

Conduct, Model Rules of Professional *See* Model Rules of Professional Conduct.

conduct, unethical *See* unethical conduct.

confabulation Unconscious filling in of gaps in memory with fabricated facts and experiences, commonly seen in organic amnesic syndromes. Patients so affected have no intent to deceive and believe the fabricated memories to be real. *Synonym*: fabrication. *See also* memory.

conference A meeting for consultation or discussion. *See also* clinicopathologic conference; conference call; morbidity and mortality conference; summation conference.

Conference of Actuaries in Public Practice *See* Conference of Consulting Actuaries.

conference call A conference by telephone in which three or more persons in different locations participate by means of a central switching unit.

conference, chief executive officer exit *See* chief executive officer exit conference.

conference, clinicopathologic *See* clinicopathologic conference.

conference committee, joint *See* joint conference committee.

Conference of Consulting Actuaries (CCA) A national organization founded in 1950 composed of 1,010 full-time consulting actuaries or governmental actuaries. Its committees focus on health issues and life issues. Formerly (1991) Conference of Actuaries in Public Practice. *See also* actuarial analysis; actuarial science; actuary.

Conference of Educational Administrators Serving the Deaf (CEASD) A national organization founded in 1868 composed of 355 executive heads of public, private, and denominational schools for the deaf in the United States and Canada. It coordinates research on the problems of deafness. Formerly (1980) Conference of Executives of American Schools for the Deaf. *See also* deaf; deaf-mute.

Conference of Executives of American Schools for the Deaf *See* Conference of Educational Administrators Serving the Deaf.

Conference of Local Health Officers, United States *See* United States Conference of Local Health Officers.

conference, morbidity and mortality *See* morbidity and mortality conference.

Conference of Podiatry Executives (COPE) A national organization founded in 1960 composed of 22 executive directors of state podiatry associations. Its purpose are to facilitate communication among member associations and their executives and to promote the exchange of information. *See also* executive; podiatric medicine.

Conference on Precision Electromagnetic Measurements (CPEM) A conference of the National Institute of Standards and Technology composed of scientists and engineers from industry, universities, and government interested in electromagnetic measurements, including microwaves and lasers. *See also* magnetic resonance.

Conference of Public Health Laboratorians (COPHL) A national organization founded in 1920 composed of 286 individuals directing or assisting in directing public health, military, hospital, and research laboratories. Its purposes include promoting the development, improvement, and effectiveness of public health laboratory services. *See also* laboratorian; public health.

Conference of Radiation Control Program Directors (CRCPD) A national organization founded in 1968 composed of 437 state and local radiological program directors and individuals from related federal protection agencies. It serves as a forum for the interchange of experience, concerns, developments, and recommendations among radiation control programs and related agencies. It promotes radiological health and uniform radiation control laws and regulations. *See also* radiation.

Conference of State and Territorial Directors of Public Health Education *See* Association of State and Territorial Directors of Public Health Education.

conference, summation *See* summation conference.

conference, tele- *See* teleconference.

confidence coefficient The probability that a confidence interval will contain the true value of the population parameter (for example, the population mean). For example, if the confidence coefficient is .95, 95 percent of the confidence intervals so calculated for each of a large number of random samples will contain the parameter and 5 percent will not. *Synonym*: coefficient of confidence. *See also* coefficient; confidence interval.

confidence interval (CI) In statistics, an interval or a range of values based on a random sample for which there is a stated probability (for example, 90%, 95%, or 99%) that the population parameter (for example, the population mean) is contained within this interval. The endpoints of the confidence interval are called confidence limits. *See also* confidence coefficient; confidence limit.

confidence limit The upper and lower boundaries of a confidence interval. *See also* confidence interval.

confidential Private or secret, as in referring to information and practices; something treated with trust, resulting in a feeling of security that information will not be disclosed to other parties. *See also* confidentiality; confidentiality and disclosure policy.

confidentiality An individual's right, within the law, to personal and informational privacy, including his or her medical record. *See also* Freedom of Information Act; medical record; patient bill of rights; patient rights; right of privacy.

confidentiality and disclosure policy   A policy of the Joint Commission on Accreditation of Healthcare Organizations dealing with information received or developed during the accreditation process. The following information is treated as confidential: information obtained from a health care organization before, during, and/or following the accreditation survey that relates to compliance with specific accreditation standards; all materials that may contribute to the accreditation decision (for example, survey report forms); written staff analyses and Accreditation Committee minutes and agenda materials; and the official accreditation decision report. The following information is subject to public release (disclosure) upon request: current accreditation status of a health care organization; hospital-specific performance data, provided certain conditions are met; for organizations surveyed in 1994 or later, the number of type I recommendations and, at the grid level, the nature of these recommendations; the date(s) of a survey after a health care organization been notified; the status of a health care organization in the accreditation decision process; applicable standards under which an accreditation survey was conducted; health care organizational and operational components included in the accreditation survey; applicable standards areas involved in a Joint Commission complaint review; the number and nature of substantive written complaints filed against an accredited health care organization since its last triennial survey that have been substantiated by the Joint Commission; for a tailored survey, the organizational component(s) that contributed to a decision of conditional accreditation or denial of accreditation; and whether, at the time a health care organization withdrew from accreditation, there were any type I recommendations for which the Joint Commission had no or insufficient evidence of resolution, and, after 1993, the nature of these recommendations at the grid element level. The Joint Commission reserves the prerogative to publish, or otherwise release publicly, aggregate performance data that are not organization specific. *See also* accreditation; confidentiality; Joint Commission on Accreditation of Healthcare Organizations; performance data; policy; performance data; type I recommendation.

confidentiality as a patient right   A patient's right, within the law, to personal and informational privacy, including his or her medical record. *See also* confidentiality; patient; right.

confinement   *See* labor.

conflict of interest   A situation in which regard for one duty leads to disregard of another, or might reasonably be expected to do so; for example, when a family of an incompetent patient has wishes that are not in the patient's best interest; when more profit may be achieved by less health care given to a patient by physicians in prepaid health plans; when a government employee's personal or financial interest conflicts or appears to conflict with his or her official responsibilities; or when a fiduciary of an organization votes on a matter that may affect his or her own personal or financial affairs. *See also* duty; fiduciary.

conformance   **1.** Agreement in form or character, as in an affirmative judgment that a product or service has met the requirements of the relevant specifications, contract, or regulation. **2.** The state of meeting requirements of the relevant specifications, contract, or regulation. *See also* compliance.

confounding variable   A factor that distorts the true relationship of a study's variables of interest by being related to the outcome of interest but extraneous to the study question and unequally distributed among the groups being compared. For example, age might confound a study of the effect of a toxin on longevity if individuals exposed to the toxin were older than those not exposed to the toxin. The presence of a confounding factor can either hide a true correlation or give the appearance of a correlation when none actually exists. *See also* scatter diagram; variable.

congenital   Existing at or before birth, as a result of either hereditary or environmental influences, as in congenital cleft palate or congenital port wine stain.

congestive heart failure (CHF)   A clinical syndrome characterized by distinctive symptoms and signs resulting from disturbances in cardiac output or from increased venous pressure. Most often applied to myocardial failure with increased pressures distending the ventricle (high end-diastolic pressure) and a cardiac output inadequate for the body's needs; often subclassified as right-sided or left-sided heart failure depending on whether the systemic or pulmonary veins are predominantly distended. *See also* heart; syndrome.

Congress of County Medical Societies (CCMS) A national organization founded in 1966 that seeks to improve communications among county medical associations. *See also* medical association; medical society.

Congressional budget In the federal budget, the budget as set forth by Congress in a concurrent resolution of both Houses. These resolutions specify the appropriate level of total budget outlays and of total new budget authority; an estimate of budget outlays and new budget authority for each major functional category, for contingencies, and for undistributed intragovernmental transactions (based on allocations of the appropriate level of total budget outlays and of total new budget authority); the amount, if any, of the surplus or deficit in the budget; the recommended level of federal revenues; and the appropriate level of the public debt. *See also* budget; president's budget.

Congressional Budget Office (CBO) A nonpartisan organization established by the Congressional Budget Act of 1974, which provides the US Congress with budget-related information and with analyses of alternative fiscal, budgetary, and program issues, including those related to health matters and programs under its Human Resources and Community Development Division. *See also* budget; congressional budget.

Congressional Record A publication issued daily when Congress is in session, containing the proceedings of Congress. Publication of the *Congressional Record* began in 1873.

Congress of Lung Association Staff (CLAS) A national organization founded in 1912 composed of 800 executives and staff members of the American Lung Association. It sponsors network opportunities, staff development, and training programs. *See also* American Lung Association; lung.

Congress Watch (CW) A congressional lobby founded in 1971 that represents consumer interests, specifically citizens' access to government decision making, campaign finance reform, the savings and loan crisis, consumer class actions, food and product safety, and protection of public health through environmental legislation. *See also* consumer; lobbying; public health.

conjoined twins *See* Siamese twins.

connective tissue The supporting cells and noncellular components of tissues and organs; for example, fibrous tissue or collagen. *See also* adipose tissue; tissue.

consciousness The state of being aware of one's own existence, sensations, thoughts, surroundings, and other phenomena; fully alert, awake, and oriented. Levels of consciousness refer to clinically differentiated degrees of awareness and alertness, variably classified and defined. For instance, one classification is alert (the state of wakefulness, oriented to people, place, and time); confused (the state of being awake but disoriented to people, place, and time); somnolent (the state of being drowsy and frequently falling asleep when alone); stuporous (the state of partial or nearly complete unconsciousness, manifested by response only to vigorous stimulation); and comatose (a state of unconsciousness from which an individual cannot be aroused, even by powerful stimulation). *See also* coma; Glasgow coma scale; lethargy; subconscious; unconscious.

conscious, sub- *See* subconscious.

conscious, un- *See* unconscious.

consecutive sample A sample in which the units are chosen on a strict "first come, first chosen" basis. For example, all individuals who are eligible for a clinical study in which consecutive sampling is employed should be included as they are seen. *Synonym*: sequential sample. *See also* sample.

consensus Agreement, especially in opinion. *See also* expert consensus.

consensus, expert *See* expert consensus.

consent Authorization for an act by one who has the authority to provide it; voluntary agreement, as in a patient's authorization to undergo a medical procedure or treatment. Consent evolves from common-law principles of personal autonomy and battery. *See also* age of consent; autonomy; battery; common law; implied consent; informed consent; presumed consent.

consent, age of *See* age of consent.

consent, implied *See* implied consent.

consent, informed *See* informed consent.

consent, patient *See* informed consent.

consent, presumed *See* presumed consent.

consequential damages Losses or injuries that are the consequence of some act but are not the direct and immediate result of that act. *Synonym*: special damages. *See also* damages; general damages.

console **1.** To comfort, as in consoling a mother of

an injured infant. **2.** The portion of a computer or peripheral that houses the apparatus used to operate the machine manually and provides a means of communication between the computer operator and the central processing unit, often in the form of a keyboard. *Synonym*: keyboard. *See also* computer terminal; input device.

Consolidated Omnibus Budget Reconciliation Act of 1985 (COBRA) Legislation that includes protection of patients against hospital "dumping" because of suspicion that hospitals with emergency services were limiting access to save money (enacted April 7, 1986). *See also* patient dumping.

Consolidated Standards Manual *See Accreditation Manual for Mental Health, Chemical Dependency, and Mental Retardation/Developmental Disabilities Services.*

consolidation A combination of two or more entities into a single new entity so that the previous entities cease to exist; for example, the formal combination of two or more hospitals into a single new legal entity that has an identity separate from any of the preexisting hospitals. *Compare* merger.

consortium A formal voluntary alliance of individuals or organizations (such as hospitals, associations, or societies), usually from the same geographic area, for a specific purpose, usually to promote a common objective or engage in a project of benefit to all members. A consortium functions under a set of bylaws or other written rules to which each member agrees to abide and that may or may not be incorporated and in which control of assets resides with each member, except as prescribed in the bylaws. *See also* bylaws.

conspect reliability *See* interobserver reliability.

conspiracy A combination of two or more persons by concerted action to accomplish an unlawful purpose, or some purpose not in itself unlawful by unlawful means, as in a conspiracy to monopolize. It is essential there are two or more conspirators because one cannot conspire with himself or herself.

constancy of purpose One of W. Edwards Deming's Fourteen Points that maintains a radical new definition of a company's role: rather than making money, it is to stay in business and provide jobs through innovation, research, constant improvement, and maintenance. *See also* Deming's Fourteen Points; Deming, W. Edwards.

constipation Difficult, incomplete, or infrequent

evacuation of dry, hardened feces from the bowels. *See also* feces; intestine; obstipation.

constraint, resource *See* resource constraint.

construct An idea or concept created or synthesized (constructed) from available information (facts and opinions) and used to seek further knowledge through scientific investigation, or to develop beliefs and values. *See also* construct validity.

construct validity The degree to which a study measures and/or manipulates what a researcher claims it does. For instance, if, on theoretical grounds, an occurrence rate for some phenomenon should change with increasing age, a measurement with construct validity would reflect this change. If construct validity has been established for a measure, it may be used as a criterion standard (gold standard) against which other measures (tests, indicators) are evaluated. *See also* construct; criterion standard; external validity; gold standard; validity.

constructed beds The total number of beds that a health care organization, such as a hospital, is constructed to accommodate. *See also* bed.

consultant An individual or an organization with expertise providing professional advice or services to another individual or organization for a fee. *Compare* employee. *See also* health care consultant; hospital consultant; image consultant; independent contractor; medical consultant; outsourcing; public relations consultant.

consultant dietitian A registered dietitian qualified by experience in administrative or clinical dietetic practice who provides counsel or supervision of dietary activities. *See also* administrative dietitian; clinical dietitian; consultant; dietitian; registered dietitian.

Consultant Dietitians in Health Care Facilities (CDHCF) A national organization founded in 1975 composed of 5,000 dietitians employed in extended care facilities, nursing homes, and other health-care-related food service operations. *See also* consultant dietitian; dietitian.

consultant, health care *See* health care consultant.

consultant, hospital *See* hospital consultant.

consultant, image *See* image consultant.

consultant, medical *See* medical consultant.

Consultant Pharmacists, American Society of *See* American Society of Consultant Pharmacists.

consultant, public health *See* public health consultant.

consultant, public relations *See* public relations

consultant.

Consultants, American Association of Dental *See* American Association of Dental Consultants.

Consultants, American Association of Healthcare *See* American Association of Healthcare Consultants.

Consultants, American Association of Legal Nurse *See* American Association of Legal Nurse Consultants.

Consultants, American Association of Medico-Legal *See* American Association of Medico-Legal Consultants.

Consultants, American Association of Nutritional *See* American Association of Nutritional Consultants.

Consultants, American Board of Professional Disability *See* American Board of Professional Disability Consultants.

Consultants to the Armed Forces, Society of Medical *See* Society of Medical Consultants to the Armed Forces.

Consultants Association, Nurse *See* Nurse Consultants Association.

Consultants, Institute of Certified Professional Business *See* Institute of Certified Professional Business Consultants.

Consultants, Society of Professional Business *See* Society of Professional Business Consultants.

consultation The process of requesting advice from another person, as in a physician requesting advice from another physician (the consultant) regarding the diagnosis and/or treatment of a patient. The consultant usually reviews the history, examines the patient, and then provides his or her written or oral opinion to the requesting practitioner. Referral for consultation is distinguished from referral for services, because responsibility for patient care is not usually delegated to a consultant. The opinion and advice of a consultant are not usually binding on the referring individual. *See also* medical consultation; referral.

consultation, medical *See* medical consultation.

consultation report In medicine, a component of a medical record consisting of a written opinion by a consultant that reflects, when appropriate, an examination of the patient and the patient's medical record(s). *See also* consultant; consultation; medical record.

consultative recommendation *See* supplemental recommendation.

Consulting Actuaries, Conference of *See* Confer-

ence of Consulting Actuaries.

consumer 1. In economics, one who buys goods and services for personal use rather than for manufacture. The consumer is the ultimate user of a product or service. *See also* monopoly. **2.** In health care, one who may or does receive health services. Although persons do at times consume health services, a "consumer," as the term is used in health legislation and programs, is someone who is not a provider, that is, one who is not involved or associated directly or indirectly with the provision of health services. The definition of "consumer" is important in public health programs, in which a majority of consumers may be required on a governing body. *See also* health care consumer.

Consumer Affairs of the American Hospital Association, National Society of Patient Representation and *See* National Society of Patient Representation and Consumer Affairs of the American Hospital Association.

Consumer Alert (CA) A national public interest organization founded in 1977 composed of 6,000 members opposing excessive regulations and supporting free enterprise, consumer rights, and freedom of choice for individual consumers. It examines current and proposed regulations in terms of demonstrated need and ultimate cost in areas where it believes consumer interests are being abused. If the regulation is deemed excessive, the organization develops proposals to change or abolish it or inform the public about its cause and effects. *See also* consumer; consumerism.

consumer, health care *See* health care consumer.

Consumer Information Center (CIC) A department of the General Services Administration, established by Presidential Order in 1970 to assist federal agencies to develop, promote, and distribute information of interest to consumers and to increase public awareness of this information. *See also* consumer; consumerism; General Services Administration.

consumerism A political movement that seeks to expand the protection of consumers of goods and services through government regulation of the quality and safety of these goods and services and through improved consumer awareness. *See also* consumer.

Consumer Organization, National Insurance *See* National Insurance Consumer Organization.

consumer price index (CPI) A measure of change

in consumer prices, as determined by a monthly survey of the Bureau of Labor Statistics of the US Department of Labor. This CPI statistic measures the change in average prices of the goods and services purchased by urban wage earners and clerical workers and their families. It is widely used as an indicator of changes in the cost of living, as a measure of inflation and deflation in the economy, and as a means for studying trends in prices of various goods and services. *Synonym:* cost-of-living index. *See also* index; medical consumer price index.

consumer price index, medical *See* medical consumer price index.

Consumer Product Safety Commission (CPSC) A federal commission created to protect the public against unreasonable risks of injury from consumer products; to assist consumers in evaluating the comparative safety of consumer products; to develop uniform safety standards for consumer products and minimize conflicting state and local regulations; and to promote research and investigation into the causes and prevention of product-related deaths, illnesses, and injuries. *See also* consumer; consumerism.

Consumers Association, American *See* American Consumers Association.

Consumers and Health Care Information, Center for Medical *See* Center for Medical Consumers and Health Care Information.

Consumers League, National *See* National Consumers League.

consumer terrorism *See* tamper.

consumption An obsolescent term for pulmonary tuberculosis. *See also* tuberculosis.

contact **1.** A coming together or touching, as of people, objects, or surfaces, as in direct contact as a mode of transmission of infection. *See also* contact isolation; direct contact; epidemiology; indirect contact. **2.** A person or an animal that has been in association with an infected person or animal or a contaminated environment so that he or she has had the opportunity to acquire the infection. *See also* infection; primary contact; secondary contact.

contact, direct *See* direct contact.

contact, indirect *See* indirect contact.

contact isolation A category of patient isolation, intended for less transmissible or serious infections, to prevent the spread of diseases or conditions that disseminate primarily by close or direct contact. A private room in a hospital is indicated but patients infected with the same pathogen may share a room. Masks are indicated for those who come close to the patient, gowns are indicated if soiling is likely, and gloves are indicated for touching infectious material. *See also* direct contact; isolation.

contact lens A thin plastic or glass lens that is fitted over the cornea of the eye to correct various vision defects. Plural: contact lenses. *See also* ophthalmology; opticianry; optometry.

Contact Lens Association of Ophthalmologists (CLAO) A national organization founded in 1962 composed of 2,000 active and resident ophthalmologists and osteopathic physicians specializing in ophthalmology. Its objective is to disseminate scientific information on ophthalmology and provide for the sharing of techniques and expertise. *See also* contact lens; ophthalmology.

Contact Lens Examiners, National *See* National Contact Lens Examiners.

Contact Lens Manufacturers Association (CLMA) A national organization founded in 1962 composed of 140 firms, corporations, or individuals who make finished contact lenses. *See also* contact lens.

Contact Lens Society of America (CLSA) A national organization founded in 1955 composed of 1,750 contact lens fitters and manufacturers of products associated with contact lenses. Its purposes are to share knowledge of contact lens technology and to foster the growth and ability of contact lens technicians. *See also* contact lens.

contact, primary *See* primary contact.

contact, secondary *See* secondary contact.

contagion **1.** Disease transmission by direct or indirect contact. **2.** A disease that is or may be transmitted by direct or indirect contact. *See also* contact; direct contact; indirect contact.

contagious Transmissible from person to person by direct or indirect contact. *See also* contact; infectious.

contaminate To make impure or unclean by contact or mixture, as in tainting a sterile condition with microorganisms or introducing biased data, inappropriate procedures, or incorrect logic that may distort the results of research or study.

Contemporary Medicine and Surgery, American Society of *See* American Society of Contemporary Medicine and Surgery.

Contemporary Ophthalmology, American Society of *See* American Society of Contemporary Ophthalmology.

content expert An individual who possesses a high degree of skill and/or knowledge in a subject or an area; for example, a trauma care expert or a billing expert. *See also* expert.

content validity The degree to which a sample of items is representative of the universe it was intended to represent. *See also* external validity; validity.

contingency fee The charge made by an attorney dependent on a successful outcome in the case; it is often agreed to be a percentage of the party's recovery (usually amounting to about one-third). Such fee arrangements are often used in negligence cases (such as malpractice cases) and other civil actions. It is unethical for an attorney to charge a criminal defendant a fee substantially contingent upon the result in the case. *Synonym:* contingent fee. *See also* fee.

contingency fund A sum of money set aside or budgeted for an organization to cover possible unknown future expenses. *See also* contingency reserves; fund.

contingency planning The process of developing alternative plans for achieving an objective. *See also* planning.

contingency reserves Reserves set aside by an insurance company for unforeseen or unplanned circumstances and expenses apart from the losses normally incurred for insured policy holders. *See also* contingency fund.

continual Recurring regularly or frequently, as in the continual need to pay health insurance premiums. *See also* continuous.

continued-stay review Periodic evaluation throughout a patient's hospitalization to determine the medical necessity and appropriateness of continued inpatient treatment. A continued-stay review may be conducted by the health care team providing the patient's care, the hospital utilization review committee, a third-party payer, or an external utilization review organization. *See also* concurrent review; review.

continuing care Care of all levels and intensity (for example, skilled nursing care, intermediate care) provided to patients in various settings (such as hospitals or nursing homes) over an extended period of time. *See also* care; intermediate care; level of care; nursing home; skilled nursing care.

continuing care retirement community A community that provides services and housing options to meet the needs of the elderly. It provides independent and congregate living and personal, intermediate, and skilled nursing care and attempts to create an environment that allows each resident to participate in the community's life to whatever degree desired. *See also* community; life care; retirement; retirement center.

continuing education In health care, education beyond initial professional preparation that is relevant to the type of care delivered in an organization and that provides current knowledge relevant to an individual's field of practice. *See also* continuing medical education.

Continuing Education, American College for *See* American College for Continuing Education.

Continuing Education, Association for *See* Association for Continuing Education.

continuing medical education (CME) Continuing education as it applies to physicians. CME may occur through taking courses, reading medical journals and texts, attending teaching programs, and taking self-study courses. CME programs are provided by organizations including medical schools, professional organizations, and hospitals. *See also* Accreditation Council for Continuing Medical Education; continuing education; medical education.

Continuing Medical Education, Accreditation Council for *See* Accreditation Council for Continuing Medical Education.

Continuing Medical Education, Network for *See* Network for Continuing Medical Education.

continuity In health care, a performance dimension addressing the degree to which the care/intervention for a patient is coordinated among practitioners, among organizations, and over time. *See also* care; dimensions of performance; primary care center.

Continuity of Care, American Association for *See* American Association for Continuity of Care.

continuous Uninterrupted in time, sequence, substance, or extent, as in continuous improvement. *See also* continual; frequent; intermittent; occasional; periodic; sporadic; successive.

continuous ambulatory peritoneal dialysis (CAPD) *See* peritoneal dialysis.

continuous data Data with a potentially infinite number of possible values along a continuum. An example of continuous data is the number of pounds a patient who is receiving total parenteral nutrition weighs over time or the number of minutes spent by prehospital personnel at a prehospital trauma scene. *Compare* discrete data. *See also* continuous; continuous variable; continuous variable indicator; continuum; data; quantitative data.

continuous flow The process by which survey reports from the Joint Commission on Accreditation of Healthcare Organizations move smoothly through the accreditation decision process and can be made according to a straightforward application of rules. *See also* accreditation; accreditation decision processing; continuous; Joint Commission on Accreditation of Healthcare Organizations.

continuous improvement *See* continuous quality improvement.

continuous probability distribution *See* probability distribution.

continuous quality improvement (CQI) In health care, a management approach to the continuous study and improvement of the processes of providing health care services to meet the needs of patients and other persons. Continuous quality improvement focuses on making an entire system's outcomes better by constantly adjusting and improving the system itself, instead of searching out and getting rid of "bad apples" (outliers). *Synonyms and near-synonyms*: continuous improvement (CI); hospital quality improvement (HQI); quality improvement (QI); and total quality management (TQM). *Compare* acceptable quality level. *See also* facilitator; improvement; outlier; process improvement; quality improvement; total quality management.

continuous variable A variable that, when measured, has a potentially infinite number of possible values along a continuum. *Compare* discrete variable. *See also* continuous data; continuum; variable.

continuous variable indicator An aggregate data indicator in which the value of each measurement can fall anywhere along a continuous scale (for example, the length of many sticks in inches). *Compare* rate-based indicator. *See also* aggregate data indicator; continuous variable; indicator.

continuum A continuing extent, succession, or whole, no part of which can be distinguished from neighboring parts except by arbitrary division, as in the continuum of body temperature.

contraception Intentional prevention of conception or impregnation through the use of various devices, agents, drugs, sexual practices, or surgical procedures. *Compare* conception. *See also* birth con-

trol; coitus interruptus; contraceptive sterilization; family planning; oral contraceptive; safe period; sponge.

Contraception, Association for Voluntary Surgical *See* Association for Voluntary Surgical Contraception.

contraception, rhythm method of *See* safe period.

contraceptive, oral *See* oral contraceptive.

contraceptive sterilization A surgical procedure performed to prevent conception, as in tubal ligation or vasectomy. *See also* ligation; sterilization.

contract 1. A formal agreement between two or more parties, especially one that is written and enforceable by law. A contract specifies the services, personnel, products, and/or space to be provided by, to, or on behalf of the parties and the consideration to be expended in exchange. *See also* aleatory contract; contracting; contract physician; contract services; exclusive contract; group contract; rescission; terminable-at-will; terms. **2.** To bring on oneself, or to be affected with, as in contracting pneumonia.

contract, aleatory *See* aleatory contract.

contract authority *See* backdoor authority.

contract, exclusive *See* exclusive contract.

contract, group *See* group contract.

contracting The process of establishing or undertaking a business relationship by contract. *See also* contract.

contract management of departments Performance of day-to-day management of one or more departments, units, services, or functions of a health care organization by another organization under contract to the facility. The health care organization retains overall administrative responsibility as well as accountability for evaluating the contractor's performance. *See also* contract; department; management.

contract management of an organization Performance of day-to-day management of a health care organization by another organization under contract to the governing body or owners who retain legal responsibility and ownership of the organization's assets and liabilities. *See also* contract; management.

contractor One that contracts or is a party to a contract. *See also* independent contractor; piece work.

contractor, independent *See* independent contractor.

contract physician A physician who, under a full-time or a part-time contract, provides care in a hospital or other type of health care organization and whose payment as defined in the contract may be an institutional responsibility, or on a fee or another agreed-on basis. *See also* contract; physician.

contract practice Individual health care provider, such as a physician or dentist, under contract to an employer group or other organization for the provision of services to its members and dependents. *See also* contract; practice.

contract, risk management *See* risk management contract.

contract services Services rendered to or on behalf of an organization under contract with an organization, agency, or individual under terms listed in a contract. Examples include laundry services, laboratory services, and emergency services. *Synonym:* contracted service. *See also* contract management of departments; contract management of an organization.

contract, social *See* social contract.

contractual adjustment Accounting adjustment made by a health care provider to reflect uncollectible differences between established charges for services rendered to insured persons and rates payable for those services under contracts with third-party payers. *See also* adjustment.

contraindication A factor or condition that renders the administration of a drug or agent or the performance of a procedure or other practice inadvisable, improper, and/or undesirable. For example, severe colitis, possible perforated organ, and acute severe diverticulitis are three contraindications to performing colonoscopy. *Compare* indication. *See also* package insert.

contralateral Situated on, pertaining to, or affecting the opposite side, as in the blunt trauma to the head caused equal injury to the contralateral side of the brain. *Compare* ipsilateral.

contrast To limit a description of items being compared to mentioning their differences, as in the excellence of the hospital contrasted sharply with the poor performance of its competitors. Compare means to describe items while noting both similarities and differences, as in comparing the good and bad features of health plans before making a decision. *Compare* compare. *See also* contrast medium.

contrast enema *See* barium enema.

contrast material *See* contrast medium.

contrast medium A substance, such as barium sulphate, used in diagnostic imaging to increase the contrast of an image. A positive contrast medium absorbs x-rays more strongly than the tissue of the structure (such as the colon) being examined; a neg-

ative contrast medium, less strongly. *See also* barium enema; radiopaque dye.

contrast resolution The number of bits per pixel in a graphic computer display; used to measure the ability to distinguish screen or print-out intensity levels. *See also* bit; computer; resolution.

contributory insurance Group health insurance in which part or all of the premium is paid by the employee and the remaining part, if any, is paid by the employer or union. *Compare* noncontributory insurance. *See also* group insurance; insurance.

contributory negligence A portion of the responsibility for a compensable injury or loss ascribed to the plaintiff due to his or her own fault. *See also* negligence; plaintiff.

control 1. To exercise authority or influence over, as in controlling output or damage control. 2. That aspect of management concerned with the comparison of actual versus planned performance, as well as the development and implementation of procedures to improve performance. *See also* management. 3. Categories of health care organizations based on responsibility for establishing policy concerning the overall operation of the organization. For instance, there are four major categories of control used by the American Hospital Association in classifying hospitals: nonfederal government-controlled hospitals; nongovernmental, not-for-profit hospitals; investor-owned (for-profit hospitals); and federal government hospitals. Within each major category are further subdivisions.

control, birth *See* birth control.

control center, poison *See* poison control center.

Control Centers, American Association of Poison *See* American Association of Poison Control Centers.

control chart A graphic display of data in the order that they occur with statistically determined upper and lower limits of expected common-cause variation. A control chart is used to indicate special causes of variation, to monitor a process for maintenance, and to determine if process changes have had the desired effect. *See also* chart; run; special cause; special-cause variation; statistical control.

control, damage *See* damage control.

control experiment An experiment that isolates the effect of one variable on a system by holding constant all variables but the one under observation. *See also* control group; experiment; variable.

control group A group used as a standard of comparison in a control experiment. This group does not receive the experimental treatment and is compared to the treatment group to determine whether the treatment had an effect. *See also* control experiment.

controllability In the federal budget, the ability of the Congress or President to control monetary outlays during a given fiscal year and under existing laws. The legislation for some health programs, such as Medicare and Civilian Health and Medical Program of the Uniformed Services (CHAMPUS), establishes health benefits as entitlements, rendering such programs uncontrollable without changing laws. *See also* budget; Civilian Health and Medical Program of the Uniformed Services; entitlement; entitlement program; Medicare.

controlled substances Drugs whose general availability is restricted in the United States under jurisdiction of the Controlled Substances Act of 1970 because of their potential for abuse or addiction. These drugs include narcotics, stimulants, depressants, hallucinogens, and cannabis. *See also* cannabis; Controlled Substances Act of 1970; DEA number; depressants; hallucinogen; narcotics; schedule I substances; schedule II substances; schedule III substances; schedule IV substances; schedule V substances; stimulant; tranquilizer.

Controlled Substances Act of 1970 A federal law establishing controls over drugs of abuse and narcotics. It classifies abused substances and subjects their use to restrictions. The act also provides financing for program development for the treatment and rehabilitation of addicted persons, study of the causes and effects of addiction, and health education related to drugs and their effects. *See also* addiction; controlled substances; drug.

controlled substances, schedule of *See* schedule of controlled substances.

controller Chief accountant of an organization; an officer who audits accounts and supervises the financial affairs of a corporation or of a governmental body. *Synonym*: comptroller. *See also* chief financial officer.

control limit In statistics, an expected limit of common-cause variation, sometimes referred to as either an upper or a lower control limit. Variation beyond a control limit is evidence that special causes are affecting a process. Control limits are calculated from process data and are not to be confused with engineering specifications or tolerance limits. Con-

trol limits are typically plotted on a control chart. *See also* common-cause variation; control chart; special-cause variation; specification; statistical control.

control, medical *See* medical control.

control, operational *See* operational control.

control plan A Blue Cross or Blue Shield Plan that sells a health plan to a local company having employees in other states or areas and arranges for other Blue Cross and Blue Shield Plans in those locations to provide the same benefits. The other plans function as subcontractors to the control plan. *See also* host plan; participating plan.

control, quality *See* quality control.

Control Society, Statistical Process *See* Statistical Process Control Society.

control, spin *See* spin control.

control, statistical *See* statistical control.

control, statistical process *See* statistical process control.

control, statistical quality *See* statistical quality control.

control trial, nonrandomized *See* nonrandomized control trial.

contusion A bruise. *Compare* abrasion; laceration. *See also* bruise.

convalescence Gradual return to health after illness or injury. *See also* convalescent center.

convalescent center A skilled nursing facility or an intermediate care facility providing health services to patients recovering from severe or debilitating illnesses or injuries. *See also* convalescence; intermediate care facility; skilled nursing facility.

convenience sample Individuals or groups selected at the convenience of an investigator or primarily because they were available at a convenient time or place. *See also* sample.

Convention and Exhibitors Association, Healthcare *See* Healthcare Convention and Exhibitors Association.

Convention, United States Pharmacopeial *See* United States Pharmacopeial Convention.

convergent validity A demonstration of the validity of a measure by correlations among two or more purported measures of a concept. Convergent validity does not, however, presuppose that one measure is a standard against which other measures should be evaluated. *See also* criterion standard; validity.

convulsion A violent involuntary contraction or series of contractions of the voluntary muscles caused by many factors ranging from high fever to uremia to brain abscesses. *Synonyms:* fit; seizure. *See also* epilepsy.

COO *See* chief operating officer.

Cooperative Health Statistics System (CHSS) A program of the National Center for Health Statistics in which federal, state, and local governments cooperated in collecting health statistics. The CHSS collected data in seven areas, including health manpower, health facilities, hospital care, and long term care. The program was terminated in 1981. The Vital Statistics Cooperative Program, a former component of CHSS, continues to collect information on births, deaths, causes of death, marriages, divorces, abortions, and other events. *See also* health statistics; National Center for Health Statistics; vital statistics.

cooperative services *See* shared services.

Coordinated Transfer Application System (COTRANS) A system begun in 1979 by the Association of American Medical Colleges to evaluate US citizens receiving undergraduate medical education outside of the United States and to sponsor those it deems qualified for Part I of the national medical board examinations. Students who take and pass the national board examinations with COTRANS sponsorship may then apply to US medical schools for completion of their training with advanced standing. Some students obtain sponsorship for the board examinations from a medical school without using COTRANS. *See also* Association of American Medical Colleges; national board examination.

Coordinating Council on Medical Education *See* Council for Medical Affairs.

coordination of benefits (COB) Provisions and procedures used by insurers to avoid duplicate payment for losses insured under more than one insurance policy. Some people, for instance, have a duplication of benefits (in their automobile and health insurance policies) for their medical costs arising from an automobile accident. A coordination of benefits or antiduplication clause in one or the other policy will prevent double payment for the expenses by making one of the insurers the primary payer and ensuring that no more than 100% of the costs are covered. *See also* benefits; duplication of benefits; primary payer.

coordinator, DRG *See* DRG coordinator.

coordinator, health unit *See* health unit coordinator.

coordinator, nurse *See* nurse coordinator.

Coordinators, National Association of Health Unit *See* National Association of Health Unit Coordinators.

coordinator, utilization review *See* utilization review coordinator.

copayment In a health insurance policy, a form of cost sharing in which a fixed amount of money is paid by the insured with each health service provided. *See also* ancillary charge; coinsurance; cost sharing; deductible; health services.

COPD *See* chronic obstructive pulmonary disease.

COPE *See* Conference of Podiatry Executives.

COPHL *See* Conference of Public Health Laboratorians.

coprolalia The compusive or obsessive use in speech of words relating to feces. *See also* compulsion; feces.

coprophagia The eating of feces. *See also* coprolalia; feces.

copyright Protection by statute or by the common law, giving artists and authors exclusive right to publish their works or to determine who may publish the work. The legal life of a copyright is the author's life plus 50 years or a flat 75 years for a copyright held by a company. Copyrights are registered in the Copyright Office of the Library of Congress.

cord, spinal *See* spinal cord.

cord, umbilical *See* umbilical cord.

core memory The random-access portion of the main memory of a computer that can be accessed directly by the central processing unit. *See also* central processing unit; computer; memory; random access memory.

coronary **1.** Pertaining to the arteries or veins of the heart. *See also* coronary artery; heart; vein. **2.** A heart attack. *See also* acute myocardial infarction.

coronary angiography An invasive procedure in which radiopaque substances are injected into coronary arteries so that diagnostic x-rays of these blood vessels may be made. *See also* angiography; coronary artery; invasive procedure; radiopaque.

coronary artery Either of two arteries that originate in the aorta and supply blood to the muscular tissue of the heart. *See also* acute myocardial infarction; angina pectoris; artery; coronary; heart.

coronary artery bypass graft (CABG) procedure A surgical procedure in which a vein or an artery is used to bypass a constricted portion of a coronary artery. *Synonym:* coronary bypass surgery. *See also* coronary artery; invasive procedure.

coronary artery bypass graft (CABG) procedure,

emergent   A CABG procedure performed due to the instability in the clinical status of the patient, which requires immediate intervention. *See also* coronary artery bypass graft procedure.

coronary artery disease (CAD)   *See* arteriosclerosis; atherosclerosis.

coronary bypass surgery   *See* coronary artery bypass graft procedure.

coronary care unit (CCU)   *See* cardiac care unit.

coronary occlusion   The partial or complete blockage of blood flow in a coronary artery, as by a thrombus or the progressive buildup of atherosclerotic plaque. *See also* atherosclerosis; coronary artery; occlusion; thrombus.

coronary thrombosis   A blood clot (thrombosis) blocking a coronary artery and causing a heart attack (myocardial infarction). *See also* acute myocardial infarction; blood clot; thrombosis.

coroner   An elected or appointed public official responsible for investigating and providing official opinions about the causes and circumstances of deaths that occur in any one or a combination of the following circumstances: without explanation; without apparent natural causes and/or explained with conflicting causes; suddenly; violently; or potentially due to foul play. A coroner investigates deaths that occur within his or her jurisdiction. *Compare* medical examiner. *See also* coroner's jury.

coroner's jury   A panel of citizens that officially reviews the circumstances, manner, and evidence in a death that appears to be due to natural causes. *See also* coroner; jury.

corporate   Pertaining to or belonging to a corporation, as in corporate liability.

corporate alliance   According to the Health Security Act (1993), a health alliance sponsored by an eligible large employer, multiemployers, rural electric cooperative, or rural telephone cooperative association, that contracts with a corporate alliance health plan. *See also* corporate alliance employer; corporate alliance health plan; health alliance; health plan; Health Security Act; large employer; large employer alliance; regional alliance.

corporate alliance eligible individual   According to the Health Security Act (1993), an eligible individual for whom a corporate alliance is the applicable health plan. *See also* corporate alliance; health plan; Health Security Act; regional alliance eligible individual.

corporate alliance employer   According to the Health Security Act (1993), an employer of an individual who is a participant in a corporate alliance health plan. *See also* corporate alliance; employer; health alliance; health plan; Health Security Act; regional alliance employer.

corporate alliance health plan   According to the Health Security Act (1993), a health plan offered by a corporate alliance. *See also* corporate alliance; health plan; Health Security Act; regional alliance health plan.

corporate dentistry   Company-owned and operated facilities providing dental services to employees and sometimes to their dependents. This approach to dental services delivery involves a closed panel arrangement in which the beneficiaries must utilize the specified dentists and facilities. *See also* closed panel group practice; dentistry.

corporate diversification   The process by which an organization, such as a hospital, broadens the sources of revenue-generating activities and services through the establishment of corporations, limited partnerships, foundations, and joint ventures to provide services, such as home care, primary care, and long term care. *See also* corporate foundation; integrated provider; joint venture; limited partnership.

corporate foundation   A private foundation created by and usually financially supported by a single corporation for the purpose of targeting the corporation's grant funds on programs, usually with high public visibility and in geographical areas where the company operates or has subsidiaries. *See also* foundation; private foundation.

corporate liability   Legal responsibility of a corporation, as opposed to individual or professional liability. In health care, this phrase often denotes a specific responsibility, such as the responsibility of a hospital as an institution to exercise reasonable care in carrying out processes of credentialing and privilege delineation of its medical staff members. A hospital may be liable to a patient injured by a physician, for example, if the hospital knew or should have known that the physician was not competent to perform the procedure involved or otherwise treat the patient, and did not reasonably act to protect the patient by, for instance, restricting the physician's privileges or by requiring supervision. *See also* corporate; liability.

corporate medicine   *See* corporate practice of medicine.

corporate planning A management process involving the determination of the basic immediate and long-term objectives of the organization and the adoption of specific action plans for attaining these objectives. *See also* corporate; management; planning.

corporate practice of medicine The business or an entity other than a physician that defines itself as a provider of health care. *See also* corporate; health care provider; physician; practice.

corporate restructuring Reorganization of a corporation, as in restructuring the traditional single-organization hospital corporate structure through the establishment of holding companies or foundations in order to protect assets, achieve greater accountability and efficiency, maximize cash flow, and allow capital accumulation. *See also* corporate; restructuring.

corporate seal A round, embossed symbol used to indicate the authenticity of an organization's formal documents.

corporate structure The setup of an organization, as in departments, agencies, and other units, and the distribution and delegation of functional responsibilities throughout an organization. The modern organization, including health care organizations, has become very complex, usually having many departments with a wide array of functions and responsibilities. *See also* corporate; organization; structure.

corporate veil The assumption in law that a corporation as a whole, rather than particular individuals or entities, is responsible for acts executed by or on behalf of its owners during normal corporate performance. *See also* corporation; organization.

corporation A legal entity, chartered by a state or the federal government, separate and distinct from the persons who own it, and regarded by the courts as an "artificial person." It may own property, incur debts, sue, or be sued. Its three chief distinguishing features are limited liability (owners can lose only when they invest); easy transfer of ownership through the sale of shares of stock; and continuity of existence. *See also* organization.

corporation, dental service *See* dental service corporation.

corporation, professional *See* professional corporation.

corporatization of health care The trend in which US community hospitals are restructuring themselves into new corporate forms, typically consisting of a holding company and several subsidiaries. Renal dialysis, home health care, rehabilitation, ambulatory surgery, and health promotion activities are increasingly being provided by large, corporately owned organizations. *See also* corporation; health promotion; hemodialysis; holding company; home health care; integrated provider; network.

Corporeal Technology, American Society of Extra- *See* American Society of Extra-Corporeal Technology.

corps An organized body or group of individuals, as in medical corps or nurse corps.

Corps Association, Retired Army Nurse *See* Retired Army Nurse Corps Association.

corpse A human body in the early period after death. *See also* cadaver.

Corps, Nurse *See* Nurse Corps.

correct **1.** To remove the errors or mistakes from. **2.** To punish for the purpose of reforming or improving. **3.** To adjust so as to meet a required standard or condition. *See also* overcorrect.

Correctional Health Care, National Commission on *See* National Commission on Correctional Health Care.

Correctional Psychology, American Association for *See* American Association for Correctional Psychology.

Corrections, American Association of Mental Health Professionals in *See* American Association of Mental Health Professionals in Corrections.

correct, over- *See* overcorrect.

correlation A statistical measure of the degree to which one phenomenon or random variable is associated with or can be predicted from another, that is, the strength of the relationship between two variables. *See also* association; correlation coefficient; negative correlation; positive correlation.

correlation coefficient A statistical measure of the degree to which the movements of two variables are related. This coefficient, represented by the letter R, can vary between +1 and -1. *Synonym:* coefficient of correlation. *See also* correlation; interobserver reliability coefficient; negative correlation; positive correlation.

correlation, negative *See* negative correlation.

correlation, positive *See* positive correlation.

corticosteroid *See* cortisol; cortisone.

cortisol A hormone produced by the adrenal glands that helps increase the level and availability of glucose to provide energy for the brain, heart, and muscles. *See also* cortisone; hormone; immunosuppressive.

cortisone The pharmaceutical name for cortisol. *See* cortisol; immunosuppressive; pharmaceutical.

COS *See* Clinical Orthopaedic Society.

cosmetic Serving to modify or improve the appearance of a physical feature, defect, or irregularity, as in cosmetic surgery or cosmetic dentistry. *See also* cosmetic dentistry; cosmetic surgery.

cosmetic dentistry Dental services provided for improving an individual's appearance. *See also* cosmetic; dentistry.

Cosmetic Ingredient Review (CIR) A cosmetic industry self-regulatory organization founded in 1976 sponsored by the Cosmetic, Toiletry, and Fragrance Association. It seeks to ensure the safety of ingredients used in cosmetics. It reviews scientific data on the safety of ingredients used in cosmetics and documents the validity of tests used to study ingredients. It maintains a database of safety information, including information on possible effects from misuse or use by hypersensitive individuals. *See also* cosmetic.

cosmetic surgery Surgery serving to modify or improve the appearance of a physical feature, defect, or irregularity. *See also* cosmetic; liposuction surgery; plastic surgery.

Cosmetic Surgery, American Academy of *See* American Academy of Cosmetic Surgery.

COSSMHO *See* National Coalition of Hispanic Health and Human Services Organizations.

cost An amount of money paid or required in payment to acquire something; the total expenses incurred to produce a good or service. *See also* allowable cost; appraisal cost; average cost; capital cost; direct cost; failure cost; fixed cost; indirect cost; marginal cost; pass-through cost; per diem cost; prevention cost; reasonable cost; variable cost; value.

cost accounting The branch of accounting concerned with providing detailed information on the cost of producing a product or a service. *See also* accounting.

cost allocation The assignment, to each of several organizational units, of an equitable proportion of the costs of activities that serve all of them and that cannot be assigned to any specific cost center. *See also* cost; allocation.

cost, allowable *See* allowable cost.

cost, appraisal *See* appraisal cost.

cost, average *See* average cost.

cost-based reimbursement Payment based on the costs of health care delivery in which all allowable costs (as determined by the insurer) incurred by a hospital or other health care organization in providing services are covered by the plan or program. It is a method still used by some insurers to pay health care providers; increasingly, however, cost-based reimbursement is being replaced by prospective reimbursement. *Compare* prospective pricing system. *See also* cost; reimbursement.

cost-benefit analysis A method of measuring the benefits expected from a decision, calculating the costs of the decision, then determining whether the benefits outweigh the costs. Corporations use this method in deciding whether to buy a piece of equipment, and the government uses it in determining whether government programs are achieving their goals or proposed programs are worthwhile. In health care, cost-benefit analysis involves comparing the costs of medical care with the economic benefits of the care, with both costs and benefits expressed in units of currency. The benefits typically include reductions in future health care costs and increased earnings due to the improved health of those receiving the care. *See also* analysis; cost-effectiveness analysis.

cost, capital *See* capital cost.

cost center An accounting device whereby all related costs attributable to some center within an organization, such as an activity, department, or program (for example, a hospital burn center), are segregated for accounting or reimbursement purposes. It contrasts with segregating costs of different types, such as nursing, medications, or laundry, regardless of which center incurred them. *See also* cost.

cost containment The process of maintaining organizational costs within a specified budget; restraining expenditures to meet organizational or project financial targets, as in cost containment in health care. *See also* budget; cost.

cost control Regulation and constraint of costs, such as price controls imposed by the federal government. *See also* cost.

cost, differential *See* marginal cost.

cost effective An expenditure for which total benefits exceed total costs, in which case the expenditure is considered cost effective. *See also* cost-effectiveness analysis.

cost-effectiveness analysis A form of analysis that seeks to determine the costs and effectiveness of an activity, or to compare similar alternative activities to determine the relative degree to which they will obtain the desired objectives or outcomes. For example, health care cost-effectiveness analysis might compare alternative programs, services, or interventions in terms of the cost per unit clinical effect (cost per life saved, cost per millimeter of mercury of blood pressure lowered, or cost per quality-adjusted life-year gained). The preferred action is one that requires the least cost to produce a given level of effectiveness or provides the greatest effectiveness for a given level of cost. *See also* analysis; cost-benefit analysis; cost effective; effectiveness.

Cost-Effectiveness, Physicians for Research in *See* Physicians for Research in Cost-Effectiveness.

cost, failure *See* failure cost.

cost, fixed *See* fixed cost.

cost, incremental *See* incremental cost.

cost, indirect *See* indirect cost.

cost-of-living adjustment (COLA) Adjustment of wages designed to offset changes in the cost of living, usually as measured by the consumer price index. COLAs are important bargaining issues in labor contracts and are politically sensitive elements of social security payments and federal pensions because they affect millions of people. *See also* adjustment; consumer price index.

cost-of-living index *See* consumer price index.

cost, marginal *See* marginal cost.

cost, opportunity *See* opportunity cost.

cost outlier In prospective payment systems of reimbursement for health care services, a patient whose cost of treatment exceeds greater than 200% of the federal rate for the diagnosis-related group (DRG) into which the patient is assigned, or $15,000. *See also* diagnosis-related groups; outlier; prospective payment.

cost, pass-through *See* pass-through cost.

cost, per diem *See* per diem cost.

cost, prevention *See* prevention cost.

cost of quality The expense of nonconformance; the cost of doing things wrong. Cost of quality results from prevention, appraisal, and failure costs. *See also* appraisal cost; failure cost; prevention cost; rework.

cost, reasonable *See* reasonable cost.

costs, base-year Medicare *See* base-year Medicare costs.

cost sharing Provision of a health insurance policy that requires the insured or otherwise covered individual to pay some portion of his or her covered medical expenses. Several forms of cost sharing are used, including deductibles, copayments, and coinsurance. *Compare* premium. *See also* copayment; coinsurance; deductible; health insurance.

cost shifting 1. The practice of charging certain patients or groups or classes of patients higher rates to recoup losses sustained when a hospital or other type of health care organization receives inadequate reimbursement for other patients or groups of patients. *See also* bad debt. **2.** A financial management strategy used by governments or employers in which payment methods are established that do not meet the full cost of care delivered by a provider, thus forcing the provider to cover these costs through higher charges to other patients. *See also* cost.

costs, out-of-pocket *See* out-of-pocket payments.

costs, personnel *See* personnel costs.

cost, variable *See* variable cost.

COTH *See* Council of Teaching Hospitals.

COTRANS *See* Coordinated Transfer Application System.

cough Forcible expulsion of air from the lungs and air passages with a characteristic noise. A cough is initiated by an expiratory effort against a closed glottis and completed when the glottis is abruptly opened, releasing air under pressure together with any matter present in the air passages. Coughing may be voluntary or reflexively induced. *See also* antitussive; expectorant; schedule V substances.

Council on Accreditation *See* Council on Accreditation of Services for Families and Children.

Council on Accreditation of Nurse Anesthesia Educational Programs/Schools An organization founded in 1975 to provide accreditation and evaluate nurse anesthesia programs. It functions within the framework of the American Association of Nurse Anesthetists. It conducts on-site reviews and educational workshops. *See also* accreditation; American Association of Nurse Anesthetists; nurse anesthetist.

Council for Accreditation in Occupational Hearing Conservation (CAOHC) An organization founded in 1973 composed of professional associations in the industrial health field that establish and maintain standards for the training of industrial audiometric technicians. It approves courses in occupational hearing conservation and certifies individuals who pass these courses. *See also* accreditation; audiometrician; certification; hearing; industrial audiometric technician.

Council on Accreditation of Services for Families and Children (COA) A national accrediting body founded in 1977 to establish an independent, objective process of agency review in the field of mental health and human services. It establishes, through a process of consensus building in the field, requirements for accreditation that include all aspects of an agency's administration, organization, and program. It is supported by seven national organizations representing a broad spectrum of the human service and mental health community: the Association of Jewish Family and Children's Agencies, Catholic Charities USA, the Child Welfare League of America, Family Service America, Lutheran Society Ministry System, the National Council for Adoption, and the National Association of Homes and Services for Children. *See also* accreditation; human services.

Council on Anxiety Disorders (CAD) A national organization founded in 1988 concerned with educating the public about anxiety disorders and advocating appropriate treatment. It sponsors seminars for health professionals and local support groups for persons with obsessive-compulsive and panic disorders. *See also* anxiety; disorder; obsessive compulsive; panic.

Council on Arteriosclerosis of the American Heart Association (CAAHA) A national organization founded in 1946 composed of 1,014 physicians and other individuals interested in cardiovascular diseases, especially arteriosclerosis. *See also* American Heart Association; arteriosclerosis; cardiovascular medicine.

Council for Biomedical Communications Associations An organization founded in 1970 composed of the Association of Biomedical Communication Directors, Association of Medical Illustrators, Biological Photographic Association, Guild of Natural Science Illustrators, and Health Sciences Communications Association. Its purpose is to explore areas of mutual concern in the health sciences communications field. Formerly (1984) Federation of Biocommunications Societies. *See also* Association of Medical Illustrators; communication; Health Sciences Communications Association.

Council on Certification of Nurse Anesthetists (CCNA) A national organization founded in 1975 that sets certification standards and policies and confers certification upon competent entry-level nurse anesthetists. *See also* certification; certified registered nurse anesthetist; nurse anesthetist.

Council for Children with Behavioral Disorders (CCBD) A division of the Council for Exceptional Children founded in 1962 composed of 8,200 members concerned with promoting the education and welfare of children and youth with behavioral and emotional disturbances. *See also* behavior; behavioral medicine.

Council on Chiropractic Education (CCE) A national council founded in 1971 composed of 23 representatives of member colleges. It acts as national accrediting agency for chiropractic colleges. *See also* accreditation; chiropractic.

Council on Chiropractic Orthopedics (CCO) A national organization founded in 1967 composed of 891 licensed chiropractic physicians who have completed 300 hours of postgraduate courses in orthopedics and other chiropractic physicians with an interest in orthopedics. It maintains the American Board of Chiropractic Orthopedists, which serves as an examining body for certification. Certified orthopedists comprise the Academy of Chiropractic Orthopedists. *See also* certification; chiropractic.

Council on Chiropractic Physiological Therapeutics (CCPT) A national organization founded in 1920 composed of 200 chiropractors who use physiotherapy in their practice and are interested in furthering the extended use of physiotherapy in the chiropractic field. Formerly (1985) American Council on Chiropractic Physiotherapy. *See also* chiropractic; physical therapy.

Council on Clinical Classifications (CCC) A nonprofit organization formed in 1975 to develop the *International Classification of Diseases, Ninth Revision, Clinical Modification* based on the World Health Organization's *International Classification of Diseases, Ninth Revision.* The sponsoring groups included the Commission on Professional and Hospital Activities, the American Academy of Pediatrics, the American College of Obstetricians and Gynecologists, the American College of Physicians, the American College of Surgeons, and the American Psychiatric Association. *See also* classification of diseases; classification system; *International Classification of Diseases,*

Ninth Revision, Clinical Modification; World Health Organization.

Council on Clinical Optometric Care (CCOC) A national organization founded in 1967 to accredit optometric clinics and centers. Its members are appointed by the president of the American Optometric Association with the consent of the board of trustees. It establishes and seeks to enforce standards relating to clinical practice and serves as a consultation resource for existing facilities on standards of practice. It conducts site visitations and examines facilities. *See also* accreditation; American Optometric Association; optometry.

Council of Community Blood Centers (CCBC) A national organization founded in 1962 composed of 40 independent, nonprofit, federally licensed blood centers serving defined geographic areas whose purpose is to provide an optimal supply of blood, blood components, and blood derivatives to people who need them. *See also* blood; blood components; blood derivative; community blood bank.

Council on Diagnostic Imaging A national organization founded in 1936 composed of 4,500 chiropractic roentgenologists, educators, students, and chiropractors interested in radiology. Its committees include the American Chiropractic Board of Radiology and the American Chiropractic Board of Thermography. *See also* chiropractic; imaging; radiology.

Council of Economic Advisers An organization within the executive office of the president of the United States, concerned with broad economic policy issues. Issues on health matters are staffed by a senior staff economist on health. *See also* adviser; economic.

Council on Education for Public Health (CEPH) A nonmembership council founded in 1974 composed of professional associations representing public health practice (American Public Health Association) and public health education (Association of Schools of Public Health). It seeks to strengthen educational programs in schools of public health and graduate public health programs through accreditation, consultation, research, and other services. *See also* accreditation; American Public Health Association; Association of Schools of Public Health; public health.

Council on Electrolysis Education (CEE) A national organization founded in 1972 that sponsors educational programs and research in the field of electrolysis and establishes criteria for accreditation and certification. *See also* accreditation; certification; electrolysis.

Council on Family Health (CFH) A national organization founded in 1966 composed of 80 manufacturers of prescription and over-the-counter medications. It provides the public and interested organizations with information on proper usage of medications and other family health concerns, such as safety in the home. *See also* medication; over-the-counter drug.

Council for Learning Disabilities (CLD) A national organization founded in 1967 composed of 4,500 professionals interested in the study of learning disabilities. It works to promote the education and welfare of individuals having specific learning disabilities by improving teacher preparation programs and resolving important research issues. Formerly (1981) Division for Children With Learning Disabilities. *See also* dyslexia; learning disability.

Council on Licensure, Enforcement and Regulation (CLEAR) An organization founded in 1980 composed of state and territorial licensing regulation officials. It provides for the exchange of state licensing information and serves as a clearinghouse of licensing activities and programs. It works to improve management and enforcement practices of state licensure officials and trains state officials. It sponsors the National Disciplinary Information System, which provides information on sanctions taken by state boards against licensed practitioners. It conducts the National Certified Investigator/Inspector Training Program. It maintains a library on state regulation issues including examinations, enforcement practices, licensing structures, and fraudulent credentials. Formerly (1991) National Clearinghouse on Licensure, Enforcement, and Regulation. *See also* certification; clearinghouse; licensure.

Council for Medical Affairs (CFMA) An organization founded in 1980 serving as a forum in which representatives of the Association of American Medical Colleges, American Board of Medical Specialties, American Hospital Association, American Medical Association, and the Council of Medical Specialty Societies can exchange information on matters relating to medical education. Each organization is represented by a chief executive officer and the two highest elected officials. Formerly (1979) Coordinating Council on Medical Education. *See also* medical education.

Council on Medical Education of the American Medical Association (CME-AMA) A council of the American Medical Association that participates in the accreditation of and provides consultation to medical school programs, graduate medical educational programs, and educational programs for a number of allied health occupations. It provides information on medical and allied health education at all levels. It publishes the *Directory of Graduate Medical Education Programs* and *Allied Health Education Directory. See also* accreditation; allied health professional; American Medical Association; graduate medical education; medical education; medical school.

Council of Medical Specialty Societies (CMSS) An association founded in 1965 composed of 23 national medical specialty societies representing 320,000 physicians. It provides a forum for discussion by specialty societies of national issues affecting the practice and teaching of medicine. It promotes communication among specialty organizations involved in the principal disciplines of medicine. *See also* specialty societies.

Council for the National Register of Health Service Providers in Psychology (CNRHSPP) A national organization founded in 1974 composed of 16,000 registrant psychologists who are licensed or certified by a state/provincial board of examiners of psychology and who have met council criteria as health service providers in psychology. *See also* psychology.

Council on Optometric Education (COE) A national accrediting body founded in 1930 for professional optometric degree (OD) programs, paraoptometric training programs, and optometric residency programs. *See also* accreditation; optometry.

Council on Podiatric Medical Education (CPME) A national organization founded in 1918 to accredit colleges of podiatric medicine, podiatric residency programs, podiatric assistant programs, and continuing education programs in podiatry. *See also* accreditation; continuing education; podiatric assistant; podiatric medicine.

Council on Professional Standards in Speech-Language Pathology and Audiology A national organization founded in 1959 that defines standards for clinical certification and for the accreditation of graduate education and professional services. It monitors the interpretation and application of these standards to individuals and organizations. It arbitrates appeals regarding certification and accreditation. Formerly (1980) American Boards of Examiners in Speech Pathology and Audiology. *See also* accreditation; American Speech-Language-Hearing Association; audiologist; certification; speech pathology; standard.

Council of Rehabilitation Specialists (CRS) A national organization founded in 1979 composed of 100 rehabilitation and social service professionals and other individuals interested in the establishment of academic and professional standards in the field of rehabilitation. It advocates adequate rehabilitation services for all blind and visually impaired persons. *See also* rehabilitation; specialist; visually impaired.

Council on Resident Education in Obstetrics and Gynecology (CREOG) A semiautonomous nonregulatory organization founded in 1967 by the American College of Obstetricians and Gynecologists and composed of national specialty organizations. It works to promote and maintain high standards of resident training in obstetrics and gynecology. It provides consultative site visits to residency programs, a clearinghouse for residency positions, conferences, a resident data bank, and a national in-training examination. *See also* American College of Obstetricians and Gynecologists; clearinghouse; obstetrics and gynecology; residency.

Council for Responsible Genetics (CRG) A national organization founded in 1983 composed of scientists, health and medical professionals, trade unionists, feminists, and peace activists interested in monitoring and analyzing the biotechnology industry including the moral and ethical issues of genetic engineering. Its areas of interest include military uses of biological research and genetic discrimination. Formerly (1989) Committee for Responsible Genetics. *See also* biotechnology; genetic engineering; genetics.

Council for Responsible Nutrition (CRN) A national organization founded in 1973 composed of 60 manufacturers, distributors, and other companies involved in the production and sale of nutritional supplements, including vitamins and minerals. It seeks an improvement in the general health of the US population through responsible nutrition, including the appropriate use of nutritional supplements. It acts as a liaison between vitamin and mineral products manufacturers and government regulatory agencies, such as the Food and Drug Administration and the Federal Trade Commission. *See also* nutrition; vitamin.

Council for Sex Information and Education (CSIE) A national clearinghouse founded in 1977 for information on sexuality and related topics. *See also* clearinghouse.

Council on Social Work Education (CSWE) A national organization founded in 1952 composed of 5,000 graduate and undergraduate programs of social work education; national, regional, and local social welfare agencies; libraries; and individuals. It formulates criteria and standards for all levels of social work education; accredits graduate and undergraduate social work programs; and provides consulting to social work educators on curriculum, faculty recruitment, and faculty development. *See also* accreditation; social work.

Council of State Administrators of Vocational Rehabilitation (CSAVR) A national organization founded in 1940 composed of 83 administrators of state vocational rehabilitation agencies. It serves as an advisory body to federal agencies and the public in the development of policies affecting rehabilitation of disabled persons. *See also* rehabilitation; vocational rehabilitation.

Council of State and Territorial Epidemiologists (CSTE) A national organization founded in 1951 composed of 65 state and territorial epidemiologists interested in establishing closer working relationships among members, providing technical advice and assistance to the Association of State and Territorial Health Officials, and consulting with and advising disciplines in other health agencies. *See also* Association of State and Territorial Health Officials; epidemiology.

Council of Teaching Hospitals (COTH) A national organization founded in 1965 composed of 400 medical-school-affiliated or university-owned teaching hospitals. It distributes communications analyzing congressional activities, executive branch actions, court decisions affecting teaching hospitals, and teaching-hospital reimbursement regulations. It disseminates special interest bibliographics, surveys of housestaff policies, and comparative hospital financial data. Its parent organization is the Association of American Medical Colleges. *See also* Association of American Medical Colleges; housestaff; medical

school; teaching hospital.

counsel **1.** Advice or guidance, especially as solicited from a knowledgeable person, as in a therapist counseling a couple. **2.** A group of counselors, or lawyers, conducting a case in court. *See also* counselor; lawyer. **3.** To advise, as in counseling a client or patient.

Counsel for Children, National Association of *See* National Association of Counsel for Children.

counseling The act or process of providing advice or guidance, as in family or marriage counseling. *See also* counsel; counselor; sex therapy.

Counseling, American Board of Examiners in Pastoral *See* American Board of Examiners in Pastoral Counseling.

Counseling Association, American *See* American Counseling Association.

Counseling Association, American Rehabilitation *See* American Rehabilitation Counseling Association.

Counseling, Association for Death Education and *See* Association for Death Education and Counseling.

Counseling, Association for Gay, Lesbian, and Bisexual Issues in *See* Association for Gay, Lesbian, and Bisexual Issues in Counseling.

Counseling Association, National Rehabilitation *See* National Rehabilitation Counseling Association.

counseling, genetic *See* genetic counseling.

counseling, individual marriage and family *See* individual marriage and family counseling.

counseling, marital *See* marital counseling.

counseling, pregnancy *See* pregnancy counseling.

counseling, preretirement *See* preretirement counseling.

counseling psychology The branch of psychology dealing with the study of people as individuals to help them develop as fully and effectively as possible. A counseling psychologist may use the interview technique with high school and college students, employees, persons needing vocational rehabilitation, and people in general who have problems concerning personal, social, educational, and vocational development and adjustment. In addition to the interview technique, counseling psychologists may use tests and observational methods to collect additional information about their clients as individuals, in groups, and in the environments in which they live and work. *See also* counseling; psychology.

counseling services Professional services for individuals, groups, or families dealing with problems due to personal relationships or stress. *See also* marital counseling; stress.

counselor   **1.** A person who gives counsel; an adviser, as in a mental health counselor, rehabilitation counselor, or an alcoholism and drug abuse counselor. *See also* advice; adviser; clinical pastoral counselor; rehabilitation counselor. **2.** A person who conducts a legal case in court, usually, but not always, a lawyer. *See also* attorney; lawyer.

counselor aide, rehabilitation   *See* rehabilitation counselor aide.

counselor, certified   *See* certified counselor.

counselor, clinical pastoral   *See* clinical pastoral counselor.

Counselor Credentialing Bodies, National Commission on Accreditation of Alcoholism and Drug Abuse   *See* National Commission on Accreditation of Alcoholism and Drug Abuse Counselor Credentialing Bodies.

counselor-at-law   A lawyer who conducts a case in court. *See also* lawyer.

counselor, rehabilitation   *See* rehabilitation counselor.

Counselors, American Association of Pastoral   *See* American Association of Pastoral Counselors.

Counselors Association, American Mental Health   *See* American Mental Health Counselors Association.

Counselors and Family Therapists, National Academy of   *See* National Academy of Counselors and Family Therapists.

Counselors, National Association of Alcoholism and Drug Abuse   *See* National Association of Alcoholism and Drug Abuse Counselors.

Counselors, National Board for Certified   *See* National Board for Certified Counselors.

Counselors, National Society of Genetic   *See* National Society of Genetic Counselors.

Counselors and Therapists, American Association of Sex Educators,   *See* American Association of Sex Educators, Counselors and Therapists.

counselor, vocational rehabilitation   *See* rehabilitation counselor.

count, bed   *See* bed count.

count, blood   *See* blood count.

count, complete blood   *See* complete blood count.

counterclaim   A claim brought by a defendant against a plaintiff in the same suit, and which asserts an independent cause of action. The claim may be based on the same transaction or any other occurrence giving rise to a right of recovery by the defendant against the plaintiff. For example, a physician sued for malpractice may counterclaim for payment of his or her bill. *See also* claim.

count, sponge   *See* sponge count.

County Health Facility Administrators, National Association of   *See* National Association of County Health Facility Administrators.

County Health Officials, National Association of   *See* National Association of County Health Officials.

county hospital   A hospital that is controlled by an agency of county government. *See also* hospital.

County Medical Societies, Congress of   *See* Congress of County Medical Societies.

coupler, acoustic   *See* acoustic coupler.

court   The branch of government responsible for the resolution of disputes arising under the laws of the government. A court system is usually divided into parts specializing in hearing different types of cases. *See also* appellate court; civil court; criminal court; matrimonial court; surrogate's court; trial court; tribunal; vacate; witness; witness stand.

court of appeals   *See* appellate court.

court, appellate   *See* appellate court.

court, civil   *See* civil court.

court, criminal   *See* criminal court.

court, intermediate appellate   *See* appellate court.

court, matrimonial   *See* matrimonial court.

court-ordered emancipation   *See* emancipated minor.

court, supreme appellate   *See* supreme appellate court.

court, surrogate's   *See* surrogate's court.

court, trial   *See* trial court.

covariance   A statistical term for the correlation between two variables multiplied by the standard deviation for each of the variables. A positive covariance indicates that the two variables tend to move up and down together; a negative covariance indicates that when one moves higher, the other tends to go lower. *See also* standard deviation; variable.

COVD   *See* College of Optometrists in Vision Development.

coverage   The guarantee against specific losses provided under the terms of an insurance policy. Coverage is sometimes used interchangeably with benefits or protection, and is also used to mean insurance or an insurance contract. *See also* adequacy of coverage;

claims-incurred coverage; claims-made coverage; commencement of coverage; full coverage; insurance coverage; occurrence-based coverage; out-of-area coverage; tail coverage; umbrella coverage.

coverage, adequacy of *See* adequacy of coverage.

coverage, claims-incurred *See* claims-incurred coverage.

coverage, claims-made *See* claims-made coverage.

coverage, commencement of *See* commencement of coverage.

coverage, first-dollar *See* first-dollar coverage.

coverage, full *See* full coverage.

coverage, insurance *See* insurance coverage.

coverage, occurrence-based *See* occurrence-based coverage.

coverage, out-of-area *See* out-of-area coverage.

coverage, tail *See* tail coverage.

coverage, umbrella *See* umbrella coverage.

covered charge A charge for services provided to an insured patient that is recognized as payable by a third-party payer. *See also* charge; third-party payer.

covered services Services provided by a physician to a member of a health plan at no charge other than the applicable copayment or deductible. *See also* copayment; deductible; health plan.

CPA *See* certified public accountant.

CPAM *See* certified patient account manager.

CPBE *See* certified professional bureau executive.

CPEM *See* Council on Precision Electromagnetic Measurements.

CPHA *See* Commission on Professional and Hospital Activities.

CPI *See* consumer price index.

CPM *See* Cesarean Prevention Movement.

CPME *See* Council on Podiatric Medical Education.

CPQA *See* certified professional in quality assurance.

CPR *See* cardiopulmonary resuscitation.

CPRI *See* Computer-Based Patient Record Institute.

CPSC *See* Consumer Product Safety Commission.

CPT *See Physicians' Current Procedural Terminology.*

CPT-4 *Physicians' Current Procedural Terminology - Fourth Edition.*

CQI *See* continuous quality improvement.

crack A highly addictive, crystalline form of cocaine made by heating a mixture of it with baking powder and water until it is hard and breaking it into small pieces that are burned and smoked for their stimulating effect. *See also* addiction; cocaine.

CRAHCA *See* Center for Research in Ambulatory Health Care Administration.

Cranial Academy (CA) A national organization founded in 1946 composed of 800 osteopathic physicians interested in the study and development of osteopathic cranial concepts and the techniques of diagnosis and treatment in structural manipulation of the body. Members have taken a course through the academy or through Sutherland Cranial Teaching Foundation, an osteopathic college. The Cranial Academy is a society of the American Academy of Osteopathy. *See also* American Academy of Osteopathy; osteopathic medicine; skull.

cranioscopy Visual inspection of the head. *See also* inspection; physical examination; skull.

cranium *See* skull.

crash Accidental or catastrophic shutdown of a computer due to user error or hardware. *See also* computer.

crash cart A wheeled vehicle containing supplies, such as medications, and equipment, such as laryngoscopes and syringes, that may be necessary for cardiopulmonary resuscitation of patients. *Synonym:* resuscitation cart. *See also* cart; cardiopulmonary resuscitation.

CRCPD *See* Conference of Radiation Control Program Directors.

creaming *See* skimming.

credentialing The process of assessing and validating the qualifications of a licensed independent practitioner to provide services in a health care organization. The determination is based on an evaluation of the individual's current license, education, training, experience, competence, and professional judgment. The process is the basis for making appointments to the professional staff of the health care organization. The process also provides information for granting clinical privileges to licensed independent practitioners. *See also* clinical privileges; economic credentialing; credentialism; license; licensed independent practitioner; physician credentialing; recredentialing.

Credentialing Bodies, National Commission on Accreditation of Alcoholism and Drug Abuse Counselor *See* National Commission on Accreditation of Alcoholism and Drug Abuse Counselor Credentialing Bodies.

Credentialing Commission (CC) An autonomous organization founded in 1962 for certifying medical technologists, laboratory technicians, and physician office laboratory technicians. *See also* credentialing; medical technologist.

credentialing, economic *See* economic credentialing.

credentialing, medical staff *See* physician credentialing.

credentialing, physician *See* physician credentialing.

credentialing, re- *See* recredentialing.

credentialism **1.** An emphasis on paper manifestations of qualification, such as college degree diplomas, instead of the actual ability to perform a job. **2.** The formalized practice of requiring education and training that is perceived legally or socially to be excessive for the performance of certain services. *See also* credentialing; credentials.

credentials Evidence of an individual's license, education, training, experience, competence, health status, and judgment. Examples of physician credentials include a diploma from medical school, a state license to practice medicine and surgery, and a board-certification document. *See also* board certified; competence; credentials committee; license.

credentials committee A group of physicians and other professionals in a hospital or other type of health care organization who are charged with the responsibility of reviewing applications for staff membership and providing reports or comments leading to a decision on the selection of medical staff members. *See also* closed staff; credentials; medical staff; open staff.

credible Believable, reliable, as in credible performance data.

credit **1.** Evidence for trust or confidence in an individual's ability to pay a debt. *See also* credit bureau; credit card; debt. **2.** To attribute to some person.

credit bureau An organization that gathers and distributes information about the credit used by individuals and organizations and on their reported financial reliability. *See also* credit.

credit card An indication to sellers that the person who received the card from an issuer has a satisfactory credit rating and that if credit is extended, the issuer of the card will pay for the merchandise delivered (or see that the seller receives payment). Most credit cards are made of plastic with raised letters to facilitate creation of machine-readable sales slips. *See also* credit.

credit rating The determination of an individual's or organization's credit history and capability of repaying obligations. Dun & Bradstreet and other

companies investigate, analyze, and maintain records on the credit responsibility of individuals and businesses. The ability of an organization to sell its bonds is often a function of its credit rating. This credit rating translates into a rating for each bond issue, which in turn determines the level of interest the organization must pay to entice buyers. The two major bond rating services are Standard and Poor's Corporation and Moody's Investors Service. *See also* credit; rating.

credit risk Financial and moral risk that an obligation will not be paid and a loss will result. *See also* credit; risk.

credit standing Reputation one earns for paying debts. Credit rating tends to be more quantitative than credit standing. *See also* credit rating.

cremation The burning or incineration of dead bodies.

CREOG *See* Council on Resident Education in Obstetrics and Gynecology.

CRG *See* Council for Responsible Genetics.

crib death *See* sudden infant death syndrome.

cricothyreotomy An incision through the cricoid and thyroid cartilages in the front part of the neck to secure a patent airway for emergency relief of acute upper airway obstruction. *Synonym*: cricothyroidotomy. *See also* airway; cricothyrotomy; tracheotomy.

cricothyrotomy An incision through the skin and cricothyroid membrane in the front part of the neck to secure a patent airway for emergency relief of acute upper airway obstruction. *See also* airway; cricothyreotomy; tracheotomy.

criminal court A trial court that hears prosecutions under the criminal laws. *Compare* civil court. *See also* civil court; court.

criminal law The body of law that deals with crimes, and their punishment, that are prosecuted by the state. *See also* law.

Crippled Children, Shriners Hospitals for *See* Shriners Hospitals for Crippled Children.

crisis An unstable condition, as in political, social, or economic affairs, involving an impending abrupt or decisive change. *See also* identity crisis; management by crisis; midlife crisis; sickle cell crisis.

crisis, identity *See* identity crisis.

Crisis Interveners, American Academy of *See* American Academy of Crisis Interveners.

crisis, midlife *See* midlife crisis.

crisis management *See* management by crisis.

crisis, sickle cell   *See* sickle cell crisis.

criteria   Expected levels of achievement or specifications against which performance or quality may be compared. For example, criteria for appropriate initial care of a patient with a headache may be measurement of body temperature and blood pressure and performance of a neurological examination. *See also* criteria set; evaluation criteria; explicit criteria; implicit criteria; occurrence criteria; outcome criteria; review criteria.

criteria, clinical   *See* practice guideline.

criteria, evaluation   *See* evaluation criteria.

criteria, explicit   *See* explicit criteria.

criteria, implicit   *See* implicit criteria.

criteria, occurrence   *See* occurrence criteria.

criteria, outcome   *See* outcome criteria.

criteria, review   *See* review criteria.

criteria set   A series of related criteria addressing the same patient sample; for example, a criteria set applied to patients presenting to the emergency department with chest pain or a different set applied to patients undergoing a cesarean section for failure to progress in labor. *See also* criteria.

criteria of survey eligibility   Conditions necessary for health care organizations to be surveyed for accreditation by the Joint Commission on Accreditation of Healthcare Organizations. The criteria address the structure, functions, and services of health care organizations. *See also* Joint Commission on Accreditation of Healthcare Organizations.

criterion   Singular form of criteria. *See* criteria.

criterion standard   In health care, a method having established or widely accepted accuracy for determining a diagnosis, providing a standard to which a new screening or diagnostic test can be compared. The method need not be a simple procedure but could include follow-up of patients to observe the evolution of their conditions or the consensus of an expert panel of clinicians, as is frequently used in the study of psychiatric conditions. Criterion standards can also be used in studies of the quality of care to indicate a level of performance, agreed to by experts or peers, to which individual practitioners or organizations can be compared. For example, in health care, a radiologist's interpretation of an x-ray is considered to be the criterion standard for accuracy in x-ray interpretation. Any nonradiologist physician interpreting the same x-ray would be compared to this criterion standard. *See also* gold standard; standard.

critical   Life-threatening, especially pertaining to a patient's condition.

critical care medicine   A medical subspecialty primarily involved with all aspects of management of the critically ill patient in an intensive (special) care unit. The medical specialties of anesthesiology, internal medicine, neurological surgery, obstetrics and gynecology, pediatrics, and surgery currently offer subspecialty certificates in critical care medicine. *See also* critical illness; pediatric critical care medicine; surgical critical care.

critical care medicine, pediatric   *See* pediatric critical care medicine.

Critical Care Medicine, Society of   *See* Society of Critical Care Medicine.

critical care nurse   A registered nurse who is qualified by advanced training to care for critically ill patients, typically in a hospital intensive care unit. *See also* certified critical care nurse; registered nurse.

Critical-Care Nurses, American Association of   *See* American Association of Critical-Care Nurses.

critical care physician   An anesthesiologist, internist, neurological surgeon, obstetrician-gynecologist, pediatrician, surgeon, or other physician who subspecializes in critical care medicine. *See also* critical care medicine; pediatric critical care specialist.

Critical Care, Society of Neurosurgical Anesthesia and   *See* Society of Neurosurgical Anesthesia and Critical Care.

critical care specialist, pediatric   *See* pediatric critical care specialist.

critical care, surgical   *See* surgical critical care.

critical care unit (CCU)   *See* special care unit.

critical illness   An illness that is immediately life-threatening and that may cause serious and irreversible functional disabilities or death. *See also* critical care medicine; illness.

critical path method   *See* critical pathway method.

critical pathway   **1.** The longest sequential series of tasks in a project. **2.** Minimum necessary tasks to accomplish an objective or meet a goal. **3.** In health care, a treatment protocol, based on a consensus of clinicians, that includes only those few vital components or items proved to affect patient outcomes, either by the omission or commission of the treatment or the timing of intervention. *Synonym*: critical path. *See also* clinical pathway; critical pathway method; path; practice parameter.

critical pathway method   A planning and control

technique that reduces variation and cost by optimizing the order of steps in a process. Manufacturing industries use this method to plan and control the complete process of material deliveries, paper work, inspections, and production. *Synonym*: critical path method. *See also* critical pathway; method; Program Evaluation and Review Technique.

CRN *See* Council for Responsible Nutrition.

CRNA *See* certified registered nurse anesthetist.

Crosby, Philip B. Quality management expert, consultant, and author (b. 1926) whose books include *Quality Is Free*, *Quality Without Tears*, and *Running Things*. He developed the "Zero Defects" system and other improvement programs and teaches that quality control happens in the management office, as well as on the manufacturing line. *See also* management; quality improvement; zero defects.

cross claim A claim brought by coplaintiffs or codefendants against each other rather than against a party on the opposite side of the litigation. *See also* claim.

cross-examination An examination of a witness by an adverse party, that is, a party other than the one that has called the witness to render the testimony. The cross-examination follows the direct examination and is the primary tool for testing the accuracy of direct testimony. *See also* direct examination; examination; witness.

crossfunctional Pertaining to processes or groups that are organized along system or process lines, rather than along departmental lines, as in a cross-functional team. *See also* crossfunctional team.

crossfunctional team A group of people from two or more areas of an organization that address an issue that affects the operations of each area. For example, the process of distributing laboratory results might be addressed by a team involving clinical laboratory staff, information management staff, nursing staff, and medical staff. *See also* functional team; team.

crossmatching The process of testing the compatibility of donor and recipient blood prior to a blood transfusion. *See also* blood transfusion; blood typing; major crossmatching; matching; minor crossmatching.

crossmatching, major *See* major crossmatching.

crossmatching, minor *See* minor crossmatching.

crossover trial In research, a method of comparing two or more treatments or interventions in which subjects or patients, on completion of the course of one treatment, are switched to another. Typically allocation to the first treatment is by random process. Participants' performance in one period is used to judge their performance in other periods, usually reducing variability. *See also* before-after trial; clinical trial; trial.

crown **1.** In dentistry, the part of a tooth that is covered by enamel and projects beyond the gum line. **2.** In dentistry, an artificial substitute for the natural crown of a tooth, as a gold crown. *See also* dentistry; prosthodontics.

CRS *See* Council of Rehabilitation Specialists.

CRT *See* cathode ray tube.

CRTI *See* Center for the Rights of the Terminally Ill.

crude death rate *See* mortality rate.

crutch A support with a cross-piece for the armpit and another for the hand, designed to take the weight of the body off an injured leg while walking. *See also* cane; walker; wheelchair.

cryobank A bank in which sperm and other cells and tissues are stored for future use. *See also* bank.

cryobirth The thawing out of a frozen embryo. *See also* birth; frozen embryo.

cryobiology The study of the effects of very low temperatures on living organisms. *See also* biology.

Cryobiology, Society for *See* Society for Cryobiology.

Cryogenic Engineering Conference (CEC) A national organization founded in 1954 composed of 4,000 academic, industrial, and government researchers and managers involved in basic and applied work in cryogenics. It provides a forum for a four-day presentation of papers and seminars concerning advances in the science and technology of cryogenics in areas, such as superconductivity, heat transfer, insulation, instrumentation, cryo-health services, and cryobiology. *See also* cryobiology; cryogenics; cryonics; cryosurgery.

cryogenics The production of extremely low temperatures or the study of extremely low temperature phenomena. *Synonym*: cryogeny. *See also* cryobiology; cryonics.

Cryogenic Society of America (CSA) A national organization founded in 1964 composed of 400 individuals and organizations engaged in cryogenic work. It encourages the dissemination of information on low temperature processes and techniques and increases public awareness of the usefulness of cryogenic technology. *See also* cryogenics.

cryogeny *See* cryogenics.

cryonics The practice of freezing a clinically dead person in hopes of bringing the person back to life when resuscitation or reconstruction is possible. *See also* death.

Cryonics Society, American *See* American Cryonics Society.

cryosurgery Application of extreme cold to tissues, often via a probe containing liquid nitrogen, to destroy or eliminate abnormal cells. *See also* cryobiology; cryogenics; cryotherapy; surgery.

Cryosurgery, American College of *See* American College of Cryosurgery.

cryotherapy The local or general use of low temperatures in medical therapy, as in cryosurgery. *See also* cryosurgery.

CS *See* central service department; cesarean section.

CSA *See* Center for the Study of Aging; Cryogenic Society of America.

CSAVR *See* Council of State Administrators of Vocational Rehabilitation.

CSB Controlled Substance Board. *See* controlled substances; Controlled Substances Act of 1970.

CSCR *See* Central Society for Clinical Research.

CSD *See* Coalition on Sexuality and Disability.

CSF *See* cerebrospinal fluid.

CSH *See* Coalition on Smoking or Health.

CSICOP *See* Committee for the Scientific Investigation of Claims of the Paranormal.

CSIE *See* Council for Sex Information and Education.

CSP *See* certified safety professional.

CSPI *See* Center for Science in the Public Interest.

CSPTE *See* Center for the Study of Pharmacy and Therapeutics for the Elderly.

CSS *See* Cognitive Science Society.

CSTE *See* Council of State and Territorial Epidemiologists.

CSWE *See* Council on Social Work Education.

CT Abbreviation for computerized tomography. *See* computerized axial tomography.

CT scan *See* CAT scan.

CT scanner *See* CAT scanner.

cued speech Utilization of hand shapes and placements to clarify lipreading and aid hearing-impaired persons in visually perceiving spoken language. It is used by families and professionals working with hearing-impaired persons. Speech pathologists also use it with hearing persons in teaching phonetics, phonics, the sounds of second languages, and in therapy for articulation and language disor-

ders. *See also* hearing impaired; speech; speech pathology.

culdoscopy The inspection of the female pelvic organs by means of an endoscope introduced into the pelvic cavity through the posterior vaginal fornix. *See also* endoscope.

cultural shock *See* culture shock.

culture **1.** The acquired and shared beliefs, value, and attitudes of a social group manifested in shared judgments, symbols, rituals, sanctions, and behavior. *See also* collaborative culture; school; religion; worldview. **2.** The propagation of microorganisms or of living tissue cells in special media conducive to their growth, as in a blood culture. *See also* blood culture; culture medium; Petri dish; subculture.

Culture Association, Tissue *See* Tissue Culture Association.

culture, blood *See* blood culture.

culture, collaborative *See* collaborative culture.

Culture Collection, American Type *See* American Type Culture Collection.

Culture Collections, US Federation for *See* US Federation for Culture Collections.

culture, enterprise *See* enterprise culture.

culture medium A liquid or gelatinous substance or preparation used for the cultivation of living cells, as in Thayer-Martin agar or MacConkey agar. *See also* culture; Petri dish; tissue culture.

Culture Organization, Tissue *See* Tissue Culture Organization.

culture, organizational *See* organizational culture.

culture shock The discontinence or discomfort felt when an individual experiences a social or cultural setting widely different from his or her usual social or cultural environment. *See also* culture; spaced-out.

culture, sub- *See* subculture.

culture, tissue *See* tissue culture.

cure To heal, remedy, or otherwise set right an undesirable or unhealthy condition. *See also* heal; lost chance of cure.

cure, lost chance of *See* lost chance of cure.

current asset Property that can be readily converted into cash, such as marketable securities, accounts receivable (goods or services sold but not paid for), and inventories (raw materials, work in progress, and finished goods intended for future sales). *See also* asset.

current, sinusoidal *See* sinusoidal current.

curettage The removal of growths or other material from the wall of a cavity or other surface by scraping with a curette, as in curettage after cervical dilatation, of uterine contents. *See also* curette; dilation and curettage; uterus.

curette A surgical instrument shaped like a scoop or spoon, used to remove tissue or growths from a body cavity. *See also* curettage.

Current Procedural Terminology (CPT) *See Physicians' Current Procedural Terminology.*

curriculum A regular and established course of study, as in a nursing curriculum.

cursor Symbol on a computer terminal screen that shows where on the screen the next character to be typed will appear. Cursors often appear as blinking dashes or rectangles. *See also* joystick; mouse; computer terminal.

CUSH *See* Computer Users in Speech and Hearing.

custodial care Care in which board, room, and other nonmedical personal assistance are provided, generally on a long-term basis to, for example, mentally retarded individuals. *See also* care; residential care; residential community care.

customary, prevailing, and reasonable charge The dollar amount a physician or other practitioner normally or usually charges the majority of his or her patients. Such fees vary by specialty, geographic area, and physicians and are under scrutiny by many third-party payers, including Medicare. Under Medicare, a customary charge is the median charge used by a particular physician for a specified type of service during the calendar year preceding the fiscal year in which a claim is processed. There is, therefore, an average delay of a year and a half in recognizing any increase in actual charges. Customary charges in addition to actual and prevailing charges are taken into account in determining reasonable charges under Medicare. *See also* charge; Medicare; third-party payer.

customary, prevailing, reasonable fee *See* customary, prevailing, and reasonable charge.

customer 1. One that regularly, customarily, or repeatedly makes purchases of, or has business dealings with, a provider of a product or services. **2.** A receiver or beneficiary of an output of a process (service or product), either internal or external to an organization, such as a hospital. *See also* external customer; immediate customer; internal customer; rework; supplier; ultimate customer.

customer, external *See* external customer.

customer, immediate *See* immediate customer.

customer, internal *See* internal customer.

customer service A department or function of an organization that responds to inquiries or complaints from customers of that organization. *See also* customer; customer service representative.

customer service representative An employee responsible for maintaining goodwill between an organization and its customers by answering questions, solving problems, and providing advice or assistance in utilizing the goods or services of the organization. *See also* customer service.

customer-supplier sundial A graphic representation of an organization or a component of an organization and those served by it. The supplier is in the middle and each customer is at the end of a spoke projecting outward.

customer, ultimate *See* ultimate customer.

cutaneous Pertaining to the skin, as in a cutaneous rash (skin rash). *See also* skin.

Cutaneous Oncology, American College of Mohs Micrographic Surgery and *See* American College of Mohs Micrographic Surgery and Cutaneous Oncology.

cutting edge *See* leading edge.

CV *See* cardiovascular; coefficient of variation.

CVA *See* cerebrovascular accident.

CVP *See* central venous pressure.

CW *See* Congress Watch.

CWBHP *See* Center for the Well-Being of Health Professionals.

CWI *See* Child Welfare Institute.

CWLA *See* Child Welfare League of America.

cyanide A highly poisonous substance that interferes with the oxygen uptake of cells by combining with cytochrome oxidase, an enzyme necessary for cellular oxygen transport. The fatal dose of cyanide is about 250 milligrams. *See also* laetrile; poison.

cyanosis A bluish discoloration, especially of the skin and mucous membranes, due to excessive concentration of reduced hemoglobin in the blood. *See also* blue babies; hemoglobin; skin.

cybernetics The theoretical study of communication and control processes in biological, mechanical, and electronic systems, especially the comparison of these processes in biological and artificial systems. *See also* communication; cyborg; medical cybernetics.

Cybernetics, American Society for *See* American Society for Cybernetics.

Cybernetics Foundation, Medical *See* Medical Cybernetics Foundation.

cybernetics, medical *See* medical cybernetics.

cyborg A human being who has certain physiological processes aided or controlled by mechanical or electronic devices. *See also* cybernetics.

cycle A round or succession of observable phenomena, recurring usually at regular intervals and in the same sequence, as in menstrual cycle or accreditation cycle. *See also* accreditation cycle; billing cycle; collection cycle; Plan-Do-Check-Act cycle; record cycle; turnaround.

cycle, accreditation *See* accreditation cycle.

cycle, billing *See* billing cycle.

cycle, collection *See* collection cycle.

cycle, Deming *See* Plan-Do-Check-Act cycle.

cycle, Plan-Do-Check-Act *See* Plan-Do-Check-Act cycle.

cycle, record *See* record cycle.

Cycle Research, Society for Menstrual *See* Society for Menstrual Cycle Research.

cycle, Shewhart *See* Plan-Do-Check-Act cycle.

cyclotron An apparatus for accelerating charged particles of atomic magnitudes by imparting to them energies of several million electron volts. The charged particles are subjected to an oscillating electric field while held in spiral orbit by a constant magnetic field. *See also* magnetic; radiation therapy.

cyst Any hollow formation, particularly one containing fluid. *See also* sebaceous cyst.

cystic fibrosis An inherited fatal disease among children and young adults, characterized by a thick mucus that clogs the lungs, creating breathing difficulties and high susceptibility to infection. The disease also affects the digestive system and other organs.

cystitis Inflammation of the bladder, occurring more frequently in women than men. *Synonyms:* acute cystitis; hematuria; inflammation; urinary tract infection.

cystoscope An endoscope for examining and treating lesions of the urinary bladder, ureter, and kidney. It consists of an outer sheath with a lighting system, a viewing device, and a passage for catheters and operative devices. *See also* endoscope.

cystoscopy The process of visualizing the urinary tract by means of a cystoscope inserted in the urethra. Cystoscopy is also used for obtaining biopsies of tumors and for the removal of polyps. *See also* cystoscope.

cyst, sebaceous *See* sebaceous cyst.

cytogenetics The branch of biology that deals with the study of heredity and variation by the methods of both cytology and genetics; the study of chromosomes. *See also* chromosome; clinical cytogenetics; cytology; genetics.

cytogeneticist, clinical *See* clinical cytogeneticist.

cytogenetics, clinical *See* clinical cytogenetics.

Cytogenetic Technologists, Association of *See* Association of Cytogenetic Technologists.

cytology The branch of biology dealing with the formation, structure, and function of cells. *See also* biology; clinical laboratory; cytopathology; microscopic anatomy.

Cytology, American Society of *See* American Society of Cytology.

cytopathologist A pathologist who subspecializes in cytopathology. *See also* cytopathology; pathologist.

cytopathology The branch of medicine and subspecialty of pathology dealing with the diagnosis of human disease by means of the study of cells. The cells are obtained from body secretions and fluids by scraping, washing or sponging the surface of a lesion, or aspirating a tumor mass or body organ with a fine needle. The cells are studied using special stains and chemical analyses. *See also* cytology; pathology; stain.

cytotechnologist An allied health professional who works with pathologists to detect changes in body cells obtained from various body sites (such as the female reproductive tract, the oral cavity, the lung, or any body cavity or lesion shedding cells) that may be important in the early diagnosis of cancer and other diseases. This is done primarily with the microscope to screen slide preparations of body cells for abnormalities in structure, indicating either benign or malignant conditions. Cytotechnologists are one type of allied health professional for which the Committee on Allied Health Education and Accreditation has accredited education programs. *See also* allied health professional; cytology; cytopathology; technologist.

Cytotechnology, American Society for *See* American Society for Cytotechnology.

cytotoxic Pertaining to an agent that poisons or damages cells.

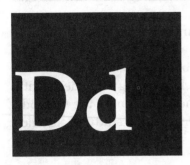

Dd

DAEEP *See* Division of Applied Experimental and Engineering Psychologists.

daily service charge The dollar amount charged by a hospital or other health care organization for a day's stay in an inpatient care unit. *See also* charge; inpatient care unit.

daisy wheel A circular plastic typehead for a letter-quality printer. *See* daisy wheel printer.

daisy wheel printer A printer using a rotating plastic wheel as a type element. It prints relatively slowly (10 to 55 characters per second) compared to a line printer, dot-matrix printer, or laser printer; the print is letter quality. *See also* dot-matrix printer; ink jet printer; laser printer; printer.

damage Impairment of the usefulness or value of a person or property; harm. *See also* damages.

damage control The action or process of minimizing the damage to one's cause (usually a political cause) after an accident or mistake has occurred. *Synonym*: damage limitation. *See also* control.

damage limitation *See* damage control.

damages In law, monetary compensation or indemnity that may be recovered in the courts by any person who has suffered loss, detriment, or injury, whether to his or her person, property, or rights, through the unlawful act or commission of negligence of another individual. Damages is the sum of money awarded to a person injured by the tort of another. *See also* apportionment of damages; apportionment of fault; compensation; compensatory damages; consequential damages; foreseeability; lost chance of cure; lost chance of survival; measure of damages; nominal damages; punitive damages; recovery; tort.

damages, apportionment of *See* apportionment of damages

damages, compensatory *See* compensatory damages.

damages, consequential *See* consequential damages.

damages, exemplary *See* punitive damages.

damages, future *See* future damages.

damages, general *See* general damages.

damages, measure of *See* measure of damages.

damages, nominal *See* nominal damages.

damages, noneconomic *See* noneconomic damages.

damages, punitive *See* punitive damages.

damages, special *See* consequential damages.

damper A mechanical device used to open, control, restrict, or close openings created by buildings' duct systems.

DANA *See* Drug and Alcohol Nursing Association.

DANB *See* Dental Assisting National Board.

Dance Medicine, Center for *See* Center for Dance Medicine.

dance therapist An individual who specializes in dance therapy. *See also* dance therapy.

dance therapy The use of dance to rehabilitate and restore patients' physical and emotional health. *See also* art therapy; drama therapy; manual arts therapy; music therapy; poetry therapy; recreational therapy.

Dance Therapy Association, American *See* American Dance Therapy Association.

D and C *See* dilation and curettage.

Darling case A landmark decision (*Darling v. Charleston Community Hospital*, 211 NE 2nd 53, Illinois [1965]), which first admitted state department of public health regulations, hospital bylaws and rules, and standards for hospital accreditation of the Joint Commission on Accreditation of Healthcare Organizations as evidence of the standards for health care services and their delivery. The evidence was used to establish the standard of care that the hospital should have delivered, which the jury found the hospital and physician in charge of the case had failed to provide. The case established the responsibility of hospitals for the care they provide to patients and the accountability of the medical staff to the hospital for care provided by medical staff members. *See also* accountability; Joint Commission on Accreditation of Healthcare Organizations; standard; standard of care.

data The collection of material or facts on which a discussion or an inference is based, such as data in a patient's medical record or indicator data. Data are the product of measurement. The word "data" is the plural of datum. *Compare* information. *See also* analog data; attribute data; data element; discrete data; infobit; inform; information; measurement data; performance data; primary data; process data; variables data.

Data Access, Fellowship and Residency Electronic Interactive *See* Fellowship and Residency Electronic Interactive Data Access.

data accuracy The degree to which data are free of errors or mistakes. *See also* accuracy of a measurement; accurate; error.

data, aggregate survey *See* aggregate survey data.

data, analog *See* analog data.

data analysis The process of interpreting data and drawing valid conclusions leading to a decision or judgment. *See also* tampering.

data, attribute *See* attribute data.

data, autopsy *See* autopsy data.

data bank *See* database.

Data Bank, National Practitioner *See* National Practitioner Data Bank.

database An organized collection of data, text, references, or pictures in a standardized format, typically stored in a computer system so that any particular item or set of items can be extracted or organized as needed. Databases may vary in content, type of information contained, and design. A database is a collection of one or more data sets. *Synonym*: data bank. *See also* clinical database; database management; data set; performance database; registry.

database, clinical *See* clinical database.

database management A methodology of storing, manipulating, and retrieving data in a database. Aspects of database management may include entering, classifying, modifying, and updating data

and presenting output reports. *See also* database; data management; management.

database management system A computer software package that manages, updates, secures, and gains computer access to databases; for example, dBase II, dBase III, Dataflex. *See also* computer software; management; update.

database, on-line *See* on-line database.

database, performance *See* performance database.

database producers Private companies or government organizations that determine subject content of a database; select data, text, references, or pictures for inclusion in the database; establish the database structure and format; establish indexing terms; and determine indexing rules and the process for searching. *See also* database services.

database, reference *See* reference database.

database services Private companies or government organizations that lease tapes from database producers; store databases on mainframe computers (on-line) or onto compact disk (CD-ROM); generate computerized indexes for each database; and provide user-friendly software to interact with the databases. On-line services issue passwords and bill users for on-line use, and CD services bill a flat fee for CD-ROM databases acquired. Examples of database services include Dialog, BRS, Paper Chase, and Prodigy. *See also* database producers; on-line searching.

data capture The process of transferring information from a written, paper format to machine-readable form on a computer. *Synonym*: capture. *See also* electronic text; machine readable.

data, claims *See* claims data.

data, clinical *See* clinical data.

data collection The process of gathering facts on how a process works or is working. Data collection is driven by knowledge of the process and guided by statistical principles. *See also* concurrent data collection; prospective data collection; retrospective data collection.

data collection, concurrent *See* concurrent data collection.

data collection logic, indicator *See* indicator data collection logic.

data collection, prospective *See* prospective data collection.

data collection, retrospective *See* retrospective data collection.

data completeness The degree to which desired

data exist and are available for use. *See also* data.

data, continuous   *See* continuous data.

data dictionary   A description of all the data fields within an information system; for example, name of patient, name of test, test result. *See also* data.

data, digital   *See* digital data.

data disclosure acts/initiatives   *See* state data initiatives.

data, discrete   *See* discrete data.

data dredging   Analysis of data already collected, performed without a prestated hypothesis. This approach is sometimes employed when data have been collected on a large number of variables and hypotheses are suggested by study of the data. The validity of data dredging is usually unacceptable. *See also* data; data analysis.

data element   A discrete piece of data, such as patient name or principal diagnosis. Data elements may be aggregated with other data elements to identify occurrences of an indicator event targeted for measurement. *See also* field; indicator; valid value.

Dataflex   *See* database management system.

data indicator, aggregate   *See* aggregate data indicator.

data initiatives, state   *See* state data initiatives.

data management   All the functions necessary for the computerized organizing, cataloging, locating, retrieving, storing, and maintaining of data. *See also* data; database management; management.

data, measurement   *See* measurement data.

data, nominal   *See* nominal data.

data noise   *See* noise in data.

data, operational   *See* operational data.

Data Organizations, National Association of Health   *See* National Association of Health Data Organizations.

data, outcome   *See* outcome data.

data parity   *See* parity; parity check.

data pattern   An identifiable arrangement of data that suggests a systematic design or orderly formation relative to a data set. *See also* data; data set; pattern.

data, performance   *See* performance data.

data, primary   *See* primary data.

data, process   *See* process data.

data processing   Conversion of data into a usable form, usually by means of a computer and a computer program. *See also* data processing department; electronic data processing.

data processing, automatic   *See* electronic data processing.

data processing department   In health care, a department providing integrated, computer-assisted recording, classifying, summarizing, transmitting, storing, and retrieving of clinical and management information. *See also* data processing; department.

data processing, electronic   *See* electronic data processing.

Data Processing Management Association (DPMA)   A national organization founded in 1951 composed of 40,000 managerial personnel, educators, and individuals interested in the management of information resources. It founded the certificate in data processing examination program, administered by the Institute for Certification of Computer Professionals. Its activities include sponsoring courses and videotaped management development seminars. *See also* data processing; management information system.

data processor, certified   *See* certified data processor.

data, raw   *See* raw data.

data reliability   The degree to which data resulting from a data collection process are accurate and complete. *See also* data validity; indicator reliability; reliability.

data, qualitative   *See* qualitative data.

data, quantitative   *See* quantitative data.

data, secondary   *See* secondary data.

data set   An aggregation of uniformly defined and classified data or items of information that describe an element, episode, or aspect of health care, as in the Uniform Hospital Discharge Data Set. *See also* discharge abstract; minimum data set; ordered data set; Uniform Clinical Data Set; Uniform Hospital Discharge Data Set.

data set, minimum   *See* minimum data set.

data set, ordered   *See* ordered data set.

data set, uniform basic   *See* minimum data set.

Data Set, Uniform Clinical   *See* Uniform Clinical Data Set.

Data Set, Uniform Hospital Discharge   *See* Uniform Hospital Discharge Data Set.

data source   Place(s) of origin, such as a medical record, from which data come. *See also* source document.

data, structural   *See* structural data.

data, subjective   *See* subjective data.

data, table of   *See* table.

data trend   One type of data pattern consisting of the general direction of data measurements; for example, a trend on a run chart or control chart is the continued rise or fall of a series of points. *See also* pattern; trend.

data validity The degree to which data are a reasonable representation of the phenemona they are collected to measure. *See also* data reliability; indicator validity; validity.

data, variables *See* variables data.

data verification process A process in which data are verified for accuracy and completeness. *See also* data; process; verification.

date, best-before *See* best-before date.

date, open *See* open date.

date, pack *See* pack date.

date rape Rape perpetrated by a victim's social escort. *See also* rape.

Date Rape, National Clearinghouse on Marital and *See* National Clearinghouse on Marital and Date Rape.

date, retroactive *See* retroactive date.

date, use-by *See* use-by date.

DATTA *See* Diagnostic and Therapeutic Technology Assessment Program.

datum *See* data.

datum, sense *See* sense datum.

day bed A bed regularly maintained by a health care organization for use during the day by patients who require partial hospitalization. *See also* bed; partial hospitalization.

day care (daycare) for adults *See* adult day care.

day care (daycare) center A facility offering services in a group setting ranging from active rehabilitation to social and health care. *See also* adult day care; day care for children.

day care (daycare) for children Personal care to substitute for or supplement the child rearing provided by the child's parent(s), especially to enable parents to work.

Daycare, National Institute on Adult *See* National Institute on Adult Daycare.

day hospital A facility or dedicated part of a facility providing a full range of hospital services, except that its patients return home or to alternative living arrangements in the evening. *See also* hospital; night hospital.

day hospitalization *See* partial hospitalization.

days, patient *See* patient days.

day treatment Structured services for individuals with mental health problems. Treatment may be devoted to teaching of living skills, or rehabilitation, therapy, and social skills. *See also* treatment.

DBA *See* Doctor of Business Administration.

dBase A popular commercial database management software package that allows access to multiple files in a database simultaneously and design of screen fields that are user-specific. *See also* database management system.

dBase II *See* database management system.

dBase III *See* database management system.

DC *See* Doctor of Chiropractic.

DCAT *See* Drug, Chemical and Allied Trades Association.

DDA *See* Dental Dealers of America.

DDNC *See* Digestive Disease National Coalition.

DDP *See* Doctors for Disaster Preparedness.

DDPA *See* Delta Dental Plans Association.

DDS *See* Doctor of Dental Surgery.

DEA *See* Drug Enforcement Agency.

deaf Lacking the sense of hearing or having profound hearing loss. *See also* deafness; hearing impaired.

Deaf, Conference of Educational Administrators Serving the *See* Conference of Educational Administrators Serving the Deaf.

deaf-mute A person who is unable to hear or speak. *See also* deaf; hearing impaired; speech.

Deaf, National Association of the *See* National Association of the Deaf.

deafness Lack of the sense of hearing, or profound hearing loss. Moderate loss of hearing is often called hearing loss. *See also* deaf; deaf-mute; hearing loss; sign language.

Deafness, National Information Center on *See* National Information Center on Deafness.

Deafness and Rehabilitation Association, American *See* American Deafness and Rehabilitation Association.

Deaf, Registry of Interpreters for the *See* Registry of Interpreters for the Deaf.

DEA number A number assigned to an individual or entity (a physician, a pharmacist, a hospital, a pharmacy, or some other qualified "business activity") by the federal government Drug Enforcement Agency showing that the individual or entity is authorized to dispense controlled substances. The Bureau of Narcotics and Dangerous Drugs (BNDD), the DEA's precursor agency, formerly issued a BNDD number (now called the DEA number). *See also* BNDD number; controlled substances; Drug Enforcement Agency.

death A permanent cessation of all vital functions;

the end of life; expiration. The Uniform Determination of Death states that an individual who has sustained either irreversible cessation of circulatory and respiratory function or irreversible cessation of the entire brain, including the brainstem, is dead. An example of brain death would be a patient whose lungs are being activated by a respirator but whose respiratory centers in the brain stem are destroyed. *See also* brain death; cryonics; death certificate; death with dignity; euthanasia; hospice; rigor mortis; thanatology; wrongful death.

death acts, natural   *See* natural death acts.

death, brain   *See* brain death.

death, cerebral   *See* vegetative state.

death certificate   A vital record signed by a licensed physician in the United States that includes cause of death, decedent's name, sex, birthdate, and place of residence and of death. Occupation, birthplace, and other information may also be included. The immediate cause of death is followed by conditions giving rise to the immediate cause; the underlying cause(s) is last. Causes of death are diseases, morbid conditions, or injuries that either resulted in or contributed to death. Underlying cause of death is the disease or injury that initiated the chain of events leading to death or the circumstances of the accident or violence that produced the fatal injury. *Compare* birth certificate. *See also* certificate; death; fetal death certificate; mortality statistics; vital records.

death certificate, fetal   *See* fetal death certificate.

death-delaying procedure   *See* death-prolonging procedure.

death with dignity   The obligation to care for the dying patient sensitively, compassionately, and ethically, including respect for the dying patient's wishes to refuse further medical care when therapy becomes futile. *See also* futility; informed refusal.

death, discharge by   *See* discharge by death.

Death Education and Counseling, Association for   *See* Association for Death Education and Counseling.

Death Education and Research, Center for   *See* Center for Death Education and Research.

death, maternal   *See* maternal death.

death, mega-   *See* megadeath.

death-prolonging procedure   Any procedure or intervention, such as artificial ventilation, that prolongs the dying process when death will occur with-

in a short time. In the Missouri living will, this does not include the performance of any procedure to provide nutrition or hydration. *Synonym*: death-delaying procedure. *See also* life-sustaining procedure; living will.

death rate   *See* mortality rate.

death rate, child   *See* child death rate.

death rate, disease-specific   *See* disease-specific death rate.

death rate, fetal   *See* fetal death rate.

death rate, hospital   *See* hospital death rate.

death rate, infant   *See* infant mortality rate.

death rate, maternal   *See* maternal mortality rate.

death rate, neonatal   *See* neonatal death rate.

Death Syndrome Clearinghouse, National Sudden Infant   *See* National Sudden Infant Death Syndrome Clearinghouse.

death, wrongful   *See* wrongful death.

debt   An obligation of goods, services, or money owed by one person or organization to another person or organization, as in a state's growing debt. *See also* bad debt; credit.

debt, bad   *See* bad debt.

debug   The act of reviewing a system to uncover and correct any errors. With a complicated computer program, for example, it may take longer to correct all the errors than it did to write the program. *See also* bug; computer program; demonstration model.

decedent   A deceased (dead) person. *See also* death.

decentralization   The distribution of administrative functions or powers of a central authority among several local authorities, as in distributing decision-making powers and policy formulation to several locations throughout an organization. The objective is to give decision-making authority to those most directly responsible for the outcome of those decisions, with first-hand experience and knowledge about the issues involved.

decentralized laboratory testing   Analytical testing performed at sites in a health care organization but physically located outside the organization's central laboratory. The testing sites are either under the jurisdiction of the organized pathology and clinical laboratory or another department or service. Examples of this testing include bedside testing and on-unit testing, such as occult-blood testing, serological screens (for example, mononucleosis), urinalysis, Gram's stains, and glucose meter testing. *See* *also* decentralized pharmaceutical services; decentralized services; laboratory; testing.

decentralized pharmaceutical services Storing, preparing, and dispensing of drugs performed at sites physically located outside a health care organization's central pharmacy. *Synonym:* satellite pharmacy. *See also* decentralized services; drug dispensing; pharmaceutical services.

decentralized services Services performed in several locations to improve efficiency, reduce cost, or both; for example, decentralized pharmaceutical or laboratory testing services. The alternative is centralized services, that is, the performance of services at or from a single location; for example, central service department. *See also* decentralized laboratory testing; decentralized pharmaceutical services.

deceptive advertising Advertising that makes false claims, misleading statements, or false impressions. Deceptive practices include false promises, unsubstantiated claims, incomplete descriptions, false testimonials or comparisons, small-print qualifications of advertisement, partial disclosure, or visual distortion of products or services. *See also* advertise; comparative advertising; competitive advertising; false advertising; image advertising; informative advertising.

decibel A unit used to express relative difference in power or intensity, usually between two acoustic or electric signals, equal to ten times the common logarithm of the ratio of the two levels. *See also* deaf; hearing; hearing impaired.

Decibel Society, American Diopter and *See* American Diopter and Decibel Society.

decile *See* quantile.

decision The passing of judgment on an issue under consideration, as in a making an accreditation decision. *See also* determination; judgment; opinion.

decision, accreditation *See* accreditation decision.

decision aggregation, accreditation *See* accreditation decision aggregation.

decisional capacity The capacity of an individual to understand the ramifications of a decision that must be made, consider the benefits and burdens of various choices, and communicate his or her choices either verbally or non-verbally. In general, individuals with decisional capacity are regarded as capable of providing informed consent to medical treatment. *See also* competence; decision; informed consent.

decision analysis A derivative of operations research and game theory that involves identifying all available choices and potential outcomes of each choice in a series of decisions that are made about diagnostic procedures, therapeutic regimens, prognostic expectations, and other important aspects of patient care. The choices are often plotted on a decision tree and at each branch, or decision node, the probabilities of each outcome that can be predicted are displayed. The decision tree shows the choices available to those responsible for patient care and the probabilities of each outcome that will follow the choice of a particular action or strategy in patient care. *See also* clinical decision analysis; decision; decision tree; utility.

decision analysis, clinical *See* clinical decision analysis.

decision maker An individual making judgments or determinations, especially one in a position of authority or power. *See also* decision.

decision making, shared *See* shared decision making.

decision node *See* decision analysis; decision tree.

decision symbol A graphic symbol in a flow chart or decision analysis, indicating the need to make a judgment about a course of action. *See also* decision analysis; symbol.

decision tree A device used in decision analysis, developed to express alternative choices in quantitative terms that can be made in the process of thinking through a problem. A series of decision options are represented as branches, and subsequent possible outcomes are represented as further branches. The junction where a decision must be made is called a decision node. *See also* decision analysis.

decisive Having the power to decide; resolute.

decoding The process of translating a code (usually a number) back into the term (such as a diagnosis) that the code represents. *Compare* coding; encoding.

decompensation A failure of an organ or system to compensate for a functional overload imposed by disease, used especially with respect to the heart, as in cardiac decompensation. *See also* cardiac decompensation.

decompensation, cardiac *See* cardiac decompensation.

decubitus **1.** The manner or posture of lying in bed. **2.** A bedsore. *See also* pressure sore.

decubitus ulcer *See* pressure sore.

deduce To apply a general rule to a specific situation, that is, make an inference from the general to the specific. For instance, the following is deductive reasoning: all people treated like *b* turn out *c*; person *a* is being treated like *b*; therefore person *a* will turn out *c*. Induce, by contrast, is to derive general principles from particular facts or instances. *Compare* induce. *See also* a priori; deductive reasoning.

deductible In a health insurance policy, a form of cost sharing in which a set amount must be paid by the insured before any payment of benefits occurs. It is often a feature of traditional indemnity insurance plans in order to reduce premiums. *See also* benefits; coinsurance; copayment; cost sharing; insured; premium.

deduction **1.** The amount that is or may be subtracted, as in deductible expenses or a tax deduction. *See also* medical deduction; payroll deduction; tax deduction. **2.** Reasoned argument proceeding from the general to the particular. *Compare* induction. *See also* deduce.

deduction, medical *See* medical deduction.

deduction, payroll *See* payroll deduction.

deduction, tax *See* tax deduction.

deductive reasoning Logical way of reaching a conclusion based on deducing from facts what to do. An example is a manager who considers the competition, customer demand, company financial status, and economic conditions in formulating a business policy. *Compare* inductive reasoning. *See also* a priori; deduce; implied; reasoning.

deemed status Status conferred by the Health Care Financing Administration (HCFA) on a health care provider when that provider is judged or determined to be in compliance with relevant Medicare conditions of participation because it has been accredited by a voluntary organization whose standards and surveying process are determined by HCFA to be equivalent to those of the Medicare program. Under the authority of Section 1865 of the Social Security Act, hospitals accredited by the Joint Commission on Accreditation of Healthcare Organizations or the American Osteopathic Association are automatically "deemed" to meet all the health and safety requirements for participation in Medicare except the utilization review requirement and the special staffing and record-keeping requirements for psychiatric hospitals. As a result of this deemed status provision, most hospitals participating in Medicare do so by meeting the standards of a private body. *See also* American Osteopathic Association; conditions of participation; Joint Commission on Accreditation of

Healthcare Organizations; Medicare.

de facto Latin phrase meaning "a right or obligation established as a matter of custom or common conduct and not founded upon a statute of common law." *Compare* de jure.

defamation The publication of a statement (communication to a third person) that injures the reputation of another person. Written defamation is called libel; oral defamation, slander. Both libel and slander are torts for which the defamer may face liability. *See also* liability.

defect The lack of something necessary or desirable for perfection or excellence, as in birth defect or an organization striving for zero defects. *Synonym*: deficiency. *See also* zero defects.

Defect and Clinical Genetic Society, Birth *See* Birth Defect and Clinical Genetic Society.

defects, zero *See* zero defects.

defendant In civil proceedings, the party responding to the complaint, that is, the one who is sued and called upon to make satisfaction for a wrong complained of by another party called the plaintiff. In criminal proceedings, the defendant is also called the accused. *Compare* plaintiff. *See also* complaint; malicious prosecution.

defense **1.** In legal proceedings, a denial, answer, or plea opposing the truth or validity of a plaintiff's case. This may be accomplished by cross-examination or by demurrer, but is more often done by introducing testimony or other evidence designed to refute all or part of the allegations of the plaintiff's case. *See also* defendant; plaintiff. **2.** The act of defending against attack, danger, or injury. **3.** A military, governmental, and industrial complex, especially as it authorizes and manages weaponry production. *See also* Department of Defense.

defense, affirmative *See* affirmative defense.

Defense, Department of *See* Department of Defense.

defense mechanism *See* mechanism.

defense panel *See* screening panel.

defensive medicine Alteration of modes of practice, induced by the threat of liability, for the principal purposes of forestalling the possibility of malpractice suits by patients and providing a good legal defense in the event of such lawsuits. *See also* lawsuit; malpractice; professional liability.

deferred retirement age The age beyond automatic retirement age that is usually not accompanied with an increase in benefits. *See also* automatic retirement age; benefit; retirement age.

defibrillation Cessation of fibrillation of the heart muscle, usually by means of electroshock. *See also* defibrillator; fibrillation; ventricular fibrillation.

defibrillator An electronic apparatus used to counteract atrial or ventricular fibrillation by the application of brief electroshock to the heart, either directly or through electrodes or paddles placed on the chest wall. *See also* defibrillation.

deficiency Lack or insufficient amount of something essential, as in nutritional deficiency, performance deficiency, or immunodeficiency. *See also* acquired immunodeficiency syndrome; defect.

deficiency syndrome, acquired immuno- *See* acquired immunodeficiency syndrome.

deficit **1.** The result of an expenditure in excess of income, as in the federal deficit. *See also* Deficit Reduction Act of 1984; deficit spending; federal deficit. **2.** The lack or impairment in a functional capacity, as in peripheral neurological deficit. *See also* peripheral neurological deficit.

deficit, federal *See* federal deficit.

deficit, peripheral neurological *See* peripheral neurological deficit.

Deficit Reduction Act of 1984 A complex federal law containing a large number of cost-containment and reimbursement-reform provisions for Medicare and Medicaid. Examples include development of a prospective payment hospital wage index, changes in payment for skilled nursing facilities, payment for clinical psychologist services, expansion of Medicaid coverage to qualified pregnant women and children, establishment of selective waivers of requirement for health maintenance organizations, and provisions leading to the development of different payment allowances for participating versus nonparticipating physicians. *See also* deficit; health maintenance organization; Medicaid; Medicare; prospective payment; skilled nursing facility.

deficit spending The spending of funds obtained by borrowing rather than by taxation. *See also* deficit; federal deficit.

definition, operational *See* operational definition.

definition of terms, indicator *See* indicator definition of terms.

deformity Malformation or distortion of part of the body, congenital or acquired. *See also* birth defect.

defraud To take something by fraud; to swindle, as

in a provider defrauding the government. *Compare* good faith. *See also* fraud and abuse.

degree **1.** The certificate of achievement that a school, college, or university gives to a student who completes a specified course of study or curriculum. *See also* associate degree; baccalaureate degree program; bachelor's degree; certificate; degree nurse; degree program; master's degree. **2.** A unit of measure, as of temperature; for example, Celsius degree.

degree, associate *See* associate degree.

degree, bachelor's *See* bachelor's degree.

degree, master's *See* master's degree.

degree program, baccalaureate *See* baccalaureate degree program.

degree nurse A nurse whose nursing education is obtained in an educational institution that grants an academic degree, as in a Bachelor of Science in Nursing (BSN). *Compare* diploma nurse. *See also* bachelor's degree; degree program.

Degree Nursing, National Organization for Associate *See* National Organization for Associate Degree Nursing.

degree program An educational organization's program that results in the conferring of a degree following successful completion, in contrast to institutions and programs conferring a diploma; for instance, a nursing degree program. *Compare* diploma school. *See also* associate degree; baccalaureate degree program; degree.

dehydration **1.** Loss or removal or water. **2.** The condition resulting from excessive water loss.

deinstitutionalization The removal of individuals from institutional settings and returning them to community life, as in the discharge of mental patients from mental health care organizations, with continued care provided in the community. The movement of mental patients back into the community was made possible in part by the development of psychotropic drugs capable of positively modifying patients' behavior so that they can function in the community. *See also* psychotropic drug.

de jure Latin phrase meaning "as a matter of law." *Compare* de facto.

delegation To appoint a person to act as one's representative or agent in a specified matter, as in the delegation of authority.

deliberate immunosuppression Immunosuppression with drugs, such as corticosteroids, to help prevent rejection of organ transplants. *See also* cortisone; immunosuppression; incidental immunosuppression.

delineated clinical privileges *See* delineation of clinical privileges.

delineation of clinical privileges The process of defining the clinical privileges a member of the medical staff or the organized professional staff of a health care organization may be granted. *See also* clinical privileges; medical staff; organized professional staff.

delirium The state of acute and severe confusion, in which an individual has little or no contact with reality. There is mental excitement, with illusions, delusions and hallucinations, and physical restlessness. Delirium is characteristic of severe toxic and febrile states. *Compare* dementia. *See also* delirium tremens; delusion; hallucination; illusion.

delirium tremens (DTs) A neuropsychiatric disorder due to acute withdrawal from prolonged abuse of alcohol. Symptoms include low-grade fever, hallucinations, confusion, nausea, and trembling. *See also* delirium; hallucination.

deliverable Capable of showing a tangible output or end product.

delivery In medicine, the process of childbirth, in particular the second and third stages of labor, during which the infant and the placenta are expelled from the uterus. *See also* breech delivery; cesarean section; labor; normal delivery; obstetrics; premature delivery; sick baby; spontaneous delivery; vaginal delivery.

delivery, abdominal *See* cesarean section.

delivery, breech *See* breech delivery.

delivery, cesarean *See* cesarean section.

delivery, forceps *See* forceps delivery.

delivery, normal *See* normal delivery.

delivery, premature *See* premature delivery.

delivery room A unit in a hospital or other health care facility for obstetric delivery and initial infant care, including resuscitation. *See also* delivery.

delivery, spontaneous *See* spontaneous delivery.

delivery system, alternative *See* alternative delivery system.

delivery, vaginal *See* vaginal delivery.

delphi method A procedure for forecasting events or selecting organizational or program goals. Experts are asked to write their best judgment about the probability of a specific event and implications of its occurrence or nonoccurrence. The results are collated and then returned to the original experts for their

interpretation, along with an opportunity to revise their own predictions. Revisions with supporting arguments are then recirculated. In theory, this feedback, which is repeated, continues to narrow the range of predictions and, in the end, a group judgment will have been reached while minimizing the possibility of distortion by personal contact, leadership influence, or the pressures of group dynamics. *Synonyms*: delphi study; delphi technique.

delphi study *See* delphi method.

delphi technique *See* delphi method.

Delta Dental plan The franchise name for any one of the statewide prepaid dental service plans that were developed through sponsorship by dental professional societies and use principles similar to those in Blue Shield medical and surgical plans. The plans are nonprofit service corporations established under state law. *See also* Blue Shield plan; dentistry; not-for-profit carrier.

Delta Dental Plans Association (DDPA) A national organization founded in 1965 composed of 47 active state dental service corporations, inactive state dental service corporations, state dental societies, and foreign dental services concerned with state dental service corporations providing prepaid dental benefits coverage to local, multistate, and national group accounts (largely employment-based groups). Formerly National Association of Dental Service Plans. *See also* Delta Dental plan; dental service corporation.

delusion A false opinion or belief, contrary to fact and unassailable by evidence or reason. It is usual to exclude from this definition articles of religious faith or other beliefs shared by persons of similar culture. *Compare* hallucination; illusion. *See also* delusions of grandeur; nihilism; religion.

delusions of grandeur Delusions involving an exaggerated concept of one's importance, power, or knowledge, or the belief that one is, or has a special relationship with, a deity or a famous person. *See also* megalomania.

demand for health services Willingness and/or ability to seek, use, and, in some settings, pay for health services. Expressed demand is equated with use, and potential demand with need. *Compare* need.

demand, law of supply and *See* law of supply and demand.

demand, on *See* on demand.

demand pacemaker An implanted artificial cardiac pacemaker in which the generator stimulus is inhibited for a set interval by a signal, thus minimizing the risk of pacemaker-induced ventricular fibrillation. *Compare* fixed-rate pacemaker. *See also* artificial cardiac pacemaker; pacemaker; ventricular fibrillation.

dementia A deterioration of intellectual function that causes changes in behavior and personality, associated with pathological changes in the brain. Dementia does not include loss of intellectual functioning caused by clouding consciousness, as in delirium, nor that caused by depression or other functional mental disorders. Dementia may be caused by a large number of conditions, some reversible and some progressive, including the most common dementia, Alzheimer's disease. Other dementias are multi-infarct dementia secondary to cerebrovascular disease, Wernicke-Korsakoff syndrome, normal-pressure hydrocephalus, and neurological diseases, such as multiple sclerosis and Parkinson's disease. *Compare* delirium. *See also* Alzheimer's disease; multi-infarct dementia; multiple sclerosis; Parkinson's disease; senile dementia.

dementia, multi-infarct *See* multi-infarct dementia.

dementia, senile *See* senile dementia.

Deming cycle *See* Plan-Do-Check-Act (PDCA) cycle.

Deming's Fourteen Points The Fourteen Points are the foundation of W. Edwards Deming's message to management. They include a blend of leadership, management theory, and statistical concepts that highlight the responsibilities of management while enhancing the capacities of employees, as together they seek to build the knowledge and application of the knowledge for improvement. *See also* cease dependence on mass inspection; constancy of purpose; Deming, W. Edwards; drive out fear; leadership; management.

Deming, W. Edwards A statistics educator, consultant, and patriarch (d. 1993) of total quality management who was responsible for the first sampling program in the United States used on the 1940 census. Deming taught statistical quality control to engineers and inspectors during World War II and then took the methods to Japan where they were in part responsible for the post-World War II revitalization of Japanese industry. *See also* acceptable quality level; Deming's Fourteen Points; statistical quality control; total quality management.

demographics Statistics showing an area's population characteristics, such as age, income, and education. *Synonym*: demographic characteristics.

demography The study of the characteristics of human populations and population segments, such as size, growth, density, distribution, and vital statistics.

demonstration model In health services, an experimental health care program, system, or organization that measures important aspects, such as costs per unit of service, rates of use by patients or clients, and clinical outcomes of encounters between providers and users. The aim of using demonstration models is to determine and, when necessary, improve on the efficiency, effectiveness, and other dimensions of performance and quality *before* the system, program, or organization is broadly implemented. *See also* debug; dimensions of performance.

demotion Assignment of an employee to a job of lower status, responsibility, or pay. *See also* disciplinary demotion; involuntary demotion; voluntary demotion.

demotion, disciplinary *See* disciplinary demotion.

demotion, involuntary *See* involuntary.

demotion, voluntary *See* voluntary demotion.

demurrer A formal objection by one of the parties to a lawsuit that the evidence presented by the opponent is insufficient to justify the lawsuit. Federal Rules of Civil Procedure, Rule 12 (b)(6), allows a party to move for dismissal because of the other party's failure to state a claim upon which relief can be granted. *See also* claim; dismissal with prejudice; dismissal without prejudice; lawsuit.

denial of accreditation *See* not accredited.

denominator The lower part of a fraction used to calculate a rate, proportion, or ratio. For instance, the denominator of a clinical indicator is the population (or population experience, as in women giving birth) at risk in the calculation of a rate. *Compare* numerator. *See also* proportion; rate; ratio.

dentacare A group dental plan similar to a health maintenance organization in which a fixed monthly payment (capitation) made to a group of dentists ensures needed dental care to enrolled members. Traditional dental insurance processes and pays dental claims on the basis of fees charged for services (fee for service). *See also* capitation; dentistry; fee for service.

dental appliance *See* orthodontic appliance.

dental assistant An individual who assists a dentist in providing direct care to patients, such as seating patients and preparing them for treatment, retrieving their dental records, preparing tray setups for dental procedures, giving the dentist necessary instruments and materials, keeping the patient's mouth clear by the use of suction and other devices, and performing selected dental x-ray and laboratory work. *See also* dentistry.

Dental Assistants Association, American *See* American Dental Assistants Association.

Dental Assistants Association, National *See* National Dental Assistants Association.

Dental Assistants, National Association of *See* National Association of Dental Assistants.

Dental Assisting National Board (DANB) A national board founded in 1948 that administers examinations to and certifies dental assistants. Formerly Certifying Board of the American Dental Assistants Association. *See also* board; certification; dental assistant.

Dental Association, American *See* American Dental Association.

Dental Association, Holistic *See* Holistic Dental Association.

Dental Association, Indian *See* Indian Dental Association.

Dental Association, National *See* National Dental Association.

Dental Association, National Medical and *See* National Medical and Dental Association.

dental audit A qualitative or quantitative evaluative review of dental services rendered or proposed by a dentist. *See also* audit; medical audit; nursing audit.

dental caries *See* caries.

dental chair A specially equipped and adjustable chair for patients undergoing dental surgery.

dental clinic Premises equipped for the dental examination and treatment of patients. Dental clinics may be situated within hospitals. *See also* clinic; dentistry.

Dental Consultants, American Association of *See* American Association of Dental Consultants.

Dental Dealers of America (DDA) A national organization founded in 1943 composed of 70 wholesale dealers of dental instruments, equipment, and supplies. *See also* dentistry.

Dental Directors, Association of State and

Territorial *See* Association of State and Territorial Dental Directors.

dental drill A powered cutting instrument employed in dental surgery, particularly in the conservative treatment of caries. *See also* caries.

Dental Editors, American Association of *See* American Association of Dental Editors.

Dental Electrosurgery, American Academy of *See* American Academy of Dental Electrosurgery.

Dental Examiners, American Association of *See* American Association of Dental Examiners.

dental extender A dental assistant or dental hygienist who, under a dentist's supervision, performs patient services not requiring the skills of a dentist. *See also* dental assistant; dental hygienist.

dental foundation A legal entity that provides dental services, education, and research on behalf of participating dentist members.

dental geriatrics The branch of dentistry dealing with dental disorders and diseases of the aged. *See also* geriatric medicine.

Dental Gold Institute (DGI) A national organization founded in 1981 composed of 15 suppliers of major precious metals to the dental profession. It provides dental professionals with information regarding current research and literature in the industry, and it works to counteract the economic effects brought about by increased use of base metals in dental work due to the sharp rise in the cost of gold. It encourages classification of alloys and the establishment of appropriate and standardized terminology. *See also* dentistry.

Dental Group Management Association (DGMA) A national organization founded in 1951 composed of 200 dental group business managers and other persons interested in group practice management. *See also* dentistry; group practice; management.

Dental Group Practice, American Academy of *See* American Academy of Dental Group Practice.

dental health The state of normality and functional efficiency of the teeth and supporting structures, the surrounding parts of the oral cavity, and the various structures related to mastication and the maxillofacial complex. *See also* dentistry; health.

dental health services All services designed or intended to promote, maintain, or restore dental health, including educational, preventive, and therapeutic services; all procedures that dentists are licensed to perform. *See also* dentistry; health services.

Dental-Hospital Bureaus of America, Medical- *See* Medical-Dental-Hospital Bureaus of America.

dental hygiene 1. The practice of keeping the mouth, teeth, and gums clean and healthy to prevent disease, as by regular brushing and flossing and visits to a dentist. *Synonym:* oral hygiene. *See also* hygiene. **2.** The work performed by a dental hygienist. *See also* dental hygienist.

dental hygiene accreditation An accreditation process in which the Commission on Dental Accreditation evaluates and, when appropriate, accredits dental hygiene programs. *See also* accreditation; dental hygiene.

dental hygienist An oral health specialist who, under the supervision of dentist, helps people prevent tooth decay and gum disease and maintain oral health. A dental hygienist may examine teeth and gums, clean deposits and stains from teeth, treat teeth with fluorides and other decay-preventive agents, take impressions of teeth, remove sutures, and take and develop x-rays. He or she instructs patients in dental health and may also provide dental health education for school children and other members of the community. *See also* public health dental hygienist.

dental hygienist, public health *See* public health hygienist.

Dental Hygienists' Association, American *See* American Dental Hygienists' Association.

dental implantology *See* implant dentistry.

dental insurance Insurance that covers the costs of specified aspects of dental care, ranging from coverage of basic diagnostic, preventive, and restorative services to coverage that includes oral surgery and orthodontics. *Synonym:* dental plan. *See also* insurance.

dental jurisprudence *See* forensic dentistry.

Dental Laboratories, National Association of *See* National Association of Dental Laboratories.

Dental Laboratories, National Board for Certification of *See* National Board for Certification of Dental Laboratories.

dental laboratory technician An individual who constructs a variety of dental appliances that conform to a dentist's specifications, including the construction of dentures (complete or partial), orthodontic appliances, bridgework, crowns, and inlays. The majority of dental technicians work in commercial dental laboratories. *Synonym:* dental technician.

See also technician.

dental laboratory technology accreditation An accreditation process in which the Commission on Dental Accreditation of dental laboratory technology education programs evaluates and, when appropriate, accredits dental laboratory technology programs. *See also* accreditation; American Dental Association; dental laboratory technician.

Dental Manufacturers of America (DMA) A national organization founded in 1932 composed of 170 manufacturing firms of dental equipment and supplies. *See also* dentistry.

Dental Materials, Academy of *See* Academy of Dental Materials.

dental plan *See* dental insurance.

Dental plan, Delta *See* Delta Dental plan.

Dental Plans Association, Delta *See* Delta Dental Plans Association.

dental practice act A state, commonwealth, or territorial statute or law delineating the legal scope of the practice of dentistry within the geographic boundaries of the jurisdiction. *See also* dentistry; medical practice act; nurse practice act.

Dental Practice Administration, American Academy of *See* American Academy of Dental Practice Administration.

dental public health *See* public health dentistry.

Dental Public Health, American Board of *See* American Board of Dental Public Health.

Dental Research, American Association for *See* American Association for Dental Research.

dental resident An dentist undergoing specialty training by carrying out actual duties under supervision in a dental residency program in a health care organization, typically a hospital. *See also* dentistry; resident.

dental school An educational institution offering programs leading to the Doctor of Dental Medicine (DMD) or Doctor of Dental Surgery (DDS) degrees. *See also* dental student; dentistry.

Dental Schools, American Association of *See* American Association of Dental Schools.

dental service An organizational unit, such as a hospital department that provides ambulatory and inpatient dental services including preventive care, diagnosis, and treatment. *See also* dentistry; service.

dental service corporation A nonprofit corporation organized by the dental profession to provide prepaid dental care coverage to the public on a group basis. *See also* corporation.

Dental Society of Anesthesiology, American *See* American Dental Society of Anesthesiology.

Dental Society, Christian *See* Christian Dental Society.

Dental Society, Christian Medical and *See* Christian Medical and Dental Society.

Dental Society, Medical Group Missions of the Christian Medical and *See* Medical Group Missions of the Christian Medical and Dental Society.

dental specialist *See* dentist, specialist.

dental specialties Eight areas of expertise in dentistry recognized by the American Dental Association: endodontics, oral and maxillofacial surgery, oral pathology, orthodontics, pediatric dentistry (pedodontics), periodontics, prosthodontics, and public health dentistry. *See also* American Dental Association; endodontics; oral and maxillofacial surgery; oral pathology; orthodontics; pedodontics; periodontics; prosthodontics; public health dentistry; specialty.

dental student An individual who is enrolled in a dental school program of study to fulfill the requirements for a doctor of dental medicine or doctor of dental surgery degree. *See also* clinical clerk; clinical clerkship; dental school.

dental surgery *See* dentistry.

dental technician *See* dental laboratory technician.

Dental Technology, National Board for Certification in *See* National Board for Certification in Dental Technology.

Dental Trade Association, American *See* American Dental Trade Association.

dental unit The equipment used in providing dental care, including a worktable, operating lights, drills, suction tube, and aerator. *See also* chairside; dental drill.

dentist An individual qualified by education and authorized by law to practice dentistry. *See* dentist, generalist; dentist, specialist.

dentist, generalist A dentist who has received the degree of Doctor of Dental Surgery (DDS) or Doctor of Medical Dentistry (DMD), who is licensed to practice dentistry and who brings his or her skills in oral diagnosis, prevention, and rehabilitation directly to the patient. *See also* dentist, specialist.

dentist, public health *See* public health dentist.

dentistry The branch of the healing arts and sci-ences devoted to maintaining the health of the teeth, gums, and other hard and soft tissues of the oral cavity. *Synonyms*: dental medicine; dental surgery. *See also* amalgam; corporate dentistry; caries; crown; filling; forensic dentistry; franchise dentistry; implant dentistry; plaque.

Dentistry, Academy of General *See* Academy of General Dentistry.

Dentistry, Academy of Operative *See* Academy of Operative Dentistry.

Dentistry, Academy for Sports *See* Academy for Sports Dentistry.

Dentistry, American Academy of the History of *See* American Academy of the History of Dentistry.

Dentistry, American Academy of Implant *See* American Academy of Implant Dentistry.

Dentistry, American Academy of Pediatric *See* American Academy of Pediatric Dentistry.

Dentistry, American Academy of Restorative *See* American Academy of Restorative Dentistry.

Dentistry, American Association of Public Health *See* American Association of Public Health Dentistry.

Dentistry, American Board of Pediatric *See* American Board of Pediatric Dentistry.

Dentistry, American Society for Advancement of Anesthesia in *See* American Society for Advancement of Anesthesia in Dentistry.

Dentistry, American Society for Geriatric *See* American Society for Geriatric Dentistry.

Dentistry for Children, American Society of *See* American Society of Dentistry for Children.

dentistry, corporate *See* corporate dentistry.

dentistry, forensic *See* forensic dentistry.

dentistry, franchise *See* franchise dentistry.

Dentistry for the Handicapped, Academy of *See* Academy of Dentistry for the Handicapped.

dentistry, implant *See* implant dentistry.

dentistry, public health *See* public health dentistry.

dentistry, retail store *See* retail store dentistry.

Dentists, American Association of Entrepreneurial *See* American Association of Entrepreneurial Dentists.

Dentists, American Association of Hospital *See* American Association of Hospital Dentists.

Dentists, American Association of Women *See* American Association of Women Dentists.

Dentists, American College of *See* American College of Dentists.

Dentists, American Society of Retired *See* American Society of Retired Dentists.

Dentists, National Association of Seventh-Day Adventist Dentists (NASDAD) A national organization founded in 1979 composed of 600 Seventh-Day Adventist dentists. *See also* dentistry.

Dentists, National Association of VA Physicians and *See* National Association of VA Physicians and Dentists.

dentist, specialist A dentist who specializes in one of eight areas of expertise in dentistry recognized by the American Dental Association. Specialist dentists typically receive an additional two to four years of training in their specialty area and often limit their practice to their specialty. After they have completed training, they are eligible to take examinations that can allow them to become board certified in their specialty. Dental specialties recognized by the American Dental Association include public health dentistry, endodontics, oral pathology, oral and maxillofacial surgery, orthodontics, pediatric dentistry, periodontics, and prosthodontics. *See also* board certified; dental specialties; dentist, generalist; specialist.

Dentists, Union of American Physicians and *See* Union of American Physicians and Dentists.

dentition 1. The teeth considered as a set, that is, their number, type, and arrangement. *See also* tooth. 2. The process of tooth development, growth, and extrusion.

denture A set of artificial or prosthetic replacement teeth for missing natural teeth and adjacent tissues. *See also* denturism; denturist; prosthodontics.

denturism The practice of making and fitting of dentures by dental technologists without benefit of a dentist's expertise. *See also* denture.

denturist A dental technologist who provides dentures for patients without the benefit of a dentist's services. Denturists are not recognized by the American Dental Association and are illegal in some states. They are relatively common in Canada, especially in the Province of Ontario. *See also* denture.

Denturist Association, National *See* National Denturist Association.

deontological ethics An ethical theory or system that holds that right or wrong is not determined by assessment of consequences, as opposed to utilitarian ethics. Deontological ethics is based on the assumption that value is inherent in the principle or duty. The Golden Rule is an example. *Compare* utilitarianism. *See also* ethics.

deoxyribonucleic acid (DNA) A large molecule, shaped like a double helix and found primarily in the chromosomes of a cell's nucleus, that contains the genetic information of a cell. *See also* cell; molecular genetics; mutation; plasmid; recombinant DNA; ribonucleic acid.

department A functional or administrative division of an organization. In health care organizations, such as hospitals, departments are frequently organized according to medical specialty, such as a pediatrics department or radiology department. A hospital also contains supporting departments, such as dietary, central supply, housekeeping, engineering and maintenance, nursing, and pharmacy departments. There is no standard departmental organization for health care organizations. A department is not a separate legal entity. *Synonym*: service(s). *See also* admitting department; clinical department; clinical engineering department; foodservice department; hospital department; laundry department; security department.

department, admissions *See* admitting department.

department chair (of a clinical service) A physician or other qualified individual who has primary responsibility for administration and quality control in a given clinical department. He or she monitors physician performance to see that standards are maintained and to take corrective action when they are not. A department chair's functions might typically include accountability for all clinical and administrative activities of the department; service on the medical executive committee; continuing review of the professional performance of all practitioners with clinical privileges in the department; appropriate follow-up action on performance issues, including the use of education, counseling, proctoring, limitation of privileges, and revocation of privileges in order to ensure the quality of medical care; enforcement of the medical staff bylaws as they pertain to department activity; participation in administration of the department through cooperation with hospital management and the nursing service; and service as presiding officer at departmental meetings. *Synonyms*: chief of service; department chief. *See also* department.

department chief *See* department chair.

department, clinical *See* clinical department.

department, clinical engineering *See* clinical engineering department.

Department of Commerce (DOC) A principal department of the executive branch of the US government, with certain health-related bureaus and laboratories, including the Bureau of the Census (provides demographic data), Bureau of Economic Analysis, National Institute of Standards and Technology, Environmental Research Laboratories within the National Oceanic and Atmospheric Administration, and National Technical Information Service.

department, data processing *See* data processing department.

Department of Defense (DOD) A principal department of the executive branch of the US government with substantial health-related accountabilities that are organized under the Office of the Assistant Secretary for Health Affairs. Functions include providing staff support to the Secretary of Defense on military medical resources and facilities, supervising the administration of the Civilian Health and Medical Program of the Uniformed Services (CHAMPUS) and the Active Duty Dependents Dental Plan, providing guidance and policy support on medical professional affairs and quality assurance, providing planning and policy support and oversight on medical readiness (defense preparedness), developing programs and initiatives in defense medical systems, and administering the Defense Health Council and Uniform Services Health Benefits Council, the Uniformed Services University of Health Sciences, the Armed Forces Institute of Pathology, the Armed Forces Epidemiological Board, and the Worldwide Aeromedical Evacuation System.

Department of Education (DOE) A principal department of the executive branch of the US government with accountabilities for special education programs, the Rehabilitation Services Administration, and the National Institute on Disability and Rehabilitation Research. The Department was created in 1979 when the Department of Health, Education and Welfare was divided into two departments: the Department of Health and Human Services and the Department of Education.

Department of Energy (DOE) A principal department of the executive branch of the US government

with certain health-related accountabilities including responsibilities of the Office of the Assistant Secretary for Environment, Safety, and Health and the Office of Civilian Radioactive Waste Management.

Department of Environmental and Drug-Induced Pathology *See* Department of Environmental and Toxicologic Pathology.

Department of Environmental and Toxicologic Pathology (DETP) An organization founded in 1966, affiliated with the Armed Forces Institute of Pathology, that evaluates biopsy and autopsy material on adverse drug-reaction cases and environment-related diseases. It has collected over 13,000 such cases. It functions in areas of consultation, investigation, and education. Formerly (1990) Department of Environmental and Drug-Induced Pathology. *See also* Armed Forces Institute of Pathology; medical toxicology; pathology.

department, foodservice *See* foodservice department.

Department of Health and Human Services (DHHS) A principal department of the executive branch of the US government with major health-related accountabilities, including the responsibilities of the Public Health Service, Health Care Financing Administration, the Office of Human Development Services, and the Social Security Administration. *See also* Health Care Financing Administration; Public Health Service; Social Security Administration.

Department of Health, Education and Welfare A former department of the executive branch of the US government that was, on October 17, 1979, divided into two departments: the Department of Health and Human Services and the Department of Education. *See also* Department of Education; Department of Health and Human Services.

department, hospital *See* hospital department.

department, housekeeping *See* housekeeping department.

department, human resources *See* personnel department.

Department of Justice (DOJ) A principal department of the executive branch of the US government that enforces certain federal laws, including antitrust laws concerned with provision of health care in federal prisons. *See also* antitrust laws; justice.

Department of Labor (DOL) A principal department of the executive branch of the US government with certain health-related accountabilities including the Mine Safety and Health Administration, Occupational Safety and Health Administration, and the National Institute of Standards and Technology. *See also* labor certification; Occupational Safety and Health Administration.

department, laundry *See* laundry department.

department, medical record *See* medical record department.

department, patient education *See* patient education department.

department, personnel *See* personnel department.

department, pharmacy *See* pharmacy department.

department, purchasing *See* purchasing department.

departments, contract management of *See* contract management of departments.

department, security *See* security department.

Departments of Psychiatry, American Association of Chairmen of *See* American Association of Chairmen of Departments of Psychiatry.

Department of State A principal department of the executive branch of the US government that advises the president in the formulation and execution of foreign policy. The Department of State's primary objective in the conduct of foreign relations is to promote the long-range security and well-being of the United States. The department determines and analyzes the facts relating to American overseas interests, makes recommendations on policy and future action, and takes the necessary steps to carry out established policy. It engages in continuous consultations with the American public, the Congress, other United States departments and agencies, and foreign governments; negotiates treaties and agreements with foreign nations; speaks for the United States in the United Nations and in more than 50 major international organizations in which the United States participates; and represents the United States at more than 800 international conferences annually.

department, surgery *See* surgery department.

Department of Transportation (DOT) A principal department of the executive branch of the US government concerned with transportation, including emergency medical services and health care for members of the US Coast Guard and their families. *See also* emergency medical services system.

Department of the Treasury A principal department of the executive branch of the US government concerned with formulating and recommending econom-

ic, financial, tax, and fiscal policies; serving as financial agent for the United States government; enforcing the law; and manufacturing coins and currency.

Department of Veterans Affairs A principal department of the executive branch of the US government that operates programs to benefit veterans and members of their families. Benefits include compensation payments for disabilities or death related to military service; pensions; education and rehabilitation; home loan guaranty; burial; and a medical care program incorporating nursing homes, clinics, and medical centers. It operates the largest health care system in the United States. Formerly Veterans Administration.

dependability The state of being counted on or trusted. *See also* dependence.

dependence **1.** The state of being dependent, of requiring support, as in the relationship between two tasks when one task depends on the completion of another. **2.** The state of being determined or controlled by something else. **3.** A compulsive or chronic need, as in drug dependence.

dependence, physical *See* physical dependence.

dependency *See* dependence.

dependency, chemical *See* chemical dependency.

Dependent Children, Aid to Families with *See* Aid to Families with Dependent Children.

dependent variable A variable whose value is dependent on the effect of independent variable(s) in the relationship under study. In statistics, the dependent variable is the one predicted by a regression equation. *Compare* independent variable. *See also* regression analysis; variable.

deployment, quality function *See* quality function deployment.

deposition A method of pretrial discovery consisting of a statement of a witness under oath, taken in question-and-answer form, as it would be in court, with opportunity given to the adversary to be present and cross-examine, with all this reported and transcribed stenographically. The information is obtained for preparation prior to trial; part or all of it may itself be admissible (allowed as evidence) at the trial, depending on the jurisdiction. *See also* discovery; evidence; interrogatory; trial; witness.

depreciation, capital *See* capital depreciation.

depressants **1.** Any agent tending to decrease the function or activity of a body or a body system. **2.** A class of controlled substances, including barbiturates and tranquilizers. These drugs are used to produce sedation, to induce sleep, to combat anxiety, and to treat epilepsy. Excessive doses cause a drunkenlike state and have side effects similar to alcohol, including a hangover. *See also* barbiturate; controlled substances.

depression   A mental state of depressed mood characterized by feelings of sadness, despair, and discouragement. Depression ranges from normal feelings of "the blues" to major depression. The diagnosis of major depressive disorder can be made in the presence of at least five of the following symptoms during the same period; at least one of the first two symptoms also must be present. The symptoms must be present most of the day, nearly daily, for at least two weeks. They include depressed mood, markedly diminished interest or pleasure in virtually all activities, significant weight gain or loss, insomnia or hypersomnia, psychomotor agitation or retardation, fatigue or loss of energy, feelings of guilt or worthlessness, indecisiveness or impaired ability to concentrate, and recurrent thoughts of death or suicide. *See also* antidepressant; electroconvulsive therapy; melancholia; suicide.

depressive illness, manic-   *See* manic-depressive illness.

depressive psychosis, manic-   *See* manic-depressive illness.

depressor, tongue   *See* tongue depressor.

dermatitis   Any skin condition in which inflammation is part of the pathology. *See also* dermatology; neurodermatitis; skin.

dermatitis, neuro-   *See* neurodermatitis.

Dermatological Association, American   *See* American Dermatological Association.

Dermatologic Surgery, American Society for   *See* American Society for Dermatologic Surgery.

dermatologist   A physician who specializes in dermatology. *See also* dermatology.

dermatologist, immuno-   *See* immunodermatologist.

dermatology   The branch of medicine and medical specialty dealing with the diagnosis and treatment of pediatric and adult patients with benign and malignant disorders of the skin, mouth, external genitalia, hair and nails. Dermatopathology and immunodermatology are two subspecialties of dermatology. *See also* alopecia; dermatitis; dermatopathology; immunodermatology; psoriasis; rash; skin.

Dermatology, American Academy of   *See* American Academy of Dermatology.

Dermatology, American Board of   *See* American Board of Dermatology.

Dermatology, American Osteopathic College of   *See* American Osteopathic College of Dermatology.

Dermatology, American Society of Podiatric   *See* American Society of Podiatric Dermatology.

dermatology, immuno-   *See* immunodermatology.

Dermatology Nurses' Association (DNA)   A national organization founded in 1982 composed of 1,600 dermatology nurses. It addresses professional issues involving dermatology nurses; develops standards of dermatologic nursing care; and conducts educational meetings. *See also* dermatology; nurse; skin.

Dermatology, Society for Investigative   *See* Society for Investigative Dermatology.

Dermatology, Society for Pediatric   *See* Society for Pediatric Dermatology.

dermatology technician   An individual skilled in preparing and administering materials prescribed by a physician for use in the care and treatment of skin problems. He or she works under the supervision of a dermatologist or other physician specializing in skin disorders. *See also* dermatology; technician; skin.

dermatopathologist   A pathologist who subspecializes in dermatopathology. *See* dermatopathology; pathologist.

dermatopathology   The branch of medical science and subspecialty of dermatology and pathology dealing with microscopic anatomic pathology of the skin. *See also* dermatology; pathology; skin.

Dermatopathology, American Society of   *See* American Society of Dermatopathology.

dermis   The sensitive connective tissue layer of the skin located below the epidermis. It contains nerve endings, sweat and sebaceous glands, and blood and lymph vessels. *See also* epidermis; skin.

descriptive statistics   Quantifying or summarizing data without implying or inferring anything beyond the sample. *Compare* inferential statistics. *See also* data; statistics.

descriptive study   A study concerned with and designed only to describe the existing distribution of variables. There is no attempt to make causal or other hypotheses. An example is a survey used to determine practitioner practice patterns relating to use of a certain technology.

descriptor In computer science, a word, a phrase, or an alphanumeric character used to identify an item in an information storage and retrieval system.

desensitization A treatment of allergy by the injection of gradually increasing amounts of the allergen responsible for the allergy. *See also* allergy; desensitize.

desensitization, failure *See* failure desensitization.

desensitize **1.** To render insensitive or less sensitive, as by long exposure or repeated shocks. **2.** In immunology, to make an individual nonreactive or insensitive to an antigen. *See also* desensitization; immunology.

designer drug A drug deliberately synthesized to circumvent antidrug regulations, using a structure that is not yet illegal but which mimics the chemistry and effects of an existing, banned drug; hence, any recreational drug with an altered structure. For example, China White, popular in the 1970s and 1980s, is an example of designer "look alikes" of heroin. *See also* drug.

design review A formal, documented, comprehensive, and systematic examination of a design to evaluate the design requirements and the capability of the design to meet these requirements, identify problems, and propose solutions.

desirable indicator An outcome or a process indicator that measures a desirable activity or result of care; for example, patient survival or successful vaginal delivery after previous cesarean section are two desirable indicators. *See also* indicator.

desirable weight The weight range for height and body build associated with the lowest frequency of disease and death. *See also* weight.

desk-top A personal computer that fits on the top surface of a desk (short for desk-top computer). Also, desk-top refers to using a desk-top computer system to produce printed documents to a publishable standard of typesetting and layout; especially in the phrase "desk top publishing." *See also* computer.

desk-top computer *See* desk-top.

desmoteric Pertaining to prison.

detailer *See* detail person.

detailing *See* academic detailing; detail person.

detailing, academic *See* academic detailing.

detail person A sales representative of a pharmaceutical manufacturer or medical supply company who promotes prescription drugs and medical supplies for use by physicians, dentists, and pharma-

cists. Detailing includes personally presenting products, advertising, and providing drug samples, supplies, and educational materials (prepared by the manufacturer) to professionals in their offices or places of work. *Synonyms:* detailer; drug rep; drug sales representative; medical representative; pharmaceutical representative. *See also* academic detailing.

detection A past-oriented strategy that attempts to identify unacceptable output after it has been produced and separate it from the acceptable output. *Compare* prevention. *See also* inspection.

determination **1.** The process of arriving at a decision, and a decision so reached. *See also* decision. **2.** Firmness of purpose; resolve. *See also* resolve; tough-minded. **3.** The settling of a question or case by authoritative decision or pronouncement, especially by a judicial body, as in a judicial determination. **4.** The ascertaining or fixing of the quantity, quality, position, or character of something, as in a determination of a hospital's compliance with performance standards, and the result of such ascertaining. *See also* authorship determination. **5.** In logic, the defining of a concept through its constituent elements.

determination, authorship *See* authorship determination.

determination, blood gas *See* blood gas determination.

determination, coefficient of *See* coefficient of determination.

deterministic Completed determined by known factors. *Compare* random. *See also* determination.

detoxification The treatment of a person for alcohol or drug dependence, such as under a medically supervised program, designed to rid the body of intoxicating or addictive substances. *See also* medical detoxification; social detoxification; withdrawal symptoms.

detoxification, medical *See* medical detoxification.

detoxification, social *See* social detoxification.

DETP *See* Department of Environmental and Toxicologic Pathology.

development **1.** The process of growing by degrees into a more advanced or mature state. *See also* developmental disability; research and development. **2.** The planned promotion of understanding, participation, and support among potential donors to an organization, such as a hospital. Development is often used broadly, consisting of planning, cultivation, and solicitation. *See also* director of development; fundraising.

development agency, state health planning and *See* state health planning and development agency.

developmental age A measure of a child's developmental progression, for example, body size, motor skills, or psychological functioning, expressed as an age. *Compare* chronological age; mental age. *See also* age.

Developmental Biology, Society for *See* Society for Developmental Biology.

Developmental Disabilities, Accreditation Council on Services for People with *See* Accreditation Council on Services for People with Developmental Disabilities.

Developmental Disabilities, American Association of University Affiliated Programs for Persons with *See* American Association of University Affiliated Programs for Persons with Developmental Disabilities.

Developmental Disabilities Councils, National Association of *See* National Association of Developmental Disabilities Councils.

developmental disability A mental or physical limitation affecting major life activities, arising before adulthood and usually lasting throughout life. Developmental disabilities can be grouped into four major categories: autism, cerebral palsy, epilepsy, and mental retardation. *See also* autism; cerebral palsy; development; disability; epilepsy; major life activities; mental retardation.

Developmental Medicine, American Academy for Cerebral Palsy and *See* American Academy for Cerebral Palsy and Developmental Medicine.

developmental psychology The branch of psychology dealing with the emotional, intellectual, and social changes that occur across the life span of human beings. Many developmental psychologists specialize in the study of children or adolescents. *See also* psychology.

Developmental Treatment Association, Neuro- *See* Neurodevelopmental Treatment Association.

development, director of *See* director of development.

development form, indicator *See* indicator development form.

development, management *See* management development.

Development, Multidisciplinary Institute for Neuropsychological *See* Multidisciplinary Institute for Neuropsychological Development.

development, organizational *See* organizational development.

development program, staff *See* staff development program.

development, research and *See* research and development.

Development Services, Office of Human *See* Office of Human Development Services.

deviation **1.** An abnormality or departure, as in deviation from the norm. **2.** Deviant behavior or attitudes. **3.** In statistics the difference, especially the absolute difference, between one number in a set and the mean of the set. *See also* number; standard deviation; statistics; variant.

deviation, standard *See* standard deviation.

device **1.** In health care, a nondrug item or apparatus, ranging from cotton swabs to artificial heart valves, used for diagnosis, treatment, or prevention of disease. A device specifically does not achieve its purpose through chemical action on or within the body, as compared to drugs. Devices are regulated by the federal Food and Drug Administration. *See also* medical device; Safe Medical Devices Act of 1990. **2.** A contrivance or a means serving a particular purpose, as in a medical device or an input device. *See also* input device.

device, input *See* input device.

device, medical *See* medical device.

Devices Act of 1990, Safe Medical *See* Safe Medical Devices Act of 1990.

DGI *See* Dental Gold Institute.

DGMA *See* Dental Group Management Association.

DHHS *See* Department of Health and Human Services.

DHS *See* Dinshah Health Society.

DIA *See* Drug Information Association.

diabetes *See* diabetes mellitus.

diabetes, adult-onset *See* adult-onset diabetes.

Diabetes Association, American *See* American Diabetes Association.

diabetes, brittle *See* type I diabetes mellitus.

Diabetes Center, Joslin *See* Joslin Diabetes Center.

Diabetes Educators, American Association of *See* American Association of Diabetes Educators.

diabetes, gestational *See* gestational diabetes.

diabetes, insulin-dependent *See* type I diabetes mellitus.

diabetes, juvenile *See* type I diabetes mellitus.

diabetes, juvenile-onset *See* type I diabetes mellitus.

diabetes, maturity-onset *See* type II diabetes mellitus.

diabetes, non-insulin-dependent *See* type II diabetes mellitus.

diabetes mellitus (DM) A complex disorder of carbohydrate, fat, and protein metabolism that is primarily a result of a relative or complete lack of insulin secretion by the pancreas or of defects of the insulin receptors. *See also* diabetic ketoacidosis; glycosuria; glucose; insulin; pancreas; recombinant human insulin; type I diabetes mellitus; type II diabetes mellitus.

diabetes mellitus, type I *See* type I diabetes mellitus.

diabetes mellitus, type II *See* type II diabetes mellitus.

diabetic **1.** A person with diabetes. **2.** Pertaining to diabetes.

diabetic coma *See* diabetic ketoacidosis.

diabetic ketoacidosis (DKA) An acute, life-threatening complication of uncontrolled diabetes mellitus in which urinary loss of water and electrolytes results in abnormally low circulating blood volume, electrolyte imbalance, elevated blood glucose levels, and breakdown of free fatty acids causing acidosis, often with coma (diabetic coma). *See also* blood gas determination; diabetes mellitus; Kussmaul breathing.

diagnosis The determination of and the conclusion arrived at through perception or scrutiny of findings, applied to an individual, family, group, or community. In health care, diagnosis is the process of recognizing the presence of a disease or condition from its symptoms, signs, laboratory findings, and other data, such as responses to therapy. Abbreviated dx. *See also* admitting diagnosis; bedside diagnosis; discharge diagnosis; misdiagnosis; physical diagnosis; physical examination.

diagnosis, admitting *See* admitting diagnosis.

Diagnosis Association, North American Nursing *See* North American Nursing Diagnosis Association.

diagnosis, bedside *See* bedside diagnosis.

diagnosis, clinical *See* clinical diagnosis.

diagnosis, codable *See* codable diagnosis.

diagnosis code A numerical classification system for diseases, conditions, and injuries, used, for instance, in coding patients' admitting and discharge diagnoses. *See also* International Classification of Diseases, Ninth Revision, Clinical Modification.

diagnosis, community *See* community diagnosis.

diagnosis, discharge *See* discharge diagnosis.

diagnosis, electro- *See* electrodiagnosis.

diagnosis, major *See* major diagnosis.

diagnosis, mis- *See* misdiagnosis.

diagnosis, office *See* bedside diagnosis.

Diagnosis, Organization of Teachers of Oral *See* Organization of Teachers of Oral Diagnosis.

diagnosis, other *See* other diagnosis.

diagnosis, physical *See* physical diagnosis.

diagnosis, principal *See* principal diagnosis.

Diagnosis, Radiology, and Medicine, Academy of Oral *See* Academy of Oral Diagnosis, Radiology, and Medicine.

diagnosis-related groups (DRGs) Groupings of diagnostic categories drawn from the *International Classification of Diseases, Ninth Revision, Clinical Modification* and modified by the presence of criteria, such as patient age and presence or absence of significant comorbidities or complications. DRGs are the case-mix measure mandated for Medicare's prospective hospital payments system by the Social Security Amendments of 1983. A major goal of DRGs is to "contain" health costs. *See also* ambulatory visit group; case mix; complication; comorbidity; cost outlier; diagnosis-related groups reimbursement system; Medicare; Social Security Amendments of 1983; uniform capital factor.

diagnosis-related groups (DRGs) reimbursement system A system created by the Social Security Amendments, signed by President Ronald Reagan in April 1983, that established the form of a prospective payment system to be used to reimburse hospitals. Previously, payment to all hospitals was made on a reasonable cost basis. The amount paid under the PPS is based on the average cost of treating a particular condition and DRG into which a discharge is classified, regardless of the number of services received or the length of the patient's stay in the hospital. *See also* cost outlier; diagnosis-related groups (DRGs); prospective payment system; reasonable cost.

diagnosis, secondary *See* other diagnosis.

diagnosis, sero- *See* serodiagnosis.

diagnostic category, major *See* major diagnostic category.

diagnostic image *See* image.

diagnostic imaging *See* imaging.

Diagnostic Imaging, Council on *See* Council on Diagnostic Imaging.

diagnostic journey The sequence of problem-solving steps in which an individual or a team of people moves from the symptoms of a problem to the root causes of the problem. *See also* diagnosis.

diagnostic laboratory immunology The branch of medical science and subspecialty of internal medicine in which laboratory tests and complex procedures are used to diagnose and treat disorders characterized by defective response of the body's immune systems. *See also* immunology; internal medicine.

Diagnostic Manufacturers, Association of Microbiological *See* Association of Microbiological Diagnostic Manufacturers.

diagnostic medical sonographer An allied health professional who uses medical ultrasound under the supervision of a physician responsible for the use and interpretation of ultrasound procedures. A sonographer obtains, reviews, and integrates pertinent patient history and supporting clinical data to improve diagnostic results; performs appropriate procedures and records anatomical, pathological, and/or physiological data for interpretation by a physician; records and processes sonographic data and other pertinent observations made during the procedure for presentation to the interpreting physician; exercises discretion and judgment in the performance of sonographic services; and provides patient education related to medical ultrasound. Diagnostic medical sonographers are one type of allied health professional for which the Committee on Allied Health Education and Accreditation has accredited education programs. *See also* accreditation; allied health professional; ultrasound; ultrasound imaging.

Diagnostic Medical Sonographers, American Registry of *See* American Registry of Diagnostic Medical Sonographers.

Diagnostic Medical Sonographers, Society of *See* Society of Diagnostic Medical Sonographers.

Diagnostic Medical Sonography, Joint Review Committee on Education in *See* Joint Review Committee on Education in Diagnostic Medical Sonography.

diagnostic profile A physician, hospital, or population profile subcategorized by specific condition or diagnosis. *See also* diagnostic profiling; profile; profiling.

diagnostic profiling A process of subcategorizing by specific condition or diagnosis a physician, hospital, or population. *See also* diagnostic profile; profile; profiling.

diagnostic radiological physics The branch of medical physics that deals with the diagnostic applications of roentgen rays (x-rays), gamma rays from sealed sources, of ultrasonic radiation, and radio-frequency radiation, and with the equipment associated with their production and use. *See also* radiological physics.

diagnostic radiology The branch of radiology that deals with the utilization of all modalities of radiant energy in medical diagnoses and therapeutic procedures using radiologic guidance. This includes, but is not restricted to, imaging techniques and methodologies utilizing radiation emitted by x-ray tubes, radionuclides, and ultrasonographic devices and the radiofrequency electromagnetic radiation emitted by atoms. *See also* radiology.

diagnostic service, ultrasonic *See* ultrasonic diagnostic service.

Diagnostics, National Foundation for Non-Invasive *See* National Foundation for Non-Invasive Diagnostics.

Diagnostic and Statistical Manual of Mental Disorders (Third Edition - Revised) A manual published by the American Psychiatric Association that provides a classification of mental disorders; often referred to as *DSM-III-R*. *See also* American Psychiatric Association.

diagnostic study Any investigative procedure, such as physical examination, x-rays, or laboratory tests, requested or performed by a physician to help establish the identity, severity, nature, and extent of a patient's disease or condition. *Synonym*: diagnostic test. *See also* diagnosis; test.

diagnostic test *See* diagnostic study.

Diagnostic and Therapeutic Technology Assessment (DATTA) Program A program run by the American Medical Association for assessing medical technology, with the purpose of providing authoritative information to physicians on the appropriate use of specific medical technology. *See also* American Medical Association; technology assessment.

diagram A plan, sketch, drawing, outline, graph, or chart designed to demonstrate or explain how something works or to clarify the relationship between the parts of a whole. *See also* affinity diagram; cause-and-effect diagram; scatter diagram.

diagram, affinity *See* affinity diagram.

diagram, cause-and-effect *See* cause-and-effect diagram.

diagram, Ishikawa *See* cause-and-effect diagram.

diagram, scatter *See* scatter diagram.

dialysis The separation of smaller molecules from larger molecules or of dissolved substances from colloidal particles in a solution by selective diffusion through a semipermeable membrane, as in hemodialysis. *See also* hemodialysis; peritoneal dialysis.

dialysis disease A collective name for the disorders, such as bone disease due to disturbance of calcium metabolism and anemia, arising during the management of chronic renal failure by prolonged intermittent kidney dialysis. It is thought to be attributable to the method of treatment rather than to the primary kidney condition. *See also* hemodialysis.

dialysis, hemo- *See* hemodialysis.

dialysis, peritoneal *See* peritoneal dialysis.

dialysis technician An individual trained in operating and maintaining the dialysis equipment used in the treatment of kidney disease, who works under the direction of a physician. *Synonym*: nephrology technician. *See also* hemodialysis; technician.

Dialysis and Transplantation, North American Society for *See* North American Society for Dialysis and Transplantation.

Diamond Foundation, The Aaron *See* The Aaron Diamond Foundation, Inc.

diaphoretic Pertaining to sweating.

diarrhea Excessive and frequent evacuation of watery feces, usually a symptom of gastrointestinal distress or disorder. *See also* antidiarrheal; feces; gastroenteritis; traveler's diarrhea.

diarrhea, traveler's *See* traveler's diarrhea.

diathermy Heat treatment in body tissues by high-frequency currents that are insufficiently intense to destroy tissues or to impair their vitality. Diathermy is used in treating chronic arthritis, bursitis, fractures, and other conditions.

dichotomous Dividing or divided into two parts or classifications. *See also* dichotomous scale.

dichotomous scale A scale that arranges items into either of two mutually exclusive categories, for example, a neonate sustains or does not sustain birth trauma. *Synonym*: dichotomous measurement scale. *See also* dichotomous; scale.

dicta The commentary of a judge in a written opinion that indicates his or her feelings on the matters under discussion but that is not necessary to the decision in the case. Dicta are not binding on courts in subsequent cases. *See also* judge.

dictation The act or process of saying or reading aloud material to another person for transcription. *See also* digital dictation; transcription.

dictation, digital *See* digital dictation.

Die, Choice in Dying - The National Council for the Right to *See* Choice in Dying - The National Council for the Right to Die.

diener An individual who maintains morgue equipment and facilities and, under the supervision of a pathologist, assists in performing autopsies. *See also* autopsy; morgue.

diet **1.** The items a person usually eats and drinks. **2.** Special food and drink planned to meet specific requirements of an individual, as in a modified diet or a low-sodium diet. *See also* nutrition.

dietary allowances, recommended *See* recommended dietary allowances.

dietary department *See* foodservice department.

dietary intakes, recommended *See* recommended dietary intakes.

Dietary Managers Association (DMA) A national organization founded in 1960 composed of 12,000 dietary managers interested in competency and quality in dietary departments and their management. *See also* foodservice department.

Dietary Support Coalition, American Celiac Society/ *See* American Celiac Society/Dietary Support Coalition.

dietetic assistant An individual who assists in providing foodservice supervision and nutritional care services under the guidance of a registered or consultant dietitian or administrator. Services may include preparing food menus from dietary instructions, maintaining sanitary conditions for food, and ordering and maintaining food and foodservice inventories. *See also* diet; dietetics; foodservice department.

Dietetic Association, American *See* American Dietetic Association.

Dietetic Association, Seventh-Day Adventist *See* Seventh-Day Adventist Dietetic Association.

dietetic educator An individual who is responsible for creating and presenting the curriculum for dietetic practitioners and for nutrition education for medical, nursing, dental, and allied health personnel. Dietetic educators usually work in a medical center, university, or college setting. *See also* curriculum; dietetics.

dietetic technician An individual who assists

dietetic assistants, foodservice supervisors, or dietitians in planning, implementing, and evaluating food programs, teaching nutrition, and providing dietary counseling. *See also* dietetics; technician.

dietetics The science dealing with the relationships of foods and nutrition to human health. *See also* nutrition.

dietitian An individual qualified by training to use his or her knowledge of nutrition to help people maintain or recover good health. *See also* administrative dietitian; clinical dietitian; consultant dietitian; nutritionist; registered dietitian; research dietitian.

dietitian, administrative *See* administrative dietitian.

dietitian, clinical *See* clinical dietitian.

dietitian, consultant *See* consultant dietitian.

dietitian, registered *See* registered dietitian.

dietitian, research *See* research dietitian.

Dietitians in Health Care Facilities, Consultant *See* Consultant Dietitians in Health Care Facilities.

diet, ketogenic *See* ketogenic diet.

differential cost *See* marginal cost.

digestion The process by which food is converted into substances that can be absorbed and assimilated by the body. It is accomplished in the alimentary canal by the mechanical and enzymatic breakdown of foods into simpler chemical compounds. *See also* alimentary tract; digestive gland; digestive system; saliva.

Digestive Disease National Coalition (DDNC) A national organization founded in 1979 composed of 30 professional medical and lay organizations interested in digestive diseases. Its objectives are to inform the public and the health care community about digestive diseases and related nutrition and seek federal funding for research, education, and training. Formerly (1986) Coalition of Digestive Disease Organizations. *See also* digestive system; gastroenterology.

Digestive Diseases Information Clearinghouse, National *See* National Digestive Diseases Information Clearinghouse.

digestive gland A gland, such as the liver or pancreas, that secretes into the alimentary canal substances necessary for digestion. *See also* digestion; digestive system; gland; liver; pancreas.

digestive system The alimentary canal and digestive glands regarded as an integrated system responsible for the ingestion, digestion, and absorption of food. *See also* alimentary tract; digestion; gas-

troenterology; pediatric gastroenterology.

digestive tract *See* alimentary tract.

digit One of ten Arabic numerical symbols, 0 through 9.

digital **1.** Expressed in digits, especially for use by a computer. **2.** Using or giving a reading in digits, as in digital data. *See also* digital data.

digital computer The most common type of business and scientific computer that performs calculations and logical operations with quantities expressed directly as digits, usually in the binary number system. *Compare* analog computer. *See also* computer.

digital conversion, analog-to- *See* analog-to-digital conversion.

digital data Data expressed in digits especially for use by a computer. Digital data is represented by discrete individual numbers (for example, a digital watch) rather than by a continuous flow of information, as with analog data. *Compare* analog data. *See also* analog-to-digital conversion; data.

digital dictation An approach to creating a medical record that, instead of representing sound (speech) as an electromagnetic wave (as in a tape recorder), stores it as large groups of numbers (digits) representing the amplitude (loudness) and frequency (pitch) of the source (speech). These numbers are specific for a file (such as one dictated medical record) and are stored on tape, computer disk, or laser disk. The file can be randomly or instantly retrieved and played back before, during, or after transcription. *See also* automated speech recognition; dictation; transcription.

digitalis A drug prepared from the seed and dried leaves of the plant genus *Digitalis*, which includes foxglove. The drug acts as a cardiac stimulant. *See also* chelation therapy; congestive heart failure; drug; heart.

dilation and curettage (D and C) A surgical procedure in which the cervix is expanded using a dilator and the uterine lining is scraped with a curette, performed for the diagnosis and treatment of various uterine conditions. *See also* curettage; curette; gynecology; uterus.

dimension An aspect or element, as in the dimensions of performance. *See also* dimensions of performance.

dimensional, multi- *See* multidimensional.

dimensions of performance Attributes of organizational performance that are related to organizations "doing the right things" (that is, appropriateness, availability, and efficacy) and "doing things well" (that is, continuity, effectiveness, efficiency, respect and caring, safety, and timeliness). Performance dimensions are definable, measurable, and improvable. *See also* appropriateness; availability; continuity; effectiveness; efficacy; multidimensional; respect and caring; safety; timeliness.

diminishing marginal return   An economic principle stating that as more units of a product or service are consumed, the marginal benefit decreases. *See also* economics.

diminishing returns   A phenomenon that beyond a certain point, adding additional units of resources to a production process will provide successively smaller increments of additional product. This is often due to crowding or adding less experienced or less appropriate resources. *Synonym*: law of diminishing returns.

Dinshah Health Society (DHS)   An organization founded in 1976 composed of 300 health professionals and other individuals who use and promote chromotherapy. *See also* chromotherapy.

diopter   A unit of measurement of the refractive power of lenses equal to the reciprocal of the focal length measured in meters; it is commonly used in measuring ocular refraction. *See also* dioptometer.

Diopter and Decibel Society, American   *See* American Diopter and Decibel Society.

dioptometer   An instrument used for measuring ocular refraction. *See also* diopter.

diphtheria   An acute infectious disease, primarily of young children, affecting the nose, throat, larynx, and skin. It is due to the bacterium *Corynebacterium diphtheriae*, which produces a powerful toxin. The toxin is carried in the circulation to affect the heart and peripheral nervous system causing heart failure and variable paralysis. Active immunization has reduced the incidence of the disease in the past 40 years. *See also* active immunization; DPT; infectious diseases; toxin.

diploma   A document issued by an educational institution, such as a university or a nursing school, testifying that the recipient has earned a degree or has successfully completed a course of study. *See also* certificate; diploma nurse; diploma school.

diploma nurse   A nurse whose education was obtained in a hospital school of nursing which granted a diploma rather than an academic degree. *Compare* degree nurse. *See also* diploma school; nursing.

diploma school   A school that is hospital owned and administered and that provides diplomas on the successful completion of required courses or assignment, rather than degrees. Typically, classroom courses and laboratory instruction are provided by nearby colleges, or credit is given for courses taken elsewhere. Diploma programs include nursing, laboratory technology, and x-ray technology. *See also* associate degree school of nursing; baccalaureate degree program; nursing.

diplomate   An individual who has received a diploma, such as a physician certified by a medical specialty board; for example, a diplomate of the American Board of Emergency Medicine. *See also* board certified.

Diplomates of the American Board of Orthodontics, College of   *See* College of Diplomates of the American Board of Orthodontics.

dipsomania   *See* potomania.

direct access   *See* random access.

direct cause   A cause that sets in motion a chain of events that brings about a result without the intervention of any other independent source. *See also* cause.

direct contact   A mode of transmission of infection between an infected host and a susceptible host. It occurs when skin or mucous surfaces touch, as in shaking hands, kissing, and sexual intercourse. *Compare* indirect contact. *See also* contact; infection; syphilis.

direct cost   The cost that is directly identifiable with a particular service or area, such as the operating room. *See also* cost.

directed verdict   An order of the court that may be issued at the request of either party at the conclusion of the opposing party's presentation of evidence or at the conclusion of the trial. It is a determination by the trial judge that the evidence or law so clearly favors one party that it is pointless for the trial to proceed. The judge decides that one side or the other is entitled to a judgment as a matter of law, taking the issue out of the hands of the jury. The conclusion of the judge should be so obvious that reasonable minds could not arrive at a differing conclusion. For example, a defendant physician, at the conclusion of the plaintiff's case, may move for a verdict in his or her favor (a directed verdict) based on an assertion that the plaintiff has failed to present sufficient evidence upon which a jury could return a verdict for the plaintiff. *See also* court; evidence; judge; jury; trial; verdict.

direct evidence   Means of proof that tends to show the existence of a fact in question, without the intervention of the proof of any other fact. Direct evidence is distinguished from circumstantial. *Compare* circumstantial evidence. *See also* evidence.

direct examination   In torts, the questioning of a witness by the party that has called the witness to render testimony. It is generally the first interrogation and is followed by a cross-examination conducted by the opposing party. *See also* cross-examination; examination; leading question; witness.

direct food additives   Substances that are intentionally added to food to improve flavor, texture, or color or to prevent spoilage. *Compare* indirect food additives. *See also* additive.

directives, advance   *See* advance directives.

director   **1.** A person who directs, controls, supervises, or manages an organization or a component thereof. **2.** A member of a governing body, as in a board of directors. *See also* governing body.

director of buildings and grounds   *See* administrative engineer.

director of development   An individual charged with soliciting contributions and finding contributors, including the planning, implementation, communications, liaison, and reporting work associated with this. *Synonym*: philanthropy director. *See also* development.

director, education   *See* education director.

director, funeral   *See* funeral director.

director of medical affairs   *See* chief of staff; medical director.

director, medical education   *See* medical education director.

director of nursing   *See* chief of nursing; nurse executive.

director, outside   *See* outside director.

director, public relations   *See* public relations director.

director, purchasing   *See* purchasing director.

director of quality assurance, physician   *See* physician director of quality assurance.

Directors of America, Association of Life Insurance Medical   *See* Association of Life Insurance Medical Directors of America.

Directors, Association of Academic Health Sciences Library   *See* Association of Academic Health Sciences

Library Directors.

Directors Association, American Medical   *See* American Medical Directors Association.

Directors Association, State Medicaid   *See* State Medicaid Directors Association.

Directors, Association of State and Territorial Dental   *See* Association of State and Territorial Dental Directors.

directors, board of   *See* governing body.

Directors in Internal Medicine, Association of Program   *See* Association of Program Directors in Internal Medicine.

Directors of Medical Education, Academy of Osteopathic   *See* Academy of Osteopathic Directors of Medical Education.

Directors, National Association of State EMS   *See* National Association of State EMS Directors.

Directors, National Association of State Mental Health Program   *See* National Association of State Mental Health Program Directors.

Directors, National Association of State Mental Retardation Program   *See* National Association of State Mental Retardation Program Directors.

Directors of Nursing Administration in Long Term Care, National Association of   *See* National Association of Directors of Nursing Administration in Long Term Care.

Directors of Nursing, Association of State and Territorial   *See* Association of State and Territorial Directors of Nursing.

directors' and officers' (D & O) liability insurance   Insurance for corporate directors and officers against claims based on negligence and failure to disclose. Such insurance provides coverage against expenses, and to a limited extent, fines, judgments, and amounts paid in settlement. *See also* corporate; indemnification; insurance.

Directors of Psychiatric Residency Training, American Association of   *See* American Association of Directors of Psychiatric Residency Training.

Directors of Public Health Education, Association of State and Territorial   *See* Association of State and Territorial Directors of Public Health Education.

Directors, Society for Hospital Social Work   *See* Society for Hospital Social Work Directors.

Directors of Volunteer Services, American Society of   *See* American Society of Directors of Volunteer Services.

Directory of Residency Training Programs An annual publication of the Accreditation Council for Graduate Medical Education of the American Medical Association. It provides medical students anticipating residency training and other persons with an official listing of accredited programs in postgraduate medical training, requirements for accreditation of residency programs, and board certification requirements for individual medical specialties. Also known as the "Green Book" because of the color of its cover. *See also* Accreditation Council for Graduate Medical Education; American Medical Association; board certified; medical specialties; medical student; residency; residency program.

Disabilities, Accreditation Council on Services for People with Developmental *See* Accreditation Council on Services for People with Developmental Disabilities.

Disabilities Act of 1990, Americans with *See* Americans with Disabilities Act of 1990.

Disabilities, American Association of University Affiliated Programs for Persons with Developmental *See* American Association of University Affiliated Programs for Persons with Developmental Disabilities.

Disabilities, Council for Learning *See* Council for Learning Disabilities.

Disabilities Councils, National Association of Developmental *See* National Association of Developmental Disabilities Councils.

Disabilities, National Information Center for Children and Youth with *See* National Information Center for Children and Youth with Disabilities.

disability Any restriction or limitation resulting from an impairment of ability to perform an activity in a manner or with the range considered normal for a human being, according to the *International Classification of Impairments, Disabilities, and Handicaps* first published in 1908 by the World Health Organization. The term disability reflects the consequences of impairment. *See also* developmental disability; handicap; impairment; learning disability; nonservice-connected disability; occupational disability; partial disability; permanent disability; service-connected disability; temporary disability; total disability; unemployment compensation disability.

Disability, Coalition on Sexuality and *See* Coalition on Sexuality and Disability.

disability compensation Compensation made to disabled employees. *See also* unemployment compensation disability.

Disability Consultants, American Board of Professional *See* American Board of Professional Disability Consultants.

disability, developmental *See* developmental disability.

Disability Evaluating Physicians, American Academy of *See* American Academy of Disability Evaluating Physicians.

Disability Evaluating Professionals, National Association of *See* National Association of Disability Evaluating Professionals.

Disability Examiners, National Association of *See* National Association of Disability Examiners.

Disability Information, Clearinghouse on *See* Clearinghouse on Disability Information.

disability insurance Insurance designed to compensate individuals who lose wages because of illness or injury. *See also* worker's compensation insurance; unemployment compensation disability.

disability insurance, state *See* unemployment compensation disability.

Disability Insurance Training Council (DITC) The educational arm of the National Association of Health Underwriters founded in 1951 composed of 11,000 members. It provides institutional advanced disability income and health insurance research seminars as well as marketing and underwriting clinics. It maintains the Health Insurance Training Council, Disability Training Insurance Council, and Registered Health Underwriters. *See also* disability insurance; National Association of Health Underwriters.

Disability Law, Commission on Mental and Physical *See* Commission on Mental and Physical Disability Law.

disability, learning *See* learning disability.

Disability, National Organization on *See* National Organization on Disability.

disability, nonservice-connected *See* nonservice-connected disability.

disability, occupational *See* occupational disability.

disability, partial *See* partial disability.

disability, permanent *See* permanent disability.

Disability and Rehabilitation Research, National Institute on *See* National Institute on Disability and Rehabilitation Research.

disability retirement Retirement made necessary

by the physical or mental inability to perform a job. *See also* disability; retirement.

disability, service-connected   *See* service-connected disability.

disability, temporary   *See* temporary disability.

disability, total   *See* total disability.

disability, unemployment compensation   *See* unemployment compensation disability.

disabled   **1.** Impaired, as in physical or mental functioning. **2.** Physically or mentally impaired persons considered as a group.

disabled veteran   A veteran of the armed services who has a service-connected disability and is considered to be disabled to an extent of 10 percent or greater by the Veterans Administration. *See also* Department of Veterans Affairs; veteran.

disaster   An occurrence causing widespread destruction and distress; a catastrophe. *See also* disaster drill; emergency preparedness plan/program.

disaster drill   A simulation of a disaster to assess and improve the effectiveness of a health care organization's or system's disaster preparedness plan. *See also* disaster preparedness plan; emergency preparedness plan/program.

disaster plan   *See* disaster preparedness plan.

Disaster Preparedness, Doctors for   *See* Doctors for Disaster Preparedness.

disaster preparedness plan   A formal written plan of action for coordinating the response of a hospital staff in the event of a disaster within the hospital or the community. *See also* disaster; emergency preparedness plan/program.

disc   *See* hard disk.

discharge   In health care, the form of release of a patient from a provider's care. *See also* admitting department; against medical advice; discharge abstract; discharge by death; discharge by transfer; disposition; patient discharge.

discharge abstract   A summary description of data abstracted from a hospitalized patient's medical record that usually includes specific clinical data, such as diagnostic and procedure codes, as well as other information about the patient, the physician, and insurance and financial status. An example of a discharge abstract is the Uniform Hospital Discharge Abstract. *See also* hospital discharge abstract system; Uniform Hospital Discharge Data Set.

discharge abstract system, hospital   *See* hospital discharge abstract system.

discharge against medical advice   *See* against medical advice.

discharge coordinator   *See* discharge planner.

discharge by death   The form of discharge occurring when a patient dies in a hospital or other type of health care organization. *See also* death; discharge.

discharge diagnosis   A diagnosis supplied by the attending physician at the time of the discharge of a patient from a hospital or other health care organization. The discharge diagnosis is likely to be the principal diagnosis. *See also* attending physician; diagnosis; principal diagnosis.

discharge instructions   The list of instructions given to a patient on discharge, as in how to take medications and when and from whom to obtain continuing care. *See also* discharge.

discharge, patient   *See* patient discharge.

discharge planner   An individual whose duties include planning for patients' continuing and follow-up care. *Synonym*: discharge coordinator. *See also* discharge planning.

discharge planning   A formalized process in a health care organization through which a program of continuing and follow-up care is planned and carried out for each patient. Discharge planning is a documented sequence of tasks and activities designed to achieve, within projected timeframes, stated goals that lead to the timely release of patients to either their homes or to facilities or programs with a lower level of care. Discharge planning is undertaken to ensure that patients stay in a hospital or other type of health care organization only for as long as medically needed. *See also* American Association for Continuity of Care; discharge planner; social work discharge planning.

discharge planning, social work   *See* social work discharge planning.

discharge summary   *See* clinical resume.

discharge by transfer   A transfer of a patient from one health care organization to another where the patient is admitted. *See also* discharge by death; transfer.

disciplinary action   Any action short of dismissal taken by an employer against an employee for violation of policy. *See also* dismissal; state medical boards' disciplinary actions.

disciplinary actions by state medical boards   *See* state medical boards' disciplinary actions.

disciplinary demotion A demotion resulting when an employee persists in some kind of misconduct or disruptive behavior having been repeatedly warned to stop. *See also* demotion.

discipline 1. A branch of teaching or knowledge, as in the disciplines of medicine or nursing. *See also* multidisciplinary; subdiscipline. 2. Punishment intended to correct or train. *See also* disciplinary action; disciplinary demotion.

discipline, sub- *See* subdiscipline.

discount A deduction from a specified sum, as in to reduce a usual fee or charge for health care services.

discoverable Pertaining to information that may be legally obtained by a party to a lawsuit, from the adverse party. Not all such information is admissible during a trial, however; the rules concerning discoverable information are much broader than the rules of admissibility. *See also* admissible evidence; lawsuit.

discovery The modern pretrial procedure by which one party gains information held by another party. The scope of material available for discovery is broad under the Federal Rules of Civil Procedure. *See also* deposition; discovery rule.

discovery rule A provision in some jurisdictions' statutes of limitations that requires a plaintiff to file certain types of lawsuits within a specific time after a wrongful act is discovered or should have been discovered if the plaintiff was reasonably alert to the problem. In some jurisdictions, application of the discovery rule is limited to cases involving a foreign object left in the body of a patient. *See also* discovery; rule; statute of limitations.

discrepancy Disagreement or divergence, as between facts or findings. *See also* nonconformities.

discrete Constituting a separate thing; distinct, as in discrete data. *See also* discrete data.

discrete data Data that can be arranged into naturally occurring or arbitrarily selected groups or sets of values, as opposed to continuous data, which have no naturally occurring breaks. An example of discrete data is the number of medical records that are complete and incomplete per given measurement period. *Compare* continuous data. *See also* data; discrete; discrete variable; probability distribution.

discrete probability distribution *See* probability distribution.

discrete variable A measurement that is limited to discrete options (for example, yes/no/unknown; less than or equal to 20 minutes/greater than 20 minutes). *Compare* continuous variable. *See also* discrete data; variable.

discrete variable indicator *See* rate-based indicator.

discriminant validity A demonstration of the validity of a measure by the lack of correlation among two or more supposedly unrelated measures of a concept. *See also* validity.

discrimination 1. The ability or power to make a clear distinction. 2. Treatment or consideration based on class or category rather than individual merit; partiality or prejudice. *See also* price discrimination.

discrimination, price *See* price discrimination.

disease A pathological or abnormal condition of a part, an organ, or a system of an organism resulting from one or more causes, such as an infection and/or a genetic defect, and characterized by an identifiable group of signs or symptoms. *See also* acute disease; chronic disease; health; illness; incubation period; notifiable disease; self-limited; sickness; staging.

disease, acute *See* acute disease.

Disease Association, American Venereal *See* American Venereal Disease Association.

Disease, Association for Research in Nervous and Mental *See* Association for Research in Nervous and Mental Disease.

disease, Alzheimer's *See* Alzheimer's disease.

disease, black lung *See* black lung disease.

disease, celiac *See* celiac disease.

disease, chronic *See* chronic disease.

Disease Clinics, National Coalition of Black Lung and Respiratory *See* National Coalition of Black Lung and Respiratory Disease Clinics.

disease, communicable *See* communicable disease.

disease, dialysis *See* dialysis disease.

disease, end stage renal *See* end stage renal disease.

disease, fatty liver *See* fatty liver disease.

disease, genetic *See* genetic disease.

disease, Graves' *See* Graves' disease.

disease, Hansen's *See* leprosy.

disease, Hodgkin's *See* Hodgkin's disease.

disease, iatrogenic *See* iatrogenic disease.

disease, industrial *See* occupational disease.

disease insurance, specified *See* specified disease insurance.

disease, malignant *See* malignant disease.

disease, metabolic   *See* metabolic disease.

Disease, National Association for Sickle Cell   *See* National Association for Sickle Cell Disease.

Disease National Coalition, Digestive   *See* Digestive Disease National Coalition.

disease, natural history of   *See* natural history of disease.

disease, notifiable   *See* notifiable disease.

disease, occupational   *See* occupational disease.

disease, organic   *See* organic disease.

disease, Parkinson's   *See* Parkinson's disease.

disease, pediatric infectious   *See* pediatric infectious disease.

disease, pelvic inflammatory   *See* pelvic inflammatory disease.

disease, periodontal   *See* periodontal disease.

disease, peripheral vascular   *See* peripheral vascular disease.

Disease Prevention and Health Promotion, Office of   *See* Office of Disease Prevention and Health Promotion.

disease, renal   *See* renal disease.

disease, reportable   *See* notifiable disease.

disease, sacred   *See* epilepsy.

Diseases, American Association for the Study of Liver   *See* American Association for the Study of Liver Diseases.

diseases, classification of   *See* classification of diseases.

disease, sexually transmitted   *See* sexually transmitted disease.

diseases, infectious   *See* infectious diseases.

Diseases Information Clearinghouse, National Arthritis and Musculoskeletal and Skin   *See* National Arthritis and Musculoskeletal and Skin Diseases Information Clearinghouse.

Diseases Information Clearinghouse, National Digestive   *See* National Digestive Diseases Information Clearinghouse.

Diseases Information Clearinghouse, National Kidney and Urologic   *See* National Kidney and Urologic Diseases Information Clearinghouse.

disease, social   *See* sexually transmitted disease.

Disease, Society for the Study of Breast   *See* Society for the Study of Breast Disease.

disease specialist, pediatric infectious   *See* pediatric infectious disease specialist.

disease-specific death rate   The number of deaths caused by a disease in relation to a given population over a given period, usually expressed as the number of deaths per 100,000 persons. *See also* child death rate; fetal death rate; hospital death rate; infant death rate; maternal mortality rate; mortality rate; neonatal death rate.

Diseases Society of America, Infectious   *See* Infectious Diseases Society of America.

disease staging   *See* staging.

diseases unit, respiratory   *See* respiratory diseases unit.

disease, surveillance of   *See* surveillance of disease.

disease, venereal   *See* venereal disease.

disincentive   A negative incentive. *See also* incentive.

disinfect   To cleanse so as to destroy or prevent the growth of pathogenic microorganisms. *See also* disinfectant.

disinfectant   An agent, such as heat, radiation, or a chemical, that disinfects by destroying, neutralizing, or inhibiting the growth of pathogenic microorganisms. *See also* antisepsis; lysol; microorganism.

disinterest   Freedom from selfish bias or self-interest, as in a disinterested ethicist who had nothing to gain or lose from the outcome of a case. Disinterest does not imply a lack of interest. *See also* dispassion; ideal ethical observer.

disk   *See* hard disk.

disk, compact   *See* compact disk.

disk drive   A computer device that holds and "plays" a disk that spins at high speeds, equipped with a head that allows electric impulses to be written onto and read from the electromagnetic surface. A disk drive allows random access to information on a disk. *Synonym:* computer disk drive. *See also* computer; diskette; random access.

diskette   A flexible plastic, oxide-coated disk, contained in a special square jacket, for use in a computer disk drive. It is used on a small computer for magnetically storing information. A standard-sized diskette is 5 1/4 inches, while a microfloppy disk is 3 1/2 inches. *Synonyms:* flexible disk; floppy; floppy disk. *See also* disk drive; jacket; microfloppy disk.

disk, hard   *See* hard disk.

disk, laser   *See* laser disk.

disk, magnetic   *See* magnetic disk.

disk, microfloppy   *See* microfloppy disk.

disk operating system (DOS)   A set of hardware instruction programs stored on a disk that a computer reads in order to know how to run application programs, such as an accounts payable program or a mailing list. *See also* MS-DOS; operating environment.

disk, optical *See* compact disk.

dismissal 1. The removal by an organization's management of an employee from employment. **2.** The termination of a lawsuit. *See also* dismissal with prejudice; dismissal without prejudice.

dismissal with prejudice The termination of a lawsuit without the right to reinstitute the proceeding. *See also* demurrer; lawsuit.

dismissal without prejudice The termination of a lawsuit that reserves the right to reinstitute the proceedings. *See also* lawsuit.

disorder An abnormal physical or mental condition, as in eating disorder or a personality disorder.

disorder, affective *See* affective disorder.

disorder, attention-deficit *See* attention-deficit disorder.

disorder, eating *See* eating disorder.

disorder, major affective *See* major affective disorder.

disorder, manic-depressive *See* manic-depressive disorder.

disorder, narcissistic personality *See* narcissistic personality disorder.

disorder, obsessive-compulsive personality *See* obsessive-compulsive personality disorder.

disorder, passive-aggressive personality *See* passive-aggressive personality disorder.

disorder, personality *See* personality disorder.

disorder, posttraumatic stress *See* posttraumatic stress disorder.

disorder, sadistic personality *See* sadistic personality disorder.

Disorders Association, American Sleep *See* American Sleep Disorders Association.

Disorders, Council on Anxiety *See* Council on Anxiety Disorders.

Disorders, Council for Children with Behavioral *See* Council for Children with Behavioral Disorders.

disorder, seasonal affective *See* seasonal affective disorder.

Disorders, National Coalition on Immune System *See* National Coalition on Immune System Disorders.

Disorders, National Coalition for Research in Neurological *See* National Coalition for Research in Neurological Disorders.

dispassion Freedom from passion or bias. Dispassion does not imply lack of feeling or emotion. *Synonym:* objectivity. *See also* disinterest; ideal ethical observer.

dispensary A place where medical or dental care is dispensed, as in a school or other institution.

Dispensing Audiologists, Academy of *See* Academy of Dispensing Audiologists.

dispensing, drug *See* drug dispensing.

dispensing fee The fee charged by a pharmacist for filling a prescription. Dispensing fees are the same in a given pharmacy for all prescriptions, and therefore represent a larger percentage markup on the cost of an inexpensive drug or small prescription than on the cost of an expensive drug or large prescription. The fixed dispensing fee reflects the identical nature of the pharmacist's service whatever the cost of the drug being dispensed. A dispensing fee is one of two ways in which pharmacists charge for filling prescriptions, the other being a standard percentage markup on the acquisition cost of drugs. Some pharmacists combine the two approaches, using a percentage markup with a minimum dispensing fee. *See also* fee; pharmacist; prescription.

dispensing, medication *See* medication dispensing.

dispensing optician *See* optician.

disposition 1. An act of transferring to another, as in appropriate disposition of a patient. *See also* against medical advice; discharge; patient discharge. **2.** An individual's nature or temperament. **3.** The act of arranging, managing, or putting affairs into order.

dissect To cut apart piece by piece and examine in detail, as in a medical examiner or coroner's dissection of a body. *See also* autopsy; cadaver; resect.

dissent To differ in opinion or belief; to disagree, as in a person cast the lone dissenting vote. *Compare* concur.

dissonance, cognitive *See* cognitive dissonance.

distal Remote; farther from any point of reference, as in the wrist is distal to the elbow (point of reference, the shoulder). *Compare* proximal.

distress syndrome, respiratory *See* respiratory distress syndrome.

distribution In statistics, the complete summary of the frequencies of the values or categories of measurement made on a group of persons or other entities. The distribution tells either how many or what proportion of the group was found to have each value (or each range of values) out of all the possible values that the quantitative measure can have. A bell-shaped curve or normal distribution is an example of a distribution in which the greatest number of observations fall in the center with fewer and fewer observations falling evenly on either side of the average. *Synonym*: frequency distribution. *See also* bimodal distribution; normal distribution; probability distribution; *t*-distribution.

distribution, Bernouille *See* binomial distribution.

distribution, bimodal *See* bimodal distribution.

distribution, blood *See* blood distribution.

distribution, chi-square *See* chi-square distribution.

distribution, frequency *See* distribution.

distribution, normal *See* normal distribution.

distribution, Poisson *See* Poisson distribution.

distribution, probability *See* probability distribution.

distribution, *t*- *See* *t*-distribution.

Distributors Association, Health Industry *See* Health Industry Distributors Association.

Distributors Association, Independent Medical *See* Independent Medical Distributors Association.

district A political jurisdiction with geographic boundaries, as in a hospital, ambulance, fire, or sanitation district. Districts are created to finance and organize special functions. *See also* district hospital.

district hospital A type of hospital that is controlled by a political subdivision of a state; this subdivision is created solely for the purpose of establishing and maintaining health care organizations. *See also* district; hospital.

districting The process of establishing a district's geographic boundaries. *See also* district.

DITC *See* Disability Insurance Training Council.

diuresis An increased excretion of urine. *See also* diuretic.

diuretic A substance that causes the body to excrete urine. *See also* diuresis.

diversification The trend of corporations, including health care organizations, such as hospitals, to enter different business areas in an effort to obtain revenue from a variety of sources and remain solvent. The organization is typically restructured in the process of diversification, and foundations, holding companies, and other entities may result. *See also* corporatization of health care; holding company; network; restructuring.

diverticula *See* diverticulum.

diverticulitis A condition in which diverticula (sacs which bulge outward from the walls of the intestine or other organs or cavities) become inflamed, which can result in bleeding, pain, and perforation. *See also* diverticulosis; diverticulum; inflammation; intestine.

diverticulosis A condition in which diverticula (sacs which bulge outward from the walls of the intestine or other organs or cavities) form. *See also* diverticulitis; diverticulum; intestine.

diverticulum A blind sac-like enlargement of the wall of a larger cavity. Diverticula of the colon caused by herniation of the mucous and submucous intestinal layers through areas of weakness in the muscular wall are common in the second half of adult life. This condition is called diverticulosis and is asymptomatic unless inflammation, called diverticulitis, occurs. *See also* diverticulitis; diverticulosis; intestine.

Divinity, Master of *See* Master of Divinity.

Division of Ambulatory Care A division of the American Hospital Association founded in 1970 composed of 2,000 hospitals and other health providers with interests in ambulatory care, emergency services, home care, health maintenance organizations, and hospices. Formerly (1990) Division of Ambulatory Care and Health Promotion. *See also* ambulatory health care; American Hospital Association.

Division of Ambulatory Care and Health Promotion *See* Division of Ambulatory Care.

Division of Applied Experimental and Engineering Psychologists (DAEEP) A division of the American Psychological Association founded in 1957 composed of 600 individuals whose principal fields of study, research, or work are within the area of general engineering psychology. It promotes research on psychological factors in the design and use of environments and systems within which human beings work and live. *See also* American Psychological Association; engineering psychology.

Division of Family Psychology (Div. 43) A division of the American Psychological Association founded in 1984 composed of 1,500 psychologists interested in family, marital, and sex psychology. *See also* American Psychological Association; family; psychology.

Division of Psychotherapy of the American Psychological Association A division of the American Psychological Association founded in 1964 composed of 5,000 psychologists and psychotherapists interested in exchanging scientific and technical information about psychotherapy. *See also* American Psychological Association; psychotherapy.

DKA *See* diabetic ketoacidosis.

DM *See* diabetes mellitus.

DMA *See* Dental Manufacturers of America; Dietary Managers Association.

DMD *See* Doctor of Dental Medicine.

DME *See* durable medical equipment.

DNA *See* deoxyribonucleic acid; Dermatology Nurses' Association.

DNA fingerprinting *See* genetic fingerprinting.

DNA, recombinant *See* recombinant DNA.

DNR *See* do-not-resuscitate order.

DO *See* Doctor of Osteopathy.

DOA Abbreviation for dead on arrival.

DOB Abbreviation for date of birth.

DOC *See* Department of Commerce.

doctor A physician, dentist, podiatrist, chiropractor, scientist, administrator, businessperson, theologian, or other person holding a doctoral degree awarded by a recognized academic or professional school. Abbreviated *Dr. See also* chiropractor; dentist; doctorate; physician; podiatrist; witch doctor.

doctorate The degree or status of a doctor as conferred by a university, as in Doctor of Dental Medicine. *See also* bachelor's degree; master's degree; postdoctoral; university.

Doctor of Business Administration (DBA) The title for an individual holding a doctoral degree in business administration. *See also* administration; doctor; doctorate; Master of Business Administration.

Doctor of Chiropractic (DC) The title for an individual holding a doctoral degree in chiropractic. *See also* chiropractor; doctor; doctorate.

Doctor of Dental Medicine (DMD) The title for an individual holding a doctoral degree in dental medicine (in Latin, *Dentariae Medicinae Doctor*). *See also* dentist; doctor; Doctor of Dental Surgery; doctorate.

Doctor of Dental Surgery (DDS) The title for an individual holding a doctoral degree in dentistry. *See also* dentist; doctor; Doctor of Dental Medicine; doctorate.

Doctor of Education (EdD) The title for an individual holding a doctoral degree in education. *See also* doctor; doctorate; education.

Doctor of Jurisprudence (JD) The title for an individual holding a Juris Doctor degree. *See also* attorney; doctorate; lawyer.

Doctor of Medicine (MD) The title for an individual holding a doctoral degree in medicine (in Latin, *Medicinae Doctor*). *See also* allopathy; doctor; doctorate; physician.

Doctor of Naturopathic Medicine (ND) The title for an individual holding a doctoral degree in naturopathic medicine. *See also* doctor; doctorate; naturopath.

Doctor of Optometry (OD) The title for an individual holding a doctoral degree in optometry. *See also* doctor; doctorate; optometry.

Doctor of Osteopathy (DO) The title for an individual holding a doctoral degree in osteopathic medicine. *See also* doctor; doctorate; osteopathic physician.

doctor-patient privilege *See* physician-patient privilege.

doctor-patient relationship *See* patient-physician relationship.

Doctor of Pharmacy (PharD or PharmD) The title for an individual holding a doctoral degree in pharmacy. *See also* doctor; doctorate; pharmacist; pharmacology.

Doctor of Philosophy (PhD) The title for an individual holding a doctoral degree in philosophy. *See also* doctor; doctorate.

Doctor of Podiatric Medicine (DPM) The title for an individual holding a doctoral degree in podiatric medicine. *See also* doctor; doctorate; podiatric medicine.

Doctor of Psychology (PsyD) The title for an individual holding a doctoral degree in psychology. *See also* doctor; doctorate; psychologist.

Doctor of Public Administration (DPA) The title for an individual holding a doctoral degree in public administration. *See also* doctor; doctorate; public administration.

Doctor of Public Health (DPH or DrPH) The title for an individual holding a doctoral degree in public health. *See also* doctor; doctorate; public health.

Doctors Association, Mission *See* Mission Doctors Association.

Doctor of Science (ScD) The title for an individual holding a doctoral degree in science. *See also* doctor; doctorate; science.

Doctors for Disaster Preparedness (DDP) A national organization founded in 1982 composed of 200 physicians and other health professionals interested in preparing health professionals and the public for medical response in the case of natural or human-caused disaster. It supports civil defense measures and maintains no position on specific military or foreign policy measures, weapons systems, or arms controls. *See also* disaster preparedness plan.

doctor, spin *See* spin doctor.

doctor, witch *See* witch doctor.

doctrine **1.** A principle or body of principles presented for acceptance or belief, as by a scientific or medical group. *See also* tenet. **2.** A rule or law, especially when established by precedent, as in substituted judgment doctrine. *See also* substituted judgment doctrine. **3.** A statement of official government policy, especially in foreign affairs and military strategy.

doctrine, captain of the ship *See* captain of the ship doctrine.

doctrine, substituted judgment *See* substituted judgment doctrine.

document Any written, spoken, or visual record, including such items as medical records and x-rays. *See also* source document.

documentation In health care, the process of recording information in the medical record and other source documents. *See also* medical record; quality of documentation; source document.

documentation, quality of *See* quality of documentation.

document, source *See* source document.

DOD *See* Department of Defense.

DOE *See* Department of Education; Department of Energy.

DOJ *See* Department of Justice.

DOL *See* Department of Labor.

domain **1.** A territory over which rule or control is exercised. **2.** A sphere of activity, concern, or function, as in public domain. *See also* public domain. **3.** In nursing, one of the three distinct areas of nursing practice: clinical practice, professional practice, and administrative practice. *See also* nursing.

domain, public *See* public domain.

Domestic Policy Council A group within the executive office of the president of the United States concerned with the establishment of broad policy in domestic affairs, including health and human services, which is usually represented by the Secretary of Health and Human Services.

Domestic Violence, National Coalition Against *See* National Coalition Against Domestic Violence.

domicile Legal home or permanent residence. An individual can have many transient residences where he or she may temporarily be found, but only one legal domicile, which is the residence to which he or she always intends to return and to remain indefinitely.

domiciliary Pertaining to one's permanent residence. *See also* domiciliary care.

domiciliary care Residential care including those services necessary for maintaining a secure home-like environment, given a patient's condition. The services may be provided either in a care facility, such as a nursing home, in an alternative living residence, such as a rest home or retirement center, or in a patient's home. Board, lodging, supervision, personal care, and home leisure activities are included. Health services are excluded. *See also* residential care.

Donabedian, Avedis A physician, health care quality expert, and author (b. 1919) whose books include *The Definition of Quality and Approaches to Its Assessment, The Criteria and Standards of Quality, the Methods and Findings of Quality Assessment and Monitoring,* and *Striving for Quality in Health Care.* He developed the framework of structure, process, and outcome for quality assurance in health care. *See also* quality; outcome; process; quality assurance; structure.

do no harm *See* Hippocratic oath.

donor **1.** An individual from whom blood, tissues, or an organ is taken for use in a transfusion or transplant. *See also* blood donor; organ donor; professional blood donor; replacement blood donor; tissue donor; voluntary blood donor. **2.** A person who provides a gift or charitable contribution of money, stocks, property, or something else of value to an individual or organization.

donor, blood *See* blood donor.

donor insemination *See* artificial insemination - donor.

donor, organ *See* organ donor.

donor, professional blood *See* professional blood donor.

Donor Program, Medic Alert Organ *See* Medic Alert Organ Donor Program.

Donor Program, National Marrow *See* National Marrow Donor Program.

donor, replacement blood *See* replacement blood donor.

donor, tissue *See* tissue donor.

donor, voluntary blood *See* voluntary blood donor.

do-not-resuscitate (DNR) order An order placed in a patient's medical record by an attending physician, with patient or surrogate consent, that directs hospital personnel not to revive the patient if cardiopulmonary arrest occurs. The decision is based on the patient's overall condition and values. *Compare* code blue. *See also* attending physician; cardiac arrest; cardiopulmonary resuscitation.

door, revolving   *See* revolving door.

DOS   *See* disk operating system.

dosage   The regulated administration of doses of therapeutic agents, expressed as amounts per units of time. *See also* dose; posology.

dose   A specified amount of a therapeutic agent, such as a drug or radiation, prescribed to be taken at one time or at stated intervals. *See also* dosage; megadose; overdose; posology; unit-dose medication system.

dose medication system, unit-   *See* unit-dose medication system.

dose, mega-   *See* megadose.

dose, over-   *See* overdose.

DOT   *See* Department of Transportation.

dot matrix   A system that uses combinations of dots to form, display, or print characters, such as letters and numbers. *See* dot-matrix printer.

dot-matrix printer   A printer that forms characters as a pattern of dots. It is faster than a daisy wheel printer, but its output is normally not of letter quality. Dot-matrix printers are used frequently with computers when letter-quality printing is not needed. *See also* daisy wheel printer; printer.

double-blind study   *See* double-blind technique.

double-blind technique   A method of studying a drug, device, or procedure in which both subjects and investigators are kept unaware of (blind to) who is actually getting which specific treatment. This is done to reduce both subject and researcher biases. In a triple-blind study, data analyzers are also kept unaware of the treatment used. *Synonyms*: double-blind study; double-mask study; double-mask technique. *See also* clinical trial; triple-blind study.

double-effect principle   An action that may have both a positive and a negative effect. The negative effect may be tolerated if the negative was not intended but is simply a by-product of the good, or positive, effect. The positive effect must outweigh the negative effect. *See also* nonmaleficence; principle.

double-mask study   *See* double-blind technique.

double-mask technique   *See* double-blind technique.

downgrading   Assignment of an employee to a position having a lower rate of pay and/or fewer responsibilities. *See also* demotion; employee.

download   To transfer data or programs from a central computer to a peripheral computer or device. *Compare* upload. *See also* computer.

Down syndrome   A chromosomal disorder charac-

terized by a small and flattened skull, a short and flat-bridged nose, epicanthal folds, short fingers, widened spaces between first and second fingers and toes, and mild to severe mental retardation. *Synonym*: Down's syndrome. *See also* amniocentesis; genetic counseling; syndrome.

Down's syndrome   *See* Down syndrome.

DPA   *See* Doctor of Public Administration.

DPH or DrPH   *See* Doctor of Public Health.

DPM   *See* Doctor of Podiatric Medicine.

DPMA   *See* Data Processing Management Association.

DPT   A triple-antigen vaccine immunizing human beings against diphtheria, pertussis, and tetanus. *See also* diphtheria; tetanus; vaccine.

Dr   *See* doctor.

drainage/secretion precautions   A category of patient isolation intended to prevent infections transmitted by direct or indirect contact with purulent material or drainage from an infected body site. A private room and masking are not indicated. Gowns should be used if soiling is likely and gloves used for touching contaminated materials. *See* direct contact; indirect contact; infection; isolation.

Drama, American Society of Group Psychotherapy and Group Psycho-   *See* American Society of Group Psychotherapy and Group Psychodrama.

drama, psycho-   *See* psychodrama.

drama therapist   An individual who specializes in drama therapy. *See also* drama therapy.

drama therapy   The intentional use of drama and theatrical processes to achieve the therapeutic goals of symptom relief, emotional and physical integration, and personal growth. It is used with individuals, groups, and families to maintain health and to treat emotional disorders, learning difficulties, geriatric problems, and social maladjustments. *See also* art therapy; dance therapy; manual arts therapy; music therapy; poetry therapy; recreational therapy.

Drama Therapy, National Association for   *See* National Association for Drama Therapy.

dream   A series of images, ideas, emotions, and sensations occurring involuntarily in the mind during certain states of sleep. *See also* mind; oneirology; sleep.

Dreams, Association for the Study of   *See* Association for the Study of Dreams.

dredging, data   *See* data dredging.

dressing   Any protective covering for a wound.

DRG   *See* diagnosis-related groups.

DRG coordinator The hospital employee who establishes the DRG (diagnosis-related group) category for a patient, informing the attending physician of the usual length of stay for that particular DRG, the medical procedures allowed in the DRG, and their allowed cost, and who assists in planning the patient's discharge and generating reports and information from the computer-based information system containing the data on the mix of inpatient cases experienced by the hospital. *See also* diagnosis-related groups.

DRG creep The phenomenon in which the distribution of patients among diagnosis-related groups (DRGs) changes without a real change in the distribution of patients treated in the hospital. This results when hospitals and physicians alter their record keeping and reporting so that more patients appear in higher-priced DRGs, resulting in increased hospital income without a corresponding increase in cost. DRG creep is often inappropriately used to refer to natural growth in case-mix severity and efforts to provide more accurate and descriptive coding. *See also* diagnosis-related groups.

DRG payment system *See* prospective payment system.

DRGs *See* diagnosis-related groups.

DRG weight Index number that reflects the relative resource consumption associated with each diagnosis-related group. *See also* diagnosis-related groups; weight.

Drinking Water Administrators, Association of State *See* Association of State Drinking Water Administrators.

drip Any infusion (usually intravenous), the rate of which is controlled by adjusting the frequency of drops in a drip-chamber. *See also* infusion.

drive Computer hardware components necessary for transferring data to and from a floppy disk (diskette). *See also* computer hardware; data; diskette.

drive out fear One of W. Edwards Deming's Fourteen Points emphasizing the need for people to feel secure in order to improve quality and productivity. Many employees are afraid to ask questions or to take a position, even when they do not understand what the job is or what is right or wrong. People continue to do things in the wrong way or not do them at all. The economic loss from fear is high. *See also* Deming's Fourteen Points; Deming, W. Edwards.

drive, tape *See* tape drive.

dropsy An abnormal accumulation of fluid in the tissue spaces; edema. *See also* edema.

drug Any chemical compound, not including food, that may be used on or administered to persons as an aid in the diagnosis, treatment, or prevention of disease or other abnormal condition. All substances recognized in the *United States Pharmacopeia, Homeopathic Pharmacopeia of the United States,* and the *National Formulary* are defined as drugs. *Compare* biological. *See also Homeopathic Pharmacopeia of the United States;* medication; *National Formulary;* posology; *United States Pharmacopeia.*

drug abuse Persistent or sporadic drug use inconsistent with or unrelated to acceptable medical or cultural practice. *See also* abuse; impaired health care provider; substance abuse.

Drug Abuse Counselor Credentialing Bodies, National Commission on Accreditation of Alcoholism and *See* National Commission on Accreditation of Alcoholism and Drug Abuse Counselor Credentialing Bodies.

Drug Abuse Counselors, National Association of Alcoholism and *See* National Association of Alcoholism and Drug Abuse Counselors.

Drug Abuse Directors, National Association of State Alcohol and *See* National Association of State Alcohol and Drug Abuse Directors.

Drug Abuse, National Certification Reciprocity Consortium/Alcoholism and Other *See* National Certification Reciprocity Consortium/Alcoholism and Other Drug Abuse (NCRC/AODA).

Drug Abuse Problems, National Association of *See* National Association of Drug Abuse Problems.

drug addiction *See* alcoholism and other drug dependence.

drug, addictive *See* addictive substance.

drug administration The act in which a single dose of an identified drug is given to a patient. *See also* administration; dose.

Drug Administration, Food and *See* Food and Drug Administration.

drug adverse reaction An undesirable response associated with use of a drug that either compromises therapeutic efficacy, enhances toxicity, or both. *See also* drug side effect.

Drug and Alcohol Nursing Association (DANA) A national organization founded in 1979 composed of 340 registered nurses, licensed practical nurses, and other health professionals involved in the treatment, prevention, and control of drug and/or alcohol addictions. It purposes include promoting and maintaining the participation of the nursing profession in the treatment of addictions and ensuring that addicted patients and their families receive high quality nursing care. *See also* addiction; alcoholism; nursing.

drug allergy A state of hypersensitivity induced by exposure to a particular antigen, resulting in harmful immunologic reactions on subsequent drug exposures, such as penicillin drug allergy. *See also* allergy; drug.

drug application, abbreviated new *See* abbreviated new drug application.

drug application, new *See* new drug application.

Drug Association, Parenteral *See* Parenteral Drug Association.

drug benefit list, additional *See* additional drug benefit list.

Drug, Chemical and Allied Trades Association (DCAT) A national organization founded in 1890 composed of 500 manufacturers of drugs, chemicals, and related products (packaging, cosmetics, essential oils), and publications, advertising agencies, agents, brokers, and importers. Its activities include monitoring federal regulation relating to drug and chemical manufacturing. *See also* drug; pharmaceutical.

drug compendium *See* compendium.

drug dispensing The issuance of one or more doses of a prescribed medication by a pharmacist or other authorized person to another person responsible for administering it. See also dispensing fee; drug; drug administration.

drug dependence *See* alcoholism and other drug dependence.

Drug Dependence, National Council on Alcoholism and *See* National Council on Alcoholism and Drug Dependence.

drug, designer *See* designer drug.

Drug Education, American Council for *See* American Council for Drug Education.

Drug Efficacy Study A study undertaken in 1966 by the National Research Council of the National Academy of Sciences to evaluate all the drugs the Food and Drug Administration had approved as safe before 1962, when Congress first required that drugs had to be proved effective before they could be marketed. The Drug Efficacy Study Group evaluated nearly 4,000 individual drug products, finding many ineffective or of only possible or probable effectiveness. The vast majority of the study's recommendations have been implemented, although there are a substantial number of administrative hearings pending on recommendations that have not yet been implemented. *See also* drug; efficacy; National Academy of Sciences.

Drug Enforcement Agency (DEA) The federal agency responsible for regulating and enforcing statutes dealing with controlled substances. The DEA, for instance, sets the licensing standards for physicians and hospitals for the handling of controlled substances, such as narcotics. Its predecessor organization was the Bureau of Narcotics and Dangerous Drugs (BNDD). *See also* controlled substances; DEA number.

drug error *See* medication error.

drug, fertility *See* fertility drug.

drug formulary A list of drugs, usually by their generic names, and indications for their use. A formulary is intended to include a sufficient range of medicines to enable physicians, dentists, and, as appropriate, other practitioners to prescribe all medically appropriate treatment for all reasonably common illnesses. *See also* formulary; hospital formulary.

Drug Information Association (DIA) A national organization founded in 1965 composed of 6,000 persons who handle drug information in government, industry, medical and pharmaceutical professions, and allied fields. It seeks to provide mutual instruction on the technology of drug information processing in all areas, including collecting, selecting, abstracting, indexing, coding, vocabulary building, terminology standardizing, computerizing data storage and retrieval, tabulating, correlating, computing, evaluating, writing, editing, reporting, and publishing. It conducts workshops and seminars. *See also* drug; information.

Drug Law Institute, Food and *See* Food and Drug Law Institute.

druggist 1. A person who operates a drug store. 2. A pharmacist who operates or works in a drug store. *See also* apothecary; drugstore; NARD; pharmacist; pharmacy.

Druggists' Association, National Wholesale *See* National Wholesale Druggists' Association.

drug, legend *See* legend drug.

drug level, serum *See* serum drug level.

drug maintenance list *See* additional drug benefit list.

Drug Manufacturers Association, Nonprescription *See* Nonprescription Drug Manufacturers Association.

Drug Marketing Associates, Chain *See* Chain Drug Marketing Associates.

drug, "me too" *See* "me too" drug.

drug, miracle *See* miracle drug.

drug monograph A document specifying the types and amounts of ingredients a drug or class of related drugs may contain, the conditions for which the drug may be given or prescribed, the directions for its use, and warnings and other information that must appear on labels for the drug's containers. Drug monographs established by the federal Food and Drug Administration (FDA) state the conditions under which specific drugs may be marketed as safe and effective. Once a monograph is promulgated, anyone who meets its requirements can market the drug without seeking approval from the FDA. *See also* Food and Drug Administration; new drug application.

drug, new *See* new drug.

drug, not new *See* not new drug.

Drug Officials, Association of Food and *See* Association of Food and Drug Officials.

drug, orphan *See* orphan drug.

drug, over-the-counter *See* over-the-counter drug.

drug, prescription *See* prescription drug.

Drug Price Competition and Patent Term Restoration Act of 1984 The act that amended the federal Food, Drug and Cosmetic statute to provide additional patent protection and patent extensions for prescription drugs and eased the requirements and procedures for making generic, equivalent drugs available when the patents on a drug run out. The act also establishes requirements for abbreviated new drug applications and their approval. *See also* abbreviated new-drug application; generic equivalents; new-drug application.

Drug Problems, National Catholic Council on Alcoholism and Related *See* National Catholic Council on Alcoholism and Related Drug Problems.

Drug Programs, National Council for Prescription *See* National Council for Prescription Drug Programs.

drug, proprietary *See* proprietary drug.

drug, psychotropic *See* psychotropic drug.

drug rep *See* detail person.

drug sales representative *See* detail person.

drug screening Testing used to determine the presence of drugs and to measure the amount of drugs in an individual. *See also* drug; screening.

drug side effect A consequence other than the one(s) for which a drug is used, as in the adverse effects produced by a drug, especially on a tissue or organ system other than the one sought to be benefited by the drug's administration. *See also* drug adverse reaction.

drugstore (drug store) A store where prescriptions are filled and drugs and other articles are sold. *See also* druggist; prescription.

Drug Stores, National Association of Chain *See* National Association of Chain Drug Stores.

drug therapy *See* chemotherapy.

Drug Trade Conference, National *See* National Drug Trade Conference.

drug usage evaluation A health care organization's medical staff responsibility in cooperation with other relevant departments/services of the organization that entails measuring, assessing, and improving the appropriate and effective use of drugs in the health care organization. Drug usage evaluation may be performed retrospectively, prospectively, or concurrently and can either address a process, such as adhering to a protocol, or an outcome, such as determining the effectiveness of parenteral nutritional support for patients. *Synonym*: drug utilization review.

drug utilization review *See* drug usage evaluation.

drug, wonder *See* wonder drug.

dry gangrene Gangrene in which the affected extremity becomes cold and dry and eventually turns black. It is a characteristic of diabetes mellitus that is already complicated by arteriosclerosis. *See also* arteriosclerosis; diabetes mellitus; gangrene; moist gangrene.

DSM-III-R *See Diagnostic and Statistical Manual of Mental Disorders (Third Edition - Revised)*.

DTs *See* delirium tremens.

dual choice The practice of giving people a choice of more than one health insurance to pay for or provide their health services. *See also* health insurance.

dual coverage *See* duplication of benefits.

due care The extent of care that should be reasonably expected to be exercised by the average person when the issue of liability arises. The legal principle of due care applies to any person acting or failing to act in any circumstance or environment in which that person may be held responsible for a function or condition.

due process of law The right of fundamental fairness in proceedings that are judicial in nature. *Substantive due process* means that all legislation should (or must) be in furtherance of a legitimate governmental objective, and *procedural due process* guarantees procedural fairness when the government would deprive an individual of his or her property or liberty. This requires that notice and right to a fair hearing be accorded before a deprivation. The phrase, "due process of law," was first expressed in the Fifth Amendment to the Constitution, which provides that "nor [shall any person] be deprived of life, liberty, or property, without due process of law." The phrase was expanded from actions of the federal government to individual states with the adoption of the Fourteenth Amendment, which states that "Nor shall any State deprive any person of life, liberty or property, without due process of law." One requirement for granting of immunity to a health care entity is that the peer review action is justified by the facts *after satisfying due process of law.*

dues The money that must be periodically paid by associations and members in order for them to remain in good standing. Dues payments are used to finance the activities of the organization.

Duke Endowment, The *See* The Duke Endowment.

dumb *See* mute.

dumb terminal A visual display terminal and keyboard of a computer with minimal input/output capability and no processing capability. *Compare* intelligent terminal. *See also* computer; computer terminal.

dumping, patient *See* patient dumping.

duodenum The first part of the small intestine. *See also* biliary tract surgery; duodenal ulcer; intestine; peptic ulcer.

duodenal ulcer An open sore in the duodenum (small intestine). *See also* ulcer.

duplication of benefits The situation in which a person covered under more than one health or accident insurance policy collects, or may collect, payments for the same hospital or medical expenses from more than one insurer. *Synonym*: dual coverage. *See also* benefits; health insurance.

durable medical equipment (DME) Medical equipment, such as a respirator or home dialysis system, that is prescribed by a physician for a patient's use and that is usable for an extended period of time. *See also* medical equipment.

durable power of attorney for health care An advance directive wider in scope than a living will that designates a family member or friend to make decisions about a patient's care should the patient become unable to do so. This type of power of attorney, in contrast to ordinary power of attorney, remains or becomes effective when the principal becomes incompetent to act for herself or himself. *See also* advance directives; living will; Patient Self Determination Act; power of attorney.

duration A period of existence or persistence, as in the duration of accreditation. *See also* accreditation duration.

duration, accreditation *See* accreditation duration.

duty Obligatory conduct owed by a person to another person. For purposes of civil liability, duty is distinguishable from a moral obligation, which is not generally enforceable at law. In health care, duty is the obligation of the caregiver owed to a patient. Duty may be established by statute, contract, or oath or may be voluntarily undertaken or ethically implied. The duty "to do no harm" and the duty of "beneficence" are the most important obligations of a physician. In tort law, duty is a legally sanctioned obligation the breach of which results in the liability of the actor. Thus under the law of negligence, if an individual owes another a duty of care, he or she must conduct himself or herself so as to avoid negligent injury to them. *See also* altruism; beneficence; breach of duty; conflict of interest; due care; negligence; obligation; responsibility.

duty, breach of *See* breach of duty.

Duty, Children's Healthcare Is a Legal *See* Children's Healthcare Is a Legal Duty.

dwarf An abnormally small person, sometimes having other distinguishing features, such as shortened extremities in an achondroplastic dwarf. *Compare* giant; gigantism. *See also* midget.

DWI Abbreviation for driving while intoxicated.

dx *See* diagnosis.

dye, radiopaque *See* radiopaque dye.

dynamite instruction Further instruction given by a trial judge to a jury when the jury has reported an inability to agree on a verdict in a criminal case. The judge advised them of their obligation to consider the opinions of their fellow jurors and to yield their own views when possible. *See also* hung jury; judge; trial; verdict.

Dying-The National Council for the Right to Die, Choice in *See* Choice in Dying - The National Council for the Right to Die.

dysentery Any condition associated with inflammation and irritation of the large intestine, giving rise to bloody diarrhea. Bacillary dysentery is usually due to *Shigella*, and amoebic dysentery due to the protozoan *Entamoeba histolytica*.

dysfunction Any impairment of function of a part, organ, tissue, or system. *See also* speech dysfunction.

dysfunction, speech *See* speech dysfunction.

dyslexia Difficulty in reading or spelling not explained by low intelligence and assumed to be associated with a specific central nervous system defect. *See also* learning disability.

dyspepsia *See* indigestion.

dyspnea Difficult or disordered breathing; shortness of breath.

dysrhythmia *See* arrhythmia.

dystocia Abnormally slow progress of labor during the process of childbirth. *See also* labor.

dysuria Pain and/or difficulty urinating. *See also* strangury.

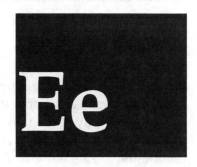

EAI *See* Emphysema Anonymous, Inc.

EAP *See* employee assistance program.

Early and Periodic Screening Diagnosis and Treatment Program (EPSDT) A program mandated by Medicaid for eligible people under 21 years of age to assess the presence of physical or mental effects and ensure treatment for them. *See also* Medicaid.

early retirement age An earlier-than-usual retirement age associated with a proportionate reduction in benefits. *See also* benefits; retirement age.

early survey option (ESO) survey A two-part survey by the Joint Commission on Accreditation of Healthcare Organizations conducted for health care organizations in operation less than six months. The initial survey assesses only organizational structure. A mandatory follow-up survey is conducted six months from the date of the initial survey to assess the process of care or service delivery through review of established performance records and implementation of policies and procedures. *See also* accreditation survey; Joint Commission on Accreditation of Healthcare Organizations; provisional accreditation.

Ear Hospitals, American Association of Eye and *See* American Association of Eye and Ear Hospitals.

earned income Wages or earnings from employment. *Compare* unearned income. *See also* income.

earnings, real *See* real earnings.

Ear, Nose, and Throat Advances in Children, Society for *See* Society for Ear, Nose, and Throat Advances in Children.

ear, nose, and throat doctor/physician/specialist/ surgeon *See* otolaryngologist-head and neck surgeon.

East Coast Migrant Health Project (ECMHP) A project founded in 1970 sponsored by the National Migrant Workers Council that provides health ser-

vices for migrant and seasonal farm workers and their families in Delaware, Florida, Georgia, Maine, Maryland, New York, New Jersey, North Carolina, Pennsylvania, South Carolina, Tennessee, Virginia, and West Virginia.

Easter Seal Society, National *See* National Easter Seal Society.

eating disorder An abnormal mental and/or physical condition related to eating; for example, anorexia nervosa, bulimia. *See also* anorexia nervosa; bulimia nervosa.

EBAA *See* Eye Bank Association of America.

EBSR *See* Eye-Bank for Sight Restoration.

ECF *See* extended care facility.

ECFMG *See* Educational Commission for Foreign Medical Graduates.

ECG *See* electrocardiogram.

echocardiogram The record produced by echocardiography. *See also* echocardiography.

echocardiography A method of graphically recording the position and motion of the heart walls or the internal structures of the heart and neighboring tissue by the echo obtained from beams of ultrasonic waves directed through the chest wall. *Synonym*: ultrasonic cardiography. *See also* heart; ultrasound imaging.

Echocardiography, American Society of *See* American Society of Echocardiography.

echogram *See* sonogram.

eclampsia The occurrence of one or more convulsions (seizures), or coma, not attributable to other cerebral conditions, such as epilepsy or cerebral hemorrhage, in a patient with preeclampsia. *See also* preeclampsia; pregnancy.

eclampsia, pre- *See* preeclampsia.

ECMA *See* Embalming Chemical Manufacturers

Association.

ECMHP   *See* East Coast Migrant Health Project.

E coli   *See Escherichia coli.*

e-com   *See* electronic computer-originated mail.

econometrics   The application of statistical methods to the study of economic data and problems. *See also* economics; measurement; metrology; statistics.

economic   **1.** Relating to the production, development, and management of material wealth, as of a country, household, or business enterprise. **2.** Pertaining to either the economy or the study of economics. *See also* economics.

Economic Advisors, Council of   *See* Council of Economic Advisors.

economic credentialing   The use of economic performance data and information in determining a practitioner's qualifications for membership and privileges on a hospital medical staff or in establishing eligibility to participate in a health care network or managed care plan. *See also* credentialing; managed care; medical staff; network; performance data; physician credentialing; practice pattern analysis.

economic evaluation   Comparative analysis of alternative courses of action in terms of both their costs and consequences. *See also* economic; evaluation.

economic freedom   Freedom from regulation or other dictates from government or other authority in economic (business) matters. In a capitalist system, economic freedom is supposed to lead to efficient allocation of resources.

economic growth   Increase, from period to period, of the real value of an economy's production of goods and services, commonly expressed as an increase in gross national product (GNP). *See also* gross national product.

economic indicator   **1.** A quantitative measure used to monitor performance and change in the economy. *See also* economy; indicator. **2.** A statistical value that provides an indication of the condition or change in direction over time of the state of the economy. *See also* lagging economic indicator; leading economic indicator.

economic indicator, lagging   *See* lagging economic indicator.

economic indicator, leading   *See* leading economic indicator.

Economic Policy Council   A group within the executive office of the president of the United States concerned with the establishment of broad economic policy, including major economic initiatives in health care. *See also* economic; policy.

Economic Recovery Tax Act of 1981 (ERTA)   Tax-cutting legislation including an across-the-board tax cut, which took effect in three stages, ending in 1983. The act included indexing of tax brackets to the inflation rate; lowering of top rates on long-term capital gains; lowering of marriage penalty tax; expansion of individual retirement accounts; creation of the All-Savers Certificate; deductions for reinvesting public utility dividends; reductions in estate and gift taxes; lowering of rates on the exercise of stock options; and change in rules on accelerated depreciation and investment credit. Many of these provisions were altered by the Tax Reform Act of 1986. *See also* tax.

economics   The study of the means by which societies allocate scarce resources. It includes the study of production, distribution, exchange, and consumption of goods and services. *See also* economy; inflation; Keynesian economics; laissez-faire; macroeconomics; microeconomics; neoclassical economics; new economics; social science; supply-side economics.

economic sanctions   Internationally, restrictions on trade and financial dealings that a country imposes on another for political reasons, usually as punishment for following policies of which the sanctioning country disapproves. *See also* sanction.

economics, Keynesian   *See* Keynesian economics.

economics, macro-   *See* macroeconomics.

economics, micro-   *See* microeconomics.

economics, neoclassical   *See* neoclassical economics.

economics, new   *See* new economics.

Economic Stabilization Program (ESP)   A 1971 federal program established by law to control wages and prices. On August 15, 1971, all wages and prices in the United States were frozen for 90 days during which time a system of wage and price controls, administered through a Cost of Living Council, was implemented. The controls continued until April 1974 when the legislative authority for them expired. Wages and prices in the health care industry were controlled through a specialized series of regulations. The 32-month period during which the controls were in effect was the only period before 1984 in which increases in US medical care fees slowed markedly since the enactment of Medicare and Medicaid.

economics, supply-side   *See* supply-side economics.

economies of scale Cost savings resulting from the aggregation of resources and/or mass production. *See also* centers of excellence; economy.

economy Recognizable and cohesive group of economic performers (producers, labor, consumers) who interact with one another. Economies usually are recognized geographically (countries, states) or, occasionally, as worldwide industries. *See also* managed economy; mature economy; mixed economy; overheating; pump priming; recession; recovery; service economy; underground economy.

economy, managed *See* managed economy.

economy, mature *See* mature economy.

economy, mixed *See* mixed economy.

economy, service *See* service economy.

economy, underground *See* underground economy.

ECRI A national organization founded in 1955 composed of 2,500 members interested in improving the safety, performance, reliability, and cost-effectiveness of health care technology through objective investigation and testing and publication of results. It provides technical consulting and accident investigation and educational programs. It functions as an information clearinghouse for hazards and deficiencies in medical devices. *See also* medical device; safety; technology.

ECT *See* electroconvulsive therapy.

ectopic pregnancy The implantation and subsequent development of a fertilized ovum outside the uterus, as in a fallopian tube. *See also* ovum; pregnancy.

ED *See* emergency department.

edema Swelling caused by retention of fluid in any part of the body, but especially the legs, ankles, and feet. *See also* dropsy.

Editors, American Association of Dental *See* American Association of Dental Editors.

Editors Association, Optometric *See* Optometric Editors Association.

Edna McConnell Clark Foundation, The *See* The Edna McConnell Clark Foundation.

EDP *See* electronic data processing.

education The knowledge and/or skill obtained or developed by a learning process. *See also* continuing education; continuing medical education; graduate medical education; in-service education; medical education; patient education.

Education, Academy of Osteopathic Directors of Medical *See* Academy of Osteopathic Directors of Medical Education.

Education and Accreditation, Committee on Allied Health *See* Committee on Allied Health Education and Accreditation.

Education, Accreditation Council for Continuing Medical *See* Accreditation Council for Continuing Medical Education.

Education, Accreditation Council for Graduate Medical *See* Accreditation Council for Graduate Medical Education.

Education Act of 1984, Comprehensive Smoking *See* Comprehensive Smoking Education Act of 1984.

Education, Advisory Council for Orthopedic Resident *See* Advisory Council for Orthopedic Resident Education.

Educational Administrators Serving the Deaf, Conference of *See* Conference of Educational Administrators Serving the Deaf.

Educational Commission for Foreign Medical Graduates (ECFMG) An organization founded in 1956 composed of the American Hospital Association, American Medical Association, American Board of Medical Specialties, National Medical Association, Federation of State Medical Boards of the United States, Association of American Medical Colleges, and Association for Hospital Medical Education that screens graduates of foreign medical schools to verify their qualifications for admittance to residency or fellowship training in US programs. It examines credentials, tests knowledge of medical matters, and tests facility with the English language. Those who successfully meet these criteria are eligible to apply for residencies in the United States. *See also* fifth pathway; foreign medical graduate; labor certification; medical school; physician; residency.

Educational Programs for the EMT-Paramedic, Joint Review Committee on *See* Joint Review Committee on Educational Programs for the EMT-Paramedic.

Educational Programs/Schools, Council on Accreditation of Nurse Anesthesia *See* Council on Accreditation of Nurse Anesthesia Educational Programs/Schools.

Educational Programs in Surgical Technology, Accreditation Review Committee for *See* Accreditation Review Committee for Educational Programs in Surgical Technology.

educational psychology The branch of psychology that attempts to improve teaching methods and materials, solve learning problems, and measure learning ability and educational progress. Researchers in this field may devise achievement tests, develop and evaluate teaching methods, or investigate how children learn at different ages. *See also* learning; psychology.

Educational Trust, Hospital Research and *See* Hospital Research and Educational Trust.

Education, American Association for Cancer *See* American Association for Cancer Education.

Education, American College for Continuing *See* American College for Continuing Education.

Education, American Council for Drug *See* American Council for Drug Education.

Education, American Council on Pharmaceutical *See* American Council on Pharmaceutical Education.

Education of the American Medical Association, Council on Medical *See* Council on Medical Education of the American Medical Association.

Education of the American Osteopathic Association, Bureau of Professional *See* Bureau of Professional Education of the American Osteopathic Association.

Education, Association for the Advancement of Health *See* Association for the Advancement of Health Education.

Education, Association of Black Nursing Faculty in Higher *See* Association of Black Nursing Faculty in Higher Education.

Education, Association for Clinical Pastoral *See* Association for Clinical Pastoral Education.

Education, Association for Continuing *See* Association for Continuing Education.

Education, Association for Hospital Medical *See* Association for Hospital Medical Education.

Education Association, Nutrition *See* Nutrition Education Association.

Education, Association of State and Territorial Directors of Public Health *See* Association of State and Territorial Directors of Public Health Education.

Education, Association for Surgical *See* Association for Surgical Education.

education, continuing *See* continuing education.

education, continuing medical *See* continuing medical education.

Education, Coordinating Council on Medical *See* Coordinating Council on Medical Education.

Education, Council on Chiropractic *See* Council on Chiropractic Education.

Education, Council on Electrolysis *See* Council on Electrolysis Education.

Education, Council on Optometric *See* Council on Optometric Education.

Education, Council on Podiatric Medical *See* Council on Podiatric Medical Education.

Education, Council for Sex Information and *See* Council for Sex Information and Education.

Education, Council on Social Work *See* Council on Social Work Education.

Education Council of the US, Sex Information and *See* Sex Information and Education Council of the US.

Education, Department of *See* Department of Education.

education department, patient *See* patient education department.

Education in Diagnostic Medical Sonography, Joint Review Committee on *See* Joint Review Committee on Education in Diagnostic Medical Sonography.

education director An individual who directs employee orientation, on-the-job training, and continuing education and, for some health care organizations, patient community education programs. *See also* continuing education; medical education director.

education director, medical *See* medical education director.

education, family life *See* family life education.

education, graduate medical *See* graduate medical education.

education, health *See* health education.

Education, Health Media *See* Health Media Education.

Education for Health Services Administration, Accrediting Commission on *See* Accrediting Commission on Education for Health Services Administration.

education, in-service *See* in-service education.

Education Institute, Hospice *See* Hospice Education Institute.

Education, Institute for Hospital Clinical Nursing *See* Institute for Hospital Clinical Nursing Education.

Education, Liaison Committee on Graduate Medical *See* Liaison Committee on Graduate Medical Education.

Education, Liaison Committee on Medical *See* Liaison Committee on Medical Education.

Education and Licensure, Federation for Accessible Nursing *See* Federation for Accessible Nursing Education and Licensure.

Education in Maternal and Child Health, National Center for *See* National Center for Education in Maternal and Child Health.

education, medical *See* medical education.

Education, National Association for Perinatal Addiction Research and *See* National Association for Perinatal Addiction Research and Education.

Education, National Association of Supervisors and Administrators of Health Occupations *See* National Association of Supervisors and Administrators of Health Occupations Education.

Education, National Center for Health *See* National Center for Health Education.

Education, National Council on Patient Information and *See* National Council on Patient Information and Education.

Education, National Council on Rehabilitation *See* National Council on Rehabilitation Education.

Education, Network for Continuing Medical *See* Network for Continuing Medical Education.

Education Network, Physicians *See* Physicians Education Network.

Education in Obstetrics and Gynecology, Council on Resident *See* Council on Resident Education in Obstetrics and Gynecology.

Education in Pathology, Universities Associated for Research and *See* Universities Associated for Research and Education in Pathology.

education, patient *See* patient education.

Education for Physician Assistants, Accreditation Review Committee on *See* Accreditation Review Committee on Education for Physician Assistants.

Education for Public Health, Council on *See* Council on Education for Public Health.

Education in Radiologic Technology, Joint Review Committee on *See* Joint Review Committee on Education in Radiologic Technology.

Education Schools, Accrediting Bureau of Health *See* Accrediting Bureau of Health Education Schools.

Education and Service, National Association for Practical Nurse *See* National Association for Practical Nurse Education and Service.

Education, Society for Nutrition *See* Society for Nutrition Education.

Education, Society for Public Health *See* Society for Public Health Education.

education, undergraduate medical *See* undergraduate medical education.

Education and Welfare Association, Presbyterian Health, *See* Presbyterian Health, Education and Welfare Association.

educator, dietetic *See* dietetic educator.

educator, public health *See* public health educator.

Educators, American Association of Diabetes *See* American Association of Diabetes Educators.

Educators, American Society of Childbirth *See* American Society of Childbirth Educators.

Educators Association, National Standards *See* National Standards Educators Association.

Educators, Association of Optometric *See* Association of Optometric Educators.

Educators, Counselors and Therapists, American Association of Sex *See* American Association of Sex Educators, Counselors and Therapists.

Educators, Institute of Electrology *See* Institute of Electrology Educators.

EEG *See* electroencephalogram.

EEG technician/technologist *See* electroencephalographic technician/technologist.

effect The result of a cause or an agent. *See also* halo effect; Hawthorne effect; placebo effect.

effect, halo *See* halo effect.

effect, Hawthorne *See* Hawthorne effect.

effectiveness In health care, a performance dimension addressing the degree to which the care/intervention is provided in the correct manner, given the current state of knowledge, in order to achieve the desired/projected outcome for a patient. Effectiveness is not synonymous with efficiency; a consideration of cost is not required. *Compare* ineffective. *See also* care; dimensions of performance; efficacy; efficiency; intervention.

Effectiveness in Health Care, Office of the Forum for Quality and *See* Office of the Forum for Quality and Effectiveness in Health Care.

Effectiveness, Physicians for Research in Cost- *See* Physicians for Research in Cost-Effectiveness.

Effectiveness Research, Center for Medical *See* Center for Medical Effectiveness Research.

effect, placebo *See* placebo effect.

efficacy **1.** In health care, a performance dimension addressing the degree to which the care/intervention for a patient has been shown to accomplish the desired/projected outcome(s). *See also* care; dimensions of performance; intervention. **2.** The extent to which a specific intervention, procedure, regimen, or service produces a beneficial result under ideal conditions. Efficacy is often used as a synonym for effectiveness in health care delivery. Efficacy is sometimes distinguished from effectiveness to mean the results of actions undertaken under ideal circumstances, with the term "effectiveness" meaning the results of actions under usual or normal circumstances. *Compare* inefficacious. *See also* effectiveness.

efficiency In health care, a performance dimension addressing the relationship between the outcomes (results of the care/intervention) and the resources used to deliver the care/intervention. The ultimate measure of efficiency is the cost of achieving a goal to the benefit achieved by the goal. *See also* care; dimensions of performance; effectiveness; efficacy; intervention; outcome; patient health outcome.

EKG *See* electrocardiogram.

elder care Home care of the aged by relatives. *See also* aged person.

elderly *See* aged person.

Elderly, Center for the Study of Pharmacy and Therapeutics for the *See* Center for the Study of Pharmacy and Therapeutics for the Elderly.

elective Subject to the choice or decision of a patient or a physician, as applied to procedures that are advantageous to the patient but not urgent or emergent; for example, elective repair of an inguinal hernia. *Compare* emergency. *See also* elective admission; elective surgery; urgent.

elective admission The formal acceptance by a health care organization of a patient whose condition permits adequate time to schedule the availability of a suitable accommodation. *Compare* emergency admission. *See also* admission; elective; urgent admission.

elective surgery Surgery that does not have to be performed immediately in order to prevent death or serious disability. If surgery can be scheduled at some future date, it is, by definition, elective. Elective surgery may result in correction of a medical problem, such as inguinal hernia repair or removal of a bunion, or it may be performed in response to patient desires, for example, cosmetic surgery. *Compare* emergency surgery. *See also* elective; surgery.

electrical distribution system A system comprised of transformers, main breakers, breaker panels, and receptacles that is used to supply electricity throughout a building.

electric convulsive therapy *See* electroconvulsive therapy.

electric nerve stimulation, transcutaneous *See* transcutaneous electric nerve stimulation.

electric shock therapy *See* electroconvulsive therapy.

electrocardiogram (ECG, EKG) A graphic tracing of the variations in electrical potential caused by the stimulation of the heart muscle and detected at the body surface. The normal electrocardiogram show deflections resulting from atrial and ventricular activity. *Synonym*: cardiogram. *See also* heart.

electrocardiographic technician An individual who operates and maintains electrocardiographic machines that record and produce tracings for use by physicians in diagnosis and treatment. *See also* electrocardiography; technician.

electrocardiography The making of graphic records of the variations in electrical potential caused by excitation of the heart muscle and detected at the body surface. Electrocardiography is a method for studying the action of the heart muscle and making cardiac diagnoses, such as acute myocardial infarction, based on the data obtained. *See also* electrocardiogram; heart.

electroconvulsive therapy (ECT) A treatment for mental disorders, primarily depression, in which convulsions and loss of consciousness are induced by application of low-voltage alternating current to the brain via scalp electrodes for a fraction of second. A muscle relaxant is used to prevent injury during the seizure. The coma lasts about five minutes and is followed by an acute confusional state lasting about an hour; some memory impairment may be present for several weeks after treatment. ECT produces a therapeutic response in a majority of cases of major depression. *Synonyms*: electric convulsive therapy; electric shock therapy; electroshock therapy; shock therapy. *See also* depression; electromedicine.

electrocution Death caused by an electric shock, as in being struck by lightening, or execution by means of electricity.

electrodiagnosis Any diagnostic method employing an electrical or electronic apparatus. *See also* diagnosis; physical medicine and rehabilitation.

Electrodiagnostic Medicine, American Association of *See* American Association of Electrodiagnostic Medicine.

electroencephalogram (EEG) A recording on which the electrical activity of the brain cells is traced from electrodes placed on the scalp. The test provides information about the status and function of the cerebral cortex (cerebrum). Variations in wave characteristics correlate well with neurological conditions and so have been useful as diagnostic criteria. A *flat EEG* is one in which no brain waves are recorded, indicating a complete lack of brain (cerebral) activity. This indicates drug overdose, low body temperature, or cerebral death. The EEG does not test the brain stem's activity. *See also* brain; cerebrum; death; electroencephalography.

Electroencephalographic Association, American Medical *See* American Medical Electroencephalographic Association.

Electroencephalographic and Evoked Potentials Technologists, American Board of Registration of *See* American Board of Registration of Electroencephalographic and Evoked Potentials Technologists.

Electroencephalographic Society, American *See* American Electroencephalographic Society.

electroencephalographic technician/technologist (EEG technician/technologist) A technician or technologist who specializes in electroencephalography. *Synonym:* encephalographic technician/technologist. *See also* electroencephalography; technician.

electroencephalography The recording of the electric currents in the brain, by means of electrodes applied to the scalp or the surface of the brain or placed within the substance of the brain. Electroencephalography is a method for making neurological diagnoses based on data obtained from the electroencephalogram. *See also* brain; electroencephalogram; epilepsy.

electrohydraulic lithotripsy *See* lithotripsy.

electrologist An individual who specializes in electrology (hair removal). *See also* electrology; electrolysis.

Electrologist Certification, National Commission for *See* National Commission for Electrologist Certification.

Electrologists, Society of Clinical and Medical *See* Society of Clinical and Medical Electrologists.

electrology The field of removal of superfluous hair by galvanic blend or short-wave methods for cosmetic and medical purposes. *See also* electrolysis.

Electrology Association, American *See* American Electrology Association.

Electrology Educators, Institute of *See* Institute of Electrology Educators.

electrolysis Destruction of living tissue, especially of hair roots, by means of an electric current applied with a needle-shaped electrode. *See also* electrology.

Electrolysis Education, Council on *See* Council on Electrolysis Education.

electrolytes Substances that, when dissolved, separate into ions capable of conducting electricity. In the body, the elements sodium, potassium, magnesium, and chloride are electrolytes that are instrumental in transmitting nerve impulses, contracting muscles, and maintaining a proper fluid level and acid-base balance of fluids.

Electromagnetic Measurements, Conference on Precision *See* Conference on Precision Electromagnetic Measurements.

Electro-Magnetics Institute, Bio- *See* Bio-Electro-Magnetics Institute.

electromagnetics Society, Bio- *See* Bioelectromagnetics Society.

Electromedical Information, National Institute of *See* National Institute of Electromedical Information.

electromedicine The application of electric currents in the prevention and treatment of diseases. *See also* electroconvulsive therapy; electrotherapy; transcutaneous electric nerve stimulation.

electromyogram (EMG) The recording produced by electromyography. *See* electromyography.

electromyography The study of the intrinsic electrical properties of skeletal muscle by means of surface or needle electrodes. The procedure is useful for study of several aspects of neuromuscular function, neuromuscular conduction, extent of nerve lesion, and reflex response through evoking electrical activity in a muscle by electrical stimulation of its nerve. *See also* American Association of Electrodiagnostic Medicine; electromyogram; muscle.

electroneurodiagnostic technologist An allied health professional who records, studies, and interprets the electrical activity of the brain and nervous system in collaboration with an electroencephalographer. He or she may take and abstract histories; apply adequate recording electrodes and use electroencephalography (EEG) and evoked potential (EP) techniques; document the clinical condition of patients; understand and employ the optimal utilization of EEG and EP equipment; understand the interface between EEG and EP equipment and other electrophysiological devices; recognize and understand EEG and EP activity displayed; manage medical emergencies in the laboratory; prepare a descriptive report of recorded activity for the electroencephalographer; and manage the laboratory and supervise EEG technicians. Electroneurodiagnostic technologists are one type of allied health professional for which the Committee on Allied Health Education and Accreditation has accredited education programs. *See also* allied health professional; electroencephalography; evoked potentials; technologist; technology.

Electroneurodiagnostic Technologists, American Society of *See* American Society of Electroneurodiagnostic Technologists.

electronic **1.** Of, relating to, or using devices constructed or working by the methods or principles of electronics. **2.** Existing as data that must be read by a computer, as in electronic mail, electronic medical record, or electronic publishing. *See also* electronic data interchange; electronic mail; electronic medical record; electronic data interchange; electronic data processing; electronic publishing; electronic striped card; electronic text.

electronic computer-originated mail (e-com) A special service offered by the US Postal System at certain post offices, consisting of computer-generated messages sent to another post office, printed into letters, inserted in special envelopes, and delivered as first-class mail.

electronic data interchange The process whereby orders, invoices, and sometimes money are transferred electronically between customers' and vendors' computers, replacing traditional paper, mail, and phone transmission of these items.

electronic data processing (EDP) The manipulation of data by a computer. The recording of data for translation into machine-readable characters and numbers is called *input*; the manipulation of the data is the *processing* stage; and the transfer of information to a printer, terminal, or other readout device is termed the *output*. *Synonyms*: automatic data processing; computing. *See also* data processing.

electronic hearing aid *See* hearing aid.

Electronic Interactive Data Access, Fellowship and Residency *See* Fellowship and Residency Electronic Interactive Data Access.

electronic mail (email or e-mail) **1.** In computer science, the transfer of messages or files of data in machine-readable form from one user to one or more other users by means of a computer network. **2.** The messages that are sent and received using this facility. The message is stored until the receiver chooses to read it. *Synonyms*: electronic message system.

Electronic Mail Association (EMA) A national organization founded in 1983 composed of 270 corporations promoting the electronic mail industry. Its goals are to support the development of technical standards and provide information concerning technical and public policies; to minimize the restrictions on the flow of transborder information; to monitor state legislation and regulatory developments; and to represent the industry in Washington, DC. *See also* electronic mail.

electronic medical record A medical record that is created in an electronic format, such as with digital dictation or automated speech recognition, so that it can be stored, transmitted, referenced, and audited electronically. *See also* digital dictation; medical record; voice input/output technology.

electronic message system *See* electronic mail.

electronic publishing **1.** The publication of text in machine-readable form (on tape, disks, CD-ROM, and so forth) rather than on paper. **2.** Texts published in this way. *See also* electronic.

electronic striped card A smart card that provides about 8,000 bytes of data and is the most flexible type of smart card, since a software program is placed into the card, permitting decisions to be made internal to the card. *See also* smart card; smart card in health care.

electronic text (etext) The machine-readable version of a text, which is created by data capture. *See also* data capture; electronic.

electron microscope A microscope that uses a beam of electrons to scan and produce an image of an object. *See also* light microscope; microscope; operating microscope.

electron microscopy Microscopy that employs a beam of electrons instead of a beam of light to illuminate the object under study. *See also* microscopy.

Electron Microscopy Society of America *See* Microcopy Society of America.

Electro-Optics Manufacturers' Association, Laser and *See* Laser and Electro-Optics Manufacturers' Association.

Electro-Optics Society, IEEE Lasers and *See* IEEE Lasers and Electro-Optics Society.

electrophysiology The study of the mechanisms of the production of electrical phenomena and their consequences in the living organism, as in cardiac electrophysiology. *See also* clinical cardiac electrophysiology; physiology.

electrophysiology, clinical cardiac   *See* clinical cardiac electrophysiology.

Electrophysiology, North American Society of Pacing and   *See* North American Society of Pacing and Electrophysiology.

electroshock therapy   *See* electroconvulsive therapy.

Electrosurgery, American Academy of Dental   *See* American Academy of Dental Electrosurgery.

electrotherapy   Medical therapy using electric currents. *Synonym*: electrotherapeutics. *See also* diathermy; electromedicine; galvanic current; transcutaneous electrical nerve stimulation.

eleemosynary   Related to charity or charitable donations. *See also* charity.

element, data   *See* data element.

elements, trace   *See* trace elements.

eligibility worker   A social worker or other qualified individual who interviews applicants or recipients to determine eligibility for public assistance and authorizes the amount of money payment, food stamps, medical care, or other general assistance. *See also* caseworker; eligible; social worker.

eligible   Qualified or entitled to be chosen; for example, in insurance, whether an individual is entitled to benefits under a specified insurance plan, governmental program, or other health care plan. *See also* insurance.

eligible, board   *See* board prepared.

EMA   *See* Electronic Mail Association; Environmental Management Association; Environmental Mutagen Society.

email or e-mail   *See* electronic mail.

emancipated minor   A minor who has authority for making health care treatment decisions. There are three categories of emancipated minors: court-ordered emancipation (for example, teenagers living separately from their parent(s) who petition the court to be treated as though they have reached legal majority); statutorily-defined emancipation (for example, married minors or minors who are parents); or medical emancipation (for example, minors seeking treatment for a specific medical condition, such as a sexually-transmitted disease). *See also* mature minor; minor.

embalming   The treatment of the dead body with antiseptics and preservatives to prevent or delay putrefaction (rotting). *See also* funeral home.

Embalming Chemical Manufacturers Association

(ECMA)   A national organization founded in 1951 composed of companies that manufacture embalming chemicals. *See also* embalming.

embolism   A blockage of a blood vessel, especially an artery, by a thrombus, air bubble, fat globule, or other material that has travelled to the point of blockage from elsewhere via the bloodstream. Treatment depends on the nature of the material causing the blockage (embolus), the degree of obstruction, and the blood vessels affected. *See also* embolus; ischemia; thromboembolism; thrombosis; thrombus.

embolus   A clot of blood (thrombus), foreign object, bit of tissue, or air or gas bubble that moves through the bloodstream until it becomes lodged in a vessel, causing an embolism. *See also* embolism.

embryo   In humans, the prefetal developing organism from the time it implants in the uterus through the eighth week of development. A fetus is the developing organism from about the eighth week after implantation until birth. *See also* embryology; fetus; frozen embryo; preembryo; pregnancy; teratology.

embryo, frozen   *See* frozen embryo.

embryology   The branch of biology that deals with the formation and development of the embryo. *See also* embryo.

embryo, pre-   *See* preembryo.

EMBS   *See* IEEE Engineering in Medicine and Biology Society.

EMCRO   *See* experimental medical care review organization.

emergency   An unexpected or sudden occasion, as in emergency surgery needed to prevent death or serious disability. *Compare* elective. *See also* acuity; level of acuity; urgent.

emergency admission   The formal acceptance by a health care organization of a patient who requires immediate medical intervention as a result of severe, life-threatening, or potentially disabling conditions. Generally, such a patient is admitted through a hospital's emergency department. *Compare* elective admission. *See also* admission; emergency; emergency department admission; urgent admission.

emergency care   Immediate evaluation of and intervention in illnesses or injuries that may be life-threatening or limb-threatening. *See also* emergency services.

emergency center, freestanding   *See* freestanding emergency center.

emergency department (ED) The component of a health care organization that provides emergency care services. An emergency department is typically supervised by physicians experienced and often specializing in emergency medicine and operates 24 hours per day, 365 days per year. *Synonyms*: casualty ward; emergency medical service(s); emergency room (ER); emergency service(s); emergency unit; emergency ward. *See also* emergency admission; emergency department admission; emergency nurse; emergency patient; emergency physician; emergency services.

emergency department admission The formal acceptance by a health care organization of an emergency department patient whose condition requires prompt inpatient attention or treatment. *Synonym*: emergency outpatient admission. *See also* admission; emergency admission.

emergency department physician *See* emergency physician.

Emergency Management Association, National *See* National Emergency Management Association.

Emergency Management, National Coordinating Council on *See* National Coordinating Council on Emergency Management.

emergency medical responder (EMR) A trained individual who arrives on the scene of a medical emergency and administers assistance prior to the arrival of emergency medical technicians or paramedics. *Synonym*: first responder. *See also* ambulance; emergency medical technician; emergency medical technician-paramedic.

Emergency Medical Service Physicians, National Association of *See* National Association of Emergency Medical Service Physicians.

emergency medical services system (EMSS) An integrated system of health manpower, facilities, and equipment, that provides all necessary emergency care in a defined geographic area. *See also* ambulance; Emergency Medical Services System Act of 1973; medical control.

Emergency Medical Services System (EMSS) Act of 1973 A federal law that established funding and systematic requirements for emergency medical services systems including sufficient trained manpower to ensure the availability of care at all times; regional training programs for all levels of personnel; emergency medical communications systems; specialized facilities; transportation; disaster plans;

integration with public safety agencies; regional and interregional mutual assistance pacts; critical care units; patient transfer continuity; consumer participation; consumer education; standard medical records; care accessibility and availability; and ongoing review and evaluation. Federal funding for the EMSS program has been eliminated.

Emergency Medical Services Training Coordinators, National Council of State *See* National Council of State Emergency Medical Services Training Coordinators.

emergency medical technician (EMT) An individual trained to render immediate basic life-support care to ill and injured individuals, under the direction of a physician, and to safely transport them in a monitored environment to health care facilities. *See also* allied health professional; basic cardiac life support; BLS unit; emergency medical technician-paramedic; emergency services; technician.

emergency medical technician-paramedic (EMT-paramedic or EMT-P) An allied health professional who, working under the direction of a physician, administers advanced emergency medical services, principally in advanced life support units. Emergency medical technician-paramedics are one type of allied health professional for which the Committee on Allied Health Education and Accreditation has accredited education programs. *See also* advanced cardiac life support; allied health professional; ALS unit; basic trauma life support; emergency medical technician; mobile intensive care unit; paramedic.

Emergency Medical Technicians, National Association of *See* National Association of Emergency Medical Technicians.

Emergency Medical Technicians, National Registry of *See* National Registry of Emergency Medical Technicians.

emergency medicine The branch of medicine and medical specialty that deals with the recognition, stabilization, evaluation, treatment, and disposition of an undifferentiated population of patients with acute illness or injury. Emergency care is episodic and handles a full spectrum of physical and behavioral conditions. Pediatric emergency medicine, sports medicine, and medical toxicology are three subspecialties of emergency medicine. A physician who specializes in emergency medicine is called an emergency physician. *See also* emergency; emergency department; emergency physician; medical toxicology; medicine; pediatric emergency medicine; sports medicine; triage.

Emergency Medicine, American Board of *See* American Board of Emergency Medicine.

Emergency Medicine, American Osteopathic Board of *See* American Osteopathic Board of Emergency Medicine.

Emergency Medicine Association, National *See* National Emergency Medicine Association.

emergency medicine, pediatric *See* pediatric emergency medicine.

emergency medicine physician *See* emergency physician.

Emergency Medicine, Residency Review Committee for *See* Residency Review Committee for Emergency Medicine.

Emergency Medicine Residents' Association (EMRA) A national organization founded in 1974 composed of 2,200 medical students and physicians enrolled in emergency medicine residency training programs. Its purposes are to provide a unified voice for emergency medicine residents, encourage high standards in training and continuing education for emergency physicians, study socioeconomic aspects of emergency medicine, and promote education of patients and the public. *See also* emergency medicine; resident.

Emergency Medicine, Society for Academic *See* Society for Academic Emergency Medicine.

emergency nurse A registered nurse, licensed practical nurse, or licensed vocational nurse engaged or interested in the care of emergency patients. *See also* licensed practical nurse; licensed vocational nurse; registered nurse.

Emergency Nurses Association (ENA) A national organization founded in 1970 composed of 20,000 registered nurses, licensed practical nurses, licensed vocational nurses, emergency medical technicians and other individuals engaged or interested in emergency patient care. *See also* emergency nurse; emergency medical technician.

emergency outpatient admission *See* emergency department admission.

emergency patient An outpatient with a potentially disabling or life-threatening condition who receives initial evaluation and medical, dental, or other health-related services in an emergency department or a freestanding emergency center. *See*

also emergency; emergency department; freestanding emergency center.

emergency physician A physician who specializes in emergency medicine. *Synonyms:* emergency department physician; emergency medicine physician; emergency room doctor (outdated); emergency room physician (outdated). *See also* emergency medicine.

emergency physician, pediatric *See* pediatric emergency physician.

Emergency Physicians, American College of *See* American College of Emergency Physicians.

Emergency Physicians, American College of Osteopathic *See* American College of Osteopathic Emergency Physicians.

emergency preparedness plan/program A component of a health care organization's safety management program designed to manage the consequences of natural disasters or other emergencies that disrupt the organization's ability to provide care. *See also* disaster preparedness plan.

emergency privileges Temporary authorization granted by the governing body of a health care organization to a licensed practitioner to provide patient care services in the organization in an emergency situation, within limits based on the individual's professional license and without regard to regular service assignment or staff status. *Compare* clinical privileges. *See also* temporary privileges.

emergency room An outdated term for emergency department. *See* emergency department.

emergency room doctor An outdated term for emergency physician. *See* emergency physician.

emergency room physician An outdated term for emergency physician. *See* emergency physician.

emergency services 1. Health services that are provided after the onset of a medical condition that manifests itself by symptoms of sufficient severity, including severe pain, that the absence of immediate medical attention could reasonably be expected by a prudent layperson, who possesses an average knowledge of health and medicine, to result in placing the patient's health in serious jeopardy; serious impairment to bodily functions; or serious dysfunction of any bodily organ or part. **2.** The component of a health care organization responsible for delivery of emergency services, as in the emergency department or emergency service(s) of a hospital. *See also* ambulance; emergency care; out-of-area coverage; service.

emergency services levels of care (I-IV) A classification, based on specific and general requirements, that describes the capability of a health care organization to provide a range of emergency services for patients who need them. For example, a hospital with Level I emergency services offers the most comprehensive emergency care services, while a hospital with Level IV emergency services provides the least comprehensive care.

emergency services, psychiatric *See* psychiatric emergency services.

emergency surgery Surgery that a physician has determined must be performed without delay in order to prevent death or serious disability. Trauma surgery is a good example of emergency surgery. *Compare* elective surgery. *See also* surgery.

emergency unit *See* emergency department.

emergicenter *See* freestanding emergency center.

emetic Any drug, substance, or procedure that induces vomiting, as in taking an emetic after ingestion of a toxic or potentially toxic substance. *Compare* antiemetic. *See also* nausea; vomit.

EMG *See* electromyogram.

EMI scan An outdated term for CAT scan. The first computerized axial tomography (CAT) scanners were made by the British firm EMI. *See also* CAT scan.

emotion Any strong feeling, such as excitement, distress, happiness, sadness, love, hate, fear, or anger. *See also* affect; mind; mood; tears.

emotional overlay An emotionally determined addition superimposed on an existing organic symptom or physical disability. *Synonym:* psychogenic overlay. *See also* emotion; overlay; psychosomatic illness.

empathy Intellectual and emotional awareness and understanding of another person's thoughts, feelings, and behavior, even those that are distressing and disturbing. Empathy emphasizes understanding, while sympathy emphasizes sharing, of another person's feelings and experiences. *Compare* sympathy.

emphysema A condition of the lung characterized by abnormal permanent enlargement of air spaces distal to the terminal bronchiole, accompanied by the destruction of their walls and with obvious fibrosis. *See also* chronic obstructive pulmonary disease; pulmonary medicine; smoking.

Emphysema Anonymous, Inc (EAI) A national organization founded in 1965 composed of 18,000

physicians, persons suffering from emphysema, and other individuals interested in helping people with emphysema through education, encouragement, and nonmedical counseling for patients and their families. *See also* emphysema.

empirical Based directly on experience, for example, by observation or experiment, rather than on reasoning or subjective arguments alone. *See also* logical empiricism; scientific empiricism; scientific method.

empiricism, logical *See* logical empiricism.

empiricism, scientific *See* scientific empiricism.

employed, self- *See* self-employed.

employed, under- *See* underemployed.

employee A person who works for another by providing stipulated services in return for financial or other compensation. An employee may work on a per-hour, a per-diem, or an annual wage basis. Employees are persons engaged in the regular work of an organization in a hired relationship, as opposed to consultants, who are independent business persons engaged to provide advice or guidance used to support and advance the work of the organization. *Compare* consultant; employer. *See also* associate; resignation; subordinate; underemployed.

employee assistance program (EAP) A formal occupational health service program designed to assist employees with personal problems through internal counseling and referral to outside counseling or treatment resources. *See also* employee.

employee benefit program The set of benefits other than salary provided for workers by an employer, such as health insurance, disability income insurance, life insurance, Social Security benefits, a retirement pension, medical clinic services, a health and wellness program, substance abuse program, children's day care center, dental insurance and other benefits. *Synonym:* fringe benefits package. *See also* benefits; employee.

employee health benefit plan An organization's insurance plan for health benefits for its employees and their dependents, provided by the employer as a benefit not included in the employees' gross salaries. The benefit plan usually requires employees to pay a percentage of the premium and to share in the cost of services covered under the plan through payment of a deductible and a percentage of the charges for at least some of the services. *See also* employee.

employee health service A service providing pre-employment medical screening and health care services to employees. *See also* employee; health services.

Employee Retirement Income Security Act (ERISA) A 1974 federal act that exempts self-insured health plans from state laws governing health insurance, including contribution to risk pools, prohibitions against disease discrimination, and other state health reforms. *See also* group health plan.

employer An individual or organization that creates worker positions, selects and hires workers, provides training and supervision, holds and exercises discipline and dismissal authority with respect to workers and work actions, and provides and manages the resources and processes of work. *Compare* employee. *See also* corporate alliance employer; large employer; large employer alliance; mandated employer insurance; pay or play; regional alliance employer.

employer alliance, large *See* large employer alliance.

employer, corporate alliance *See* corporate alliance employer.

employer insurance, mandated *See* mandated employer insurance.

employer, large *See* large employer.

employer, regional alliance *See* regional alliance employer.

Employers on Health Care Action, National Association of *See* National Association of Employers on Health Care Action.

employment The work in which one is engaged; occupation. *Compare* unemployment. *See also* employee; employer; scope of employment.

employment, scope of *See* scope of employment.

Employment Standards Administration (ESA) An agency of the US Department of Labor that administers laws and regulations relating to employment including, for instance, the laws and regulations concerning the provision of compensation to workers injured on their jobs. One of its major divisions is the Office of Workers' Compensation. *See also* workers' compensation.

employment, un- *See* unemployment.

empower To invest with power, especially legal power or official authority. In total quality management, empowerment is a principle saying that employees should be given the authority and

resources necessary to continuously improve the processes they use to the overall benefit of the organization and its customers. *See also* enabling; individualism; total quality management.

empowerment *See* empower.

empowerment, patient *See* shared decision making.

empty calories Calories from sources, such as fats, sweets, and alcohol, that are largely devoid of essential nutrients, including vitamins and minerals. *See also* calorie; vitamin.

EMR *See* emergency medical responder.

EMRA *See* Emergency Medicine Residents' Association.

EMS Abbreviation for emergency medical services. *See* emergency medical services system.

EMSA *See* Microscopy Society of America.

EMS Directors, National Association of State *See* National Association of State EMS Directors.

EMS Pilots Association, National *See* National EMS Pilots Association.

EMSS *See* emergency medical services system.

EMT *See* emergency medical technician.

EMT-P *See* emergency medical technician-paramedic.

EMT-paramedic *See* emergency medical technician-paramedic.

EMT-Paramedic, Joint Review Committee on Educational Programs for the *See* Joint Review Committee on Educational Programs for the EMT-Paramedic.

ENA *See* Emergency Nurses Association.

enable To remove barriers or constraints and stimulate action in order to achieve desired objectives. *See also* enabling.

enabling Providing the means, opportunity, power, or authority for an individual to take action. *See also* authority; empower; enable; power.

ENC *See* Enteral Nutrition Council.

encephalitis Inflammation of the brain, occurring in association with central nervous system infections, especially by certain viruses. The most common form of mild encephalitis is due to the mumps virus. *See also* central nervous system; inflammation; meningitis; mumps; virus.

encephalographic technician/technologist *See* electroencephalographic technician/technologist.

Encephalographic Technicians and Technologists, American Board of Certified and Registered *See* American Board of Certified and Registered Encephalographic Technicians and Technologists.

encephalopathy A generalized decrease in cerebral function when the brain has been insulted by a disease or injury of another organ system, as in hepatic encephalopathy. *See also* brain; hepatic encephalopathy; hypertensive encephalopathy.

encephalopathy, hepatic   *See* hepatic encephalopathy.

encephalopathy, hypertensive   *See* hypertensive encephalopathy.

encoding   Converting information into a code. *Compare* decoding. *See also* code; coder; coding.

encounter   In health care, a contact between a patient and a health professional in which a health service is provided. In managed care, an encounter is a face-to-face meeting between a covered person and a health care provider in which services are provided. The number of encounters per member per year is calculated as the total number of encounters per year divided by the total number of members per year. *See also* health service; managed care.

endarterectomy   A surgical procedure in which the thickened, inner layer of an artery is removed, as in carotid artery endarterectomy. *See also* artery; carotid endarterectomy.

endarterectomy, carotid   *See* carotid endarterectomy.

endemic   Pertaining to a disease or agent with a low morbidity rate that is always present in a geographical area or a population, as in diseases endemic to the tropics. *Compare* epidemic; pandemic.

endocrine   Pertaining to glands that are ductless, secreting their active products (hormones) directly into the blood or other body fluids. The major endocrine organs include the pituitary gland, thyroid gland, parathyroid glands, adrenal glands, pancreas, and gonads. *Compare* exocrine. *See also* gland; hormone; pituitary gland; thyroid gland.

Endocrine Society (ES)   A national organization founded in 1918 composed of 6,050 physicians and researchers interested in the study of internal secretions. *See also* endocrinology; Women's Caucus of the Endocrine Society.

Endocrine Society, Women's Caucus of   *See* Women's Caucus of the Endocrine Society.

endocrinologist   An internist who subspecializes in endocrinology. *See also* endocrinology.

endocrinologist, pediatric   *See* pediatric endocrinologist.

endocrinologist, reproductive   *See* reproductive endocrinologist.

Endocrinologists, Society of Reproductive   *See* Society of Reproductive Endocrinologists.

endocrinology   The branch of medicine and sub-

specialty of internal medicine dealing with disorders of the internal (endocrine) glands, such as the thyroid and adrenal glands; disorders, such as diabetes and metabolic and nutritional disorders; pituitary diseases; and menstrual and sexual problems. *See also* internal medicine; pediatric endocrinology; reproductive endocrinology.

endocrinology, pediatric   *See* pediatric endocrinology.

endocrinology, reproductive   *See* reproductive endocrinology.

endodontics   The branch of dentistry and dental specialty dealing with the causes, diagnosis, prevention, and treatment of diseases of the pulp and other dental tissues that affect the vitality of the teeth. *See also* dental specialties; endodontist.

Endodontics, American Board of   *See* American Board of Endodontics.

Endodontic Society, American   *See* American Endodontic Society.

endodontist   A dentist who specializes in endodontics. *See* endodontics.

Endodontists, American Association of   *See* American Association of Endodontists.

endogenous   Developing or originating from within an organism, or arising from causes within the organism, as in endogenous obesity. *Compare* exogenous. *See also* endogenous infection; endogenous obesity.

endogenous cause   *See* common cause.

endogenous-cause variation   *See* common-cause variation.

endogenous infection   Infection due to reactivation of previously dormant organisms, as occurs in tuberculosis, histoplasmosis, and other diseases. *See also* infection.

endogenous obesity   Obesity due to metabolic (endocrine) abnormalities. *Compare* exogenous obesity. *See also* obesity.

endometriosis   A disorder in which fragments resembling the uterine mucous lining (endometrium) are also found in other locations in the body, usually the abdomen. The tissue fragments are subject to the same variations in phase with the menstrual cycle, giving rise to extremely painful menstruation, infertility, painful sexual intercourse, and heavy or irregular bleeding. *See also* laparoscopy; menses; uterus.

endometritis   Inflammation of the endometrium, the mucous lining of the uterus. *See also* inflammation; uterus.

endorphin A naturally occurring substance produced by the pituitary gland in the brain and acting on the central and the peripheral nervous systems to raise the threshold to pain (reduce pain). Endorphins produce pharmacologic effects similar to morphine. *See also* enkephalin; morphine; pituitary gland.

endorsement in professional licensure The recognition by one jurisdiction of a license given by another jurisdiction, when the qualifications and standards required by the licensing jurisdiction are equivalent to or higher than those of the endorsing jurisdiction. Endorsement relieves licensees of the burden of obtaining a second license in the endorsing jurisdiction. Endorsement does not necessarily require reciprocity between the two states. *See also* license; licensure; reciprocity.

endoscope An illuminated optic instrument for visualization of the inside of a body cavity or organ. An endoscope may be introduced through a natural opening in the body or through a surgical incision. Types of endoscopes for viewing specific areas of the body include the bronchoscope, colonoscope, cystoscope, gastroscope, laparoscope, otoscope, proctoscope, proctosigmoidoscope, and sigmoidoscope. *See also* bronchoscope; colonoscope; cystoscope; endoscopy; fiberoptics; gastroscope; laparoscope; otoscope; proctoscope; proctosigmoidoscope; sigmoidoscope.

Endoscopic Surgeons, Society American Gastrointestinal *See* Society American Gastrointestinal Endoscopic Surgeons.

endoscopy Visual inspection of a body cavity by means of an endoscope, as in gastrointestinal endoscopy. *See also* culdoscopy; endoscope; fiberoptics.

Endoscopy, American Society for Gastrointestinal *See* American Society for Gastrointestinal Endoscopy.

endostomy *See* enterostomy.

endostomy therapist *See* enterostomal therapist.

endotracheal Within or through the trachea, as in endotracheal intubation. *See also* endotracheal intubation; endotracheal tube; nasotracheal intubation.

endotracheal intubation The process of inserting an endotracheal tube into the trachea. *See also* intubation; mechanical airway; nasotracheal intubation.

endotracheal tube A tube, often surrounded by an inflatable cuff, inserted into the trachea (windpipe) for administration of anesthesia, maintenance of an airway, ventilation of the lungs, and/or prevention of entrance of foreign material, such as stomach contents, into the tracheobronchial tree. An endotracheal tube may be passed through the mouth or the nose, depending on clinical circumstances. *See also* airway; endotracheal intubation; trachea.

endowment 1. The act of providing with property, income, or a source of income. **2.** The funds or property donated to an institution, an individual, or a group as a source of income, as in The Duke Endowment.

Endowment, The Duke *See* The Duke Endowment.

end point A point of termination; for example, a health event that leads to completion or termination of follow-up of an individual in a clinical trial or study, such as death or major morbidity, particularly related to the study question. *See also* outcome.

end product The result of a completed series of processes or changes. *See also* end point; outcome; process.

end result *See* outcome.

end stage kidney disease *See* end stage renal disease.

end stage renal disease (ESRD) Kidney disease in which the kidneys can no longer function well enough to sustain life, requiring dialysis or renal transplant. Medicare, the primary source for paying for long-term hemodialysis, extends certain benefits to patients with end stage renal disease. *Synonym*: end stage kidney disease. *See also* disease; hemodialysis; kidney; Medicare; nephrology; renal.

enema A liquid injected or to be injected into the rectum. *See also* barium enema; contrast enema.

enema, barium *See* barium enema.

enema, contrast *See* barium enema.

Energy and Commerce, Committee on *See* Committee on Energy and Commerce.

Energy, Department of *See* Department of Energy.

Energy Institute, Health and *See* Health and Energy Institute.

Energy and Natural Resources, Committee on *See* Committee on Energy and Natural Resources.

Enforcement Agency, Drug *See* Drug Enforcement Agency.

Enforcement and Regulation, Council on Licensure, *See* Council on Licensure, Enforcement and Regulation.

engage To retain or enter into an agreement or relationship, as in the hospital engaged the consultant's services.

engineer A person who is trained or professionally engaged in a branch of engineering. *See also* administrative engineer; bioengineer; chief engineer; clinical engineer; engineering; hospital engineer; industrial engineer; public health engineer.

engineer, administrative *See* administrative engineer.

engineer, bio- *See* bioengineer.

engineer, chief *See* chief engineer.

engineer, clinical *See* clinical engineer.

engineer, hospital *See* hospital engineer.

engineer, industrial *See* industrial engineer.

engineering The application of scientific and mathematical principles to practical ends, such as the design, manufacture, and operation of efficient and economical structures, machines, processes, and systems. *See also* genetic engineering; quality assurance engineering; quality engineering; reliability engineering.

Engineering, American Society of Sanitary *See* American Society of Sanitary Engineering.

Engineering (of AHA), American Society for Hospital *See* American Society for Hospital Engineering (of AHA).

engineering, computer-aided software *See* computer-aided software engineering.

Engineering Conference, Cryogenic *See* Cryogenic Engineering Conference.

engineering department, clinical *See* clinical engineering department.

engineering, genetic *See* genetic engineering.

engineering and maintenance department *See* maintenance department.

Engineering in Medicine and Biology Society, IEEE *See* IEEE Engineering in Medicine and Biology Society.

Engineering, National Institute for Rehabilitation *See* National Institute for Rehabilitation Engineering.

Engineering Professors, Association of Environmental *See* Association of Environmental Engineering Professors.

Engineering Psychologists, Division of Applied Experimental and *See* Division of Applied Experimental and Engineering Psychologists.

engineering psychology The branch of psychology dealing with the design and use of equipment through the "human factors" approach. Engineering psychology answers questions, such as, "What kind of lighting best combines visibility with restfulness? What is the best arrangement of office machines for their most effective use in transcription, reproduction, and distribution?" Engineering psychologists sometimes join with personnel and organizational psychologists, who focus more on individuals and groups than on equipment. *See also* engineering; ergonomics; human factors; psychology.

engineering, quality *See* quality engineering.

engineering, quality assurance *See* quality assurance engineering.

engineering, reliability *See* reliability engineering.

Engineering Society, Biomedical *See* Biomedical Engineering Society.

engineer, medical *See* bioengineer.

engineer, public health *See* public health engineer.

Engineers, American Academy of Environmental *See* American Academy of Environmental Engineers.

Engineers, American Society of Safety *See* American Society of Safety Engineers.

engineer, sanitary *See* sanitary engineer.

Engineers, Institute of Electrical and Electronics *See* Institute of Electrical and Electronics Engineers.

Engineers, Society of Fire Protection *See* Society of Fire Protection Engineers.

enkephalin A naturally occurring opiate involved in the perception of pain and the integration of emotional experiences. *See also* emotion; endorphin; opiate; pain; pituitary gland.

enriched A legal labeling definition for foods indicating the addition of nutrients either to replace those that are lost in processing or to add nutrients the food does not naturally contain. *Synonym:* fortified. *See also* labeling.

enroll In the insurance field, to agree to participate in a contract for benefits from an insurance company or health maintenance organization. *See also* enrollment.

enrollment 1. The total number of individuals enrolled with an insurance company or health maintenance organization. 2. The process by which a health plan signs up groups and individuals for membership, or the number of enrollees who sign up in any one group. *See also* conditions of enrollment; enrollment period; health maintenance organization; health plan; open enrollment.

enrollment, conditions of *See* conditions of enrollment.

enrollment, open *See* open enrollment.

enrollment period In the insurance field, the period during which individuals may enroll for insurance or health maintenance organization benefits. *See also* enrollment.

ENT doctor/physician/specialist *See* otolaryngologist-head and neck surgeon.

enteral Having to do with the intestine, as in enteral feeding. *See also* intestine.

enteral feeding Food that is supplied directly to the intestine through a tube rather than by being eaten. *See also* enteral and parenteral nutrition and infusion therapy services; intestine.

enteral formula Foods for special dietary use, primarily for nutritional management of patients with various medical conditions, that necessitate nasogastric feeding or supplementation. *See also* enteral feeding; intestine; nasogastric feeding.

Enteral Nutrition, American Society for Parenteral and *See* American Society for Parenteral and Enteral Nutrition.

Enteral Nutrition Council (ENC) A national council founded in 1983 composed of seven manufacturers and marketers of enteral formulas. Its purpose is to provide for communication between manufacturers and marketers of enteral nutrition products and government and regulatory bodies. *See also* enteral feeding; enteral formula; nutrition.

enteral and parenteral nutrition and infusion therapy services Services for the provision of nutrients or therapeutic agents to patients by administration into the intestine or by intravenous infusion for the purpose of improving or maintaining an individual's nutritional status or health condition. *See also* enteral feeding; nutrition; parenteral nutrition; total parenteral nutrition.

enteric Pertaining to inside the intestines, as in using enteric precautions to prevent transmission of disease. *See also* enteric precautions; intestine.

enteric fever *See* typhoid fever.

enteric precautions A category of patient isolation intended for infections transmitted by direct or indirect contact with feces. Specifications include use of a private room if patient hygiene is poor. Masks are not indicated but gowns are used if soiling is likely. Gloves are used for touching contaminated materials. *See also* enteric; isolation.

enteritis Any condition involving inflammation or irritation of part of the intestine. *See also* inflammation; intestine.

enterostomal therapist A registered nurse qualified by an accredited training program in enterostomal therapy, who provides wound drainage services to patients who need them. *See also* enterosto-

my; registered nurse; therapist.

enterostomy A surgical procedure that produces a permanent opening into the intestines through the abdominal wall, as in a colostomy or ileostomy. *See also* colostomy; enterostomal therapist; ileostomy; intestine.

enterprise culture A capitalist society in which entrepreneurial activity and initiative are explicitly encouraged; a culture founded on an individualistic, go-getting economic ethic. *See also* culture; entrepreneur.

enterprise, joint *See* joint enterprise.

enterprise liability A plan relating to tort reform in which medical liability is shifted from physicians to health plans (for example, health maintenance organizations). Patients would sue the health plans rather than physicians, thereby providing physicians immunity from medical liability. Some observers contend that this approach could further erode physician autonomy by giving nonphysicians more reasons to dictate how physicians do their work. In theory, these nonphysicians would be closely examining the care provided by physicians to prevent lawsuits. *See also* health plan; lawsuit; physician; professional liability.

enterprise zone An area in which a government seeks to stimulate new enterprise by creating financial incentives, such as tax concessions, for businesses. Enterprise zones are generally found in derelict inner urban districts that have experienced serious employment declines.

enthesis The use of artificial material in the repair of a defect or deformity of the body.

entitlement A benefit that an individual has a right or a claim to, such as veterans' pensions and civil-service retirement pay. *See also* Civilian Health and Medical Program of the Uniformed Services (CHAMPUS); Civilian Health and Medical Program of the Veterans Administration (CHAMPVA); controllability; entitlement authority; entitlement program.

entitlement authority Legislation that requires the payment of entitlements to any person or government meeting the requirements established by law. Examples of mandatory entitlements are veterans' pensions, social security benefits, and uniformed services health benefits (including Civilian Health and Medical Program of the Uniformed Services [CHAMPUS] for dependents of military personnel on active duty, retirees, and retiree dependents). The Congressional Budget and Impoundment Control

Act of 1974 placed restrictions on the enactment of new federal entitlement authority. *See also* authority; backdoor authority; Civilian Health and Medical Program of the Uniformed Services; controllability; entitlement; open-ended programs.

entitlement program A government program, such as Social Security or Medicare, that guarantees and provides benefits to a particular group of people, such as individuals over the age of 65 years. *See also* backdoor authority; entitlement; entitlement authority; Medicare; open-ended programs.

entity An independently existing thing; a reality.

entrepreneur An individual who organizes, operates, and assumes the risk for a new business venture. *Compare* intrapreneur. *See also* enterprise culture.

Entrepreneurial Dentists, American Association of *See* American Association of Entrepreneurial Dentists.

environment **1.** The circumstances or conditions of one's surroundings. **2.** The natural world viewed as a unified whole with interrelationship and balance among the parts that must be conserved.

environmental **1.** Relating to the conditions of one's surroundings. **2.** Concerned with the conservation of the environment, hence serving this cause. *See also* environment.

Environmental Engineering Professors, Association of *See* Association of Environmental Engineering Professors.

Environmental Engineers, American Academy of *See* American Academy of Environmental Engineers.

Environmental Geochemistry and Health, Society for *See* Society for Environmental Geochemistry and Health.

environmental health The health profession dealing with detecting, identifying, controlling, and managing physical and social conditions affecting the health of populations, such as workers in factories or residents of communities. Practitioners of environmental health include, among others, sanitarians, inspectors, and environmentalists. *Synonym:* industrial health. *See also* industrial hygienist; occupational health; sanitarian.

Environmental Health Administrators, National Conference of Local *See* National Conference of Local Environmental Health Administrators.

Environmental Health Association, National *See* National Environmental Health Association.

environmental health practitioner *See* industrial hygienist; sanitarian.

Environmental Health Science and Protection, National Accreditation Council for *See* National Accreditation Council for Environmental Health Science and Protection.

Environmental Health/Sciences Centers, Association of University *See* Association of University Environmental Health/Sciences Centers.

Environmental Health, Society for Occupational and *See* Society for Occupational and Environmental Health.

environmental health specialist *See* industrial hygienist; sanitarian.

Environmental Management Association (EMA) A national organization founded in 1957 composed of 1,200 individuals administering environmental sanitation maintenance programs in industrial plants, commercial and public buildings, institutions, and governmental agencies. It conducts educational programs and presents awards. Subsidiaries include the Food Sanitation Institute; Buildings-Grounds; and the Health Care Institute.

Environmental Medicine, American Academy of *See* American Academy of Environmental Medicine.

Environmental Medicine, American Board of *See* American Board of Environmental Medicine.

Environmental Medicine, American College of Occupational and *See* American College of Occupational and Environmental Medicine.

Environmental Mutagen Society (EMA) A national organization founded in 1969 composed of 1,100 bioscientists in universities, governmental agencies, and industry interested in promoting basic and applied studies of mutagenesis. *See also* mutagen; mutagenesis.

environmental pollution *See* pollution.

Environmental Protection Agency (EPA) A federal agency created to allow for coordinated and effective governmental action to protect the environment through the abatement and control of pollution on a systematic basis. The EPA is responsible for various research, monitoring, standard-setting, and enforcement activities and controlling air pollution, water pollution, hazardous waste disposal, and other threats to the environment. Its health-related responsibilities are managed by its Offices of Air Quality Planning and Standards, Radiation Programs, Pesticide Programs, Toxic Substances, Health and Environmental Assessment, Health Research, Emergency and Remedial Response, Solid Waste, Drinking Water, Ground-Water Protection, Municipal Pollution Control, and Water Regulations and Standards. *See also* backdoor authority; hazardous waste; pollution.

environmental services Ancillary services, such as housekeeping, laundry, maintenance, and liquid and solid waste control, performed to improve safety, sanitation, and efficiency of the operation of a hospital or other type of health care organization. *See also* ancillary services.

Environmental Services of the American Hospital Association, American Society for Healthcare *See* American Society for Healthcare Environmental Services of the American Hospital Association.

Environmental Services, American Society for Healthcare *See* American Society for Healthcare Environmental Services of the American Hospital Association.

Environmental and Toxicologic Pathology, Department of *See* Department of Environmental and Toxicologic Pathology.

environment, operating *See* operating environment.

enzyme A protein molecule that is a specific catalyst for many of the chemical reactions that take place in the body. *See also* biochemistry; protein.

EOB *See* explanation of benefits.

EOMB *See* Explanation of Medicare Benefits.

EP *See* evoked potentials.

EPA *See* Environmental Protection Agency.

epidemic A disease, such as influenza, that breaks out, spreads rapidly, attacks many people in a geographical area, causes a high death rate, and then subsides. Epidemic applies especially to infectious diseases, as in an epidemic of cholera, but is also applied to any disease, injury, or other health-related event occurring in outbreaks, as in an epidemic of teenage suicide. *Synonym:* outbreak. *Compare* endemic; pandemic. *See also* behavioral epidemic; cholera; infectious diseases; influenza.

epidemic, behavioral *See* behavioral epidemic.

Epidemiological Society, American *See* American Epidemiological Society.

Epidemiologic Research, Society for *See* Society for Epidemiologic Research.

epidemiologist An investigator who studies the occurrence of disease or other health-related conditions or events in defined populations, such as a community or medical facility. *See also* hospital epi-

demiologist; medical epidemiologist; nurse epidemiologist.

epidemiologist, hospital *See* hospital epidemiologist.

epidemiologist, medical *See* medical epidemiologist.

epidemiologist, nurse *See* nurse epidemiologist.

Epidemiologists, Council of State and Territorial *See* Council of State and Territorial Epidemiologists.

epidemiology The study of the distribution and determinants of health-related conditions or events in specified populations and the application of this study to control of health problems. *See also* epidemiologist; population; vector; vital statistics.

Epidemiology, American College of *See* American College of Epidemiology.

epidermis The outer protective layer of the skin, covering the dermis. *See also* dermis; skin; tissue.

epidural anesthesia Injection of local anesthesia into the epidural space of the spinal column to achieve regional anesthesia of the abdominal, genital, or pelvic area. It is widely used in vaginal childbirth, cesarean delivery, and gynecologic surgery. *See also* anesthesia; local anesthesia; regional anesthesia.

epilepsy Paroxysmal transient disturbances of brain function that may be manifested as episodic impairment or loss of consciousness, abnormal motor phenomena, psychic or sensory disturbances, or disturbance of the autonomic nervous system. *Synonyms:* sacred disease; seizure disorder. *See also* barbiturate; convulsion; developmental disability.

Epilepsy Society, American *See* American Epilepsy Society.

Episcopal Coalition on Alcohol and Drugs, National *See* National Episcopal Coalition on Alcohol and Drugs.

episiotomy A surgical incision of the perineum and vagina performed during labor in order to enlarge the outlet of the birth canal and prevent spontaneous tearing of these tissues. *See also* delivery; labor; obstetrics.

episode An occurrence or incident that is part of a progression or a larger sequence, as in a period in which a disease or other health problem exists, measured from its onset to its resolution; for example, a major depressive episode. *See also* incident; occurrence.

EPO *See* exclusive provider organization.

eponym The name of a person used as part of the name of a disease, syndrome, finding, anatomical feature, device, or procedure, as in Pott's fracture, Swan-Ganz catheter, or Bright's disease. The physician or physicians associated with an original description or invention are the most frequent to be honored with an eponym, but a few diseases are named after patients; for example, Christmas disease is named after Mr Christmas.

EPSDT   *See* Early and Periodic Screening Diagnosis and Treatment Program.

epsom salts   Hydrated magnesium sulphate used as an osmotic laxative, particularly when rapid bowel evacuation is desired. A popular source of medicinal magnesium sulphate was the mineral springs at Epsom, Surrey. *See also* laxative.

Equilibration Society, American   *See* American Equilibration Society.

equipment, durable medical   *See* durable medical equipment.

equipment management   A component of a health care organization's plant, technology, and safety management program designed to assess and limit the clinical and physical risks of fixed and portable equipment used for the diagnosis, treatment, monitoring, and care of patients and the risks of other fixed and portable electrically powered equipment. *See also* home equipment management services; management; plant, technology, and safety management.

equipment management services, home   *See* home equipment management services.

equipment, medical   *See* medical equipment.

Equipment Suppliers, National Association of Medical   *See* National Association of Medical Equipment Suppliers.

Equipment Technicians, Society of Biomedical   *See* Society of Biomedical Equipment Technicians.

equity   **1.** Measure of fairness in the consumption of goods and services. **2.** Freedom from bias or favoritism.

equivalence, bio-   *See* bioequivalence.

equivalence, chemical   *See* chemical equivalence.

equivalence, pharmaceutical   *See* pharmaceutical equivalence.

equivalency   Evidence that compliance with the intent of a standard has been achieved in a manner other than as prescribed by the standard. The concept is employed, for example, in the selection of pharmaceuticals and in the determination of qualifications in educational, professional, and organizational certifications. *See also* certification; compliance; standard.

equivalents, therapeutic   *See* therapeutic equivalents.

equivalents, generic   *See* generic equivalents.

ER   Abbreviation for emergency room (outdated). *See* emergency department.

ER doctor   Abbreviation for emergency room doctor (outdated). *See* emergency physician.

ergonomics   The study of humans in their working environment, particularly in relation to the principles governing the efficient use of human energy. *See also* engineering psychology; human factors.

ERISA   *See* Employee Retirement Income Security Act.

ER physician   Abbreviation for emergency room physician (outdated). *See* emergency physician.

error   A mistake; for example, a false or mistaken result obtained in a study or experiment. *See also* accounting error; medication error; probable error; random error; sampling error; standard error; systematic error; type I error; type II error.

error, accounting   *See* accounting error.

error, alpha   *See* type I error.

error, beta   *See* type II error.

error, conclusion   *See* statistical conclusion validity.

error, drug   *See* medication error.

error, measurement   *See* measurement error.

error, medication   *See* medication error.

error, probable   *See* probable error.

error, random   *See* random error.

error, refractive   *See* refractive error.

error, sampling   *See* sampling error.

error, standard   *See* standard error.

error, trial and   *See* trial and error.

error, type I   *See* type I error.

error, type II   *See* type II error.

ERTA   *See* Economic Recovery Tax Act of 1981.

erythrocyte   *See* red blood cell.

ES   *See* Endocrine Society.

ESA   *See* Employment Standards Administration; Exer-Safety Association.

Escherichia coli (E coli)   A species of gram-negative bacteria that normally inhabits the large intestine. Under certain conditions some strains can be pathogenic, particularly when transferred to other sites, such as the urinary tract. The bacillus has been extensively employed as an experimental system in genetic engineering. *Synonym:* coliform bacillus. *See also* bacteria; genetic engineering; intestine.

escort service, patient   *See* patient escort service.

ESO   *See* early survey option survey.

esophageal reflux   *See* gastroesophageal reflux.

esophageal reflux, gastro- *See* gastroesophageal reflux.

esophagitis, reflux *See* reflux esophagitis.

Esophagological Association, American Broncho- *See* American Broncho-Esophagological Association.

esophagology The study of diseases and injuries of the respiratory tract and upper digestive tract. *See also* esophagus; gastroenterology.

esophagus The muscular, membranous tube for the passage of food from the pharynx to the stomach. *See also* alimentary tract; esophagology; gastroenterology; gastroesophageal reflux; reflux esophagitis.

ESP *See* Economic Stabilization Program.

ESRD *See* end stage renal disease.

essential nutrient A nutrient necessary for health that one must obtain in food or through dietary supplements because the body either does not make it at all or does not make enough of it. *See also* nutrient.

established name The name given to a drug or pharmaceutical product by the United States Adopted Names Council, as required by the federal Food, Drug and Cosmetic Act. Established names are usually shorter and simpler than chemical names and are most commonly used in the scientific literature. Most physicians and pharmacists learn about drug products using the products' established names; for example, penicillin. *Compare* chemical name. *See also* name.

established patient A patient for whom a physician or other provider has a medical record. *See also* medical record; patient.

estimate **1.** A measurement or a statement about the value of some quantity that is known, believed, or suspected to contain a degree of error. *See also* error. **2.** A single value (point) or interval (range) of an unknown population parameter based on a sample of the population. *See also* parameter.

estrogen A sex hormone made in both sexes, but in much greater quantities in women. It is produced by the ovaries, adrenal glands, the placenta, and by the enzyme aromatase in fatty tissue. It is responsible for the development and maintenance of female secondary sex characteristics. *Compare* testosterone. *See also* hormone; ovary; sex hormone.

ESWL Abbreviation for extracorporeal shock wave lithotripsy. *See* lithotripsy.

etext *See* electronic text.

ethanol Ethyl alcohol that is produced by the fermentation of sugars. The pharmacological effects of alcohol, chiefly central nervous system depression and peripheral vasodilatation, are mostly employed for social and recreational purposes. The medical importance of alcohol centers on its roles as a drug of addiction and as a general tissue poison. *See also* addiction; alcohol; alcoholism.

ether An anesthetic agent rarely used because of its inflammability and irritant effect on the respiratory tract. *See also* anesthetic.

ethical In accordance with the principles of right and wrong that govern the conduct of a business or profession. *Compare* unethical. *See also* ethics.

ethical dilemma A situation in which acting on one moral conviction or belief means breaking another. *See also* ethical; principle of the least advantaged.

Ethical Hypnosis, Association to Advance *See* Association to Advance Ethical Hypnosis.

ethical observer, ideal *See* ideal ethical observer.

ethicist One who can classify, diagnose, and suggest solutions for moral problems; for example, in a hospital, an ethicist provides staff education, aids in policy formation, and consults on clinical cases. *See also* ethics.

ethics The branch of philosophy that deals with systematic approaches to moral issues, such as the distinction between right and wrong and the moral consequences of human actions. Ethics involves a system of behaviors, expectations, and morals composing standards of conduct for a population or a profession. *See also* bioethics; biomedical ethics; code of ethics; deontological ethics; ethicist; ethics committee; medical ethics; morality; moral law; organ procurement; utilitarianism.

ethics, code of *See* code of ethics.

ethics committee A multidisciplinary committee of a health care organization that provides case consultation designed to help resolve moral conflicts that arise in difficult medical cases; educates institutional personnel in the ways in which ethics affect their job responsibilities; and develops institutional policies on various ethical issues. The committee typically includes physicians, nurses, chaplains, social workers, consumer representatives, and professionals with expertise in moral decision making. *See also* ethics; ethics committee model for reviewing cases; euthanasia.

ethics committee model for reviewing cases Four models defined by whether case review is mandatory and whether an attending physician must abide by an ethics committee's recommendation regarding a case: **1.** optional/optional (most cases): case review is optional and the physician need not abide by the recommendations; **2.** optional/mandatory (least common): case review is optional and the physician must abide by the recommendations; **3.** mandatory/optional: case review is mandatory for specified cases and the physician need not abide by the recommendations; **4.** mandatory/mandatory: case review is mandatory for specified cases and the physician must abide by the recommendations. *See also* ethics committee; physician.

ethics, deontological *See* deontological ethics.

ethics, medical *See* medical ethics.

ethics, normative *See* normative ethics.

ethics, situation *See* situation ethics.

ethnobiology The study of the plant and animal lore of a specific people or region, including the study of the medicinal uses of plant and animal products.

Ethnobiology, Society of *See* Society of Ethnobiology.

etiology The science of causes; causality, as in the etiology of coma. *See also* causality; cause; pathogenesis.

eugenics The science of increasing the frequency of desirable genes and decreasing the frequency of undesirable genes. *See also* eugenic sterilization; gene.

eugenic sterilization Sterilization performed to prevent inheritance of a mental or physical disability or disease. *See also* eugenics; sterilization.

euphemism The act or an example of substituting a mild, indirect, or vague term for one considered harsh, blunt, or offensive; for example, birth control as a euphemism for contraception, even though birth control properly embraces other methods of population limitation, such as infanticide, abortion, and moral restraint. *See also* bureaucratese; jargon; language; legalese.

euphoria An exaggerated feeling of physical and mental well-being, especially when the feeling is not justified by external reality. Euphoria may be induced by drugs, such as the opium derivatives, amphetamines, and alcohol; it is also a feature of mania. *See also* alcohol; amphetamines; heroin; intoxication; mania; opiate.

euthanasia The act or practice of painlessly terminating the life of a person or an animal. As applied to persons, it is accepted in some cultures but in the United States is treated as criminal, subjecting those responsible to prosecution under the homicide statutes. An exception has been developed in some jurisdictions, however, in which the termination of an incurably ill patient is no longer treated as criminal if done by a guardian or immediate family member after consultation with an ethics committee of a hospital, and if accomplished by the negative means of withdrawing life support systems or extraordinary medical care rather than by some affirmative act. *See also* active euthanasia; ethics; ethics committee; passive euthanasia.

euthanasia, active *See* active euthanasia.

euthanasia, passive *See* passive euthanasia.

euthanize To subject to euthanasia. *See also* euthanasia.

euthenics The study of the improvement of human functioning and well-being by improvement of living conditions. *See also* ergonomics.

Evaluating Professionals, National Association of Disability *See* National Association of Disability Evaluating Professionals.

evaluation **1.** The process or act of examination and careful judgment, as in the measurement and assessment of the performance of a hospital, practitioner, or program. *See also* drug usage evaluation; economic evaluation; evaluation criteria; qualitative evaluation; quantitative evaluation. **2.** In mathematics, the calculation of the numerical value of something.

evaluation of care The process of measuring and assessing the degree to which health care processes and outcomes meet accepted standards or norms. *See also* evaluation.

evaluation committee, product *See* product evaluation committee.

evaluation criteria Standards or guidelines for measuring and assessing the degree to which desired objectives are met. *See also* criteria; evaluation.

evaluation, drug usage *See* drug usage evaluation.

evaluation, economic *See* economic evaluation.

evaluation, monitoring and *See* monitoring and evaluation.

Evaluation, National Advisory Council for Health Care Policy, Research, and *See* National Advisory Council for Health Care Policy, Research, and Evaluation.

Evaluation, Office of Health Planning and *See* Office of Health Planning and Evaluation.

evaluation, performance-based quality-of-care *See* performance-based quality-of-care evaluation.

evaluation, qualitative *See* qualitative evaluation.

evaluation, quantitative *See* quantitative evaluation.

Evaluation and Review Technique, Program *See* Program Evaluation and Review Technique.

evaporated milk Milk that has been heated, vacuum concentrated, homogenized, and canned. *See also* milk.

event Something that takes place or comes to pass, usually a notable occurrence. *Synonyms:* episode; happening; incident; occurrence. *See also* adverse event; episode; incident; life events; occurrence; sentinel event.

event, adverse *See* adverse event.

event indicator, sentinel *See* sentinel event indicator.

event, sentinel *See* sentinel event.

events, life *See* life events.

evidence 1. Information helpful in forming a conclusion or making a judgment. 2. In law, the documentary or oral statements and the material objects admissible as testimony in a court of law. *See also* admissible evidence; burden of proof; circumstantial evidence; direct evidence; medical evidence; preponderance of the evidence.

evidence, admissible *See* admissible evidence.

evidence, circumstantial *See* circumstantial evidence.

evidence, direct *See* direct evidence.

evidence, medical *See* medical evidence.

evidence, preponderance of the *See* preponderance of the evidence.

evident, tamper *See* tamper evident.

evoked potentials (EP) In electroneurodiagnostic testing, the sum of the stimulus-evoked bioelectrical potentials from the peripheral nerve, retina, or cochlear mechanism, from the spinal cord or central conduction pathways, and from cortical and subcortical structures. *See also* electroneurodiagnostic technologist.

Evoked Potentials, American Society for Clinical *See* American Society for Clinical Evoked Potentials.

Evoked Potentials Technologists, American Board of Registration of Electroencephalographic and *See* American Board of Registration of Electroencephalographic and Evoked Potentials Technologists.

evolution 1. Development according to natural laws and by means of natural processes. 2. Differentiation into species from common ancestors. *See also* natural selection.

exacerbation An increase in the severity of a disease or any of its symptoms, as in an exacerbation of asthma.

examination 1. A set of questions or exercises testing knowledge or skill, as in certification examination. *See also* certification examination; specialty board examination. 2. The process of testing or checking the condition or health of, as in examination of a patient. *See also* physical examination.

examination, certification *See* certification examination.

Examination Committee, Foreign Pharmacy Graduate *See* Foreign Pharmacy Graduate Examination Committee.

examination, cross- *See* cross-examination.

examination, direct *See* direct examination.

examination, national board *See* national board examination.

examination, pelvic *See* pelvic examination.

examination, physical *See* physical examination.

examination, specialty board *See* specialty board examination.

examine To observe carefully or critically in order to determine condition or quality, as in examining a patient for signs of abuse. *See also* examination; inspect; investigate.

examiner, medical *See* medical examiner.

Examiners, American Association of Dental *See* American Association of Dental Examiners.

Examiners, American Association of Osteopathic *See* American Association of Osteopathic Examiners.

Examiners, American Council of Hypnotist *See* American Council of Hypnotist Examiners.

Examiners, National Association of Disability *See* National Association of Disability Examiners.

Examiners, National Board of Medical *See* National Board of Medical Examiners.

Examiners, National Board of Osteopathic Medical *See* National Board of Osteopathic Medical Examiners.

Examiners, National Board of Podiatric Medical *See* National Board of Podiatric Medical Examiners.

Examiners, National Contact Lens *See* National Contact Lens Examiners.

Examiners for Nursing Home Administrators, National Association of Boards of *See* National Association of Boards of Examiners for Nursing Home Administrators.

Examiners–Nursing and Technology, Board of Nephrology *See* Board of Nephrology Examiners–

Nursing and Technology.

Examiners in Optometry, National Board of *See* National Board of Examiners in Optometry.

Examiners in Pastoral Counseling, American Board of *See* American Board of Examiners in Pastoral Counseling.

Examiners of Psychodrama, Sociometry, and Group Psychotherapy, American Board of *See* American Board of Examiners of Psychodrama, Sociometry, and Group Psychotherapy.

examiners, state board of medical *See* state board of medical examiners.

excellence, centers of *See* centers of excellence.

excipient An inert substance mixed with a medicinal compound to act as a vehicle and facilitate administration. *Synonym*: vehicle. *See also* lactose; linctus; pharmaceutical necessity; pill; tablet.

exclusions In the insurance area, specific hazards, perils, or conditions listed in an insurance or medical-care-coverage policy for which the policy does not provide benefit payments. Preexisting conditions are usually exclusions, including heart disease, diabetes, hypertension, and pregnancies that existed before a policy was in effect. Other examples are self-inflicted injuries, combat injuries, cosmetic surgery, custodial care, and injuries covered by workers' compensation. Exclusions often prevent persons who have a serious condition or disease from securing insurance coverage, either for the particular disease or in general. *See also* general exclusion; preexisting condition; waiver.

exclusive contract An agreement that gives a physician or group of physicians the right to provide all administrative and clinical services required for the operation of a hospital department and precludes other physicians from practicing that specialty in that institution for the period of the contract. *Compare* open staff. *See also* closed staff; contract.

exclusive dealing arrangement An arrangement in which a buyer agrees not to deal in any goods or services that compete with those of the seller.

exclusive provider organization (EPO) Identical to a preferred provider organization from which the phrase was derived, except that persons enrolled in the plan are eligible to receive benefits only when they use the services of the contracting providers. No benefits are available when non-contracting providers are used except in certain emergency situations. Technically, many health care organizations can be described as exclusive provider organizations. *See also* preferred provider organization.

execute To carry out or put into effect; to perform, as in executing the surgical procedure well. *See also* accomplish; perform.

executed Fully accomplished or performed; leaving nothing unfulfilled.

executive A person having administrative or managerial authority in an organization, such as a hospital, nursing home, or other type of health care organization. *See also* chief executive officer; executive housekeeper; physician executive.

executive committee A standing committee of the governing body of an organization, the functions and authority of which vary among organizations. For instance, an executive committee may function as the governing body between board meetings and have full authority to make binding decisions for the governing body on a broad range of issues. Alternatively, the executive committee may be restricted to routine functions, such as creating meeting agendas and recommending committee appointments. *See also* executive; medical staff executive committee; standing committee.

executive committee, medical staff *See* medical staff executive committee.

executive director *See* chief executive officer.

Executive Directors, Association of Osteopathic State *See* Association of Osteopathic State Executive Directors.

executive, health care *See* executive.

executive housekeeper A housekeeping director certified by the National Executive Housekeepers' Association. *See also* housekeeping director.

executive information system A computer system process developed to give top and middle management information they need for decision making. *See also* information system; middle management.

executive, nurse *See* nurse executive.

executive order A rule or regulation issued by a chief administrative authority.

executive oversight The sum of the processes by which an executive attempts to exercise control and direction of an organization and to hold individual managers responsible for the implementation of their programs. *See also* executive; oversight.

executive, physician *See* physician executive.

Executive Recruiters, National Association *See* National Association of Executive Recruiters.

Executives, American Association of Medical Society *See* American Association of Medical Society Executives.

Executives, American College of Healthcare *See* American College of Healthcare Executives.

Executives, American College of Physician *See* American College of Physician Executives.

Executives, American Organization of Nurse *See* American Organization of Nurse Executives.

Executives, College of Osteopathic Healthcare *See* College of Osteopathic Healthcare Executives.

Executives, Conference of Podiatry *See* Conference of Podiatry Executives.

executive search firm *See* headhunter.

executive session A meeting of a board, commission, or legislative group or subgroup that is not open to the public.

Executives, National Association of Health Services *See* National Association of Health Services Executives.

Executives, National Council of State Pharmacy Association *See* National Council of State Pharmacy Association Executives.

executive vice president *See* chief executive officer.

exemplary damages *See* punitive damages.

exercise Any physical activity engaged in for reasons of health, recreation, sport, or training. *Compare* sedentary. *See also* aerobics; fitness; passive exercise; workout.

exercise, passive *See* passive exercise.

Exer-Safety Association (ESA) A national organization founded in 1980 composed of 4,000 fitness instructors, personal trainers, health spas, YMCAs, community recreation departments, and hospital wellness programs, whose purposes are to improve the qualifications of exercise instructors, to train instructors to develop safe exercise routines that will help people avoid injury while exercising, and to prepare instructors for national certification. *See also* certification; fitness; wellness.

exhaustion A state of extreme fatigue, with no further energy reserves available. *See also* prostration.

exhaustion of remedies A legal doctrine that requires a plaintiff to exhaust all nonjudicial remedies (for example, administrative hearings and appeals) before pursuing a lawsuit. *See also* lawsuit; plaintiff; remedy.

exhibitionism A public genital exposure, usually with intent to shock or alarm and so to gain sexual gratification. This sexual deviation occurs almost exclusively in males and may be compulsive. *See also* genitalia; obsessive-compulsive.

Exhibitors Association, Healthcare Convention and *See* Healthcare Convention and Exhibitors Association.

exit conference *See* chief executive officer exit conference.

exocrine Pertaining to a gland from which the secretion is removed by means of a duct, rather than directly by the blood circulation as is the case with endocrine (ductless) glands. *Compare* endocrine. *See also* gland.

ex officio Latin phrase meaning "by virtue or because of an office." Many individuals hold positions on boards, commissions, advisory groups, councils, or other bodies because of an office that they currently occupy. For example, the mayor of a city may be an ex officio member of the board of directors of a hospital in his or her city.

exogenous Derived or developed from outside the body, as in exogenous infection. *Compare* endogenous. *See also* exogenous infection.

exogenous cause *See* special cause.

exogenous-cause variation *See* special-cause variation.

exogenous infection Infection caused by organisms not normally present in the body but which have gained entrance from the environment, as in meningococcal meningitis. *See also* endogenous; infection.

exogenous obesity Obesity due to overeating. *Compare* endogenous obesity. *See also* endogenous; obesity.

expected morbidity The predicted incidence of illness or injury in a defined population over a defined time interval. *See also* expected mortality; morbidity; morbidity rate.

expected mortality The predicted incidence of death in a defined population over a defined time interval. *See also* expected morbidity; mortality; mortality rate.

expectorant Any medicinal agent that promotes the ejection by coughing of material accumulated in the air passages. Most expectorants are mild irritants that stimulate the secretion of mucus. *See also* antitussive; cough.

expeditious evacuation *See* load and go.

expenditure, capital *See* capital expenditure.

experience rating In insurance, the process of setting rates based partly or wholly on the previous claims experience of various groups and subgroups of subscribers, members, or beneficiaries, and then projecting required revenues for a future policy year for a specific group or pool of groups. Premiums vary with the health experience of different groups and subgroups or with such variables as age, sex, and health status. Experience rating is the most common method of determining premiums for health insurance in private programs. *Compare* community rating. *See also* group insurance; insurance; rating.

experiment A study or inquiry in which an investigator or group of investigators intentionally alters one or more factors under controlled conditions in order to study the effects of so doing. *See also* animal experimentation; control experiment; experimental method; red bead experiment.

Experimental Biology and Medicine, Society for *See* Society for Experimental Biology and Medicine.

experimental medical care review organization (EMCRO) The forerunner of the professional services review organization (PSRO) program; the PSRO was, in turn, a forerunner of the peer review organization (PRO). The EMCRO was established to help medical societies create formal organizations and procedures for reviewing the quality and use of medical care in hospitals, nursing homes, and offices. Ten EMCROs were initially supported by federal funds; only some of these organizations actually did review health care services. The use of explicit criteria and standard definitions was required of all EMCROs, but particular approaches to organizing reviews were determined by individual organizations. *See also* peer review organization; professional services review organization.

experimental method An approach to a question in which an investigator intentionally alters one or more factors under controlled conditions in order to study the effects of so doing. *See also* method; scientific method; survey.

Experimental Psychologists, Association of *See* Society of Experimental Psychologists.

experimental psychology The branch of psychology dealing with the processes of sensation, perception, learning, and motivation. The work of experimental psychologists may involve studying how people attend to and use different kinds of visual and auditory information and how this processing of information is affected by what they are looking or listening for. *See also* psychology.

Experimental Therapeutics, American Society for Pharmacology and *See* American Society for Pharmacology and Experimental Therapeutics.

experimentation, animal *See* animal experimentation.

experiment, control *See* control experiment.

experiment, red bead *See* red bead experiment.

expert An individual who has acquired a high degree of skill or knowledge in a subject or an area, as in a content expert or a methodology expert. *See also* authority; content expert; expert witness; methodology expert.

expert consensus Agreement in opinion of experts.

expert, content *See* content expert.

expert, methodology *See* methodology expert.

expert panel A group of experts convened to accomplish one or more objectives, such as a task force convened for indicator development. *See also* committee; panel; task force.

expert system A type of artificial intelligence in which the decision practices and principles of well-regarded specialists in a field are built into the computer program. The program then guides users to sound conclusions in situations similar to those covered by the system, such as in medical diagnosis or treatment. *See also* artificial intelligence.

expert task force for indicator development A group of experts in specific fields (for example, anesthesia care, obstetrics care, trauma care, cardiovascular care, oncology care, infection surveillance and control, medication usage) convened by the Joint Commission on Accreditation of Healthcare Organizations to draft indicator sets as part of the Agenda for Change. *See also* Agenda for Change; Joint Commission on Accreditation of Healthcare Organizations.

expert witness An individual who has special knowledge of the subject about which he or she is to testify, and whose input is obtained by a plaintiff who is trying to demonstrate that he or she has been injured. *See also* expert; medical evidence; witness.

expiration date **1.** A date stamped on a product to indicate the last date on which it should be used. **2.** The time established in a contract or by a collective bargaining agreement for the contract or agreement to terminate; for example, the date that a health insurance policy terminates.

explanation of benefits (EOB) A notice describing the actions relating to payment (or nonpayment) of an insurance claim, issued by the insurance company to the beneficiary after each claim has been processed. *See also* benefits; Explanation of Medicare Benefits.

Explanation of Medicare Benefits (EOMB) A notice printed by a Medicare carrier or fiscal intermediary that identifies what services were actually covered, what charges were actually approved, how much of the allowed charges were credited toward the yearly deductible, and the amount Medicare actually paid. Each Medicare beneficiary receives this notice after each Medicare claim has been processed. *See also* benefits; explanation of benefits; Medicare.

explicit Specifically stated, as in explicit criteria. *Compare* implicit. *See also* explicit criteria; explicit review.

explicit criteria In health care, criteria that are specified in advance of a medical review process. *Compare* implicit criteria. *See also* criteria; explicit review.

explicit review Review of the processes and outcomes of patient care using explicit criteria specified in advance. *Compare* implicit review. *See also* explicit criteria.

Exploration of Psychotherapy Integration, Society for the *See* Society for the Exploration of Psychotherapy Integration.

exploratory panel *See* screening panel.

exponentially In mathematics, the rate of change in which the numbers increase according to the value of an exponent. In an exponential progression with an exponent of 2, the progression would be, 2, 4, 16, 256, and so forth. *Compare* arithmetically; geometrically. *See also* linear; logarithmic.

express **1.** To set forth in words. **2.** To show, as with a gesture. **3.** To make known feelings or opinions.

expressed demand (for health services) *See* demand (for health services).

Expression, American Society of Psychopathology of *See* American Society of Psychopathology of Expression.

expressive aphasia *See* motor aphasia.

extended benefits Supplemental insurance coverage for services, such as mental health services. *See also* benefits.

extended care Care provided in a skilled treatment facility rather than a hospital or home when acute care is not required but skilled nursing care is necessary. *See also* extended care facility; skilled nursing care; skilled nursing facility.

extended care facility (ECF) An outdated term (since 1972 when the Social Security statute was amended) for skilled nursing facility. *See also* extended care unit; skilled nursing facility.

extended care services Under Medicare, carefully delineated services provided in a skilled nursing facility for a limited time after a hospital stay and for the same condition as the hospital stay. *See also* extended care.

extended care unit A unit of a hospital that provides treatment for inpatients who require convalescent, rehabilitative, or long-term skilled nursing care. *See also* skilled nursing facility; unit.

extended family Two or more generations of family living in close proximity and maintaining close contact, but not living under one roof. *Compare* nuclear family. *See also* family.

Extension Program Foundation, Optometric *See* Optometric Extension Program Foundation.

extension survey A survey of limited scope conducted by the Joint Commission on Accreditation of Healthcare Organizations to ensure that a previously demonstrated level of compliance is being maintained following an organizational change. *See also* accreditation survey; Joint Commission on Accreditation of Healthcare Organizations; survey.

external benchmarking *See* benchmarking.

external customer A customer who buys a product or a service but who is not a member of the organization that produces the product or service; for example, a patient and a third-party payer are external customers of a hospital or a physician. *See also* customer.

external environmental factor An environment-related variable, such as the number of nursing beds available in a community or payer reimbursement policies, that may influence a health care organization's performance data. These factors often are not within the organization's or practitioner's control but can affect organizational performance and outcomes achieved. *See also* factor; organization factor; patient factor; practitioner factor.

externality In health economics, something that results from an encounter between a consumer and provider and that confers benefits or imposes costs on other people but is not reflected in any charge for the transaction. For example, an externality of immunizations (vaccinations) is the protection provided to other people who have not been immunized. The protection is not considered when an individual immunization is priced. *See also* immunization.

external review Review in which criteria and standards are set or ratified by persons or organizations other than the individuals or organizations undergoing evaluation. *Compare* internal review. *See also* criteria; evaluation; medical review; utilization review.

external validity The extent to which an experimental finding can be projected to a population at large. In health care, the extent to which the results of a study may be generalized beyond the subjects of a study to other settings, providers, procedures, and diagnoses. An experiment has high external validity when the sample is representative of the population and simulates real-life conditions. *See also* construct validity; content validity; face validity; predictive validity; validity.

extracorporeal oxygenator *See* heart-lung machine.

extracorporeal shock wave lithotripsy (ESWL) *See* lithotripsy.

extracorporeal technologist *See* perfusionist.

ExtraCorporeal Technology, American Society of *See* American Society of ExtraCorporeal Technology.

extraction Removal (particularly of teeth, lens, and fetuses) by drawing out.

extramural birth A newborn born in a nonsterile environment. *See also* birth.

extraordinary care **1.** Use of advanced technology in medical treatment to keep a patient alive, for example, mechanical ventilation. **2.** Care that involves life-supporting medical interventions that offer no significant health improvement or that cannot be administered without excessive pain. *Compare* ordinary care.

extrapolate To infer, estimate, or predict by extending or projecting known information. For instance, in mathematics, to extrapolate is to estimate a value of a variable outside a known range from values within a known range by assuming that the estimated value follows logically from the known values. *Compare* interpolate.

extrapolation The inference, estimate, or prediction resulting from extrapolating. *Compare* interpolation. *See also* extrapolate.

extrasystemic cause *See* special cause.

extrasystemic-cause variation *See* special-cause variation.

Eye Bank Association of America (EBAA) A national organization composed of 97 eye banks promoting eye banking. It makes possible over 40,000 eye transplants annually and establishes standards for the procurement and distribution of eyes. *See also* tissue bank.

Eye-Bank for Sight Restoration (EBSR) A national organization founded in 1944 that collects and distributes healthy corneal tissue obtained from individuals who have arranged to donate their eyes, or whose relatives have authorized such donation, at the time of death. It provides speakers to explain the eye-bank program to hospital and professional groups. *See also* tissue bank.

Eye and Ear Hospitals, American Association of *See* American Association of Eye and Ear Hospitals.

eyeglasses *See* spectacles.

Eye Hospital Annual Conference, Wills *See* Wills Eye Hospital Annual Conference.

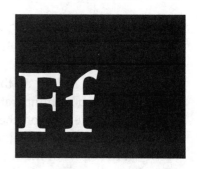

F Abbreviation for Fahrenheit degree. *See also* Fahrenheit scale.

FAAFP *See* Fellow of the American Academy of Family Physicians.

FAAN *See* Fellow of the American Academy of Nursing.

FAAO-HNS *See* Fellow of the American Academy of Otolaryngology-Head and Neck Surgery.

FAAOS *See* Fellow of the American Academy of Orthopaedic Surgeons.

FAANaOS *See* American Academy of Neurological and Orthopaedic Surgeons.

FAAP *See* Fellow of the American Academy of Pediatrics.

fabrication *See* confabulation.

FACA *See* Fellow of the American College of Angiology.

FACC *See* Fellow of the American College of Cardiology.

FACCP *See* Fellow of the American College of Chest Physicians.

FACD *See* Fellow of the American College of Dentists.

FACEP *See* Fellow of the American College of Emergency Physicians.

face validity Intelligibility; the degree to which a measure or test makes sense, or appears to be a reasonable reflection of some variable, to an informed user. Face validity is the most superficial type of validity; nevertheless, it often contributes to the presumed legitimacy of a test and is, therefore, an important consideration in gaining acceptance of a measure or test. *Synonym*: faith validity. *See also* measure; test; validity.

FACFS *See* Fellow of the American College of Foot Surgeons.

FACHE *See* Fellow of the American College of Healthcare Executives.

Facial and Neck Pain and TMJ Orthopedics, American Academy of Head, *See* American Academy of Head, Facial and Neck Pain and TMJ Orthopedics.

Facial Plastic, and Reconstructive Surgery, American Academy of *See* American Academy of Facial Plastic and Reconstructive Surgery.

facilitate To make easy or easier.

facilitator In quality improvement, a person who has developed special expertise in the quality improvement process. He or she does not belong to a quality improvement team but helps it achieve results by helping to focus its efforts, teaching quality improvement methods, consulting to the team leader, and helping connect the work to the knowledge necessary for improvement. *See also* adviser; continuous quality improvement; quality improvement team.

facility A physical entity, such as the physical plant, equipment, and supplies of a hospital, that is required to carry out the purpose of an organization. *See also* ambulatory surgical facility; community residential facility; extended care facility; freestanding ambulatory surgical facility; health facility; long term care facility; skilled nursing facility; substance abuse facility.

facility, ambulatory surgical *See* ambulatory surgical facility.

facility, community living *See* halfway house.

facility, community residential *See* community residential facility.

facility, extended care *See* extended care facility.

facility, freestanding ambulatory surgical *See* freestanding ambulatory surgical facility.

facility, health *See* health facility.

facility, long term care *See* long term care facility.

facility manager *See* administrative engineer.

facility, skilled nursing   *See* skilled nursing facility.

facility, substance abuse   *See* substance abuse facility.

FACMGA   *See* Fellow of the American College of Medical Group Administrators.

FACOG   *See* Fellow of the American College of Obstetricians and Gynecologists.

FACP   *See* Fellow of the American College of Physicians.

FACPE   *See* Fellow of the American College of Physician Executives.

FACPM   *See* Fellow of the American College of Preventive Medicine.

FACR   *See* Fellow of the American College of Radiology.

FACS   *See* Fellow of the American College of Surgeons.

facsimile   *See* fax.

facsimile machine   *See* fax machine.

FACSM   *See* Fellow of the American College of Sports Medicine.

fact   An objective statement of reality that can be verified by observation or judged reasonably likely because of documentary evidence. For example, a historic fact would be the attempted assassination of President Reagan on March 30, 1981. This fact can be verified by checking records written by observers. A scientific fact would be the temperature at which water boils. It can be rechecked at any time and its validity established. *Compare* factoid. *See also* fact finder; fact-finding; inform; issue of fact.

fact finder   The person or group of persons in a judicial or administrative proceeding that has the responsibility of determining the facts relevant to decide a controversy; for example, the judge in a nonjury trial, a jury, a hearing officer, or a hearing body. *See also* fact; judge; jury.

fact-finding   Discovery or determination of facts or accurate information. *See also* fact.

fact, historic   *See* fact.

faction   An informal group operating within an organization and often opposing a larger group. A faction forms through voluntary membership of people who believe they share common goals.

factoid   Unverified or inaccurate information that is presented as factual, often as part of a publicity effort, and that is then accepted as true because of constant repetition. *Compare* fact.

factor   **1.** Something that produces or influences a result. **2.** In statistics, an independent variable used to identify membership of qualitatively different groups. A causal role may be implied; for instance, a faulty hospital medical staff credentialing process may be a factor in a malpractice case. *See also* external environmental factor; independent variable; multifactorial; occupancy factor; organization factor; patient factor; practitioner factor; risk factor; variable.

factor analysis   The mathematical process by which a large amount of data are reduced into a structure that can be more easily studied. Factor analysis summarizes information contained in a large number of variables and condenses it into a smaller number of factors containing variables that are interrelated. For instance, two variables of weight and height of men could be condensed into one variable: size. *See also* analysis; factor.

factor, external environmental   *See* external environmental factor.

factorial, multi-   *See* multifactorial.

factor, occupancy   *See* occupancy factor.

factor, organization   *See* organization factor.

factor, organization-based   *See* organization factor.

factor, patient   *See* patient factor.

factor, patient-based   *See* patient factor.

factor, practitioner   *See* practitioner factor.

factor, practitioner-based   *See* practitioner factor.

factor, Rh   *See* Rh factor.

factor, rhesus   *See* Rh factor.

factor, risk   *See* risk factor.

factors, indicator underlying   *See* indicator underlying factors.

Factors Society, Human   *See* Human Factors Society.

factor, uniform capital   *See* uniform capital factor.

fact, scientific   *See* fact.

fact sheet   A document used in media relations and development that provides a concise statement about an organization or a program. *See also* development; public relations.

factor VIII   A substance in blood that is essential to the coagulation process and is deficient in some hemophiliacs. *Synonym*: antihemophilic factor. *See also* coagulopathy; hemophilia.

faculty   **1.** All of the members of a learned profession, as in medical school faculty. *See also* professor. **2.** Any of the divisions or comprehensive branches of learning at a college or university, as in the faculty of law.

Faculty in Higher Education, Association of Black

Nursing *See* Association of Black Nursing Faculty in Higher Education.

Faculty in the Medical Humanities, Association for *See* Association for Faculty in the Medical Humanities.

faculty practice plan *See* medical practice plan.

FADE process A quality improvement process composed of focus, analyze, develop, and execute steps, developed by Organizational Dynamics, Inc. *See also* continuous quality improvement; FOCUS-PDCA; Plan-Do-Check-Act cycle.

FAF *See* Financial Accounting Foundation.

Fahrenheit scale A temperature scale still used in the United States in which the interval between Fahrenheit's two original fixed points, which are the lowest temperature attainable by a freezing mixture of ice and salt (0 degrees) and the normal temperature of the human body (96 degrees originally), is divided into 96 degrees. Fresh water freezes at about 32° F and boils at about 212° F. The scale was developed by Gabriel Daniel Fahrenheit (1686-1736), a German physicist. The Fahrenheit scale is an example of an interval scale. *See also* Celsius scale; interval scale; scale; temperature; thermometer.

FAHS *See* Federation of American Health Systems.

failed vaginal birth after cesarean section *See* vaginal birth after cesarean section.

failure The condition or fact of not achieving the desired end or ends. *Compare* success. *See also* congestive heart failure; failure cost; failure desensitization; liver failure; renal failure; respiratory failure.

failure, congestive heart *See* congestive heart failure.

failure cost The cost associated with services or products that have been found not to conform or perform to their requirements, including the evaluation, disposition, and consumer-affairs aspects of such failures. Failure cost includes, for example, the cost associated with redesign, rework, scrap, warranty, and product liability. *See also* appraisal cost; cost; cost of quality; prevention cost; rework.

failure desensitization A situation in which individuals have worked with a flawed system for so long that they come to believe failures of the system are normal. *See also* desensitize; system.

failure, liver *See* liver failure.

failure, renal *See* renal failure.

failure, respiratory *See* respiratory failure.

faint *See* syncope.

faith **1.** Confident belief in the truth, value, or trustworthiness of a person, an idea, or a thing. *See also* good faith. **2.** A belief that does not rest on logical proof or material evidence. **3.** In theology, the virtue defined as secure belief in God and a trusting acceptance of God's will. *See also* religion.

faith, good *See* good faith.

faith healer One who treats disease with prayer.

faith validity *See* face validity.

falling out *See* unconscious.

false Contrary to fact or truth, as in false advertising. *Compare* true. *See also* false advertising; false negative; false positive; falsify; lie.

false advertising Advertising that describes goods, services, or real property in a misleading fashion. *See also* advertise; comparative advertising; competitive advertising; deceptive advertising; image advertising; informative advertising.

falsehood *See* lie.

false negative A negative result in a person or a case that actually has the condition or characteristic for which the test was conducted; for example, a false negative occurs when a pregnancy test is negative for a woman who is pregnant. *See also* false positive; sensitivity of a test; specificity of a test; test.

false positive A positive result in a person or a case that does not have the condition or characteristic for which the test was conducted; for example, a false positive occurs when a pregnancy test is positive for a nonpregnant woman. *See also* false negative; HCFA generic quality screens; sensitivity of a test; specificity of a test; test.

falsification of information The fabrication, in whole or in part, of any information provided by an applicant or accredited organization to the Joint Commission on Accreditation of Healthcare Organizations. This includes, but is not limited to, any redrafting, reformatting, or content deletion of documents. *See also* falsify; forgery; Joint Commission on Accreditation of Healthcare Organizations.

falsify To change something that is true. It may be statements, representations, or acts made to deceive other persons through distortion, such as an unauthorized altering of the contents of a medical record or quality assurance documents. *See also* falsification of information.

Families and Children, Council on Accreditation of Services for *See* Council on Accreditation of Services for Families and Children.

Families with Dependent Children, Aid to *See* Aid to Families with Dependent Children.

family   **1.** A fundamental social group typically consisting of a man and woman and their offspring. *See also* sibling. **2.** Two or more people who share goals and values, have long-term commitments to one another, and reside usually in the same dwelling place. *See also* significant other. **3.** A group of persons sharing common ancestry. **4.** In epidemiology, a group of two or more persons united by blood, adoptive or marital ties, or the common law equivalent; the family may include members who do not share the household but are united to other members by blood, adoptive or marital, or equivalent ties. *See also* extended family; nuclear family; patient's family.

family caseworker   *See* family counselor.

family counseling, individual marriage and   *See* individual marriage and family counseling.

family counselor   A social worker, usually with a bachelor's or a master's degree from a school of social work or other qualified individual, who works with families having problems in family relationships or other social problems. Family counselors perform counseling for married couples, parents and their children, and unwed parents and may also help in home management, work adjustment, vocational training, or the need for financial assistance. Family counselors may help clients use agency services, such as homemaker and day care services, as well as other community resources, and help determine clients' eligibility for financial assistance. *See also* caseworker; social worker.

family doctor   *See* family physician.

family, extended   *See* extended family.

Family Foundation, The Henry J. Kaiser   *See* The Henry J. Kaiser Family Foundation.

family ganging   The practice of requiring or encouraging a patient to return for care to a health program with his or her entire family, even when the rest of the family does not need care, so that the program or provider can charge the patient's third-party payer for care given to each member of the family. The practice and the term originated and is most common in Medicaid mills, which frequently have the mother of a sick child bring in all her other children for care whether or not they need it. *See also* Medicaid mill.

Family and Health Section   *See* Family and Health Section of the National Council on Family Relations.

Family and Health Section of the National Council on Family Relations (FHS)   A section of the National Council on Family Relations founded in 1984 composed of health and education professionals. It serves as a forum for all professionals involved in interdisciplinary work in the family and health fields. Formerly (1991) Family and Health Section. *See also* National Council on Family Relations.

family history   Part of a patient's medical history in which questions are asked about the incidence and prevalence of specific diseases and disorders in his/her family in an attempt to determine whether the patient has a hereditary or familial tendency toward a particular disease or condition, as in the patient has a family history of heart disease. *See also* history; medical history.

family life education   Presentations or workshops given by social workers or other qualified individuals about marriage, parenting, and family or couple communications. *See also* education; social worker.

Family Medicine, Society of Teachers of   *See* Society of Teachers of Family Medicine.

Family, National Institute for the   *See* National Institute for the Family.

family, nuclear   *See* nuclear family.

family, patient's   *See* patient's family.

family physician   A physician specializing in family practice. *Synonyms*: family doctor; family practitioner. *Compare* general practitioner. *See also* family practice.

Family Physicians, American Academy of   *See* American Academy of Family Physicians.

Family Physicians, Uniformed Services Academy of   *See* Uniformed Services Academy of Family Physicians.

family planning   Social, educational, or medical services and supplies to help individuals determine family size or prevent unplanned pregnancies. This may include birth control counseling and referral, pregnancy testing, sterilization counseling, venereal disease referrals, public education service, and infertility counseling and referrals. *See also* birth control; contraception; family; planning.

Family Planning, American Academy of Natural   *See* American Academy of Natural Family Planning.

family planning, natural   *See* natural family planning.

Family Planning and Reproductive Health Association, National   *See* National Family Planning and Reproductive Health Association.

family practice (FP)   The branch of medicine and

medical specialty dealing with the prevention, diagnosis, and treatment of a wide variety of ailments in patients of all ages. Geriatric medicine and sports medicine are two subspecialties of family practice. *See also* family; geriatric medicine; sports medicine.

Family Practice, American Board of *See* American Board of Family Practice.

family practitioner *See* family physician.

family, pro- *See* pro-family.

Family Psychology (Div. 43), Division of *See* Division of Family Psychology (Div. 43).

Family Relations, National Council on *See* National Council on Family Relations.

family therapist An individual who specializes in family therapy. *See also* family therapy.

Family Therapists, National Academy of Counselors and *See* National Academy of Counselors and Family Therapists.

family therapy A form of psychotherapy that focuses on the individual as a family member; it involves examination of the interrelationships of family members while all members are together in group sessions, in order to identify and alleviate the problems of one or more members of the family. *See also* group therapy; psychotherapy.

Family Therapy, American Association for Marriage and *See* American Association for Marriage and Family Therapy.

Family Therapy Association, American *See* American Family Therapy Association.

Family Therapy Network (FTN) A network founded in 1976 composed of 50,000 members interested in promoting the exchange of ideas and information among family therapists. *See also* family therapy.

Family Therapy Section of the National Council on Family Relations A section of the National Council on Family Relations founded in 1955 composed of practicing family therapists and family therapy supervisors, educators, and researchers. It seeks to improve the practice of family therapy through the development of theory, research, and training. Formerly (1991) National Council on Family Relations Family Therapy Section. *See also* family; family therapy.

Family Violence Information, Clearinghouse on *See* Clearinghouse on Family Violence Information.

Family Violence, National Council on Child Abuse and *See* National Council on Child Abuse and Family Violence.

FANEL *See* Federation for Accessible Nursing Education and Licensure.

FAOTA *See* Fellow of the American Occupational Therapy Association.

FAPA *See* Fellow of the American Psychiatric Association; Fellow of the American Psychological Association.

FAPHA *See* Fellow of the American Public Health Association.

faradic electrical current A form of low-voltage electric current used in the physical treatment of disease; for example, in podiatric medicine. A farad is a unit of capacitance that increases the potential difference between the plates of a capacitor by one volt with a charge of one coulomb (the meter-kilogram-second unit of electrical charge equal to the quantity of charge transferred in one second by a stead current of one ampere). *See also* podiatric medicine.

faradism The therapeutic application of a faradic electrical current. *See also* faradic electrical current.

FARB *See* Federation of Associations of Regulatory Boards.

farmer's lung A respiratory disorder caused by occupational exposure to fungal spores from moldy stored hay that has not been properly dried. *See also* lung; pulmonary medicine.

FASA *See* Federated Ambulatory Surgery Association.

FASB *See* Financial Accounting Standards Board.

FASEB *See* Federation of American Societies for Experimental Biology.

fast To go without food. *See also* anorexia nervosa.

fat Any of the simple lipids, that is, triglycerides of fatty acids, particularly oleic, palmitic, and stearic acids. It is contained in the cells of fatty (adipose) tissue, where it functions as the principal energy store of the body. *See also* lard; lipid; saturated fat.

fat, saturated *See* saturated fat.

fatality A death resulting from an accident or a disaster, as in highway fatalities. *See also* fatality rate.

fatality rate The number of deaths during a given period for a stipulated population; for example, the percentage of people in the United States who die of lung cancer or trauma in one year. *See also* mortality rate; rate.

fat-soluble vitamin Vitamin A, D, E, or K, which the body absorbs with the aid of fat and then stores in fat. Each of these vitamins is a chemical, as well as a vitamin, and megadoses can be harmful. *Compare* water-soluble vitamin. *See also* vitamin; vitamin A; vitamin D; vitamin E; vitamin K.

fatty liver disease A condition in which fat collects in the cells of the liver, distorting it. It can result from excessive alcohol intake, kwashiorkor (protein malnutrition), diabetes mellitus, Reye's syndrome, and toxicity of some drugs. *See also* disease.

fatty tissue *See* adipose tissue.

fauces The passage between the mouth and the pharynx, containing the tonsils. *See also* tonsils.

fault, apportionment of *See* apportionment of fault.

favorable selection *See* skimming.

fax **1.** Facsimile telegraphy, a system allowing documents to be scanned, digitized, and transmitted to a remote destination using a telephone network. *Synonym*: telefacsimile. **2.** A copy of a document transmitted in this way. *Synonym*: facsimile. *See also* fax machine; telefacsimile.

fax machine A machine capable of performing facsimile telegraphy. *Synonym*: facsimile machine. *See also* fax.

FBA *See* Federal Bar Association.

FBPCS *See* Federation of Behavioral, Psychological and Cognitive Sciences.

FCAP *See* Fellow of the College of American Pathologists.

FDA *See* Food and Drug Administration.

FDLI *See* Food and Drug Law Institute.

feasibility Practicability; for instance, in the context of evaluations of performance indicators, whether use of a certain indicator to convey information to the public about performance is feasible. *See also* feasibility study.

feasibility study A preliminary study to determine practicability of a proposed program or process and to appraise the factors, such as cost, that may influence its practicability. *See also* feasibility; pilot study.

febrile Characterized by an elevated body temperature (fever). *See also* fever; temperature.

FEC *See* freestanding emergency center.

feces Excrement discharged from the alimentary canal through the anus, consisting of undigested food, a mass of bacteria, shed intestinal cells, mucus, water, bile pigment, and other secretions. *See also* constipation; coprolalia; coprophagia; diarrhea; dysentery; meconium; obstipation; stool.

Federal Agency for Health Care Policy and Research *See* Agency for Health Care Policy and Research.

federal assistance programs Programs available to state and local governments including country, city, metropolitan, and regional governments; schools, colleges, and universities; health care organizations; nonprofit and profit-making organizations; and individuals and families. Current federal assistance programs are listed in the *Catalogue of Federal Domestic Assistance* published annually.

Federal Bar Association (FBA) A national organization founded in 1920 composed of 15,000 attorneys employed by the federal government as legislators, judges, lawyers, or members of quasi-judicial boards and commissions, and other persons with an interest in federal law who practice before a federal court or agency. *See also* attorney; bar.

federal component Under Medicare, the applicable federal rate, based on regional and national rates published in the *Federal Register* and dependent on the hospital's location, as part of the prospective pricing (payment) system. *See also* Federal Register; Medicare; prospective payment system.

federal deficit Shortfall that results when the federal government spends more in a fiscal year than it receives in revenue. To cover the shortfall, the government must borrow from the public by floating long-term and short-term debt. *See also* deficit; Gramm-Rudman-Hollings amendment.

Federal Emergency Management Agency (FEMA) The federal agency responsible for emergency preparedness and response by private, nonprofit, and public organizations and for natural, humanmade, and nuclear emergencies.

Federal Employees Health Benefits Program (FEHBP) The largest employer-sponsored contributory group health insurance program in the world. It is voluntary for federal employees, and about 72 percent of those eligible are covered. It was established under the Federal Employees Health Benefits Act of 1959, began operation in July 1960, and is administered by the Office of Personnel Management. Each employee can choose from a variety of health plans approved in each locality. *See also* Office of Personnel Management.

federal government hospital A hospital that is managed by an agency or department of the federal government, such as the Department of Defense, the Department of Veterans Affairs, and the Indian Health Service. *See also* government hospital; nonfederal government hospital.

Federal Health Insurance Plan (FHIP) A comprehensive health insurance plan included as one of three health insurance plans in the Ford Administration's 1974 proposal for national health insurance. The FHIP would have replaced Medicare for providing health insurance coverage for persons 65 years old and older. *See also* national health insurance.

Federal Insurance Contributions Act (FICA) The statute establishing the Social Security tax, and, through amendments over the years, the tax rates for employers and employees. *See also* Social Security Act; Society Security Administration.

Federal Physicians Association (FPA) A national organization founded in 1978 composed of 250 civil service physicians employed by or retired from the federal government. Its objectives are to improve the health care of patients served by federal civil service physicians; to advance the practice of medicine within the federal government; and to better the working conditions and benefits of federal civil service physicians. Formerly (1982) American Academy of Federal Civil Service Physicians. *See also* physician.

Federal Register An official daily publication of the federal government providing a uniform system for making available to the public proposed and final rules, legal notices, and similar proclamations, orders, and documents having general applicability and legal effect. The *Federal Register* publishes material from all federal agencies. *See also* rule.

Federal Trade Commission (FTC) A federal agency created in 1914 to protect consumers against unfair methods of competition and deceptive business practices, including sales fraud and violation of the antitrust laws. For instance, the FTC is responsible for ensuring that preferred provider organizations and other competitive medical plans do not cause price fixing among most or all physicians in a locality. The agency's Bureau of Competition is responsible for the enforcement of the antitrust laws. The Bureau of Consumer Protection protects consumers against sales fraud and any other unfair or deceptive business practices. The Bureau of Economics performs economic analysis both for informational purposes and for use in litigation by the trial staff.

Federated Ambulatory Surgery Association (FASA) A national organization founded in 1974 composed of 1,200 physicians, nurses, health administrators, and other individuals representing more than 400 outpatient surgery facilities. It promotes the concept of freestanding ambulatory (outpatient) surgical care. Formerly (1986) Freestanding Ambulatory Surgery Association. *See also* ambulatory surgical facility.

Federation for Accessible Nursing Education and Licensure (FANEL) An organization founded in 1983 composed of registered nurses, licensed practical nurses, educators, health care organizations, schools, and hospital administrators seeking to maintain licensure through current education programs for registered nurses and licensed practical nurses. *See also* licensed practical nurse; licensure; registered nurse.

Federation of American Health Systems (FAHS) A national organization founded in 1966 composed of 1,000 privately-owned or investor-owned (for-profit) hospitals. It maintains a speakers' bureau, compiles statistics on the investor-owned hospitals industry, and bestows awards. Formerly (1985) Federation of American Hospitals. *See also* investor-owned hospital.

Federation of American Hospitals *See* Federation of American Health Systems.

Federation of American Societies for Experimental Biology (FASEB) A federation founded in 1913 composed of 7 scientific societies with a total of 30,000 members. These societies are the American Physiological Society; American Society for Biochemistry and Molecular Biology; American Society for Pharmacology and Experimental Therapeutics; American Association of Pathologists; American Institute of Nutrition; American Association of Immunologists; and American Society of Cell Biology. It maintains a placement service and bestows awards.

Federation of Associations of Health Regulatory Boards *See* Federation of Associations of Regulatory Boards.

Federation of Associations of Regulatory Boards (FARB) A federation founded in 1973 composed of 20 state regulatory board associations concerned with exchanging information and engaging in programs and joint activities relating to the education and licensing of professionals. Formerly (1985) Federation of Associations of Health Regulatory Boards. *See also* licensure; regulatory agency.

Federation of Behavioral, Psychological and Cognitive Sciences (FBPCS) A national federation founded in 1980 composed of 15 scientific societies representing 90,000 research scientists. It promotes research in behavioral, psychological, and cognitive sciences, their physiological bases, and applications in health, education, and human development. *See also* cognitive science.

Federation of Biocommunications Associations *See* Council for Biomedical Communications Associations.

Federation for Culture Collections, US *See* US Federation for Culture Collections.

Federation of Feminist Women's Health Centers (FFWHC) A national organization founded in 1975 composed of 163 women's health clinics and individuals interested in working to secure reproductive rights for women and men, educating women about the normal functions of their bodies, and improving the quality of women's health care. *See also* feminism.

Federation Licensing Examination (FLEX) The standardized examination for state licensure of physicians. Developed by the Federation of State Medical Boards of the United States, the examination is based on National Board of Medical Examiners test materials. *See also* Federation of State Medical Boards of the United States; national board examination; National Board of Medical Examiners.

Federation of Nurses and Health Professionals (FNHP) An AFL-CIO federation founded in 1978 composed of 35,000 registered nurses, licensed practical nurses, and other professional and technical employees in the health field. It is a division of the American Federation of Teachers. *See also* licensed practical nurse; registered nurse.

Federation of Podiatric Medical Boards (FPMB) An organization founded in 1936 composed of state boards of podiatry examiners. It serves as a repository for information relating to common problems among boards of podiatry examiners and promotes competency examinations with national standards used by examining boards, among other activities. *See also* podiatric medicine.

Federation of Prosthodontic Organizations (FPO) A national organization founded in 1965 composed of 16 organizations of dentists. It improves prosthodontic service rendered to the public and improves communication among members and other organizations. *See also* prosthodontics.

Federation of State Medical Boards of the United

States (FSMB) An organization founded in 1912 composed of 67 state medical examining and licensing boards, including 12 osteopathic boards. It maintains a disciplinary actions data bank and an examinations data bank. *See also* state medical boards.

Federation of Straight Chiropractic Organizations (FSCO) An organization founded in 1978 composed of 1,200 individuals and organizations in the chiropractic field interested in promoting the practice of straight (traditional) chiropractic medicine. It conducts lobbying and educational programs. *See also* chiropractic.

fee The dollar amount charged for a service. *See also* contingency fee; dispensing fee; fee for service; fixed fee; honorarium.

fee, contingency *See* contingency fee.

feedback **1.** The return of a portion of the output of a process or system to the input, especially when used to maintain performance or to control a system or process. **2.** The portion of the output so returned. *See also* biofeedback; input; negative feedback; output; process; system.

feedback, bio- *See* biofeedback.

feedback, negative *See* negative feedback.

feeding, enteral *See* enteral feeding.

feeding, nasogastric *See* nasogastric feeding.

fee, dispensing *See* dispensing fee.

fee, fixed *See* fixed fee.

fee maximum In health insurance, the maximum amount a participating health care provider may be paid for a specific service provided to plan members under a specific contract. A comprehensive listing of fee maximums used to reimburse physicians or other providers on a fee-for-service basis is called a fee schedule. *See also* fee schedule; maximum.

fee schedule A list of charges (maximum charges) or allowances for health services. *See also* fee maximum.

fee for service (FFS) An arrangement under which patients pay physicians, hospitals, or other health care providers for each encounter or service rendered, as contrasted with salary, per capita, or prepayment systems in which the payment is not changed with the number of services actually used or if no services are used. *See also* alternative delivery system; capitation; fee-for-service plan; prepayment plan.

fee-for-service plan A type of prepaid health care plan similar to a health care insurance plan in which health care providers are reimbursed for each encounter or service rendered. *See also* fee for service.

fee splitting   An unethical practice by a health care specialist or consultant involving the return of part of his or her fee to another health professional who referred the patient in the first place.

FEHBP   *See* Federal Employees Health Benefits Program.

Feigenbaum, Armand   A statistician and management specialist generally credited with coining the terms *total quality control* and *total quality management*. He teaches that all quality approaches are synergistic and a combination of them is better than any one plan. Feigenbaum followed W. Edwards Deming and Joseph M. Juran to Japan in the 1950s. *See also* Deming, W. Edwards; Juran, Joseph M; total quality management.

fellow   **1.** An individual who has been granted status or fellowship higher than that of membership by an association, usually after meeting additional requirements for education and performance, as in "Fellow of the American College of Cardiology," abbreviated FACC. **2.** An individual whose position is supported by special stipends for advanced study and research, as in a "fellow in toxicology." *See also* fellowship.

Fellow of the American Academy of Family Physicians (FAAFP)   A family physician who has achieved the rank of fellow after meeting additional requirements beyond those required for membership in the American Academy of Family Physicians. Evidence of this distinction is a credential. *See also* American Academy of Family Physicians; credentials; family physician; fellow.

Fellow of the American Academy of Nursing (FAAN)   A registered nurse who has achieved the rank of fellow after meeting additional requirements beyond those required for membership in state nurses' associations, which are constituent members of the American Nurses' Association. Evidence of this distinction is a credential. *See also* American Academy of Nursing; American Nurses' Association; credentials; fellow; registered nurse.

Fellow of the American Academy of Orthopaedic Surgeons (FAAOS)   An orthopaedic surgeon who has achieved the rank of fellow after meeting additional requirements beyond those required for membership in the American Academy of Orthopaedic Surgeons. Evidence of this distinction is a credential. *See also* American Academy of Orthopaedic Surgeons; credentials; fellow; orthopaedic/orthopedic surgeon.

Fellow of the American Academy of Otolaryngology-Head and Neck Surgery (FAAO-HNS)   An otolaryngologist-head and neck surgeon who has achieved the rank of fellow after meeting additional requirements beyond those required for membership in the American Academy of Otolaryngology-Head and Neck Surgery. Evidence of this distinction is a credential. *See also* American Academy of Otolaryngology-Head and Neck Surgery; credentials; fellow; otolaryngologist-head and neck surgeon.

Fellow of the American Academy of Pediatrics (FAAP)   A pediatrician who has achieved the rank of fellow after meeting additional requirements beyond those required for membership in the American Academy of Pediatrics. Evidence of this distinction is a credential. *See also* American Academy of Pediatrics; credentials; fellow; pediatrician.

Fellow of the American College of Angiology (FACA)   An angiologist who has achieved the rank of fellow after meeting additional requirements beyond those required for membership in the American College of Angiology. Evidence of this distinction is a credential. *See also* American College of Angiology; angiology; blood vessel; credentials; fellow.

Fellow of the American College of Cardiology (FACC)   A cardiologist who has achieved the rank of fellow after meeting additional requirements beyond those required for membership in the American College of Cardiology. Evidence of this distinction is a credential. *See also* American College of Cardiology; cardiologist; cardiovascular medicine; credentials; fellow.

Fellow of the American College of Chest Physicians (FACCP)   A chest physician who has achieved the rank of fellow after meeting additional requirements beyond those required for membership in the American College of Chest Physicians. Evidence of this distinction is a credential. *See also* American College of Chest Physicians; credentials; fellow.

Fellow of the American College of Dentists (FACD)   A dentist who has achieved the rank of fellow after meeting additional requirements beyond those required for membership in the American College of Dentists. Evidence of this distinction is a credential. *See also* American College of Dentists; credentials; dentist; fellow.

Fellow of the American College of Emergency Physicians (FACEP) An emergency physician who has achieved the rank of fellow after meeting additional requirements beyond those required for membership in the American College of Emergency Physicians. Evidence of this distinction is a credential. *See also* American College of Emergency Physicians; credentials; emergency physician; fellow.

Fellow of the American College of Foot Surgeons (FACFS) A podiatrist who has achieved the rank of fellow after meeting additional requirements beyond those required for membership in the American College of Foot Surgeons. Evidence of this distinction is a credential. *See also* American College of Foot Surgeons; credentials; fellow; podiatrist.

Fellow of the American College of Healthcare Executives (FACHE) A health care executive who has achieved the rank of fellow after meeting additional requirements beyond those required for membership in the American College of Healthcare Executives. Evidence of this distinction is a credential. *See also* American College of Healthcare Executives; administrator; credentials; fellow.

Fellow of the American College of Medical Group Administrators (FACMGA) A medical group administrator who has achieved the rank of fellow after meeting additional requirements beyond those required for membership in the American College of Medical Group Administrators. Evidence of this distinction is a credential. *See also* American College of Medical Group Administrators; administrator; credentials; fellow.

Fellow of the American College of Obstetricians and Gynecologists (FACOG) An obstetrician-gynecologist who has achieved the rank of fellow after meeting additional requirements beyond those required for membership in the American College of Obstetricians and Gynecologists. Evidence of this distinction is a credential. *See also* American College of Obstetricians and Gynecologists; credentials; fellow; obstetrician-gynecologist.

Fellow of the American College of Physician Executives (FACPE) A physician executive who has achieved the rank of fellow after meeting additional requirements in the American College of Physician Executives. Evidence of this distinction is a credential beyond those required for membership. *See also* American College of Physician Executives; credentials; executive; fellow; physician.

Fellow of the American College of Physicians (FACP) An internist who has achieved the rank of fellow after meeting additional requirements beyond those required for membership in the American College of Physicians. Evidence of this distinction is a credential. *See also* American College of Physicians; credentials; fellow; internist.

Fellow of the American College of Preventive Medicine (FACPM) A physician specializing in preventive medicine who has achieved the rank of fellow after meeting additional requirements beyond those required for membership in the American College of Preventive Medicine. Evidence of this distinction is a credential. *See also* American College of Preventive Medicine; credentials; fellow; preventive medicine.

Fellow of the American College of Radiology (FACR) A radiologist who has achieved the rank of fellow after meeting additional requirements beyond those required for membership in the American College of Radiology. Evidence of this distinction is a credential. *See also* American College of Radiology; credentials; fellow; radiologist.

Fellow of the American College of Sports Medicine (FACSM) A physician specialist in sports medicine who has achieved the rank of fellow after meeting additional requirements beyond those required for membership in the American College of Sports Medicine. Evidence of this distinction is a credential. *See also* American College of Sports Medicine; credentials; fellow; sports medicine.

Fellow of the American College of Surgeons (FACS) A surgeon who has achieved the rank of fellow after meeting additional requirements beyond those required for membership in the American College of Surgeons. Evidence of this distinction is a credential. *See also* American College of Surgeons; credentials; fellow; surgeon.

Fellow of the American Occupational Therapy Association (FAOTA) A specialist in occupational therapy who has achieved the rank of fellow after meeting additional requirements beyond those required for membership in the American Occupational Therapy Association. Evidence of this distinction is a credential. *See also* American Occupational Therapy Association; credentials; fellow; occupational therapist.

Fellow of the American Psychiatric Association (FAPA) A psychiatrist who has achieved the rank of fellow after meeting additional requirements beyond those required for membership in the American Psychiatric Association. Evidence of this distinction is a credential. *See also* American Psychiatric Association; credentials; fellow; psychiatrist.

Fellow of the American Psychological Association (FAPA) A psychologist who has achieved the rank of fellow after meeting requirements beyond those required for membership in the American Psychological Association. Evidence of this distinction is a credential. *See also* American Psychological Association; credentials; fellow; psychologist.

Fellow of the American Public Health Association (FAPHA) A specialist in public health who has achieved the rank of fellow after meeting requirements beyond those required for membership in the American Public Health Association. Evidence of this distinction is a credential. *See also* American Public Health Association; credentials; fellow; public health.

Fellow of the College of American Pathologists (FCAP) A pathologist who has achieved the rank of fellow after meeting additional requirements beyond those required for membership in the College of American Pathologists. Evidence of this distinction is a credential. *See also* College of American Pathologists; credentials; fellow; pathologist.

fellow servant A coworker, defined for the purpose of the fellow servant rule, which absolves an employer of liability for injury to a worker resulting from the negligence of a coworker. Fellow servants, who were said to assume the risk of each other's negligence, are employees engaged in the same common pursuits under the same general control, serving the same master, engaged in the same general business, and deriving authority and compensation from a common source. Employer's Liability Acts and Workers' Compensation statutes have abrogated the fellow servant doctrine. *See also* workers' compensation acts.

fellow servant doctrine *See* fellow servant.

fellowship The period of training for a subspecialty, which occurs after completion of a residency. It is becoming increasingly common, however, to call this period of training a residency, instead of a fellowship. For example, a physician interested in becoming a certified cardiologist would complete three years of general residency in internal medicine and then three more years of residency (formerly fellowship) in cardiovascular disease (cardiology). *See also*

fellow; medical education; medical subspecialist.

Fellowship for Medicine in Israel, American Physicians *See* American Physicians Fellowship for Medicine in Israel.

Fellowship and Residency Electronic Interactive Data Access (FRIEDA) An electronic database sponsored by the American Medical Association with information about each residency program. The database is made available to medical schools and hospitals. *See also* American Medical Association; fellowship; residency.

Fellowships, National Medical *See* National Medical Fellowships.

felon A small abscess or boil, particularly underneath a fingernail or toe nail. *See also* abscess; boil.

FEMA *See* Federal Emergency Management Agency.

feminism **1.** Belief in the social, political, and economic equality of the sexes. **2.** The movement organized around this belief.

feminist A person whose beliefs and behavior are based on feminism. *See also* feminism.

Feminist Women's Health Centers, Federation of *See* Federation of Feminist Women's Health Centers.

fertility The capacity to conceive or induce conception. *Compare* infertility. *See also* artificial insemination-donor; artificial insemination - husband; fertility drug; fertility rate; noncoital reproduction.

fertility drug Any drug administered to induce ovulation and pregnancy in patients with infertility caused by not ovulating; for example, clomiphene. Hyperstimulation may lead to multiple ovulation and multiple pregnancy. *See also* drug; fertility; ovulation.

fertility rate A measure of human reproduction calculated as the number of live births per 1000 women aged 15 through 44 years. *See also* fertility; rate.

Fertility Society, American *See* American Fertility Society.

fertilization Union of the male and female sex cells to form a single cell or zygote that then divides to eventually form the embryo and then fetus. *See also* frozen embryo; in-vitro fertilization; preembryo; preembryo transfer.

fertilization, in-vitro *See* in-vitro fertilization.

fetal alcohol syndrome A pattern of fetal maldevelopment with characteristic cardiovascular, limb, and craniofacial defects and mental disability caused by the mother's alcohol consumption while pregnant. The fetus may also be stillborn as a result.

See also alcoholism; syndrome; teratogen.

fetal death   *See* stillbirth.

fetal death certificate   A vital record registering a fetal death or stillbirth. Some health jurisdictions require the use of a fetal death certificate for all products of conception, whereas other jurisdictions require its use only in cases in which gestation has reached a particular duration, usually the 20th or the 28th week. *See also* certificate; death certificate.

fetal death rate   The number of fetal deaths in relation to total births, that is, live births and fetal deaths combined, usually expressed as the number of fetal deaths per 1,000 total births. *See also* child death rate; disease-specific death rate; hospital death rate; infant mortality rate; live birth; mortality rate; neonatal death rate; stillbirth.

fetal distress   Compromised or abnormal condition of the fetus, usually characterized by abnormal heart rhythm and discovered during pregnancy or labor, sometimes through the use of a fetal monitor. Fetal distress may necessitate emergency cesarean delivery. *See also* cesarean section; fetal monitor.

fetal medicine, maternal-   *See* maternal-fetal medicine.

fetal medicine specialist, maternal-   *See* maternal-fetal medicine specialist.

fetal monitor   A device used during pregnancy, labor, and childbirth to observe the fetal heart rate and maternal uterine contractions in order to monitor for the development of fetal distress. *See also* fetal distress; monitor.

fetishism   A sexual deviation, almost exclusive to males, in which erotic feelings are aroused by inanimate objects, such as articles of clothing. *See also* transvestism.

fetus   A postembryonic developing organism from approximately the end of the eighth week after conception to birth, as distinguished from the embryo and the newborn. *Compare* embryo. *See also* teratogen; teratology; viable.

fever   Elevation in the temperature of the body above normal caused by severe stress, strenuous exercise, dehydration, and, most importantly, infection or other disease. *Synonym:* pyrexia. *See also* febrile; hyperpyrexia; malignant hyperpyrexia; pyrogen.

fever, childbed   *See* puerperal fever.

fever, hay   *See* hay fever.

fever, puerperal   *See* puerperal fever.

fever, typhoid   *See* typhoid fever.

FFS   *See* fee for service.

FFWHC   *See* Federation of Feminist Women's Health Centers.

FH   *See* Floating Hospital.

FHCE   *See* Foundation for Health Care Evaluation.

FHIP   *See* Federal Health Insurance Plan.

FHS   *See* Family and Health Section of the National Council on Family Relations.

FHSR   *See* Foundation for Health Services Research.

FI   *See* fiscal intermediary.

fiber   **1.** Food substances, such as bran, that are not broken down by the process of digestion. *See also* bran. **2.** A slender, elongated, threadlike object or structure, as in fiberoptics. *See also* fiberoptics.

fiberoptics   The development and application of image transmission along flexible transparent fibers made of glass or plastic. *See also* endoscopy; fiber; keyhole surgery; optics.

fibrillation   Recurrent, involuntary, and abnormal muscular contraction in which a single or a small number of fibers act separately rather than as a coordinated unit, especially in the heart, as in atrial or ventricular fibrillation where   caused primarily by ischemia of the heart muscle. One treatment of fibrillation is defibrillation by means of electroshock. *See also* defibrillation; heart; ischemia; ventricular fibrillation.

fibrillation, ventricular   *See* ventricular fibrillation.

FICA   *See* Federal Insurance Contribution Act.

fiduciary   **1.** Relating to or founded upon trust, confidence, responsibility, or obligation, as in a physician has a fiduciary relationship with a patient, and a hospital trustee with a hospital. **2.** A person having a legal duty, created by his or her understanding, to act primarily for the benefit of another in matters connected with his or her undertaking. *See also* privileged communication.

field   **1.** In computer science, a defined area of a storage medium, such as a set of bit locations or a set of adjacent columns on a punch card, used to record a type of information consistently. *See also* bit; computer. **2.** An element of a database record in which one piece of information (data element) is stored. *See also* database; data element.

field investigator, public health   *See* public health field investigator.

field theory of motivation   A theory explaining how motivation depends on the organizational environment because human behavior is not based solely on the unique personality of the employee, but also on organizational forces in the midst of which he or she operates. *See also* motivation.

fifth pathway One way in which an individual with all or part of his or her undergraduate medical education abroad can enter graduate medical education in the United States. The fifth pathway consists of a period of supervised clinical training sponsored by a US medical school to such students who, upon successful completion of the training, then become eligible for an approved internship or residency. *See also* Educational Commission on Foreign Medical Graduates; foreign medical graduate; graduate medical education; labor certification.

file In computer science, a collection of stored information. The data in a computer file is stored so that a computer can both read information from the file or write information to the file. Personal computers can store files on magnetic tape, floppy disks, or hard disk. *See also* flat file; record; relational file.

file, circular *See* round file.

file, flat *See* flat file.

file, relational *See* relational file.

file, round *See* round file.

filling Material used to provide a temporary or permanent filling for a tooth cavity, such as gold, amalgam, and various synthetic compounds. *See also* amalgam; dentistry.

film badge A photographic film packet, sensitive to ionizing radiation, used for estimating the exposure of personnel working with x-rays and other radioactive sources. *See also* radiation.

finance The science of the management of money and other assets.

finance committee A standing committee responsible for overseeing an organization's financial operations and status. *See also* finance; standing committee.

Finance, Committee on *See* Committee on Finance.

financial accounting An accounting system that provides balance sheet and income statement results. *See also* accounting; accounting system.

Financial Accounting Foundation (FAF) An organization founded in 1972 that established and maintains the Financial Accounting Standards Board and Financial Accounting Standards Advisory Council. *See also* Financial Accounting Standards Board.

Financial Accounting Standards Board (FASB) An independent board established and maintained by the Financial Accounting Foundation, responsible for establishing and interpreting generally accepted accounting principles. These principles are generally recognized as authoritative by the American Institute of Certified Public Accountants and the Securities and Exchange Commission. The FASB was formed in 1973 to succeed and continue the activities of the Accounting Principles Board. *See also* accounting; Financial Accounting Foundation; generally accepted accounting principles; principle.

financial audit An independent audit conducted to determine the degree to which an organization's financial reports reflect its financial status. *See also* audit; independent audit.

financial director *See* chief financial officer.

Financial Management Association, Healthcare *See* Healthcare Financial Management Association.

financial officer, chief *See* chief financial officer.

financial statement A report of financial status and activity. The two most common types of financial statements are the balance sheet and the operating statement. *See also* balance sheet; operating statement.

financing The process of acquiring money for a purpose. Most health care financing uses debt financing (borrowing money), donations (charitable contributions), equity financing (selling ownership), or tax financing (the use of tax revenues). *See also* capital financing.

Financing Administration, Health Care *See* Health Care Financing Administration.

financing, capital *See* capital financing.

Financing Study Group, Healthcare *See* Healthcare Financing Study Group.

financing system, alternative *See* alternative financing system.

finding In clinical care, a discrete piece of information about a patient that can be elicited during patient assessment, such as a physical finding (for example, a heart murmur or an enlarged spleen) or a laboratory finding (for example, a high hemoglobin level or a negative test for acquired immunodeficiency syndrome virus). Findings include both signs and symptoms. *See also* sign; symptom.

finesse Skillful, subtle handling of a situation, as in an experienced manager finessing a successful resolution to the dilemma. *See also* maneuver.

fire-extinguishing system, automated *See* automated fire-extinguishing system.

Fire Protection Association, National *See* National Fire Protection Association.

Fire Protection Engineers, Society of *See* Society of Fire Protection Engineers.

firmware Computer software that has been programmed into the circuitry of a computer. *Compare* computer hardware; computer software.

first-dollar coverage Insurance or prepayment coverage under which the third-party payer assumes liability for covered services as soon as the first dollar or expense for such services is incurred, without requiring the insured to pay a deductible. *See also* coverage; full coverage.

first generation type I recommendation The first opportunity a surveyed health care organization has to correct a type I recommendation issued by the Joint Commission on Accreditation of Healthcare Organizations, either through a written progress report or through a focused survey (the first follow-up to a full team survey). *See also* focused survey; Joint Commission on Accreditation of Healthcare Organizations; type I recommendation; written progress report.

first responder *See* emergency medical responder.

First Responders, National Association of *See* National Association of First Responders.

fiscal Pertaining to the administering of financial affairs (debt, taxation, revenues, and expenditures) of a public or private organization, as in a hospital's fiscal year. *Compare* monetary. *See also* fiscal year.

fiscal agent *See* fiscal intermediary.

fiscal intermediary (FI) A person or an organization that serves as another's financial agent. In health care, a fiscal intermediary processes claims, provides services, and issues payments on behalf of certain private, federal, and state health benefit programs or other insurance organizations. For instance, providers of health care select public or private fiscal intermediaries, which enter into an agreement with the Secretary of Health and Human Services under Part A of Medicare, to pay claims and perform other functions. Blue Cross or private insurance companies are usually, but not always, the intermediary in these arrangements. *Synonyms:* fiscal agent; intermediary; third-party administrator.

fiscal policy Use of government spending and taxation policies to achieve desired goals.

fiscal year (FY) Any twelve month period for which an organization plans the use of its funds; for instance, the fiscal year of the federal government is from October 1 to September 30. *Compare* calendar year.

fishbone *See* cause-and-effect diagram.

fishbone chart *See* cause-and-effect diagram.

fishbone diagram *See* cause-and-effect diagram.

fishing expedition Exploratory inquiry to find clues and leads for further study. *See also* data dredging.

fitness The state of being physically fit, especially as the result of exercise and proper nutrition. *See also* exercise; nutrition; physical fitness program; wellness; workout.

Fitness Association, American (1) *See* American Fitness Association.

Fitness Association, American (2) *See* American Fitness Association.

Fitness in Business, Association for *See* Association for Fitness in Business.

Fitness, Positive Pregnancy and Parenting *See* Positive Pregnancy and Parenting Fitness.

fitness program, physical *See* physical fitness program.

fittest, survival of the *See* survival of the fittest.

fixed asset Property used for production of goods and services, such as a hospital's buildings, land, and equipment, which is not bought or sold in the normal course of business. *See also* asset; plant.

fixed charge A charge that remains the same regardless of the extent of use. For example, rent and property insurance are often fixed charges that are unaffected by the production level of a health care organization or professional practice. *See also* charge.

fixed cost A cost that remains the same regardless of sales volume. Fixed costs include, for example, executives' salaries, interest expense, rent, depreciation, and insurance expenses. They contrast with variable costs, such as the cost of supplies, which vary, but not necessarily in direct relation to sales. *See also* cost.

fixed fee A set price for the completion of a project. For a contractor, setting a fixed fee entails the risk of absorbing higher than anticipated costs before a project is complete, but for the customer a fixed fee is more easily budgeted. *See also* fee.

fixed income An income that is not adjusted to reflect changes in prices. Interest on most bonds and income from most annuities and some pensions are fixed incomes. *See also* income.

Fixed Prosthodontics, American Academy of *See* American Academy of Fixed Prosthodontics.

fixed-rate pacemaker An implanted artificial cardiac pacemaker in which the generator stimulates the heart at a predetermined rate, regardless of the heart's rhythm. *Compare* demand pacemaker. *See also* artificial cardiac pacemaker; pacemaker.

fixed-wing aircraft *See* ambulance.

fixing, price *See* price fixing.

flat EEG *See* electroencephalogram.

flat file In computer science, a record (such as a medical record) transcribed on a word processor that is not indexed according to its content but, rather, exists as a collection of unrelated words at a particular spot on a computer disk. In a large collection of flat files, each containing one record (such as a medical record), it would be impossible to ask: "How many records contain the diagnosis of sprained ankle?" *Compare* relational file. *See also* field; file; medical record.

flatulence Air or gas in the intestinal tract. *See also* indigestion; flatus.

flatus Gas expelled from the digestive tract. *See also* burp; flatulence.

FLEX *See* Federation Licensing Examination.

flexible sigmoidoscope A flexible illuminated endoscope for performing sigmoidoscopy. *See also* sigmoidoscope.

flexible sigmoidoscopy Sigmoidoscopy performed with a flexible endoscope with appropriate illumination for examining the sigmoid colon. *See also* sigmoidoscopy.

flexible spending account (FSA) An account managed by an employer that allows employees to set aside pretax funds for health care, legal, and day-care services. *See also* account.

flexible working hours A flexible work schedule in which workers can, within a prescribed range of time in the morning and afternoon, start and finish their workday at their own discretion as long as they complete the total number of hours required for a given work period, usually a month. *Synonyms:* flexitime; flextime.

flexitime *See* flexible working hours.

flextime *See* flexible working hours.

Flight Nurses Association, National *See* National Flight Nurses Association.

Flight Paramedics Association, National *See* National Flight Paramedics Association.

Flight Surgeons, Society of United States Air Force *See* Society of United States Air Force Flight Surgeons.

Floatation Tank Association (TANK) A national organization founded in 1982 composed of 200 medical and other health professionals using flotation tanks in conjunction with other patient treatments; academicians and scientific researchers studying the effect of using tanks; tank manufacturers and proprietors of public tank facilities; and other individuals interested in the use of tanks for relaxation and treatment of smoking, hypertension, chronic pain, and obesity. Flotation tanks are also known as sensory deprivation tanks, relaxation tanks, and isolation tanks. They are believed to be capable of bringing about changes in physiology and providing access to the unconscious mind.

Floating Hospital (FH) An organization founded in 1866 that provides medical and dental services, screening tests, social services, and health education for parents, children, and senior citizens in a recreational setting on a ship that cruises New York waters as it provides its services. Formerly (1980) St John's Guild - The Floating Hospital.

float nurse A nurse who is assigned to patient care duty when needed, usually to assist in times of unusually heavy workloads or to assume the duties of absent nursing personnel. *See also* nurse.

floor nurse A nurse working on, but not in charge of, a patient care unit. *Compare* nursing supervisor.

floppy *See* diskette.

floppy disk *See* diskette.

flowchart (flow chart) A pictorial summary that shows with symbols and words the steps, sequence, and relationship of the various operations involved in the performance of a function or a process. A flowchart completely describes an algorithm. *Synonym:* flow diagram. *See also* algorithm; flowcharting; matrix flowchart.

flowcharting The process of creating a flowchart for a function or a process. *See also* flowchart.

flowchart, matrix *See* matrix flowchart.

flow diagram *See* flowchart.

flu *See* influenza.

fluoridation of water A process in which the essential trace mineral, fluoride, is added to the water supply to reduce the frequency of dental cavities.

fluoroscope A device used for examining deep structures by means of roentgen rays. A fluoroscope is used, for example, to produce images during a barium enema procedure. *Synonym:* roentgenoscope. *See also* barium enema; radiology.

FMC Foundation for medical care. *See* medical foundation.

FMG *See* foreign medical graduate.

FNB *See* Food and Nutrition Board.

FNHP *See* Federation of Nurses and Health Professionals.

focused survey A survey conducted by the Joint Commission on Accreditation of Healthcare Organizations during the accreditation cycle to assess the degree to which a health care organization has improved its level of compliance relating to specific recommendations issued by the Joint Commission. The subject matter of the survey is typically an area(s) of performance identified as a deficiency in compliance; however, other performance areas may also be assessed by a surveyor(s), even though they may not be an immediate concern. *See also* accreditation survey; compliance level; Joint Commission on Accreditation of Healthcare Organizations; type I recommendation.

FOCUS-PDCA A quality improvement strategy that helps build knowledge of process, customer, and small-scale improvement using the scientific method. The acronym stands for Find a process to improve; Organize a team that knows the process; Clarify current knowledge of the process; Understand sources or process variation; Select the process improvement; Plan the improvement and continued data collection; Do the improvement, data collection and analysis; Check and study the results; Act to hold the gain and to continue improving the process. *See also* continuous quality improvement; FADE process; Plan-Do-Check-Act (PDCA) cycle.

folk medicine The use of home remedies and procedures handed down by tradition. *See also* medicine.

follow-up survey A survey of a health care organization conditionally accredited by the Joint Commission on Accreditation of Healthcare Organizations, conducted within six months following Joint Commission staff approval of findings of correction to determine the degree to which deficiencies have been corrected and whether full accreditation should be awarded. *See also* accreditation; conditional accreditation; Joint Commission on Accreditation of Healthcare Organizations; survey.

fomite An article that is capable of conveying infection to other people because it has been contaminated by pathogenic organisms. Examples include eating utensils, drinking glasses, and handkerchiefs.

See also indirect contact; infection.

font In computer science, a complete set of characters in a particular typeface style and size. *See also* computer.

food Any mixture of fats, proteins, carbohydrates, water, minerals, vitamins, and nonabsorbable elements, such as cellulose and fiber, which, when eaten, maintains life and growth by providing energy to build and repair tissues. *See also* additive; alimentation; food grades; food poisoning; food supplement; health foods; imitation food; junk food; natural food; substitute food.

food additive *See* additive.

food additives, indirect *See* indirect food additives.

Food Associates, Natural *See* Natural Food Associates.

Food and Drug Administration (FDA) The US federal agency within the US Public Health Service, Department of Health and Human Services, responsible for enforcing the provisions of the US Food, Drug, and Cosmetic Act, which include implementing and administering federal statutes and regulations established to provide protection for the public against poisoning and contamination or other health hazards in foods, food substances, and food additives. The FDA also seeks to ensure the safety and effectiveness of drugs and drug substances through controlling the sale and legal use of drugs, including the licensing of new drugs and the identification and facilitation of orphan drugs. Its principal divisions include the Office of the Commissioner, Center for Devices and Radiological Health, Center for Drugs and Biologics, Center for Food Safety and Applied Nutrition, Center for Veterinary Medicine, and National Center for Toxicological Research. *See also* medical device; orphan drug.

Food, Drug and Cosmetic Act *See* Food and Drug Administration.

Food and Drug Law Institute (FDLI) A national organization founded in 1949 composed of 380 manufacturers and distributors of food, drugs, cosmetics, and devices, and law firms interested in promoting the development of knowledge about the laws that regulate the research, production, and sale of food, drugs, medical devices, and cosmetics. It provides a forum for the discussion of issues pertaining to food and drug laws.

Food and Drug Officials, Association of *See* Association of Food and Drug Officials.

food grades A system by which the US Department of Agriculture (USDA) measures the quality of appearance, uniformity, texture, and sometimes taste of some meat, poultry, eggs, dairy products, and fresh or canned produce.

food, health *See* health foods.

Food and Health Policy, Public Voice for *See* Public Voice for Food and Health Policy.

food, imitation *See* imitation food.

food, junk *See* junk food.

food, natural *See* natural food.

Food and Nutrition Board (FNB) A division of the National Academy of Sciences - Institute of Medicine founded in 1940 to evaluate and offer advice concerning the relationship between food consumption, nutritional status, and public health. *See also* Institute of Medicine; National Academy of Sciences; nutrition.

food poisoning Acute illness caused by eating food containing toxic substances or organisms, such as bacteria and fungi, and the toxins they produce. Bacteria commonly responsible for food poisoning are campylobacter, *Clostridium botulinum*, *Salmonella*, and *Staphyloccoccus*. *See also* botulism; campylobacter.

food preservative *See* preservative.

Food Sanitation Institute *See* Environmental Management Association.

Foods Association, African-American Natural *See* African-American Natural Foods Association.

food service *See* foodservice.

foodservice The business of making, transporting, and serving or dispensing prepared foods, as in a restaurant or a hospital. *See also* foodservice department.

Food Service Administrators, American Society for Hospital *See* American Society for Hospital Food Service Administrators.

foodservice department The department of a health care organization, such as a hospital, that provides food preparation and service to patients and staff and also provides nutritional care to patients. *Synonym*: dietary department. *See also* department; foodservice.

foods, health *See* health foods.

food stamps Stamps that are purchased for a certain amount of money and then exchanged for a larger quantity of food at grocery stores. For example, $60 worth of food stamps may be bought for only $20, but these stamps may be exchanged at the store for $60 worth of food.

food, substitute *See* substitute food.

food supplement A concentrate of one or more nutrient substances, used to supplement a nutritionally inadequate diet. Some "food supplements" are, in fact, "unsafe food additives," by the definition of US law. *See also* additive.

Foot and Ankle Society, American Orthopaedic *See* American Orthopaedic Foot and Ankle Society.

footer The bottom margin of a printed document, which repeats on every page. Some computer programs can also include text, pictures, automatic consecutive page numbers, date, and time. *See also* header; word processing.

footing Totaling a column of numbers.

foot orthopedics *See* podiatric orthopedics.

Foot Orthopedists, American College of *See* American College of Foot Orthopedists.

foot specialist *See* podiatrist.

foot surgeon *See* podiatrist.

Foot Surgeons, American College of *See* American College of Foot Surgeons.

Foot Surgeons, National College of *See* National College of Foot Surgeons.

Foot Surgery, Academy of Ambulatory *See* Academy of Ambulatory Foot Surgery.

"for cause" unannounced survey *See* unannounced survey.

force-field analysis A method for understanding competing forces that increase or decrease the likelihood of successfully implementing change. *See also* analysis; force-field theory; present state.

force-field theory A theory maintaining that creative problem solving can best be accomplished by a group working with objective data rather than relying on intuition. Such groups require a leader to keep them from straying from the topic and to limit discussion to a reasonable amount of time. *See also* force-field analysis; theory.

force, task *See* task force.

forceps An instrument with two blades and a handle for compressing, grasping, handling, or pulling tissues in operations and for handling sterile dressing and other surgical supplies, as in mosquito forceps (a small hemostatic forceps). *See also* clamp; forceps delivery; obstetric forceps.

forceps delivery Extraction of an infant from the birth canal by applying obstetric forceps to the infant's head and then pulling gently. *See also* delivery; forceps; obstetric forceps.

forceps, obstetric *See* obstetric forceps.

Ford Foundation, The   *See* The Ford Foundation.

forecasting   The process of estimating future trends that relies on extrapolation of existing trends. An example of forecasting is extrapolation of mortality trends in 1990-1991 for coronary artery disease in women suggesting that mortality rates will continue to rise in the future. *See also* extrapolation; prediction; projection; scenario building.

foreclosure   Termination of all rights of a mortgage. A foreclosed property may be sold to satisfy a debt.

foreign medical graduate (FMG)   A physician who graduates from a medical school outside the United States and Canada. In order to practice in the United States, an FMG must meet certain requirements, such as certification by the Educational Commission for Foreign Medical Graduates (ECFMG). An American citizen who graduates from medical schools outside the United States is called a *United States foreign medical graduate* or *USFMG*. A citizen of another nation who is a graduate of a foreign medical school is called an *alien foreign medical graduate* or *alien FMG*. *See also* Educational Commission on Foreign Medical Graduates; fifth pathway; labor certification. *See also* certification; medical school; physician.

Foreign Nursing Schools, Commission on Graduates of   *See* Commission on Graduates of Foreign Nursing Schools.

Foreign Pharmacy Graduate Examination Committee (FPGEC)   An organization founded in 1982 that provides information to foreign pharmacy graduates concerning entry into the United States' pharmacy profession and health care system. It evaluates qualifications of foreign pharmacy graduates, gathers and disseminates data on foreign graduates, and maintains information on foreign pharmacy schools to produce an examination that measures academic competence against United States pharmacy school standards. *See also* pharmacy.

forensic   Applying the knowledge of a particular subject, such as medicine or dentistry, to the law through the process of legal action and judgment. *See also* forensic chemistry; forensic dentistry; forensic medicine; forensic mental health services; forensic pathology; forensic psychiatry.

forensic chemistry   The use of chemical knowledge in the solution of legal problems. *See also* chemistry; forensic.

forensic dentistry   The branch and specialty of dentistry dealing with the investigation, preparation,

preservation, and presentation of dental evidence and opinion in courts and other legal, correctional, and law-enforcement settings. *Synonyms:* dental jurisprudence; forensic odontology. *See also* dentistry; forensic.

forensic medicine   The branch of medicine that interprets or establishes the medical facts in civil or criminal law cases. Subspecialties of forensic medicine include forensic pathology, forensic psychiatry, forensic toxicology, and forensic biochemistry. *Synonym:* medical jurisprudence. *See also* forensic; medicine; murder.

Forensic Medicine, Milton Halpern Institute of   *See* Milton Halpern Institute of Forensic Medicine.

forensic mental health services   Psychiatric services provided to patients diagnosed with a mental illness and hospitalized on an order issued by a criminal/juvenile justice system. *See also* forensic; mental health services; mental illness.

forensic odontology   *See* forensic dentistry.

Forensic Odontology, American Society of   *See* American Society of Forensic Odontology.

forensic pathologist   A pathologist who subspecializes in forensic pathology. The forensic pathologist serves the public as coroner or medical examiner or by performing medicolegal autopsies for such officials. *See also* forensic pathology.

forensic pathology   The branch of medicine and subspecialty of pathology dealing with the investigation and evaluation of specific classes of death defined by law, such as cases of sudden, unexpected, suspicious, and violent death. *See also* forensic pathologist; pathology.

forensic psychiatrist   A psychiatrist who subspecializes in forensic psychiatry. *See also* forensic psychiatry.

forensic psychiatry   The branch and subspecialty of psychiatry dealing with the legal evaluation of patients with sexual disorders, antisocial personality disorders, paranoid disorders, and addictive disorders. Forensic psychiatry also may involve observing persons for malingering, using ancillary information, such as police reports, interviewing relatives and witnesses, reviewing prior medical records, and testifying in court. *See also* psychiatry.

Forensic Psychiatry, American Board of   *See* American Board of Forensic Psychiatry.

Forensic Psychology, American Academy of   *See* American Academy of Forensic Psychology.

forensic sciences   The application of any science to

the law, as in forensic toxicology, forensic psychiatry, forensic anthropology. *See also* genetic fingerprinting.

Forensic Sciences, American Academy of *See* American Academy of Forensic Sciences.

Forensic Toxicologists, Society of *See* Society of Forensic Toxicologists.

foreseeability A test used in law to measure the extent of damages for which one may be responsible. Every act will set a series of events in motion that extend to eternity; however, in most jurisdictions, a defendant is only responsible for those results that would be reasonably forseeable. For example, it is reasonably foreseeable that a result of negligent surgery will be the patient's pain and suffering. *See also* damages; tortfeasor.

forgery Illegal production of something counterfeit; the fraudulent making or altering of a writing with the intent to infringe on the rights of another. *See also* authentication; falsification of information; falsify.

format Arrangement of data or method of presenting data. In computers, format is the method of arranging information that is to be stored or displayed. Format can refer to how information is stored on a computer disk or making the computer record a pattern of reference marks on a disk. A brand-new disk must always be formatted before it can be used. Formatting a used disk erases any information previously recorded on it.

form, indicator development *See* indicator development form.

Forms 1007 and 1008 Forms used in the Medicare prospective payment system to calculate a hospital's adjustments to its base year Medicare costs. *See also* base year Medicare costs; prospective payment system.

formula A liquid food for infants, containing most of the nutrients in human milk.

Formula Council, Infant *See* Infant Formula Council.

formula, enteral *See* enteral formula.

formulary A book or other collection of stated and fixed forms, as in a drug formulary. *See also* drug formulary; hospital formulary; *National Formulary*.

formulary, drug *See* drug formulary.

formulary, hospital *See* hospital formulary.

form, uniform claim *See* uniform claim form.

for-profit hospital *See* investor-owned hospital.

fortified *See* enriched.

FORTRAN Acronym for formula translation, a computer language developed by IBM in the late 1950s. It was the first language allowing program-

mers to describe calculations by means of mathematical formulas.

Fortune 500 An annual listing by *Fortune* magazine of the 500 largest US industrial (manufacturing) corporations. *Fortune* also publishes the Fortune Service 500, which ranks the 500 largest US nonmanufacturing companies.

FORUM *See* Forum for Medical Affairs.

Forum for Death Education and Counseling *See* Association for Death Education and Counseling.

Forum for Health Care Planning, The *See* The Forum for Health Care Planning.

Forum for Medical Affairs (FORUM) A national organization founded in 1944 composed of 800 presidents, presidents-elect, and past presidents of state medical associations, members of the American Medical Association (AMA) and the House of Delegates, editors of state medical association journals, executive directors of state medical associations, and representatives of AMA-recognized medical specialty societies. *See also* American Medical Association; medical association.

for your information (FYI) A notation on a memorandum that indicates that no action is required on the contents.

for your interest (FYI) *See* for your information.

foster care home A facility that provides custodial care (housekeeping and meals) for individuals who need it. *See also* custodial care.

foster care services for adults Twenty-four-hour supervised living arrangements for adults in a family setting with access to social services and community resources. *See also* foster care services for children.

foster care services for children Twenty-four-hour substitute family or group home care for a planned period of time. This home provides experiences and conditions that promote normal growth. The child, his or her family, and the foster parents are provided with casework services and other treatment or community services. *See also* foster care services for adults.

foundation The establishment of an institution with provisions for continuing existence; for example, a nonprofit organization with private funds (usually from a single source, either an individual, a family, or a corporation) whose program is managed by its own trustees or directors, established to maintain or aid social, educational, charitable, religious, or other activities serving the common welfare primarily through making grants. *See also* corporate foundation; dental foundation; grant; grant proposal; medical foundation; private foundation.

foundation, corporate *See* corporate foundation.

foundation, dental *See* dental foundation.

Foundation, G. Harold and Leila Y. Mathers Charitable *See* G. Harold and Leila Y. Mathers Charitable Foundation.

Foundation for Health Care Evaluation (FHCE) A national organization founded in 1971 composed of 3,500 physicians interested in ensuring the availability of quality health care at reasonable costs. It evaluates health care services at hospitals, retirement homes, and other facilities; develops health care standards for hospitals; and offers consultation services to operators of health care facilities to improve efficiency in services.

Foundation for Health Services Research (FHSR) A national organization founded in 1981 composed of 1,400 members. It conducts professional and educational activities beneficial to the field of health services research. *See also* health services research.

Foundation, Kansas Health *See* Kansas Health Foundation.

foundation, medical *See* medical foundation.

foundation for medical care *See* medical foundation.

foundation, private *See* private foundation.

Foundation, Richard King Mellon *See* Richard King Mellon Foundation.

Foundation, Robert W. Woodruff *See* Robert W Woodruff Foundation, Inc.

Foundations, The Champlin *See* The Champlin Foundations.

Foundation of Thanatology *See* American Institute of Life Threatening Illness and Loss, (Division of Foundation of Thanatology).

Foundation, The Aaron Diamond *See* The Aaron Diamond Foundation, Inc.

Foundation, The David and Lucile Packard *See* The David and Lucile Packard Foundation.

Foundation, The Edna McConnell Clark *See* The Edna McConnell Clark Foundation.

Foundation, The Ford *See* The Ford Foundation.

Foundation, The Henry J. Kaiser Family *See* The Henry J. Kaiser Family Foundation.

Foundation, The John A. Hartford *See* The John A. Hartford Foundation, Inc.

Foundation, The John D. and Catherine T. MacArthur *See* The John D. and Catherine T. MacArthur Foundation.

Foundation, The Kresge *See* The Kresge Foundation.

Foundation, The Robert Wood Johnson *See* The Robert Wood Johnson Foundation.

Foundation, The William K. Warren *See* The William K. Warren Foundation.

Foundation, WM Keck *See* WM Keck Foundation.

Foundation, WK Kellogg *See* WK Kellogg Foundation.

Fourteen Points, Deming's *See* Deming's Fourteen Points.

fourth party Business and industry purchasers of health care services (for example, employers and business coalitions) who are interested in managing health care costs. The first party is the patient, the second party is the health care provider, and the third party is the third-party payer. The fourth party as a purchaser of health care services may contract with a third party. *See also* health care provider; patient; third-party payer.

FP *See* family practice.

FPA *See* Federal Physicians Association.

FPGEC *See* Foreign Pharmacy Graduate Examination Committee.

FPMB *See* Federation of Podiatric Medical Boards.

FPO *See* Federation of Prosthodontic Organizations.

fractionation **1.** The act or process of charging separately for several services or component services that were previously subject to a single charge or not billed at all, usually resulting in an increase in the total charge. Fractionation is often a response by health care providers to limitations made by third-party payers on increases in specific charges, changed medical practices, or advances in medical technology. *See also* unbundling. **2.** The process of separating blood components of whole blood. *See also* blood components.

fracture A break, rupture, or crack, especially in bone or cartilage. *See also* stress fracture; traction; wound.

Fracture Association, American *See* American Fracture Association.

fracture, stress *See* stress fracture.

franchise dentistry A system for marketing dental practice, usually under a trade name, where permitted by state law and regulations. Participating dentists receive the benefits of media advertising, a national referral system, and financial and management consultation support in return for financial investment or other consideration. *See also* dentistry.

fraternal insurance A cooperative insurance plan provided by an organization to its members. *See also* insurance.

fraternal twins Twins resulting from the simultaneous fertilization of two ova. *Compare* identical twins. *See also* genetics; twin.

fraud and abuse *Fraud* is a false statement, willfully made, for material gain and with the intent to deceive; for example, acts, such as misrepresenting eligibility or need for health services, claiming reimbursement for services not rendered or for nonexistent patients. *Abuse* is an exaggerated statement, willfully made, for material gain and with the intent to confuse. Fraud and abuse is a criminal (felony) misuse of the Medicare system. *See also* defraud; safe harbor regulations.

Fraud Association, National Health Care Anti- *See* National Health Care Anti-Fraud Association.

Fraud, National Council Against Health *See* National Council Against Health Fraud.

frauds, statute of *See* statute of frauds.

free choice of physician *See* free choice of provider.

free choice of provider The view that any health care financing mechanism should preserve the ability of a patient or client to choose any provider of care in the marketplace without being restrained by economic sanctions of insurers and other third-party payers. *See also* health care provider.

free clinic A neighborhood clinic or health program that provides health services in a relatively informal setting to students, transient youth, and minority groups. Care is provided free or a nominal charge by staff members who are predominantly volunteers. *See also* clinic.

Freedom of Choice in Medicine, Committee for *See* Committee for Freedom of Choice in Medicine.

Freedom of Information Act Enacted by Congress in 1966, the act requires federal agencies to make certain information available to the public. Medical records are exempt. *See also* confidentiality; medical record.

free radical A byproduct of oxygen metabolism that can attack cell components and irreversibly damage them. Necessary for health in small qualities; harmful in large quantities.

freestanding Refers to a health care facility that is separate from a hospital or other health care organi-

zation. Freestanding does not necessarily indicate separate ownership; a hospital may operate a freestanding facility or a facility may be owned by a separate organization.

freestanding ambulatory care center A facility with an organized professional staff that provides various health treatments on an outpatient basis only and that may be, depending on the level of care it is equipped to provide, a freestanding emergency center, freestanding urgent care center, or primary care center. *Compare* hospital-based ambulatory care center. *See also* freestanding emergency center; freestanding urgent care center; primary care center.

Freestanding Ambulatory Surgery Association *See* Federated Ambulatory Surgery Association.

freestanding ambulatory surgical facility A health care facility, physically or geographically separate from a hospital, that provides surgical services to outpatients who do not require hospitalization. Offices of private physicians or dentists are not included in this category unless the offices have a distinct area that is used solely for outpatient surgical treatment on a routine, organized basis. *Synonyms*: freestanding surgicenter; surgical center; surgicenter. *See also* ambulatory surgical facility.

freestanding emergency center (FEC) A facility that is designed, organized, equipped, and staffed to provide health care on a 24-hour-per-day basis for injuries and illness, including those that are life-threatening, that provides laboratory and radiologic services and has established arrangements for transporting critical patients or patients requiring hospitalization once stabilized, and that does not provide continuity of care but treats episodic, emergency, and primary care cases. *See also* freestanding ambulatory care center.

Freestanding Radiation Oncology Centers, Association of *See* Association of Freestanding Radiation Oncology Centers.

freestanding surgicenter *See* freestanding ambulatory surgical facility.

freestanding urgent care center A facility that provides primary and urgent care treatment on a less than 24-hour-per-day basis and that is supported by laboratory and radiology services but does not receive patients transported by ambulance, is not equipped to treat true medical emergencies, such as heart attack or stroke victims, and does not provide continuity of care. *Synonyms*: urgent care center;

urgicenter. *See also* freestanding ambulatory care center; urgent.

frequency In general, the number of times something occurs within a specified period of time, such as the number of heartbeats occurring in one minute. *See also* occurrence.

frequency distribution *See* distribution.

frequency polygon A graphic display of a frequency distribution made by joining a set of points, for each of which the abscissa is the midpoint of the class and the ordinate, or height, is the frequency.

frequent Occurs often, at short intervals. *See also* continuous; intermittent; occasional; periodic; sporadic.

FRIEDA *See* Fellowship and Residency Electronic Interactive Data Access.

friendly visit Regular visits to isolated, homebound, or institutionalized elderly people to reduce their isolation and loneliness. *See also* visit.

Friends of Wine, Society of Medical *See* Society of Medical Friends of Wine.

frigid **1.** Lacking warmth of feeling; stiff. **2.** Persistently averse to sexual intercourse. *See also* impotence; sex therapy.

fringe benefit *See* perquisite.

fringe benefits package *See* employee benefit program.

frivolous In law, clearly lacking in substance or clearly insufficient as a matter of law. For example, a claim is frivolous if it is not supported by the facts or it is one for which the law recognizes no remedy.

frontal lobotomy *See* prefrontal lobotomy.

frozen embryo An egg fertilized and then frozen before introduction into the uterus. Such eggs are obtained from women who are taking fertility drugs, thus producing more than the usual one egg per month. Fertilization is carried out in vitro (outside the body). *See also* cryobirth; cryotherapy; embryo; fertilization.

FSA *See* flexible spending account.

FSCO *See* Federation of Straight Chiropractic Organizations.

FSMB *See* Federation of State Medical Boards of the United States.

FT *See* American Institute of Life Threatening Illness and Loss, (Division of Foundation of Thanatology).

FTC *See* Federal Trade Commission.

FTE *See* full-time equivalent.

FTN *See* Family Therapy Network.

full coverage Insurance that pays for every dollar of a loss with no maximum and no deductible amount. *See also* coverage; first-dollar coverage.

full team survey The accreditation survey conducted by the Joint Commission on Accreditation of Healthcare Organizations every three years by a full complement of surveyors. *See also* accreditation survey; Joint Commission on Accreditation of Healthcare Organizations; survey; triennial survey.

full-time Employed for or involving a customary number of hours of working time, as in a full-time worker. *Compare* part-time. *See also* full-time equivalent; full-time worker.

full-time equivalent (FTE) A work force equivalent of one individual working full-time for a specific period, which may be made up of several part-time individuals or one full-time individual. For example, three part-time nurses working a combined total of 60 hours equal 1.5 FTEs when the normal full-time work week for a single individual is 40 hours. *See also* staffing ratio.

full-time worker According to the Bureau of Labor Statistics, a person employed at least thirty-five hours per week. *Compare* part-time worker.

function **1.** A goal-directed, interrelated series of processes, such as the patient assessment or information management functions of an accredited health care organization. *See also* high-risk function; high-volume function; important function. **2.** A quality, trait, or fact that is so related to another as to be dependent on and to vary with this other, as in the success of the endeavor is a function of the commitment of management and employees to continuously improving performance and the quality of services. **3.** The actions and activities expected of a person or a thing, as in a pharmacist's function(s) in the hospital or the function of the gallbladder. *Compare* morphology; structure.

function, admitting *See* admitting function.

functional age Age defined by ability and performance rather than chronologically. *See also* age; chronological age; developmental age; mental age.

functional illiterate A person whose reading and writing skills are so poor that he or she cannot function effectively in the most basic business, office, or factory employment. Such individuals may have earned a high school diploma, making this credential less valid as a predictor of performance.

functional benchmarking *See* benchmarking.

functional integration The state in which two entities share common management, support, and clinical services. *See also* integration.

functionalism **1.** The doctrine that the function of an object should determine its design and materials. **2.** A doctrine stressing purpose, practicality, and utility.

functional organization The structure of an organization based on functional performance. Organizational departments are created to fulfill organizational functions, such as marketing, finance, and personnel or, in a health care organization, patient admission, patient assessment, patient treatment, and patient discharge. *See also* function; organization.

Functional Orthodontics, American Association for *See* American Association for Functional Orthodontics.

Functional Neurosurgery, American Society for Stereotactic and *See* American Society for Stereotactic and Functional Neurosurgery.

functional team A group of people addressing an issue in which any recommended changes would not be likely to affect people outside the specific area. *See also* crossfunctional team; team.

function deployment, quality *See* quality function deployment.

function, governmental *See* governmental function.

function, high-risk *See* high-risk function.

function, high-volume *See* high-volume function.

function, important *See* important function.

function, invisible patient care *See* invisible patient care function.

function laboratory, special *See* special function laboratory.

function, line *See* line function.

function, visible patient care *See* visible patient care function.

fund A sum of money or other resources set aside for a specific purpose, as in a pension fund. *See also* contingency fund; general fund; restricted fund; trust fund; unrestricted fund.

fund, contingency *See* contingency fund.

fund, general *See* general fund.

Funding, Coalition for Health *See* Coalition for Health Funding.

fundoscope *See* ophthalmoscope.

fundoscopy *See* ophthalmoscopy.

fundraising Organized activities for soliciting con-

tributions, gifts, grants, requests, and other donations to provide support for programs and services, as in fundraising for charitable organizations or political campaigns. *See also* development.

fund, restricted *See* restricted fund.

Fund, The Commonwealth *See* The Commonwealth Fund.

fund, trust *See* trust fund.

fund, unrestricted *See* unrestricted fund.

funeral The ceremonies held in connection with the burial or cremation of a dead person.

funeral director A person, usually an embalmer, whose business is to arrange for the burial or cremation of the dead and assist at the funeral rites. *Synonyms*: mortician; undertaker. *See also* funeral home.

funeral home An establishment where dead people are prepared for burial or cremation and wakes and funerals may be held. *See also* embalming.

fungitrol machine A box-like apparatus with ultraviolet lights for treating foot diseases and conditions. *See also* fungus; machine.

fungus A microscopic parasitic plant causing a spongy, granular growth on tissues, as in fungus growing on the skin of the foot. *See also* microorganism; mycology; ringworm.

furuncle *See* boil.

futility In patient care, a situation in which a patient's condition is hopeless, and the results of treatment would only be temporary and fleeting and thus not be beneficial. *Synonym*: medically futile. *See also* Baby Doe regulations; death with dignity.

future damages The loss or injury expected to occur in the future for which the law allows recovery. In most jurisdictions, with the exception of noneconomic damages, such as future pain and suffering, the amount awarded is reduced to its present money value. *See also* damages; noneconomic damages.

future state In an organizational transformation, the vision of where the organization will be after it is transformed. For the transformation to continuous quality improvement, the future state includes constancy of purpose, leaders who model the new way, collaboration, customer mindedness, and a process focus. *See also* continuous quality improvement.

FY *See* fiscal year.

FYI *See* for your information.

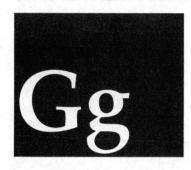

GAAP *See* generally accepted accounting principles.

GAAS Acronym for generally accepted auditing standards, as established by the American Institute of Certified Public Accountants. *See* American Institute of Certified Public Accountants; generally accepted accounting principles.

gag **1.** To retch. *See also* vomit. **2.** A device to keep the jaws separated during surgical procedures. *See also* surgery.

gag reflex A normal neural reflex elicited by touching the soft palate or posterior pharynx, the response being elevation of the palate, retraction of the tongue, and contraction of the pharyngeal muscles. The reflex, frequently performed with a tongue depressor, is used as a test of the integrity of the vagus and glossopharyngeal cranial nerves. *See also* reflex; tongue depressor.

gains, capital *See* capital gains or losses.

gait Manner of walking, including rhythm, cadence, and speed.

Galen (130?-200? AD) A Greek anatomist, physician, and writer whose theories formed the basis of European medicine until the Renaissance.

gallbladder The pear-shaped sac connected to the liver that stores and concentrates bile, the mixture of acids and salts the liver produces to help digest fat in the small intestine. *See also* bile; cholecystectomy; laparascopic cholecystectomy.

gallstone A small rounded mass composed chiefly or cholesterol of bilirubin and calcium that forms in the gallbladder or in the gallbladder's ducts. *See also* bilirubin; gallbladder.

galvanic current Low-voltage direct current used in the physical treatment of disease by podiatrists and other health professionals. Named after Luigi Galvani, an Italian physiologist born in 1737. *See also* galvanism; transcutaneous electric nerve stimulation.

galvanism The therapeutic application of electricity in the form of direct current. *See also* electromedicine; galvanic current; transcutaneous electric nerve stimulation.

galvanometer An instrument for detecting, measuring, or comparing small electric currents. *See also* galvanism.

gaming The unethical or illegal manipulation of a process or system for the purpose of unwarranted gain or advantage, as in "gaming the system"; for example, gaming the diagnosis-related groups reimbursement system. *See also* diagnosis-related groups reimbursement system.

gangrene The death and putrefaction (enzymatic and bacterial decomposition) of a mass of tissue, usually associated with obstruction of arterial blood supply. The extremities are most often affected, but gangrene can occur in the intestines and gallbladder. *See also* dry gangrene; gas gangrene; moist gangrene.

gangrene, dry *See* dry gangrene.

gangrene, gas *See* gas gangrene.

gangrene, moist *See* moist gangrene.

GAO *See* US General Accounting Office.

GAP *See* Group for the Advancement of Psychiatry.

GAPP *See* General Administrative Policies and Procedures.

garbage in, garbage out *See* GIGO.

gas A substance, neither liquid nor solid, whose physical state is characterized by occupying the whole of the space in which it is contained. *See also* burp; carbon monoxide; flatus; gas chamber; gas gangrene; nerve gas.

gas chamber A device for judicial and other executions, usually employing hydrocyanic acid gas. *See also* gas.

gas gangrene A complication of extensive wounds, particularly when contaminated with soil, due to anaerobic infection with toxin-producing *Clostridia*. The condition causes muscle decay and death and gas formation locally and systemic toxemia and shock. *Synonym*: clostridial myonecrosis. *See also* complication; gangrene.

gas, nerve *See* nerve gas.

gastric juice Secretions of the glands in the wall of the stomach. The major components of gastric juice are mucus, the digestive enzyme pepsin, hydrochloric acid, and a protein called intrinsic factor that promotes absorption of vitamin B_{12}. *See also* enzyme; stomach.

gastric lavage Irrigation of the stomach usually carried out with a large-bore tube and diluted saline solution. It is a traditional emergency measure in cases of poisoning. *See also* lavage; stomach.

gastric ulcer A sore that forms in the stomach. *See also* peptic ulcer; ulcer.

gastritis Inflammation of the lining of the stomach, characterized by loss of appetite, nausea, vomiting, and discomfort after eating. *See also* inflammation; stomach.

gastroenteritis Inflammation of the stomach and intestine; the diagnosis is usually associated with the familiar syndrome of diarrhea and vomiting or "stomach flu." *See also* diarrhea; enteritis; inflammation; intestine; stomach.

Gastroenterological Association, American *See* American Gastroenterological Association.

gastroenterologist An internist who subspecializes in gastroenterology. *See also* hepatologist; gastroenterology; pediatric gastroenterologist.

gastroenterologist, pediatric *See* pediatric gastroenterologist.

gastroenterology The branch of medicine and subspecialty of internal medicine dealing with the digestive organs, including the stomach, bowel, liver, and gallbladder, and disorders, such as abdominal pain, ulcers, diarrhea, cancer, and jaundice. *See also* alimentary tract; digestive system; esophagology; gastroenterologist; internal medicine; malabsorption.

Gastroenterology, American College of *See* American College of Gastroenterology.

Gastroenterology Nurses and Associates, Society of *See* Society of Gastroenterology Nurses and Associates.

Gastroenterology and Nutrition, North American Society for Pediatric *See* North American Society for Pediatric Gastroenterology and Nutrition.

gastroenterology, pediatric *See* pediatric gastroenterology.

gastroesophageal reflux A disorder in which the lower esophageal sphincter does not stay closed when the stomach is full or under pressure, with the result that food and acidic digestive juices back up (or reflux) into the esophagus, causing heartburn. *Synonym*: esophageal reflux. *See also* antacid; esophagus; heartburn; reflux; reflux esophagitis.

gastrointestinal (GI) Pertaining to the stomach and the intestines, as in gastrointestinal upset or gastrointestinal bleeding. *See also* alimentary tract; digestive system; GI series; intestine.

Gastrointestinal Endoscopic Surgeons, Society American *See* Society American Gastrointestinal Endoscopic Surgeons.

Gastrointestinal Endoscopy, American Society for *See* American Society for Gastrointestinal Endoscopy.

Gastrointestinal Pathology Club *See* Gastrointestinal Pathology Society.

Gastrointestinal Pathology Society (GIPS) A national organization founded in 1979 composed of 145 physicians, researchers with doctoral degrees, and other individuals interested in disseminating information and increasing knowledge about the pathology of the gastrointestinal tract. It presents research and educational programs at annual meetings. Formerly (1987) Gastrointestinal Pathology Club. *See also* alimentary tract; gastroenterology; pathology.

gastroscope An endoscope for examining the interior of the stomach. *See also* endoscope; gastroscopy; stomach.

gastroscopy The process of visualizing the interior of the stomach by means of a gastroscope inserted through the esophagus. *See also* gastroscope; stomach.

gastrostomy A surgical procedure in which a tube is placed through the abdominal wall directly into the stomach for feeding. *See also* nutritional support; stomach.

gastrostomy tube *See* nutritional support.

Gantt chart A calendar graph that displays task scheduling and status.

gatekeeper An individual who monitors and/or oversees the actions of other persons, as in a physician who determines health services to be provided to a patient and coordinates provision of the services by other persons. *See also* gatekeeper mechanism.

gatekeeper mechanism In health care, an arrangement whereby a patient is assigned to or chooses from a selected group of primary care physicians, and the primary care physician assumes responsibility for, reviews, and approves all health services the patient receives, including care from specialists. *Compare* open access. *See also* gatekeeper; health services; mechanism; patient; primary care physician.

gatekeeper model *See* closed panel group practice.

Gaussian distribution *See* normal distribution.

gay **1.** Relating to or sharing the life-style and concerns of the homosexual community. **2.** A homosexual person. *See also* American Association of Physicians for Human Rights; homosexuality; lesbianism.

Gay Alcoholism Professionals, National Association of Lesbian/ *See* National Association of Lesbian/Gay Alcoholism Professionals.

Gay and Bisexual People in Medicine, Lesbian, *See* Lesbian, Gay and Bisexual People in Medicine.

Gay Caucus of Public Health Workers, Lesbian and *See* Lesbian and Gay Caucus of Public Health Workers.

Gay Issues, National Association of Social Workers Committee on Lesbian and *See* National Association of Social Workers Committee on Lesbian and Gay Issues.

Gay Issues, Society for the Psychological Study of Lesbian and *See* Society for the Psychological Study of Lesbian and Gay Issues.

Gay, Lesbian, and Bisexual Issues in Counseling, Association for *See* Association for Gay, Lesbian, and Bisexual Issues in Counseling.

Gay and Lesbian Psychiatrists, Association of *See* Association of Gay and Lesbian Psychiatrists.

Gay and Lesbian Scientists and Technical Professionals, National Organization of *See* National Organization of Gay and Lesbian Scientists and Technical Professionals.

Gay Men's Health Crisis (GMHC) A social service agency for the clinical treatment of acquired immunodeficiency syndrome (AIDS). It provides support and therapy groups for AIDS patients and their families and sends volunteer crisis counselors to work with AIDS patients. *See also* acquired immunodeficiency syndrome; gay.

Gay Public Health Workers Caucus *See* Lesbian and Gay Caucus of Public Health Workers.

GB *See* governing body.

GCS *See* Glasgow coma scale.

gender Sexual identity, especially in relation to society or culture, as in gender gap. *See also* gender gap; gender identity; gender neutral; gender role; sex change.

gender gap A disproportionate difference, as in attitudes and voting preferences, between the sexes. *See also* gender.

gender identity Awareness of knowing to which sex (female of male) one belongs; this awareness normally begins in infancy, continues through childhood, and is reinforced during adolescence. *See also* adolescence; gender; sex change.

gender neutral Free of explicit or implicit reference to gender or sex, as in the term "chair" instead of "chairman." *See also* gender.

gender role Sexual identity that a person assumes and presents to other people. *See also* gender; sex change.

gene A hereditary unit consisting of a linear segment of deoxyribonucleic acid (DNA) forming part of a chromosome and determining a particular characteristic in an organism. *See also* chromosome; eugenics; gene therapy; genotype; heredity; oncogene; sociobiology.

gene, onco- *See* oncogene.

General Accounting Office, US *See* US General Accounting Office.

General Administrative Policies and Procedures (GAPP) A term used by the Joint Commission on Accreditation of Healthcare Organizations to describe its offer to provide an accreditation survey and an accreditation decision to a health care organization. Each accreditation manual published by the Joint Commission is introduced by a General Administrative Policies and Procedures section, which embodies a comprehensive program-specific description of the accreditation process and the terms and conditions for an entity's participation in it. *See also* accreditation; Joint Commission on Accreditation of Healthcare Organizations.

general anesthesia An agent, usually given by inhalation or intravenous injection, that produces unconsciousness and complete loss of sensation throughout the body. *See also* anesthesia; general anesthetic; local anesthesia; major surgery; regional anesthesia.

general anesthetic An anesthetic, such as

halothane, that produces general anesthesia. *See also* anesthetic; general anesthesia.

General Constituency Section for Small or Rural Hospitals (SSRH)　A section of the American Hospital Association founded in 1976 composed of 4,000 community hospitals that have fewer than 100 acute care beds, are located outside a standard metropolitan statistical area, or admit 4,000 or fewer patients per year. *See also* American Hospital Association; hospital.

general damages　The compensatory damages that one would reasonably expect to result from an act; for example, pain and suffering and disfigurement could all reasonably be expected to result from unnecessary surgery. General damages are distinguishable from consequential (special) damages, which do not necessarily result from such an act. *See also* consequential damages; damages.

general duty nurse　*See* staff nurse.

general exclusion　A provision in a health insurance contract or health service plan that stipulates a type of specific service that is not covered as a benefit. *See also* exclusions.

general fund　Unrestricted monies and other liquid assets that are available for an organization's general use. *See also* fund.

general hospital　A hospital whose primary functions are to provide diagnostic and therapeutic services to patients for short-term acute surgical and nonsurgical conditions. Some specialized treatment and some longer term chronic care may also be provided. *See also* hospital.

general internal medicine　*See* internal medicine.

General Internal Medicine, Society of　*See* Society of General Internal Medicine.

general liability insurance　Insurance covering the risk of loss for most accidents and injuries to third parties (the insured and its employees are not covered), which arise from the actions or negligence of the insured and for which the insured may have legal liability, except those injuries directly related to the provision of professional health services, which are usually separately covered by professional liability insurance. One situation in which general liability insurance would pay, for instance, is if a hospital visitor slips and falls on a wet floor. *Synonym:* liability insurance. *See also* insurance; liability.

generalist　One whose knowledge and skills are not restricted to a particular field. *Compare* specialist. *See also* dentist, generalist.

generalized lymphadenopathy, persistent　*See* persistent generalized lymphadenopathy.

generally accepted accounting principles (GAAP)　Conventions, rules, and procedures that define accepted accounting practice. Since the 1930s, the Securities and Exchange Commission has had the authority to establish accounting standards but has never done so. Instead, it has allowed the accounting profession to establish its own guidelines, first through the Committee on Accounting Principles (from 1939 to 1959), and later through the Accounting Principles Board (from 1959-1973), both belonging to the American Institute of Certified Public Accountants. In 1973, the Accounting Principles Board was superseded by the Financial Accounting Standards Board. *See also* accounting; American Institute of Certified Public Accountants; Financial Accounting Standards Board.

generally recognized as effective (GRAE)　A condition that a drug must fulfill if it is not to be considered a new drug and thus not be the subject of premarket approval requirements of the Federal Food, Drug, and Cosmetic Act. To qualify as GRAE, a drug must be so considered by experts qualified by scientific training and experience to evaluate the safety and effectiveness of drugs and must have been used to material extent or for a material time. *See also* generally recognized as safe; new drug.

generally recognized as safe (GRAS)　A condition that a drug must fulfill if it not to be considered a new drug, or a food must fulfill if it is not to be considered a food additive. A drug that is GRAS and GRAE (generally recognized as effective) does not require the premarket approval prescribed for new drugs in the Food, Drug, and Cosmetic Act. Safety is determined by experts qualified by scientific training and experience to evaluate the safety and effectiveness of drugs. *See also* generally recognized as effective; new drug.

general partner　A member of a partnership who has authority to make decisions binding on the partnership, shares in the profits, and has unlimited liability for losses. A partnership has at least one general partner and may have limited and other general partners. *See also* junior partner; limited partner; partner; partnership.

general practice　The provision of comprehensive medical care as a continuing responsibility regardless of age of the patient or of the condition that may temporarily require the services of a specialist. *See also* American College of Medicine; American Osteopathic Board of General Practice; general practitioner; practice.

General Practice, American Osteopathic Board of *See* American Osteopathic Board of General Practice.

general practitioner (GP) A physician whose practice is not oriented to a specific medical specialty but instead covers a variety of medical problems in patients of all ages. A general practitioner is not a specialist, as is, for example, a family physician or general surgeon. *Compare* family physician. *See also* practice; medical specialties.

General Practitioner, American Academy of Orthodontics for the *See* American Academy of Orthodontics for the General Practitioner.

General Practitioners in Osteopathic Medicine and Surgery, American College of *See* American College of General Practitioners in Osteopathic Medicine and Surgery.

general revenue Government revenues raised without regard to the specific purpose for which they might be used. For instance, federal general revenues come from personal and corporate income taxes and some excise taxes. The government cost of many health care programs, such as Medicaid, is financed from general revenues. *See also* revenue.

General Services Administration (GSA) The federal agency that manages the federal government's property and records, including the construction and operation of buildings; procurement and distribution of supplies; utilization and disposal of property; transportation, traffic, and communications management; stockpiling of strategic materials; and management of the governmentwide automatic data-processing resources program. *See also* Consumer Information Center.

general support grant A grant made to generally support an area of concern or interest to the grant-making organization. *Compare* project grant. *See also* grant.

general surgeon A physician who specializes in general surgery. *See also* general surgery; surgeon.

general surgery The branch of medicine and medical specialty dealing with the management of a broad spectrum of surgical conditions affecting almost any area of the body. Management includes diagnosis and provision of preoperative, operative,

and postoperative care to surgical patients. Surgery also involves management of trauma and critically ill patients. Four subspecialties of surgery are general vascular surgery, pediatric surgery, surgical critical care, and surgery of the hand. *See also* pediatric surgery; surgery; surgery of the hand; surgical critical care; vascular surgery.

general vascular surgeon *See* vascular surgeon.

general vascular surgery *See* vascular surgery.

generalist dentist *See* dentist, generalist.

generation **1.** All of the offspring that are at the same stage of descent from a common ancestor. **2.** A class of objects derived from a preceding class, as in a new generation of computers. **3.** The number of times a health care organization receives a type I recommendation from the Joint Commission on Accreditation of Healthcare Organizations within one accreditation cycle. *See also* first generation type I recommendation; Joint Commission on Accreditation of Healthcare Organizations; second generation type I recommendation; type I recommendation.

generation type I recommendation, first *See* first generation type I recommendation.

generation type I recommendation, second *See* second generation type I recommendation.

generic **1.** Relating to or descriptive of an entire group or class. **2.** Pertaining to the descriptive or nonproprietary (nontrade) name of a drug or other product; for example, diazepam is the generic name for *Valium*.

generic drug law Modern statutes enacted by many states that permit or require pharmacists in certain circumstances to substitute a drug with the same active ingredients and of the same generic type for the drug prescribed by the physician. *See also* generic; generic equivalents.

generic equivalents Drugs not protected by a trademark and sold under generic names with the same active chemical ingredients as those sold under proprietary brand names. Generic equivalents are not necessarily therapeutic equivalents. *Compare* brand name; chemical name. *See also* antisubstitution laws; generic name; therapeutic equivalents.

generic name The descriptive or nonproprietary (nontrade) name of a drug or other product; for example, acetaminophen is the generic name for *Tylenol*. Each drug is licensed under a generic name and also may be given a brand name by its manufacturer. *Compare* brand name; chemical name;

trademark. *See also* name.

Generic Pharmaceutical Industry Association (GPIA) A national organization founded in 1981 composed of 22 manufacturers, distributors, and retailers of generic drugs interested in increasing the availability of equivalent generic pharmaceuticals on the market. It promotes the recognition, acceptance, and use of generic prescription drug products. *See also* generic; generic equivalents.

generic screen *See* HCFA generic quality screens; screening.

gene splicing A method for recombining the chemical structures of a gene. *See also* gene; genetic engineering; recombinant DNA; transduction.

gene therapy The technique or process of introducing normal genes into cells in place of defective or missing ones in order to correct genetic disorders. For instance, if a patient's body does not produce needed enzymes, gene therapy would introduce healthy cells capable of producing the enzymes in the body of the patient. *See also* gene; therapy.

genetic Pertaining to a gene or heredity, or to origin, birth, or development. *See also* gene; genetics.

Genetic Association, American *See* American Genetic Association.

genetic code The sequence of nucleotides in the deoxyribonucleic acid (DNA) molecule of a chromosome that specifies the amino acid sequence in the synthesis of proteins. This code is the basis of heredity. *See also* chromosome; deoxyribonucleic acid; gene.

genetic counseling The process of determining the risk of a particular genetic disorder, such as sickle cell anemia, hemophilia, or Tay-Sachs disease occurring within a family, and providing information and advice to parents based on that determination. *See also* counseling; genetic counselor.

genetic counselor A person qualified by training to advise patients about the origin, transmission, and development of genetic disorders. *See also* genetic disease.

Genetic Counselors, National Society of *See* National Society of Genetic Counselors.

genetic disease A disease or abnormality that results from inherited factors; for example, sickle cell disease and hemophilia. *See also* disease; genetics.

genetic engineering Techniques by which genetic material is deliberately altered by recombinant DNA so as to change or improve the hereditary properties of microorganisms, plants, and animals. *Synonym:* recombinant DNA technology. *See also* *Escherichia coli;* gene splicing; plasmid; recombinant DNA; therapeutic genetics; transduction.

genetic father *See* genetic parent.

genetic fingerprinting The analysis of genetic information from a blood sample, semen sample, or other small piece of human material as an aid to the identification of a person. It has revolutionized the forensic sciences. *Synonym:* DNA fingerprinting. *See also* forensic sciences.

genetic mapping The process of assigning individual genes to particular chromosomes and to particular chromosomal locations. *See also* chromosome; gene.

genetic mother *See* genetic parent.

genetic parent A parent who furnishes the sperm (the genetic father) or the ovum (the genetic mother) to an embryo. *See also* gestational parent; noncoital reproduction; parent; rearing parent.

genetics The science of biological variation. *See also* biology; clinical genetics; human genetics; medical genetics; molecular genetics.

Genetics, American Board of Medical *See* American Board of Medical Genetics.

Genetics, American Society of Human *See* American Society of Human Genetics.

Genetics Association, Behavior *See* Behavior Genetics Association.

genetics, clinical *See* clinical genetics.

genetics, clinical biochemical *See* clinical biochemical genetics.

genetics, clinical cyto- *See* clinical cytogenetics.

genetics, clinical molecular *See* clinical molecular genetics.

Genetics, Council for Responsible *See* Council for Responsible Genetics.

genetic screening The process of testing and analyzing a defined population of people to detect the presence of or susceptibility to a particular disease or diseases; for example, screening for sickle cell disease among high-risk groups. *See also* genetic counseling; screening.

genetics, human *See* human genetics.

genetics, immuno- *See* immunogenetics.

genetics, medical *See* medical genetics.

genetics, molecular *See* molecular genetics.

Genetics Society of America (GSA) A national organization founded in 1931 composed of 3,700 individuals and organizations interested in the field of genetics. It provides facilities for associations and conferences of students in the field of genetics. *See also* genetics.

Genetic Society, Birth Defect and Clinical *See* Birth Defect and Clinical Genetic Society.

genetics, therapeutic *See* therapeutic genetics.

Genetic Support Groups, Alliance of *See* Alliance of Genetic Support Groups.

genital herpes *See* herpes simplex.

genitalia The organs of reproduction. *See also* exhibitionism; organ; ovary; penis; reproduction; testis.

Genito-Urinary Surgeons, American Association of *See* American Association of Genito-Urinary Surgeons.

genome The totality of the genes in a complete haploid set of chromosomes. *See also* chromosome; gene.

genotype The genetic makeup of an individual organism. *Compare* phenotype. *See also* artificial selection; gene; identical twins; selection.

genu valgum *See* knock-knee.

geochemistry The chemistry of the composition and alterations of the solid matter of the earth or a celestial body. *See also* chemistry.

Geochemistry and Health, Society for Environmental *See* Society for Environmental Geochemistry and Health.

geometrically In mathematics, the rate of change in which each number in a progression of numbers is multiplied by a constant. For instance, a geometrical progression beginning with 6 and with a constant of 2 would be 6, 12, 24. *Compare* arithmetically; exponentially. *See also* linear; logarithmic.

geometric mean A mean calculated by taking the nth root of n values in a sample multiplied together. The geometric mean is used most often in change and index calculations, such as the change in costs of health services in a geographic area from one year to the next. *See also* mean.

geriatric Pertaining to elderly people. *See also* geriatric care worker; geriatric medicine.

Geriatric Care Managers, National Association of Private *See* National Association of Private Geriatric Care Managers.

geriatric care worker An individual trained in meeting the physical and social needs of elderly patients, primarily in an institutional setting.

Geriatric Dentistry, American Society for *See* American Society for Geriatric Dentistry.

geriatrician An internist, family physician, or other physician who specializes in the health, care, social welfare, and diseases (such as incontinence, falls, Parkinson's disease, and Alzheimer's disease) of elderly people. *See also* geriatric medicine.

geriatric medicine The branch of medicine and subspecialty of family practice and internal medicine dealing with the prevention, diagnosis, treatment, and rehabilitation of disorders common to elderly people. *Synonym*: geriatrics. *See also* family practice; gerontology; internal medicine; medicine; osteoporosis.

geriatric nurse A registered nurse qualified by education and training to provide nursing care to the elderly. *See also* registered nurse.

geriatric psychiatrist A psychiatrist who subspecializes in geriatric psychiatry. *See also* geriatric psychiatry.

geriatric psychiatry The branch and subspecialty of psychiatry dealing with the diagnosis and treatment of mental, addictive, and emotional disorders of the elderly. *See also* psychiatry.

Geriatric Psychiatry, American Association for *See* American Association for Geriatric Psychiatry.

geriatrics *See* geriatric medicine.

geriatrics, dental *See* dental geriatrics.

Geriatrics Society, American *See* American Geriatrics Society.

Geriatrics Society, National *See* National Geriatrics Society.

germ **1.** A small mass of living substance that can develop into an animal or a plant, usually referring to a microorganism that can cause disease, such as a bacterium or a virus. *See also* bacterium/bacteria; virus. **2.** Any primary source from which growth and development can occur, as in the germ of an idea.

German measles *See* rubella.

gerodentistry *See* gerodontics.

gerodontics An area of dentistry dealing with research, diagnosis, and treatment of dental diseases of the elderly. *Synonym*: gerodentistry. *See also* dental geriatrics.

Gerontological Society of America (GSA) A national organization founded in 1945 composed of 7,000 physicians, physiologists, psychologists, anatomists, biochemists, economists, sociologists, social workers, botanists, pharmacologists, nurses, and other individuals interested in improving the well-being of elderly people by promoting scientific study of the aging process, publishing information for professionals about aging and bringing together groups interested in research on aging. It sponsors fellowship programs in applied gerontology. *See also* fellowship; gerontology.

gerontology The branch of science dealing with the nature of the aging process and old age. *See also* geriatric medicine.

Gerontology, The Center for Social *See* The Center for Social Gerontology.

gerontophobia 1. A morbid dislike of old people. 2. A dread of growing old. *See also* phobia.

gestalt A physical, psychological, or symbolic configuration or pattern of elements so unified as a whole that its properties cannot be derived from a simple summation of its parts. *Synonym:* pattern. *See also* gestaltism.

gestaltism A school of psychology that maintains that building up images by piece-by-piece association is not the only basis of perceptual processes, but that patterns, configurations, and forms ("gestalt" is the German word for "form") can be recognized as integrated entities on the basis of previous experience. For example, in the trick drawing that can be recognized either as a vase or as two separate human profiles, which image is immediately perceived is determined by such experience. *Synonym:* gestalt psychology. *See also* gestalt; gestalt therapy.

gestaltist A person who adheres to or practices the principles of gestalt psychology. *See also* gestaltism.

gestalt psychology *See* gestaltism.

gestalt therapy A form of psychotherapy that emphasizes treating a person as an integrated whole by focusing on perceptual structures and patterns and interrelationships with other people and the environment. *See also* gestaltism; psychotherapy.

gestation 1. The period of development of the fertilized ovum in the uterus from conception to birth. *See also* pregnancy. 2. The conception and development of an idea or plan in the mind.

gestational diabetes Diabetes mellitus that appears during some pregnancies, triggered by the increase in hormones during pregnancy, which partially blocks the action of insulin. *See also* diabetes mellitus; insulin; pregnancy.

gestational mother *See* gestational parent.

gestational parent The woman who bears a child.

The gestational mother may also be the genetic mother, the rearing mother, or neither. *See also* genetic parent; noncoital reproduction; parent; rearing parent.

GHAA *See* Group Health Association of America.

G. Harold and Leila Y. Mathers Charitable Foundation A private foundation established in 1975 that focuses its giving in the field of medical research performed at various hospitals, medical research institutes, and universities throughout the United States. *See also* foundation; private foundation.

GI *See* gastrointestinal.

giant In medicine, an adult taller than 80 inches (6 feet, 8 inches), or a child who exceeds the mean height for his or her age by three standard deviations. Such individuals either represent the extreme end of the normal distribution curve or suffer from an endocrine abnormality, usually pituitary gigantism. *Compare* dwarf; midget. *See also* growth hormone; height; pituitary gland.

gigantism Height of more than 6 feet, 8 inches in an adult. *Compare* dwarf; midget. *See also* giant; growth hormone; height.

gigabyte In computer science, storage of one billion bits in a computer. *See also* bit; byte; megabyte.

GIGO Acronym in computer science meaning "garbage in, garbage out," that is, the integrity and quality of output is dependent on the integrity and quality of the input. *See also* input; output.

GIMS *See* Graduates of Italian Medical Schools.

gingiva The mucous membrane and fibrous tissue encircling the neck of each tooth. *Synonym:* gums. *See also* gingivitis; periodontics.

gingivitis Inflammation of the gums (gingiva). *See also* inflammation.

GIPS *See* Gastrointestinal Pathology Society.

GI series Abbreviation for gastrointestinal series, a sequence of diagnostic imaging tests of the gastrointestinal tract, especially the stomach and intestines. *See also* barium enema; gastrointestinal; intestine; series; stomach.

G-Jo *See* acupressure.

gland Any specialized structure that produces and secretes or excretes chemical substances, whose action or function takes place elsewhere than in the gland itself. The primary classification of glands is into exocrine and endocrine. *See also* endocrine; exocrine; mammary gland; pancreas; pituitary gland; salivary glands; sebaceous gland; thyroid gland.

gland, mammary   *See* mammary gland.

gland, pituitary   *See* pituitary gland.

gland, sebaceous   *See* sebaceous gland.

glands, salivary   *See* salivary glands.

gland, thyroid   *See* thyroid gland.

glasses   *See* spectacles.

glaucoma   A disease of the eye in which elevated eye pressure, due to obstruction of the outflow of aqueous humor (the watery fluid surrounding the eye's lens), damages the optic nerve and causes visual defects. *See also* ophthalmology.

Glasgow coma scale (GCS)   In trauma care, a scoring instrument used to quantify depth and duration of impaired consciousness based on a patient's eye opening, verbal performance, and motor responsiveness. The GCS was developed to allow for reliable assessment and recording of changing states of altered neurological status over time. The 15-point scale demonstrates better neurological function with higher numbers. It has limited utility in estimating prognosis or outcome. *See also* coma; consciousness; scale; score; Trauma Score.

global budget   In health care, a nationwide limit or cap on categories of private and public health care spending. *See also* budget; top-down global budgeting.

global budgeting, top-down   *See* top-down global budgeting.

globus hystericus   A feeling of a lump in the throat that cannot be swallowed, often accompanying anxiety or an emotional experience. *See also* anxiety.

glomerulonephritis   Inflammation of the glomerulus, the tuft of blood capillaries in the kidneys. *See also* kidney.

glottis   The opening of the larynx, comprising the vocal cords and the space between them. *See also* larynx.

glucagon   A hormone stored and released by the pancreas, that raises the blood sugar by stimulating the breakdown of glycogen in the liver. Its action opposes the action of insulin. *See also* glycogen; insulin; pancreas.

glucose   A monosaccharide (simple sugar) that the body uses directly for energy. It is the major energy source in the body and is monitored in the blood in many disorders, including diabetes mellitus. *Synonym*: sugar. *See also* blood glucose; diabetes mellitus; glycogen; glycosuria; hyperglycemia; hypoglycemia.

glucose, blood   *See* blood glucose.

glue sniffing   A practice most common among adolescents in which a solvent, such as toluene, is squeezed onto a piece of cloth and its vapors are inhaled from a plastic bag. The intoxication is similar to intoxication with alcohol, causing excitement and uninhibited and aggressive behavior. *See also* addiction.

gluten   A protein that makes up 8% to 15% of wheat flour. Gluten is important in the pathogenesis of celiac disease and nontropical sprue (a chronic disease affecting food absorption that causes anemia and gastrointestinal disorders). *See also* celiac disease; gastroenterology.

glycogen   Large chains of glucose molecules that are stored in the liver and muscles for future energy use, when they will be converted back to glucose for the body's direct energy needs. *See also* glucose; glycogen.

glycosuria   Sugar (glucose) in the urine; a major sign of diabetes mellitus. *See also* diabetes mellitus; glucose.

GME   *See* graduate medical education.

GMHC   *See* Gay Men's Health Crisis.

GMP   Acronym for good manufacturing practice, the medical-device-manufacturing industry's version of total quality management. *See also* medical device; total quality management.

gnathic   Of or relating to the jaw, as in gnathologic orthopedics.

Gnathologic Orthopedics, American Academy of   *See* American Academy of Gnathologic Orthopedics.

GND   *See* gross national debt.

gnotobiotics   The study of germ-free animals and the techniques involved in rearing laboratory animals entirely free from microorganisms or whose microflora can be precisely specified. *See also* animal experimentation; microorganism.

Gnotobiotics, Association for   *See* Association for Gnotobiotics.

GNP   *See* gross national product.

goal   A statement of a desired future state, condition, or purpose; for example, a health care organization's goal might be a postsurgical-wound-infection rate of zero. A goal differs from an objective by having a broader (if any) deadline, and usually by being long range (more than a year) rather than short range (within a year or less). *See also* management; mission statement; objective; target.

GOG   *See* Gynecologic Oncology Group.

goiter Enlargement of the thyroid gland located at the front of the neck. Goiter may be caused by dietary iodine deficiency, tumor, or overactivity (hyperthyroidism) or underactivity (hypothyroidism) of the thyroid gland. Treatment is based on the cause and often involves removal of all or part of the gland. *See also* hyperthyroidism; hypothyroidism; thyroid gland.

golden handcuffs Benefits provided by an employer to make it difficult or unattractive for the employee to leave and work elsewhere. *See also* benefits.

golden hour In trauma care, the concept that mortality rates are lowest when trauma victims are provided with definitive care within one hour after injury. *See also* advanced trauma life support; basic trauma life support; trauma; traumatology.

golden parachute An employment agreement that guarantees an upper-level executive a lucrative severance benefit when and if control of a company is transferred to another organization, or when a company desires to replace an executive with another person.

Gold Foil Operators, American Academy of *See* American Academy of Gold Foil Operators.

Gold Institute, Dental *See* Dental Gold Institute.

gold standard A method, procedure, or measurement that is widely accepted as being the best available. It provides a reference point against which the performance of other methods, procedures, or measurements can be measured. Originally, gold standard was the monetary system under which units of currency were converted into fixed amounts of gold. Such a system is said to be anti-inflationary. The United States was taken off the gold standard in 1933. *See also* benchmark; criterion standard; standard.

gonadotropin Any hormone that stimulates the gonads to produce the male and female sex hormones. *See also* gonads; hormone; human chorionic gonoadotrophin; sex hormone.

gonadotropin, human chorionic *See* human chorionic gonadotropin.

gonads Gamete-producing organs. In humans, they are the ovaries (female) and testes (male), producing respectively ova (eggs) and spermatozoa (sperm). *See also* ovum; spermatozoa.

gonorrhea A common venereal disease caused by the bacterium *Neisseria gonorrheae* and transmitted through contact with an infected person or with secretions containing the bacteria. *Synonym:* clap. *See also* bacteria; pelvic inflammatory disease; sexually-transmitted disease; venereology.

good faith **1.** Compliance with standards of decency and honesty. *See also* faith. **2.** In law, the total absence of intention to seek unfair advantage of or to defraud another party and the honest intention to fulfill one's obligations. *Compare* defraud.

goodness-of-fit test A statistical procedure, such as the chi-square test, that tests the hypothesis that a particular probability distribution fits an observed set of data. *See also* chi-square test; hypothesis; test.

goods Material items that are the product of any economy, as in a color television set or a piece of x-ray equipment. *See also* economy; product; service.

Good Samaritan A compassionate person who unselfishly helps other people. *See also* Good Samaritan laws.

Good Samaritan laws Statutes in all states that, although varied in their detail, generally provide some form of immunity to those who, without a duty to act, nevertheless render aid in an emergency. *See also* Good Samaritan; immunity.

googol **1.** The number 10 raised to the 100th power. It is written out as a number 1 followed by 100 zeros. The term was coined at the age of nine years by Milton Sirotta, nephew of the American mathematician Edward Kasner (1878-1955). **2.** Any very large number. *See also* number.

goods *See* product.

goose bumps A condition in which the hairs on the skin stand straight up, often as a response to cold, fright, or stress. *Synonym:* gooseflesh.

gooseflesh *See* goose bumps.

gout A disorder producing excessive uric acid, some of which forms as crystals around joints, causing pain and inflammation. *Synonym:* podagra. *See also* joint; rheumatology.

govern **1.** To exercise political authority. **2.** To have or exercise a determining influence.

governance **1.** The process, act, or power of governing. *See also* self-governance. **2.** Government. *See also* govern; government.

governance, self- *See* self-governance.

governing board *See* governing body.

governing body (GB) In health care, the individual(s), group, or agency having ultimate authority and responsibility for establishing policy, maintaining patient care quality, and providing for organizational management and planning. The governing body represents the community and is the policy-making body of the institution. *Synonyms:* administrative board; board; board of commissioners; board of directors; board of governors; board of trustees; governing board; partners. *See also* chief executive officer; outside director; trustee.

governing body bylaws   Rules that establish the roles and responsibilities of the governing body. *See also* bylaws; governing body.

governing instrument   A document describing the structure and processes that govern an organization's actions. The Internal Revenue Service identifies two types of governing instruments: creating documents, such as articles of organization, and operating documents, such as bylaws. *See also* articles of organization; bylaws.

government   The exercise of authority in the administration of the affairs of a state, community, or society. In the United States, the federal and state governments operate under a written constitution from which their sovereignty and authority emanate. *See also* politics.

governmental function   An activity performed for the general public good, such as operating a police department or conducting safety inspections. When a jurisdiction engages in a governmental function, the jurisdiction is generally immune from tort liability for its actions unless a lawsuit is specifically permitted by statute. *See also* function; government; sovereign immunity.

government hospital   A hospital that is owned by either the local, state, or federal government. *See also* federal government hospital; hospital; nonfederal government hospital.

government hospital, federal   *See* federal government hospital.

government hospital, nonfederal   *See* nonfederal government hospital.

Governmental Industrial Hygienists, American Conference of   *See* American Conference of Governmental Industrial Hygienists.

government relations unit   A body, such as a standing committee, often found in health care organizations. A government relations unit collects, analyzes, and maintains current information about proposed legislation that may affect the organization and recommends legislative policy positions. *See also* unit.

GP   *See* general practitioner.

GPIA   *See* Generic Pharmaceutical Industry Association.

GPWW   *See* group practice without walls.

graduate   An individual who has attained a given academic degree, such as a medical school or nursing school graduate, or has been certified as completing an education program not leading to a degree. *See also* certification; diplomate; foreign medical graduate; graduate medical education; United States medical graduate.

Graduate Examination Committee, Foreign Pharmacy   *See* Foreign Pharmacy Graduate Examination Committee.

graduate medical education (GME)   Medical education after receipt of the Doctor of Medicine (MD) or equivalent degree, including the education received as an intern, resident, or fellow, and continuing medical education. *See also* continuing education; continuing medical education; fellow; fifth pathway; intern; medical education; resident; undergraduate medical education.

Graduate Medical Education, Accreditation Council for   *See* Accreditation Council for Graduate Medical Education.

Graduate Medical Education, Liaison Committee on   *See* Liaison Committee on Graduate Medical Education.

Graduates, Educational Commission for Foreign Medical   *See* Educational Commission for Foreign Medical Graduates.

Graduates of Italian Medical Schools (GIMS)   A national organization founded in 1966 composed of 500 physicians of any national origin who graduated from schools in Italy. It maintains a placement service and charitable program. *See also* medical school.

graduate training   *See* graduate medical education.

graduate, United States medical   *See* United States medical graduate.

graduate year one   *See* PGY-1.

GRAE   *See* generally recognized as effective.

graft   *See* transplant.

graft, skin   *See* skin graft.

Gramm-Rudman-Hollings amendment   Federal legislation passed in 1986 that sets budget deficit goals and mandates reductions in federal expenditures if Congress does not meet the annual goals. *See also* budget; deficit; federal deficit.

gram-negative bacteria   *See* Gram's stain.

gram-positive bacteria *See* Gram's stain.

Gram's stain An empirical method of identifying and classifying bacteria according to color. They turn red or blue when a stain is applied to them. Red-staining or pink-staining bacteria are gram-negative bacteria; violet-staining or blue-staining bacteria are gram-positive bacteria. The method was described by the Danish physician, Hans Christian Joachim Gram (1853-1938). *See also* bacteria; empirical; microbiology; stain.

grandfather clause A provision of policy or law that allows persons, engaged in a certain business before the passage of an act regulating that business, to receive a license or prerogative without meeting all the criteria that new entrants into the field would have to fulfill. For example, the Food, Drug, and Cosmetic Act exempts certain drugs from its pre-market approval requirements on the basis of their long use. Or, a medical specialty board establishes new and higher standards required for board certification, such as the requirement for completing an accredited residency program in the specialty. The specialty board might exempt for a period of years a category of physicians who did not meet the requirement, such as those individuals completing a residency program in another specialty. The statement of exemption would be a grandfather clause. *See also* board certified; license.

grand jury A body of persons summoned and sworn to determine whether the facts and accusations presented by the prosecutor warrant an indictment and eventual trial of the accused. It is called "grand" because of the relatively large number of jurors impaneled (traditionally 23 members), as compared with a petit jury. *Compare* petit jury. *See also* impanel; indictment; jury; trial.

grand rounds A weekly meeting held in medical schools and teaching and other hospitals in which one or more important medical cases and relevant educational material are presented to health professionals, especially the members of the medical staff, as a learning experience. *See also* medical staff; morbidity and mortality conference; physician; rounds.

grant A financial award, gift, or bestowal made by a foundation, governmental agency, or other organization to support a project, program, individual, or organization. *See also* capitation grant; foundation; general support grant; grant proposal; matching grant; project grant.

grant, capitation *See* capitation grant.

grantee A recipient of grant funds. *See also* grant.

grant, general support *See* general support grant.

grant, matching *See* matching grant.

grant, project *See* project grant.

grant proposal A written document submitted to a foundation or government agency requesting grant funds. *Synonym:* grant request. *See also* foundation; grant.

grant request *See* grant proposal.

grantsmanship The art of writing successful grant proposals. *See also* grant; grant proposal.

granulocyte *See* white blood cell.

grapevine Unofficial path of verbal communication. Rumors or "scuttlebutt" are spread from person to person through an informal information network.

graph A visual display of the relationship between variables. The values of one set of variables are plotted along the horizontal, or x, axis and the values of a second variable, along the vertical, or y, axis. Typical relationships between x and y are linear, exponential, or logarithmic. *See also* axis; bar graph; chart; exponentially; linear; line graph; logarithmic; plot; table; variable.

graph, bar *See* bar graph.

graph, grouped bar *See* grouped bar graph.

graph, line *See* line graph.

graph, stacked bar *See* stacked bar graph.

GRAS *See* generally recognized as safe.

gratis Free, as in medical care provided gratis to patients who cannot afford to pay.

gratuitous Unasked for item or service voluntarily given without expectation of reward or consideration.

grave robber A person who plunders valuables from tombs or graves or who steal corpses after burial, as for illicit dissection. *See also* corpse; dissect.

Graves' disease A condition in which the thyroid becomes hyperactive, causing increased metabolism. *See also* disease; thyroid gland.

graveyard shift Work shift in the middle of the night, for example, from 11 PM to 7 AM.

gravidity The number of pregnancies, completed or incomplete, experienced by a woman. *See also* pregnancy.

Gravitational Strain Pathology, Institute for *See* Institute for Gravitational Strain Pathology.

Great Depression The period from the end of 1929 until the onset of World War II, during which economic activity slowed and unemployment was very high. *See also* economy; New Deal.

Great Society A set of economic and social programs advocated by President Lyndon Johnson, with the objectives of eradicating poverty, increasing employment, improving environmental and urban conditions, and fostering rapid economic growth.

Green Book *See Directory of Residency Training Programs.*

grid *See* accreditation decision grid.

grid element *See* accreditation decision grid.

grid element score *See* accreditation decision grid.

gridlock A complete lack of movement or progress resulting in a backup or stagnation, as in political gridlock in Washington, DC.

grid score *See* accreditation decision grid.

grieve *See* mourn.

gross anatomy The study of the organs or parts of the body large enough to seen with the unaided eye (that is, without the aid of a microscope). *Synonym:* macroscopic anatomy. *Compare* microscopic anatomy. *See also* anatomy.

gross autopsy rate *See* autopsy rate.

gross and flagrant violation In health care, a violation that presents an imminent danger to the health, safety, or well-being of a Medicare beneficiary or that unnecessarily places the beneficiary at risk of substantial and permanent harm. Utilization and quality control peer review organizations (PROs) identify potential violations and recommend sanctions, but the Office of the Inspector General of the US Department of Health and Human Services makes the final decision as to whether to impose sanctions. *Compare* substantial violation. *See also* peer review organization.

gross national debt (GND) The total amount of debt in existence within an economy, both public and private. *See also* national debt.

gross national product (GNP) The total monetary measure of a nation's annual production of goods and services during one year. Economists consider the GNP to be one of the most important concepts in economic science, and the United States and other nations expend considerable effort collecting, analyzing, and publishing GNP statistics. *See also* economic growth; no-growth; recession.

gross negligence In health care, the failure to use even slight care in the provision of health services or of an expected duty. In the law of torts, the degrees of negligence are, in general, slight negligence,

which is failure to use great care; ordinary negligence, which is failure to use ordinary care; and gross negligence. Gross negligence occurs when an individual knows the harmful consequences of his or her actions and is indifferent to these consequences. *See also* negligence.

ground ambulance *See* ambulance.

group An assemblage of persons or objects gathered or located together, as in pressure group.

Group Administrators, American College of Medical *See* American College of Medical Group Administrators.

Group for the Advancement of Psychiatry (GAP) A national organization founded in 1946 composed of 300 psychiatrists organized in working committees interested in applying the principles of psychiatry toward the study of human relations. It investigates topics, such as school desegregation, use of nuclear energy, religion, psychiatry in the armed forces, mental retardation, and medical uses of hypnosis. *See also* psychiatry.

group contract An insurance contract made with an employer or other entity that covers a group of persons identified by their employment, dependent relationship to employees, or by some other relationship to the contracting entity. *See also* contract; group.

group dynamics The forces and characteristics of a group's interaction process through which creative contributions occur. *See also* group.

grouped bar graph A bar graph in which the bars are classified by two variables. One variable classifies the groups and the other variable defines the bars within each of the groups. *See also* bar graph; variable.

GROUPER software Computer software used by Medicare fiscal intermediaries or other third-party payers to assign patient discharges to the appropriate diagnosis-related groups (DRGs) using the following information abstracted from the inpatient financial bill: patient's age, sex, and principal diagnosis; principal procedures performed; and discharge status. The GROUPER uses the Uniform Hospital Discharge Data Set (UHDDS), with up to five diagnoses and four procedures coded by the *International Classification of Diseases, Ninth Revision, Clinical Modification. See also* diagnosis-related groups; fiscal intermediary; Uniform Hospital Discharge Data Set.

Group Health Association of America (GHAA) An association founded in 1959 composed of 1,000 group practice prepayment health plans and related organizations that support health maintenance organizations. It was formed by the merger of American Labor Health Association and Group Health Federation of America. *See also* group practice; health maintenance organization.

group health plan According to the Health Security Act recently (1993) introduced to Congress, an employee welfare benefit plan (as defined in the Employee Retirement Income Security Act of 1974) providing medical care to participants or beneficiaries directly or through insurance, reimbursement, or otherwise. *See also* Employee Retirement Income Security Act; health plan; Health Security Act.

group insurance Any insurance plan, such as health insurance, that covers individuals by means of a single-group agreement, contract, or policy issued to an employer or association with which the insured individuals are affiliated. Group insurance is usually much lower in cost than comparable individual insurance. Group insurance is usually experience rated. *See also* experience rating; insurance.

Group Management Association, Dental *See* Dental Group Management Association.

Group Management Association, Medical *See* Medical Group Management Association.

group medicine *See* group practice.

group model HMO A health maintenance organization (HMO) that predominantly contracts with one independent group practice to provide health services, usually in HMO-owned or HMO-managed facilities. *See also* health maintenance organization.

group, multispecialty *See* multispecialty group.

group practice A formal association of three or more physicians, dentists, podiatrists, or other health professionals providing services, with income from the medical practice pooled and redistributed to the members of the group according to a prearranged plan. *Synonym*: group medicine. *See also* closed panel group practice; group practice without walls; multispecialty group; open panel group practice; practice; prepaid group practice.

Group Practice, American Academy of Dental *See* American Academy of Dental Group Practice.

Group Practice Association, American *See* American Group Practice Association.

group practice, closed panel *See* closed panel group practice.

group practice, multispecialty *See* multispecialty group practice.

group practice, open panel *See* open panel group practice.

group practice, prepaid *See* prepaid group practice.

group practice, single specialty *See* single specialty group practice.

group practice without walls (GPWW) A network of physicians who have merged into one legal entity but maintain individual practice locations. The assets of the individual practices have been acquired by a larger group, but some autonomy is retained at each site. The central management owns both the facility and the equipment and provides administrative services. Links to hospitals vary widely. *Synonym*: group without walls. *See also* group practice; integrated provider; management services organization; physician hospital organization.

group, pressure *See* pressure group.

group psychotherapy *See* group therapy.

Group Psychotherapy, American Board of Examiners of Psychodrama, Sociometry, and *See* American Board of Examiners of Psychodrama, Sociometry, and Group Psychotherapy.

Group Psychotherapy Association, American *See* American Group Psychotherapy Association.

Group Psychotherapy and Psychodrama, American Society of *See* American Society of Group Psychotherapy and Psychodrama.

group, public interest *See* public interest group.

group purchasing In health care, a shared service combining the purchasing power of individual hospitals in order to obtain lower prices for equipment, supplies, and services. *See also* purchasing department.

group, special interest *See* special interest.

group, splinter *See* splinter group.

group, sub- *See* subgroup.

group, support *See* support group.

group therapy A form of psychotherapy involving approximately six to eight people and a therapist; the interactions of the group members are considered an important part of the therapy. *Synonym*: group psychotherapy. *See also* psychotherapy.

group think The psychological pressure for consensus at any cost, which tends to suppress both dissent and the appraisal of alternatives in decision-making groups. Group think connotes deterioration of mental efficiency and moral judgment due to in-group pressures.

group without walls *See* group practice without walls.

group worker, social *See* social group worker.

growth hormone A hormone synthesized and released by the pituitary gland that stimulates the growth of long bones in the limbs and increases protein synthesis and the use of fats for energy. Excessive production results in gigantism or acromegaly, enlargement of the bones of the head, feet, and hands. Deficient production results in dwarfism. *See also* giant; gigantism; hormone; pituitary gland; recombinant DNA.

Growth Society, Bioelectrical Repair and *See* Bioelectrical Repair and Growth Society.

GSA *See* General Services Administration; Genetics Society of America; Gerontological Society of America.

guardian In law, a person appointed by a court to administer the personal affairs or property of an individual who is not capable of such duties; for example, a guardian for an elderly person or a dependent child. A guardian may be a parent, trustee, committee, conservator, or other person empowered by law to act as a guardian. *Synonym:* legal guardian. *See also* ad litem.

guardian ad litem An individual charged by a court with the authority and duty to represent the interests of a minor or an incompetent adult in a legal action. *See* ad litem.

guard, security *See* security guard.

guide A manual or other model outlining policies or procedures used to instruct a sequence of actions.

Guide to the Health Care Field, AHA *See* AHA *Guide to the Health Care Field.*

guideline A statement or other indication of policy or procedure by which to determine a course of action. *See also* practice guideline; scoring guideline.

guideline, practice *See* practice guideline.

guideline, scoring *See* scoring guideline.

guidelines, health planning *See* health planning guidelines.

Guild of Hypnotherapists, American *See* American Guild of Hypnotherapists.

Guild of the United States, National Catholic Pharmacists *See* National Catholic Pharmacists Guild of the United States.

gums *See* gingiva.

gun-control law A law restricting or regulating the sale, purchase, or possession of firearms or establishing a system of licensing, registration, or identification of firearms or their owners or users. *See also* law; trauma; traumatology.

gurney A wheeled cot used for moving patients. *See also* cart; litter; patient; stretcher.

Gynecological Laparoscopists, American Association of *See* American Association of Gynecological Laparoscopists.

Gynecological and Obstetrical Society, American *See* American Gynecological and Obstetrical Society.

Gynecologic Investigation, Society for *See* Society for Gynecologic Investigation.

gynecologic nurse practitioner, obstetric- *See* obstetric-gynecologic nurse practitioner.

gynecologic oncologist A gynecologist who subspecializes in gynecologic oncology. *See* gynecologic oncology.

Gynecologic Oncologists, Society of *See* Society of Gynecologic Oncologists.

gynecologic oncology The branch of medicine and subspecialty of obstetrics and gynecology dealing with the health care of women with gynecologic cancer; for example, ovarian or vulvar cancer. *See also* gynecology; oncology.

Gynecologic Oncology Group (GOG) A national organization founded in 1970 composed of 39 institutions and teaching hospitals conducting research in gynecological oncology. *See also* gynecologic oncology.

gynecologist A physician who specializes in gynecology. *See* gynecology.

gynecologist, obstetrician- *See* obstetrician-gynecologist.

Gynecologists, American College of Obstetricians and *See* American College of Obstetricians and Gynecologists.

Gynecologists, American College of Osteopathic Obstetricians and *See* American College of Osteopathic Obstetricians and Gynecologists.

gynecology The branch of medicine and specialty dealing with the health care of women, including the function and diseases of the female genital tract. It encompasses both medical and surgical concerns and is usually practiced in combination with obstetrics. *See also* hysterectomy; obstetrics and gynecology; oophorectomy; Pap smear.

Gynecology, American Board of Obstetrics and *See* American Board of Obstetrics and Gynecology.

Gynecology, Council on Resident Education in Obstetrics and *See* Council on Resident Education in Obstetrics and Gynecology.

gynecology, obstetrics and *See* obstetrics and gynecology.

Gynecology and Obstetrics, Association of Professors of *See* Association of Professors of Gynecology and Obstetrics.

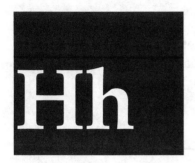

Hh

HA *See* Health Academy.

HAA *See* Hospice Association of America.

habeus corpus The procedure to challenge the legality of detention or custody.

habilitation Medical, educational, and other measures undertaken for individuals born with limited functional abilities. Rehabilitation, by contrast, refers to similar measures for individuals who have lost abilities because of injury or disease. *See also* rehabilitation; vocational habilitation.

habilitation, re- *See* rehabilitation.

habilitation, vocational *See* vocational habilitation.

habit Automatic response or pattern of behavior learned by frequent repetition. *See also* addiction.

habitual abortion Repeated spontaneous expulsion of the products of conception in three or more pregnancies, often for no known cause. *See also* abortion; spontaneous abortion.

habitus **1.** The general physical build of a person, as in a tall and slender habitus. *See also* physique. **2.** Constitution, especially as related to predisposition to disease.

HAI *See* Hospital Audiences.

hair Slender filaments of dense keratin made up of cornefied epidermal cells enclosing a variable amount of pigment. Each filament arises from a depression known as a hair follicle and is associated with a sebaceous gland. Body hair distribution is largely controlled by the sex hormones and can have diagnostic significance in endocrine disorders. *See also* hirsutism; sebaceous gland; skin; trichology.

Hair Loss Council, American *See* American Hair Loss Council.

Haitian Coalition on AIDS (HCA) A national organization founded in 1983 composed of 70 community centers; professional groups of physicians, jour-

nalists, lawyers, nurses, and social workers; and civil rights and media representatives. Its purpose is to educate the public concerning what the coalition believes is the discriminatory classification of Haitians as an ethnic group that runs a high risk of contracting acquired immunodeficiency syndrome (AIDS). *See also* acquired immunodeficiency syndrome; discrimination.

Haitian Physicians Abroad, Association of *See* Association of Haitian Physicians Abroad.

half-life A measure of the rate of exponential decay of the radioactivity of a radioisotope (radioactive isotope). It is the time taken for the activity to be reduced by one half, that is, for one half of the atoms present to disintegrate. Half-lives of differing isotopes vary between less than a millionth of a second to more than a million years. *See also* biological half-life; radioisotope.

half-life, biological *See* biological half-life.

halfway house A residence that uses community resources to assist persons who have left highly structured institutions for treatment of mental illness or substance abuse, to adjust and reenter society. The facility emphasizes emotional growth through confrontation and support. *Synonym:* community living facility. *See also* residential community-based care.

Halfway House Alcoholism Programs of North America, Association of *See* Association of Halfway House Alcoholism Programs of North America.

hallucination A false visual, auditory, olfactory, gustatory, or tactile perception. Hallucinations are a symptom of severe mental illness, such as schizophrenia, but also occur in other conditions, such as from use of hallucinogens or during delirium tremens. *Compare* illusion. *See also* delirium tremens;

hallucinogen; psychedelic.

hallucinogen A substance that induces hallucinations. Examples are lysergic acid diethylamide (LSD), mescaline, and phencyclidine. *See also* controlled substances; hallucination; lysergic acid; mescaline; PCP; psychedelic; schedule I substances.

halo effect **1.** Generalization from the perception of one outstanding personality trait to an overly favorable evaluation of the whole personality. **2.** The beneficial effect of an interview or other encounter, as may occur in the course of a research project or a patient visit. The halo effect cannot be attributed to the content of the interview or to any specific act or treatment; it is the result of indefinable interpersonal factors present in the interaction. *See also* effect; Hawthorne effect; placebo effect.

Hammurabi, Code of *See* Code of Hammurabi.

Hand, American Society for Surgery of the *See* American Society for Surgery of the Hand.

handicap According to the *International Classification of Impairment, Disabilities, and Handicaps,* a disadvantage for a given individual, resulting from an impairment or a disability, that limits or prevents the fulfillment of a role that is normal, depending on age, sex, and social and cultural practices, for that individual. *See also* disability; impairment.

Handicapped, Academy of Dentistry for the *See* Academy of Dentistry for the Handicapped.

handicapped individual, qualified *See* qualified handicapped individual.

Handicapped, National Council on the *See* National Council on the Handicapped.

handicapped person Any person who has a physical or mental impairment that substantially limits one or more of the person's major life activities; has a record of such an impairment; or is regarded as having such an impairment. *See also* qualified handicapped individual.

Handicapped Physicians, American Society of *See* American Society of Handicapped Physicians.

hand massage A type of physical therapy in which the hand is massaged to stimulate circulation. *See also* massage; physical therapy.

hand surgeon A general surgeon, an orthopedic surgeon, or a plastic surgeon subspecializing in hand surgery. *See also* hand surgery; surgeon.

hand surgery The subspecialty of general surgery, orthopaedic surgery, and plastic surgery dealing with the investigation, preservation, and restoration by medical, surgical, and rehabilitative means of all structures of the upper extremity directly affecting the form and function of the hand and wrist. *See also* general surgery; orthopaedic surgery; plastic surgery.

Hand Surgery, American Association for *See* American Association for Hand Surgery.

Hand Surgery, American Board of *See* American Board of Hand Surgery.

Hand Therapists, American Society of *See* American Society of Hand Therapists.

hand vibrator An instrument used to massage and stimulate circulation to restore motion. *See also* hand massage; physical therapy.

HANES *See* Health and Nutrition Examination Survey.

hanging Death due to suspension by the neck. In judicial hanging, death results from compression of the medulla oblongata owing to immediate dislocation at the upper end of the cervical spine. *See also* death.

hangnail A torn shred of skin beside a fingernail. *See also* paronychia; skin.

Hansen's disease *See* leprosy.

HAP *See* Hospital Accreditation Program.

hard copy Any readable output from a computer that is produced on paper or another permanent medium, as contrasted with the information shown on a cathode ray tube screen. *See also* cathode ray tube; printer; printout.

hard disk In computer science, a computer data-storage medium that consists of a rigid disk with an electromagnetic coating allowing information to be transcribed on it and from it. Usually permanently mounted in a dust-proof container, a hard disk has a storage capacity approximately 10 to 100 times that of a diskette. *See also* diskette; magnetic disk.

hard knocks, school of *See* school of hard knocks.

hard line A firm, uncompromising policy, position, or stance, as in the leadership took a hard line on the need to restructure the organization.

hard sell Aggressive, high-pressure selling or promotion, as in the pharmaceutical drug representative's hard sell of the new drugs. *Compare* soft sell.

hardware *See* computer hardware.

hare lip A congenital groove or cleft in the upper lip, which may be associated with a similarly cleft palate, due to failure of developmental fusion of the two sides. *See also* cleft palate; plastic surgery.

harm, do no *See* Hippocratic oath.

harrassment, sexual   *See* sexual harrassment.

Harrison Anti-Narcotic Act   A federal statute restricting the use and distribution of dangerous drugs, such as opiates and their derivatives and many stimulants, including lysergic acid (LSD). *See also* controlled substances; lysergic acid; narcotics; opiate.

Hartford Foundation, Inc, The John A   *See* The John A Hartford Foundation, Inc.

Harvey Society (HS)   A national organization founded in 1905 composed of 1,600 persons with a Doctor of Philosophy (PhD) or a Doctor of Medicine (MD) degree active or interested in making contributions to the literature of medical and biological science. It sponsors a series of public lectures delivered by persons active in the field. It is named after William Harvey. *See also* Harvey, William.

Harvey, William   (1578-1657)   An English physician whose inductive reasoning and experiments led him, among other discoveries, to the discovery of the circulation of the blood. *See also* Harvey Society; inductive reasoning.

Hastings Center (HC)   An organization founded in 1969 composed of 11,500 physicians, nurses, lawyers, administrators, public policymakers, and other academic and health professionals interested in medical and professional ethics. *See also* ethics.

HAV   Abbreviation for hepatitis A virus, the etiologic agent causing hepatitis A. *See also* hepatitis; infectious hepatitis.

hay fever   A seasonal allergic rhinitis. *See also* allergy; rhinology; sneezing.

Hawthorne effect   The effect (usually beneficial) that an encounter has on an individual, a group of people, or the function of a system being studied. The Hawthorne effect is similar to the placebo effect, but is not obtained intentionally and is the effect of the encounter on, for example, the person doing the encountering rather than of what other persons in the encounter are doing for that person. The name comes from classic industrial management experiments at the Hawthorne (Illinois) plant of the Western Electric Company. *See also* halo effect; placebo; placebo effect.

hazard   A situation or event that introduces or increases the probability of a loss arising from a danger or peril, or that increases the extent of a loss. Examples of hazards include infectious waste, slippery floors, and unqualified individuals providing health services. *See also* biohazard; moral hazard; occupational hazard; peril; risk.

hazard, bio-   *See* biohazard.

Hazard Control Management, Academy of   *See* Academy of Hazard Control Management.

Hazard Control Management, Board of Certified   *See* Board of Certified Hazard Control Management.

hazard, moral   *See* moral hazard.

hazard, occupational   *See* occupational hazard.

hazardous materials   Substances, such as radioactive or chemical materials, that are dangerous to humans and other living organisms. *See also* safety management.

Hazardous Materials Advisory Council (HMAC)   An organization founded in 1978 composed of 280 shippers, carriers, and container manufacturers of hazardous materials, substances, and wastes. It is concerned with promoting safe transportation of these materials, answering regulatory questions, guiding appropriate governmental resources, and advising establishment of corporate compliance and safety programs. *See also* hazardous materials; hazardous waste.

Hazardous Materials Control Research Institute   *See* Hazardous Materials Control Resources Institute.

Hazardous Materials Control Resources Institute (HMCRI)   An organization founded in 1976 composed of 5,000 corporations, engineers, scientists, government and corporate administrators, and other individuals interested in the safe management of hazardous materials and waste prevention, control, and cleanup. Its activities include disseminating information about technical advances and institutional requirements in hazardous waste disposal and conducting training programs on toxic and hazardous materials control and management. *See also* hazardous materials; hazardous waste.

Hazardous Materials Research, Center for   *See* Center for Hazardous Materials Research.

hazardous waste   Waste materials, such as biologic waste that can transmit disease (also called infectious waste), radioactive materials, and toxic chemicals, that are dangerous to living organisms and require special precautions for disposal. *Synonym:* biological waste. *See also* safety management; waste.

Hb   *See* hemoglobin.

HBC   *See* Human Biology Council.

HBV   Abbreviation for hepatitis B virus, the etiologic agent causing hepatitis B. *See also* hepatitis; infectious hepatitis.

HC *See* Hastings Center.

HCA *See* Haitian Coalition on AIDS.

HCEA *See* Healthcare Convention and Exhibitors Association.

HCFA *See* Health Care Financing Administration.

HCFA generic quality screens The list of occurrences that are applied by utilization and quality control peer review organizations (PROs) to select medical cases that may have quality problems and that merit scrutiny. Because these screens generate a large amount of false positives, their application is only the first step in a multistage review process. *See also* false positive; occurrence criteria; occurrence reporting; occurrence screening; peer review organization.

HCG *See* human chorionic gonadotropin.

HCMMS *See* Health Care Material Management Society.

HCQIA *See* Health Care Quality Improvement Act of 1986.

HCS *See* Membership Section for Health Care Systems.

HDA *See* Holistic Dental Association.

HDL *See* high-density lipoprotein.

HDS *See* Hospital Discharge Survey.

headache A pain in the head. *Synonym*: cephalagia. *See also* cluster headache; migraine.

Headache, American Association for the Study of *See* American Association for the Study of Headache.

header The top margin of a printed document, which repeats on every page. Some computer programs can also include text, pictures, automatic consecutive page numbers, date, and time. *See also* footer; word processing.

head, eye, ear, nose, and throat (HEENT) *See* otolaryngology.

Head, Facial and Neck and TMJ Orthopedics, American Academy of *See* American Academy of Head, Facial and Neck and TMJ Orthopedics.

headhunter An individual or private employment agency specializing in recruiting professional and managerial personnel. *Synonym*: executive search firm. *See also* recruitment.

head louse A species of lice closely related to the body louse but whose habitat is restricted to the hair of the head. The active parasites are easily recognized with the naked eye, as are their eggs or nits, which are firmly adhered to hair shafts. *See also* body louse; nits; parasite; pediculosis.

Head/Neck Nurses, Society of Otorhinolaryngology and *See* Society of Otorhinolaryngology and Head/Neck Nurses.

head and neck surgeon *See* otolaryngologist-head and neck surgeon.

Head and Neck Surgeons, Society of *See* Society of Head and Neck Surgeons.

Head and Neck Surgeons, Society of Military Otolaryngologists - *See* Society of Military Otolaryngologists - Head and Neck Surgeons.

Head and Neck Surgeons, Society of University Otolaryngologists - *See* Society of University Otolaryngologists - Head and Neck Surgeons.

Head and Neck Surgery, American Academy of Otolaryngology - *See* American Academy of Otolaryngology - Head and Neck Surgery.

Head and Neck Surgery, American Society for *See* American Society for Head and Neck Surgery.

head nurse The clinical and administrative leader of the nurses working in a given area of a health care organization, such as a floor, ward, or unit. The head nurse is continuously responsible for the activities of the unit. *See also* nurse; nurse manager.

heal To become or make well or healthy. *See also* cure.

Healing Association, American *See* American Healing Association.

Healing, Center for Attitudinal *See* Center for Attitudinal Healing.

health A state of complete physical, mental, and social well-being and not merely the absence of disease or infirmity, according to the World Health Organization. *See also* environmental health; holistic health; World Health Organization.

Health Academy (HA) A national organization founded in 1989 composed of 600 public relations consultants and senior public relations professionals working in many health care settings including hospitals, multihospital systems, medical and dental organizations, and insurance companies and health maintenance organizations. *See also* public relations.

Health Accreditation Program, Community *See* Community Health Accreditation Program.

Health Act, Child *See* Child Health Act.

Health Act of 1970, Occupational Safety and *See* Occupational Safety and Health Act of 1970.

Health Activation Networks, Wellness and *See* Wellness and Health Activation Networks.

health administration The management of

resources, procedures, and systems that operate to meet patients' needs and wants in the health care system. *Synonyms*: health care administration; health care management. *See also* administrator; Master of Health Administration.

Health Administration, American College of Mental *See* American College of Mental Health Administration.

Health Administration, Association of University Programs in *See* Association of University Programs in Health Administration.

Health Administration, Master of *See* Master of Health Administration.

Health Administration, Occupational Safety and *See* Occupational Safety and Health Administration.

health administrator, public *See* public health administrator.

Health Administrators, Association of Mental *See* Association of Mental Health Administrators.

Health Administrators, National Conference of Local Environmental *See* National Conference of Local Environmental Health Administrators.

health aide program A program of the Indian Health Service in which members of a target population assist physicians, public health nurses, sanitarians, medical social workers, and other persons in clinical and field health programs. *See also* Indian Health Service.

Health Agencies, American Federation of Home *See* American Federation of Home Health Agencies.

Health Agencies, National Voluntary *See* National Voluntary Health Agencies.

health agency, home *See* home health agency.

health agency, voluntary *See* voluntary health agency.

health aide, home *See* home health aide.

health alliance As defined in the Health Security Act (1993), a regional alliance or a corporate alliance. *Synonyms*: health care alliance; health insurance purchasing cooperative (HIPC); purchasing alliance. *See also* corporate alliance; regional alliance.

Health, American Board of Dental Public *See* American Board of Dental Public Health.

Health, American Council on Science and *See* American Council on Science and Health.

Health Associated Representatives *See* Health Industry Representatives Association.

Health Association of America, Group *See* Group Health Association of America.

Health Association, American College *See* American College Health Association.

Health Association, American Public *See* American Public Health Association.

Health Association, American Protestant *See* American Protestant Health Association.

Health Association, American School *See* American School Health Association.

Health Association, American Social *See* American Social Health Association.

Health, Association for the Care of Children's *See* Association for the Care of Children's Health.

Health Association, Mennonite *See* Mennonite Health Association.

Health Association, National Environmental *See* National Environmental Health Association.

Health Association, National Family Planning and Reproductive *See* National Family Planning and Reproductive Health Association.

Health Association, National Mental *See* National Mental Health Association.

Health Association, National Minority *See* National Minority Health Association.

Health Association, National Rural *See* National Rural Health Association.

Health Association, New Professionals Section of the American Public *See* New Professionals Section of the American Public Health Association.

Health Association, Nutrition for Optimal *See* Nutrition for Optimal Health Association.

Health Association, Respiratory *See* Respiratory Health Association.

Health, Association of Schools of Public *See* Association of Schools of Public Health.

Health, Association of Teachers of Maternal and Child *See* Association of Teachers of Maternal and Child Health.

Health Association of the United States, Catholic *See* Catholic Health Association of the United States.

Health Association, United States - Mexico Border *See* United States - Mexico Border Health Association.

health behavior Conduct or manner demonstrated by a person to maintain, attain, or regain health and to prevent illness. Health behavior often reflects a person's health beliefs. *See also* behavior; health belief model.

health belief model A paradigm that describes a person's health behavior as an expression of health beliefs. Components of the model include the person's perception of his or her susceptibility to disease; the severity of the consequence of contracting the disease; the perceived benefits of care and barriers to preventive behavior; and the internal or external stimuli that result in health behavior by the person. *See also* belief; health behavior.

health benefit plan, employee *See* employee health benefit plan.

health benefits *See* benefits; comprehensive benefit package.

health, board of *See* board of health.

Health Board, National *See* National Health Board.

Health Board, National Indian *See* National Indian Health Board.

health card An identification card, similar to a credit card, proposed in several national health insurance bills, that would be issued to each covered individual or family unit. This card would be presented at the time of services and would be rendered in lieu of any cash payment. The individual would subsequently receive a bill for any cost-sharing not covered under the insurance plan. Health cards, some argue, would simplify eligibility determination, billing and accounting, and the study of use of services. *Synonym*: health security card. *See also* optical-stripe card; smart care; smart card in health care.

health care (healthcare) Care provided to individuals or communities by agents of the health services or professions for the purpose of promoting, maintaining, monitoring, or restoring health. Health care is broader than, and not limited to, medical care, which implies therapeutic action by or under the supervision of a physician. *See also* comprehensive health care; medical care.

Healthcare Access Management, National Association of *See* National Association of Healthcare Access Management.

health care account, individual *See* individual health are account.

Health Care, Accreditation Association for Ambulatory *See* Accreditation Association for Ambulatory Health Care.

Health Care Action, National Association of Employers on *See* National Association of Employers on Health Care Action.

health care administration *See* health administration.

Health Care Administration, Center for Research in Ambulatory *See* Center for Research in Ambu-

latory Health Care Administration.

Health Care Administrators, American College of *See* American College of Health Care Administrators.

health care alliance *See* health alliance.

Healthcare, Alliance for Alternatives in *See* Alliance for Alternatives in Healthcare.

health care, ambulatory *See* ambulatory health care.

Health Care Anti-Fraud Association, National *See* National Health Care Anti-Fraud Association.

Health Care Association, American *See* American Health Care Association.

Health Care Association, American Indian *See* American Indian Health Care Association.

Health Care Association, Managed *See* Managed Health Care Association.

Healthcare Central Service Personnel, American Society for *See* American Society for Healthcare Central Service Personnel.

health care coalition An organization composed of provider, business, and consumer representatives, and sometimes representatives of government, interested in health care issues, such as cost. *See also* business health care coalition; coalition.

health care coalition, business *See* business health care coalition.

Health Care, Coalitions for *See* Coalitions for Health Care.

health care, community *See* community health care.

health care, comprehensive *See* comprehensive health care.

health care consumer One who may receive or is receiving health services. While all people at times consume health services, a consumer, as the term is used in health legislation and programs, is usually someone who is never a provider, that is, not associated in any direct or indirect way with the provision of health services. The distinction has become important in programs in which a consumer majority on the governing body is required, as is the case with community health centers and health systems agencies assisted under the Public Health Service Act. *See also* consumer; consumerism; health care provider.

health care consultant An individual who provides professional advice and services to health care organizations, often about management and planning issues, for a fee. *See also* consultant; health care organization.

Healthcare Consultants, American Association of
See American Association of Healthcare Consultants.

Healthcare Convention and Exhibitors Association (HCEA) A national organization founded in 1930 composed of 500 manufacturers and distributors of products or services used or prescribed by health professionals who exhibit at conventions. Associate members are manufacturers or other organizations that provide products or services to health care conventions. It works to increase the efficiency and effectiveness of health care conventions and exhibits as a marketing and educational medium and provides for the professional development of convention and exhibit personnel, especially exhibit managers. Formerly (1990) Health Care Exhibitors Association. *See also* marketing.

health care delivery system, comprehensive *See* comprehensive health care delivery system.

Healthcare Education and Training of the American Hospital Association, American Society of *See* American Society of Healthcare Education and Training of the American Hospital Association.

Health Care Environmental Services of the American Hospital Association, American Society for *See* American Society for Healthcare Environmental Services of the American Hospital Association.

Health Career Schools, National Association of *See* National Association of Health Career Schools.

Health Care Exhibitors Association *See* Healthcare Convention and Exhibitors Association.

health care executive *See* administrator; executive.

Healthcare Executives, American College of *See* American College of Healthcare Executives.

Healthcare Executives, College of Osteopathic *See* College of Osteopathic Healthcare Executives.

Health Care Facilities, Consultant Dietitians in *See* Consultant Dietitians in Health Care Facilities.

Healthcare Financial Management Association (HFMA) A national organization founded in 1946 composed of 27,000 financial management professionals employed by hospitals and long term care facilities, public accounting and consulting firms, insurance companies, government agencies, and other organizations. *See also* UB-92.

Health Care Financing Administration (HCFA) A component of the US Department of Health and Human Services that administers the Medicare program and certain aspects of state Medicaid programs. *See also* Department of Health and Human Services; Medicaid; Medicare; UB-92.

Healthcare Financing Study Group (HFSG) An organization founded in 1973 composed of 40 investment banking, law, consulting, and accounting firms involved in providing capital financing for health care organizations. It analyzes legislative and regulatory proposals from the viewpoint of the health care financial community. Formerly (1981) Hospital Financing Study Group. *See also* financing.

Healthcare Forum, The *See* The Healthcare Forum.

Healthcare Human Resources Administration, American Society for *See* American Society for Healthcare Human Resources Administration.

health care industry The branch of business concerned with all aspects of providing health care services to health care consumers. Services range from those provided by physicians and hospitals to those provided by medical equipment manufacturers, health insurance companies, and pharmaceutical companies. *See also* health care consumer; industry.

health care informatics *See* medical informatics.

Health Care Information, Center for Medical Consumers and *See* Center for Medical Consumers and Health Care Information.

Healthcare Information and Management Systems Society (HIMSS) A national organization founded in 1961 composed of 3,800 persons engaged in the analysis, design, and operation of hospital telecommunications, management, and information systems. *See also* clinical information system; hospital information system; management information system.

health care institution *See* health care organization.

Healthcare Internal Audit Group *See* Association of Healthcare Internal Auditors.

Healthcare Internal Auditors, Association of *See* Association of Healthcare Internal Auditors.

Healthcare Leadership, Academy for Catholic *See* Academy for Catholic Healthcare Leadership.

Healthcare Is a Legal Duty, Children's *See* Children's Healthcare Is a Legal Duty.

health care management *See* health administration.

health care, managed *See* managed care.

health care manager *See* administrator.

Health Care Marketing and Public Relations, American Society for *See* American Society for Health Care Marketing and Public Relations.

Health Care Material Management Society (HCMMS) A national organization founded in

1975 composed of 1,500 materials management personnel in health care and hospital fields concerned with advancing health care management. It administers a certification program and develops audiovisual programs on topics, such as hospital costs, distribution, logistics, life-cycle costs, and recycling management of inventory. *See also* certification; materials management department.

Health Care, National Commission on Correctional *See* National Commission on Correctional Health Care.

Health Care, National Committee for Quality *See* National Committee for Quality Health Care.

health care network *See* network.

Health Care Networks, Accreditation Manual for *See Accreditation Manual for Health Care Networks.*

Health Care Network Accreditation Program The survey and accreditation program of the Joint Commission on Accreditation of Healthcare Organizations for eligible health care networks. *See also* accreditation; *Accreditation Manual for Health Care Networks*; Joint Commission on Accreditation of Healthcare Organizations; network; survey.

Health Care, Office of the Forum for Quality and Effectiveness in *See* Office of the Forum for Quality and Effectiveness in Health Care.

health care organization A generic term used to describe many types of organizations that provide health care services. *Synonym*: health care institution. *See also* health care; organization.

Healthcare Organizations, Joint Commission on Accreditation of *See* Joint Commission on Accreditation of Healthcare Organizations.

Healthcare Philanthropy, Association for *See* Association for Healthcare Philanthropy.

Health Care Planning, The Forum for *See* The Forum for Health Care Planning.

Healthcare Planning and Marketing of the American Hospital Association, Society for *See* Society for Healthcare Planning and Marketing of the American Hospital Association.

health care plan, prepaid *See* prepaid health plan.

Health Care Policy, National Council on Alternative *See* National Council on Alternative Health Care Policy.

Health Care Policy, Research, and Evaluation, National Advisory Council for *See* National Advisory Council for Health Care Policy, Research, and Evaluation.

health care professional *See* health professional.

health care provider A health professional or health care organization, or group of health professionals or health care organizations, that provides health services to patients. Examples include a physician, dentist, nurse, or allied health professional, or an organization, such as a physician-hospital organization, skilled nursing facility, or home health agency. *Synonyms*: health provider; health service provider; health services provider; provider. *See also* capitation; corporate practice of medicine; group practice; group practice without walls; health services; impaired health care provider; integrated provider; nonparticipating provider; participating physician; physician-hospital organization; primary care provider; referral provider.

health care provider, impaired *See* impaired health care provider.

Health Care Quality Improvement Act (HCQIA) of 1986 Federal legislation that authorizes the National Practitioners Data Bank and provides immunity from liability, including antitrust liability, for peer review decisions by hospitals and other health facilities regarding physicians and dentists, provided requirements of the act are satisfied. *See also* National Practitioner Data Bank.

Healthcare Quality, National Association for *See* National Association for Healthcare Quality.

Healthcare Radiology Administrators, American *See* American Healthcare Radiology Administrators.

Healthcare Recruitment, National Association for *See* National Association for Healthcare Recruitment.

Health Care, Reform American Council for *See* American Council for Health Care Reform.

Healthcare Resources, Quality *See* Quality Healthcare Resources.

Healthcare Risk Management, American Society for *See* American Society for Risk Management.

health care, skimming in *See* skimming in health care.

health care system *See* health system.

Health Care System, Lutheran General *See* Lutheran General Health Care System.

Health Care Systems, Membership Section for *See* Membership Section for Health Care Systems.

health care team A group of health professionals who provides coordinated services to increase the probability that desired outcomes will be achieved, as in a cardiovascular health care team. *See also* team.

health care technology The application of science to health care objectives, as in devices for extracorporeal oxygenation during open-heart surgery. *See also* health care; technology.

Health Care Technology Assessment, National Center for Health Services Research and *See* National Center for Health Services Research and Health Care Technology Assessment.

health center, academic *See* academic medical center.

health center, community *See* community health center.

health center, community mental *See* community mental health center.

Health Centers, Association of Academic *See* Association of Academic Health Centers.

Health Centers, Federation of Feminist Women's *See* Federation of Feminist Women's Health Centers.

Health Centers, National Association of Community *See* National Association of Community Health Centers.

Health Centers, National Council of Community Mental *See* National Council of Community Mental Health Centers.

Health Clearinghouse, National Maternal and Child *See* National Maternal and Child Health Clearinghouse.

Health Club Association, National *See* National Health Club Association.

Health, Coalition on Smoking or *See* Coalition on Smoking or Health.

health coordinating council, statewide *See* statewide health coordinating council.

Health Council, American Industrial *See* American Industrial Health Council.

Health, Council on Education for Public *See* Council on Education for Public Health.

Health, Council on Family *See* Council on Family Health.

Health Council, National *See* National Health Council.

Health Council, Silicones *See* Silicones Health Council.

Health Counselors Association, American Mental *See* American Mental Health Counselors Association.

Health Crisis, Gay Men's *See* Gay Men's Health Crisis.

health data disclosure acts *See* state data initiatives.

Health Data Organizations, National Association of *See* National Association of Health Data Organizations.

health decision The actual choice made by health care practitioners or recipients of care when confronted by a defined health problem. A specific decision is a choice between a primary scenario and an alternative scenario(s). *See also* decision.

health, dental *See* dental health.

health, dental public *See* public health dentistry.

health dentistry, public *See* public health dentistry.

health economics The social science dealing with the demand for and supply of health care resources and the impact of health services on the health of a population. *See also* economics.

health education Providing information to the general public or of special group, such as school children, that increases awareness and favorably influences behavior in such a way as to promote health and prevent disease. *See also* education; patient education.

Health Education and Accreditation, Committee on Allied *See* Committee on Allied Health Education and Accreditation.

Health Education, Association for the Advancement of *See* Association for the Advancement of Health Education.

Health Education, Association of State and Territorial Directors of Public *See* Association of State and Territorial Directors of Public Health Education.

Health Education, National Center for *See* National Center for Health Education.

Health Education Resource Organization (HERO) A nonmembership organization founded in 1983 that provides patient services and preventive education regarding acquired immunodeficiency syndrome (AIDS) to Maryland residents and disseminates information on AIDS prevention and treatment nationwide. *See also* acquired immunodeficiency syndrome.

Health Education Schools, Accrediting Bureau of *See* Accrediting Bureau of Health Education Schools.

Health Education, Society for Public *See* Society for Public Health Education.

Health, Education and Welfare Association, Presbyterian *See* Presbyterian Health, Education and Welfare Association.

Health, Education, and Welfare, Department of *See* Department of Health, Education, and Welfare.

Health and Energy Institute (HEI) A national organization founded in 1978 composed of 7,000 members concerned about the impact of nuclear energy on health and the environment, with an emphasis on radiation law, radiation danger to women, and nuclear technology. It conducts research and educational programs on the effects of food irradiation and nuclear development for electric power or weapons. Formerly (1983) Health and Energy Learning Project.

Health and Energy Learning Project *See* Health and Energy Institute.

health, environmental *See* environmental health.

Health Evaluation, Acute Physiology and Chronic *See* Acute Physiology and Chronic Health Evaluation.

health facility Health or medical institution, such as hospitals, nursing homes, rehabilitation centers, reproductive health centers, independent clinical laboratories, hospices, and ambulatory surgical centers, whose primary function is to provide health services. *See also* facility; health care organization.

Health Facility Administrators, National Association of County *See* National Association of County Health Facility Administrators.

health facility licensing agency, state *See* state health facility licensing agency.

Health Facility Survey Agencies, Association of *See* Association of Health Facility Survey Agencies.

health fair A community health education event that focuses on prevention of disease and promotion of health through such activities as audiovisual exhibits and free diagnostic services.

Health Federation, National *See* National Health Federation.

HEALTH FILE An on-line computerized database counterpart to the *Hospital Literature Index*, including citations to the literature dealing with nonclinical aspects of health care delivery from 1975 to the present. *See also Hospital Literature Index.*

health foods Articles of food on sale to the public, often from dedicated retail outlets, which by virtue of their ingredients or methods of manufacture are claimed to be more healthful than their conventional equivalents; for example, foods with a high content of dietary fiber, such as raw carrots or whole-wheat bread. *See also* food.

Health Foundation, Kansas *See* Kansas Health Foundation.

Health Fraud, National Council Against *See* National Council Against Health Fraud.

Health Funding, Coalition for *See* Coalition for Health Funding.

health history *See* medical history.

health, holistic *See* holistic health.

Health and Human Services Assembly, Protestant *See* Protestant Health and Human Services Assembly.

Health and Human Services, Department of *See* Department of Health and Human Services.

Health and Human Services Organizations, National Coalition of Hispanic *See* National Coalition of Hispanic Health and Human Services Organizations.

Health and Human Values, Society for *See* Society for Health and Human Values.

Health Industry Bar Code Council *See* Health Industry Business Communications Council.

Health Industry Business Communications Council (HIBCC) A national group founded in 1984 composed of 1,000 individuals and companies in the health care industry concerned with improving the quality and economic efficiency of health care by instituting and overseeing a uniform system of computer bar coding for identification of health care equipment and by promoting the use of this and other automated technologies in the health care industry. Formerly (1987) Health Industry Bar Code Council. *See also* bar code.

Health Industry Distributors Association (HIDA) A national organization founded in 1902 composed of 725 distributors of medical, laboratory, surgical, and home health care equipment and supplies to hospitals, physicians, nursing homes, and industrial medical departments. Formerly (1982) American Surgical Trade Association.

Health Industry Manufacturers Association (HIMA) A national organization founded in 1974 composed of 300 domestic manufacturers of medical devices, diagnostic products, and health care information systems. It develops programs and activities on economic, technical, medical, and scientific matters affecting the industry. It gathers and disseminates information concerning national and international developments in legislative, regulatory, scientific, or standards-making areas. *See also* medical device.

Health Industry Representatives Association (HIRA) A national organization founded in 1978 composed of 200 manufacturers' representatives who operate independent marketing firms under contract to manufacturers of noncompeting lines and manufacturers within the health care industry who market through independent marketing firms. Formerly (1986) Health Associated Representatives.

Health Information Center, ODPHP National *See* ODPHP National Health Information Center.

Health Information Council (HIC) A national organization founded in 1988 composed of 750 corporations and organizations in the health industry and other groups interested in promoting healthy life-styles as a method of preventing illness and abuse. It directs programs related to the family unit and wellness of individuals. *See also* wellness.

health information infrastructure A communications network consisting of computer-based patient record systems, computerized knowledge-based systems, and reference databases, all of which are connected through high-speed communications links using common definitions, codes, and forms. *See also* infrastructure; national information infrastructure.

Health Information Management Association, American *See* American Health Information Management Association.

Health, Institute for Reproductive *See* Institute for Reproductive Health.

health insurance Insurance against loss by disease or accidental bodily injury. Health insurance usually covers some of the medical costs of treating a disease or injury, may cover other losses (such as loss of present or future earnings) associated with disease or injury, and may be either individual or group insurance. *See also* commercial health insurance; cost sharing; dual choice; duplication of benefits; group insurance; individual health insurance; insurance; recurring clause; waiting period.

Health Insurance for the Aged and Disabled, Title XVIII *See* Medicare.

Health Insurance Association of America (HIAA) A national organization founded in 1956 composed of 300 accident and health insurance firms concerned with the development of voluntary insurance against loss of income and financial burdens resulting from injury and illness. *See also* health insurance; insurance; UB-92.

Health Insurance Benefits Advisory Council (HIBAC) An advisory council of the Department of Health and Human Services that provided gener-

al policy advice and recommendations in the administration of Medicare and Medicaid. The Omnibus Deficit Reduction Act of 1984 terminated the Council. The Council consisted of 19 nongovernmental experts in health-related fields who were selected by the Secretary of Health and Human Services and held office for terms of four years.

Health Insurance, Bureau of *See* Bureau of Health Insurance.

health insurance claim number (HICN) An identification number of a Medicare beneficiary (often his or her Social Security number), consisting of seven or nine digits and an alphabetical prefix or suffix. Medicare requires that the HICN number appear on all documents related to a beneficiary. *See also* health insurance; Medicare.

health insurance, commercial *See* commercial health insurance.

Health Insurance, Committee for National *See* Committee for National Health Insurance.

health insurance, comprehensive *See* comprehensive health insurance.

health insurance, individual *See* individual health insurance.

health insurance, national *See* national health insurance.

Health Insurance Plan, Comprehensive *See* Comprehensive Health Insurance Plan.

Health Insurance Plan, Federal *See* Federal Health Insurance Plan.

health insurance purchasing cooperative (HPIC) *See* health alliance.

health insurance, supplemental *See* supplemental health insurance.

health intervention Any action taken to modify the health of an individual or group. The intervention may pertain to disease prevention, detection, diagnosis, or management. *See also* allopathic physician; allopathy; intervention.

Health Interview Survey (HIS) A survey conducted annually by the National Center for Health Statistics to collect health-related information, such as illness and injury recall, health conditions and related disabilities, hospitalization, and physician visits, on a sampling of American households. *See also* interview; National Center for Health Statistics.

health IRA (individual retirement account) A tax-preferred plan that would encourage saving for future medical expenses. *Synonym:* medical IRA. *See* *also* individual retirement account.

Health Laboratorians, Conference of Public *See* Conference of Public Health Laboratorians.

Health Laboratory Services, National Council on *See* National Council on Health Laboratory Services.

health law An area of law dealing with health fields, including medical, dental, nursing, and hospital administration. *See also* hospital law; law.

Health Law Program, National *See* National Health Law Program.

Health Law Project, Mental *See* Mental Health Law Project.

Health Lawyers Association, National *See* National Health Lawyers Association.

health maintenance Preservation of the physical, mental, and social well-being of a person. *See also* health maintenance organization.

health maintenance organization (HMO) A health care organization that, in return for prospective per capita (capitation) payments, acts as both insurer and provider of comprehensive but specified medical services. A defined set of physicians provide services to a voluntarily enrolled population. *See also* enrollment; group model HMO; Health Maintenance Organization Act of 1973; independent practice association model HMO; network; network model HMO; staff model HMO.

Health Maintenance Organization Act of 1973 A federal statute that sets standards of qualifications for health maintenance organizations (HMOs) and mandates that employers of 25 or more persons who currently offer a medical benefit plan must also offer the option of joining a qualified HMO if one exists in the area. *See also* health maintenance organization.

health manpower *See* health personnel.

Health Media Education (HME) An organization founded in 1974 composed of 150 members interested in producing and distributing materials that provide consumers and health personnel with information needed to plan and implement community health programs. *See also* media; public health.

health, mental *See* mental health.

Health, National Association of Nurse Practitioners in Reproductive *See* National Association of Nurse Practitioners in Reproductive Health.

Health, National Association for Rural Mental *See* National Association for Rural Mental Health.

Health, National Institute for Occupational Safety and *See* National Institute for Occupational Safety and Health.

Health, National Institutes of *See* National Institutes of Health.

health network *See* network.

health network, community *See* community health network.

Health Network, National Women's *See* National Women's Health Network.

health nurse, occupational *See* occupational health nurse.

Health Nurses, American Board for Occupational *See* American Board for Occupational Health Nurses.

Health and Nutrition Examination Survey (HANES) A survey conducted every four years by the National Center for Health Services Research and Health Care Technology Assessment. The survey gathers data in many areas, such as medically defined illnesses and population distributions based on blood pressure, serum cholesterol levels, and nutritional status. *See also* National Center for Health Services Research and Health Care Technology Assessment.

Health, Obstetric, and Neonatal Nurses, Association of Women's *See* Association of Women's Health, Obstetric, and Neonatal Nurses.

health, occupational *See* occupational health.

Health Occupations Education, National Association of Supervisors and Administrators of *See* National Association of Supervisors and Administrators of Health Occupations Education.

Health Officials, Association of State and Territorial *See* Association of State and Territorial Health Officials.

Health Officials, National Association of County *See* National Association of County Health Officials.

Health Officers, United States Conference of Local *See* United States Conference of Local Health Officers.

Health Organization, Pan American *See* Pan American Health Organization.

Health Organization, World *See* World Health Organization.

health outcome, patient *See* patient health outcome.

health personnel Collectively, all people working in the provision of health services whether as individual practitioners or employees of health care organizations and programs; they may or may not be professionally trained and/or subject to public regulation. *See also* human resources.

Health Personnel in Ophthalmology, Joint Commission on Allied *See* Joint Commission on Allied Health Personnel in Ophthalmology.

Health Physicians, American Association of Public *See* American Association of Public Health Physicians.

health physicist A physicist who directs research, training, and monitoring programs to protect patients and laboratory personnel from radiation hazards and who sometimes computes the dosage and treatment plan for radiation therapy. *See also* health physics; radiation.

health physics The profession that deals with radiation protection and safety. *See also* physics.

Health Physics, American Board of *See* American Board of Health Physics.

Health Physics Society (HPS) A national organization founded in 1956 composed of 6,890 persons engaged in some form of activity in the field of health physics. *See also* health physicist; health physics; radiation.

health physics technician A technician skilled in monitoring radiation levels, giving instruction in radiation safety, labeling radioactive materials, and assisting a health physicist. *See also* health physicist; technician.

health plan **1.** In health insurance, a specific set of benefits packaged for general offering for the needs of a specific purchaser. *See also* additional drug benefit list; Blue Cross/Blue Shield plan; enrollment; incentive benefit plan; plan; prepaid health plan; state health plan. **2.** According to the Health Security Act (1993), a plan that provides the comprehensive benefit package and meets other requirements. *See also* appropriate self-insured health plan; basic health services; comprehensive benefit package; corporate alliance health plan; Health Security Act; primary care network; state-certified health plan.

health plan, appropriate self-insured *See* appropriate self-insured health plan.

health plan, Clinton *See* Health Security Act.

health plan, corporate alliance *See* corporate alliance health plan.

health plan, group *See* group health plan.

health plan, incentive benefit *See* incentive benefit plan.

health plan, prepaid *See* prepaid health plan.

health planner In public health, an individual who

is involved in studying and administering programs to develop needed health resources for an area, a population, a type of health service, or a health program. *See also* health planning; public health.

health planning Planning concerned with improving health, undertaken comprehensively for a whole community or for a particular population, type of health service, or health program. Some definitions include all activities undertaken for the purpose of improving health (such as education and nutrition); other definitions are limited to including conventional health services and programs, public health, or personal health services. Federal participation in the funding of health planning ended on September 30, 1986. *See also* health planning guidelines; planning.

Health Planning Association, American *See* American Health Planning Association.

health planning and development agency, state *See* state health planning and development agency.

Health Planning and Evaluation, Office of *See* Office of Health Planning and Evaluation.

health planning guidelines Guidelines for directing health-planning functions and policies mandated by the Health Planning and Resources Development Act of 1974 and issued by the US Department of Health and Human Services for use by state and local planning agencies. The termination of federal funding for health planning has essentially resulted in the continued use of the guidelines in most states as a reference source for their own planning. *See also* guideline; health planning.

Health Planning and Resources Development Act of 1974, National *See* National Health Planning and Resources Development Act of 1974.

health plan, state *See* state health plan.

health plan, state-certified *See* state-certified health plan.

health policy **1.** A statement of a decision regarding a goal in health care and a plan for achieving that goal. *See also* policy. **2.** A field of study and practice in which the priorities and values underlying health resource allocation are determined.

Health Policy Advisory Center (Health/PAC) A national organization founded in 1968 that monitors and interprets the health system to change-oriented groups of health workers, consumers, professionals, and students. It seeks to create a health system that provides low-cost, high-quality services, emphasizes prevention of illness, and is accountable to the communities that receive its care and the workers who provide it. *See also* health policy; policy.

Health Policy Forum, National *See* National Health Policy Forum.

Health Policy Project, Intergovernmental *See* Intergovernmental Health Policy Project.

Health Policy, Public Voice for Food and *See* Public Voice for Food and Health Policy.

health practitioner Any person who implements a health intervention; for example, a physician, podiatrist, or public health officer. *See also* health intervention; health professional.

health professional Any person who has completed a course of study and is skilled in a field of health, such as a nurse, occupational therapist, or osteopathic physician. Health professionals are often licensed by a government agency and/or certified by a professional organization. *Synonym:* health care professional. *See also* allied health professional; professional.

health professional, allied *See* allied health professional.

health professional, mental *See* mental health professional.

Health Professionals, American Board of Urologic Allied *See* American Board of Urologic Allied Health Professionals.

Health Professionals, Association of Reproductive *See* Association of Reproductive Health Professionals.

Health Professionals, Center for the Well-Being of *See* Center for the Well-Being of Health Professionals.

Health Professionals, Federation of Nurses and *See* Federation of Nurses and Health Professionals.

Health Professions, American Society of Allied *See* American Society of Allied Health Professions.

Health Professions Association, Arthritis *See* Arthritis Health Professions Association.

Health Professions, National Association of Advisors for the *See* National Association of Advisors for the Health Professions.

Health Professions, National Center for the Advancement of Blacks in the *See* National Center for the Advancement of Blacks in the Health Professions.

Health Professions Schools, Association of Minority *See* Association of Minority Health Professions Schools.

Health Program Directors, National Association of State Mental *See* National Association of State Mental Health Program Directors.

Health Programs, Association of Maternal and Child *See* Association of Maternal and Child Health Programs.

Health Project, East Coast Migrant *See* East Coast Migrant Health Project.

Health Project, National Black Women's *See* National Black Women's Health Project.

health promotion Efforts to change people's behavior in order to promote healthy lives and to help prevent illnesses and accidents. *See also* corporatization of health care; wellness; wellness program.

Health Promotion Institute A program, founded in 1985, of the National Council on the Aging, composed of 600 professionals who are interested in developing and implementing a health promotion programs for senior citizens. Formerly (1991) National Center for Health Promotion and Aging. *See also* health promotion; National Council on the Aging.

Health Promotion, Office of Disease Prevention and *See* Office of Disease Prevention and Health Promotion.

health promotion program *See* wellness program.

health provider *See* health care provider.

health, public *See* public health.

health record *See* medical record.

health record analyst *See* medical record analyst.

health record, patient *See* medical record.

health record, patient's *See* medical record.

Health Research Group, Public Citizen *See* Public Citizen Health Research Group.

Health Research, Melpomene Institute for Women's *See* Melpomene Institute for Women's Health Research.

Health Resource Center, National Women's *See* National Women's Health Resource Center.

health resources Personnel, facilities, funds, and technology used or that could be made available in providing health services. *See also* resources.

Health Resources and Services Administration (HRSA) A federal agency within the Public Health Service responsible for administering federal health programs, such as health services scholarships, maternal and child health, and Indian health. The principal divisions of the agency are the Bureau of Health Care Delivery and Assistance, Bureau of

Resources Development, and Bureau of Health Professions. *See also* Public Health Service.

Health Review Commission, Occupational Safety and *See* Occupational Safety and Health Review Commission.

health risk A disease precursor associated with a higher than average morbidity or mortality. Disease precursors include patient-based factors, such as age, sex, comorbidities, and severity of illness. For instance, a patient who smokes, has high blood pressure, and whose father died of a heart attack at age 40 years is at risk for experiencing a heart attack. *See also* comorbidity; health risk appraisal; risk; severity of illness.

health risk appraisal A process of gathering, analyzing, and comparing an individual's prognostic characteristics of health with a standard age group, thereby predicting the likelihood that a person may develop prematurely a health problem associated with a high morbidity and mortality rate. One purpose of health risk appraisal is to prescribe measures and programs to counter detected risks. *Synonym*: health risk assessment. *See also* health risk.

health risk assessment *See* health risk appraisal.

Health Roundtable, Women and *See* Women and Health Roundtable.

Health and Safety, Association of University Programs in Occupational *See* Association of University Programs in Occupational Health and Safety.

health, school *See* school health.

Health Science and Protection, National Accreditation Council for Environmental *See* National Accreditation Council for Environmental Health Science and Protection.

Health/Sciences Centers, Association of University Environmental *See* Association of University Environmental Health/Sciences Centers.

Health Sciences Communications Association (HESCA) A national organization founded in 1959 composed of 600 media managers, graphic artists, biomedical librarians, producers, faculty members of health science schools, health organizations, and industry representatives that acts as a clearinghouse for information used by professionals engaged in health science communications. *See also* clearinghouse; communication.

Health Sciences Consortium (HSC) A cooperative founded in 1971 composed of 1,000 health science institutions concerned with publishing effec-

tive instructional materials at a low cost. It develops sales training and continuing education instructional materials for pharmaceutical companies.

health sciences librarian A librarian responsible for providing services to meet the needs of health sciences personnel and health professionals. *See also* health sciences library; librarian.

health sciences library A library responsible for providing services to meet the informational, educational, and research-related needs of health sciences personnel and health professionals. *See also* health sciences librarian; library.

Health Sciences Library Directors, Association of Academic *See* Association of Academic Health Sciences Library Directors.

Health Section of the National Council on Family Relations, Family and *See* Family and Health Section of the National Council on Family Relations.

Health Security Act A health reform bill introduced to Congress in 1993 that ensures individual and family security through health care coverage for all Americans in a manner that contains the rate or growth in health care costs and promotes responsible health insurance practices, to promote choice in health care, and to ensure and protect the health care of all Americans. *Synonyms*: American Health Security Act; Clinton health plan. *See also* comprehensive benefit package; corporate alliance; health alliance; health plan; National Health Board; regional alliance.

Health Security Action Council (HSAC) A national organization founded in 1969 composed of individuals and organizations concerned with increasing grass-roots support for national health insurance and progressive health plans through publicity and education. *See also* national health insurance; security.

health security card *See* health card; regional alliance.

health service *See* health services.

health service area (HSA) A defined geographic region designated under the National Health Planning and Resources Development Act of 1974, covering such factors as geography, political boundaries, population, and health resources, for the effective planning and development of health services. *See also* catchment area; Medicare locality; medically underserved area.

Health Service, Commissioned Officers Association of the United States Public *See* Commissioned Officers Association of the United States Public Health Service.

Health Service Corps, National   *See* National Health Service Corps.

health service, employee   *See* employee health service.

health service, national   *See* national health service.

health service provider   *See* health care provider.

Health Service Providers in Psychology, Council for the National Register of   *See* Council for the National Register of Health Service Providers in Psychology.

health services   Services that are performed by health professionals, or by other persons under their direction, for the purpose of promoting, maintaining, monitoring, or restoring health. *See also* basic health services; community health services; dental health services; encounter; industrial health services; occupational health services; patient; personal health services; preventive health services; quality of care.

Health Services Administration, Accrediting Commission on Education for   *See* Accrediting Commission on Education for Health Services Administration.

health services administrator   *See* administrator; health administration.

Health Services Association, American Correctional   *See* American Correctional Health Services Association.

health services, basic   *See* basic health services.

health services, community   *See* community health services.

health services, demand for   *See* demand for health services.

health services, dental   *See* dental health services.

health services, employee   *See* employee health services.

Health Services Executives, National Association of   *See* National Association of Health Services Executives.

health services, industrial   *See* industrial health services.

Health Services Marketing, Academy for   *See* Academy for Health Services Marketing.

Health Services, National Consortium for Child Mental   *See* National Consortium for Child Mental Health Services.

health services, occupational   *See* occupational health services.

health services, personal   *See* personal health services.

health services, preventive   *See* preventive health services.

health services research   Research concerned with the organization, financing, administration, effects, and other aspects of health services. Health services research is often concerned with the relationships among need, demand, supply, use, and outcomes of health services. Structure, process, and outcome of health services may be evaluated. Evaluation of structure is concerned with resources, facilities, and manpower; process, with matters, such as where, by whom, and how health care is provided; and outcome, with the results of the services (such as the degree to which individuals receiving health services actually experience measurable benefits). *See also* health services; indicator measurement system; outcome; process; research; structure.

Health Services Research, Association for   *See* Association for Health Services Research.

Health Services Research, Foundation for   *See* Foundation for Health Services Research.

Health Services Research and Health Care Technology Assessment, National Center for   *See* National Center for Health Services Research and Health Care Technology Assessment.

Health and Social Welfare Organizations, National Assembly of National Voluntary   *See* National Assembly of National Voluntary Health and Social Welfare Organizations.

Health Society, Dinshah   *See* Dinshah Health Society.

Health, Society for Environmental Geochemistry and   *See* Society for Environmental Geochemistry and Health.

Health, Society for Occupational and Environmental   *See* Society for Occupational and Environmental Health.

health standard, occupational safety and   *See* occupational safety and health standard.

Health Standards and Quality Bureau (HSQB) An organizational element within the Health Care Financing Administration that is responsible for carrying out the quality assurance provisions of the Medicare and Medicaid programs, implementation of health and safety standards for providers of care in their programs, and the professional review provision of Medicare and Medicaid programs. *See also* Health Care Financing Administration; peer review organization.

health statistician *See* biostatistician.

health statistics Aggregated data describing and enumerating attributes, events, occurrences, and structures, processes, and outcomes relating to health, disease, and health services. The data may be derived from survey instruments, medical records, administrative documents, and other source documents. Vital statistics are a subset of health statistics. *See also* statistics; vital statistics.

Health Statistics, Association for Vital Records and *See* Association for Vital Records and Health Statistics.

Health Statistics, National Center for *See* National Center for Health Statistics.

Health Statistics System, Cooperative *See* Cooperative Health Statistics System.

health status An individual's or a population's state of health. *See also* health status indicator.

health status indicator A tool used to quantify various aspects of a population's health status. *See also* health status; indicator.

health system The network of organizations and individuals who provide health services in a defined geographic area. A health system is established, according to the American Hospital Association, when a single hospital owns, leases, or contract-manages nonhospital, preacute, and/or postacute health-related facilities (for example, wellness services, mental health services, outpatient services, employer health services, long term care); or two or more hospitals are owned, leased, sponsored, or contract-managed by a central organization. In the latter instance, a single holding company board of directors has the programmatic and fiscal responsibilities to promote the health of the community. *Synonym*: health care system. *See also* community; holding company; multihospital system; network.

Health System, Coalition for a National *See* Coalition for a National Health System.

health systems agency (HSA) A not-for-profit organization or unit of local government designated under the National Health Planning and Resources Development Act of 1974 to perform various health planning functions within a defined geographic area, develop the areawide health systems plan, conduct certificate-of-need reviews, and review the proposed use of some federal health funds. *See also* National Health Planning and Resources Development Act of 1974.

Health Systems, Federation of American *See* Federation of American Health Systems.

Health Technicians, National Association of Air National Guard *See* National Association of Air National Guard Health Technicians.

Health Technology Assessment, Office of *See* Office of Health Technology Assessment.

Health Underwriters, National Association of *See* National Association of Health Underwriters.

health unit clerk *See* health unit coordinator.

health unit coordinator An individual who coordinates nonclinical nursing unit activities; for example, performing routine clerical and reception duties, scheduling appointments and patient-service requirements, monitoring the location of technical and professional people assigned to the unit, ordering supplies, updating patient chart information, and transcribing physician's orders. *Synonyms*: unit clerk; unit health clerk; unit secretary; ward clerk. *See also* unit.

Health Unit Coordinators, National Association of *See* National Association of Health Unit Coordinators.

health unit, mobile *See* mobile health unit.

Health and Welfare Ministries, United Methodist Association of *See* United Methodist Association of Health and Welfare Ministries.

health, wholistic *See* holistic health.

hearing **1.** The sense by which sound is perceived. **2.** The capacity for sound perception. *See also* active listening; deaf; deaf-mute; hearing aid; hearing impaired; hearing loss; listen. **3.** In law, a formal proceeding with issues of fact or law to be tried in which parties have a right to be heard. It is similar to a trial and may result in a final order. *See also* trial.

hearing aid A small electronic apparatus that amplifies sound and is worn in or behind the ear to compensate for impaired hearing. *Synonyms*: auditory substitutional device; electronic hearing aid. *See also* audiology; hearing; hearing impaired; otolaryngology.

hearing aid, electronic *See* hearing aid.

Hearing Aid Society, National *See* National Hearing Aid Society.

hearing aid specialist *See* National Hearing Aid Society.

Hearing Association, American Speech-Language- *See* American Speech-Language-Hearing Association.

Hearing, Computer Users in Speech and *See* Computer Users in Speech and Hearing.

Hearing Conservation Association, National *See* National Hearing Conservation Association.

Hearing Conservation, Council for Accreditation in Occupational *See* Council for Accreditation in Occupational Hearing Conservation.

hearing impaired **1.** Pertaining to a diminished or defective sense of hearing, although not deaf from birth, to such an extent as to have to rely on aids, such as lip reading in order to understand speech. *See also* cued speech; hearing aid; lip reading. **2.** A deaf person. *See also* deaf.

Hearing Industries Association (HIA) A national organization founded in 1957 composed of 40 companies engaged in the manufacture and/or sale of electronic hearing aids, their component parts, and related products and services on a national basis. It cooperates in and contributes toward efforts to promote the number of hearing aid users, collects trade statistics, and conducts market research activities, investigations, and experiments with hearing aids. *See also* hearing aid.

hearing loss A partial or complete loss of sound perception. *See also* deafness; hearing.

hearing therapy aide, speech and *See* speech and hearing therapy aide.

heart The muscular pump situated in the chest that maintains circulation of the blood. The right and left sides of the heart are separate functional units, each comprising a filling chamber, or atrium, and a much thicker and more muscular ventricle. *See also* acute myocardial infarction; cardiovascular medicine; carditis; congestive heart failure; echocardiography; electrocardiography; heart rate; open-heart surgery; palpitation.

Heart Association, American *See* American Heart Association.

Heart Association, Council on Arteriosclerosis of the American *See* Council on Arteriosclerosis of the American Heart Association.

Heart Association, Peruvian *See* Peruvian Heart Association.

heart attack Familiar term for myocardial infarction. *See also* acute myocardial infarction; heart.

heartburn A painful, burning sensation in the chest below the sternum resulting from irritation in the esophagus, most often due to backflow of acidic stomach contents into the esophagus. *Synonym:* pyrosis. *See also* gastroesophageal reflux; indigestion; reflux esophagitis.

heart failure *See* congestive heart failure.

heart failure, congestive *See* congestive heart failure.

heart-lung machine An apparatus, consisting of a blood pump and blood oxygenator, used during heart surgery that temporarily takes over the functions of the heart and lungs. A heart-lung machine is used to allow a cardiovascular surgeon to operate on a dry, nonbeating heart, as for coronary artery bypass graft procedures. *Synonym:* extracorporeal oxygenator. *See also* American Society of Extra-Corporeal Technology; heart; machine; open-heart surgery; perfusionist.

heart muscle *See* muscle.

heart palpitation *See* palpitation.

heart rate The number of heart contractions (beats) per unit of time. *See also* heart; rate.

Heart Research, National *See* National Heart Research.

Heart Savers Association, National *See* National Heart Savers Association.

heart seizure A layperson's term for heart attack. *See also* acute myocardial infarction.

heart surgery, open- *See* open-heart surgery.

heart transplant An operation in which the heart of a human donor is transplanted into a patient deemed to have irreversible heart disease and otherwise negligible chances of survival. The transplanted heart is connected to the recipient's circulatory system and takes over the functions of the diseased heart. *See also* donor; transplantation.

hedonism A doctrine that pleasure is the highest good. *See also* materialism; narcissism.

HEENT Acronym for head, eye, ear, nose, and throat. *See* otolaryngology.

HEI *See* Health and Energy Institute; Hospice Education Institute.

height Vertical measurement, or tallness. *See also* dwarf; giant; gigantism; measurement; midget; weight.

Heimlich maneuver A subdiaphragmatic abdominal thrust that is recommended for relieving foreign-body airway obstruction. Named after Dr Harry J. Heimlich (b. 1920) who developed the procedure. *Synonyms:* abdominal thrust; subdiaphragmatic abdominal thrust. *See also* airway; maneuver.

helicopter *See* ambulance.

heliotherapy Treatment of disease by exposure to sunshine.

helminth   Any parasitic worm. *See also* parasitology.

Helpern Institute of Forensic Medicine, Milton   *See* Milton Helpern Institute of Forensic Medicine.

hemapheresis   *See* apheresis.

hematemesis   Vomiting of blood, indicating rapid upper gastrointestinal bleeding from esophageal swollen or dilated blood vessels, peptic ulcer or other lesions. *See also* anemia; blood; esophagus; hemorrhage; vomit.

hematochezia   The passage of blood through the rectum, usually from bleeding in the colon or rectum, but sometimes from higher in the digestive tract. Hematochezia usually results from cancer, colitis, or ulcers. *Compare* melena. *See also* anemia; hemorrhage.

hematocrit   A measure of the packed cell volume of red blood cells, expressed as a percentage of the total blood volume. The normal range is between 43% and 49% in men and between 37% and 43% in women. *See also* blood count; hemoglobin.

hematologist   An internist, a pathologist, or a pediatrician who subspecializes in hematology. *See also* hematology; internist; pathologist; pediatric hematologist-oncologist.

hematologist-oncologist, pediatric   *See* pediatric hematologist-oncologist.

hematology   The branch of medicine and subspecialty of internal medicine, pathology, and pediatrics dealing with diseases of the blood, spleen, and lymph glands. The scope of hematology includes disorders, such as anemia, clotting conditions, sickle cell disease, hemophilia, leukemia, and lymphoma. *See also* anemia; hematology/pathology; hemophilia; internal medicine; leukemia; lymphoma; pathology; pediatric hematology-oncology; sickle cell anemia.

Hematology, American Society of   *See* American Society of Hematology.

hematology laboratory   A laboratory for examination of blood specimens by means of serologic and other tests. *See also* clinical laboratory; hematology.

Hematology/Oncology, American Society of Pediatric   *See* American Society of Pediatric Hematology/Oncology.

hematology-oncology, pediatric   *See* pediatric hematology-oncology.

hematology/pathology   The branch of medicine and subspecialty of pathology dealing with laboratory diagnosis of anemias, leukemias, lymphomas, bleeding disorders, and blood clotting disorders. *See*

also hematology; pathology.

hematology technologist   A medical technologist who specializes in the performance of blood tests for use by physicians in the diagnosis and treatment of diseases of the blood and bone marrow. *See also* medical technologist; technologist.

hematoma   Localized collection of blood, usually clotted, in an organ, space, or tissue. It results from the escape of blood from a blood vessel, often as the result of trauma. When the hematoma occurs near the skin surface, it causes discoloration, that is, a bruise. *See also* bruise.

Hematopathology, Society for   *See* Society for Hematopathology.

hematuria   The presence of blood in the urine. *See also* blood; cystitis; urination.

hemicrania   Headache on one side of the head. *See also* headache; migraine.

Hemlock Society (HS)   A national organization founded in 1980 composed of 42,000 individuals supporting the option of active voluntary euthanasia for the advanced terminally ill and seriously incurably ill. It promotes a climate of public opinion tolerant of the terminally ill individual's right to end his or her own life in a planned manner. It works to improve existing laws on assisted suicide. It does not encourage suicide for any primary reason other than terminal illness and approves suicide prevention work. It believes that the final decision to terminate one's life should be one's own. *See also* active euthanasia; euthanasia; hopelessly ill; suicide.

hemocytometer   An apparatus in which blood cells are counted. *See also* blood count; hematocrit; red blood cell.

hemodialysis   A procedure in which wastes are removed directly from a patient's blood by an artificial kidney machine called a dialyzer or hemodialyzer. Hemodialysis is used in patients with renal insufficiency or failure from many causes. Arteriovenous fistulas or external shunts provide access to a patient's bloodstream. *Synonyms*: dialysis; renal dialysis. *See also* dialysis; corporatization of health care; end stage renal disease; home hemodialysis; kidney; peritoneal dialysis.

hemodialysis, home   *See* home hemodialysis.

hemodialysis technician   A registered nurse or other qualified individual who is skilled in the operation of hemodialysis equipment and treatment of patients with kidney disorders requiring hemodialysis. *See also* hemodialysis; technician.

hemodialyzer *See* hemodialysis.

hemoglobin (Hb) A complex protein-iron molecule in the blood that carries oxygen from the lungs to the cells that need it and carbon dioxide away from the cells to the lungs. The normal concentrations of hemoglobin in the blood are 12 to 16 grams per deciliter in women and 13.5 to 18 grams per deciliter in men. *See also* blood count; cyanosis; hemoglobinometer.

hemoglobinometer Any of various types of instruments for measuring the hemoglobin concentration of blood. *See also* blood; hemoglobin.

hemophilia A group of hereditary bleeding disorders in which there is a deficiency of one of the factors required for blood to clot. Hemophilia A (classic hemophilia, factor VIII deficiency) is a chromosome X-linked disorder due to deficiency of coagulation factor VIII. Hemophilia B (factor IX deficiency, Christmas disease) is also a chromosome X-linked disorder due to deficiency of coagulation factor IX. The clinical severity of the disorder varies markedly with the extent of the deficiency. *See also* factor VIII; hematology; blood transfusion.

hemoptysis Coughing up blood from the respiratory tract, as in hemoptysis secondary to tuberculosis of the lungs. *See also* cough.

hemorrhage Excessive loss of blood characterized by profuse bleeding from the blood vessels. *Compare* hemostasis. *See also* abruptio placenta; hematemesis; hematochezia.

hemorrhoid An itching or painful mass of dilated veins in swollen anal tissue. *Synonym*: piles. *See also* colon and rectal surgery.

hemostasis The arrest of hemorrhage by intrinsic physiological mechanisms or by surgical or pharmacological intervention. *Compare* hemorrhage.

Henry J. Kaiser Family Foundation, The *See* The Henry J. Kaiser Foundation.

heparin A naturally occurring acid mucopolysaccharide (complex carbohydrate) that has potent anticoagulant properties. It is used in the prevention and treatment of disorders in which there is excessive or undesirable clotting, such as thrombophlebitis, pulmonary embolism, and certain cardiac conditions. It is administered intravenously or subcutaneously. *See also* anticoagulant.

hepatic encephalopathy An encephalopathy (disease of the brain) due to advanced disease of the liver. It is characterized by disturbances of consciousness that may progress to deep coma (hepatic coma) and psychiatric changes of varying degrees. *See also* encephalopathy; jaundice; liver failure.

hepatitis Inflammation of the liver, usually due to viral infection, but also the result of alcohol and drug abuse or certain bacterial infections. Hepatitis A virus is found in fecal matter and is spread by improper food handling or by contaminated seafood. Hepatitis B virus is spread by direct blood contact, such as with blood transfusions or use of contaminated needles. Hepatitis C, or non-A, non-B hepatitis, is also transmitted through blood contact. *See also* infectious hepatitis; jaundice; liver failure; serum hepatitis; tatooing.

hepatitis, infectious *See* infectious hepatitis.

hepatitis, serum *See* serum hepatitis.

hepatologist A physician specializing in diseases of the liver. *See also* cirrhosis of the liver; gastroenterologist.

herbalism A type of alternative medicine based on remedies of plant origin. *See also* alternative medicine; herbs.

herbs Vascular nonwoody plants, that is, leafy plants with no permanent parts above the ground, used in medicine or cooking. *See also* herbalism.

hereditary Transmitted or capable of being transmitted from parent to offspring. *See also* heredity.

heredity **1.** The transmission of characteristics from parent to offspring. *See also* inheritance. **2.** The genetic make-up of an individual. *See also* gene; genetics; genotype.

hernia Any abnormal protrusion of one anatomical structure, or part of it, through another. The most common variety is herniation of part of the intestine through a weakness in the abdominal wall. *Synonym*: rupture. *See also* hiatal hernia; inguinal hernia; truss.

hernia, hiatal *See* hiatal hernia.

hernia, inguinal *See* inguinal hernia.

HERO *See* Health Education Resource Organization.

heroin A highly addictive, powerful chemical derivative of morphine made from the opium poppy. People inject, snort, or ingest it for its euphoric effects. *See also* euphoria; junkie; methadone; narcotics; opiate.

herpes simplex A virus that causes many human disorders, ranging from the familiar recurrent "cold sore" around the lips to encephalitis. Herpes infection is either primary or recurrent. Most infections of the lips, mouth, pharynx, eye, and central nervous system are caused by herpes simplex virus type I (HSV type I). Genital and neonatal infections are usually caused by herpes simplex virus type II (HSV type II). *Compare* HIV. *See also* virus.

herpes zoster An acute infectious disease caused by the varicella-zoster virus. It is due to reactivation of the virus latent in sensory nerve ganglia following a previous infection, usually chickenpox. It causes pain in a specific sensory distribution followed by virus multiplication in the same area of skin with the production of crops of characteristic skin lesions that look like blisters. *Synonym*: shingles. *See also* chickenpox; virus.

HESCA *See* Health Sciences Communications Association.

heterosexuality Sexual attraction to persons of the opposite sex. *Compare* bisexuality; homosexuality; transsexuality.

heuristics **1.** A method of solving problems involving intelligent trial and error. By contrast, an algorithmic method of solving problems is a clearly specified procedure that is guaranteed to give the correct answer. **2.** In computer science, heuristic pertains to using a problem-solving technique in which the most appropriate solution of several found by alternative methods is selected at successive stages of a program for use in the next step of the program. *Compare* algorithm. *See also* trial and error.

HEW *See* Department of Health, Education, and Welfare.

HFMA *See* Healthcare Financial Management Association.

HFS *See* Human Factors Society.

HFSG *See* Healthcare Financing Study Group.

HHA *See* home health agency.

HHS *See* Department of Health and Human Services.

HI Abbreviation for Hospital Insurance Program. *See* Medicare, Part A.

HIA *See* Hearing Industries Association.

HIAA *See* Health Insurance Association of America.

hiatal hernia A condition in which a portion of the stomach protrudes through the diaphragm into the chest. *See also* hernia; stomach.

HIBAC *See* Health Insurance Benefits Advisory Council.

HIBCC *See* Health Industry Business Communications Council.

HIBR *See* Huxley Institute for Biosocial Research.

HIC *See* Health Information Council.

hiccup Spasmodic contraction of the diaphragm, either isolated or occurring in short-lived repetitive bursts. There is usually no obvious cause, but hiccups are sometimes due to a pathological process irritating the diaphragm.

HICN *See* health insurance claim number.

HIDA *See* Health Industry Distributors Association.

hidden agenda A secret or unannounced motivation or bias behind a statement or policy of a person or group when participating in an activity. *See also* agenda.

high-density lipoprotein (HDL) The smallest and densest of the lipoproteins. The cholesterol on them is nicknamed "good" cholesterol. They retrieve cholesterol from the body's tissues and transport it to the liver, which excretes much of it in the bile. *See also* cholesterol; lipoprotein.

Higher Education, Association of Black Nursing Faculty in *See* Association of Black Nursing Faculty in Higher Education.

high ground A position of superiority or advantage, especially one which is likely to accord with public opinion, in a debate, conflict, or election campaign.

high-mortality outlier A health care provider, such as an individual hospital, with mortality rates that are higher than expected after adjustment for patient-based factors, such as age, comorbidities, and severity of illness. *Compare* low-mortality outlier. *See also* outlier.

high-risk function An important function that exposes individual patients to a greater chance of undesirable occurrences if not carried out effectively and appropriately; also applies to services that are inherently risky, even when effectively and appropriately performed, because of certain patient attributes and/or newness of the service. *See also* function; important function.

high-risk nursery *See* neonatal intensive care unit.

high-risk pool A fund set up to offer health insurance to small groups and individuals who have been denied coverage or whose medical history makes rates too high. *See also* health insurance; risk; risk pool.

high-risk process An important process, procedure, or activity that exposes individual patients to a greater chance of undesirable outcomes if not carried out effectively and appropriately; also applies to activities and procedures that are inherently risky, even when effectively and appropriately performed, because of certain patient attributes and/or newness of the activity or procedure. *See also* important process; process.

high tech Products or services using advanced technology; for example, microelectronics and computers are considered to be high tech. *Compare* low tech. *See also* technology.

high-volume function A function that is performed frequently or affects large numbers of patients; for example, discharge planning is an organizational function that is performed frequently and may affect large numbers of patients. *See also* function; important function; volume.

high-volume process An important process, procedure, or activity that is performed frequently or affects large numbers of patients; for example, some diagnostic radiology and clinical laboratory tests are high-volume processes in most hospitals. *See also* important process; process; volume.

Hill-Burton Act Legislation, and the programs under that legislation, for federal assistance in construction and modernization of hospitals and other health facilities, beginning with the Hospital Survey and Construction Act of 1946. *See also* hospital.

HIMA *See* Health Industry Manufacturers Association.

HIMSS *See* Healthcare Information and Management Systems Society.

HIPC Acronym for health insurance purchasing cooperative. *See* health alliance.

hip joint The joint formed by the rounded upper end (head of the femur) and the socket (acetabulum) of the hip bone. *See also* hip replacement; joint.

Hippocrates of Cos (460-circa 370 BC) A Greek physician who is generally regarded as the father of medicine. An oath that appears in the body of work attributed to Hippocrates and his school, and known as the Hippocratic oath, has been the ethical guide of the medical profession since those days. *See also* code of ethics; Hippocratic oath; neohippocraticism.

Hippocratic oath A statement, attributed to the ancient Greek physician Hippocrates, that serves as an ethical guide for physicians and is incorporated into the graduation ceremonies at many medical schools. The duties "to do no harm" and of confidentiality are based in the Hippocratic oath. It reads as follows: "I swear by Apollo the physician, by Aesculapius, Hygeia, and Panacea, and I take to witness all the gods, and all the goddesses, to keep according to my ability and my judgment the following Oath: To consider dear to me as my parents him who taught me this art; to live in common with him and if necessary to share my goods with him; to look upon his children as my own brothers, to teach them this art if they so desire without fee or written promise; to impart to my sons and the sons of the master who taught me and disciples who have enrolled themselves and have agreed to the rules of the profession, but to these alone, the precepts and the instruction. I will prescribe regimen for the good of my patients according to my ability and my judgment and never do harm to anyone. To please no one will I prescribe a deadly drug, nor give advice which may cause his death. Nor will I give a woman a pessary to procure abortion. But I will preserve the purity of my life and my art. I will not cut for stone, even for patients in whom the disease is manifest; I will leave this operation to be performed by practitioners (specialists in this art). In every house where I come I will enter only for the good of my patients, keeping myself far from all intentional ill-doing and all seduction, and especially from the pleasures of love with women or with men, be they free or slaves. All that may come to my knowledge in the exercise of my profession or outside of my profession or in daily commerce with men, which ought not to be spread abroad, I will keep secret and will never reveal. If I keep this oath faithfully, may I enjoy my life and practice my art, respected by all men and in all times; but if I swerve from it or violate it, may the reverse be my lot." *See also* Aesculapius; Hygeia; Panacea; code of ethics.

hip replacement An operation frequently undertaken in patients disabled by osteoarthritis or other disorders of the hip, in which the joint is totally replaced by a ball-and-socket device made of artificial materials. *See also* hip joint; orthopaedic/orthopedic surgery.

HIRA *See* Health Industry Representatives Association.

hirsutism An abnormal degree of hairiness. *See also* hair.

HIS *See* Health Interview Survey; hospital information system.

Hispanic Health and Human Services Organizations, National Coalition of *See* National Coalition of Hispanic Health and Human Services Organizations.

Hispanic National Bar Association (HNBA) A national organization founded in 1972 composed of

3,800 members of 19 local and eight state bar associations concerned with cultivating the science of jurisprudence; promoting reform in the law; facilitating the administration of justice; advancing the standing of the legal profession; and promoting high standards among Hispanic lawyers. Formerly (1980) La Raza National Bar Association. *See also* attorney; bar; lawyer.

Hispanic Nurses, National Association of *See* National Association of Hispanic Nurses.

Histochemical Society (HS) A national organization founded in 1950 composed of 550 physicians and scientists who employ histochemical and cytochemical techniques in their research. *See also* histochemistry; histology.

histochemistry An extension of microscopical staining techniques whereby known chemical reactions are used in order to identify particular compounds or types of compounds in the tissues and structures under examination. *See also* chemistry; histology; pathology; stain.

histocompatibility A state of mutual tolerance that allows some tissues to be grafted effectively to other tissues or blood to be transfused without rejection by a recipient. *See also* blood transfusion; histocompatibility antigen; transplantation.

histocompatibility antigen (HLA) Any of various antigens on the surface of cell membranes that serve to identify a cell as self or nonself. These antigens determine whether a tissue graft or blood transfusion will be accepted or rejected by a recipient. *See also* antigen; blood transfusion; histocompatibility; transplantation.

Histocompatibility and Immunogenetics, American Society for *See* American Society for Histocompatibility and Immunogenetics.

histogram A graphic display, using a bar graph, of the frequency distribution of a variable. Rectangles are drawn so that their bases lie on a linear scale representing different intervals, and their heights are proportional to the frequencies of the values within each of the intervals. A bell-shaped distribution is considered normal; skewed results represent problems or inefficiencies or may signal that unexpected processes are occurring. *See also* bar graph; variable.

histologic technician An allied health professional skilled in processing sections of body tissue by fixation, dehydration, embedding, sectioning, decalcification, microincineration, mounting, and routine and special staining. Histologic technicians are one type of allied health professional for which the Committee on Allied Health Education and Accreditation has accredited education programs. *Synonym*: histotechnician. *See also* allied health professional; histologic technologist; histology; medical technologist; technician.

histologic technologist An allied health professional who performs all functions of a histotechnician as well as the more complex procedures for processing tissues. A histotechnologist identifies tissue structures, cell components, and their staining characteristics, and relates them to physiological functions. Histologic technologists are one type of allied health professional for which the Committee on Allied Health Education and Accreditation has accredited education programs. *Synonym*: histotechnologist. *See also* allied health professional; histology; medical technologist.

histologist A medical scientist, such as a pathologist, biologist, or laboratory technologist, who specializes in the examination and study of cells and tissues. *See also* histology.

histology The branch of biology dealing with the microscopic identification of cells and tissue and the organization of cells into various body tissues. *See also* biology; histochemistry; microscopic anatomy.

histopathologist A pathologist or other qualified individual who specializes in the study of changes in diseased tissues. *See also* histologist; histology; pathology.

histopathology laboratory A laboratory in which tissues are microscopically examined. *See also* clinical laboratory; laboratory; microscope.

Historical Society, Optometric *See* Optometric Historical Society.

historic fact *See* fact.

history A chronological record of events, as of the life or development of an institution, often including an explanation of those events. *See also* accreditation history; case history; family history; legislative history; medical history; psychohistory; social science.

history, accreditation *See* accreditation history.

history, case *See* case history.

History of Chiropractic, Association for the *See* Association for the History of Chiropractic.

History of Dentistry, American Academy of the *See* American Academy of the History of Dentistry.

history of disease, natural *See* natural history of disease.

history, family *See* family history.

history, legislative *See* legislative history.

history, medical *See* medical history.

History of Medicine, American Association for the *See* American Association for the History of Medicine.

History of Nursing, American Association for the *See* American Association for the History of Nursing.

History of Pharmacy, American Institute of the *See* American Institute of the History of Pharmacy.

history, psycho- *See* psychohistory.

History Research, Society for Life *See* Society for Life History Research.

History of Technology, Society for the *See* Society for the History of Technology.

histotechnologist *See* histologic technologist.

Histotechnology, National Society for *See* National Society for Histotechnology.

HIV Acronym for human immunodeficiency virus, which can cause a breakdown of the body's immune system, leading in some cases to the development of acquired immunodeficiency syndrome (AIDS). Previously called HTLV III (human T lymphotropic virus, type III). *See also* acquired immunodeficiency syndrome; retrovirus.

HIV/AIDS Program A national AIDS (acquired immunodeficiency syndrome) awareness program founded in 1983 of the United States Conference of Mayors. It acts as a forum for information exchange among members and provides policy information to the media. *See also* acquired immunodeficiency syndrome; HIV.

HIV infection The presence of human immunodeficiency virus (HIV) in the blood and body secretions of an individual who is capable of infecting other people if the infected individual's blood or secretions comes in contact with another person's blood (sharing needles, blood transfusions), cavity linings (vagina, rectum), or broken skin (cuts, abrasions). *See also* acquired immunodeficiency syndrome; AIDS-related complex; asymptomatic HIV infection; HIV; persistent generalized lymphadenopathy.

HIV infection, asymptomatic *See* asymptomatic HIV infection.

HLA *See* histocompatibility antigen.

HMAC *See* Hazardous Materials Advisory Council.

HMCRI *See* Hazardous Materials Control Resources Institute.

HME *See* Health Media Education.

HMO *See* health maintenance organization.

HMO, network model *See* network model HMO.

HMO, staff model *See* staff model HMO.

HNA *See* Hospice Nurses Association.

HNBA *See* Hispanic National Bar Association.

Hodgkin's disease A malignant disease of the lymphoid and reticuloendothelial systems that was described by Thomas Hodgkin, a British Quaker physician, in 1832. *Synonym*: Hodgkin's lymphoma. *See also* lymphoma; hematology-oncology; reticuloendothelial system.

Hodgkin's lymphoma *See* Hodgkin's disease.

holding A court's decision on the specific question under consideration in a hearing. The holding has precedential significance. Sometimes the term is used more broadly to indicate any ruling of the court. *See also* court.

holding company A corporate entity organized for the purpose of owning stock in and managing one or more corporations. Holding companies traditionally own many corporations in widely different business areas. *See also* company; corporatization of health care; network; parent company.

Holistic Dental Association (HDA) A national organization founded in 1980 composed of 200 dentists, chiropractors, dental hygienists, physical therapists, and physicians interested in a holistic approach to better dental care for patients. It expands techniques, medications, and philosophies that pertain to extractions, anesthetics, fillings, crowns, and orthodontics. In addition to conventional treatments, it encourages use of homeopathic medications, acupuncture, cranial osteopathic medicine, nutritional techniques, and physical therapy in treating patients. *See also* dentistry; holistic health.

holistic health The belief that the whole individual, his or her own responsibility for his or her well-being, and a variety of influences (for example, social, psychological, environmental) affect health, including nutrition, exercise, and mental relaxation. *Synonym*: wholistic health. *See also* fitness; health promotion; preventive medicine; wellness.

Holistic Medical Association, American *See* American Holistic Medical Association.

holistic medicine A doctrine of preventive and therapeutic medicine that emphasizes the importance of regarding a person as a whole being within his or her social, cultural, and environmental context rather than as a patient with isolated malfunction of a particular system or organ. *See also* holistic health; medicine.

Holistic Nurses Association, American *See* American Holistic Nurses Association.

home for the aged A residential care facility that provides health-related, personal, social, and recreational services to elderly persons. *See also* aging; residential care facility.

home care *See* home health care.

Home Care, Accreditation Manual for *See Accreditation Manual for Home Care.*

Home Care Accreditation Program The survey and accreditation program of the Joint Commission on Accreditation of Healthcare Organizations for eligible home health care organizations. *See also* accreditation; *Accreditation Manual for Home Care*; home health care; Joint Commission on Accreditation of Healthcare Organizations; survey.

Home Care, National Association for *See* National Association for Home Care.

home care program An organizational entity that provides home health care. *See also* home health care; hospital-based home care program.

home care program, hospital-based *See* hospital-based home care program.

home dialysis *See* home hemodialysis.

home equipment management services Services, including the selection, delivery, setup, and maintenance of equipment, to meet a patient's or client's needs in his or her place of residence, and the education of patients or clients in the use of such equipment. *See also* home health care; home infusion services; home pharmaceutical services.

home, foster care *See* foster care home.

home, funeral *See* funeral home.

Home Health Agencies, American Federation of *See* American Federation of Home Health Agencies.

home health agency (HHA) A public or private organization that provides home health care. To be certified under Medicare an agency must provide skilled nursing services and at least one additional therapeutic service (physical therapy, speech therapy, occupational therapy, medical social services, or home health aide services) in the home, under a plan established and periodically reviewed by a physician. *See also* agency; home health care; visiting nurse association.

home health aide A nursing assistant who provides personal care and home management services to allow patients to live in their own homes. A home health aide works under the supervision of a physician or registered nurse and may help patients bathe, exercise, and dress. He or she may check the patient's temperature, blood pressure, and pulse and respiration rates; give massages; and help give medications. *See also* aide; homemaker; nursing assistant; personal care; visiting nurse association.

home health care Services provided by health professionals in an individual's place of residence on a per-visit or per-hour basis to patients or clients who have or are at risk of an injury, an illness, or a disabling condition or who are terminally ill and require short-term or long-term intervention by health professionals. These services may include dental, medical, nursing, occupational therapy, physical therapy, speech-language pathology and audiology, social work, and nutrition counseling services. *Synonyms:* home care; home health services; in-home care. *See also* home infusion services; intensive home health care; intermediate care; intermediate home health care; intermittent care; maintenance home health care; skilled nursing care.

home health care agency *See* home health agency.

home health care aide *See* home health aide.

home health care, intensive *See* intensive home health care.

home health care, intermediate *See* intermediate home health care.

home health care, maintenance *See* maintenance home health care.

home health services *See* home health care.

home hemodialysis Long-term hemodialysis performed in the home. *See also* hemodialysis.

home infusion services Home health services, home pharmaceutical services, and home equipment management services directly related to the administration of drug therapy by continuous or intermittent infusion to patients or clients in their place of residence. *See also* home health care; home equipment management services; home pharmaceutical services.

Homelessness and Mental Illness, National Resource Center on *See* National Resource Center on Homelessness and Mental Illness.

homemaker In home health care, an aide who mainly performs light housekeeping, shopping for groceries and household supplies, planning and making meals, changing bed linens, and doing laundry. *See also* home health aide; homemaker services.

homemaker services Nonmedical support services, such as bathing and cooking, given to homebound individuals who are unable to perform these tasks. Homemaker services are intended to preserve independent living and normal family life for the aged, disabled, sick, or convalescent. *See also* homemaker.

home management services Chore services, such as routine housekeeping tasks, minor household repairs, shopping, lawn care, and snow shoveling; homemaking services, which provide for and teach child care, personal care, and home management to individuals and families; housing services, which help individuals get, keep, and improve housing and modify existing housing; and money management services, which help set up workable budgets and deal with debts. *See also* home health care.

home nursing Nursing care provided to patients in their homes by members of the family. *See also* nursing.

Homeopathic Pharmacists, American Association of *See* American Association of Homeopathic Pharmacists.

Homeopathic Pharmacopeia of the United States One of three official compendia of drugs and medications in the United States recognized in the Federal Food, Drug, and Cosmetic Act. The other two are the *United States Pharmacopeia* and the *National Formulary*. *See also* compendium; *National Formulary*; *United States Pharmacopeia*.

homeopathy A system of medicine described by Samuel Hahnemann based on the simile phenomenon; that is, that disease is treated by administering minute doses of a drug that in massive amounts produces the symptoms in healthy individuals similar to those of the disease itself. This was said to stimulate bodily defense against the signs and symptoms. The Hahnemann Medical College now trains allopathic, rather than homeopathic physicians. *Compare* allopathy; osteopathic medicine; naprapathy; naturopathy.

Homeopathy, American Institute of *See* American Institute of Homeopathy.

Homeopathy, National Center for *See* National Center for Homeopathy.

homeostasis A steady state in the internal environment of the body maintained by feedback and control mechanisms, involving primarily the nervous and endocrine systems. *See also* biology;

endocrinology.

home pharmaceutical services Services that procure, prepare, preserve, compound, dispense, and/or distribute pharmaceutical products to meet a patient's or client's needs in his or her place of residence, and that monitor a patient's or client's clinical status while in his or her place of residence. *See also* home equipment management services; home health care; home infusion services; pharmaceutical services.

home plan In Blue Cross and Blue Shield reciprocity programs, the particular Blue Cross organization that provides a subscriber's coverage. Reciprocity is a mutual agreement and business process in which Blue Cross and Blue Shield organizations process claims for services rendered by providers in their respective jurisdictions against coverage plans written by other Blue Cross and Blue Shield organizations. *See also* Blue Cross plan; host plan.

home, rest *See* rest home.

Homes for the Aging, American Association of *See* American Association of Homes for the Aging.

home and school visitor *See* school social worker.

Homes and Hospitals Association, American Baptist *See* American Baptist Homes and Hospitals Association.

Homes and Services for Children, National Association of *See* National Association of Homes and Services for Children.

Homes Society, Lutheran Hospitals and *See* Lutheran Hospitals and Homes Society.

home visit *See* visit.

homicide *See* murder.

homogenization A process by which the particles in a fluid are broken up and evenly distributed. It usually refers to milk in which the fat globules are broken up and dispersed to prevent the cream from separating from the milk. *See also* nutrition.

homograft *See* allograft.

homophobia Fear or dislike of homosexuals and homosexuality. *See also* homosexuality; phobia.

homosexuality Sexual attraction to persons of the same sex. *Compare* bisexuality; heterosexuality; transsexuality. *See also* gay; homophobia; lesbianism; pederasty.

honorarium A payment given to a professional person for services for which fees are not legally or traditionally required. *See also* fee.

hopelessly ill Suffering from an incurable illness.

See also terminal illness.

horizontal agreement An agreement between or among direct competitors. *See also* agreement.

horizontal integration Organizing or relating together of like entities performing at the same functional level; for example, two or more hospitals sharing the same medical staff or sharing the same nursing staff with a single nurse executive. The purpose of horizontal integration is to improve the degree to which resources are used efficiently and to increase purchasing power and marketing and management capacity. *Compare* vertical integration. *See also* integration.

hormone A substance produced by one tissue and conveyed by the bloodstream to another to cause physiological activity, such as growth or metabolism. Examples of hormones include human growth hormone, human follicle stimulating hormone, human luteinizing hormone, and human thyroid stimulating hormone. *See also* cortisol; endocrinology; estrogen; gonadotropin; growth hormone; hormone replacement therapy; insulin; protein; sex hormone.

hormone, growth *See* growth hormone.

Hormone and Pituitary Program, National *See* National Hormone and Pituitary Program.

hormone replacement therapy A technique designed to relieve some of the unpleasant symptoms experienced by women during and after menopause, by boosting estrogen levels artificially. *See also* hormone; menopause; replacement therapy.

hormone, sex *See* sex hormone.

Horney Clinic, Karen *See* Karen Horney Clinic.

Horticultural Therapy Association, American *See* American Horticultural Therapy Association.

horticulture The cultivation of a garden including fruits, vegetables, flowers, and/or ornamental plants.

hoshin Japanese word meaning "focus like the arrow on a compass." *See also* hoshin planning; kaizen.

hoshin planning A planning and management technique with seven specific tools designed to help an organization target one or two "breakthrough goals," rather than trying to accomplish too many things at once. *See also* hoshin; planning.

hospice A concept, originated in England, of caring for the terminally ill and their families in a manner that enables the patient to live as fully as possible, makes the entire family the unit of care, and centers the caring process in the home whenever appropri-

ate. Inpatient facilities are available for patients unable to be cared for at home. The hospice team includes nurses, social workers, chaplains, and volunteers, as well as physicians. *See also* terminal care; terminal illness.

Hospice Association of America (HAA) A national organization founded in 1985 composed of 1,300 hospices, home health agencies, community cancer centers and health professionals concerned with promoting the concept of hospice. *See also* hospice.

Hospice Organization, National *See* National Hospice Organization.

hospice benefit A Medicare benefit that pays for hospice care for beneficiaries with a life expectancy of six months or less. Hospices authorized under Medicare must provide nursing care, social services, physician care, and counseling services. *See also* benefit; Medicare.

Hospice Education Institute (HEI) A nonmembership organization founded in 1985 that provides educational and informational services to health professionals and the public on subjects, such as hospice care, death and dying, and bereavement counseling. *See also* hospice.

Hospice, National Institute for Jewish *See* National Institute for Jewish Hospice.

Hospice Nurses Association (HNA) A national organization founded in 1985 composed of 400 registered nurses involved in hospice care. It promotes high professional standards in hospice nursing. *See also* hospice; nurse.

Hospice Organization, National (NHO) *See* National Hospice Organization.

hospital A health care organization that has a governing body, an organized medical staff and professional staff, and inpatient facilities and provides medical, nursing, and related services for ill and injured patients twenty-four hours per day, seven days per week. For licensing purposes, each state has its own definition of hospital. *See also* governing body; health care organization; Hill-Burton Act; medical staff.

hospital accreditation *See* accreditation.

Hospital Accreditation Program (HAP) The survey and accreditation program of the Joint Commission on Accreditation of Healthcare Organizations for eligible hospitals. *See also* accreditation; *Accreditation Manual for Hospitals*; hospital; Joint Commission on Accreditation of Healthcare Organizations; survey.

Hospital Activities, Commission on Professional and *See* Commission on Professional and Hospital Activities.

hospital, acute care *See* acute care hospital.

hospital administrator *See* administrator.

hospital, affiliated *See* affiliated hospital.

hospital affiliation A contractual agreement between a health plan and one or more hospitals whereby the hospital provides the inpatient benefits offered by the health plan. *See also* health plan.

Hospital Annual Conference, Wills Eye *See* Wills Eye Hospital Annual Conference.

hospital, associate *See* medical control.

Hospital Association of America, Lutheran *See* Lutheran Hospital Association of America.

Hospital Association, American *See* American Hospital Association.

Hospital Association, American Osteopathic *See* American Osteopathic Hospital Association.

Hospital Association, American Society for Healthcare Education and Training of the American *See* American Society for Healthcare Education and Training of the American Hospital Association.

Hospital Association, Baptist *See* Baptist Hospital Association.

Hospital Association, National Society of Patient Representation and Consumer Affairs of the American *See* National Society of Patient Representation and Consumer Affairs of the American Hospital Association.

hospital attorney A lawyer employed by a hospital, who manages the legal affairs of the hospital. *See also* attorney; hospital; hospital law.

Hospital Attorneys, American Academy of *See* American Academy of Hospital Attorneys.

Hospital Audiences (HAI) An organization founded in 1969 to promote the cultural enrichment of mentally and physically disabled individuals, primarily in hospitals, nursing homes, mental health and retardation facilities, and shelters for the homeless. It arranges for individuals to attend cultural events and brings cultural events and art workshops into institutions for those unable to leave.

hospital autopsy An autopsy performed by a pathologist or other member of the medical staff on the body of a person who had at some time been a patient of the hospital. *See also* autopsy; hospital.

hospital auxiliary *See* auxiliary.

hospital, back-up *See* back-up hospital.

hospital-based ambulatory care center An organized hospital facility providing nonemergency medical and/or dental services to patients who are not assigned to a bed as inpatients during the time services are rendered. An emergency department in which services are provided to nonemergency patients does not constitute an organized ambulatory care center. *Compare* freestanding ambulatory care center. *See also* ambulatory health care; hospital.

hospital-based home care program A home care program sponsored by a hospital. *See also* home care program; home health care; hospital.

hospital-based physician A physician who spends the predominant part of his or her practice time within one or more hospitals instead of in an office setting or provides services to one or more hospitals or their patients. Hospital-based physicians often have a special financial arrangement with the hospital (salary or percentage of fees collected), and frequently include pathologists, anesthesiologists, radiologists, and emergency physicians. *See also* anesthesiologist; emergency physician; hospital; pathologist; radiologist.

hospital base year Hospital fiscal year ending on or after September 30, 1982, for which costs are used to determine the unadjusted target rate per discharge used to establish the hospital-specific component of the diagnosis-related group price used in prospective payment systems of Medicare and other third parties. *See also* diagnosis-related groups; hospital component; Medicare.

hospital bed An accommodation including lodging, food, and routine medical and nursing services provided in a hospital. *See also* bed; hospital; hospital corner.

hospital benefits Benefits provided under a health insurance policy or plan providing coverage for hospital charges incurred by an insured person because of illness or injury. *See also* benefits; hospital.

hospital blood bank A blood bank that is owned and operated by a hospital primarily to meet the needs of its own patients. *See also* blood bank; hospital.

hospital board *See* governing body.

Hospital Bureaus of America, Medical-Dental- *See* Medical-Dental-Hospital Bureaus of America.

hospital, certified *See* certified hospital.

hospital chain *See* multihospital system.

hospital, charitable *See* charitable hospital.

hospital, children's *See* children's hospital.

hospital, chronic disease   *See* chronic disease hospital.

hospital, city   *See* municipal hospital.

Hospital Clinical Nursing Education, Institute for   *See* Institute for Hospital Clinical Nursing Education.

hospital closure   The closing of a hospital or of any special care units or departments within a hospital.

hospital, community   *See* community hospital.

Hospital and Community Psychiatry, Institute on   *See* Institute on Hospital and Community Psychiatry.

hospital component   In Medicare, the hospital-specific target rate per discharge, reflecting the hospital's average base-year experience in treating patients under the cost-based reimbursement methodology used prior to prospective pricing. *See also* hospital base year; Medicare.

hospital consultant   A person who, as an independent contractor, provides advice on organization and management to hospitals. *See also* consultant; independent contractor.

hospital corner   A tight-fitting triangular fold made by tucking a sheet and blanket securely under a mattress at the foot of the bed and along each side. *See also* hospital bed.

hospital, county   *See* county hospital.

hospital, day   *See* day hospital.

hospital death rate   The number of deaths of hospital inpatients in relation to the total number of inpatients over a given period. *See also* disease-specific death rate; hospital; inpatient; mortality rate.

Hospital Dentists, American Association of   *See* American Association of Hospital Dentists.

hospital department   A division of a hospital, such as pharmacy, housekeeping, dietary, and nursing departments, which often supports clinical departments, such as pediatrics and surgery departments. *See also* clinical department; department; hospital.

hospital discharge abstract   *See* discharge abstract.

hospital discharge abstract system   A system for abstracting a minimum data set from hospital medical records for the purpose of producing summary statistics about hospitalized patients; for example, the hospital inpatient enquiry (HIPE) and professional activity study (PAS). The statistical tabulations commonly include length of stay by final diagnosis, surgical operations, and specified hospital services, and also give outcomes, such as "death" and "discharged alive from hospital." This system is usually considered inadequate for performance-based quality-of-care evaluation and epidemiologic

purposes because it is not possible to infer representativeness or to generalize; this is because the data usually lack a defined denominator and the same person may be counted twice or more in the event of two or more hospital discharges during the period of inquiry. *See also* discharge abstract; professional activity study (PAS); hospital.

Hospital Discharge Survey (HDS)   Since 1965 an annual national survey conducted by the National Center for Health Statistics, monitoring admissions and discharges of patients to and from a sample of short-stay general and specialty hospitals. Data are collected on, for example, diagnoses, procedures, and lengths of stay. *See also* National Center for Health Statistics.

hospital, district   *See* district hospital.

hospital emergency department   *See* emergency department.

hospital engineer   An individual who is responsible for the operation of a hospital's physical plant and equipment. *See also* engineering; hospital.

Hospital Engineering (of AHA), American Society for   *See* American Society for Hospital Engineering.

hospital epidemiologist   A physician, nurse, or other qualified individual typically responsible for conducting a hospital's infection control program. *See also* epidemiologist; hospital; infection control.

hospital, federal government   *See* federal government hospital.

Hospital Financing Study Group   *See* Healthcare Financing Study Group.

Hospital Food Service Administrators, American Society for   *See* American Society for Hospital Food Service Administrators.

hospital formulary   A list of all the drugs routinely stocked by a hospital's pharmacy. *See also* drug formulary; formulary; hospital.

hospital, for-profit   *See* investor-owned hospital.

hospital, general   *See* general hospital.

hospital, government   *See* government hospital.

hospital hospitality house   A temporary residential facility for patients and their families.

Hospital Hospitality Houses, National Association of   *See* National Association of Hospital Hospitality Houses.

hospital indemnity   A form of insurance that provides a stated weekly or monthly payment while the insured is hospitalized regardless of expenses incurred or other insurance. *See also* hospital; indemnity.

hospital infection   *See* nosocomial infection.

hospital information system (HIS)   An integrated, computer-assisted system designed to store, manipulate, and retrieve information dealing with administrative and clinical aspects of providing health services within the hospital. *See also* clinical information system; information system; management information system.

Hospital Insurance Program (HI)   *See* Medicare, Part A.

hospital, investor-owned   *See* investor-owned hospital.

hospitalism   The effects of lengthy or repeated hospitalization or institutionalization on patients, especially infants and children (in whom the condition may be characterized by social regression, personality disorders, and stunted growth) and the elderly (in whom the condition may be characterized by disorientation).

hospitality house, hospital   *See* hospital hospitality house.

Hospitality Houses, National Association of Hospital   *See* National Association of Hospital Hospitality Houses.

hospitalization   The act of placing a person in a hospital as a patient or the condition of being hospitalized. *See also* hospital; partial hospitalization; weekend hospitalization.

Hospitalization, American Association for Partial   *See* American Association for Partial Hospitalization.

hospitalization, day   *See* partial hospitalization.

hospitalization, night   *See* partial hospitalization.

hospitalization, partial   *See* partial hospitalization.

hospitalization services, partial   *See* partial hospitalization services.

hospitalization, weekend   *See* weekend hospitalization.

hospitalize   To place in a hospital for diagnosis and treatment. *See also* hospitalization.

Hospitalized Veterans Writing Project (HVWP)   An organization founded in 1946 composed of individuals and organizations interested in encouraging hospitalized US veterans to write for pleasure and rehabilitation during their hospital stay. *See also* veteran; writer.

hospital law   A subspecialty of medical law dealing with the legal aspects of hospital administration and hospital legal liability. *See also* health law; hospital attorney; law; medical law.

hospital, licensed   *See* licensed hospital.

Hospital Literature Index   A quarterly index to English-language journal articles in health administration, planning, organization, economics, legislation, accreditation and licensure, and health insurance. *See also* HEALTH FILE.

hospital, long-term   *See* long-term hospital.

hospital marketing   The marketing of hospital services to the community served by the hospital. *See also* hospital; marketing.

Hospital Materials Management, American Society for   *See* American Society for Hospital Materials Management.

Hospital Medical Education, Association for   *See* Association for Hospital Medical Education.

hospital, mental   *See* psychiatric hospital.

hospital mortality rate   Number of deaths as a proportion of the total number of hospital patients or admissions. *See also* mortality rate; proportion.

hospital, municipal   *See* municipal hospital.

hospital, night   *See* night hospital.

hospital, nonfederal government   *See* nonfederal government hospital.

hospital, not-for-profit   *See* not-for-profit hospital.

Hospital Nursing Education, Institute for Clinical   *See* Institute for Clinical Hospital Nursing Education.

hospital organization, physician-   *See* physician-hospital organization.

Hospital Pharmacists, American Society of   *See* American Society of Hospital Pharmacists.

hospital-physician independent contractor relationship   As applied to a hospital-physician contract, the relationship in which a hospital is presumed to control only the result to be accomplished by a physician under contract, not the methods by which a physician exercises professional judgment in fulfillment of contractual obligations. *See also* independent contractor.

Hospital Podiatrists, American Association of   *See* American Association of Hospital Podiatrists.

hospital, prison   *See* security hospital.

hospital, private   *See* private hospital.

hospital privileges   *See* admitting privileges.

hospital profile   A longitudinal or cross-sectional statistical summary of hospital-specific objective health care data used to assess and improve health care delivery. *See also* hospital; hospital profiling; profile; profiling.

hospital profiling   Aggregating and analyzing health care data representing distinctive features or characteristics of a hospital. *See also* hospital; hospital profile; profile; profiling.

hospital, proprietary *See* investor-owned hospital.

hospital, psychiatric *See* psychiatric hospital.

hospital, public *See* public hospital.

hospital, registered *See* registered hospital.

hospital, rehabilitation *See* rehabilitation hospital.

Hospital Research and Educational Trust (HRET) An organization founded in 1944 that encourages and engages in educational, research, and demonstration activities to improve the management of hospitals and health services. *See also* hospital; research.

hospital, resource *See* medical control.

Hospitals *See Hospitals and Health Networks.*

Hospitals, Accreditation Manual for *See Accreditation Manual for Hospitals.*

Hospitals, American Association of Eye and Ear *See* American Association of Eye and Ear Hospitals.

Hospitals of America, Voluntary *See* Voluntary Hospitals of America.

Hospitals Association, American Baptist Homes and *See* American Baptist Homes and Hospitals Association.

hospital, satellite *See* satellite hospital.

Hospitals, Children in *See* Children in Hospitals.

Hospitals, Council of Teaching *See* Council of Teaching Hospitals.

Hospitals for Crippled Children, Shriners *See* Shriners Hospitals for Crippled Children.

hospital, security *See* security hospital.

hospital, self-insured *See* self-insured hospital.

Hospitals, General Constituency Section for Small or Rural *See* General Constituency Section for Small or Rural Hospitals.

Hospitals and Health Networks The monthly publication of the American Hospital Association. Formerly (1993) *Hospitals. See also* American Hospital Association.

Hospitals and Homes Society, Lutheran *See* Lutheran Hospitals and Homes Society.

hospital, short-stay *See* short-term hospital.

hospital, short-term *See* short-term hospital.

Hospitals, National Association of Private Psychiatric *See* National Association of Private Psychiatric Hospitals.

Hospitals, National Association of Public *See* National Association of Public Hospitals.

Hospitals, National Council of Community *See* National Council of Community Hospitals.

Hospital Social Work Directors, Society for *See* Society for Hospital Social Work Directors.

hospital social worker *See* medical/hospital social worker.

hospital, specialty *See* specialty hospital.

Hospitals and Programs, Section for Rehabilitation *See* Section for Rehabilitation Hospitals and Programs.

Hospitals, Section for Metropolitan *See* Section for Metropolitan Hospitals.

Hospitals and Related Institutions, National Association of Children's *See* National Association of Children's Hospitals and Related Institutions.

hospital staff The body of hospital employees. *Compare* medical staff. *See also* staff.

Hospital Statistics, AHA *See AHA Hospital Statistics.*

Hospital Survey and Construction Act *See* Hill-Burton Act.

Hospitals, Volunteer Trustees of Not-For-Profit *See* Volunteer Trustees of Not-For-Profit Hospitals.

hospital, teaching *See* teaching hospital.

hospital, tertiary care *See* tertiary care hospital.

hospital, university *See* university hospital.

hospital utilization The number of hospital stays or hospital days per 1,000 persons; for example, 150 hospital stays for every 1,000 persons in one year. *See also* utilization.

hospital volume The number of a particular procedure (such as coronary artery graft bypass procedure) performed or condition (such as congestive heart failure) treated in a hospital over a specified time period. A high-volume procedure or condition often provides the basis for performance measurement, assessment, and improvement. *See also* hospital; volume.

hospital, voluntary *See* voluntary hospital.

Hospital Workers Union, Independent *See* Independent Hospital Workers Union.

host plan A Blue Cross reciprocity program in which one Blue Cross plan pays the claims of an individual who is a subscriber to a different Blue Cross plan. *See also* Blue Cross plan; control plan; home plan; plan.

house call A professional visit made to a home, especially by a physician. *See also* visit.

house, hospital hospitality *See* hospital hospitality house.

House, Nurses' *See* Nurses' House.

house officer *See* housestaff.

housestaff Individuals, licensed as appropriate, who are graduates of medical, dental, osteopathic, or podiatric schools; who are appointed to a health care organization professional graduate training program that is approved by a nationally recognized accrediting body approved by the US Department of Education; and who participate in patient care under the direction of licensed independent practitioners of the pertinent clinical disciplines who have clinical privileges in the organization and are members of, or are affiliated with, the medical staff. *Synonyms*: house officer; house staff. *See also* teaching hospital.

Housestaff Organizations, National Federation of *See* National Federation of Housestaff Organizations.

housekeeper, executive *See* executive housekeeper.

housekeeping department In health care, a division of an organization providing for cleaning of premises and furnishings, including control of pathogenic organisms. *See also* department; executive housekeeper; housekeeping director.

housekeeping director An individual who manages the hospital's housekeeping program. *See also* housekeeping department.

Howard Hughes Medical Institute A nonprofit scientific and philanthropic organization incorporated in 1953 in Delaware, whose principal purpose is medical research and support of science education. Through its medical research program, its investigators conduct biomedical research throughout the United States in the fields of cell biology and regulation, genetics, immunology, neuroscience, and structural biology. The Institute is qualified as a medical research organization, not as a private foundation, under the federal tax code.

HPS *See* Health Physics Society.

HRET *See* Hospital Research and Educational Trust.

HRSA *See* Health Resources and Services Administration.

HS *See* Harvey Society; Hemlock Society; Histochemical Society.

HSA *See* health service area; health systems agency.

HSAC *See* Health Security Action Council.

HSC *See* Health Sciences Consortium.

HSQB *See* Health Standards and Quality Bureau.

HTLV III *See* human T lymphotropic virus, type III.

Hughes Medical Institute, Howard *See* Howard Hughes Medical Institute.

Human Behavior, Institute for the Advancement of *See* Institute for the Advancement of Human Behavior.

Human Biology Council (HBC) A national organization founded in 1974 composed of individuals who are involved in fields related to human biology, including physical anthropology, sports medicine, genetics, nutrition, physiology, and pediatrics. It promotes the study of human biology and sponsors seminars and workshops. *See also* biology.

human chorionic gonadotropin (HCG) A hormone secreted by the placenta that aids the implantation of the fertilized egg in the uterine wall. The presence of HCG in blood and/or urine is used as a positive finding for pregnancy. *See also* gonadotropin; hormone; pregnancy.

Human Development, National Institute of Child Health and *See* National Institute of Child Health and Human Development.

Human Development Services, Office of *See* Office of Human Development Services.

human engineering *See* engineering psychology.

Humane Options in Childbirth Experiences, Center for *See* Center for Humane Options in Childbirth Experiences.

human factors The branch of industrial psychology dealing with designing machines so that humans can use them effectively. *See also* engineering psychology.

Human Factors Society (HFS) A national organization founded in 1957 composed of 4,800 psychologists, engineers, industrial designers, and other scientists and practitioners who are interested in the use of human factors and ergonomics in the development of systems and devices of all kinds. It promotes the discovery and exchange of knowledge concerning human characteristics that apply to the design of systems and devices intended for human use and operation. *See also* engineering psychology; ergonomics; human factors.

human genetics The science of biological variation in humans. *See also* genetics.

Human Genetics, American Society of *See* American Society of Human Genetics.

human immunodeficiency virus *See* HIV.

human insulin, recombinant *See* recombinant human insulin.

Humanistic Psychology, Association for *See* Association for Humanistic Psychology.

humanitarian A person who is devoted to promoting human welfare and the advancement of social reforms. *See also* human rights; philanthropy.

humanities Those branches of knowledge, such as philosophy, literature, and art, that are concerned with human thought and culture. *Synonym*: liberal arts.

Humanities, Association for Faculty in the Medical *See* Association for Faculty in the Medical Humanities.

humankind *See* personkind.

Human Resource Certification Institute (PAI) A certifying body founded in 1975 that accredits professionals in personnel administration and industrial relations based on their mastery of the field. *See also* certification; human resources; human resources management.

human resource management *See* human resources management.

Human Resource Management, Society for *See* Society for Human Resource Management.

human resources All personnel available to an organization or all the workers in a society. *Synonym*: manpower. *See also* personnel; staffing.

Human Resources Administration, American Society for Healthcare *See* American Society for Healthcare Human Resources Administration.

Human Resources, Committee on Labor and *See* Committee on Labor and Human Resources.

human resources department *See* personnel department.

human resources management The field of managing people in work organizations. Personnel, like money and time, are seen as resources that require management in order for an organization to function effectively. *See also* personnel management.

human rights The basic rights and freedoms to which all humans are entitled, such as the rights to life and liberty, freedom of thought and expression, and equality before the law. *See also* humanitarian; patient rights; rights.

Human Rights, American Association of Physicians for *See* American Association of Physicians for Human Rights.

Human Rights, Bay Area Physicians for *See* Bay Area Physicians for Human Rights.

human sensing *See* sensing.

Human Services, Department of Health and *See* Department of Health and Human Services.

Human Services Organizations, National Coali-

tion of Hispanic Health and *See* National Coalition of Hispanic Health and Human Services Organizations.

human T lymphotropic virus, type III (HTLV III) The former name for the human immunodeficiency virus (HIV). *See* HIV.

Human Values, Society for Health and *See* Society for Health and Human Values.

humor That which is intended to induce laughter or amusement, as in therapeutic humor. *See also* laughter.

humoral immune response An immune response that is mediated by B lymphocytes or B cells and occurs against bacterial invasion. *See also* immune response.

humoralism The ancient theory that health and illness result from a balance or imbalance of bodily liquids called humors (phlegm, blood, black bile or gall, yellow bile or choler). The theory is associated with Hippocratic writers, but it long antedates Hippocrates. Humoralism was displaced only in 1858 by Rudolf Virchows' *Cellularpathologie*. *See also* phlegm.

Humor, American Association for Therapeutic *See* American Association for Therapeutic Humor.

Humulin *See* recombinant human insulin.

hunger A strong desire for food. *See also* cachexia; starvation.

hung jury A jury so irreconcilably divided in opinion that they cannot agree on any verdict by the required unanimity. *See also* dynamite instruction; jury; jury trial; mistrial.

Husband-Coached Childbirth, American Academy of *See* American Academy of Husband-Coached Childbirth.

Huxley Institute for Biosocial Research (HIBR) A national organization founded in 1971 composed of 3,000 physicians, psychiatrists, biochemists, scientists, and other professionals interested in promoting biomedical research and the practice of orthomolecular medicine for the prevention and treatment of chronic disorders affecting brain function. *See also* orthomolecular medicine.

HVWP *See* Hospitalized Veterans Writing Project.

hydrogenation The process of transforming a soft or liquid polyunsaturated fatty acid into a harder, more saturated fat by adding hydrogen, usually accomplished by bubbling hydrogen gas through the liquid oil. Saturated fat means hydrogenated fat. *See also* hypercholesterolemia; saturated fat.

hydrophobia Irrational fear of water. *See also* phobia. *See* rabies.

hydrotherapy The use of water to treat disorders; mostly limited to exercises in special pools for rehabilitation of paralyzed patients. Water is propelled by a pump that forces air and water in a given direction which massages the body or parts of the body. *See also* physical therapy.

hyfrecator A machine that produces a current, used by podiatrists to eliminate plantar warts (warts on the sole of the foot). *See also* verrucae.

Hygeia The goddess of health, one of the daughters of Aesculapius and sister of Panacea. *See also* Aesculapius; Hippocratic oath; hygiene.

hygiene **1.** The science dealing with the promotion and preservation of health. **2.** Conditions and practices that serve to promote or preserve health, as in personal hygiene. *Synonym:* cleanliness.

hygiene accreditation, dental *See* dental hygiene accreditation.

Hygiene, American Academy of Industrial *See* American Academy of Industrial Hygiene.

Hygiene, American Board of Industrial *See* American Board of Industrial Hygiene.

Hygiene, American Society of Tropical Medicine and *See* American Society of Tropical Medicine and Hygiene.

Hygiene Association, American Industrial *See* American Industrial Hygiene Association.

hygiene, dental *See* dental hygiene.

hygiene, oral *See* oral hygiene.

Hygiene Society, American Natural *See* American Natural Hygiene Society.

hygienist, dental *See* dental hygienist.

hygienist, public health dental *See* public health dental hygienist.

Hygienists, American Conference of Governmental Industrial *See* American Conference of Governmental Industrial Hygienists.

Hygienists' Association, American Dental *See* American Dental Hygienists' Association.

hyper- A prefix meaning over, above, beyond, excessive. *Compare* hypo-.

hyperactivity A condition characterized by excessive movement and restlessness, seen especially in children. *See also* attention-deficit disorder.

hyperbaric chamber A chamber in which the oxygen pressure is higher than in the atmosphere, used to treat carbon monoxide poisoning, decompression sickness, gangrene, and other disorders. *See also* hyperbaric medicine.

Hyperbaric Medical Society, Undersea and *See* Undersea and Hyperbaric Medical Society.

hyperbaric medicine The treatment of disease in an environment of atmospheric pressure with higher than normal oxygen. It is used to treat conditions, such as carbon monoxide poisoning, decompression sickness, and gangrene. *Synonym:* baromedicine. *See also* hyperbaric chamber; nitrogen narcosis.

hypercholesterolemia A metabolic condition, usually inherited, characterized by excessive amounts of cholesterol in the blood. High levels of cholesterol and other lipids may lead to the development of atherosclerosis (fatty deposits on the arteries' inner walls). Hypercholesterolemia may be reduced or prevented by avoiding saturated fats, which are found in red meats, eggs, and dairy products. *See also* atherosclerosis; cholesterol; hydrogenation; saturated fat.

hypergeometric distribution *See* probability distribution.

hyperglycemia A greater than normal amount of glucose in the blood usually resulting from diabetes mellitus. *Compare* hypoglycemia. *See also* blood glucose; diabetes mellitus; glucose.

hyperkalemia A greater than normal amount of potassium in the blood, commonly caused by acute renal failure. This condition, left untreated, may cause marked cardiac abnormalities, including cardiac standstill (asystole). *Compare* hypokalemia. *See also* electrolytes.

hyperlipidemia An excess of lipids in the blood plasma, including the glycolipids, lipoproteins, and the phospholipids. *See also* lipid; lipoprotein.

hypernatremia A greater than normal amount of sodium in the blood, caused by excessive water loss from the body (for example, from excessive urination, diarrhea, sweating) or inadequate water intake. *Compare* hyponatremia. *See also* electrolytes.

hyperpyrexia An extreme degree of fever, defined as being present when the body temperature reaches 41° C (106° F) or above. It may represent the upper end of the distribution of thermoregulatory response to infections and toxic and immunological agents, or it may result from damage to the central nervous system control mechanism, as with stroke. It is a danger to life if allowed to continue, as in heat stroke. *Synonym:* hyperthermia. *Compare* hypothermia. *See also* fever; malignant hyperpyrexia.

hyperpyrexia, malignant *See* malignant hyperpyrexia.

hypertension Persistently high arterial blood pressure that is associated with increased risk of morbidity and mortality from cardiovascular, cerebrovascular, and renal disease. *Compare* hypotension. *See also* antihypertensive; blood pressure; hypertensive encephalopathy; malignant hypertension; normotensive.

Hypertension, American Society of *See* American Society of Hypertension.

Hypertension Association, National *See* National Hypertension Association.

hypertension, malignant *See* malignant hypertension.

hypertensive encephalopathy An encephalopathy (disease of the brain) due to malignant hypertension. It is characterized by a complex of cerebral phenomena, including headache, convulsions, and coma. *See also* encephalopathy; malignant hypertension.

hyperthermia *See* hyperpyrexia.

hyperthermia, malignant *See* malignant hyperpyrexia.

hyperthyroidism A disorder in which the thyroid is overactive, excessively increasing metabolism. *Compare* hypothyroidism. *See also* goiter; iodine; thyroid gland.

hypnosis A passive, sleeplike state in which perception and memory are altered, and a person is more responsive to suggestion and has more recall than usual. It is used in psychotherapy and in medicine to induce relaxation and relieve pain. *See also* behavioral medicine; hypnotherapy.

Hypnosis, American Board of Psychological *See* American Board of Psychological Hypnosis.

Hypnosis, American Society of Clinical *See* American Society of Clinical Hypnosis.

Hypnosis, Association to Advance Ethical *See* Association to Advance Ethical Hypnosis.

Hypnosis Association, American *See* American Hypnosis Association.

Hypnosis and Psychotherapy, Institute for Research in *See* Institute for Research in Hypnosis and Psychotherapy.

Hypnosis, Society for Clinical and Experimental *See* Society for Clinical and Experimental Hypnosis.

Hypnotherapists, American Association of Professional *See* American Association of Professional Hypnotherapists.

Hypnotherapists, American Guild of *See* American Guild of Hypnotherapists.

hypnotherapy Therapy based on or using hypnosis, as in treatment of chronic pain. *See also* hypnosis; therapy.

hypnotic A drug that induces sleep. *See also* drug; sedative; sleep; thalidomide.

hypnotic suggestion A suggestion imparted to a person in the hypnotic state, by which she or he is induced to alter perceptions or memory or to perform actions. *See also* hypnosis; hypnotherapy; suggestion.

hypnotism The practice of inducing hypnosis. *Synonym*: mesmerism. *See also* hypnosis.

hypnotist A hypnotherapist or an entertainer. *See also* hypnosis.

Hypnotist Examiners, American Council of *See* American Council of Hypnotist Examiners.

Hypnotists' Association, American *See* American Hypnotists' Association.

hypo- A prefix meaning below, beneath, under, less than normal, deficient. *Compare* hyper-.

hypochondriasis A chronic, abnormal concern about one's own health. *See also* neurosis.

hypodermic *See* syringe.

hypodermic needle A short, slender, hollow needle used to inject drugs beneath the skin. *See also* aspirating needle; needle; syringe.

hypodermic syringe *See* syringe.

hypoglycemia A less than normal amount of glucose in the blood, usually caused by administration of too much insulin or excessive secretion of insulin by the islet cells of the pancreas. *Compare* hyperglycemia. *See also* blood glucose; glucose; pancreas.

hypokalemia A condition that may be caused by diuretic therapy and other etiologies, in which an inadequate amount of potassium, the major intracellular cation, is found in the blood. *Compare* hyperkalemia. *See also* electrolytes.

hypomania A moderate degree of elevation of mood and activity. *See also* mania.

hyponatremia A lower than normal amount of sodium in the blood that, left untreated, can produce confusion and lethargy, seizure, or coma. It may be caused by inadequate excretion of water or by excessive water intake. *Compare* hypernatremia. *See also* electrolytes.

hypotension Abnormally low blood pressure. *Compare* hypertension. *See also* blood pressure.

hypothalamus A part of the brain that activates, controls, and integrates the peripheral autonomic nervous system, endocrine processes, and bodily functions, such as sleep, sexual desire, appetite, and body temperature. *See also* brain.

hypothermia Abnormally low body temperature. *Compare* hyperpyrexia. *See also* temperature.

hypothesis **1.** A supposition or conjecture, arrived at from observation or reflection, that leads to predictions that can be proved or refuted. **2.** Any conjectured case in a form that will allow it to be tested and proved or refuted. *See also* alternative hypothesis; hypothesis testing; null hypothesis.

hypothesis, alternative *See* alternative hypothesis.

hypothesis, null *See* null hypothesis.

hypothesis testing A statistical procedure that involves stating something to be tested, collecting evidence, and then making a decision as to whether the statement should be accepted as true or rejected. *See also* hypothesis.

hypothyroidism A disorder in which the activity of the thyroid is decreased. *Synonyms*: myxedema; underactive thyroid gland. *Compare* hyperthyroidism. *See also* goiter; thyroid gland.

hysterectomy The operation of surgically removing the uterus, performed either through the abdominal wall (abdominal hysterectomy) or through the vagina (vaginal hysterectomy). *See also* partial hysterectomy; oophorectomy; radical hysterectomy; total hysterectomy; uterus; vagina.

hysterectomy, abdominal *See* hysterectomy.

hysterectomy, partial *See* partial hysterectomy.

hysterectomy, radical *See* radical hysterectomy.

hysterectomy, subtotal *See* partial hysterectomy.

hysterectomy, supracervical *See* partial hysterectomy.

hysterectomy, total *See* total hysterectomy.

hysterectomy, vaginal *See* hysterectomy.

hysteria **1.** A neurosis characterized by the presentation of a physical ailment without an organic cause. *See also* neurosis; psychogenic; psychosomatic. **2.** Uncontrollable emotion.

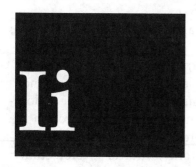

IAHB *See* Institute for the Advancement of Human Behavior.

iamatology The science of remedies. *See also* remedy.

IAR *See* Institute for Aerobics Research.

IARASM *See* Institute for Advanced Research in Asian Science and Medicine.

IASA *See* Insurance Accounting and Systems Association.

iatrogenesis Creation of an injury or an illness as a result of an activity (a procedure, therapy, or other element of care) performed by a physician or, more broadly, any health professional. *See also* cascade iatrogenesis; iatrogenic; nosocomial.

iatrogenesis, cascade *See* cascade iatrogenesis.

iatrogenic **1.** Resulting from the professional activities of physicians, or, more broadly, from the activities of health professionals. Originally applied to disorders induced in the patient by autosuggestion based on a physician's examination, manner, or discussion, the term is currently applied to any undesirable condition in a patient occurring as the result of treatment by a physician (or other health professional), especially to infections acquired by the patient during the course of treatment. **2.** Pertaining to an illness or injury resulting from a procedure, therapy, or other element of care. *See also* cascade iatrogenesis; nosocomial.

iatrogenic disease Illness or injury resulting from physicians' professional activities, or, more broadly, from the activities of health professionals. *See also* disease; iatrogenic.

iatrology The science of medicine. *See also* medicine.

iatros Greek word meaning "physician." *See also* iatrogenic; physician.

IATROS A nonmembership organization founded in 1981 composed of physicians who are interested in promoting the practice of independent Hippocratic medicine without political or governmental control. Hippocratic medicine is defined by IATROS as the private practice of medicine that contracts for service solely between the patient and his or her private doctor. The organization believes that the trend toward socialized medicine deviates from a true medical ethic and will eventually serve only the state, not the patient. *See also* Hippocrates of Cos; iatros; socialized medicine.

IBM compatible *See* PC clone.

IBM look-alike *See* PC clone.

IBS *See* Biometric Society.

IBR *See* Institutes for Behavior Resources.

ICC *See* Injury Control Center.

ICCP *See* Institute for Certification of Computer Professionals.

ICCS *See International Classification of Clinical Services.*

ICD-9-CM *See International Classification of Diseases, Ninth Revision, Clinical Modification.*

ICF *See* intermediate care facility.

ICF/MR Abbreviation for an intermediate care facility specializing in care for the mentally retarded. *See* intermediate care facility.

ICLRN *See* Interagency Council on Library Resources for Nursing.

icon In computer science, an on-screen graphic that may be used to access programs, data files, commands, or other stored or computer-embedded information. *See also* computer.

ICPBC *See* Institute of Certified Professional Business Consultants.

ICPI *See* Intersociety Committee on Pathology Information.

ICPS *See* Interamerican College of Physicians and

Surgeons.

icterus　*See* jaundice.

ICU　*See* intensive care unit.

ID　*See* identification number.

IDA　*See* Indian Dental Association.

IDDM　Acronym for insulin-dependent diabetes mellitus. *See* diabetes mellitus.

idea　An intellectual notion or conception. *See also* concept; ideation; ideology; imagination; research and development; theorem.

ideal　**1.** A thought or conception of something in its absolute perfection. **2.** Conforming to an ultimate form or standard of perfection or excellence. *See also* ideal ethical observer; idealist.

ideal ethical observer　A theory proposing that an act can be judged as "right" by ascertaining whether "an ideal moral judge" would approve of it. The ideal moral judge would have the qualities of omniscience, omniprecipience, disinterest, and dispassion. *See also* disinterest; dispassion; ethics; omniprecipience; omniscience.

idealist　A person whose conduct is influenced by ideals that often conflict with practical considerations. *Compare* pragmatism; realist. *See also* ideal.

ideation　The formation of ideas, or the ability of the mind to form ideas. *See also* idea.

identical twins　Twins derived from a single fertilized ovum and therefore possessing identical genotypes. *Synonym*: monozygotic twins. *Compare* fraternal twins. *See also* genetics; genotype; twin.

identification number (ID, ID number)　In health insurance, the insured's or subscriber's group number, individual policy or contract number, or group number and unique individual or family policy and contract number. An identification number may be a Social Security number. *See also* health insurance; number.

Identification Manufacturers, Automated　*See* Automated Identification Manufacturers.

identification system, patient　*See* patient identification system.

identify　To ascertain the origin, nature, or definitive characteristics of, as in identifying the underlying factors contributing to organizational performance. *Compare* misidentify.

identity　The aggregate of characteristics by which a thing is definitively recognizable or known. *See also* identity crisis.

identity crisis　A psychosocial state or condition of disorientation and role confusion occurring especially in adolescents as a result of conflicting pressures and expectations and often producing acute anxiety. A social structure, such as a corporation, can exhibit an analogous state of confusion. *See also* adolescence; crisis; identity.

ideologue　An advocate of a particular ideology. *See also* ideology.

ideology　A systematic scheme of ideas, usually related to society or politics, or to the conduct of a class or group, and regarded as justifying actions. An ideology is often held implicitly or is adopted as a whole and maintained, regardless of the course of events. *See also* idea; ideologue; implicit; politics; society.

idiocy　An outdated term for the severest grade of mental retardation. *See also* imbecility; mental retardation.

idiopathic　Of unknown cause, as in idiopathic disease (a disease for which there is no identifiable cause).

idiopathy　A disease of unknown cause.

idiosyncrasy　**1.** A characteristic unique to an individual or group. **2.** A peculiar or unusual variation, as in an unusual reaction to a drug, article of food, or other substance, that is not explicable on an immunological basis and not due to inherent toxicity of the substance concerned.

idiot　An outdated term for a person who is severely mentally retarded, now meaning a stupid or foolish person. *See also* mental retardation.

idiot savant　A mentally retarded person who exhibits genius in a highly specialized area, such as mathematics or music. *See also* mental retardation.

idle time　**1.** Time when an employee is unable to work because of equipment malfunction or other factors beyond the employee's control. **2.** Time during which a computer is not in use. *See also* time.

ID number　*See* identification number.

idol　A person or a thing that is blindly or excessively adored.

IDSA　*See* Infectious Diseases Society of America.

IEE　*See* Institute of Electrology Educators.

IEEE　*See* Institute of Electrical and Electronics Engineers.

IEEE Engineering in Medicine and Biology Society (EMBS)　A society of the Institute of Electrical and Electronics Engineers composed of 7,026 individuals. It is concerned with concepts and methods of the physical and engineering sciences applied in biology and medicine, including formalized mathematical theory, experimental science, technological developments, and practical clinical applications. It disseminates information on current methods and technologies used in biomedical and clinical engineering. *See also* bioengineering; Institute of Electrical and Electronics Engineers.

IEEE Lasers and Electro-Optics Society (LEOS) A society of the Institute of Electrical and Electronics Engineers that serves as a forum for discussion of quantum electronics, optoelectronic theory, and techniques and applications, and the design, development, and manufacture of systems and subsystems (such as lasers and fiberoptics). *See also* fiberoptics; Institute of Electrical and Electronics Engineers; laser; optics.

IFC *See* Infant Formula Council.

Ig *See* immunoglobulin.

IG *See* inspector general.

ignorant Lacking education or knowledge. *Compare* education; knowledge.

IGSP *See* Institute for Gravitational Strain Pathology.

IHCA *See* individual health care account.

IHCNE *See* Institute for Hospital Clinical Nursing Education.

IHCP *See* Institute on Hospital and Community Psychiatry.

IHPP *See* Intergovernmental Health Policy Project.

IHS *See* Indian Health Service.

IHWU *See* Independent Hospital Workers Union.

IIA *See* Impotence Institute of America; Information Industry Association; Intelligence Industries Association.

ILAR *See* Institute of Laboratory Animal Resources.

ileostomy A surgically created opening of the ileum on the abdominal surface, through which fecal matter is emptied. The procedure is performed in advanced or recurrent ulcerative colitis, Crohn's disease, or cancer of the large bowel. *See also* ileum; intestine; ostomy; stoma.

ileum The lower part of the small intestine. *See also* intestine.

ileus Intestinal obstruction from any cause, including that due to lack of intestinal motility. *See also* intestine; obstruction.

illation **1.** The act of inferring or drawing conclusions. *See also* infer; inference. **2.** A conclusion drawn. *See also* conclusion.

illegal Prohibited by law; for example, behavior that can result in either criminal sanctions (such as prison sentences or fines) or civil sanctions (such as liability or injunctions) is illegal. *Compare* legal; legalize.

Ill, National Alliance for the Mentally *See* National Alliance for the Mentally Ill.

illness An abnormal condition or disease, or a subjective state of a person who feels aware of not being well. *Compare* wellness. *See also* ailment; catastrophic illness; critical illness; disease; severity of illness; sickness; terminal illness.

illness, catastrophic *See* catastrophic illness.

illness, critical *See* critical illness.

Illness and Loss, (Division of Foundation of Thanatology), American Institute of Life Threatening *See* American Institute of Life Threatening Illness and Loss, (Division of Foundation of Thanatology).

illness, manic-depressive *See* manic-depressive illness.

illness, mental *See* mental illness.

Illness, National Resource Center on Homelessness and Mental *See* National Resource Center on Homelessness and Mental Illness.

illness, pedal *See* pedal illness.

illness, psychosomatic *See* psychosomatic illness.

illness, severity of *See* severity of illness.

illness, terminal *See* terminal illness.

illusion False impression or wrongful interpretation of what has been perceived by the senses. *Compare* hallucination. *See also* delirium; money illusion.

illusion, money *See* money illusion.

illustrator, medical *See* medical illustrator.

Illustrators, Association of Medical *See* Association of Medical Illustrators.

IM *See* implementation monitoring; intramuscular.

IMA *See* Islamic Medical Association.

image **1.** A picture or reproduction with a more-or-less likeness to an objective reality. **2.** The picture or representation of body structures and functions obtained through use of technologies, such as computerized axial tomography and x-ray. *Synonym:* diagnostic image. *See also* imaging.

image advertising A type of advertising directed at the creation of a specific image for an entity, such as a hospital boasting a considerable amount of technology and a large number of specialists, as distinguished from advertising directed at the specific attributes of the entity, such as the hospital's less-than-desirable location. Image advertising is frequently used in political campaigns to promote the idea of a candidate as "one of the people," rather than to point out a candidate's qualifications. *See also* advertise; comparative advertising; competitive advertising; deceptive advertising; false advertising; informative advertising.

image consultant A public relations professional who specializes in teaching executives and other persons how to project a more impressive image by dressing, speaking, socializing, and otherwise behaving in a more "executive" manner. *See also* consultant; image.

imagination The formation of a mental image of something that is neither perceived as real nor present to the senses. Also, the ability to confront and deal with reality by using the creative power of the mind. *See also* idea; mind.

imaging Use of technologies to produce pictures or images of body structures and functions, especially in radiological and ultrasound images. *Synonym:* diagnostic imaging. *See also* computerized axial tomography; image; magnetic resonance imaging; positron emission tomography; radiography; ultrasonics.

Imaging, American Society of Neuro- *See* American Society of Neuroimaging.

Imaging, Council on Diagnostic *See* Council on Diagnostic Imaging.

imaging, diagnostic *See* imaging.

imaging, magnetic resonance *See* magnetic resonance imaging.

Imaging Society, Computerized Medical *See* Computerized Medical Imaging Society.

Imaging, Society for Magnetic Resonance *See* Society for Magnetic Resonance Imaging.

imaging, ultrasound *See* ultrasound imaging.

imbecility An outdated term for mental retardation less severe than idiocy. *See also* idiocy; mental retardation.

IMD *See* institution for mental disease.

IMDA *See* Independent Medical Distributors Association.

imitation food A federal labeling definition for foods that contain a lower percentage of the food than specified by the federal government for the standard product. *See also* food.

immediate cause The nearest cause in point of time and space to a result. It is not necessarily the direct or proximate cause. *See also* cause; direct cause; proximate cause.

immediate customer A customer, such as a person or unit, that directly receives the output of a process. *See also* customer.

immune **1.** Protected from, or not susceptible, to a disease, especially infectious diseases. *See also* infectious diseases; immunization. **2.** A computer system protected against hacking or against destructive software devices, such as the virus and worm. *See also* virus; worm.

immune response A defense reaction of the body whereby an invading substance or antigen, such as a transplanted organ or bacteria, is recognized as foreign by the body. The body then produces antibodies specific against the antigen to destroy or neutralize it. There are two basic kinds of immune response: cell-mediated immune response and humoral immune response. *See also* cell-mediated immune response; humoral immune response; immunocompromised; lymphocyte.

immune response, cell-mediated *See* cell-mediated immune response.

immune response, humoral *See* humoral immune response.

immune system The organs, cells, and molecules responsible for the recognition and disposal of foreign (nonself) material that enters the body. *See also* immune response; immunology; reticuloendothelial system.

Immune System Disorders, National Coalition on *See* National Coalition on Immune System Disorders.

immunity **1.** The condition of being protected against infectious disease conferred either by the immune response generated by immunization or previous infection or by other nonimmunologic factors. *See also* immunization; natural immunity. **2.** In law, exemption from normal legal prosecution; for example, a hospital and a hospital medical staff are granted immunity from civil damage actions related to performing formal peer review if certain minimum due process rights are afforded the physician being reviewed as part of a disciplinary hearing process. *See also* charitable immunity; Good Samaritan laws; sovereign immunity.

immunity, charitable *See* charitable immunity.

immunity, natural *See* natural immunity.

immunity, sovereign *See* sovereign immunity.

immunization The induction of production against

infectious diseases. *See also* active immunization; immunity; passive immunization; toxoid.

immunization, active *See* active immunization.

immunization, acquired *See* active immunization.

immunization, passive *See* passive immunization.

immunize *See* vaccinate.

immunoassay A laboratory technique involving binding between an antigen and its homologous antibody to identify and quantify a substance in a sample. *See also* antibodies; antigen; assay; radioimmunoassay.

immunocompromised Unable to develop a normal immune response, as in an AIDS patient. *See also* immune response.

immunodeficiency The abnormal condition in which some part of the body's immune system is inadequate. As a result, resistance to infectious disease is decreased, as in AIDS and other disorders. *See also* acquired immunodeficiency syndrome; immune system; opportunistic infection.

immunodeficiency syndrome, acquired *See* acquired immunodeficiency syndrome.

immunodermatologist A dermatologist who is skilled in the subspeciality of immunodermatology. *See also* dermatologist; immunodermatology.

immunodermatology A subspecialty of dermatology dealing with the study of the cause, diagnosis, treatment, and outcome of skin diseases involving the immune system. *See also* dermatology; immune system.

immunogenetics **1.** The study of genetic control of immunity. *See also* immunity. **2.** The branch of immunology dealing with the molecular and genetic bases of the immune response. *See also* genetics; immunology.

Immunogenetics, American Society for Histocompatibility and *See* American Society for Histocompatibility and Immunogenetics.

immunoglobulin (Ig) Any of five structurally and antigenically distinct antibodies present in the blood serum and external secretions of the body. The five classes of immunoglobulins are IgA, IgD, IgE, IgG, and IgM. *See also* antibodies; immunology.

immunologist A physician or scientist specializing in immunology. *See also* allergy and immunology; immunology.

Immunologists, American Association of *See* American Association of Immunologists.

immunology The branch of biomedical science dealing with the response of an organism to antigenic challenge, the recognition of self and nonself, and all the biological (in vivo), serological (in vitro), and physical chemical aspects of immune phenomena. It encompasses the study of the structure and function of the immune system (basic immunology); immunization, organ transplantation, blood banking, and immunopathology (clinical immunology); laboratory testing of cellular and humoral immune function (laboratory immunology); and the use of antigen-antibody reactions in other laboratory tests (serology and immunochemistry). *See also* allergy and immunology; antibodies; desensitize; immune response; immune system; immunogenetics; radioimmunology; rejection; serology.

Immunology, American Academy of Allergy and *See* American Academy of Allergy and Immunology.

Immunology, American Board of Allergy and *See* American Board of Allergy and Immunology.

Immunology, American College of Allergy and *See* American College of Allergy and Immunology.

Immunology, American Osteopathic College of Allergy and *See* American Osteopathic College of Allergy and Immunology.

immunology, diagnostic laboratory *See* diagnostic laboratory immunology.

Immunology, Joint Council of Allergy and *See* Joint Council of Allergy and Immunology.

immunology, radio- *See* radioimmunology.

Immunology and Respiratory Medicine, National Jewish Center for *See* National Jewish Center for Immunology and Respiratory Medicine.

Immunology Society, American In-Vitro Allergy/ *See* American In-Vitro Allergy/Immunology Society.

Immunology Society, Clinical *See* Clinical Immunology Society.

immmunopathologist A pathologist who specializes in immunopathology. *See also* immunopathology; pathology.

immunopathology The branch of medical science and subspecialty of pathology dealing with the study of the causes, diagnoses, and prognoses of disease by the application of immunological principles to the analysis of tissues, cells, and body fluids. *See also* immunology; pathology.

immunosuppression A lowering by various agents of the body's normal immune response to the invasion of foreign substances. *See also* deliberate immunosuppression; immune response; incidental immunosuppression.

immunosuppression, deliberate *See* deliberate immunosuppression.

immunosuppression, incidental *See* incidental immunosuppresion.

immunosuppressive Drugs such as corticosteroids, biological agents, or procedures such as irradiation, which depress all or part of the immune system. *See also* cortisol; cortisone; immune system; immunosuppression; irradiation.

impact **1.** The effect or impression of one thing on another. *See also* outcome. **2.** The power of making a strong, immediate impression.

impair To diminish in strength, value, or quality, as in an impaired driver. *See also* impaired health care provider; physician impairment.

impaired health care provider A health care provider, such as a physician or nurse, who is unable to provide services with reasonable skill and safety to patients because of physical or mental illness, including alcoholism or substance dependence. *See also* drug abuse; employee assistance program; health care provider; physician impairment.

impaired physician *See* impaired health care provider; physician impairment.

Impaired Physician Program (IPP) A national organization founded in 1975 that provides assistance to physicians, other health professionals, and their spouses with problems, such as alcoholism, substance abuse, or codependence. It seeks to locate and identify persons in need of help and to provide assistance. It conducts inpatient and outpatient treatment programs and assists physicians and other health professionals in re-entering their profession. *See also* impaired health care provider; physician; physician impairment.

impairment Any loss or abnormality of psychological, physiological, or anatomical structure or function, according to the *International Classification of Impairments, Disabilities, and Handicaps* first published in 1980 by the World Health Organization. *See also* impair; disability; handicap; *International Classification of Impairments, Disabilities, and Handicaps*; physician impairment.

Impairment Bureau, Medical *See* Medical Impairment Bureau.

impairment, physician *See* physician impairment.

impanel The process by which jurors are selected and sworn in to their task. *See also* jury; jury trial; panel; voir dire.

impeachment An attempt to discredit the testimony of a witness in court. Impeachment is usually accomplished by presenting facts that either contradict the testimony or suggest that the witness is generally not worthy of belief. *See also* court; witness.

implant **1.** An object or material, such as an alloplastic or radioactive material, partially or totally inserted or grafted into the body for prosthetic, therapeutic, diagnostic, or experimental purposes; for example, a dental implant to provide support and retention to a complete denture. *See also* radioactive implant; silicone. **2.** To insert or graft an object or material into the body of a recipient, as in to implant a drug capsule. *See also* replant; transplant.

implantation The insertion or grafting into the body of biological, living, inert, or radioactive material. *See also* alloplastic; implant; organ bank; silicone; transplantation.

implant dentistry The field of dentistry dealing with the surgical insertion of dental transplants and the design and insertion of prosthodontic devices to replace missing teeth. *Synonym:* dental implantology; implant prosthodontics. *See also* dentistry; prosthodontics.

Implant Dentistry, American Academy of *See* American Academy of Implant Dentistry.

implant prosthodontics *See* implant dentistry.

Implant Prosthodontics, American Academy of *See* American Academy of Implant Prosthodontics.

implant, radioactive *See* radioactive implant.

Implants and Transplants, Academy for *See* Academy for Implants and Transplants.

implementation The process of putting into action policies, procedures, goals, objectives, and tasks; for example, the implementation of new standards. *See also* implementation monitoring.

implementation monitoring (IM) An approach used by the Joint Commission on Accreditation of Healthcare Organizations to evaluate a surveyed health care organization's progress toward compliance with new or revised standards that may require substantial time for implementation within organizations. Such standards are surveyed and scored, but resulting recommendations do not contribute to the accreditation decision. *See also* accreditation; implementation; Joint Commission on Accreditation of Healthcare Organizations; standard.

implicit Implied or understood but not directly

expressed, as in implicit criteria for assessing level of performance. *Compare* explicit. *See also* criteria; ideology; implicit criteria; implicit review.

implicit criteria In health care, criteria that are subjective and not specified in advance of a medical review process. *Compare* explicit criteria. *See also* criteria; implicit review; implied.

implicit review Review of processes or outcomes of care using subjective or implied criteria. *Compare* explicit review. *See also* implicit criteria; implied.

implied Not explicitly written or stated; determined by deduction from known facts, as in an implied contract is one created by actions but not necessarily written or spoken. *See also* deductive reasoning; implied consent.

implied consent The apparent acceptance of a proposed course of action or promise of outcome; for example, in life-threatening situations, a physician may undertake life-saving treatment without the expressed consent of a patient when the patient is unable to provide consent. Most states have a statute implying the consent of individuals who drive upon its highways to submit to some type of scientific test or tests measuring the alcoholic content of the driver's blood. Implied consent is based on the principle of beneficence, which prescribes that a person in serious need must be helped by one who can do so without harm or great inconvenience. *See also* beneficence; consent; informed consent.

important aspects of care Care activities or processes that occur frequently or affect large numbers of patients; that place patients at risk of serious consequences if not provided correctly, or if incorrect care is provided, or if correct care is not provided; and/or that tend to produce problems for patients or staff. Such activities or processes are deemed most important for purposes of continuous measurement and improvement.

important function An organizational function believed, on the basis of evidence or expert consensus, to increase the probability of achieving desired patient outcomes. Important organizational functions include, but are not limited to, patient rights and organizational ethics; entry to a setting or service; patient assessment; nutritional care; treatment of patients and operative and other invasive procedures; education of patients and family; leadership; management of information; management of human resources; management of the environment

of care; surveillance, prevention, and control of infection; and improvement of organizational performance. *See also* function; high-risk function; high-volume function.

important process A process believed, on the basis of evidence or expert consensus, to increase the probability that desired outcomes will occur. *See also* high-risk process; high-volume process; process.

impotence **1.** Weakness or ineffectualness. **2.** Inability of the male to initiate, maintain, or complete sexual intercourse. *See also* frigid; sex therapy; sexual intercourse.

Impotence Institute of America (IIA) An organization founded in 1983 composed of urologists, psychiatrists, psychologists, sex therapists and counselors, and plastic surgeons; manufacturers of penile implant devices; and hospitals and other institutions that offer assistance and meeting facilities for Impotents Anonymous and I-ANON. It informs and educates the public on the subject of impotence and its causes and treatments. *See also* impotence; sex therapy.

imprinting Rapid learning of species-specific behavior patterns that occurs with exposure to the proper stimulus at a sensitive period of early life.

improve To raise to a more desirable or more excellent quality or condition; to make better; to become better. *See also* improvement.

improvement The act or process of making or becoming better, as in continuous quality improvement, or the state of being improved, as in performance improvement. *See also* capital improvement; continuous quality improvement; performance improvement; process improvement.

improvement, capital *See* capital improvement.

improvement, continuous quality *See* continuous quality improvement.

improvement council, quality *See* quality improvement council.

Improvement in Health Care, National Demonstration Project on Quality *See* National Demonstration Project on Quality Improvement in Health Care.

improvement, performance *See* performance improvement.

improvement, process *See* process improvement.

improvement project, quality *See* quality improvement project.

improvement, quality *See* quality improvement.

improvement team, quality *See* quality improvement team.

impulse **1.** An impelling force, such as a cardiac impulse felt or seen over the chest with each heart beat. **2.** A mental urge to act in a particular way. *See also* instinct.

IMS *See* indicator measurement system; Institute of Mathematical Statistics.

IMSystem *See* indicator measurement system.

inaccurate Mistaken or incorrect, as in inaccurate data or an inaccurate conclusion. *Compare* accurate.

inadequate Not adequate to fulfill a need or meet a requirement, as in inadequate documentation. *Synonym*: insufficient. *Compare* adequate.

inadvertent Marked by unintentional lack of care, often accidentally, as in the needle was inadvertently left on the counter by the student.

inane Lacking substance or sense, as in an inane comment.

inappropriate Unsuitable or improper, given the set of circumstances, as in the course of action was inappropriate. *Compare* appropriate.

in-breeding Reproduction by the mating of individuals who are closely related and therefore have similar genotypes. In-breeding of animals is often desirable, for example, in the maintenance of genetically pure strains for laboratory purposes. In human populations, in-breeding increases the likelihood that undesirable recessive genes will find expression. Most societies forbid by custom, religion, or law unions between closely blood-related people (consanguineous relatives). *See also* gene; genotype.

incentive An expectation of a reward or fear of punishment that induces action or motivates effort. For example, the requirement that a patient pay the first dollars for a health service (a deductible) is a *negative incentive* (also called disincentive). A monetary reward to a health care organization or practitioner for decreasing hospital and practitioner costs is a *positive incentive*. *See also* incentive benefit plan; incentive pay plan; tax incentive.

incentive benefit plan A health plan that rewards beneficiaries for lowering their consumption of health services. *See also* benefit; health plan; incentive.

incentive, negative *See* incentive.

incentive pay plan A compensation program whereby wages increase as productivity increases above a set standard or base. *See also* incentive; pay; plan; wage.

incentive, positive *See* incentive.

incentive, tax *See* tax incentive.

inception The beginning of something, such as a project. *See also* inception cohort.

inception cohort A group of persons, assembled at a common time early in the development of a specific clinical disorder (for example, at the time of first exposure to a reputed cause of a disorder or at the time of initial diagnosis), who are followed thereafter in a study. *See also* cohort.

incest **1.** Sexual intercourse between close relatives, particularly those of first degree, for example, father and daughter, brother and sister. **2.** The statutory crime of sexual relations between persons who are so closely related that their marriage is illegal or forbidden by custom or law. *See also* taboo.

incidence In epidemiology, the frequency of new occurrences of a condition or disease within a defined time interval, as in the number of times a disease occurs during a year. *Synonym:* occurrence. *Compare* prevalence. *See also* epidemiology; incidence rate; incident.

incidence rate The number of new events or cases of a specified disease or condition divided by the number of people in a population at risk for the disease or condition during a specified period time, usually one year. *Compare* prevalence rate. *See also* incidence; rate.

incident An event or an occurrence that is usually unexpected and undesirable. An incident in a hospital, for example, is generally an event resulting in injury or the immediate threat of injury to a patient or other persons and for which the organization may be liable. When an incident is unexpected and occurs because of chance it is often called an accident, rather than an incident. *See also* accident; adverse patient occurrence; incident report; incident reporting.

incidental immunosuppression Immunosuppression resulting from chemotherapy or radiotherapy in cancer treatment. It may also occur in disease when the body's normal immune response is inadequate, as in AIDS. *See also* deliberate immunosuppression; immune response; immunosuppression.

incident report A written report, usually completed by a nurse and forwarded to risk management personnel, that describes and provides documentation for any unusual problem, incident, or other situation that is likely to lead to undesirable effects or that varies from established policies and procedures. *See also* incident; incident reporting; report.

incident reporting A system in many health care organizations for collecting and reporting adverse patient occurrences (APOs), such as medication errors and equipment failures. It is based on individual incident reports, usually completed by nurses who witness adverse events. For several reasons, including fear of punitive action, reluctance of nonphysicians to report incidents involving physicians, lack of understanding of what a reportable incident is, and lack of time for paperwork, the effectiveness of incident reporting is limited. Incident reporting is the central source of information in traditional risk management programs, identifying between 5% and 30% of APOs. *See also* adverse patient occurrence; occurrence reporting; occurrence screening; risk management.

incision **1.** A slit or opening made by cutting, as in an abdominal incision. *See also* thoracotomy; wound. **2.** The act of cutting.

inclusive Taking in the specified extremes as well as the area between them, as in inclusive language. *See also* inclusive language.

inclusive language Nonsexist language; language that is deliberately phrased so as to include both women and men explicitly rather than using masculine forms to cover both. *See also* inclusive; language.

incoherent **1.** Disordered, lacking logical connection or continuity, as in incoherent ideas. **2.** Unable to express oneself in an intelligible manner, as in an incoherent speaker. *Compare* coherent.

income The amount of money or its equivalent received during a period of time in exchange for labor or services, from the sale of goods or property, or as profit from financial investments. *See also* earned income; fixed income; money income; net income; real income; revenue; supplemental security income; unearned income.

income, earned *See* earned income.

income, fixed *See* fixed income.

income, money *See* money income.

income, net *See* net income.

income, real *See* real income.

Income Security Act, Employee Retirement *See* Employee Retirement Income Security Act.

income, supplemental security *See* supplemental security income.

income tax A tax based on income earned by a person or business. It is the main source of revenue for the federal government and one of the main sources for many states. *See also* tax.

income, unearned *See* unearned income.

incompetent **1.** Pertaining to a person who is legally incapable of understanding the nature and consequence of his or her actions and incapable of making a rational decision, including, for example, the mentally ill and minors. *See also* commitment; minor; non compos mentis; substituted judgment doctrine; surrogate; ward. **2.** Pertaining to a person who is unable to perform required work in an acceptable manner, as in an incompetent health professional. *Compare* competence. *See also* Peter principle.

incomplete abortion *See* abortion.

incontinence The inability to control urination or defecation. *See also* stress incontinence; urinary incontinence.

incontinence, stress *See* stress incontinence.

incontinence, urinary *See* urinary incontinence.

incorporate To legally organize under the laws of a state.

incremental cost *See* marginal cost.

incubation period The time period between exposure to a disease-causing organism, such as chickenpox, and the appearance of the symptoms and signs of the disease. *See also* disease.

incubator **1.** In hospitals, a special transparent apparatus that provides a controlled environment for premature or low-birth-weight infants. **2.** An apparatus that provides suitable conditions for the growth and development of microorganisms, cells, tissues, organs, or embryos. *See also* isolation incubator.

incubator bed A bed regularly maintained for premature and other infants who require special environmental conditions. *See also* bed; incubator.

incubator, isolation *See* isolation incubator.

incur To acquire or come into, as in insurance; to become liable for a loss, claim, or expense.

IND *See* investigational new drug.

indemnification The act of protecting against damage, loss, or injury; for example, in corporate law, the practice by which corporations pay expenses of officers or directors who are named as defendants in litigation relating to corporate affairs. *See also* directors' and officers' liability insurance; indemnify.

indemnified **1.** Insured or secured against loss or damage that may occur in the future. **2.** Reimbursed for loss or damages due to injury or harm.

indemnify   **1.** To insure or secure against loss or damage that may occur in the future. **2.** To compensate for loss or damage already suffered. *See also* indemnity.

indemnity   **1.** Security against damage, loss, or injury. **2.** Legal exemption from liability for damages. **3.** Compensation for damage, loss, or injury suffered. *See also* indemnity benefits.

indemnity benefits   Under health insurance policies, benefits in the form of cash payments rather than services. The indemnity insurance contract usually defines the maximum amounts that will be paid for the covered services. In most cases, after the provider of services has billed the patient in the usual way, the insured person submits to the insurance company proof that he or she has paid the bills and is then reimbursed by the insurance company in the amount of the covered costs, making up the difference himself or herself. In some instances, the provider of services may complete the necessary forms and submit them to the insurance company directly for reimbursement, billing the patient for costs that are not covered. *Compare* service benefits. *See also* benefits; indemnity.

indemnity, hospital   *See* hospital indemnity.

indemnity plan, managed   *See* managed indemnity plan.

independent audit   An audit conducted by an outside person or firm not connected in any way with the organization or individual being audited. *Compare* internal audit. *See also* audit.

independent contractor   An individual who is self-employed and who contracts to perform a piece of work according to his or her own methods. An independent contractor is subject to his or her employer's control only as to the end product or final result of his or her work. *See also* consultant; contractor; hospital-physician independent contractor relationship; piecework.

independent contractor relationship, hospital-physician   *See* hospital-physician independent contractor relationship.

independent events   Two or more events that do not affect each other.

Independent Hospital Workers Union (IHWU)   A national organization founded in 1980 representing hospital workers and protecting their rights to a fair salary and acceptable working conditions. *See also* labor union.

Independent Medical Distributors Association (IMDA)   A national organization founded in 1978 composed of 100 independent distributors of high-technology health care products.

independent physician association   *See* individual practice association.

independent practice association   *See* individual practice association.

independent practice association model HMO   A health maintenance organization (HMO) that contracts directly with physicians in independent practices; and/or contracts with one or more associations of physicians in independent practices; and/or contracts with one or more multispecialty group practices. The plan is predominantly organized around solo/single specialty practices. *See also* health maintenance organization; individual practice association.

independent practitioner   *See* licensed independent practitioner.

independent practitioner, licensed   *See* licensed independent practitioner.

independent variable   The characteristic being observed or measured that is hypothesized to influence an event or manifestation (the dependent variable) within the defined area of the relationships under study. The independent variable is not influenced by the event or manifestation but may cause it or contribute to its variation. In statistics, an independent variable is one of several variables that appear as arguments in a regression equation. *Compare* dependent variable. *See also* regression; regression analysis; variable.

index   **1.** A number or statistic that puts in context a condition, such as a current economic or financial state or level of performance, especially by relating it to a base year, the previous year, or some other time; for example, the consumer price index. Indexes are often used to make adjustments in rates, such as wage rates and pension benefits, set by long-term contracts. *See also* case-mix index; consumer price index; performance index. **2.** Something that serves to guide, point out, or otherwise facilitate reference, such as an alphabetized list of names, places, and subjects treated in a printed work, giving the page or pages on which each item is mentioned. *See also* Index Medicus; medical record index; therapeutic index.

index, AS-SCORE   *See* AS-SCORE index.

index case The first case, or model case, of a disease, as contrasted with subsequent cases. *See also* case.

index, case-mix *See* case-mix index.

index, consumer price *See* consumer price index.

index of leading indicators *See* economic indicator.

index, medical record *See* medical record index.

Index Medicus A monthly catalogue of the world's important biomedical literature, published since 1960 by the National Library of Medicine. A cumulative index is published annually as the *Cumulative Index Medicus*. *See also* index.

index, misery *See* misery index.

index, performance *See* performance index.

index, therapeutic *See* therapeutic index.

India, American Association of Psychiatrists from *See* American Association of Psychiatrists from India.

Indian Dental Association (IDA) A national organization founded in 1983 composed of 225 dentists in the United States who are of Asian-Indian descent. It seeks to further the professional education of members. *See also* dentistry.

Indian Health Board, National *See* National Indian Health Board.

Indian Health Care Association, American *See* American Indian Health Care Association.

Indian Health Service (IHS) A division of the US Public Health Service of the Department of Health and Human Services that is responsible for delivering public health and medical services to native American Indians throughout the United States. The federal government has a direct and permanent legal obligation to provide health services to most Indian people, undertaken in treaties written with the Indian Nations in the past two centuries. *See also* Public Health Service.

Indian Physicians, Association of American *See* Association of American Indian Physicians.

Indians Into Medicine (INMED) A nonmembership organization founded in 1973 to support American Indian students. It seeks to increase the awareness of and interest in health care professions among young American Indians; recruit and enroll American Indians in health care education programs; and place American Indian health professionals in service to American Indian communities. *See also* Native American; medicine.

Indian Social Workers Association, National *See*

National Indian Social Workers Association.

indicate 1. To point out or signify, as in the long white coat indicates an attending physician and not a medical student, or a fever indicates illness. **2.** To demonstrate the necessity, expedience, or advisability of, as in the hemorrhage from the wound indicates the need for emergency blood transfusion.

indicated In health care, a course of action that is warranted, given a certain set of circumstances; for example, an electrocardiogram is indicated for an adult patient complaining of crushing substernal chest pain. *See also* indicate; indication.

indication 1. A guideline, recommendation, or rule that specifies when certain courses of action are necessary, expedient, advisable or otherwise appropriate, as for a specific disease or condition. For example, the presence of an abnormality on barium enema, such as a filling defect, is one indication to perform colonoscopy. **2.** Something that serves to indicate, as in a fever in a week-old infant is an indication for blood cultures. *Compare* contraindication. *See also* indicate; indicated.

indicator 1. A quantitative measure used to measure and improve performance of functions, processes, and outcomes. *See also* aggregate data indicator; continuous variable indicator; indicator measurement system; outcome indicator; process indicator; rate-based indicator; sentinel event indicator. **2.** A statistical value that provides an indication of the condition or direction over time of performance of a defined process or achievement of a defined outcome. *See also* economic indicator; lagging economic indicator; leading economic indicator. **3.** A substance used to test for a particular reaction because of a predictable, easily detected change; for example, litmus paper turning pink on exposure to an acid.

indicator, aggregate data *See* aggregate data indicator.

indicator, continuous variable *See* continuous variable indicator.

indicator data collection logic An indicator information set component that describes the sequence of data element retrieval and aggregation through which numerator events and denominator events are identified by an indicator. *See also* indicator information set; logic.

indicator definition of terms An indicator information set component that explains terms used in the indicator statement. *See also* indicator information set; indicator statement.

indicator, desirable *See* desirable indicator.

indicator development form A form used to describe and record the development process for an individual indicator. *See also* indicator; indicator information set.

indicator, discrete variable *See* rate-based indicator.

indicator, economic *See* economic indicator.

indicator, health status *See* health status indicator.

indicator information set Indicator-specific information typically composed of an indicator statement, definition of terms, indicator type, rationale, description of indicator population, indicator data collection logic, and underlying factors that may explain variations in data. *See also* indicator; indicator data collection logic; indicator definition of terms; indicator rationale; indicator statement; indicator underlying factors.

indicator, lagging economic *See* lagging economic indicator.

indicator, leading economic *See* leading economic indicator.

indicator measurement system (IMSystem, IMS) A performance measurement system developed by the Joint Commission on Accreditation of Healthcare Organizations in conjunction with accredited health care organizations. It is designed to **1.** continuously collect objective performance data that are derived from the application of aggregate data indicators by health care organizations; **2.** aggregate, risk-adjust as necessary, and analyze the performance data on a national level; **3.** provide comparative data to participating organizations for use in their internal performance improvement efforts; **4.** identify patterns that may call for more focused attention by the Joint Commission at the organizational level; and **5.** provide a national performance database that can serve as a resource for health services research. Formerly (1992) indicator monitoring system. *See also* health services research; indicator; Joint Commission on Accreditation of Healthcare Organizations; performance; performance assessment; performance database; performance improvement; performance measurement.

indicator monitoring system *See* indicator measurement system.

indicator, outcome *See* outcome indicator.

indicator population An indicator information set component that describes an indicator's numerator and denominator; populations may be subcategorized to provide more homogeneous populations for subsequent data assessment. *See also* indicator information set.

indicator, process *See* process indicator.

indicator, rate-based *See* rate-based indicator.

indicator rationale An indicator information set component that explains why an indicator is useful in specifying and assessing the process or outcome care measured by the indicator. *See also* indicator information set.

indicator reliability The degree to which an indicator accurately and completely identifies occurrences from among all cases at risk of being indicator occurrences. *See also* data reliability; indicator validity; reliability.

indicator, sentinel event *See* sentinel event indicator.

indicator statement An indicator information set component that describes the function, process, or outcome being measured; for example, "patients for whom percutaneous transluminal coronary angioplasty has succeeded." *See also* indicator information set.

indicator testing process The process by which individual indicators are evaluated for many attributes, including their degrees of reliability and validity, and their feasibility. *See also* testing.

indicator threshold The level, value, or point at which indicator data signal the need for more in-depth review of the process or outcome measured by the indicator. *See also* threshold.

indicator underlying factors Indicator information set component that delineates patient, practitioner, organization, and community systems' characteristics that may explain variations in performance data and thereby direct performance improvement activities and efforts. *See also* factor; indicator information set; indicator measurement system; variation.

indicator, undesirable *See* undesirable indicator.

indicator validity The degree to which an indicator identifies events that merit further review by various individuals or groups providing, or in some way influencing, the process or outcome defined by the indicator. *See also* data validity; indicator reliability; validity.

indictment A formal written accusation, which is presented to a grand jury, charging a person with criminal conduct. *See also* grand jury.

indigent A needy or poor person or one who does not have sufficient property or income to furnish a living, nor anyone able or willing to provide support. *See also* medically indigent.

indigent medical care *See* medically indigent.

indigent, medically *See* medically indigent.

indigestion A condition associated with food or eating, for example, abdominal pain or discomfort, heartburn, flatulence, nausea, and/or vomiting. *Synonym:* dyspepsia. *See also* flatulence; heartburn; nausea; vomit.

indirect contact A mode of transmission of infection between an infected host organism and a susceptible host organism via fomites (contaminated articles or objects) or vectors (organisms that transmit diseases). Vectors may be mechanical (for example, flies) or biological (for example, the disease agent undergoes part of its life cycle in the vector species). *Compare* direct contact. *See also* contact; fomite; infection; vector.

indirect cost A cost that cannot be easily seen in the product or service. The cost of electricity, a chief executive officer's salary, and hazard insurance on hospital buildings are examples of indirect costs. *See also* cost.

indirect food additives More than 10,000 substances that unintentionally enter foods during growing, processing, packaging, or preparing; for example, chemicals in some plastic packaging that may leach into food during microwaving. *Compare* direct food additives. *See also* additive; food.

individual A single person as distinguished from a group or class. *Compare* group.

individual health care account (IHCA) A proposed method of financing health care by giving tax advantages to persons who establish and maintain personal individual health care accounts (IHCAs). An IHCA is similar in concept to an individual retirement account (IRA) in that money placed in an IHCA would be excluded from the individual's taxable income and would be invested, with principal and income to be used only for specified health services. *See also* individual retirement account.

individual health insurance Coverage of a single life, in contrast to group health insurance, which covers many lives. Individual health insurance is usually considerably more costly than group health insurance. *Compare* group insurance. *See also* health insurance; insurance.

individualism A philosophy that characterizes a manager or an employee who makes decisions and performs tasks in his or her own way or style. The advantages of encouraging individualism is that creativity and naturalism may result in greater motivation and accomplishment. The disadvantages may include employees ignoring corporate goals and policies. *See also* empower.

individual marriage and family counseling Counseling that helps with a variety of issues, including crisis situations, family violence, incest, suicide, family conflicts, parenting skills, communications, and stress management. *See also* counseling; marital counseling.

individual practice *See* solo practice.

individual practice association (IPA) A partnership, corporation, association, or other legal entity that enters into an arrangement for the provision of services with persons who are licensed to practice medicine, osteopathic medicine, and dentistry, and with other care personnel. IPAs are one source of professional services for health maintenance organizations (HMOs) and are modeled after medical foundations. IPAs may also be the primary management and financial bases for some HMOs. *Synonyms:* independent physician association; independent practice association. *See also* health maintenance organization; independent practice association model HMO; preferred provider organization.

individual practice plan A health plan offered by a medical foundation, preferred provider organization, or health maintenance organization that obtains its professional services by agreement with a network of individual practitioners from an individual practice association. Originally synonymous with medical foundation. *See also* health maintenance organization; individual practice association; medical foundation.

individual retirement account (IRA) A fund under the Tax Reform Act of 1986 into which any individual employee can contribute up to $2,000 per year. However, income level and eligibility for an employee pension plan determine whether the employee's contribution of a percentage is tax deductible. *See also* health IRA; individual health care account; retirement plan.

individual retirement account, health *See* health IRA.

individual retirement account, medical   *See* health IRA.

induce   **1.** To start, cause, or stimulate the beginning of an activity, such as to induce anesthesia or to induce labor. **2.** To derive general principles from particular facts or instances; for example, persons *a*, *b*, and *c* have exudate on their tonsils and a positive *Streptococcus* throat culture; persons *d*, *e*, and *f* do not have exudate on their tonsils and do not have a positive throat culture; therefore, all people with exudate on their tonsils will have a positive throat culture. Deduce, by contrast, means to apply a general rule to a specific situation. *Compare* deduce. *See also* inductive reasoning.

induced abortion   A termination of a pregnancy that is the result of deliberate efforts. *See also* abortifacient; abortion; induce; RU-486.

induced labor   Labor brought on by mechanical or other extraneous means, usually by the intravenous infusion of oxytocin (a hormone that stimulates uterine contractions). *See also* induce; labor; uterus.

induction   **1.** The process or act of initiating or causing to occur, as in induction into the armed services or induction of labor. *See also* induce. **2.** The process or act of deriving general principles from particular facts or instances. *Compare* deduction. **3.** The act of introducing one into possession of an office or a benefice with customary ceremonies, as in induction of an individual into a professional society. *See also* induced labor.

inductive reasoning   Adjusting a course of action based on a limited amount of information gathered. It is a process in which one starts from a specific experience and draws inferences (generalizations) from it. For example, a physician, by observing a patient's reaction to a therapeutic maneuver (for example, palpating the abdomen), may induce a patient's diagnosis (appendicitis) and what should be done to meet those needs (laparotomy). *Compare* deductive reasoning. *See also* induce; reasoning.

inductive statistics   The branch of statistics that deals with generalizations, predictions, estimations, and decisions from data initially presented. *See also* inductive reasoning; statistics.

induration   **1.** Hardness, as in skin induration overlying the carcinoma. **2.** The process of becoming hard.

industrial   **1.** Pertaining to manufacturing or productive enterprises, as in industrial (occupational) diseases. *See also* postindustrial. **2.** A classification by stock market analysts of companies that produce and distribute goods and services. Utilities, transportation companies, and financial service companies are generally excluded from this classification. *See also* industry.

industrial audiometric technician   An individual certified by the Council for Accreditation in Occupational Hearing Conservation to conduct pure-tone air conduction hearing tests and related duties as part of an occupational hearing conservation program. *See also* audiometrician; Council for Accreditation in Occupational Hearing Conservation; technician.

industrial complex, medical-   *See* medical-industrial complex.

industrial disease   *See* occupational disease.

industrial engineer   In health care, an individual who uses the techniques of human and material resources management to help a hospital or other health care organization manage its resources. An industrial engineer seeks an integrated system of workers, materials, and equipment using the mathematical, physical, and social sciences. *Synonym:* management engineer. *See also* engineering.

industrial health   *See* environmental health.

Industrial Health Council, American   *See* American Industrial Health Council.

industrial health services   An older term referring to health services provided by physicians, dentists, nurses, and other health personnel in an industrial setting for the appraisal, protection, and promotion of the health of employees at work. *Synonym:* occupational health services. *See also* occupational health services.

Industrial Hygiene, American Academy of   *See* American Academy of Industrial Hygiene.

Industrial Hygiene, American Board of   *See* American Board of Industrial Hygiene.

Industrial Hygiene Association, American   *See* American Industrial Hygiene Association.

industrial hygienist   In public health, an individual who investigates working conditions at places of employment to identify hazards that may cause disease or injury and determine their source. He or she, for example, takes samples of work materials to detect and evaluate employee exposure to toxic substances, uses ventilation-testing equipment and measuring devices to determine airflow rates, noise, lasers, and other physical factors in the work place, and measures airborne concentrations of dust, gases, and mists using air sampling instruments and collection devices. *Synonyms*: environmental health practitioner; environmental health specialist. *See also* environmental health; sanitarian.

Industrial Hygienists, American Conference of Governmental *See* American Conference of Governmental Industrial Hygienists.

industrialism An economic and social system based on the development of large-scale industries and marked by the production of large quantities of inexpensive manufactured goods and the concentration of employment in urban factories.

Industrial Management, American Association of *See* American Association of Industrial Management.

Industrial Medicine, American Society of Legal and *See* American Society of Legal and Industrial Medicine.

Industrial Medicine and Surgery, American Board of *See* American Board of Industrial Medicine and Surgery.

industrial nurse *See* occupational health nurse.

Industrial Nurses, American Association of *See* American Association of Industrial Nurses.

industrial, post- *See* postindustrial.

industrial relations Dealings of a company with employees and other individuals and groups. *See also* labor relations; personnel management.

industrial social worker A social worker who works in employer assistance programs that typically provide a social service to employees whose personal problems are interfering with their job performance. *Synonyms*: occupational social worker; personal assistance social worker. *See also* social worker.

Industrial Social Workers, American Association of *See* American Association of Industrial Social Workers.

Industries Association, Hearing *See* Hearing Industries Association.

Industries Association, Intelligence *See* Intelligence Industries Association.

Industries, National Association for Senior Living *See* National Association for Senior Living Industries.

industry 1. Commercial production and sale of goods and services. **2.** Any department or branch of art, occupation, or business conducted as a means of livelihood or for profit, especially one that uses much labor and capital and is a distinct branch of trade. *See also* health care industry.

Industry Association, Generic Pharmaceutical *See* Generic Pharmaceutical Industry Association.

Industry Association, Information *See* Information Industry Association.

Industry Association, Optical *See* Optical Industry Association.

Industry Association, Smart Card *See* Smart Card Industry Association.

Industry Distributors Association, Health *See* Health Industry Distributors Association.

industry, health care *See* health care industry.

Industry Manufacturers Association, Health *See* Health Industry Manufacturers Association.

industry, regulated *See* regulated industry.

Industry Representatives Association, Health *See* Health Industry Representatives Association.

ineffective Not producing an intended effect, as in a treatment ineffective at halting the spread of cancer. *Compare* effectiveness. *See also* inefficacious.

inefficacious Not producing a desired effect or result, as in a costly and inefficacious treatment. *Compare* efficacy. *See also* ineffective.

inert In pharmacology, not active; acting, for example, as a binder or flavoring agent in a drug. In chemistry, not taking part in a chemical reaction or acting as a catalyst.

inertia A state of inactivity or sluggishness; indisposition to change. *Compare* change.

inevitable abortion A condition in which vaginal bleeding has been profuse or prolonged and the cervix has become effaced or dilated, and termination of the pregnancy is certain to happen. *See also* abortion.

infant 1. A child in the earliest period of life, especially before he or she can walk. **2.** A child from age one month to two years. *See also* neonate; premature infant; postmature infant.

infant death *See* infant mortality.

infant death rate *See* infant mortality rate.

Infant Death Syndrome Clearinghouse, National Sudden *See* National Sudden Infant Death Syndrome Clearinghouse.

infant death syndrome, sudden *See* sudden infant death syndrome.

Infant Formula Council (IFC) A national organization founded in 1970 composed of six manufacturers and marketers of infant formula products. It supports scientific research regarding the characteristics, qualities, and uses of infant formula products;

collects scientific information on such products for dissemination to the public; keeps members informed of regulatory and legislative matters; and provides communication between infant formula manufacturers and government and regulatory bodies. *See also* formula; infant.

infanticide The killing of an infant, particularly the killing of a newborn infant by its mother, or the killing of newborn children as a societal practice, a primitive method of population control. *See also* infant.

infantile paralysis *See* poliomyelitis.

infant mortality Death of live-born children less than one year old. *Synonym:* infant death. *See also* infant; infant mortality rate; neonatal mortality; neonate.

infant mortality rate A measure of the yearly rate of deaths of live-born children less than one year old. The denominator is the number of live births in the same year. This is a common measure of health status in a community. *See also* infant mortality; rate.

infant, newborn *See* neonate.

infant, postmature *See* postmature infant.

infant, premature *See* premature infant.

infant, term *See* term infant.

infarct An area of dead tissue resulting from diminished or stopped blood flow to the tissue, as in myocardial (heart muscle) infarct. *See also* infarction.

infarction The process of tissue dying as a result of diminished or stopped blood flow to the tissue, as in myocardial infarction or cerebral infarction (stroke). *See also* acute myocardial infarction; ischemia.

infarction, acute myocardial *See* acute myocardial infarction.

infect 1. To transmit a disease-producing microorganism. *See also* infection. **2.** Entry of a computer virus or other malicious software into a computer system to contaminate the memory or data of the computer. *See also* computer; virus.

infection 1. An illness or disease produced by an infectious agent. **2.** Invasion and multiplication of pathogenic microorganisms in body tissues. *See also* inflammation.

infection, airborne *See* airborne infection.

infection, asymptomatic HIV *See* asymptomatic HIV infection.

infection, community-acquired *See* community-acquired infection.

infection control A health care organization's pro-

gram, including policies and procedures, for the surveillance, prevention, and control of infection. All patient care and patient care support departments and services are included in such a program. Examples of infection control measures include hand washing, protective clothing, isolation procedures, and ongoing measurement of performance. *See also* infection control committee; isolation.

Infection Control, Association for Practitioners in *See* Association for Practitioners in Infection Control.

infection control committee A multidisciplinary group that oversees a health care organization's infection control program including representatives from at least the medical staff, nursing, and administration and the person(s) directly responsible for management of infection surveillance, prevention, and control. *See also* committee; infection control.

infection control nurse *See* infection control practitioner/specialist.

infection control practitioner/specialist An individual who specializes in infection control. *See also* epidemiologist; infection control; infection control committee.

infection, endogenous *See* endogenous infection.

infection, exogenous *See* exogenous infection.

infection, HIV *See* HIV infection.

infection, hospital-acquired *See* nosocomial infection.

infection, nidus of *See* nidus.

infection, nosocomial *See* nosocomial infection.

infection, opportunistic *See* opportunistic infection.

infection rate *See* nosocomial infection rate.

infection rate, nosocomial *See* nosocomial infection rate.

Infection Society, Surgical *See* Surgical Infection Society.

infections, slow virus *See* slow virus infection.

infection, wound *See* wound infection.

infectious Caused or capable of being transmitted by infection, as in infectious mononucleosis. *Compare* contagious. *See also* contagious; infectious diseases.

infectious disease, pediatric *See* pediatric infectious disease.

infectious diseases 1. Diseases caused by pathogenic agents, such as bacteria or viruses. The disease may or may not be contagious. *See also* acquired immunodeficiency syndrome; communicable disease; diphtheria; epidemic; malaria; measles;

mumps; leprosy; rubella; tuberculosis. **2.** The branch of medicine and subspecialty of internal medicine dealing with the diagnosis and management of patients with infectious diseases. *See also* antibiotic; chickenpox; cholera; internal medicine; Koch's postulates; pediatric infectious disease; pox; rabies; roseola; rubella; smallpox; syphilis; tetanus; typhoid fever.

infectious disease specialist, pediatric *See* pediatric infectious disease specialist.

Infectious Diseases Society of America (IDSA) A national organization founded in 1963 composed of 3,500 physicians and microbiologists who have a career commitment to the field of infectious diseases. *See also* infectious diseases.

infectious diseases specialist An internist who specializes in infectious diseases. *See also* infectious diseases; internal medicine.

infectious hepatitis Hepatitis caused by hepatitis A virus. *See also* hepatitis.

infectious waste *See* hazardous waste.

infer To conclude from evidence or premises. *See also* illation; inference.

inference The process of passing from observations and axioms to generalizations; a deduction from the facts given. In statistics, the development of a generalization from sample data, usually with calculated degrees of uncertainty. *See also* deduction; inferential statistics; sampling statistics; statistical inference.

inference, statistical *See* statistical inference.

inferential statistics The branch of statistics dealing with the process of drawing information from samples of observations of a population and making conclusions about the population. Sampling must be conducted to be representative of the underlying population and procedures must be capable of drawing correct conclusions about the population. *Compare* descriptive statistics. *See also* inference.

infertility The condition of having diminished or absent capacity to produce offspring. Many cases of infertility can be corrected through surgery, drugs, or other medical procedures. *Compare* fertility. *See also* reproductive endocrinology; sterile; sterilization.

infestation Parasite attack, as by mites, ticks, or worms. *See also* parasite; worm.

infighting Rivalry and disagreement among members or groups within an organization.

infiltration The dissemination within a tissue or organ of another tissue, substance, or pathological

change that is not normally present in it.

infirm To be weak or sickly.

infirmary A place for care of sick or injured people, especially a small hospital or dispensary in an institution.

inflammation The response of the body's tissues to irritation or injury, characterized by pain, swelling, redness, and heat. *See also* arthritis; carditis; cellulitis; cystitis; diverticulitis; encephalitis; endometritis; enteritis; gastritis; gastroenteritis; gingivitis; meningitis; nephritis; orchitis; vaginitis.

inflammatory disease, pelvic *See* pelvic inflammatory disease.

inflation A persistent increase in the level of consumer prices or a persistent decline in the purchasing power of money, caused by an increase in available currency and credit beyond the proportion of available goods and services. *See also* economics; Phillips curve.

influence Power to sway or affect based on ability, position, prestige, or wealth; for example, personal influence. *See also* personal influence.

influence, personal *See* personal influence.

influenza An acute viral illness characterized by fever, muscle aches, and fatigue, occurring in sporadic epidemics and pandemic outbreaks. Pandemics, affecting many continents, have occurred at intervals varying from 8 to 18 years throughout the twentieth century. *Synonym:* flu. *See also* epidemic; pandemic.

info *See* information.

infobit A discrete piece of information or data. *See also* data; information.

infomania A preoccupation with or uncontrolled desire for information; the amassing of facts for their own sake. *See also* data; fact; information; mania.

infomercial A television or video commercial presented in the form of a short, informative documentary. *See also* information.

inform To relate, instruct, or provide with the facts or data, as in informing a patient about discharge. *Compare* misinform. *See also* data; fact; information.

informal leader A leader whose power and authority over a group are derived from his or her acceptance by the group rather from his or her office, position, status, or rank in the formal chain of command in the formal organization. An informal leader has earned a group leadership role by the group's acceptance. *See also* leader.

informatics The whole of information technology and its applications. *See also* information; information science; medical informatics; technology.

informatics, medical *See* medical informatics.

Informatics Association, American Medical *See* American Medical Informatics Association.

information Data that have been transformed through analysis and interpretation into a form useful for drawing conclusions and making decisions. *See also* data; information science; infobit.

Information Act, Freedom of *See* Freedom of Information Act.

Information Association, Drug *See* Drug Information Association.

Information Center for Children and Youth with Disabilities, National *See* National Information Center for Children and Youth with Disabilities.

Information Center on Deafness, National *See* National Information Center on Deafness.

Information, Center for Medical Consumers and Health Care *See* Center for Medical Consumers and Health Care Information.

Information Center, National Rehabilitation *See* National Rehabilitation Information Center.

Information Center, Non-Circumcision *See* Non-Circumcision Information Center.

Information Center, ODPHP National Health *See* ODPHP National Health Information Center.

Information Clearinghouse, National Kidney and Urologic Diseases *See* National Kidney and Urologic Diseases Information Clearinghouse.

Information Council, Health *See* Health Information Council.

Information Exchange on Young Adult Chronic Patients, The *See* The Information Exchange on Young Adult Chronic Patients.

information, falsification of *See* falsification of information.

Information Industry Association (IIA) A national organization founded in 1968 composed of 800 companies interested and involved in the generation, distribution, and use of information. It works to keep members informed about the latest technologies and marketing trends; facilitates the formation of partnerships and business alliances; and serves as a channel to customers, acquisitions, and venture capital companies. *See also* information.

information infrastructure, health *See* health information infrastructure.

information infrastructure, national *See* national information infrastructure.

Information, Intersociety Committee on Pathology *See* Intersociety Committee on Pathology Information.

information management *See* management information system.

Information Management, Association for *See* Association for Information Management.

Information Management Association, American Health *See* American Health Information Management Association.

Information Management, Society for *See* Society for Information Management.

information management system *See* management information system.

Information and Management Systems Society, Healthcare *See* Healthcare Information and Management Systems Society.

information officer, chief *See* chief information officer.

information question The precise question that a team of people (for example, a quality improvement project team) is trying to answer by collecting and analyzing data. *See also* information.

Information Resource Centers, National Organization of Circumcision *See* National Organization of Circumcision Information Resource Centers.

information science The study of the creation, use, and communication of information. *See also* informatics; information; medical informatics.

Information Science, American Society for *See* American Society for Information Science.

information science, medical *See* medical informatics.

information set, indicator *See* indicator information set.

information system Equipment and procedures used for the collection, recording, processing, storage, retrieval, and display of information for use by other people to make decisions. Information systems include information-processing methodologies, such as telecommunications and records management. *See also* clinical information system; executive information system; hospital information system; information; information science; management information system.

information system, clinical *See* clinical information system.

information system, executive *See* executive information system.

information system, hospital　*See* hospital information system.

information system, management　*See* management information system.

information systems director　*See* chief information officer.

information theory　The mathematical formulations that explain the communication of information. *See also* information; information science; theory.

informative advertising　Advertising that provides specific information about performance and quality of specific services or products. *See also* advertise; comparative advertising; competitive advertising; deceptive advertising; false advertising; image advertising.

informed consent　Agreement or permission accompanied by full notice about what is being consented to. Informed consent is constitutionally required in certain areas in which one may consent to what otherwise would be an unconstitutional violation of a right. Informed consent in tort law refers to the requirement that a patient be apprised of the nature and risks of a medical procedure before the physician or other health professional can validly claim exemption from liability for battery or from responsibility for medical complications and other undesirable outcomes. *Synonym:* patient consent. *Compare* informed refusal. *See also* autonomy; battery; consent; implied consent; patient participation; patient's right of autonomy; right of privacy; therapeutic privilege.

informed refusal　Rejection of treatment by a patient or his or her representatives after provision of full information on the treatment's benefits and risks. *Compare* informed consent. *See also* autonomy; death with dignity; refusal.

infrared　Denotes that portion of the spectrum of electromagnetic radiation with wavelengths longer than those of visible light but shorter than those of radio waves (between about 0.8 and 1000 micrometers). Infrared radiation is sometimes referred to as radiant heat or invisible heat radiation. *See also* infrared radiation therapy; thermography.

infrared radiation therapy　A type of physical therapy using the application of heat to the foot or other parts of the body by means of an infrared lamp. *See also* infrared; phototherapy; physical therapy; thermography.

infrastructure　An underlying base or foundation, especially for an organization or a system; for example, the infrastructure of a hospital consists of the basic facilities, equipment, services, and human resources needed for the hospital to function. *See also* health information infrastructure.

infrastructure, health information　*See* health information infrastructure.

infrastructure, national information　*See* national information infrastructure.

infusion　Introduction of a substance, such as normal saline or antibiotics, directly into a vein or between tissues. It is accomplished by gravity rather than by injection. *Compare* injection. *See also* drip; home infusion services.

infusion services, home　*See* home infusion services.

ingenious　Pertaining to inventive skill and imagination, as in an ingenious idea. *See also* idea.

ingenuous　**1.** Lacking in sophistication or worldliness. **2.** Openly straightforward or frank.

inguinal hernia　The most common form of hernia, in which the abdominal viscera protrude into the inguinal canal located in the groin. *See also* hernia.

inhalation　A method of administering gases or drugs in gaseous, vapor, or aerosol form by drawing them into the lungs along with inhaled air. Inhalation is used with gaseous and volatile anesthetics, volatile substances, such as amyl nitrite, and drugs in aqueous solution, which can be atomized to form a finely dispersed mist. *See also* anesthetic; inhaler.

inhalation anesthetic　An anesthetic, such as nitrous oxide, that is inhaled as a gas. *See also* anesthetic; inhalation.

inhalation therapist　*See* respiratory therapist.

inhalation therapy　*See* respiratory therapy.

inhaler　Any device for administering substances in gaseous, vapor, or aerosol form by inhalation. *See also* inhalation.

inheritance　The process of genetic transmission to offspring from parents. *See also* genetics; heredity.

inhibition　The act of influencing in a negative direction; of diminishing, restraining, or extinguishing altogether an event, action, or process.

in-home care　*See* home health care.

in-house　Pertaining to activities conducted within an organization, as opposed to being brought in or done from the outside; for example, in-house publishing or an in-house statistician.

initial　Starting at the beginning, as in an initial survey.

initialism A word formed from the initial letters or parts of a compound term and read or spoken letter by letter, for example, DRG (diagnosis-related group). *See also* abbreviation; acronym.

initial survey An accreditation survey of a health care organization not previously accredited by the Joint Commission on Accreditation of Healthcare Organizations, or an accreditation survey of an organization performed without reference to any prior survey findings. *See also* accreditation survey; Joint Commission on Accreditation of Healthcare Organizations; survey.

initiative An action of creating or starting; the characteristic or ability of originating new ideas or methods. For example, a manager with initiative possesses the aptitude to bring forth new ideas or techniques and will take action without having to wait for instructions, or a state government may support a data initiative. *See also* leadership; state data initiatives; take-charge.

initiatives, state data *See* state data initiatives.

injection The act of forcing a liquid, such as a drug, into a part. The liquid may be injected into a vein (intravenous injection), into a muscle (intramuscular injection), under the skin (subcutaneous injection), or into the skin (intradermal injection). *Compare* infusion.

injunction Judicial prohibition requiring a party to refrain from doing or continuing to do some specific activity or act. *See also* permanent injunction; preliminary injunction; trial.

injunction, permanent *See* permanent injunction.

injunction, preliminary *See* preliminary injunction.

injury Damage, harm, hurt, or impairment; trauma. *See also* antitrust injury; birth trauma; compensable injury; legal injury; medical injury; personal injury; trauma.

injury, antitrust *See* antitrust injury.

Injury Association, American Spinal See American Spinal Injury Association.

injury, compensable *See* compensable injury.

Injury Control Center (ICC) A national organization founded in 1987 composed of universities, medical centers, doctors, and research associates who support scientific research and training to improve injury control, particularly prevention activities, acute care of trauma patients, and rehabilitation of the disabled. *See also* injury; trauma.

injury, legal *See* legal injury.

injury, medical *See* medical injury.

Injury Nurses, American Association of Spinal Cord *See* American Association of Spinal Cord Injury Nurses.

injury, personal *See* personal injury.

Injury Psychologists and Social Workers, American Association of Spinal Cord *See* American Association of Spinal Cord Injury Psychologists and Social Workers.

injury scale, abbreviated *See* abbreviated injury scale.

injury severity score (ISS) In trauma care, the sum of the squares of the highest abbreviated injury scale (AIS) score for three body areas. The ISS has a high correlation with mortality and length of hospital stay and a low correlation with morbidity and disability prediction. Because of the mortality correlation, the ISS has become the gold standard for comparing the quality of care between hospitals or emergency medical services systems or following quality of care in the same institution over time. The ISS has limited utility in the field and emergency departments because it is calculated retrospectively. *See also* abbreviated injury scale; gold standard; trauma; traumatology.

ink jet printer A printer that forms characters by firing tiny dots of ink at the paper. It is usually more expensive and faster than a daisy-wheel printer. *See also* daisy wheel printer; printer.

inlier A patient who is included within the trim points, or expected length-of-stay boundaries, of a diagnosis-related group. *Compare* outlier. *See also* diagnosis-related groups.

in loco parentis Latin phrase meaning "in place of parents"; a legal doctrine that allows a "stand in" to exercise the legal rights, duties, and responsibilities a parent possesses toward a child.

INMED *See* Indians Into Medicine.

innovation 1. The act of introducing something new. **2.** Something newly introduced or a change in current methods or procedures.

inoculation The introduction of foreign material into a living organism or culture medium,, particularly of a disease agent, vaccine, serum, or microorganisms. *See also* vaccine.

inpatient An individual who receives health services while lodged in a hospital or other health care organization at least overnight. *Compare* outpatient. *See also* patient.

inpatient admission The formal acceptance by a

health care organization of a patient who is to receive lodging and continuous nursing service in an area of the facility where patients generally stay at least overnight. *See also* admission; inpatient; newborn admission.

inpatient admission, newborn *See* newborn admission.

inpatient, adult *See* adult inpatient.

inpatient, ambulatory *See* ambulatory inpatient.

inpatient bed, pediatric *See* pediatric inpatient bed.

inpatient care Health services provided to patients who have been admitted to hospitals. *Compare* outpatient care.

inpatient care unit An area of a hospital in which inpatient care is provided. Such units are often defined by socioeconomic characteristics (pediatric unit), diagnoses (oncology unit), or severity of illness (intensive care unit). *Synonym*: patient care unit. *See also* inpatient care; patient mix; unit; unit manager; ward.

inpatient census The number of inpatients in a hospital or other health care organization at a given time. *See also* ADT; census; inpatient.

inpatient, pediatric *See* pediatric inpatient.

inpatient unit, psychiatric *See* psychiatric inpatient unit.

input The service or product provided to a process. Inputs to one process are the outputs from preceding processes. *See also* electronic data processing; input measure; management by objectives; output; supplier.

input device Computer hardware, such as a keyboard or a light pen, used to enter data into a computer. *See also* computer; computer hardware; console; joystick; light pen; mouse; optical character reader.

input measure A measure of the quality of services based on structural components of an organization, such as the number and type of resources used to provide services. The number of board certified medical specialists or ownership of certain technologies are examples of input measures. Input measures provide a measure of what an organization puts into a system or expends in its operation to achieve certain results, but do not provide information about an organization's actual level of performance (output, outcomes, or results) in providing the services it is capable of providing. *See also* input;

outcome measure; process measure.

INS *See* Intravenous Nurses Society.

insanity A social and legal (but not medical) term for madness, lunacy, or unsoundness of mind. The original complete form was "insanity of mind," sanity being an archaic word for health. *Compare* sanity.

inscription *See* prescription.

insemination The deposit of seminal fluid within the female genital tract (vagina or cervix). *See also* artificial insemination.

insemination, artificial *See* artificial insemination.

insemination, donor *See* artificial insemination - donor.

in-service education Teaching or instruction taking place or continuing while one is a full-time employee. *See also* education.

insomnia Persistent inability to sleep. *See also* sleep.

inspect To examine carefully and critically, especially for abnormalities, flaws, or errors; for example, a physician inspecting a patient's mucous membranes, or personnel inspecting manufactured devices before allowing shipment. *See also* examine; inspection; investigate.

inspection 1. The process of examining carefully, as in physical diagnosis. *See also* cranioscopy; physical diagnosis. 2. Activities, such as measuring, examining, testing, or gauging one or more characteristics of a product or service and comparing these with specified requirements to determine conformity. Inspection is a past-oriented strategy that attempts to identify unacceptable output after it has been produced and separate it from the good output; for example, inspection of hospital buildings for compliance with safety standards. *Compare* prevention. *See also* appraisal cost; detection; quality inspection; Occupational Safety and Health Administration.

inspection, quality *See* quality inspection.

inspection stamp A stamp from the US Department of Agriculture that must be placed on meat, poultry, and packaged, processed meat products before sale to consumers to indicate that the food is wholesome and was prepared (slaughtered, packaged, processed) under sanitary conditions.

inspector A person who has been assigned to inspect something, especially an officer whose duties are to examine and inspect things over which he or she has jurisdiction, as in meat inspectors, building inspectors, and health inspectors. *See also* inspection; inspector general.

inspector general (IG) An officer with general investigative powers within a civil, military, or other organization, such as the inspector generals of various federal agencies whose primary function is to conduct and supervise audits and investigations relating to operations and procedures over which the agency has jurisdiction. *See also* inspector.

instinct In biology, an innate, inherited, species-typical pattern of behavior that is independent of reason, experience, and learning and which normally results in achievement of adaptive ends. True instinctive behavior is impulsive. *See also* impulse.

Institute for Advanced Research in Asian Science and Medicine (IARASM) An organization founded in 1972 whose purpose is to advance international understanding between Asia and the West in the areas of science, medical systems, and health care delivery. It serves as a clearinghouse for international scholarly efforts in the mediation of scientific and biomedical exchange with Asian countries. It assists in generating innovative curricula in medical education, translates contemporary and classical Asian scientific and medical literature, and provides training for medical professionals in acupuncture therapeutics. *See also* acupuncture.

Institute for the Advancement of Human Behavior (IAHB) A national organization founded in 1977 that provides continuing education for health care professionals on behavioral topics, such as the psychology of health care, human sexuality, the healing power of laughter and play, maintaining long-term health behaviors, and the role of imagery in health care. *See also* behavioral medicine.

Institute for Aerobics Research (IAR) An organization founded in 1970 to promote understanding of the relationship between living habits and health, to provide leadership in enhancing the physical and emotional well-being of individuals, and to promote participation in aerobics. Its activities include sponsoring weekly training courses and certification testing of fitness leaders in education, government, human services, and corporate sectors. Its divisions include behavioral sciences, computer services, continuing education, consultation, epidemiology, and exercise-physiology. *See also* aerobics; certification; exercise; fitness.

Institute for Certification of Computer Professionals (ICCP) An organization founded in 1973 that promotes the development of computer examina-

tions of high quality, directed toward information technology professionals and designed to encourage competence and professionalism. Individuals passing the examinations automatically become members of the Association of the Institute for Certification of Computer Professionals. *See also* Association of the Institute for Certification of Computer Professionals; certification.

Institute of Certified Professional Business Consultants (ICPBC) A national organization founded in 1975 composed of 270 individuals providing business advisory services to physicians, dentists, and other professionals. It maintains a code of ethics, rules of professional conduct, and a certification program. It administers an examination and conducts a review course. *See also* certification.

Institute of Electrical and Electronics Engineers (IEEE) An organization founded in 1963 composed of 274,000 engineers and scientists in electrical engineering, electronics, and allied fields concerned with the development of devices and methods to improve the utility of electricity. *See also* engineer.

Institute of Electrology Educators (IEE) A national organization founded in 1979 composed of 55 electrology schools and teachers. It instructs teachers and standardizes the curriculum and teaching of electrology. *See also* electrology.

Institute for Gravitational Strain Pathology (IGSP) A medical institute founded in 1957 to study the ill effects (backaches, postural decline, aging) of terrestrial gravity on humans and to develop ways to counteract pathology of gravitational strain. It provides instruction with a tool called the "antigravity leverage technique," designed to modify and reduce the harmful consequences of gravity.

Institute for Hospital Clinical Nursing Education (IHCNE) A national organization founded in 1967 composed of 165 hospital schools of nursing. It provides support for issues common to hospital schools of nursing and promotes advancement of schools through educational programs and other activities. Formerly (1991) Assembly of Hospital Schools of Nursing. *See also* nursing.

Institute on Hospital and Community Psychiatry (IHCP) An annual forum sponsored by the American Psychiatric Association that is open to employees of all psychiatric and related health and educational facilities. It includes lectures by experts in the field and accredited courses on problems, programs, and trends. *See also* American Psychiatric Association; psychiatry.

Institute of Laboratory Animal Resources (ILAR) A national institute founded in 1952 under the auspices of the National Academy of Sciences that acts in an advisory capacity to the federal government, upon request, and to other public and private agencies. It maintains an information center and answers inquiries concerning animal models for biomedical research, location of unique animal colonies, availability of genetically defined animals from those colonies and from animal breeders, and nonanimal alternatives. Its committees develop guidelines on breeding, conservation, and humane care and use of animals.

Institute for Lifestyle Improvement *See* National Wellness Institute.

Institute of Mathematical Statistics (IMS) A national organization founded in 1935 composed of 4,000 mathematicians and other individuals interested in mathematical statistics and probability theory. *See also* statistics.

Institute for Medical Records Economics *See* Medical Records Institute.

Institute of Medicine (IOM) A national organization formed under a charter from the National Academy of Sciences in 1970 composed of 500 clinical, academic, and health policy experts who study and inform public health policy issues. Membership in the IOM is by invitation. Formerly (1970) Board on Medicine of the National Academy of Sciences. *See also* National Academy of Sciences; public health.

Institute for Rational-Emotive Therapy (IRET) A national organization founded in 1968 that provides professional training and moderate-cost treatment services, including individual and group psychotherapy, marriage and family counseling, and crisis intervention; consultative services for mental health professionals, corporations, and community agencies; and research programs in applied psychology. Rational-emotive therapy, IRET's chief treatment approach, is a psychological theory and technique devised in 1955 based on the assumption that human beings become disturbed through acquiring irrational thoughts, beliefs, philosophies, or attitudes. Rational-emotive therapy asserts that people can be taught to change their negative and disturbed feelings and behaviors by consciously correcting the false beliefs and inaccurate perceptions that underlie and accompany these feelings. *See also* psychotherapy.

Institute for Reality Therapy (IRT) A national organization founded in 1967 composed of board-certified psychiatrists, psychologists, social workers, and consultants in a variety of related fields interested in teaching reality therapy and control theory psychology to people who are involved in the helping professions. Reality therapy is a method of working with individuals and groups emphasizing the responsibility of the individual for his or her own behavior. *See also* psychotherapy.

Institute for Reproductive Health (IRH) A national organization composed of people supporting informed, responsible health care for women and working toward the passage of regulatory legislation for informed consent. It conducts research on women's issues, including sexually-transmitted diseases and their effect on female fertility, analysis of risks and losses due to hysterectomy, and surgical abuses against women. *See also* hysterectomy; informed consent; reproduction; sexually-transmitted disease.

Institute for Research in Hypnosis *See* Institute for Research in Hypnosis and Psychotherapy.

Institute for Research in Hypnosis and Psychotherapy (IRHP) A national organization founded in 1954 composed of psychologists, psychiatrists, physicians, and social workers trained in clinical hypnosis, hypnotherapy, and hypnoanalysis. It sponsors research in clinical and experimental hypnosis, offers postgraduate training in hypnosis and its applications, and develops standards and procedures for advanced education in clinical and experimental hypnosis. Formerly (1982) Institute for Research in Hypnosis. *See also* hypnosis; hypnotherapy.

Institutes for Behavior Resources (IBR) A national organization founded in 1960 composed of 200 persons with backgrounds in psychology, education, sociology, social services, and law. It conducts basic and applied research in behavioral psychology; investigates human performance, law and behavior, and social problems; and works with agencies dealing with youth problems to stimulate them to seek alternatives to punishment in handling juvenile delinquent behaviors. *See also* behavioral science.

Institute for Victims of Terrorism *See* Institute for Victims of Trauma.

Institute for Victims of Trauma (IVT) A nonmembership organization founded in 1987 composed of professionals specializing in posttraumatic stress, crisis intervention, and the study of terrorism. It is a nonpolitical group assisting victims of terrorism, accidents, and natural and man-made disasters. It acts as a liaison with governmental and nongovernmental organizations and institutions and maintains a library on traumatic stress, victimology, and terrorism. Formerly (1988) Institute for Victims of Terrorism. *See also* posttraumatic stress disorder; terrorism.

institution An established organization or foundation, especially one dedicated to education, public service, or culture, as in health care institutions, such as hospitals or nursing homes for the care of persons who are sick, disabled, or mentally ill. *See also* health care organization; institution for mental disease.

institution, health care *See* health care organization.

institution for mental disease (IMD) A type of health care organization primarily engaged in providing diagnosis, treatment, and care for persons with mental diseases.

institutional review board (IRB) An organizational committee, mandated in 1981 and since governed by the Department of Health and Human Services, that is designated to review and approve biomedical research that involves humans as subjects. The purpose of IRBs is to provide certain protections for human subjects of research and research proposals only if conditions established by federal regulations are met. Some conditions, for example, are that the risks to which subjects are exposed are minimized, that the risks to subjects are reasonable in relation to the anticipated benefits, if any, to the subjects, and that the informed consent of all participants is sought and appropriately documented. *See also* informed consent.

Instructors, National Association of Rehabilitation *See* National Association of Rehabilitation Instructors.

instrument A tool used to perform a task, such as a measurement; for example, a clinical indicator is an instrument to measure the level of performance in carrying out an important clinical process or achieving an important clinical outcome. *See also* bioinstrumentation; bougie; calibration; governing instrument; survey instrument; tool.

Instrumentation, Association for the Advancement of Medical *See* Association for the Advancement of Medical Instrumentation.

instrumentation, bio- *See* bioinstrumentation.

instrument, governing *See* governing instrument.

instrument, survey *See* survey instrument.

insufficient *See* inadequate.

insulin A hormone produced by the beta cells of the pancreas that regulates the metabolism of carbohydrates and is necessary for the utilization of glucose in body cells with insulin receptors. Until recently all insulin for therapeutic purposes had been obtained by extraction from animal pancreatic glands. It is now possible to produce human insulin on a commercial scale by the techniques of genetic engineering. *See also* diabetes mellitus; genetic engineering; gestational diabetes; glucagon; hormone; pancreas; recombinant human insulin.

insulin-dependent diabetes *See* type I diabetes mellitus.

insulin, recombinant human *See* recombinant human insulin.

insurance The contractual relationship and benefit that exist when one party, for a consideration, agrees to reimburse another for loss to a person or thing caused by designated contingencies. The first party is the insurer; the second, the insured; the contract, the insurance policy; the consideration, the premium; the person or thing, the risk; and the contingency, the hazard or peril. Insurance is a formal social device for reducing the risk of losses for individuals by spreading the risk over groups. *See also* health insurance; McCarran-Ferguson Act; reinsurance; subrogation.

Insurance Accounting and Systems Association (IASA) A national organization founded in 1928 composed of 1,700 insurance companies writing all lines of insurance, and independent public accountants, actuarial consultants, management consultants, statisticians, and statistical organizations concerned with accounting practices and their management in the insurance industry. *See also* insurance.

Insurance for the Aged and Disabled, Title XVIII, Health *See* Medicare.

Insurance Association of America, Health *See* Health Insurance Association of America.

Insurance Benefits Advisory Council, Health *See* Health Insurance Benefits Advisory Council.

Insurance, Bureau of Health *See* Bureau of Health Insurance.

insurance, catastrophic *See* catastrophic insurance.

insurance claim number, health *See* health insurance claim number.

insurance claims review   *See* claims review.

insurance clerk   *See* reimbursement specialist.

insurance, commercial health   *See* commercial health insurance.

insurance commissioner   A state official who is charged with the enforcement of laws pertaining to insurance in each state. *See also* insurance.

Insurance, Committee for National Health   *See* Committee for National Health Insurance.

insurance company   An organization that underwrites insurance policies. There are two principal types of insurance companies: mutual and stock. *Synonym*: insurer. *See also* mutual insurance company; stock insurance company.

insurance company, captive   *See* captive insurance company.

insurance company, mutual   *See* mutual insurance company.

insurance company, stock   *See* stock insurance company.

insurance, comprehensive health   *See* comprehensive health insurance.

insurance, comprehensive major medical   *See* comprehensive major medical insurance.

Insurance Consumer Organization, National   *See* National Insurance Consumer Organization.

insurance, contributory   *See* contributory insurance.

insurance coverage   The amount of protection available and the kind of loss that would be paid for under an insurance contract with an insurer. *See also* coverage; insurance.

insurance, dental   *See* dental insurance.

insurance, group   *See* group insurance.

insurance, health   *See* health insurance.

insurance, individual health   *See* individual health insurance.

insurance, liability   *See* general liability insurance.

insurance, life   *See* life insurance.

insurance, malpractice   *See* medical malpractice insurance.

insurance, mandated employer   *See* mandated employer insurance.

insurance, medical malpractice   *See* medical malpractice insurance.

Insurance Medicine, American Academy of   *See* American Academy of Insurance Medicine.

insurance, national health   *See* national health insurance.

insurance, noncontributory   *See* noncontributory insurance.

insurance, participating   *See* participating insurance.

insurance policy   A written contract of insurance. *See also* contract; insurance; policy; policyholder.

insurance pool   An organization of insurers through which particular types of risks are shared or pooled. The risk of high loss by any particular insurance company is thus transferred to the group as a whole (the insurance pool) with premiums, losses, and expenses shared in agreed amounts. The advantage of a pool is that the size of expected losses can be predicted for the pool with much more certainty than for any individual party to it. Pooling arrangements are often used for catastrophic coverage or for certain high-risk populations like the disabled. *See also* catastrophic illness; insurance; insurance company.

insurance, professional liability   *See* professional liability insurance.

insurance, property   *See* property insurance.

insurance purchasing cooperative, health   *See* health alliance.

insurance, re-   *See* reinsurance.

insurance regulation   *See* McCarran-Ferguson Act.

insurance, self   *See* self insurance.

insurance, social   *See* social insurance.

insurance, specified disease   *See* specified disease insurance.

insurance, sponsored malpractice   *See* sponsored malpractice insurance.

insurance, state disability   *See* unemployment compensation disability.

insurance, supplemental health   *See* supplemental health insurance.

insurance, umbrella   *See* umbrella coverage.

insurance, umbrella liability   *See* umbrella coverage.

insurance, unemployment   *See* unemployment insurance.

insurance, workers' compensation   *See* workers' compensation insurance.

insured   The entity whose interests are protected by an insurance policy and who contracts for a policy of insurance that indemnifies the entity against loss of property, life, or health, or in the event of accident. *Compare* insurer. *See also* beneficiary; insurance; member; named insured; underinsured.

insured, named   *See* named insured.

insured, under-   *See* underinsured.

insurer   The party to an insurance policy who contracts to pay losses or render services. *Compare* insured. *See also* insurance company.

integrate To bring together different parts to make a whole; for example, integrating research and development with product development.

integrated circuit An electronic device consisting of many minute transistors and other circuit elements on a single silicon chip. The ultimate integrated circuit is the microprocessor, a single chip that contains the complete arithmetic and logic unit of a computer. *See also* circuit; microcircuit; microprocessor.

integrated provider A health care provider that offers a comprehensive corporate umbrella for the management of a diversified health care delivery system. The system typically includes one or more hospitals, a large group practice, a health plan, and other health care operations. Physicians practice as employees of the system or in a tightly affiliated physician group. The system has the capability to provide several levels of health care to patients in geographically contiguous areas. *See also* corporate diversification; group practice; group practice without walls; health care provider; management services organization; physician-hospital organization.

integration In health care, the linking together of components of a health care system. *See also* functional integration; horizontal integration; vertical integration.

integration, functional *See* functional integration.

integration, horizontal *See* horizontal integration.

Integration, Society for the Exploration of Psychotherapy *See* Society for the Exploration of Psychotherapy Integration.

integration, vertical *See* vertical integration.

intellect The capacity to know, perceive, and understand, in contrast to the capacity for emotion.

intelligence 1. The ability of living organisms, especially humans, to learn, to understand, to apply experience, and to make judgments. **2.** The ability of a computer to respond to different circumstances or developments. *See also* artificial intelligence; intelligence quotient.

Intelligence, American Association for Artificial *See* American Association for Artificial Intelligence.

intelligence, artificial *See* artificial intelligence.

Intelligence Industries Association (IIA) A national organization founded in 1986 composed of commercial firms involved in the production of natural language and image processing systems, micro-

electronic circuits, speech technology systems, and biosensors. Associate members are investment banking, venture capital, public accounting, and law firms. Affiliate members are national laboratories and academic research centers. *See also* artificial intelligence; biosensor; natural language processing; voice input/output technology.

intelligence quotient (IQ) Mental age expressed as a percentage of chronological age. The quotient is obtained by dividing a subject's score on intelligence tests by the average score on the same tests by individuals of the same age group and multiplying by 100. *See also* intelligence.

intelligent terminal An input/output device in which computer processing components are built into the terminal. *Compare* dumb terminal. *See also* computer; computer terminal; input device.

intelligible Pertaining to that which is stated clearly and can be understood or comprehended.

intensity 1. The amount or degree of strength, as in the intensity of light or the intensity of service provided to a patient. *See also* intensity of service. **2.** The magnitude of force or energy per unit.

intensity of service The amount or degree of service provided to a patient or a group of similar patients in a health care organization, such as the average number of laboratory tests or x-rays provided per emergency department patient or per hospitalized patient per day, subcategorized by attending physician. *See also* intensity; level of service; service.

intensive, capital *See* capital intensive.

intensive care Continuous health services provided to critically ill patients with life-threatening conditions, usually in an organizational setting where professional and supportive services are concentrated for that purpose. *See also* level of care; special care unit.

intensive care nurse *See* critical care nurse.

intensive care unit (ICU) A unit of a hospital established for patients requiring extraordinary care on a concentrated and continuous basis. *See also* special care unit.

intensive care unit, medical *See* medical intensive care unit.

intensive care unit, mobile *See* mobile intensive care unit.

intensive care unit, neonatal *See* neonatal intensive care unit.

intensive care unit, pediatric *See* pediatric intensive care unit.

intensive care unit, surgical   *See* surgical intensive care unit.

intensive home health care   Health services for persons with serious illnesses whose medical condition are unstable and who require concentrated physician and nursing management in the home. *See also* home health care.

intensive, labor   *See* labor intensive.

intensive, people   *See* people intensive.

intent   What is intended; meaning or purport; for example, legislative intent or intent of a standard. *See also* intent of standard; legislative intent.

intent, legislative   *See* legislative intent.

intent of standard   A brief explanation of the meaning, rationale, and significance of a standard, as in the intent of a Joint Commission on Accreditation of Healthcare Organizations standard. *See also* Joint Commission on Accreditation of Healthcare Organizations; legislative intent; standard.

interactive   **1.** Acting or capable of acting on each other. **2.** In computer science, pertaining to a two-way electronic or communications system in which response is direct and continual. *See also* interactive computer system.

interactive computer system   A computer system capability whereby an outside person feeds information to the computer, which can respond, as with a teaching program. *See also* computer; interactive; system.

interactive terminal   In computer science, a computer or data-processing terminal capable of providing a two-way communication with the system to which it is connected. *See also* computer terminal; interactive.

Interagency Council on Library Resources for Nursing (ICLRN)   An advisory board founded in 1960 composed of 25 representatives from agencies and organizations concerned with the library needs of nurses, including American Academy of Nursing, American Nurses' Association, Medical Library Association, American Hospital Association, American Medical Association, National League for Nursing, American Journal of Nursing Company, and US Public Health Service, Nursing Division. It promotes development and improvement of library resources and services for nurses in all health science libraries. *See also* health sciences library; library; nursing.

Interamerican College of Physicians and Sur-

geons (ICPS)   An organization founded in 1979 composed of 4,000 physicians in countries of the Americas. It encourages understanding and communication among members concerning all aspects of medical practice. It promotes health education in Hispanic communities in the Western Hemisphere and maintains a library of Spanish-language medical books. *See also* physician; surgeon.

intercourse, sexual   *See* sexual intercourse.

interdisciplinary   Relating to, or involving, two or more academic disciplines that are usually considered distinct, as in medicine and nursing. *See also* discipline; multidisciplinary.

interdisciplinary patient care plan   A plan required by federal regulations for patients in long term care facilities. The plan defines the patient's problems and needs and sets measurable goals, approaches to the care, and the profession responsible for the care. *Synonyms:* care plan; patient care plan. *See also* care plan; long term care.

interest, best   *See* best interest.

interest, conflict of   *See* conflict of interest.

interest, public   *See* public interest.

interest, special   *See* special interest.

interface   **1.** The way in which parts of a computer system link together, as in a device converting signals from one device into signals that the other device understands. **2.** The interaction between two different data processing devices or systems that handle data differently, such as different formats or codes. *See also* parallel interface; serial interface.

interface, parallel   *See* parallel interface.

interface, serial   *See* serial interface.

Intergovernmental Health Policy Project (IHPP)   A national organization founded in 1979 composed of 2,500 health policy researchers. It provides information on health legislation and programs to state executive officials, legislators, and legislative staff. It serves as an information clearinghouse and responds to specific information requests on state programs. *See also* health policy.

interim   An interval of time between one event, process, or period and another; for example, interim rate and interim report. *See also* interim rate; interim report.

interim rate   An amount of money periodically paid to a health care provider by a third-party payer under a retrospective reimbursement arrangement until a more accurate rate can be determined. The final payment is then established by adjustments to the total of the interim payments based on the determined rate. *See also* rate; retrospective reimbursement; third-party payer.

interim report　A report issued before a project or a reporting period has been completed. *See also* report.

interjudge reliability　*See* interobserver reliability.

intermediary, fiscal　*See* fiscal intermediary.

intermediate care　The second highest level of nursing care (skilled nursing care is the highest level), generally overall supervision by a registered nurse at least one shift per day. Patients receiving intermediate care can typically perform some of the activities of daily living. *Synonyms*: basic nursing care; intermediate nursing care. *See also* activities of daily living; intermediate care facility; intermediate care unit; intermediate home health care; level of care.

intermediate care facility (ICF)　A health care organization recognized under the Medicaid program that is licensed under state law to provide, on a regular basis, health services to individuals who do not require the degree of care or treatment that a hospital or skilled nursing facility is designed to provide, but who because of their mental or physical condition require services (above the level of lodging and board) that can be made available to them only through institutional facilities. *See also* intermediate care; intermediate care facility for the mentally retarded.

intermediate care facility for the mentally retarded　A public institution for care of the mentally retarded or people with related conditions. *See also* intermediate care facility.

intermediate care unit　A portion of a skilled nursing facility that is organized to provide intermediate care for patients. *See also* intermediate care; skilled nursing care; unit.

intermediate home health care　Health services provided at home for persons whose medical condition is not expected to fluctuate significantly as rehabilitation is achieved or the disease progresses. *See also* home health care.

intermediate nursing care　*See* intermediate care.

intermediate service　*See* level of service.

intermittent　Not occurring often and tending to emphasize pauses and interruptions, not occurrences. *See also* continuous; frequent; intermittent care; occasional; periodic; sporadic; successive.

intermittent care　A type of home health care that includes daily care for a two-to-three week period and thereafter under "exceptional circumstances." *See also* home health care; intermittent.

intern　In medicine, a medical school graduate fulfilling an initial resident appointment in a hospital prior to being licensed to practice medicine independently. *See also* internship; nurse intern.

internal audit　An audit performed by personnel of an organization to determine the degree to which internal procedures, operations, and accounting practices are in proper order. *Compare* independent audit. *See also* audit.

Internal Auditors, Association of Healthcare　*See* Association of Healthcare Internal Auditors.

internal consistency　The extent to which all items in a particular scale measure the same dimension. *See also* scale.

internal control number　A number assigned to an incoming claim by a third-party claims administrator that identifies the claim and matches it to any correspondence or subsequent billing or medical information received about the claim. *See also* claim; number; third-party claims administrator; third-party payer.

internal customer　A member of an organization who receives products and services supplied by other individuals within an organization with the intent of supporting the organization's mission or business objectives. For example, a medical technologist (as supplier) working in a clinical laboratory provides certain services in response to a request for a laboratory test made by a physician, who is, in this scenario, the medical technologist's internal customer. *See also* customer; supplier.

internal medicine　The branch and specialty of medicine dealing with the long-term, comprehensive management of both common and complex medical illnesses of adolescents, adults, and the elderly. Adolescent medicine, cardiovascular medicine, clinical cardiac electrophysiology, critical care medicine, diagnostic laboratory immunology, endocrinology, gastroenterology, geriatric medicine, hematology, infectious diseases, medical oncology, nephrology, pulmonary diseases, rheumatology, sports medicine, and allergy and immunology are subspecialty areas of internal medicine. Synonym: general internal medicine. *See also* American College of Physicians.

Internal Medicine, American Board of *See* American Board of Internal Medicine.

Internal Medicine, American Society of *See* American Society of Internal Medicine.

Internal Medicine, Association of Program Directors in *See* Association of Program Directors in Internal Medicine.

Internal Medicine, Society of General *See* Society of General Internal Medicine.

Internal Organs, American Society for Artificial *See* American Society for Artificial Internal Organs.

internal review Review in which practitioners are involved in setting or adopting the criteria and standards by which they evaluate themselves. *Compare* external review. *See also* medical review; utilization review.

internal validity The extent to which the design of a study contributes to the confidence that can be placed in the study's results. Internal validity is relevant to both measurement studies and studies of causal relationships; it is the extent to which the detected relationships are most likely due to factors accounted for in the study, rather than other factors. *See also* validity.

International Classification of Clinical Services (ICCS) A classification and coding system developed by the Commission on Professional and Hospital Activities for certain hospital-provided services in order to standardize patient care data and to facilitate computer handling of the data. For example, a scheme is available for anesthesia, cardiology, and respiratory therapy. *See also* Commission on Professional and Hospital Activities.

International Classification of Diseases, Ninth Revision, Clinical Modification (ICD-9-CM) The two-part classification system in current use for coding patient medical information used in abstracting systems and for classifying patients into diagnosis-related groups (DRGs) for Medicare and other third-party payers. The first part is a comprehensive list of diseases with corresponding codes compatible with the World Health Organization's list of disease codes. The second part contains procedure codes independent of the disease codes. It is currently published by the federal government. *See also* coding; Council on Clinical Classifications.

International Classification of Health Problems in Primary Care A classification of diseases, conditions, and other reasons for providing primary care. This classification may be used for labeling conditions in problem-oriented records as used by primary care health professionals. It is an adaptation of the *International Classification of Diseases, Ninth Edition, Clinical Modification (ICD-9-CM)* but makes more allowance for the diagnostic uncertainty that characterizes primary care. *See also* primary care.

International Classification of Impairments, Disabilities, and Handicaps A classification that attempts to produce a systematic taxonomy of the consequences of injury and disease; first published by the World Health Organization in 1980. *See also* disability; handicap; impairment.

internist A physician who specializes in internal medicine and its branches. *See also* internal medicine.

Internists, American College of Osteopathic *See* American College of Osteopathic Internists.

intern, nurse *See* nurse intern.

internship Any period of practical, on-the-job training that is part of a larger educational program. In medicine, osteopathic medicine, dentistry, podiatric medicine, and other health professions, internship is a one-year program of graduate medical education coming in the year after graduation. Residencies are increasingly beginning in the first year after graduation, gradually eliminating internships. *See also* medical education; residency.

Internship Centers, Association of Psychology Postdoctoral and *See* Association of Psychology Postdoctoral and Internship Centers.

Interns, National Association of Residents and *See* National Association of Residents and Interns.

Interns and Residents, Committee of *See* Committee of Interns and Residents.

interobserver reliability The degree to which different raters give similar ratings. *Synonyms*: conspect reliability; interjudge reliability; interrater reliability; scorer reliability. *See also* interobserver reliability coefficient; reliability; reliability testing.

interobserver reliability coefficient A correlation coefficient that expresses the degree to which raters agree or disagree. *See also* correlation coefficient; interobserver reliability.

interpolate To predict or estimate the value of variables within the range of observations; for example, in mathematics to interpolate is to estimate the value of a function or series between two known values. *Compare* extrapolate. *See also* variable.

interpolation The prediction resulting from the

process of interpolating. *Compare* extrapolation.

interpret To define or explain the meaning of, as in interpreting data; translate or construe. *See also* interpretation.

interpretation 1. The act or process of interpreting, for example, translating or explaining. **2.** The result of interpreting, as in differing interpretations of the data. *See also* interpret.

Interpreters for the Deaf, Registry of *See* Registry of Interpreters for the Deaf.

interrater reliability *See* interobserver reliability.

interrogatory In civil actions, such as a malpractice lawsuit, a pretrial discovery tool in which written questions put forth for consideration by one party are served on the adversary, who must answer by written replies made under oath. Although an interrogatory is not as flexible an instrument as a deposition, which includes the opportunity to cross-examine, an interrogatory is regarded as an effective and efficient means of establishing important facts held by the adversary. *See also* deposition.

interruptus, coitus *See* coitus interruptus.

Intersociety Committee on Pathology Information (ICPI) An organization founded in 1957 composed of one representative from each sponsoring society: American Association of Pathologists; American Society of Clinical Pathologists; Association of Pathology Chairmen; College of American Pathologists; and US and Canadian Academy of Pathology. It disseminates information about the medical practice and research achievements of pathology and produces career information and supplies it to schools and students. It publishes annually the *Directory of Pathology Training Programs: Anatomic, Clinical, Specialized. See also* pathology.

Interstate Postgraduate Medical Association of North America (IPMANA) An organization founded in 1916 that presents annual four-day teaching programs in various branches of medicine and medical research, aimed at the family practitioner who must keep up with new developments in a short time away from his or her practice. *See also* family practitioner.

interval The amount of time between two specified instants, events, or states, or the space between two objects, points, or parts. *See also* interval scale.

interval scale A type of ordinal scale in which values have a natural equal distance between them and in which a particular distance (interval) between two values in one region of the scale meaningfully represent the same distance between two values in another region of the scale. The zero point is arbitrary. Examples include Celsius and Fahrenheit temperature scales and date of birth. Addition and subtraction are permissible, but not multiplication or division of such scales; statistical analyses, such as the Pearson correlation, factor analysis, or discriminant analysis may be used with interval scales. *See also* Celsius scale; Fahrenheit scale; nominal scale; ordinal scale; ratio scale; scale.

Interveners, American Academy of Crisis *See* American Academy of Crisis Interveners.

intervening cause An independent act that occurs between the time of the original negligence or malpractice and the time of injury. An intervening cause will absolve the original actor of liability only if the intervening act is totally independent and not reasonably foreseeable by the original actor. For example, if a physician commits a negligent act that will ultimately result in a patient's injury and a different physician commits a later negligent act that triggers the injury, the original physician may still be held liable, as most courts hold the actions of the second physician to have been foreseeable by the first. *Synonym:* supervening cause. *See also* cause; foreseeability.

intervention Any action that is intended to interrupt or change events in progress. *See also* active euthanasia; allopathic medicine; allopathy; health intervention; medical intervention; nursing intervention; surgical intervention.

Interventional Radiology, Society of Cardiovascular and *See* Society of Cardiovascular and Interventional Radiology.

intervention, health *See* health intervention.

intervention, medical *See* medical intervention.

intervention, nursing *See* nursing intervention.

Interventions, Society for Cardiac Angiography and *See* Society for Cardiac Angiography and Interventions.

intervention, surgical *See* surgical intervention.

interview A conversation between two or more people for the purpose of yielding information for guidance, counseling, treatment, or employment. *See also* leadership interview; public information interview; structured interview; unstructured interview.

interview, leadership *See* leadership interview.

interview, public information *See* public information interview.

interview, structured *See* structured interview.

Interview Survey, Health *See* Health Interview Survey.

interview, unstructured *See* unstructured interview.

Intestinal Endoscopic Surgeons, Society American Gastro- *See* Society American Gastrointestinal Endoscopic Surgeons.

intestine The part of the alimentary tract extending between the pyloric opening of the stomach and the anus; it comprises in descending order the small intestine (duodenum, jejunum, ileum) and the large intestine (cecum, colon, rectum, anal canal). *Synonyms*: bowel; gut. *See also* alimentary tract; barium enema; colon; constipation; duodenum; enteral feeding; enteric; gastrointestinal; ileum; ileus; intussusception; jejunum; laxative; peristalsis; rectum; stomach; volvulus; worm.

intoxication The state of being poisoned, particularly, the state of being under the influence of alcohol or other euphoriant substance. *See also* alcohol; alcoholism; euphoria.

intraarterial Into or within an artery, as in an intraarterial catheter for measuring arterial blood pressure. *Compare* intravenous.

intracorporate entrepreneur *See* intrapreneur.

Intractable Pain, National Committee on the Treatment of *See* National Committee on the Treatment of Intractable Pain.

intradermal injection *See* injection.

intrahospital transfer A transfer of a patient within the same hospital, as from one patient care unit to another (for example, cardiac care unit to step-down unit), from one clinical service to another (for example, medicine service to surgery service), or from one physician to another. *See also* transfer.

intramuscular (IM) Into or within muscle, as in intramuscular injection of penicillin. *See also* injection; parenteral.

intramuscular injection *See* injection.

intraoperative Pertaining to the time during a surgical operation, as in intraoperative autotransfusion. *See also* perioperative; postoperative; preoperative.

intraoperative autotransfusion The collection, processing, and reinfusion of a patient's blood shed from a wound or body cavity during surgery. *See also* autotransfusion; blood transfusion; postoperative autotransfusion.

intrapreneur A business person who uses entrepreneurial skills from within a large corporation to revitalize and diversify its business, rather than setting up competing small businesses. *Synonym*: intracorporate entrepreneur. *Compare* entrepreneur.

intrarater reliability Consistency of judgments by a single rater. *See also* interobserver reliability; reliability.

intravenous (IV) Into or within a vein, as in intravenous fluids. *Compare* intraarterial. *See also* drip; infusion; parenteral.

intravenous anesthetic An anesthetic, such as thiopental, that is administered through a vein. *See also* anesthetic; barbiturate.

intravenous feeding tube *See* nutritional support.

intravenous injection *See* injection.

Intravenous Nurses Society (INS) A national organization founded in 1973 composed of 6,000 registered nurses involved in intravenous therapy, licensed practical nurses, and pharmacists. It conducts a certification program for intravenous nurses and an advanced studies program in intravenous nursing. *See also* certification; licensed practical nurse; pharmacist; registered nurse.

intravenous team A group of people specially trained to phlebotomize (remove blood) from patients and insert intravenous catheters for the administration of therapies, such as medication, nutrition, and fluids. *See also* phlebotomy.

intravenous therapy Administration of medication, nutrition, and other fluids via vein. *See also* intravenous; therapy.

intravenous tube *See* nutritional support.

introvert An individual whose thoughts and interests appear to be directed inward, rather than expressed by means of outward action, and who therefore seems withdrawn or reserved.

intubation Placement and maintenance of a tube in an opening, especially passage of a breathing tube into the trachea to allow passage of oxygen or anesthetic gas. *See also* airway; endotracheal intubation; nasogastric intubation; nasotracheal intubation; orotracheal intubation.

intubation, endotracheal *See* endotracheal intubation.

intubation, nasogastric *See* nasogastric intubation.

intubation, nasotracheal *See* nasotracheal intubation.

intubation, orotracheal *See* orotracheal intubation.

intuition The act of knowing or sensing without the use of rational processes. Intuition is one source of hypotheses. *See also* common sense; hypothesis;

seat-of-the-pants.

intumescence 1. The process of swelling. **2.** The state of being swollen.

intussusception The prolapse or invagination of part of the intestine into the adjoining segment, a cause of intestinal obstruction, particularly during the first year of life. *See also* intestine.

inurement To serve to the benefit of someone, as in private gain from corporate activities. For example, if a nonprofit organization, such as a hospital, provides incentives to attract individuals, such as physicians, the incentives may be considered inurement by the Internal Revenue Service and thus affect the tax-exempt status of the hospital.

invalid 1. Falsely reasoned or based, as in an invalid interpretation of the data. **2.** Suffering from disease or disability. **3.** An individual who is temporarily or permanently disabled by illness or injury. *See also* invalidism.

invalidism 1. The state of being a recognized or confirmed invalid. **2.** A state of chronic ill health. *See also* invalid.

invasive Pertaining to a medical procedure in which a part of the body is entered. *Compare* noninvasive. *See also* invasive procedure.

invasive procedure A procedure involving puncture or incision of the skin or insertion of an instrument or foreign material into the body, including, but not limited to, percutaneous aspirations and biopsies, cardiac and vascular catheterizations, endoscopies, angioplasties, and implantations and excluding venipuncture and intravenous therapy. *Compare* noninvasive. *See also* cardiac catheterization; invasive.

investigate To conduct a thorough, searching, probing, systematic inquiry, usually over a period of time. *See also* investigation; investigational new drug.

investigation The act or process of investigating, as in a clinical investigation of a new procedure. *See also* investigate.

investigational new drug (IND) A drug available solely for experimental use in order to determine its safety and effectiveness. An IND is not yet approved by the Food and Drug Administration (FDA) for marketing to the general public and only experts qualified by training and experience to investigate the drug's safety and effectiveness may prescribe it. Use of the drug in humans requires approval by the FDA of an IND application, which includes reports of animal toxicity tests with the drug, a description of proposed clinical trials, and a list of the names and qualifications of the investigators conducting these studies. *See also* new drug; new drug application.

Investigation, American Society for Clinical *See* American Society for Clinical Investigation.

Investigation of Claims of the Paranormal, Committee for the Scientific *See* Committee for the Scientific Investigation of Claims of the Paranormal.

Investigation, Society for Gynecologic *See* Society for Gynecologic Investigation.

Investigative Dermatology, Society for *See* Society for Investigative Dermatology.

investigative reporting A style of reporting used in television and radio that actively seeks to expose malpractice, injustice, or any other activity deemed to be against the public good. *See also* investigate; media.

investigator, public health field *See* public health field investigator.

investment 1. Property or other possession acquired for future financial return or benefit. **2.** A commitment, such as a time investment.

investment, capital *See* capital investment.

investor-owned hospital A hospital that is owned and operated by a corporation or an individual and that operates on a for-profit basis. *Synonyms:* for-profit hospital; proprietary hospital. *See also* hospital.

invisible patient care function A goal-directed interrelated series of processes that supports direct patient care but often is far removed from the patient's immediate experience; for example, the safety management or performance improvement functions of a hospital. *Compare* visible patient care function. *See also* function.

in vitro Latin phrase meaning "in glass," that is, outside of the living organism and in an artificial environment, such as a test tube. *Compare* in vivo. *See also* in-vitro fertilization.

In-Vitro Allergy/Immunology Society, American *See* American In-Vitro Allergy/Immunology Society.

in-vitro fertilization (IVF) The process of removing an ovum, fertilizing the ovum with sperm in a culture medium in the laboratory, and placing the fertilized ovum into the uterus. *Synonym:* test-tube baby technique. *See also* fertilization; in vitro.

in vivo Latin phrase meaning "in the living organism." *Compare* in vitro.

invoice A bill prepared by a seller of goods or services and submitted to the purchaser. The invoice lists all items or services purchased, together with amounts owed. *See also* bill; billing.

invoicing *See* billing.

involuntary commitment A court-directed admission of a patient to a mental health care facility against the patient's will. In most jurisdictions, the individual with mental illness must be incapable of taking care of himself or herself, likely to injure himself or herself, or likely to injure another person. *See also* commitment.

involuntary demotion A demotion resulting from an employee's inability to perform adequately on the job. *See also* demotion.

involuntary muscle *See* muscle.

involuntary smoking The inhalation by nonsmokers of tobacco smoke left in the air by smokers. Involuntary smoking includes both smoke exhaled by smokers and smoke released directly from burning tobacco into ambient air. The latter is called sidestream smoke, or secondhand smoke, and contains a higher proportion of toxic and other carcinogenic substances than exhaled smoke. *Synonyms*: passive smoking; secondary smoking. *See also* nicotine; sidestream smoke; smoke; smoking; tobacco.

iodine An element that is an essential component of the human diet, being required for the synthesis of the thyroid hormones. A radioactive isotope of iodine is used extensively in the diagnosis of thyroid gland conditions. and in the treatment of thyrotoxicosis and thyroid carcinoma. *See also* hormone; hyperthyroidism; radioisotope; thyroid gland.

IOM *See* Institute of Medicine.

IPA *See* individual practice association.

IPMANA *See* Interstate Postgraduate Medical Association of North America.

IPP *See* Impaired Physician Program.

ipsilateral Situated on, pertaining to, or affecting the same side. *Compare* contralateral.

IQ *See* intelligence quotient.

IRA *See* individual retirement account.

IRA, health *See* health IRA.

IRA, medical *See* health IRA.

IRB *See* institutional review board.

IRET *See* Institute for Rational-Emotive Therapy.

IRH *See* Institute for Reproductive Health.

IRHP *See* Institute for Research in Hypnosis and Psychotherapy.

iron A trace mineral essential as part of hemoglobin and myoglobin. Good sources include red meat, liver, fish, green leafy vegetables, enriched bread, dried prunes, apricots and raisins. Humans absorb the iron from animal sources on average five times better than that from plant sources. *See also* iron-deficiency anemia.

iron-deficiency anemia Anemia caused by a deficiency or iron, most often as a result of loss of blood from menstruation, ulcers, or malignancies, or as a result of increased iron needs during pregnancy or infancy. *See also* anemia; iron.

iron lung A lay term for an early design of respirator, in which artificial ventilation was maintained by applying cyclical pressure variation to the interior of a rigid metal cylinder within which the patient's body, excluding only the head, was enclosed. *See also* poliomyelitis; respirator.

irradiation Exposure or treatment by photons, electrons, neutrons, or other ionizing radiations. Artificial radioisotopes are made by irradiating stable isotopes with neutrons. In small doses irradiation is sometimes used to sterilize food, utilizing the sensitivity of biological cells to ionizing radiation. *See also* immunosuppressive; radiation; radioisotope.

irrational Not endowed with reason; marked by a lack of accord with reason or sound judgment, as in an irrational person or an irrational decision. *Compare* rational.

irrebuttable presumption A legal proposition that allows a fact finder (judge or jury) to accept a fact as true if other underlying facts are proved. The presumption becomes irrebuttable when, depending on the jurisdiction, the opposing party is not allowed to offer evidence to contradict the ultimate fact, once the underlying facts have been proved. *Compare* rebuttable presumption. *See also* fact finder; presumption.

irregular medicine *See* alternative medicine.

irrigation The process of washing out a wound, body cavity, or hollow viscus by means of a stream of water, saline, or other fluid.

irritable bowel syndrome A group of syndromes, including abdominal pain and cramping, constipation, diarrhea, bloating, and stomach distress, that emotional stress or anxiety may trigger; usually affecting young adults. *See also* syndrome.

irritant An agent that gives rise to irritation, particularly chemical irritation of the skin or mucous membranes.

IRT *See* Institute for Reality Therapy.

ischemia Decreased blood supply to a given body part, sometimes resulting from vasoconstriction, thrombosis, or embolism; for example, myocardial (heart muscle) ischemia. *See also* acute myocardial infarction; angina pectoris; cerebrovascular accident; embolism; fibrillation; infarct; thrombosis; transient ischemic attack; volvulus.

ischemic attack, transient *See* transient ischemic attack.

Ishikawa diagram *See* cause-and-effect diagram.

Ishikawa, Kaoru *See* cause-and-effect diagram.

Islamic Medical Association (IMA) A national organization founded in 1967 composed of 6,000 Muslim physicians and allied health professionals interested in assisting Muslim communities worldwide. It awards scholarships to needy students and donates books, educational and research materials, and medical supplies and equipment to charity medical institutions in Muslim countries. *See also* allied health professional; medical association.

isolate To set apart from other persons or animals or to place in quarantine, as in an inpatient with chickenpox must be isolated from patients in the obstetrics and perinatal wards. *See also* isolation; quarantine.

isolation In health care, the separation of infected persons or animals from other persons or animals to prevent or limit the direct or indirect transmission of the infectious agent from those infected to those who are susceptible or who may spread the agent to others. *Synonym*: patient isolation. *See also* blood/body fluid precautions; contact isolation; drainage/secretion precautions; enteric precautions; quarantine; respiratory isolation; strict isolation; tuberculous isolation.

isolation, AFB *See* tuberculosis isolation.

isolation bed A bed regularly maintained by a health care organization for inpatients who require isolation. *See also* bed; isolation.

isolation, contact *See* contact isolation.

isolation incubator An incubator bed regularly maintained for premature and other infants who require isolation. *See also* incubator; isolation.

isolation, patient *See* isolation.

isolation, respiratory *See* respiratory isolation.

isolation, strict *See* strict isolation.

isolation, tuberculous *See* tuberculous isolation.

isotonic saline *See* saline.

isotope An atom of the same element but differing in mass number from other isotopes of that element. The difference relates to a different number of neutrons in the nucleus. Isotopes are identical in all chemical properties and in all physical properties except those dependent on atomic mass. Almost all elements occur in nature as mixtures of several isotopes. *See also* radioisotope.

isotope, radio- *See* radioisotope.

isotope, radioactive *See* radioisotope.

Israel, American Physicians Fellowship for Medicine in *See* American Physicians Fellowship for Medicine in Israel.

ISS *See* injury severity score.

issue **1.** A point or matter of discussion, debate, or dispute, as in ethical issues relating to human organ procurement activities. **2.** A matter of public concern, as in economic issues troubling the country.

issue of fact A question regarding the existence of a fact that is generally presented for determination to the fact finder (judge or jury). *See also* fact finder; issue of law; judge; jury; jury trial.

issue of law A legal determination, made by a judge alone, requiring that the judge apply legal principles to the facts for a resolution of the matter. This may occur in a summary judgment proceeding in which one part accepts, for the purpose of argument, all facts asserted by the opposing party, but claims that, in spite of these facts, he or she is entitled under the law to a judgment in his or her favor. For example, the statute of limitations may mandate a judgment in one's favor in spite of the underlying fact that negligence occurred. *See also* issue of fact; summary judgment.

Italian Medical Schools, Graduates of *See* Graduates of Italian Medical Schools.

itch The cutaneous sensation that provokes the urge to scratch. *See also* antipruritic; pruritis.

IV *See* intravenous.

IVF *See* in-vitro fertilization.

IVT *See* Institute for Victims of Trauma.

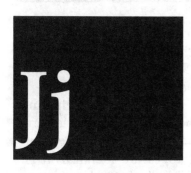

Jj

jacket   A stiff plastic encasement around a computer diskette (floppy disk). It contains holes that give the disk drive access to the information on the disk. The disk should not be removed from the jacket. *See also* diskette.

Jackson Hole approach   An approach to managed competition that advocates three major changes in the US health insurance system. Regional health insurance purchasing cooperatives (HIPCs) are formed to manage the marketplace for health care coverage, especially for small firms and individuals. Employers and HIPCs contribute the same amount of money for coverage regardless of which plan a consumer chooses. New rules are created making it more difficult for plans to avoid enrolling high-risk individuals. *See also* managed competition.

Jackson Orthopaedic Society, Ruth   *See* Ruth Jackson Orthopaedic Society.

JAMA   *See Journal of the American Medical Association.*

jargon   **1.** The specialized or technical language of a trade, profession, or similar group. *See also* terminology. **2.** Nonsensical, incoherent, or meaningless talk. *See also* bureaucratese; legalese; psychobabble.

jaundice   Yellowish discoloration of the skin, mucous membranes, and sclerae of the eyes due to excessive bilirubin (bile pigment). It is caused by many disorders, including liver diseases, biliary obstruction, and hemolytic anemias. Newborns commonly develop physiologic jaundice, which disappears after a few days. *Synonym*: icterus. *See also* bilirubin; hepatitis; kernicterus; liver.

jaw   *See* gnathic; mandible; maxilla.

JCAHO   *See* Joint Commission on Accreditation of Healthcare Organizations.

JCAHPO   *See* Joint Commission on Allied Health Personnel in Ophthalmology.

JCAI   *See* Joint Council of Allergy and Immunology.

JCSMS   *See* Joint Commission on Sports Medicine and Science.

JD   *See* Juris Doctor.

JDC   *See* Joslin Diabetes Center.

Jehovah's Witness   A member of a religious denomination founded in Pittsburgh in 1872 by Charles Taze Russell, in which active evangelism is practiced and Witnesses consider themselves a society of ministers. Civil authority is regarded as necessary and is obeyed as long as its laws do not contradict the laws of God, and Witnesses refuse to bear arms, salute the flag, or participate in secular government. Jehovah's Witnesses will undergo needed surgery but will not accept any blood transfusions even in the event of an emergency. *See also* blood transfusion.

jejunum   The second part of the small intestine. *See also* intestine.

jet lag   A temporary condition characterized by fatigue, sleep disturbances, and sluggish body functions, caused by a disruption of the body's normal circadian rhythm resulting from high-speed travel, usually through several time zones. *See also* chronobiology; circadian; lag.

Jewish Center for Immunology and Respiratory Medicine, National   *See* National Jewish Center for Immunology and Respiratory Medicine.

Jewish Hospice, National Institute for   *See* National Institute for Jewish Hospice.

Jewish Pharmaceutical Society of America (JPSA)   A national organization founded in 1950 composed of 100 Jewish pharmacists. *See also* pharmacist; pharmacy.

Jin Shin Do Foundation for Bodymind Acupressure (JSDF)   A certification, referral, and educational organization founded in 1982 composed of

200 teachers and practitioners of the Jin Shin Do acupressure method. Jin Shin Do acupressure integrates a traditional Japanese acupressure technique with classical Chinese acu-theory, Taoist philosophy and breathing methods, and Western psychology. *See also* acupressure; certification.

JIT *See* just in time.

job **1.** A regular activity performed in exchange for payment, especially as one's trade, occupation, or profession. *See also* occupation; profession; vocation; work. **2.** The position in which a person is employed. **3.** A specific project.

job description Definition of an employment position or a task including duties, responsibilities, and conditions required in the performance of the job. *See also* job.

job lock A situation in which an individual is locked into a position with his or her current employer because preexisting medical conditions make the individual uninsurable elsewhere. *See also* job; preexisting condition.

job satisfaction The sense of fulfillment and pride achieved when performing a task or working in an employment position. *See also* job; satisfaction.

job security Freedom from the fear of losing or being dismissed from one's employment. *See also* job; security.

job sharing A situation in which the responsibilities, hours, and pay of one position are divided between two or more people. Job sharing is an alternative to layoffs because two people can continue to have part-time work until economic conditions improve. *See also* job; layoff; part-time.

job specification Requirements for a particular position or task including the skills, education, and experience needed. *See also* job; specification.

Joggers Association, American Medical *See* American Medical Athletic Association.

John A. Hartford Foundation, Inc, The *See* The John A. Hartford Foundation, Inc.

John D. and Catherine T. MacArthur Foundation, The *See* The John D. and Catherine T. MacArthur Foundation.

Johnson Foundation, The Robert Wood *See* The Robert Wood Johnson Foundation.

joint **1.** A place or part at which two or more things are joined. **2.** Any articulation between two bones. *See also* arthralgia; arthritis; bunion; gout; hip joint; knock-knee; ligament; orthopaedic/orthopedic surgery; osteoarthritis; physical therapy; rheumatology; sprain; tendon; ultrasound physical therapy.

Joint Commission on Accreditation of Hospitals *See* Joint Commission on Accreditation of Healthcare Organizations.

Joint Commission on Accreditation of Healthcare Organizations (Joint Commission, JCAHO) An independent, not-for-profit, national organization founded in 1951 that develops organization standards and other performance measures, awards accreditation decisions, and provides education and consultation to the following types of organizations: hospitals; psychiatric facilities, substance abuse treatment and rehabilitation programs, community mental health centers, organizations providing services for the mentally retarded and developmentally disabled; long term care facilities; hospice programs; ambulatory health and managed care organizations; pathology and clinical laboratory programs; home care organizations; and health care networks. Its corporate members are the American College of Physicians, American College of Surgeons, American Dental Association, American Hospital Association, and American Medical Association. It is governed by a Board of Commissioners composed of representatives of corporate member organizations, public members, and an at-large-representative of the nursing profession. Formerly (1987) Joint Commission on Accreditation of Hospitals. *See also* accreditation; accreditation survey.

Joint Commission accreditation manuals *See* standards manuals.

Joint Commission Agenda for Change *See* Agenda for Change.

Joint Commission on Allied Health Personnel in Ophthalmology (JCAHPO) A national organization founded in 1969 for certifying allied health personnel in ophthalmology. Its objectives include encouraging the establishment of medically oriented programs for training allied health personnel in ophthalmology, developing standards of education and training in the field, and examining, certifying, and recertifying ophthalmic medical personnel. *See also* allied health professional; certification; ophthalmic medical technician; ophthalmic medical technologist; ophthalmology; recertification.

Joint Commission on Competitive Safeguards and the Medical Aspects of Sports *See* Joint Commission on Sports Medicine and Science.

Joint Commission Journal on Quality Improvement, The *See The Joint Commission Journal on Quality Improvement.*

Joint Commission Perspectives A bimonthly newsletter that provides current information about the Joint Commission on Accreditation of Healthcare Organizations and its accreditation programs, including all changes in the standards, policies, and procedures; explanations of standards; progress in the Agenda for Change initiatives; and announcements concerning publications and education programs. *See also* Agenda for Change; Joint Commission on Accreditation of Healthcare Organizations.

Joint Commission on Sports Medicine and Science (JCSMS) A national organization founded in 1966 composed of five organizations: American College Health Association, National Association of Intercollegiate Athletics, National Athletic Trainers Association, National Federation of State High School Associations, and National Junior College Athletic Association. It promotes communication among organizations concerned with the health and safety of individuals engaged in athletics. It establishes guidelines and standards for athletic programs and recommends rules and administration policies for athletic programs. Formerly (1988) Joint Commission on Competitive Safeguards and the Medical Aspects of Sports. *See also* sports medicine.

Joint Commission survey *See* accreditation survey; extension survey; focused survey; follow-up survey; full team survey; special survey; specialized survey; tailored survey; triennial survey; unannounced survey; validation survey.

Joint Committee on Cancer, American *See* American Joint Committee on Cancer.

joint conference committee In a health care organization, a committee with members representing the governing body, the medical staff, and the hospital administration, whose purpose is to facilitate understanding and communication about issues of mutual concern within the organization. *See also* committee; conference.

Joint Council of Allergy and Immunology (JCAI) A national organization founded in 1975 composed of 2,850 physicians specializing in allergy or clinical immunology. Members must belong to the American Academy of Allergy and Immunology or the American College of Allergy and Immunology. It serves as the political and socioeconomic arm for these organizations. *See also* allergy and immunology; American Academy of Allergy and Immunology; American College of Allergy and Immunology.

joint enterprise An enterprise or undertaking founded on consensual agreement of parties.

joint, hip *See* hip joint.

joint probability The probability that two or more specific outcomes or results will occur in an event. *See also* probability.

Joint Review Commission for Ophthalmic Medical Personnel *See* Joint Review Committee for Ophthalmic Medical Personnel.

Joint Review Committee on Educational Programs for the EMT-Paramedic (JRCEMT-P) A national organization founded in 1979 that cooperates with the Committee on Allied Health Education and Accreditation to accredit emergency medical technician-paramedic training programs across the United States. It establishes national education standards and programs for the EMT-paramedic. *See also* accreditation; allied health professional; emergency medical technician-paramedic.

Joint Review Committee on Education in Diagnostic Medical Sonography (JRCDMS) A national organization founded in 1979 composed of physicians and ultrasonographers whose purpose is to evaluate, and recommend for accreditation, educational programs in the field of diagnostic medical sonography. *See also* diagnostic medical sonographer; ultrasound imaging.

Joint Review Committee on Education in Radiologic Technology (JRCERT) A national organization founded in 1969 whose purpose is to evaluate, and recommend for accreditation, educational programs in the fields of radiography and radiation therapy technology. Its participants are physicians, radiographers, and radiation therapy technologists. *See also* radiation therapy; radiography.

Joint Review Committee on Education for the Surgical Technologist *See* Accreditation Review Committee for Educational Programs in Surgical Technology.

Joint Review Committee for Ophthalmic Medical Personnel (JRCOMP) A national organization composed of individuals from collaborating health organizations, including the Association of Technical Personnel in Ophthalmology and the Joint Commission on Allied Health Personnel in Ophthalmology, whose primary activity is to evaluate ophthalmic educational programs applying for accreditation from the American Medical Association Committee on Allied Health Education and Accreditation. It reviews and revises guidelines, maintains policies, and approves processes that comply with standards established for national accrediting agencies. It provides teams of representatives to conduct site visits of programs. Formerly (1989) Joint Review Commission for Ophthalmic Medical Personnel. *See also* accreditation; ophthalmology.

Joint Review Committee for Respiratory Therapy Education (JRCRTE) A national organization founded in 1963 composed of 13 physicians, respiratory therapists, and public representatives who develop standards and requirements for accredited educational programs of respiratory therapy for recommendation to the American Medical Association (AMA); conduct evaluations of educational programs that have applied for accreditation to the AMA and make recommendations to the AMA's Committee on Allied Health Education and Accreditation; and maintain a working relationship with other organizations interested in respiratory therapy education and evaluation. *See also* American Medical Association; respiratory therapy.

joint and several liability A rule of law that allows an individual who has suffered loss or injury as a result of the acts of more than one person to collect the entire compensation from any one of the wrongdoers without regard to his or her individual fault or contribution. *See also* joint tortfeasors; liability.

Joint Surgeons, Association of Bone and *See* Association of Bone and Joint Surgeons.

joint tortfeasors Two or more persons who have acted in concert, each negligently, in producing an injury or loss or whose separate negligent acts, though not in concert, combined to create a single injury or loss. In some jurisdictions, such activity is the basis for the imposition of joint and several liability. *See also* joint and several liability; tortfeasor.

joint underwriting association (JUA) An independent association of insurers authorized by a state to write a certain kind of insurance, especially general liability insurance, such as malpractice insurance. *See also* general liability insurance; underwriting.

joint venture A contract or agreement and a legal entity characterized by two or more parties who work on a project together, sharing profits, losses, and control. For example, in the health care field, a hospital

and members of its medical staff may create a formalized cooperative effort (such as setting up a diagnostic imaging facility) instead of being in competition with one another (as by a group of radiologists setting up a diagnostic imaging center that is in direct competition with the diagnostic imaging facilities set up by a hospital). A joint venture, which is usually limited to a single project, differs from a partnership, which forms the basis for cooperation on many projects. *Compare* partnership. *See also* affiliation; corporate diversification; safe harbor regulations.

Joslin Diabetes Center (JDC) A national organization founded in 1968 composed of 350 persons interested in advancing knowledge and improving treatment of diabetes with the goal of discovering a means of prevention and cure. It investigates new methods in the clinical treatment of diabetes; conducts research at its Elliott P. Joslin Research laboratory; and maintains a diabetes treatment unit to instruct diabetic patients in the proper management of their disease. *See also* diabetes mellitus.

journal An academic or professional periodical, such as the *Journal of the American Medical Association, New England Journal of Medicine, American Journal of Nursing,* and *American Pharmacy,* that disseminates research findings widely, cheaply, and in considerable detail. *Synonyms:* medical journal. *See also American Journal of Nursing; American Pharmacy; Journal of the American Medical Association; New England Journal of Medicine;* refereed journal; throw-away journals.

Journal of the American Medical Association (JAMA) A weekly medical journal published by the American Medical Association. The *JAMA* is composed of clinical, research, and other articles relevant to the practice of medicine. *See also* American Medical Association; journal; refereed journal.

journalism The collecting, writing, editing, and presenting news or news articles in newspapers and magazines and in radio and television broadcasts. *See also* media; New Journalism; press.

Journalism, New *See* New Journalism.

journal, refereed *See* refereed journal.

journal, throw-away *See* throw-away journal.

journey, remedial *See* remedial journey.

joystick A computer input device that is used to move the computer cursor or other object displayed on the computer screen; usually used to play video games. *See also* computer; cursor; input device.

JPSA *See* Jewish Pharmaceutical Society of America.

JRCDMS *See* Joint Review Committee on Education in Diagnostic Medical Sonography.

JRCEMT-P *See* Joint Review Committee on Educational Programs for the EMT-Paramedic.

JRCERT *See* Joint Review Committee on Education in Radiologic Technology.

JRCOMP *See* Joint Review Committee for Ophthalmic Medical Personnel.

JRCRTE *See* Joint Review Committee for Respiratory Therapy Education.

JSDF Jin Shin Do Foundation for Bodymind Acupressure.

JUA *See* joint underwriting association.

judge **1.** An appointed or elected official with the power to make decisions in a court of law. *See also* court; dicta; fact finder. **2.** To form an opinion after careful consideration. *See also* judgment; misjudge.

judge, mis- *See* misjudge.

judgment **1.** The use of one's understanding and intuition to resolve a problem. *See also* assumption; cognition; common sense; decision; judge; opinion; reasoning; value judgment. **2.** The conclusion of a court on the claims of the parties as submitted for determination. *See also* summary judgment.

judgment doctrine, substituted *See* substituted judgment doctrine.

judgment, summary *See* summary judgment.

judgment, value *See* value judgment.

junior partner A partner in a partnership who is limited as to both profits and management participation. *See also* general partner; limited partner; partner; partnership.

junk bond A bond bearing high interest and high risk, issued by a company seeking to raise a large amount of capital quickly, usually in order to finance a corporate takeover.

junk food High-carbohydrate food, such as potato chips, french fries, and sweets, that appeals to popular taste and provides many calories fast, but has little lasting nutritional value. *See also* food.

junkie **1.** A narcotics addict, especially one addicted to heroin. *See also* heroin; narcotics. **2.** Anyone who has an insatiable interest, as in a television junkie.

Juran, Joseph M. (b. 1904) An engineer and patriarch of total quality management who is credited with the idea that putting out a fire may save the building, but it does not improve it, that is, although crisis management has its uses, it does not lead to quality improvement. He has written numerous books on quality with the central theme that planning, control, and improvement lead to quality. *See also* continuous quality improvement; management by crisis.

jurisdiction **1.** A geographic or political entity governed by a particular legal system or body of laws. **2.** The power or authority of a court over the individuals or property in dispute and the subject matter of the dispute.

Juris Doctor (JD) The title for an individual who holds a Doctor of Jurisprudence degree. The title was formerly abbreviated as LLB (Bachelor of Laws) or LLD (Doctor of Laws). *See also* attorney; jurisprudence; lawyer.

jurisprudence The science of law, including the study of the structure and underlying principles of legal systems.

Jurisprudence, Society of Medical *See* Society of Medical Jurisprudence.

jurist An individual, such as a judge, lawyer, or scholar, who is expert in the field of law. *See also* judge.

juror A member of a jury. *See also* jury.

jury A group of peers or a cross-section of a community who are summoned and sworn to decide on the facts at issue in a trial. *See also* coroner's jury; grand jury; hung jury; impanel; issue of fact; jury trial; petit jury; voir dire.

jury, coroner's *See* coroner's jury.

jury, grand *See* grand jury.

jury, hung *See* hung jury.

jury, petit *See* petit jury.

jury trial The trial of an issue of fact before a jury. The parties to a suit present their evidence to the jury. The judge then instructs the jury as to how the law applies to their findings of fact, and the jury then deliberates and renders its verdict. *See also* hung jury; impanel; issue of fact; jury; trial.

justice The principle of moral rightness, that is, a duty that is called upon when there are issues concerning what is rightfully due a person, an institution, or a society. This is most commonly seen when more than one group is competing for the same resource, such as human organs for transplantation and tax money for health care services. *See also* poetic justice; tribunal.

Justice, Department of *See* Department of Justice.

justice, poetic *See* poetic justice.

just in time (JIT) A supply system organized so that the right amount of supplies is always available. In total quality management, the term is often used to describe training in specific tools and techniques that is delivered to an improvement team just in time to be used. This avoids providing team members with large amounts of pretraining, much of which may be forgotten before it is actually used. *See also* total quality management.

juvenile-onset diabetes *See* type I diabetes mellitus.

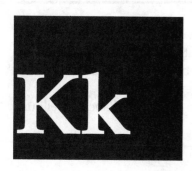

K A unit of measure (1,024 bytes) of the memory held by a computer or storage device. *See also* bit; byte; computer.

Kaiser Family Foundation, The Henry J. *See* The Henry J. Kaiser Family Foundation.

Kaiser Foundation Health Plan *See* Kaiser-Permanente Medical Care Program.

Kaiser Foundation Hospitals *See* Kaiser-Permanente Medical Care Program.

Kaiser-Permanente Medical Care Program One of the world's largest private, prepaid medical care delivery systems operating in California, Hawaii, Oregon, Washington, Colorado, and Ohio. It is composed of three cooperating organizations: the Kaiser Foundation Health Plan, a nonprofit corporation that is the membership component of the program; Kaiser Foundation Hospitals, a charitable nonprofit corporation that contracts with the Kaiser Foundation Health Plan to provide hospital services for the plan's membership; and Permanente Medical Groups, groups of physicians organized as partnerships or as professional corporations to provide medical services required by the health plan's members. *See also* prepaid health plan.

kaizen Japanese word meaning "gradual, unending improvement." *See also* hoshin.

Kansas Health Foundation Originally founded in 1978 with a primary mission of providing philanthropic support to the Wesley Medical Center, the Kansas Health Trust became independent in 1985, and in 1993, restructured as the Kansas Health Foundation. The Kansas Health Trust controls the assets of the Kansas Health Foundation. Its grant philosophy is to initiate requests for proposals and invited proposals only, instead of responding to unsolicited requests. Giving is in the areas of primary care education, public health, prevention, leadership, rural health, and enhancing Kansas' ability to keep track of who is getting sick and why. Giving is restricted to health care organizations in Kansas. *See also* foundation; private foundation.

Kansas Health Trust *See* Kansas Health Foundation.

Kaposi's sarcoma A malignant skin tumor often beginning as reddish soft swellings on the hands or feet. There is a strong association between Kaposi's sarcoma and the acquired immunodeficiency syndrome, especially in homosexual men. Named after Moriz Kohn Kaposi (1837-1902), a Hungarian dermatologist. *See also* acquired immunodeficiency syndrome; reticulosis; sarcoma.

Karen Horney Clinic (KHC) An organization founded in 1955 that promotes the psychoanalytic and psychotherapeutic treatment of individuals and groups focusing on the special problems of children, adolescents, the developmentally disabled, victims of violent crimes, adult survivors of childhood sexual abuse, and persons with psychoneurotic and emotional problems. It is named for Karen Horney (1885-1952), a German-American psychoanalyst and author of books on neurosis, psychoanalysis, and related topics. *See also* psychoanalysis.

karyology The study of the cell nucleus. *See also* cell.

Keck Foundation, WM *See* WM Keck Foundation.

Kellogg Foundation, WK *See* WK Kellogg Foundation.

keloid An overgrowth of collagen tissue during the formation of a scar, resulting in the scar being thickened and elevated. *See also* scar.

Kelvin scale An absolute temperature scale whose unit of measurement, the kelvin, is equal to 1/273.16 of the absolute temperature of the triple point of water. A kelvin unit is equal to 1° C. *See also* Celsius scale; scale; temperature.

Keogh plan A retirement plan, available since 1963, for self-employed individuals, such as private physicians and their employees; named after Eugene James Keogh, a former US representative from New York. *See also* individual retirement account.

keratorefraction A surgical procedure in which the shape of the cornea and iris is changed in order to correct nearsightedness and astigmatism. *See also* ophthalmology; procedure.

Kerato-Refractive Society (KRS) A national organization founded in 1979 composed of 2,000 ophthalmologists and scientists interested in the latest advances in keratorefractive and laser techniques. Its purpose is to keep professionals and other persons informed of the most recent advances and developments in ophthalmologic care. *See also* keratorefraction; ophthalmology.

kernicterus A condition that occurs in hemolytic disease of the newborn when the concentration of free-floating (unconjugated) bilirubin reaches such high levels that it crosses the blood-brain barrier and causes cerebral damage, such as deafness. *See also* bilirubin; jaundice.

Kerr-Mills A popular name for the Social Security Amendments of 1960, which expanded and modified the federal government's responsibility for helping states to pay for medical care for the aged poor. *Synonym*: Medical Assistance for the Aged.

ketoacidosis, diabetic *See* diabetic ketoacidosis.

ketogenic diet A diet that is high in protein and low in carbohydrates. It causes the body to produce ketones and can lead to ketosis and potentially serious side effects. *See also* carbohydrates; diet; ketosis.

ketone A byproduct of partially burned fatty acids that the body can use as energy when carbohydrates are not available. *See also* carbohydrates; ketosis.

ketosis A condition caused by deficiency or inadequate utilization of carbohydrates, in which ketones accumulate in the blood rendering it acidic. Ketosis is seen most frequently in diabetes mellitus and starvation. Untreated, it may progress to ketoacidosis, coma, and death. *See also* carbohydrates; diabetes mellitus; diabetic ketoacidosis; ketone.

keyboard *See* console.

key function *See* important function.

keyhole surgery Minimally invasive surgery, carried out through a very small incision using fiberoptic instruments; for example, laparoscopic cholecystectomy. *See also* fiberoptics; laparoscopic cholecystectomy; surgery.

key items, probes, and scoring guidelines (KIPS) KIPS are tools used in surveying the plant, technology, and safety management (PTSM) standards for the Hospital Accreditation Program of the Joint Commission on Accreditation of Healthcare Organizations. *Key items* are individual PTSM standards. A *probe* is a tool to quantify compliance with a standard. *Scoring guidelines* include a score of 1 if 91% to 100% of applicable departments/services in a hospital have a program to manage hazardous materials and hazardous wastes, a score of 2 if 76% to 90% of departments/services comply with the standard, and so on to a score of 5 if fewer than 26% of departments/services comply or if there is no such program. *See also* Hospital Accreditation Program; Joint Commission on Accreditation of Healthcare Organizations; plant, technology, and safety management; scoring guideline.

Keynesian economics A body of economic thought propounded by the British economist and government adviser, John Maynard Keynes (1883-1946). He believed that insufficient demand causes unemployment and that excessive demand results in inflation; government should therefore manipulate the level of aggregate demand by adjusting levels of government expenditure and taxation. For instance, to avoid a depression Keynes advocated increased government spending and easy money, resulting in more investment, higher employment, and increased consumer spending. *See also* economics; neoclassical economics.

keypad, numeric *See* numeric keypad.

key process variable (KPV) A component of a process that has a cause-and-effect relationship of sufficient magnitude with the key quality characteristic such that manipulation and control of the key process variable will reduce variation of the key quality characteristic and/or change its level. *See also* key quality characteristic; operational definition; variable.

keypunch A type of data entry involving punching holes into 80-column computer cards in a code that can be machine-read by a computer.

key quality characteristic (KQC) The most important quality characteristic of a service or product.

KQCs must be operationally defined by combining knowledge of the customer with knowledge of the process. KQCs are measured to understand the actual performance of a process. *See also* key process variable; operational definition; quality characteristics.

KHC *See* Karen Horney Clinic.

kidney A principal organ of excretion of water-soluble waste products and regulation of water, sodium, potassium, and hydrogen and their associated anions. Each kidney contains about a million functional units, each comprising a glomerulus and a renal tubule. Other functions of the kidney include control of the rate of red blood cell production by the bone marrow, and control of arterial blood pressure. *See also* end stage renal disease; glomerulonephritis; hemodialysis; nephrectomy; nephritis.

kidney dialysis *See* hemodialysis.

Kidney and Urologic Diseases Information Clearinghouse, National *See* National Kidney and Urologic Diseases Information Clearinghouse.

killer cells *See* lymphocyte.

killing **1.** To stop an undertaking or process, as in killing a project. **2.** Committing murder. **3.** A sudden large profit, as in making a killing on the futures market.

kin One's relatives or family. *See also* next of kin.

kinesia Movement; sometimes a synonym for motion sickness. *See also* motion sickness.

kinesiology The study of motion of the human body, particularly relevant to the fields of orthopaedic surgery and physical medicine and rehabilitation. *See also* kinesiotherapy.

kinesiotherapy A treatment by means of body movements. *See also* kinesiology.

Kinesiotherapy Association, American *See* American Kinesiotherapy Association.

kinetics The study of the rates at which chemical reactions and biological processes proceed, as in cell kinetics. *See also* cell kinetics; pharmacokinetics.

kinetics, cell *See* cell kinetics.

kin, next of *See* next of kin.

KIPS *See* key items, probes, and scoring guidelines.

kiting In health care, increasing the quantity of a drug ordered by a prescription. A pharmacist, patient, or other individual may kite the quantity of the original prescription, for example, by adding zeros to the number shown on a prescription. When done by a pharmacist, he or she then provides the patient with the quantity originally prescribed but bills a third party, such as Medicaid, for the larger quantity. A patient who kites is often dependent on the drug. *See also* fraud and abuse; shorting.

kleptomania A morbid, uncontrollable, and irrational impulse to steal. Shoplifting is the usual manifestation, though the kleptomaniac may also steal from friends' houses, fellow guests in hotels, and elsewhere.

KMAA *See* Korean Medical Association of America.

knock-knee Inward displacement of the knee joints so that they are abnormally close together. *Synonym*: genu valgum. *See also* joint.

knocks, school of hard *See* school of hard knocks.

knot, surgeon's *See* surgeon's knot.

know-how The ability to perform a particular function, as in having the necessary know-how to run a department.

knowledge **1.** The sum or range of what has been perceived, discovered, or learned. *Compare* ignorance. **2.** Specific information about a subject. *See also* education.

knowledge base The database of facts, inferences, and procedures needed for problem solving on a particular subject. *See also* knowledge-based system.

knowledge-based system In health care, a computer system that combines access to data and systematic use of logic rules and probability statements intended to help health care providers make better clinical decisions; for example, by recognizing out-of-range laboratory values or undesirable trends, associating symptoms with the correct diagnosis, or selecting the optimal treatment approach. *See also* knowledge base; system.

Koch's postulates A statement of the four criteria necessary to prove that a disease is caused by a particular microorganism, stated by Robert Koch (1843-1910), a German bacteriologist. The criteria (postulates) are the following: the organism must be observed in every case of the disease; the organism must be isolated and grown in pure culture; the organism grown in pure culture must be capable of reproducing the disease when inoculated into a suitable experimental animal; and the organism must be recovered from the experimental disease. Koch's postulates were later revised by Alfred Evans in response to expanding biomedical knowledge. *See also* infectious diseases; postulate.

Korean Medical Association of America (KMAA) A national organization founded in 1974 composed of 4,300 Korean-American physicians. Its purpose is to provide a social and scientific forum for the exchange of scholarly information among members and between Korean-Americans and Korean physicians. *See also* medical association.

KPV *See* key process variable.

KQC *See* key quality characteristic.

Kresge Foundation, The *See* The Kresge Foundation.

KRS *See* Kerato-Refractive Society.

kudos Recognition in the form of acclaim, praise, a bonus or medal, or other means, given by an entity for exceptional achievement.

Kussmaul breathing A striking form of hyperventilation, known as "air hunger," characteristic of severe metabolic acidosis. *See also* breathing; diabetic ketoacidosis.

kyphosis A deformity of the thoracic spine causing increased posterior convexity. *Compare* lordosis; scoliosis. *See also* orthopaedic/orthopedic surgery; spine.

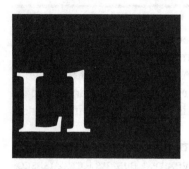

label Something that identifies, as in a drug label. *See also* labeling.

labeling Written, printed, or graphic matter displayed on or accompanying a food, drug, device, or cosmetic, or on any of their containers or wrappers, according to the federal Food, Drug, and Cosmetic Act; for example, a package insert for a prescription drug product. Labeling is regulated by the Food and Drug Administration. A label cannot contain any false or misleading statements and must include adequate instructions for use, unless a product is exempt by regulation. *See also* enriched; Food and Drug Administration; label; lite; low calorie; mandatory copy; package insert.

labor **1.** The process of giving birth, or parturition, by which a mother expels a fetus from her uterus via the birth canal at which point it becomes an infant, or newborn. The four stages of labor are the stage of dilatation, which begins with the onset of regular uterine contractions and ends when the cervical opening is completely dilated and flush with the vagina, thus completing the birth canal; the stage of expulsion, which extends from the end of the first stage until the expulsion of the infant; the placental stage, which extends from the expulsion of the infant until the placenta and membranes are expelled; and the hour or two after delivery when uterine tone is established. *Synonyms*: childbirth; confinement; delivery; parturition; travail. *See also* birth; childbearing; delivery; dystocia; induced labor; labor room. **2.** Physical or mental exertion, as in labor intensive. *See also* labor intensive. **3.** Workers considered as a group. *See also* labor union.

laboratorian An individual who devotes himself or herself to laboratory work, as distinguished from a clinician. *Compare* clinician. *See also* laboratory; surveyor.

Laboratorians, Conference of Public Health *See* Conference of Public Health Laboratorians.

Laboratories Association, Optical *See* Optical Laboratories Association.

Laboratories, National Association of Dental *See* National Association of Dental Laboratories.

Laboratories, National Board for Certification of Dental *See* National Board for Certification of Dental Laboratories.

Laboratories, National Conference of Standards *See* National Conference of Standards Laboratories.

Laboratories, Underwriters *See* Underwriters Laboratories.

laboratory **1.** In health care, a place for observation, practice, or testing, as in a cardiac catheterization laboratory. *See also* cardiac catheterization laboratory; pulmonary function laboratory. **2.** In health care, a facility in which materials from the human body are examined for the purposes of providing information about the state of health of human beings. *See also* clinical laboratory; hematology laboratory; histopathology laboratory; special function laboratory.

Laboratory Animal Care, American Association for Accreditation of *See* American Association for Accreditation of Laboratory Animal Care.

Laboratory Animal Management Association (LAMA) A national organization founded in 1984 composed of 265 laboratory animal facility managers. It evaluates and updates basic and advanced management techniques and educates laboratory animal facility managers. *See also* animal experimentation; management.

Laboratory Animal Medicine, American College of *See* American College of Laboratory Animal Medicine.

Laboratory Animal Resources, Institute of *See* Institute of Laboratory Animal Resources.

Laboratory Animal Science, American Association for *See* American Association for Laboratory Animal Science.

Laboratory Assessment, Commission on Office *See* Commission on Office Laboratory Assessment.

Laboratory Association, American Clinical *See* American Clinical Laboratory Association.

laboratory, cardiac catheterization *See* cardiac catheterization laboratory.

laboratory, clinical *See* clinical laboratory.

laboratory, hematology *See* hematology laboratory.

laboratory, histopathology *See* histopathology laboratory.

laboratory immunology, diagnostic *See* diagnostic laboratory immunology.

Laboratory Management Association, Clinical *See* Clinical Laboratory Management Association.

laboratory, medical *See* clinical laboratory.

laboratory, pulmonary function *See* pulmonary function laboratory.

Laboratory Sciences, National Accrediting Agency for Clinical *See* National Accrediting Agency for Clinical Laboratory Sciences.

Laboratory Services, National Council on Health *See* National Council on Health Laboratory Services.

laboratory services, pathology and clinical *See* pathology and clinical laboratory services.

laboratory, special function *See* special function laboratory.

Laboratory Standards, National Committee for Clinical *See* National Committee for Clinical Laboratory Standards.

laboratory technician *See* dental laboratory technician; medical laboratory technician (associate degree); medical laboratory technician (certificate).

laboratory technician (associate degree), medical *See* medical laboratory technician (associate degree).

laboratory technician (certificate), medical *See* medical laboratory technician (certificate).

laboratory technician, dental *See* dental laboratory technician.

laboratory technician, ophthalmic *See* ophthalmic laboratory technician.

laboratory technologist *See* medical technologist.

laboratory technology accreditation, dental *See* dental laboratory technology accreditation.

laboratory testing, decentralized *See* decentral-ized laboratory testing.

labor certification Certification required and provided by the US Department of Labor for certain aliens, such as foreign medical graduates. The certification may be considered for individuals with occupations for which a shortage exists in the United States (for example, physicians, nurses). *See also* certification; Department of Labor; Educational Commission for Foreign Medical Graduates; foreign medical graduate; labor.

Labor, Department of *See* Department of Labor.

Labor and Human Resources, Committee on *See* Committee on Labor and Human Resources.

labor, induced *See* induced labor.

labor intensive Requiring a high proportion of human effort relative to capital investment; for example, health services, computer programming. Labor costs are more important than capital costs in labor-intensive activities. *See also* labor; people intensive.

labor relations The manner of conducting operations between management and labor, especially on the part of a business organization with respect to the demands of its labor force. *See also* industrial relations; labor.

labor room A room or area in a health care facility regularly maintained for maternity patients in active labor. *Compare* birthing room. *See also* labor.

labor union An organization of wage earners formed for the purpose of serving members' interests with respect to wages and working conditions, as in a hospital workers' union. *See also* labor.

Lab Personnel, National Certification Agency for Medical *See* National Certification Agency for Medical Lab Personnel.

laceration A wound caused by ripping, cutting, or tearing tissue. *See also* abrasion; bruise; suture; wound.

lactase An enzyme on the surface of cells lining the small intestine necessary to digest lactose, a sugar found in milk. *See also* enzyme; intestine; lactose; lactose intolerance.

lactation Milk secretion and ejection by the breast. *See also* mammary gland; milk; nursing.

lactose The principal sugar in milk. It is frequently used as a "filler" in pharmaceutical products. *See also* excipient; lactase; lactose intolerance.

lactose intolerance The decreased ability to digest

milk sugar caused by a deficiency of lactase. *See also* lactase.

lactovegetarian A vegetarian who will not eat meat or eggs but who will eat dairy products. *See also* vegetarian.

laetrile An illegal drug derived from amygdalin which is isolated from the pits of stone-bearing fruits, such as apricots. Laetrile is 6% cyanide by weight and is purported to have antineoplastic (inhibiting the formation of tumors) properties. *See also* cyanide.

lag The delay between a stimulus and an observed reaction, or between any other two causally connected events. *See also* jet lag; lagging economic indicator.

lagging economic indicator An economic indicator that changes after a change in the economy has occurred. It is used to confirm trends. *Synonym:* lagging indicator. *Compare* leading economic indicator. *See also* economic indicator.

lagging indicator *See* lagging economic indicator.

lag, jet *See* jet lag.

laissez-faire A doctrine that government interference in business and economic affairs should be minimal. Adam Smith's *The Wealth of Nations* (1776) described laissez-faire economics in terms of an "invisible hand" that would provide for the maximum good for all, if people in business were free to pursue profitable opportunities as they saw them. *See also* economics.

LAMA *See* Laboratory Animal Management Association.

LAN *See* local area network.

landmark In law, a case that sets an important precedent.

language 1. A form of communication that has grammar and semantics, conveys meaning that can be abstract or referential (refers to actions at another time or location), and is understood by other listeners. *See also* communication; inclusive language; learning disability; linguistics; semantics; speech. 2. In computer science, a system of symbols and rules used for communication with or between computers, as in computer language.

language, body *See* nonverbal communication.

Language-Hearing Association, American Speech- *See* American Speech-Language-Hearing Association.

language, inclusive *See* inclusive language.

language, machine *See* machine language.

language, natural *See* natural language.

language processing, natural *See* natural language processing.

language, programming *See* programming language.

language, sign *See* sign language.

laparoscope An endoscope consisting of an illuminated tube with an optical system that is inserted through the abdominal wall for examining the peritoneal cavity. *Synonyms:* celioscope; peritoneoscope. *See also* endoscope; laparoscopy.

laparoscopic cholecystectomy An abdominal surgical procedure in which the gall bladder is removed by inserting instruments for visualizing inside the abdomen and instruments for manipulation, such as cutting, application of lasers, and sewing, through a small incision, often under local anesthesia. *See also* cholecystectomy; keyhole surgery; laparoscopy.

Laparoscopists, American Association of Gynecological *See* American Association of Gynecological Laparoscopists.

laparoscopy The process of examining the interior of the abdomen (peritoneal cavity) by means of a laparoscope inserted through the abdominal wall, as for examination of the liver or for the surgical treatment of endometriosis. *Synonym:* peritoneoscopy. *See also* endometriosis; peritoneal cavity.

laparotomy An abdominal incision to gain access to the peritoneal cavity. *See also* incision.

lapse 1. To fall from a previous level or standard, as of accomplishment, quality, or conduct. 2. To come to an end; for example, in insurance, the termination of an insurance policy when a policy holder fails to pay the premium within the time period required. *See also* insurance.

laptop computer *See* microcomputer.

lard The purified internal fat of the abdomen of the hog. *See also* fat.

large employer According to the Health Security Act recently (1993) introduced to Congress, an employer that has more than 5,000 full-time employees in the United States. *See also* corporate alliance; employer; Health Security Act; large employer alliance.

large-employer alliance According to the Health Security Act (1993), a large-employer sponsor of a corporate (health) alliance. *See also* corporate alliance; health alliance; Health Security Act; large employer.

Laryngological, Rhinological and Otological Society, American *See* American Laryngological, Rhinological and Otological Society.

laryngology The branch of medicine dealing with the throat, pharynx, larynx, nasopharynx, and tracheobronchial tree. *See also* otolaryngology.

Laryngology and Head/Neck Nurses, Society of Otorhino- *See* Society of Otorhinolaryngology and Head/Neck Nurses.

laryngology, oto- *See* otolaryngology.

laryngoscope An illuminated instrument for use in direct visual examination of the larynx, as in visualizing the larynx prior to intubating a patient. *See also* intubation; laryngoscopy; larynx.

laryngoscopy Examination of the interior of the larynx with a specially designed illuminated instrument (laryngoscope). *See also* laryngoscope; larynx.

larynx Part of the air passage in the throat, located between the back of the tongue and the trachea (windpipe). It contains the vocal cords. *See also* glottis; laryngoscopy.

laser Acronym for light amplification by stimulated emission of radiation. An instrument that produces a thin beam of light by converting electromagnetic radiation of mixed frequencies to one or more discrete frequencies of highly amplified and coherent ultraviolet, visible, or infrared radiation. Laser is used surgically to destroy tissue or to separate parts, as in laser angioplasty. *See also* laser angioplasty.

laser angioplasty Angioplasty (eliminating areas of blockage or narrowing in blood vessels) in which lasers are used to burn away blockages. *See also* angioplasty.

Laser Association of America *See* Laser and Electro-Optics Manufacturers' Association.

laser disk A disk on which signals or data are recorded digitally as a series of pits and bumps under a protective coating, which is read optically by a laser beam reflected from the surface. *See also* compact disk.

Laser and Electro-Optics Manufacturers' Association (LEMA) A national organization founded in 1985 composed of laser industry companies involved with laser technology. Its primary objective is to collectively represent members' interests through industrial services and government legislative advocacy, particularly at the federal level. It provides an interface between the laser industry and government with regard to matters of training, safety standards, imports and exports, and new tech-

nologies. Formerly (1990) Laser Association of America. *See also* laser.

Laser Institute of America (LIA) An organization founded in 1968 composed of 1,700 laser scientists, researchers, and manufacturers; educational and governmental institutions; and individuals and businesses. It assists in the establishment of laser health and safety standards, definitions, and methods of measurements. It seeks to advance the state of laser application technology. *See also* laser.

Laser Medicine and Surgery, American Society for *See* American Society for Laser Medicine and Surgery.

laser printer In computer applications, a laser beam that generates an image, then transfers it to paper electrostatically. Laser-printer output may be very fast, with quality that approaches that of typesetting. *Compare* daisy wheel printer; dot-matrix printer; ink jet printer. *See also* printer.

Lasers and Electro-Optics Society, IEEE *See* IEEE Lasers and Electro-Optics Society.

Laser Surgery, American Board of Neurological/ Orthopaedic *See* American Board of Neurological/ Orthopaedic Laser Surgery.

Last Word: Therapies, Inc An organization founded in 1980 composed of 700 psychiatrists, psychologists, counselors, organizations, and individuals interested in promoting past-life regression therapy as a means of helping individuals realize their capacity to change and improve their lives. It works for the establishment of clinical standards for training therapists. It registers therapists and offers training programs in past-life regression techniques. Formerly (1991) Association for Past-Life Research and Therapy. *See also* psychotherapy.

lateral Pertaining to a side, away from the center, as in the arms are lateral to the chest or the eyes are lateral to the midline of the face. *Compare* bilateral; medial; unilateral.

latitude Freedom from normal restraints, limitations, or regulations; the ability to exercise judgment without outside interference.

laughing gas *See* nitrous oxide.

laughter A physical expression (unarticulated sounds, facial contortions, and heaving body movements) characteristic of amusement and mirth, evoked by events, situations, appearances, or thoughts of a ludicrous or incongruous nature or by bodily stimuli, such as tickling. *See also* humor.

Laughter Therapy (LT) An organization founded in 1981 that supplies tapes of "Candid Camera" to patients, nursing homes, doctors, hospices, and clinics. "Candid Camera" was a regular weekly comedy series on CBS that ran from 1960-1967 and was produced by Allen Funt. The program displayed people from all walks of life and their reactions to strange or unexpected occurrences or situations. Because studies and experiences have shown that humor is one of the most useful forms of therapy, the tapes are being used for patients with terminal illness, depression, and other illnesses. *See also* humor; laughter.

laundry Soiled clothing or linens.

laundry department The unit of a hospital or other health care organization responsible for the laundering, storage, and distribution of linens, uniforms, and other textile items. *See also* environmental services; laundry manager.

laundry list An item-by-item enumeration.

laundry manager An individual who manages a health care organization's laundry activities. *See also* laundry department; manager.

lavage A washing, especially of a hollow organ, such as the stomach, as in gastric lavage. *See also* gastric lavage.

lavage, gastric *See* gastric lavage.

law **1.** Rules to guide individuals' actions in a society. **2.** The totality of rules of conduct put in force by legislative authority or court decisions or established by local custom. *See also* administrative law; civil law; common law; criminal law. **3.** In science, a constant fact or principle, as in the law of relativity.

law, adjective *See* adjective law.

law, administrative *See* administrative law.

Law, American Academy of Psychiatry and the *See* American Academy of Psychiatry and the Law.

Law, American Society for Pharmacy *See* American Society for Pharmacy Law.

law, case *See* case law.

law, civil *See* civil law.

Law, Commission on Mental and Physical Disability *See* Commission on Mental and Physical Disability Law.

law, common *See* common law.

law, criminal *See* criminal law.

law of diminishing returns *See* diminishing returns.

lawful Pertaining to any act performed within the bounds of law or authorized by law and that does not give rise to any legal liability. *See also* law; liability.

law, gun control *See* gun control law.

law, health *See* health law.

law, hospital *See* hospital law.

Law Institute, Food and Drug *See* Food and Drug Law Institute.

law, issue of *See* issue of law.

law, medical *See* medical law.

Law and Medicine, American Society of *See* American Society of Law and Medicine.

law, mistake of *See* mistake of law.

law, moral *See* moral law.

law, Murphy's *See* Murphy's law.

law, natural *See* natural law.

law, Parkinson's *See* Parkinson's law.

law of parsimony *See* Ockham's razor.

Law Program, National Health *See* National Health Law Program.

Law Project, Mental Health *See* Mental Health Law Project.

law, rape shield *See* rape shield law.

law, required request *See* required request law.

law, routine inquiry *See* required request law.

laws, antisubstitution *See* antisubstitution laws.

laws, antitrust *See* antitrust laws.

Law, Say's *See* Say's Law.

laws, Good Samaritan *See* Good Samaritan laws.

laws, license *See* license laws.

law, slip *See* slip law.

Law Society, American Psychology - *See* American Psychology - Law Society.

law, statutory *See* statutory law.

lawsuit An action brought before a court, as to recover a right or redress a grievance. *Synonym:* suit. *See also* action; ad damnum; defensive medicine; malicious prosecution.

law, sunshine *See* sunshine law.

law of supply and demand An economic proposition in a free society stating that the relationship between supply and demand determines price and the quantity produced. A change in either will lead to changes in price and amount produced in order to achieve equilibrium in the market. *See also* market; supply.

lawyer A person whose profession involves giving legal advice and assistance to clients and who is admitted to practice law in a court system. *See also* attorney; barrister; counsel; counselor; solicitor;

solicitor general.

Lawyers of America, Association of Trial *See* Association of Trial Lawyers of America.

Lawyers, American College of Trial *See* American College of Trial Lawyers.

Lawyers Association, National Health *See* National Health Lawyers Association.

Lawyers, National Association of Women *See* National Association of Women Lawyers.

Lawyers, National Conference of Black *See* National Conference of Black Lawyers.

laxative An agent that promotes evacuation of the intestines. *Synonyms*: aperient; cathartic; purgative. *See also* bulimia nervosa; epsom salts; intestine.

lay Pertaining to activities or things not associated with the professions or a specific profession, as in the lay perspective. *See also* layperson.

layman *See* layperson.

layoff The removal, either temporarily or permanently, of an employee from a payroll, not because of poor performance, but because of an economic slowdown or a production cutback. *See also* employee; job sharing; outplacement.

layperson A person who is not a member of a profession, such as medicine, law, or architecture. *Synonyms*: layman; laywoman. *See also* lay.

laywoman *See* layperson.

lazar A diseased person, as in a leper. *See also* leper.

lazaretto A hospital treating contagious diseases, especially a leprosarium. *See also* leper; leprosy.

LCAO *See* Leadership Council of Aging Organizations.

LCGME *See* Liaison Committee on Graduate Medical Education.

LCME *See* Liaison Committee on Medical Education.

LCSW Licensed clinical social worker. *See* licensed social worker.

LDL *See* low-density lipoprotein.

lead **1.** To show the way to by going in advance. *Compare* mislead. *See also* leader. **2.** A soft bluish-white metallic element that is a cumulative poison. *See also* chelation therapy; poison; saturnism.

leader An individual who leads other individuals on a course. *See also* boss; opinion leader; organization leaders; team leader.

leader, informal *See* informal leader.

leader, opinion *See* opinion leader.

leadership The capacity or ability to lead. *See also* informal leader; lead; leader; opinion leader; participative leadership; take-charge.

Leadership, Academy for Catholic Healthcare *See* Academy for Catholic Healthcare Leadership.

Leadership Coalition on AIDS, National *See* National Leadership Coalition on AIDS.

Leadership Council of Aging Organizations (LCAO) A national organization founded in 1978 composed of 34 professional groups serving elderly persons. Its objective is to further the public's understanding of the potential and needs of elderly persons. It acts as a coordinating body in reviewing and acting on public policy issues. *See also* aging.

leadership exit conference *See* chief executive officer exit conference.

leadership interview A meeting of all surveyors from the Joint Commission on Accreditation of Healthcare Organizations present on the first day of a survey with the senior leadership of a health care organization for the purpose of making an assessment of how the organization's leaders work together in performance improvement activities, the role that each of the major components of the organization play in its management, and the extent to which the standards' requirements for communication and cooperation are being met by the organization. *See also* accreditation survey; chief executive officer exit conference; interview; Joint Commission on Accreditation of Healthcare Organizations; leadership.

leadership, participative *See* participative leadership.

leadership style *See* management style.

leaders, organization *See* organization leaders.

leader, team *See* team leader.

leading economic indicator An economic indicator, such as the average workweek, weekly claims for unemployment insurance, new orders, vendor performance, stock prices, and changes in the money supply, that is often used to forecast business conditions. *Synonym*: leading indicator. *Compare* lagging economic indicator. *See also* economic indicator.

leading edge The foremost position in a trend or movement, as in a hospital on the leading edge of customer-driven quality improvement. *Synonym*: cutting edge.

leading indicator *See* leading economic indicator.

leading question A question posed by a trial lawyer that is ordinarily improper on direct examination because it suggests to the witness the answer the lawyer wants delivered. It has the effect of prompting the answer that is to be given regardless of actual memory. *See also* court; direct examination; lawyer; trial; witness.

Lead Poisoning, Alliance to End Childhood *See* Alliance to End Childhood Lead Poisoning.

League of America, Child Welfare *See* Child Welfare League of America.

League for Nursing, National *See* National League for Nursing.

learn To gain knowledge, comprehension, or mastery of subject matter through experience and/or study. *See also* knowledge; learning.

learning The act or process of gaining knowledge and/or skill. *See also* learning curve; learning disability; lesson.

learning curve A graph that depicts the rate of learning, especially a graph of progress in the mastery of a skill against the time required for achieving the mastery. *See also* graph; learning.

Learning Disabilities, Council for *See* Council for Learning Disabilities.

learning disability An abnormal condition in understanding or using spoken or written language, affecting a person of normal intelligence and not arising from emotional disturbance or impairment of sight or hearing. *See also* attention-deficit disorder; disability; dyslexia; language; learning.

learning organization An organization that practices creative learning by using certain basic principles relating to total quality management. *See also* learning; organization; total quality management.

learning psychology The branch of psychology that examines how lasting changes in behavior are caused by experience, practice, or training; for example, the importance of rewards and punishment in the learning process, the different ways individuals and species learn, and the factors that influence memory. *See also* learning; psychology.

least-effort principle A theory among advertisers that consumers will make purchases based on the least amount of effort possible and will tend to buy what is readily at hand. *See also* advertise; consumer; principle.

leave, sick *See* sick leave.

LED Acronym for light emitting diode, a semiconductor diode that converts applied voltage to light and is used in digital displays. *See also* digital.

legal **1.** Pertaining to the law, as in legal age. *See also* law. **2.** Authorized by or based on law, as in a legal right. *Compare* illegal. *See also* lawful. **3.** Applicable

to lawyers or their profession, as in legal malpractice. *See also* attorney; lawyer.

legal age The age at which an individual may by law assume the rights and responsibilities of an adult. *Compare* minor. *See also* age; age of majority; legal.

legal cap Ruled writing paper in tablet form, measuring 8 1/2 inches by 13 to 16 inches and generally used by lawyers. *See also* lawyer; legal pad.

Legal Duty, Children's Healthcare Is a *See* Children's Healthcare Is a Legal Duty.

legalese The style of language used by the legal profession, especially when the language is considered complex or abstruse. *See also* bureaucratese; jargon; officialese.

legal guardian *See* guardian.

Legal and Industrial Medicine, American Society of *See* American Society of Legal and Industrial Medicine.

legal injury Any damage resulting from a violation of a legal right, and which the law will recognize as deserving of redress; for example, antitrust injury. *See also* antitrust injury; injury.

legalize To authorize or sanction by law, as in legalizing abortion. *Compare* illegal.

legal majority *See* age of majority.

legal malpractice Failure of an attorney to use such skill, prudence, and diligence as lawyers of ordinary skill and capacity commonly possess and exercise in performance of tasks which they undertake, and when such failure proximately causes damage giving rise to an action in tort. *See also* malpractice; medical malpractice.

Legal Medicine, American College of *See* American College of Legal Medicine.

Legal Nurse Consultants, American Association of *See* American Association of Legal Nurse Consultants.

legal pad A pad of ruled, usually yellow writing paper that measures 8 and 1/2 inches by 14 inches. *See also* legal cap; legal size.

legal right An interest that the law will protect. *See also* legal wrong.

legal size Being a sheet of paper that measures approximately 8 and 1/2 inches by 14 inches. *See also* legal pad.

legal wrong Invasion or interruption of a legal right. *See also* legal right.

legend drug A prescription drug which carries the

labeling, "Caution: Federal law prohibits dispensing without prescription." *See also* drug; prescription drug.

legibility, medical record *See* medical record legibility.

legible Capable of being deciphered, as in handwriting that is legible. *See also* medical record legibility; readable.

legislate To enact laws or pass resolutions via legislation, in contrast to court-made law. *See also* legislation.

legislation 1. A law or a body of laws enacted. **2.** The act of enacting laws.

legislative intent Interpretation of the meaning of a law, usually provided by regulators and the courts, but also by a legislative history and other means. *See also* intent; intent of standard; legislative history.

legislative history A written record of the writing of a law (statute), such as an Act of Congress, including committee reports, testimony, and legislative proceedings including discussion and debate. A legislative history usually provides the most complete explanation of the meaning and intent of a law. *See also* history; intent; legislative intent.

LEMA *See* Laser and Electro-Optics Manufacturers' Association.

length of stay (LOS) The number of calendar days that elapse between an inpatient's admission and discharge in a hospital or other health care organization, used as a measure of the use of health facilities. It is typically reported as an average number of days spent in a facility per admission or discharge, calculated as follows: total number of days in the facility for all discharges and deaths occurring during a period divided by the number of discharges and deaths during the same period. In concurrent review an appropriate length of stay may be assigned each patient upon admission. Average lengths of stay vary and are measured for people with various ages, specific diagnoses, or sources of payment. *See also* average length of stay; concurrent review.

lens 1. A transparent, biconvex structure of the eye between the iris and the vitreous humor that focuses light rays entering through the pupil to form an image on the retina. *See also* ophthalmology. **2.** A ground or molded piece of glass, plastic, or other transparent material with opposite surfaces, either or both of which are curved, through which light rays are refracted so that they converge or diverge to form an image. *See also* contact lens; light micro-

scope; ophthalmology; opticianry; optometry; spectacles.

Lens Association of Ophthalmologists, Contact *See* Contact Lens Association of Ophthalmologists.

lens, contact *See* contact lens.

Lens Examiners, National Contact *See* National Contact Lens Examiners.

Lens Manufacturers Association, Contact *See* Contact Lens Manufacturers Association.

Lens Society of America, Contact *See* Contact Lens Society of America.

LEOS *See* IEEE Lasers and Electro-Optics Society.

leper A person afflicted with leprosy. *See also* leprosy.

leprosy A slowly progressive, chronic infectious disease caused by *Mycobacterium leprae* and characterized by the development of lesions in the skin, mucous membranes, nerves, bones, and viscera. It leads to the loss of sensation, paralysis, gangrene, and deformation. *Synonym:* Hansen's disease. *See also* infectious diseases; lazaretto; leper.

Leprosy Missions, American *See* American Leprosy Missions.

Lesbian, and Bisexual Issues in Counseling, Association for Gay, *See* Association for Gay, Lesbian, and Bisexual Issues in Counseling.

Lesbian/Gay Alcoholism Professionals, National Association of *See* National Association of Lesbian/Gay Alcoholism Professionals.

Lesbian, Gay and Bisexual People In Medicine (LGBPM) A national organization founded in 1976 composed of 350 physicians and physicians-in-training interested in improving the quality of health care for gay patients and improving working conditions and professional status of gay health professionals and students. Formerly (1985) Lesbian and Gay People in Medicine. *See also* bisexuality; gay; lesbianism.

Lesbian and Gay Caucus of Public Health Workers (LGCPHW) A caucus of the American Public Health Association founded in 1975 and composed of 150 public health workers in the fields of administration, government, nursing, direct care, and teaching, who are interested in disseminating information on the health needs of lesbians and gay men. It serves as a support network for gay public health workers. It believes homophobia interferes with the proper delivery of health care to gays and lesbians, restricts or eliminates their contributions as health workers, and causes physical and mental health problems. Formerly (1990) Gay Public Health Workers Caucus. *See also* American Public Health Association; gay; homophobia; lesbianism; public health.

Lesbian and Gay Issues, National Association of Social Workers Committee on *See* National Association of Social Workers Committee on Lesbian and Gay Issues.

Lesbian and Gay Issues, Society for the Psychological Study of *See* Society for the Psychological Study of Lesbian and Gay Issues.

Lesbian and Gay People in Medicine *See* Lesbian, Gay and Bisexual People in Medicine.

lesbianism Sexual attraction of women to other women. *Synonym:* sapphism. *See also* gay; homosexuality; tribadism.

Lesbian Psychiatrists, Association of Gay and *See* Association of Gay and Lesbian Psychiatrists.

Lesbian Scientists and Technical Professionals, National Organization of Gay and *See* National Organization of Gay and Lesbian Scientists and Technical Professionals.

lesion A localized change in an organ or a tissue, as in a suspicious-looking skin lesion.

lesson Something to be learned. *See also* learning.

lethargy Abnormal drowsiness or stupor; lack of energy or interest. *See also* consciousness.

letter quality Pertaining to printed characters similar in clarity to those produced by a conventional typewriter, as in a letter-quality computer printer. Daisy-wheel printers and laser printers produce letter-quality output. *See also* daisy wheel printer; laser printer.

"letting die" *See* passive euthanasia.

leukemia A form of cancer in which the leukocytes (white blood cells) proliferate and spread throughout the body. Leukemia is classified according to which type of leukocyte predominates. *See also* cancer; white blood cell.

leukocyte *See* white blood cell.

Leukocyte Biology (A Reticuloendothelial Society) Society for *See* Society for Leukocyte Biology (A Reticuloendothelial Society).

level A relative position, rank, or concentration on a scale, as in levels of consciousness, confidence level, or level of performance. *See also* acceptable quality level; level of acuity; level of care; level of service; level of significance; midlevel; scale; serum drug level.

level, acceptable quality *See* acceptable quality level.

level of acuity The degree or state of disease or injury existing in a patient prior to treatment. The greater the level of acuity, the greater the amount of health care resources (for example, health professionals, laboratory, operating rooms, special care units) required to treat the patient. *See also* acuity; emergency; severity of illness; urgent.

level of care A relative amount or intensity of care provided to a patient; for example, intermediate nursing care, skilled nursing care, tertiary care, intensive care. *See also* alternative level of care; continuing care; intermediate care; intensive care; skilled nursing care.

level of care, alternative *See* alternative level of care.

level of compliance *See* compliance level.

level of consciousness *See* consciousness.

level, mid- *See* midlevel.

level of nursing care *See* level of care.

level, poverty *See* poverty level.

level, serum drug *See* serum drug level.

level of service A relative intensity of services provided for a patient; for example, minimal, brief, limited, intermediate, extended, comprehensive, or unusually complex designations when a physician provides one-on-one services for a patient, or various levels of service provided by a health care organization, such as partial hospitalization, ambulatory surgery, tertiary services. *See also* level; level of care.

level of significance The probability of a false rejection of the null hypothesis in a statistical test. *Synonym:* significance level. *See also* p (probability) value; statistical significance.

lexicon **1.** A dictionary. **2.** A stock of terms used in a particular profession, subject, or style, as in a lexicon of health care terms. *See also;* lexikon; lexis.

lexikon Greek word meaning "word book." *See also* lexicon.

lexis Greek word meaning word. *See also* lexicon; lexikon.

Lexis A computerized on-line legal research system that enables the user to enter various search terms and receive information and cases that fit the designated query. *See also* legal; paralegal.

LGBPM *See* Lesbian, Gay and Bisexual People in Medicine.

LGCPHW *See* Lesbian and Gay Caucus of Public Health Workers.

LGHCS *See* Lutheran General Health Care System.

LHA *See* Lutheran Hospital Association of America.

LHHS *See* Lutheran Hospitals and Homes Society.

LI *See* Lifegain Institute.

LIA *See* Laser Institute of America.

liability An obligation to do or refrain from doing something, as in professional liability. *See also* corporate liability; defensive medicine; enterprise liability; joint and several liability; no-fault medical practice liability; product liability; professional liability; service liability; tort liability; vicarious liability.

Liability Alliance, The Product *See* The Product Liability Alliance.

Liability Attorneys, American Board of Professional *See* American Board of Professional Liability Attorneys.

liability, corporate *See* corporate liability.

liability, enterprise *See* enterprise liability.

liability insurance *See* general liability insurance.

liability insurance, directors' and officers' *See* directors' and officers' liability insurance.

liability insurance, general *See* general liability insurance.

liability insurance, professional *See* professional liability insurance.

liability, joint and several *See* joint and several liability.

liability limits *See* limits on liability.

liability, medical *See* professional liability.

liability, no-fault medical practice *See* no-fault medical practice liability.

liability, product *See* product liability.

liability, professional *See* professional liability.

liability, service *See* service liability.

liability, tort *See* tort liability.

liability, vicarious *See* vicarious liability.

Liaison Committee on Continuing Medical Education *See* Accreditation Council for Continuing Medical Education.

Liaison Committee on Graduate Medical Education (LCGME) A subgroup of the Council for Medical Affairs intended to serve as the accrediting agency for graduate medical education. *See also* accreditation; Council for Medical Affairs; graduate medical education; medical education.

Liaison Committee on Medical Education (LCME) A committee founded in 1942 sponsored by the American Medical Association and the Association of American Medical Colleges drawing membership from these groups and the Committee on

Accreditation of Canadian Medical Schools, two students, one federal participant, and two public members. Its principle function is to conduct accrediting activities in undergraduate medical education. *See also* accreditation; Council for Medical Affairs; medical education; undergraduate medical education.

libel Written or printed statements that injure another person's reputation. *See also* defamation; slander.

liberal arts *See* humanities.

librarian A person who specializes in library work. *See also* health sciences librarian; library; medical librarian.

librarian, health sciences *See* health sciences librarian.

librarian, medical *See* medical librarian.

librarian, medical record *See* medical record administrator.

library An information center in which materials, such as books, periodicals, newspapers, pamphlets, prints, records, and tapes, are kept for reading, reference, or lending. *See also* health sciences library; professional library.

Library Association, Medical *See* Medical Library Association.

Library Directors, Association of Academic Health Sciences *See* Association of Academic Health Sciences Library Directors.

library, health sciences *See* health sciences library.

library, medical *See* health sciences library.

Library of Medicine, National *See* National Library of Medicine.

library, professional *See* professional library.

Library Resources for Nursing, Interagency Council on *See* Interagency Council on Library Resources for Nursing.

lice Plural form of louse. *See* body louse; head louse.

license An official or a legal permission, granted by competent authority, usually public, to an individual or organization to engage in a practice, an occupation, or an activity otherwise unlawful; for example, a license to practice medicine and surgery. A license is usually needed to begin lawful practice; thus, it is usually granted on the basis of examination and/or proof of education rather than on measurement of actual performance. A license is usually permanent but may be conditioned on annual payment of a fee, proof of continuing education, or proof of competence. Grounds for revocation of a license include incompetence, commission of a crime (whether or not related to the licensed practice), or moral turpitude. There is no national licensure system for health professionals, although requirements are often so nearly standardized as to constitute a national system. *See also* competence; continuing education; licensure; state board of medical examiners.

licensed Having an official or a legal right, granted by competent authority, to engage in a practice, occupation, or activity otherwise unlawful; for example, a licensed practical nurse or a licensed independent practitioner. *See also* license.

licensed beds The total number of beds that a state licensing agency authorizes a health care organization to operate on a regular basis. *See also* bed; licensed.

licensed hospital A hospital granted the legal right by an appropriate governmental agency to operate in accordance with the requirements of the government. *See also* hospital; licensed.

licensed independent practitioner An individual who is permitted by law and by the health care organization(s) in which he or she practices to provide patient care services without direction or supervision, within the scope of the individual's license and in accordance with individually granted clinical privileges. *See also* clinical privileges; licensed; practitioner.

licensed practical nurse (LPN) A nurse who has completed a practical nursing program and is licensed by a state to provide routine patient care under the direction of a registered nurse or a physician. *See also* licensed; physician; registered nurse.

Licensed Practical Nurses Association, American *See* American Licensed Practical Nurses Association.

Licensed Practical Nurses, National Federation of *See* National Federation of Licensed Practical Nurses.

licensed vocational nurse (LVN) A licensed practical nurse who is permitted by license to practice in California or Texas. *See also* licensed practical nurse.

licensed social worker A social worker who is licensed in a particular state. Requirements for and definitions of social workers vary from state to state. *See also* license; social worker.

license laws Laws that govern the activities of occupations that require licensing, such as accountants, lawyers, physicians, nurses, and barbers. *See also* law; license.

licensing agency, state health facility *See* state health facility licensing agency.

licensing, medical *See* medical licensure.

Licensing and Registration, PR Committee for *See* PR Committee for Licensing and Registration.

licensure A legal right that is granted by a governmental agency in compliance with a statute governing the activities of a profession (such as medicine, dentistry, or nursing) or the operation of an activity (such as a hospital). *See also* license; limited licensure; mandatory licensure; medical licensure; qualify; state board of medical examiners.

licensure, endorsement in professional *See* endorsement in professional licensure.

Licensure, Enforcement and Regulation, Council on *See* Council on Licensure, Enforcement and Regulation.

Licensure Examination, National Council *See* National Council Licensure Examination.

Licensure, Federation for Accessible Nursing Education and *See* Federation for Accessible Nursing Education and Licensure.

licensure, limited *See* limited licensure.

licensure, mandatory *See* mandatory licensure.

licensure, medical *See* medical licensure.

lie A false statement deliberately presented as being true. *Synonym:* falsehood.

life The property or quality that distinguishes living organisms from dead organisms and inanimate matter, manifested by growth, reproduction, metabolism, and response to stimuli or adaptation to the environment originating from within the organism. *See also* life expectancy; quality of life; wrongful life.

life activities, major *See* major life activities.

Lifebanc A national program founded in 1986 designed to increase the number of useful body organs and tissues available for transplant by encouraging individuals to consider donating their body organs and tissues for use after death. The program includes procurement of all organs and tissues when circumstances are favorable and transplant is medically feasible. It organizes and implements public and professional education programs and coordinates recovery teams on 24-hour call from participating hospitals and other health care organizations. It also conducts training programs for hospital staff on organ donation procedures and solicitation. *See also* organ procurement.

life care · Long-term, continuing care offered by

retirement communities to their residents on a contract basis through provision of services ranging from independent living to skilled nursing care. *See also* continuing care retirement community.

Life Council, Child *See* Child Life Council.

life events Changes or disturbances in the pattern of living that may be associated with or cause changes in health. Examples include death of a spouse or other close relative, loss of a regular job, relocation, marriage, having and raising children, and divorce. *See also* event.

life expectancy The number of years a person is expected to live based on present age and sex. The figure is most often used by actuaries to determine insurance premiums. *See also* actuary.

Lifegain Institute (LI) A national organization founded in 1977 composed of 900 people who work with health promotion programs in hospitals, corporations, colleges, and communities. It promotes health practices, such as exercise, nutrition, safety, and the reduction or curtailment of smoking and alcohol consumption, through health promotion programs that provide a supportive environment in which to change unhealthy practices. *See also* health promotion.

Life History Research, Society for *See* Society for Life History Research.

life insurance Insurance that guarantees a specific sum of money to a designated beneficiary upon the death of the insured or to the insured if he or she lives beyond a certain age. *See also* insurance; Medical Impairment Bureau.

life, quality of *See* quality of life.

Life Safety Code® A set of standards for the construction and operation of buildings, intended to provide a reasonable degree of fire safety; prepared, published, and periodically revised by the National Fire Protection Association (NFPA) and referenced by the Joint Commission on Accreditation of Healthcare Organizations to evaluate health care organizations under its life safety management program. The provisions of the *LSC* relating to hospitals and nursing facilities must (except in cases when a waiver is granted) be met by facilities certified for participation under Medicare and Medicaid.* *See also* Joint Commission on Accreditation of Healthcare Organizations.

Life Safety Code® is a registered trademark of the National Fire Protection Association, Quincy, Massachusetts.

life safety management program A component of a health care organization's plant, technology, and safety management program designed to protect patients, personnel, visitors, and property from fire and the products of combustion and to provide for the safe use of buildings and grounds. *See also* Joint Commission on Accreditation of Healthcare Organizations; plan of correction, plant, technology, and safety management; plant, technology, and safety management; safety management.

Life Sciences, Association for Politics and the *See* Association for Politics and the Life Sciences.

life specialist, child *See* child life specialist.

life signs *See* vital signs.

life-style (lifestyle) The set of attitudes, behaviors, beliefs, and values that is influenced by the process of socialization, including, for instance, use of substances, such as alcohol, tobacco, and coffee; exercise; dress; recreation; dietary habits. Life-style often affects health. In marketing jargon, life-style is the sum total of the likes and dislikes of particular customers or a section of the market, as expressed in the products they buy to fit their self-image and way of life. *See also* value system.

life support, advanced *See* advanced cardiac life support.

life support, advanced cardiac *See* advanced cardiac life support.

life support, advanced pediatric *See* advance pediatric life support.

life support, advanced trauma *See* advanced trauma life support.

life support, basic *See* basic cardiac life support.

life support, basic cardiac *See* basic cardiac life support.

life support, basic trauma *See* basic trauma life support.

life support care Health services provided for patients requiring extraordinary measures in order to sustain and prolong life. *See also* life support system.

life support system Equipment (for example, a respirator), medications, and services (for example, nursing care) that create a viable environment for patients who otherwise might not survive. The phrase, "termination of life support systems," refers to discontinuing products and services that support the life of patients who are completely dependent on artificial means for survival. *See also* death-prolonging procedure; life-sustaining procedure.

life-sustaining procedure Any intervention that is judged likely to be effective in prolonging the life of a patient or that is being used to sustain the life of a patient. In law, a life-sustaining procedure is one that may be suspended on a court order or pursuant to a living will in the case of, for example, a comatose and terminally ill person. Life-sustaining procedures include mechanical or other artificial means to sustain, restore, or supplant some vital function, such as breathing, which serve to prolong the moment of death when, in the judgment of attending and consulting physicians (as reflected in the patient's medical records), death is imminent if such procedures are not used. *See also* attending physician; death-prolonging procedure; living will.

life table A statistical table exhibiting mortality and survivor characteristics of a given population. A life table may be used, for example, to compute damages resulting from injuries that destroy the earning capacity of a person. *See also* life; table.

lifetime reserve A Medicare term referring to the pool of 60 days of hospital care upon which a patient may draw after he or she has used up the maximum Medicare benefit for a single illness. *See also* Medicare; reserve.

life, wrongful *See* wrongful life.

ligament Any binding or connecting anatomical structure, usually a band of fibrous tissue between bones in the region of a joint. *See also* joint.

ligand assay A testing procedure that measures proteins, peptides, or haptens and deals with methods, such as radioimmunoassay, florescence immunoassay, and receptor assay. *See also* assay; immunoassay; radioimmunoassay.

Ligand Assay Society, Clinical *See* Clinical Ligand Assay Society.

ligation The process of tying off a blood vessel or a duct with a suture or wire, as in a surgeon ligating a torn vein to stop the bleeding, or a gynecologist ligating fallopian tubes to render a patient sterile. *See also* sterilization.

ligature Any material, such as catgut, wire, silk, or synthetic substances, used to bind, bandage, or tie a structure.

light *See* lite.

light emitting diode *See* LED.

light pen Photosensitive device used with a computer monitor and software to provide data and program commands. *See also* computer; input device.

light microscope A microscope that uses light as the source of radiation and a combination of lenses to magnify and focus an object. *See also* electron microscope; lens; microscope; operating microscope.

likelihood ratio A ratio for a screening or diagnostic test (including clinical signs or symptoms) that expresses the relative odds that a given test result would be expected in a patient with (as opposed to one without) the disorder or condition of interest. *See also* ratio.

limb, phantom *See* phantom limb.

limit The point, level, or degree beyond which something cannot or may not proceed. *See also* boundary; normal limits; parameter.

limitation of liability acts *See* limits on liability.

limitations period *See* statute of limitations.

limitations, statute of *See* statute of limitations.

limited code *See* slow code.

limited licensure Licensure restricting a physician's practice to a single health care organization, such as a mental hospital, designated by the state. Physicians with limited licenses are often foreign medical graduates. *See also* foreign medical graduate; licensure.

limited partner An individual who has been admitted to a limited partnership and who contributes capital and shares in the profits but who does not manage the business and is not personally liable for partnership debts. *See also* general partner; junior partner; limited partnership; partner.

limited partnership A type of partnership in which partners generally assume no monetary responsibility beyond the capital originally contributed. *See also* corporate diversification; limited partner; partnership.

limits on liability **1.** In insurance, limits on dollar coverage contained in an insurance policy. Malpractice insurance, for instance, generally contains, such limits on the amounts payable for an individual claim, or in the policy year. Excess coverage describes insurance with limits higher than these conventional amounts. *See also* liability. **2.** State and federal statutes that limit liability for certain types of damages, such as pain and suffering; that limit the liability of certain persons or groups, for example, the liability of corporate directors for acts of the corporation; or that limit the time period in which action can be maintained, as in statute of limitations. *Synonym*: limitation of liability acts. *See also* statute of limitations.

limits, normal *See* normal limits.

linctus A medicine made by mixing a drug with syrup, honey, or other sweet excipient (inert substance). *See also* drug; excipient.

-line A telephone service, as in a helpline, a hotline, or an AIDSline.

linear Anything that follows a straight line, as in a linear equation. *See also* arithmetically; exponentially; geometrically; graph; logarithmic.

linear regression *See* regression.

line function An interlinked group of activities, such as hospital operations or clinical services, that contributes directly to the output of an organization. *See also* function.

line graph A series of line segments connecting points of paired numerical data, representing the functional relationship between the two variables. *See also* graph; variable.

line, hard *See* hard line.

line management The administration of line functions of an organization. *See also* assistant administrator; line function; management.

line printer A high-speed computer printer that prints a line at a time rather than a character at a time. *See also* printer.

line, regression *See* regression line.

line, trend *See* trend line.

line, umbilical *See* umbilical line.

linguistics The science of the languages. *See also* language; psycholinguistics.

linguistics, psycho- *See* psycholinguistics.

liniment A liquid preparation for external application to the unbroken skin, which may contain substances that have analgesic, soothing, or other properties. *See also* lotion.

link **1.** A unit in a connected series, as in linked (or interlinked) organizational functions. **2.** A connecting element. *See also* linkage; weakest link theory.

linkage **1.** The act or process of linking together. **2.** The linking together of different issues because of the belief that progress in one area is relevant and necessary to progress in other areas. *See also* link; weakest link theory.

link theory, weakest *See* weakest link theory.

lipid A fatty substance composed of different proportions of hydrogen, carbon, and oxygen; for example, triglycerides, cortisol, and cholesterol. Together with the carbohydrates and proteins, they constitute the principal structural material of living cells. *See also* cholesterol; fat; hyperlipidemia.

lipoma A benign growth arising form adipose (fatty) tissue. *See also* adenoma; adipose tissue; myoma; neurinoma.

lipoprotein A soluble complex of a lipid (fat) and a protein. Since lipids are insoluble in water, proteins serve as the main lipid transport mechanism in plasma. Some lipoproteins transport cholesterol in the blood, as high-density (HDL), low-density (LDL), and very-low-density (VLDL) lipoproteins. *See also* high-density lipoprotein; hyperlipidemia; low-density lipoprotein; protein; very-low-density lipoprotein.

lipoprotein, high-density *See* high-density lipoprotein.

lipoprotein, low-density *See* low-density lipoprotein.

lipoprotein, very-low-density *See* very-low-density lipoprotein.

liposuction surgery A cosmetic surgical procedure consisting of removing excess fatty (adipose) tissue from the body with a vacuum pump through a tube, or cannula, inserted into a small incision in the fat. It is not meant to reduce weight but to adjust body contours. Liposuction surgery is not currently part of the ordinary medical school curriculum. *Synonym:* suction lipectomy. *See also* adipose tissue; cosmetic surgery.

Lipo-Suction Surgery, American Society of *See* American Society of Lipo-Suction Surgery.

lip reading A technique for understanding unheard speech by interpreting the lip and facial movements of the speaker. *See also* hearing impaired.

lip service A verbal expression of agreement or allegiance, that is hypocritically unsupported by real conviction or action.

liquid asset Cash. also includes other current assets that can be quickly converted into cash. *See also* asset.

list, additional drug benefit *See* additional drug benefit list.

list, check- *See* checklist.

listen To make an effort to hear something, as in she could hear but would not listen. *See also* active listening; hearing.

listening, active *See* active listening.

Listening and Mediation, Child Abuse *See* Child Abuse Listening and Mediation.

lite A food label with various meanings, including that the food contains fewer calories, less fat, or less sodium or is a lighter color than the standard product. *See also* labeling.

lithotomy position   A position formerly employed for the extraction of stones from the urinary bladder, characterized by a patient lying on his or her back with the hips and knees flexed and the thighs apart and externally rotated.

lithotripsy   Noninvasive pulverization of urinary tract stones by means of a lithotripter. Extracorporeal shock wave lithotripsy (ESWL) refers to the type of lithotripsy in which shock waves are generated in a water-filled bath in which the patient sits. Other methods of lithotripsy include electrohydraulic lithotripsy and ultrasonic lithotripsy. *See also* lithotripter.

lithotripter   A noninvasive device that pulverizes urinary tract stones by passing shock waves through a water-filled bath in which the patient sits. The device creates stone fragments small enough to be expelled in the urine. *See also* lithotripsy.

litigation   Judicial contest through which legal rights are sought to be determined and enforced, as in the medical malpractice case was in litigation for over seven years.

Litigation Group, Public Citizen   *See* Public Citizen Litigation Group.

litigious   Tending to engage in lawsuits, as in the patient's litigious nature caused health professionals to avoid him. *See also* lawsuit.

litter   A stretcher. *See also* cart; gurney.

live birth   "The complete expulsion or extraction from its mother of a product of conception, irrespective of the duration of the pregnancy, which, after such separation, breathes or shows any other evidence of life, such as beating of the heart, pulsation of the umbilical cord, or definite movement of voluntary muscles, whether or not the umbilical cord has been cut or the placenta is attached; each product of such a birth is considered live born" (World Health Organization, 1950). This definition includes no requirement that the product of conception be viable or capable of independent life and thus includes very early and patently nonviable fetuses. *See also* birth; conceptus; fetus; World Health Organization.

liver   A large, dark red organ occupying the upper right-hand portion of the abdominal cavity. Its primary functions are digestion, excretion, and protein and carbohydrate metabolism. It is essential to life. *See also* biliary tract surgery; bilirubin; cirrhosis of the liver; fatty liver disease; gastroenterology; glycogen; jaundice; liver failure; liver function tests.

liver, cirrhosis of the   *See* cirrhosis of the liver.

liver disease, fatty   *See* fatty liver disease.

liver failure   Failure of the liver usually caused by a complication of viral hepatitis, cirrhosis, or ingestion of hepatotoxic substances. It is manifested by hepatic encephalopathy or hepatic coma. *See also* hepatic encephalopathy; hepatitis; jaundice.

Liver Diseases, American Association for the Study of   *See* American Association for the Study of Liver Diseases.

liver function tests   A series of laboratory tests usually performed when liver disease is known or suspected, most of which consist of biochemical measurements made on serum or plasma. They include measurements of bilirubin, alkaline phosphatase, albumin, globulin, prothrombin, and various liver enzymes. *See also* liver.

living, activities of daily   *See* activities of daily living.

Living Bank, The   *See* The Living Bank.

living-in unit   A hospital room regularly maintained for mothers to assume care of newborns or for relatives to assist in the care of a chronically ill or other type of patient, under the supervision of nursing personnel.

living, standard of   *See* standard of living.

living will   Instructional directives in written form that indicate the author's wishes for medical treatment should he or she become incapacitated and unable to participate in medical decision-making. Many states have "living will" legislation; for example, Kansas has the Natural Death Act and Missouri, the Death-Prolonging Procedures Act. Natural death acts are pieces of legislation generally enacted to codify living wills and often contain specific examples. *Synonym:* terminal care document. *See also* advance directives; death-prolonging procedure; durable power of attorney of health care; life-sustaining procedure; natural death acts; Patient Self Determination Act; severability clause; will.

LLB   *See* Juris Doctor.

load and go   Refers to the management by prehospital personnel of trauma patients whose conditions are so critical that they may die if they do not receive definitive care within a matter of minutes. Once such a patient is recognized, he or she is immediately transported to the nearest appropriate trauma facility. *Synonym*: expeditious evacuation. *See also* ambulance; advanced trauma life support; basic trauma life support; trauma; traumatology.

loading In insurance, the amount added to the actuarial value of the coverage (expected or average amounts payable to the insured) to cover the expense to the insurer of securing and maintaining the business. *See also* premium.

lobe A major anatomical subdivision of an organ or a structure, usually having a clear boundary, as in the lobes of the liver. *See also* liver.

lobbying Any attempt by a person or a group of persons to influence federal or state legislation or a governmental official for or against a specific cause by the provision of information, argument, or other means. The term derives from the frequent presence of lobbyists in the lobbies of Congressional and other governmental chambers. *See also* advocacy; lobbyist.

lobbyist A person who is involved in the business of persuading legislators to pass laws that are favorable, and to defeat those that are unfavorable, to the interest of the lobbyist or of his or her clients. The Omnibus Budget Reconciliation Act of 1993 (OBRA '93) expanded the definition of lobbying to include efforts to influence actions or positions of certain high-level federal executive branch officials. *See also* lobbying.

lobotomy, prefrontal *See* prefrontal lobotomy.

local anesthesia Administration of a local anesthetic agent, such as lidocaine, to cause loss of sensation in a small area of the body, as for suturing of a laceration. *See also* anesthesia; general anesthesia; laceration; local anesthetic; nerve block; regional anesthesia.

local anesthetic An anesthetic, such as lidocaine, whose action is limited to an area of the body determined by the site of its application; it produces its effect by blocking nerve conduction. *See also* anesthetic; local anesthesia; nerve block.

local area network (LAN) In computer science, a system that links together electronic office equipment, such as computers, terminals, and word processors, and forms a network within an office or

a building. *See also* computer; network; networking; wide area network.

Local Environmental Health Administrators, National Conference of *See* National Conference of Local Environmental Health Administrators.

Local Health Officers, United States Conference of *See* United States Conference of Local Health Officers.

locality, Medicare *See* Medicare locality.

locality rule A legal doctrine stating that the standard of care in a malpractice lawsuit is measured by the degree to which it adheres to standards of care exercised by similar professionals within the same or a similar geographic area or locality, rather than within the world, nation, state, or profession at large. *Compare* national standard rule. *See also* rule; standard of care.

lockjaw *See* tetanus.

locum tenens Latin phrase meaning "to hold a place"; a person, such as a physician or cleric, who substitutes temporarily for another.

locus 1. The position of a point, as defined by the coordinates on a graph, or the position of a gene on a chromosome. **2.** A center or focus of great activity, as in the locus of the continuous quality improvement movement in the United States originated in industry.

log A record of the progress of an undertaking, as in a computer log or a patient-scheduling log.

logarithmic Pertaining to use of exponents, as in a logarithmic increase. *See also* arithmetically; exponentially; geometrically; graph; linear.

logic 1. The study of the principles of reasoning. *See also* logical empiricism. **2.** In computer science, the nonarithmetic operations performed by a computer, such as sorting, comparing, and matching, that involve yes-no decisions. *See also* logic bomb. **3.** Computer circuitry.

logical empiricism A philosophy asserting the primacy of observation in assessing the truth of statements of fact and holding that subjective arguments not based on observable data are meaningless. *See also* empirical.

logic bomb A set of instructions surreptitiously included in a computer program so that if a particular set of conditions ever occurs, the instructions will be put into operation, usually with disastrous results. The logic bomb is a malicious or even criminal use of computing know-how and has been used as a way of destroying evidence of a computer fraud as soon as information that might lead to the culprits is accessed; as the basis for blackmail; and as a way for a programmer to take revenge on an employer by causing the system to crash mysteriously.

logic, indicator data collection *See* indicator data collection logic.

logo A unique design or symbol used as a trademark by a group, such as a company, publishing house, or hospital.

logomachy A battle of words, as in the logomachy between the two disciplines threatened to derail efforts at improving service to customers.

log on To establish a connection from a terminal to a computer and to identify oneself as an authorized user. *See also* computer; password.

long bone Any of several elongated bones of vertebrate limbs that have a roughly cylindrical shape containing marrow; for example, in humans, the femur, tibia, humerus, and radius. *See also* bone; bone marrow.

longevity Long life, usually influenced by genetic factors. *See also* heredity.

Longevity Association, American *See* American Longevity Association.

longitudinal study A study in which the same individuals or group of individuals are examined on a number of occasions over a long period of time. *See also* cohort study.

long-range planning *See* strategic planning.

long term Being in effect for a long time, as in a long term care hospital.

long term care (LTC) The health and personal care services provided to chronically ill, aged, disabled, or retarded persons, in an institution or in the place of residence. These persons are not in an acute phase of illness but require convalescent, physical supportive, and/or restorative services on a long-term basis. Long term care is sometimes used more narrowly to refer only to long-term institutional care, such as that provided in nursing homes, homes for the retarded and mental health care organizations. Ambulatory services, like home health care, which also can be provided on a long-term basis, are seen as alternatives to long-term

institutional care. *See also* long term; Long Term Care Accreditation Program; long term care administrator; long term care facility.

Long Term Care, Accreditation Manual for *See* Accreditation Manual for Long Term Care.

Long Term Care Accreditation Program The survey and accreditation program of the Joint Commission on Accreditation of Healthcare Organizations for eligible hospital-based and freestanding long term care organizations. *See also* accreditation; *Accreditation Manual for Long Term Care*; Joint Commission on Accreditation of Healthcare Organizations; long term care; survey.

long term care administrator An administrator who manages a long term care facility, as in a nursing home administrator. *See also* administrator; long term care facility.

Long Term Care Campaign (LTCC) A national organization founded in 1987 composed of 140 organizations promoting legislation to enact social insurance, such as Social Security or Medicare, that would provide for long-term health care. It conducts lobbying on state and national levels. *See also* long term care.

long term care facility (LTCF) A facility traditionally known as a nursing home, including both skilled nursing facilities and intermediate care facilities, depending on the extent of nursing and related medical care provided. *See also* intermediate care facility; long term care; skilled nursing facility.

Long Term Care, National Association of Directors of Nursing Administration in *See* National Association of Directors of Nursing Administration in Long Term Care.

Long-Term Care, National Institute on Community-Based *See* National Institute on Community-Based Long-Term Care.

Long Term Care Services, Special Constituency Section for Aging and *See* Special Constituency Section for Aging and Long Term Care Services.

long-term hospital A hospital that treats patients who are not in an acute phase of illness, but who require an intensity of medical and skilled nursing services not available in nursing homes. *See also* chronic disease hospital; hospital.

long-term planning *See* strategic planning.

loop A set of statements in a computer program that is executed repeatedly. *See also* computer program.

loophole A technicality making it possible to circumvent a law's intent without violating its letter. *See also* law.

loop, rework *See* rework loop.

lordosis Exaggerated curvature of the spine, resulting in abnormal concavity of the lumbar region when viewed from the back. *Synonym:* swayback. *Compare* kyphosis; scoliosis. *See also* spine.

LOS *See* length of stay.

loss **1.** The condition of being deprived or bereaved of something or someone. **2.** Any diminution of quantity, quality, or value of property, resulting from the occurrence of some undesired event. **3.** In insurance, the basis for a claim under the terms of an insurance policy.

loss, capital *See* capital gains or losses.

lost chance of cure An element of damages. It allows recovery if a patient's opportunity to be cured of a disease has been reduced by another's negligence. Some jurisdictions require proof that cure was probable before the negligent act but is no longer probable as a result of the negligence. *See also* cure; damages; lost chance of survival; negligence.

lost chance of survival An element of damages. It allows recovery if a patient's opportunity to survive a disease has been reduced by another's negligence. Some jurisdictions require proof that survival was probable before the negligent act but is no longer probable as a result of the negligence. *See also* damages; lost chance of cure; negligence.

lotion An aqueous solution or suspension for external application to the skin. Lotions cools by evaporation and requires frequent reapplication. *See also* liniment.

louse, body *See* body louse.

louse, head *See* head louse.

low birth weight Weight of an infant of 2500 grams or less (5 pounds, 8.2 ounces) at birth. These babies are at risk for developing lack of oxygen during labor and low blood sugar and slow growth and development after birth. *See also* birth weight; weight.

low calorie A label applied to foods that contain no more than 40 calories per serving and no more than 0.4 calories per gram. A "serving size" can be whatever the seller chooses. This label cannot be applied to certain foods naturally low in calories, such as celery. *See also* calorie; labeling.

low-density lipoprotein (LDL) The most abundant of the lipoproteins, LDLs usually carry about 65% of the circulating cholesterol to cells. High levels are often associated with atherosclerosis. *See also* atherosclerosis; cholesterol; lipoprotein.

lower adjacent value *See* adjacent value, lower.

lower control limit *See* control limit.

low-mortality outlier A health care provider, such as an individual hospital, with mortality rates that are lower than expected after adjustment for patient and other characteristics. *Compare* high-mortality outlier. *See also* outlier.

low tech Products or services using earlier or less developed technology; for example, a gauze bandage to wrap or cover a laceration or a visit to a physician or other health professional for suture removal are considered to be low tech. *Compare* high tech. *See also* technology.

LP *See* lumbar puncture.

LPN *See* licensed practical nurse.

LSC *See Life Safety Code*®.

LSD Abbreviation for lysergic acid diethylamide. *See* lysergic acid.

LSM *See Accreditation Manual for Pathology and Clinical Laboratory Services.*

LT *See* Laughter Therapy.

LTC *See* long term care.

LTCC *See* Long Term Care Campaign.

LTCF *See* long term care facility.

Lucille P. Markey Charitable Trust A trust established in 1983 in Florida set up to distribute the entire estate of the donor by 1997. It supports and encourages basic medical research. Fields of inquiry include cellular and molecular biology, developmental biology, structural biology, neurobiology, immunology, genetics, and virology. Occasional grants are made to support summer seminars at research institutions and to fund projects that are directly related to medical research, such as the development, financing, and organization of medical research; the history of basic medical research; and the dissemination of the results of such research.

lues *See* syphilis.

lumbago A painful condition of the lower back (small of the back), occurring, for example, from a muscle strain.

lumbar puncture (LP) The insertion of a hollow needle beneath the spinal (arachnoid) membrane at the lumbar (lower back) region of the spinal cord to withdraw cerebrospinal fluid for diagnostic purposes, such as determining the presence of meningitis, or to administer medications. *Synonyms*: spinal puncture; spinal tap. *See also* cerebrospinal fluid; meningitis; spinal cord.

lumen The inner open space or cavity of a tube, such as a blood vessel, or an organ, such as the intestine.

lumpectomy The least invasive procedure for breast cancer involving removal of the lump (tumor) and a small amount of tissue through a small incision, leaving only a slight depression in the breast. *Compare* mastectomy; modified radical mastectomy; quadrantectomy. *See also* mammary gland.

lung Either of two spongy, saclike respiratory organs occupying the chest cavity together with the heart and functioning to remove carbon dioxide from the blood and provide it with oxygen. *See also* adult respiratory distress syndrome; pneumoconiosis; pulmonary; pulmonary medicine; rales; respiration; respiratory.

Lung Association, American *See* American Lung Association.

Lung Association Staff, Congress of *See* Congress of Lung Association Staff.

lung, brown *See* brown lung.

lung disease, black *See* black lung disease.

lung, farmer's *See* farmer's lung.

lung, iron *See* iron lung.

Lung and Respiratory Disease Clinics, National Coalition of Black *See* National Coalition of Black Lung and Respiratory Disease Clinics.

Lutheran General Health Care System (LGHCS) An organization composed of 10 health care corporations that promotes the philosophy that good health care involves an understanding of human ecology and must meet the emotional and spiritual, as well as physical, needs of patients. It defines human ecology as the understanding and care of human beings as whole persons in light of their relationships to God, themselves, their families, and the society in which they live. It supports the concept of holistic health care. It sponsors the Park Ridge Center, an institute for the study of health, faith, and ethics, and Parkside Alcoholic Research Foundation, which studies the cause and course of alcoholism and substance abuse. Formerly (1986) Lutheran Institute of Human Ecology. *See also* holistic health; holistic medicine; Park Ridge Center.

Lutheran Hospital Association of America (LHA) A national organization composed of 110 hospitals sponsored by a Lutheran church or bearing the title Lutheran. It offers periodic grants for the advancement of health care chaplaincy programs. *See also* chaplain; chaplaincy service; hospital.

Lutheran Hospitals and Homes Society (LHHS) An organization founded in 1938 for the purpose of operating and maintaining Lutheran hospitals, nursing homes, homes for the aged, and a hospital-school for disabled children.

Lutheran Institute of Human Ecology *See* Lutheran General Health Care System.

LVN *See* licensed vocational nurse.

lymphadenopathy, persistent generalized *See* persistent generalized lymphadenopathy.

lymph node Any of the many small (1 to 25 millimeters in diameter) bean-shaped structures that filter lymph and produce lymphocytes. Lymph nodes are concentrated in several areas of the body, such as the armpit, groin, and neck. *Synonym*: lymph gland. *See also* bubo; persistent generalized lymphadenopathy.

lymphocyte A white blood cell that normally comprises approximately 25% of the total white blood cell count but is increased in response to infection. There are two kinds of lymphocytes known as *B cells* and *T cells*. B cells, on exposure to a specific antigen, are activated and differentiate rapidly to produce plasma cells and memory cells. Plasma cells synthesize and secrete antibodies. T cells, when exposed to a specific antigen, produce large numbers of new T cells sensitized to that antigen. T cells are often "killer cells" because they secrete immunologically essential chemical compounds and assist B cells in destroying foreign protein. T cells also play a role in the body's resistance to the proliferation of cancer cells. *See also* blood cell;

immune response; reticuloendothelial system; white blood cell.

lymphoma   A solid malignant tumor of the lymphoid tissue, such as Burkitt's lymphoma and Hodgkin's disease. *See also* Hodgkin's disease; malignant.

lysergic acid (LSD)   A synthetic hallucinogen that is used as a "recreational drug." It can induce psychologic dependence and may be associated with hazards, such as panic, depression, paranoia, and prolonged psychotic episodes. *Synonyms*: acid; LSD. *See also* hallucination; hallucinogen.

lysol   A disinfectant mixture of a solution of soft soap (a mixture of the potassium salts of stearic, oleic, and palmitic acids) with cresols (the three isomers of hydroxytoluene). *See also* disinfectant.

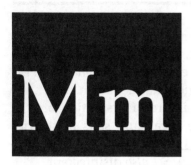

MA *See* mental age.

MacArthur Foundation, The John D. and Catherine T. *See* The John D. and Catherine T. MacArthur Foundation.

machine A system or device, such as a computer or a magnetic resonance imaging machine, that performs or assists in the performance of a human task. *See also* computer; fax machine; fungitrol machine; heart-lung machine; mechanism.

machine code *See* machine language.

machine, facsimile *See* fax machine.

machine, fax *See* fax machine.

machine, fungitrol *See* fungitrol machine.

machine, heart-lung *See* heart-lung machine.

machine language The basic language of a computer requiring no further translation. Machine language statements are written in a binary code and each statement corresponds to one machine action. Machine language programs are very flexible, but are difficult and time-consuming to write and susceptible to errors. *Synonym*: machine code. *See also* computer; language.

machine readable Pertaining to a printed pattern that can be read or scanned by a device, usually an electronic device. *See also* data capture; electronic mail; readable; scanner.

macroeconomics Study of the aggregate forces of a nation's economy as a whole, using such data as price levels, unemployment, inflation, and industrial production. *Compare* microeconomics. *See also* economics.

macroscopic anatomy *See* gross anatomy.

maggot A fly larva that may infect open sores, usually of derelict and neglected persons. *See also* myiasis.

magical thinking In psychology, a belief that thinking about an event in the external world can cause it to occur. Magical thinking is considered a normal phase in the mental development of infants and very young children. In older age groups, it can be a symptom of schizophrenia and some types of neurosis. *See also* neurosis; schizophrenia.

magic bullet A drug, therapy, or preventive therapy that cures or prevents a disease, as in there is no magic bullet against cancer.

magnetic Having the property of being surrounded by a magnetic field and either the natural or induced attraction of iron or steel. *See also* cyclotron; magnetic resonance.

magnetic bubble memory In computer science, a memory in which data are stored in the form of bubbles, or circular areas, on a thin film of magnetic silicate. Magnetic bubble memory is similar to random access memory (RAM) but does not lose the stored information when the computer is turned off. *See also* memory; random access memory.

magnetic disk A memory device covered with a magnetic coating on which information is stored by magnetization of microscopically small needles. *See also* hard disk.

Magnetic Measurements, Conference on Precision Electro- *See* Conference on Precision Electromagnetic Measurements.

magnetic resonance The phenomenon of absorption of certain frequencies of radio and microwave radiation by atoms placed in a magnetic field. The pattern of absorption reveals molecular structure. *Synonyms*: NMR; nuclear magnetic resonance. *See also* magnetic resonance imaging.

magnetic resonance imaging (MRI) The noninvasive diagnostic use of a nuclear magnetic resonance spectrometer to produce electronic images of specific atoms and molecular structures in solids, especially human cells, tissues, and organs. This approach to visualizing soft tissues of the body by applying an external magnetic field makes possible the distinction between hydrogen atoms in different environments. *Synonym*: nuclear magnetic resonance imaging. *See also* imaging; magnetic resonance.

magnetic resonance imaging scanner The machine used to carry out magnetic resonance imaging. *Synonym*: MRI; MRI scanner. *See also* magnetic resonance imaging.

Magnetic Resonance Imaging, Society for *See* Society for Magnetic Resonance Imaging.

magnetic resonance, nuclear *See* nuclear magnetic resonance.

Magnetics Institute, Bio-Electro- *See* Bio-Electro-Magnetics Institute.

Magnetics Society, Bioelectro- *See* Bioelectro-magnetics Society.

magnetic-striped card *See* single magnetic-striped card.

magnetic tape A data storage device, usually in a cassette.

magnetism The branch of physics concerned with magnets and magnetic fields. *See also* magnetic; magnetic resonance; physics.

magnification Apparent increase in size, as under a microscope. *See also* microscope.

maim To disable by a wound, typically as a result of violence. *See also* violence.

Maimonides (1135-1204) A physician, rabbi, Jewish philosopher born in Cordova, Spain, who was the physician to Saladin, under whom he wrote many medical works in Arabic, among them a commentary on the aphorisms of Hippocrates and treatises on asthma, diet, poisons, and hygiene. A prayer attributed to him is considered to rank beside the oath of Hippocrates as an ethical guide to the medical profession.

mainframe *See* mainframe computer.

mainframe computer A large, powerful computer, often serving several connected terminals and typically supporting 100 to 500 users at a time. The IBM 370 and IBM 3081 are examples of mainframe computers. It is usually kept physically separate from users, typically in a climate-controlled environment with restricted access and a sophisticated fire-extinguishing system. *Synonym*: mainframe. *See also* computer; microcomputer; on-line.

mainstream The prevailing current of thought, influence, or activity, as in mainstream morality.

maintenance The work of keeping something in proper condition; upkeep. *See also* health maintenance; health maintenance organization; maintenance department; maintenance home health care; maintenance therapy.

maintenance department Unit of a health care organization providing for repair and upkeep of its physical plant, including heating, ventilating, and air conditioning systems, utilities, telecommunications, and clinical engineering equipment. *Synonyms*: engineering and maintenance department; physical plant and maintenance department. *See also* department; maintenance.

maintenance engineer *See* chief engineer.

maintenance, health *See* health maintenance.

maintenance home health care Home health care provided to persons whose primary needs are usually for personal care and/or other supportive environmental and social services. *See also* home health care; personal care.

maintenance organization, health *See* health maintenance organization.

maintenance therapy The prescription of a drug or drugs on a long-term basis in doses sufficient to sustain a therapeutic effect that has been established initially by a different drug or drug combination or the same drug in different dosage. *See also* maintenance; therapy.

major affective disorder Any of a group of psychotic disorders not caused by organic abnormality of the brain and characterized by persistent disturbances in mood and thought processes and inappropriate emotional responses, as occur in some forms of manic-depressive illness. *See also* disorder; manic-depressive illness.

major crossmatching The act or process whereby red blood cells of a donor are placed into a recipient's serum to test for compatibility between blood types prior to blood transfusion. *Compare* minor crossmatching. *See also* blood transfusion; crossmatching.

major diagnosis Diagnosis accounting for the greatest resource consumption during a patient's stay in a health care facility. *See also* diagnosis.

major diagnostic category (MDC) A phrase used in prospective payment systems, which refers to the initial classification of each patient into a major diagnostic category based on his or her principal diagnosis. Each patient is then further classified according to age, complications, and other characteristics into one of many diagnosis-related groups (DRGs). *See also* diagnosis-related groups; major diagnosis.

majority, age of *See* age of majority.

majority, legal *See* age of majority.

major life activities The activities and conditions of self-care, language, learning, mobility, self-direction, capacity for independent living, and economic self-sufficiency. The level of these activities is used to determine eligibility for social services programs for people with handicaps, mental retardation, and developmental disabilities. *See also* developmental disability; mental retardation.

major medical insurance *See* catastrophic insurance.

major surgery Surgery in which the operative procedure is extensive or hazardous, as in entering one of the body cavities (chest, head, abdomen) or amputating above the ankle or wrist; it usually requires general anesthesia or assistance in respiration. *Compare* minor surgery. *See also* general anesthesia; operation; surgery.

makeover In business, the restructuring of a company by a new management, especially if the results seem only cosmetic.

make-work Uneconomic use of a work force for the sole purpose of creating employment; a job having no value.

malabsorption A condition in which there is inadequate intestinal absorption of one or more groups of nutrients, with the consequent loss of those nutrients in the feces and the development of nutritional deficiency syndromes; for example, celiac disease. *See also* celiac disease; feces; gastroenterology; intestine; malnutrition; nutrient.

maladjustment In psychiatry, the failure to fit one's inner needs to the environment. *See also* psychiatry.

malady Disease, illness. *See also* disease; illness.

malaise A vague feeling of weakness or discomfort, often an early symptom of illness.

malaria A tropical disease arising from infection by one or more of four species of protozoa belonging to the genus *Plasmodium*, transmitted by female mosquitoes; it is characterized by high fever, chills, anemia, and enlargement of the spleen. *See also* infectious diseases; tropical medicine.

Malcolm Baldrige National Quality Award A national award to recognize manufacturing firms, service firms, and small businesses that "excel in quality achievement and quality management." Established in 1987 and named for a former US Secretary of Commerce, the award is based on an examination of categories of organizational characteristics and operations. The Baldridge Award is the US equivalent to the Deming Award offered in Japan.

male chauvinism An attitude of superiority or dominance by men over women, regardless of all factors being constant. A male chauvinist discriminates against women by applying stereotyped ideas. *See also* chauvinism.

male climacteric *See* climacteric.

Male Psychology and Physiology, Society for the Study of *See* Society for the Study of Male Psychology and Physiology.

malformation Any abnormality of structure due to faulty development.

malfunction Failure to perform; for example, the failure of a medical device to meet any of its performance specifications or to perform as intended. *See also* device; medical device; Safe Medical Devices Act of 1990.

malice The intent, without just cause or reason, to commit a wrongful act that will result in harm to another. *See also* malicious prosecution.

malicious prosecution Legal grounds on which a defendant may countersue a plaintiff if the plaintiff's lawsuit was totally frivolous, without any merit, and was brought simply to harass the defendant. *See also* defendant; lawsuit; malice; plaintiff; prosecute; prosecution.

malignancy In pathology, a malignant tumor. *See also* cancer; malignant; pathology; seminoma.

malignant Tending to become progressively worse and to result in death, as in malignant hyperpyrexia (hyperthermia) or a malignant tumor having the properties of anaplasia (undifferentiated cells, characteristic of tumor tissue), invasion, and metastasis. *Compare* benign. *See also* malignant disease; malignant hyperpyrexia; malignant hypertension; metastasis; precancerous.

malignant disease **1.** Any disease associated with cancer. *See also* cancer. **2.** Any noncancerous condition having a rapidly progressive and virulent character; for example, malignant hypertension, malignant hyperpyrexia. *See also* malignant hypertension; malignant hyperpyrexia.

malignant hypertension A severe state of elevated blood pressure characterized by edema of the back portion of the eye with vascular hemorrhages, thickening of small arteries and arterioles, and left ventricular enlargement. It may lead to hypertensive encephalopathy (degenerative disease of the brain). *See also* hypertension; hypertensive encephalopathy; malignant disease.

malignant hyperpyrexia A rare, genetically determined complication of general anesthesia, resulting in a dangerously elevated body temperature, increased heart rate, rapid breathing, and muscle rigidity. *Synonym*: malignant hyperthermia. *See also* hyperpyrexia.

malignant hyperthermia *See* malignant hyperpyrexia.

malingerer A person who feigns illness or injury for the purpose of a consciously desired end, such as avoiding job responsibilities. *See also* malingering.

malingering The willful, deliberate, and fraudulent feigning or exaggeration of the symptoms of illness or injury, done for the purpose of achieving a consciously desired end, such as collecting insurance or avoiding work or duty. *See also* malingerer.

malnutrition Any disorder of nutrition, resulting from an inadequate, excessive, or unbalanced diet or from impaired ability to absorb and assimilate foods. *See also* malabsorption; nutrition.

malocclusion A condition in which the teeth of the opposing jaws do not contact or mesh normally; it is often corrected by orthodontics. *See also* occlusion; orthodontics.

malpractice Improper or unethical conduct or unreasonable lack of skill by a holder of a professional or official position, often applied to physicians, dentists, lawyers, and public officers to denote negligent or unskillful performance of duties when professional skills are obligatory. Malpractice is a cause of action for which damages are allowed. *See also* action; damages; defensive medicine; lawsuit; legal malpractice; medical malpractice; occurrence policy; professional liability; standard of care.

malpractice insurance *See* medical malpractice insurance.

malpractice insurance, medical *See* medical malpractice insurance.

malpractice insurance, sponsored *See* sponsored malpractice insurance.

malpractice, legal *See* legal malpractice.

malpractice, medical *See* medical malpractice.

maltreatment Treatment of a patient that is lacking in adequate skill and involves willful acts, neglect, or lack of knowledge on the part of a health care provider.

mammaplasty Reconstructive or cosmetic plastic surgery to alter the size or shape of the breast(s). *See also* cosmetic surgery; plastic surgery.

mammary gland The specialized milk-producing gland, representing a modified sweat gland, situated on the front of female mammals including human beings. In the human female, two such glands, together with connective and adipose tissue, form the two breasts. *Synonym*: breast. *See also* gland; lactation; mammaplasty; mammogram; mammography; mastectomy; mastitis; milk.

mammogram A diagnostic image (roentgenogram) of the breast. *See also* roentgenogram.

mammography A procedure in which the soft tissues of the breast (mammary gland) are radiographed to detect benign or malignant tumors. Periodic mammography is generally recommended for women thought to be at high risk for breast cancer and in certain other situations. *See also* mammary gland; radiography.

MANA *See* Midwives Alliance of North America.

manage The act or process of administering an organization's activities to achieve particular objectives. *See also* administration; management.

managed care Organizations of health care providers, such as physicians and hospitals, formed to enhance efficiency of work performed. This is accomplished by, for example, increasing beneficiary cost sharing, controlling inpatient admissions and lengths of stay, establishing cost-sharing incentives for outpatient surgery, selectively contracting with health care providers, and directly managing high-cost health care cases. A health maintenance organization (HMO) is a common form of managed care. *Synonym*: managed health care. *See also* encounter; health maintenance organization; managed competition; physician-hospital organization.

Managed Care Pharmacy Association, American *See* American Managed Care Pharmacy Association.

Managed Care Physicians, National Association of *See* National Association of Managed Care Physicians.

managed care plan *See* managed care.

Managed Care and Review Association, American *See* American Managed Care and Review Association.

managed competition A proposed system for

financing and delivering health care that attempts to blend employers into large purchasing networks to shop for the best health coverage at the lowest price. In this proposed system, the government would require any insurance company, health maintenance organization, or other health plan bidding for business to offer a standard core-benefits package. The thesis behind this proposal is that the large purchasing networks' considerable buying power would generate competition among health plans resulting in lowering prices and improving quality. All employers would be required to contribute the cost of health coverage for their employees, and the government would subsidize the cost for the low-income unemployed population. *See also* competition; health alliance; Jackson Hole approach.

managed economy An economy in which considerable government intervention takes place in order to direct economic activity. *See also* economy.

managed health care *See* managed care.

Managed Health Care Association (MHCA) A national organization founded in 1989 composed of more than 120 of the nation's largest private-sector employers working to foster a more productive, accountable, and cost-effective US health care delivery system through the expansion and improvement of managed health care. Member organizations have implemented or are considering implementing managed care programs. *See also* managed care.

managed health care insurance plan *See* managed care.

managed indemnity plan A traditional indemnity insurance plan that offers a variety of utilization review features. *See also* indemnity; utilization review.

management **1.** The setting of goals and directing an organization to the achievement of these goals. *Compare* mismanagement. *See also* goal; leadership; take-charge. **2.** The group of persons responsible for running an organization or directing human activities toward achievement of goals, including top management. *See also* administration; manager; management by crisis; management development; management by objectives; middle manager; mismanagement; organizational planning; theory x; theory y; theory z.

Management, Academy of Hazard Control *See* Academy of Hazard Control Management.

Management, Academy of Pharmacy Practice and *See* Academy of Pharmacy Practice and Management.

management and administration In health care, the activities pertaining to directing and controlling the delivery of health services of an entire organization or its components, as established by an organization's policies. *See also* administration; management.

Management Agency, Federal Emergency *See* Federal Emergency Management Agency.

Management, American Association of Industrial *See* American Association of Industrial Management.

Management, American Institute of *See* American Institute of Management.

Management, American Society for Healthcare Risk *See* American Society for Healthcare Risk Management.

Management, American Society for Hospital Materials *See* American Society for Hospital Materials Management.

Management Analysis System, Medical *See* Medical Management Analysis System.

Management Association, American *See* American Management Association.

Management Association, American Health Information *See* American Health Information Management Association.

Management Association, Clinical Laboratory *See* Clinical Laboratory Management Association.

Management Association, Data Processing *See* Data Processing Management Association.

Management Association, Dental Group *See* Dental Group Management Association.

Management Association, Environmental *See* Environmental Management Association.

Management Association, Healthcare Financial *See* Healthcare Financial Management Association.

Management Association, Laboratory Animal *See* Laboratory Animal Management Association.

Management Association, Medical Group *See* Medical Group Management Association.

Management Association, National Emergency *See* National Emergency Management Association.

Management Association, Quality and Productivity *See* Quality and Productivity Management Association.

Management Association, Radiology Business *See* Radiology Business Management Association.

Management, Association for Systems *See* Association for Systems Management.

Management, Board of Certified Hazard Control
See Board of Certified Hazard Control Management.

Management and Budget, Office of   *See* Office of Management and Budget.

management contract, risk   *See* risk management contract.

management by crisis   A reactive method of management whereby strategies are formulated as events occur. This short-sighted approach frequently leads to organizational confusion reflected in lowered levels of both performance and the achievement of desired outcomes. *Synonyms:* crisis management; "putting out fires" approach. *Compare* management by objectives. *See also* crisis; Juran, Joseph M.; management.

management, data   *See* data management.

management, database   *See* database management.

management of departments, contract   *See* contract management of departments.

management development   Any deliberate effort by an organization to provide managers with skills they need for future duties, such as providing them with the opportunity for advanced education. A manager is usually trained so that he or she can be of greater organizational value not only in present, but also in future assignments. *See also* management.

management engineer   *See* industrial engineer.

management, equipment   *See* equipment management.

management, health care   *See* health administration.

management, human resources   *See* human resources management.

management information system (MIS)   An information system consisting of a group of computer programs designed to collect, store, and transmit data to support management in planning and directing organizational operations. *See also* case-mix management information system; clinical information system; hospital information system; information system; management; system.

management information system, case-mix   *See* case-mix management information system.

management, line   *See* line management.

management, middle   *See* middle management.

management, mis-   *See* mismanagement.

Management, National Association of Healthcare Access   *See* National Association of Healthcare Access Management.

Management, National Coordinating Council on Emergency   *See* National Coordinating Council on Emergency Management.

management by objectives   An approach to management in which control is exercised by results and outputs, rather than by inputs. Performance is continuously measured in an organization, objectives are stated in measurable terms, staff participate in decision making, rewards are based on performance, and specific performance standards for management and professional personnel are set and directed at attaining the organization's overall goals. *Compare* management by crisis. *See also* management; objective.

management, office   *See* office management.

Management, Office of Personnel   *See* Office of Personnel Management.

management of an organization, contract   *See* contract management of an organization.

management, outcomes   *See* outcomes management.

management, pain   *See* pain management.

management, personnel   *See* personnel management.

management, plant, technology, and safety   *See* plant, technology, and safety management.

management, project   *See* project management.

management, program   *See* project management.

management program, life safety   *See* life safety management program.

management program, pain   *See* pain management program.

management, quality   *See* quality management.

management, records   *See* records management.

management, risk   *See* risk management.

management, safety   *See* safety management.

management science   A school of management emphasizing the use of mathematics and statistics as an aid in resolving production and operations problems. A major objective is to provide management with a quantitative basis for decisions and actions. *See also* management; science; statistics.

management services, home   *See* home management services.

management services, home equipment   *See* home equipment management services.

management services organization (MSO)   A legal entity that provides administrative and practice management services to physicians. For example, a physician-entity owned by one or more physicians may contract with an MSO for administrative, management, and support services. An MSO is usually a direct subsidiary of a hospital, which typically owns 100% of the MSO. MSOs may also be owned by investors. *See also* group practice without walls; integrated provider; physician-hospital organization.

Management, Society for Advancement of *See* Society for Advancement of Management.

Management Society, Health Care Material *See* Health Care Material Management Society.

Management, Society for Human Resource *See* Society for Human Resource Management.

Management, Society for Information *See* Society for Information Management.

Management Society, National Safety *See* National Safety Management Society.

management style The leadership style a manager uses in administering an organization or its components. Four basic leadership styles are exploitative-authoritative, benevolent-authoritative, consultative-democratic, and participative-democratic. *See also* management.

management system, database *See* database management system.

Management Systems Society, Healthcare Information *See* Healthcare Information Management Systems Society.

management, total quality *See* total quality management.

management, utilities *See* utilities management.

management, utilization *See* utilization management.

manager An individual responsible for directing the activities of an organization or one of its component thereof.

manager, business office *See* business office manager.

manager, clinic *See* clinic manager.

manager, laundry *See* laundry manager.

manager, materials *See* materials manager.

manager, matrix *See* matrix manager.

manager, middle *See* middle manager.

manager, nurse *See* nurse manager.

manager, office *See* office manager.

manager, patient account *See* patient account manager.

manager, risk *See* risk manager.

Managers Association, Dietary *See* Dietary Managers Association.

Managers, National Association of Private Geriatric Care *See* National Association of Private Geriatric Care Managers.

Managers, National Network for Social Work *See* National Network for Social Work Managers.

manager, unit *See* unit manager.

mandate A directive to do something, as in measurement mandate or mandated employer insurance.

mandated employer insurance Health insurance for employees that employers are required by law to purchase. *See also* employer; health insurance.

mandatory Required by authority, as in mandatory licensure. *See also* mandatory licensure.

mandatory copy Copy that by law must be included in the advertising and/or on the labels of some products, such as alcoholic beverages, cigarettes, and some food and drug items. *See also* labeling.

mandatory licensure The legal requirement by a state or other jurisdiction that professional practitioners, such as physicians, dentists, nurses, and lawyers, must be licensed. *See also* licensure.

mandible The bone of the lower jaw. *See also* maxilla.

maneuver **1.** Any dexterous procedure or technique, as in the Heimlich maneuver. *See also* Heimlich maneuver. **2.** Artful handling of matters, marked by manipulation to gain a desired end, as in he had no room left in which to maneuver. *See also* finesse.

maneuver, Heimlich *See* Heimlich maneuver.

mania **1.** An excessively intense enthusiasm, interest, or preoccupation, as in mania for muesli. *See also* infomania. **2.** In psychiatry, mania is a mood disorder characterized by profuse and rapidly changing ideas (flight of ideas), rapid speech, exaggerated gaiety, and excessive physical activity. As in other psychoses, a manic patient has little or no insight into his or her condition. *See also* euphoria; hypomania; manic-depressive illness; nymphomania; pharmacomania; potomania; psychosis.

mania, hypo- *See* hypomania.

mania, info- *See* infomania.

mania, nympho- *See* nymphomania.

mania, pharmaco- *See* pharmacomania.

mania, poto- *See* potomania.

manic-depressive **1.** A person whose mental state periodically swings from mania to depression. **2.** Pertaining to a mental state that periodically swings from mania to depression. *See also* manic-depressive illness.

manic-depressive illness In psychiatry, a major affective disorder marked by alternating episodes of mania and depression. *Synonyms:* bipolar disorder; bipolar illness; manic-depressive disorder; manic-depressive psychosis. *See also* depression; major affective disorder; mania.

manic-depressive psychosis   *See* manic-depressive illness.

manifest   To show clearly to the sight or understanding, as in manifesting signs of AIDS.

manipulate   **1.** To manage, influence, or control by shrewdness, sometimes deviously. **2.** To operate, work, or treat with the hands. *See* also osteopathic medicine.

manipulative medicine   The use of mechanical forces applied through the hands to diagnose and treat functional disorders of the musculoskeletal system. *See also* North American Academy of Musculoskeletal Medicine; osteopathic medicine.

manipulative treatment, osteopathic   *See* osteopathic manipulative treatment.

manner   A way of doing something, as in the manner in which a procedure is performed. *See also* method.

manpower   *See* human resources.

manpower, health   *See* health personnel.

manual arts therapist   An individual who specializes in manual arts therapy. *See also* manual arts therapy.

manual arts therapy   The use of work-related skills, such as metalworking or graphic arts, to rehabilitate and restore patients' physical and emotional health. *See also* art therapy; dance therapy; drama therapy; music therapy; poetry therapy; recreational therapy.

manual, policies and procedures   *See* policies and procedures manual.

manual, procedure-coding   *See* procedure-coding manual.

manuals, accreditation   *See* standards manuals.

manual skill   The ability to use one's hands efficiently and with great dexterity in the performance of a task or operation; for example, a surgeon should have a great deal of manual skill.

manuals, standards   *See* standards manuals.

Manufacturers of America, Dental   *See* Dental Manufacturers of America.

Manufacturers Association, Contact Lens   *See* Contact Lens Manufacturers Association.

Manufacturers Association, Health Industry   *See* Health Industry Manufacturers Association.

Manufacturers' Association, Laser and Electro-Optics   *See* Laser and Electro-Optics Manufacturers' Association.

Manufacturers, Association of Microbiological

Diagnostic   *See* Association of Microbiological Diagnostic Manufacturers.

Manufacturers Association, Nonprescription Drug   *See* Nonprescription Drug Manufacturers Association.

Manufacturers Association, Orthopedic Surgical   *See* Orthopedic Surgical Manufacturers Association.

Manufacturers Association, Pharmaceutical   *See* Pharmaceutical Manufacturers Association.

Manufacturers, Automatic Identification   *See* Automatic Identification Manufacturers.

Manufacturers, National Association of Pharmaceutical   *See* National Association of Pharmaceutical Manufacturers.

manufacturing, computer-aided   *See* computer-aided manufacturing.

Manufacturing Opticians, National Association of   *See* National Association of Manufacturing Opticians.

MAODP   *See* Medic Alert Organ Donor Program.

margin   *See* markup.

marginal benefit   In health economics, the additional benefit of consuming one extra unit of a good or service. *See also* benefit.

marginal cost   In health economics, the additional cost of producing one extra unit of a good or service. This cost varies with the volume of the operation. A hospital, for example, has a high cost for its first percutaneous transluminal coronary angioplasty procedure or its first meal served. Subsequent angioplasties and meals have lower costs each (marginal costs) until the volume becomes so large as to require improvements in facilities and increases in personnel. At this point, the marginal costs rise until a new output level is reached. *Synonyms*: differential cost; incremental cost. *See also* cost.

marginal return, diminishing   *See* diminishing marginal return.

marginal tax rate   A tax rate on an additional dollar of income. Due to the progressive rate structure of income taxes, an additional dollar of income could be taxed at a higher rate than all previous income. *See also* medical deduction; tax.

marginal utility   The additional usefulness or satisfaction a consumer receives from the consumption of one more unit of a good or service. *See also* utility.

marihuana   *See* cannabis.

marijuana   *See* cannabis.

marital counseling   Therapy used to assist married couples to realize the potential of their married lives and to resolve problems impairing their marital relationship. *See also* counseling services.

Marital and Date Rape, National Clearinghouse on *See* National Clearinghouse on Marital and Date Rape.

markdown A reduction in the original retail price of an item or a service, which was determined by adding a percentage factor, called a markup, to the cost of the merchandise or service. The term markdown does not apply unless the price is dropped below the original selling price. *See also* markup.

market 1. The geographical area in which an organization, product, or service can be or is being sold. 2. In health care, to publicize a health care organization and its services with the intention of increasing their use. *See also* buyer's market; overkill; saturation; seller's market.

marketable Easily sold, as in a hospital's executive fitness program is a highly marketable service. *See also* market.

market analysis The process of determining the characteristics of a market and the measurement of its capacity to contribute to or buy a service or product. *See also* analysis; marketing research.

market, buyer's *See* buyer's market.

market division An arrangement whereby competitors divide territories or customers among themselves. *See also* market.

marketing The processes associated with promoting goods or services for sale. The classic components of marketing are product, price, place, and promotion, that is, the selection and development of a *product*, determination of its *price*, selection and design of distribution channels (*place*), and all aspects of generating or enhancing demand for the product, including advertising (*promotion*). *See also* niche; overkill; performance; positioning.

Marketing, Academy for Health Services *See* Academy for Health Services Marketing.

Marketing of the American Hospital Association, Society for Healthcare Planning and *See* Society for Healthcare Planning and Marketing of the American Hospital Association.

Marketing Associates, Chain Drug *See* Chain Drug Marketing Associates.

Marketing Association, Biomedical *See* Biomedical Marketing Association.

marketing concept An idea or strategy for marketing a product or service, as in the philosophy of marketing a product or service that is benefit oriented

rather than product oriented. For instance, a successful marketing concept in the health care industry is that the industry is in the business of selling health, longevity, or youth, that is, the benefits to be derived from its services (surgical operations, medications), but not the services themselves. *See also* concept; marketing.

marketing, hospital *See* hospital marketing.

marketing plan A plan that details an organization's marketing effort. *Synonym:* marketing strategy. *See also* marketing; plan.

Marketing and Public Relations, American Society for Health Care *See* American Society for Health Care Marketing and Public Relations.

marketing research The gathering and evaluation of data regarding consumers' preferences for products and services and the moving of goods and services from the producer to the consumer. Marketing research typically covers three broad areas: market analysis, which yields information about the marketplace; product research, which yields information about the characteristics and desires for the product; and consumer research, which yields information about the needs and motivations of the consumer. *See also* market analysis; marketing; research.

market penetration 1. A marketing strategy used by an organization to increase the sales of a good or service within an existing market through the employment of more aggressive marketing tactics, such as hospitals that run frequent radio and television commercials on several channels over many months. *See also* market. 2. The degree to which a particular product or service is purchased in a particular market. *See also* penetration.

market power The ability to profitably maintain prices above competitive levels or restrain output, for a significant period. *See also* market; power.

market price A recent price agreed upon by buyers and sellers of a product or service, as determined by supply and demand. *See also* market; price.

market research *See* marketing research.

market share The percentage of total sales in the relevant market attributable to an individual business entity. *See also* market.

market, seller's *See* seller's market.

market, soft *See* buyer's market.

Markey Charitable Trust, Lucille P. *See* Lucille P. Markey Charitable Trust.

markup 1. Determination of a retail selling price,

based on some percentage increase in the wholesale cost. For example, a 30% markup on an item wholesaling at $100 would be $30, resulting in a retail selling price of $130. *Synonym*: margin. *Compare* markdown. **2.** A process of a congressional committee in which the committee writes law, develops policy, and makes decisions about the final language of a bill the committee will recommend to the full Congress. Markup usually takes place after public hearings on a subject. *See also* executive session.

marriage and family counseling, individual *See* individual marriage and family counseling.

Marriage and Family Therapy, American Association for *See* American Association for Marriage and Family Therapy.

marrow, bone *See* bone marrow.

Marrow Donor Program, National *See* National Marrow Donor Program.

marrow transplant, bone *See* bone marrow transplant.

mask In medicine, a covering of the face either for the purpose of preventing the exchange of airborne microorganisms between the wearer's upper respiratory tract and the surrounding air or to allow the administration of inhalational anesthetics or other gaseous mixtures. *See also* isolation.

masked *See* blinded.

masochism **1.** The act or an instance of deriving sexual gratification from being physically or emotionally abused. **2.** The tendency to seek to be offended, dominated, or mistreated. *See also* sadism; sadomasochism.

massage **1.** A form of physical therapy consisting of the rubbing, kneading, thumping, pressing, or pummeling of parts of the body to aid circulation or relax the muscles. *See also* hand massage; physical therapy; spa; vibromassage. **2.** The manipulation of figures or data, usually so as to give them a more acceptable or desirable appearance, as in the data were massaged by putting them in different places in the accounts.

massage, hand *See* hand massage.

Massage Professionals, Associated Bodywork and *See* Associated Bodywork and Massage Professionals.

Massage Therapy Association, American *See* American Massage Therapy Association.

massage, vibro- *See* vibromassage.

mass communication Informing the general public through use of widely circulating media, such as newspapers, magazines, television, and radio. *See also* communication.

mass inspection, cease dependency on *See* cease dependency on mass inspection.

mass media Radio and television broadcast stations and networks, newspapers, magazines, and outdoor advertisements designed to appeal to the general public. *See also* media; multimedia; press.

mass production Processing or manufacturing of uniform products in large quantities using interchangeable parts and machinery, as in the mass production of personal computers.

MAST Acronym for medical antishock trousers or military antishock trousers. An inflatable garment used to combat shock, stabilize fractures, stop bleeding, increase peripheral vascular resistance, and permit autotransfusion of small amounts of blood. *Synonym*: pneumatic antishock garment. *See also* autotransfusion; hemostasis.

mastectomy Surgical removal of the breast. *See also* lumpectomy; mammary gland; modified radical mastectomy; quadrantectomy.

mastectomy, modified radical *See* modified radical mastectomy.

Master of Business Administration (MBA) The title for a person holding a master's degree in business who has generally spent two years learning the body of knowledge in business and a specialty, such as accounting, business analysis, finance, management, marketing, or real estate. *See also* Doctor of Business Administration; master's degree.

Master of Divinity (MDiv) The title for a person holding a master's degree in divinity. *See also* chaplain; master's degree.

Master Facility Inventory of Hospitals and Institutions (MFI) A computerized data file, maintained by the National Center for Health Statistics, of approximately 33,000 inpatient health care facilities in the United States, including short term and long term care hospitals, nursing and related care homes, and custodial and remedial care facilities. The data are collected by the American Hospital Association's Annual Survey of Hospitals and the National Center for Health Statistics biennial mail survey of facilities other than hospitals. The data include location, ownership, major types of services, beds, patient census, admissions, discharges, deaths, staffing, and many other characteristics. *See also* American Hospital

Association; National Center for Health Statistics.

Master of Health Administration (MHA) The title for a person holding a master's degree in health administration. *See also* administrator; health care administration; master's degree.

Master of Health Services Administration (MHSA) The title for a person holding a master's degree in health services administration. *See also* administration; health services; master's degree.

Master of Hospital Administration (MHA) The title for a person holding a master's degree in hospital administration. *See also* administrator; hospital; master's degree.

Master of Pharmacy (PharM) The title for a person holding a master's degree in pharmacy. *See also* master's degree; pharmacy.

Master of Public Administration (MPA) The title for a person holding a master's degree in public administration. *See also* master's degree; public administration.

Master of Public Health (MPH) The title for a person holding a master's degree in public health. *See also* master's degree; public health.

Master of Science in Nursing (MSN) The title for an individual holding a master's degree in nursing. *See also* advanced practice nurse; master's degree; registered nurse.

master's degree An academic degree conferred by a college or university upon those who complete at least one year of prescribed study beyond the bachelor's degree, as in a Master of Social Work. *See also* bachelor's degree; degree; doctorate; university.

master and servant An employer-employee relationship that develops from an express or implied employment contract between a master, or employer, and a servant, or employee. The servant is expected to perform services, usually for a salary, and is under the master's control. Servant means, in its broadest sense, a person of any rank or position who is subject to the control of another. An independent contractor, by contrast, is not under an employer's direct control, but serves an employer only as to the results of his or her work and not as to the method by which the work is done. Under the master and servant relationship, the master will be liable for the actions of his or her servant committed while the servant was acting within the scope of his or her employment. *Compare* independent contractor. *See also* borrowed servant; captain of the ship doctrine;

respondeat superior.

Master of Social Work (MSW) The title for an individual holding a master's degree in social work. *See also* master's degree; social worker.

mastitis Inflammation of the mammary gland. *See also* mammary gland.

masturbation The production of orgasm by genital stimulation by means other than sexual intercourse. *See also* onanism; sexual intercourse.

matching 1. Comparing and selecting objects having similar or identical characteristics, as in the selection of compatible donors and recipients for blood transfusion or transplantation. *See also* crossmatching. 2. The deliberate process of making a study group and a comparison group comparable in factors that are extraneous to the purpose of the investigation but that might interfere with the interpretation of the study's findings (for example, in case-control studies, individual cases might be matched or paired with a specific control on the basis of comparable age, gender, clinical features, or a combination). *See also* clinical trial. 3. A process by which most medical students obtain an appointment for the PGY-1 (postgraduate year 1). It usually takes place through the National Resident Matching Program. *See also* National Resident Matching Program; PGY-1.

matching, cross- *See* crossmatching.

matching grant A grant made under the condition that additional funds be raised from other sources. *See also* grant.

materialism The theory or doctrine that comfort, pleasure, and worldly possessions constitute the greatest good and highest value in life. *See also* hedonism.

Material Management Society, Health Care *See* Health Care Material Management Society.

material, raw *See* raw material.

Materials Advisory Council, Hazardous *See* Hazardous Materials Advisory Council.

Materials, American Society for Testing and *See* ASTM.

Materials Control Resources Institute, Hazardous *See* Hazardous Materials Control Resources Institute.

materials, hazardous *See* hazardous materials.

Materials Management, American Society for Hospital *See* American Society for Hospital Materials Management.

materials management department A unit of a health care organization that acquires and disposes of supplies of materials, furniture, and equipment, and, in many hospitals, has responsibility for central services, laundry, and printing services. Materials management departments have become one of the common services included in joint-venture and cooperative networks serving a group of hospitals. Materials management is also structured as a central service support division in a health care corporation that includes many hospitals and other types of health care organizations. The centralization of purchasing for multiple hospitals produces savings through volume discounts and reduced shipment costs. *Synonym*: purchasing and stores. *See also* materials management department.

materials manager In health care organizations, an individual who has overall responsibility for the procurement, storage, distribution, and disposal of hospital supplies and equipment. *See also* manager; materials science.

Materials Research, Center for Hazardous *See* Center for Hazardous Materials Research.

materials science The study of the characteristics and uses of the various materials, such as metals, ceramics, and plastics, used in science and technology. *See also* science.

Materials, Society for Bio- *See* Society for Biomaterials.

materia medica **1.** The substances used in medicine, that is, drugs. **2.** The branch of science that deals with the properties and application of drugs. *See also* pharmacology.

maternal Relating to a mother or motherhood, as in maternal instinct or maternal-fetal medicine.

Maternal and Child Health, Association of Teachers of *See* Association of Teachers of Maternal and Child Health.

Maternal and Child Health Clearinghouse, National *See* National Maternal and Child Health Clearinghouse.

Maternal and Child Health, National Center for Education in *See* National Center for Education in Maternal and Child Health.

maternal and child health programs *See* maternal and child health services.

Maternal and Child Health Programs, Association of *See* Association of Maternal and Child Health Programs.

maternal and child health (MCH) services Organized health and social services for pregnant women, mothers, their children, and (rarely) fathers. Mothers and children are often considered vulnerable populations with special health needs, who will be benefited by preventive medicine and being accorded a high public priority. *See also* preventive medicine.

maternal death Death of a pregnant woman or of a woman within a specified postdelivery period, as in maternal death secondary to postdelivery infection or blood loss. The World Health Organization defines maternal death as the death of a woman while pregnant or within 42 days of termination of pregnancy, regardless of the duration of the pregnancy, from any cause related to or aggravated by the pregnancy or its management but not from accidental or incidental causes. Maternal deaths may be divided into direct obstetrical deaths, deaths resulting from preexisting disease, or conditions not due to direct obstetric causes. *Synonym*: maternal mortality. *See also* abruptio placenta; death; maternal mortality rate.

maternal deprivation The deprivation of an infant or child of the stimulation, held to be important to mental and emotional development, normally provided by mother-child interaction.

maternal-fetal medicine A subspecialty of obstetrics and gynecology involving management of patients with complications of pregnancy. *See also* maternal-fetal medicine specialist.

maternal-fetal medicine specialist An obstetrician-gynecologist who subspecializes in maternal-fetal medicine. *See also* maternal-fetal medicine; obstetrics and gynecology.

maternal mortality *See* maternal death.

maternal mortality rate A rate measuring maternal death from causes associated with childbirth. Deaths used in the numerator are those arising during pregnancy or from puerperal causes (that is deaths occurring during and/or due to deliveries, or due to complications of pregnancy, childbirth, and the puerperium). The denominator is the number of live births that occurred among the population of a given geographic area during the same year. *Synonym*: maternal death rate. *See also* maternal death; mortality rate.

maternity Pertaining to the state of being a mother, as in maternity ward or maternity benefits. *Compare* paternity.

maternity benefits Insurance coverage for the

costs of pregnancy, labor and delivery, postpartum care, complications of pregnancy, and in some plans, family planning. *See also* benefits; maternity.

Maternity Center Association (MCA) A national organization founded in 1918 composed of 600 physicians, nurses, nurse-midwives, public health workers, and laypersons interested in improvement of maternity care, maternal and infant health, and family life. It maintains two Childbearing Centers for low-risk families, sponsors research, and cosponsors the community-based Nurse-Midwifery Education Program. *See also* childbearing; childbearing center; maternity; nurse-midwife.

maternity leave The leave of absence from work granted to a mother to care for her infant. *See also* paternity leave.

maternity ward A unit of a hospital that provides care for women during pregnancy and childbirth as well as for newborn infants. *See also* maternity; ward.

Mathematical Statistics, Institute of *See* Institute of Mathematical Statistics.

Mathers Charitable Foundation, G. Harold and Leila Y. *See* G. Harold and Leila Y. Mathers Charitable Foundation.

matriarchy A social system in which the mother is head of the family and descent is traced through the mother's side of the family. *Compare* patriarchy.

matricide The act of killing one's mother. *Compare* patricide. *See also* murder.

matrimonial court A trial court responsible for hearing divorce proceedings. *See also* court; matrimony; trial court.

matrimony The act or state of being married. *See also* matrimonial court.

matrix **1.** A situation within which something else originates, develops, or is contained, as in an organizational matrix. **2.** Pertaining to a situation within which something else originates, develops, or is contained, as in a matrix organization. **3.** In mathematics, the regular formation of elements into columns and rows. **4.** In computer science, the network of intersections between input and output leads in a computer, functioning as an encoder or a decoder.

matrix manager A manager who shares with another manager formal authority over a subordinate. *See also* manager; matrix; matrix organization.

matrix organization An organization that uses a multiple command system whereby an employee

may be accountable to a particular manager for overall performance as well as to one or more leaders of particular projects. *See also* matrix; organization.

matrix flowchart A flow chart that places the activities in the diagram under columns representing the individual organization units performing the work. *Synonym:* matrix flow diagram. *See also* flowchart; matrix.

matrix flow diagram *See* matrix flowchart.

maturation The stage or process of becoming mature or fully developed, as in attainment of emotional and intellectual maturity. *See also* mature economy; mature minor.

mature economy An economy of a nation whose population has stabilized or is declining, and whose economic growth is no longer robust. A mature economy is typically characterized by a decrease in spending on roads or factories and a relative increase in consumer spending. *See also* economy.

mature minor A minor who is judged by a health care provider to have the capacity to make decisions and is allowed to authorize or consent to medical treatment. *See also* age of majority; emancipated minor; minor.

maturity-onset diabetes *See* type II diabetes mellitus.

mausoleum A grand or stately tomb. *See also* sepulchre.

max To perform to maximum ability or capacity, as in maxed out.

maxilla The bone of the upper jaw, which also forms part of the eye socket, the palate, and the nose. *See also* mandible.

maxillofacial In anatomy, relating to or involving the maxilla and the face, as in maxillofacial trauma. *See also* maxilla.

Maxillofacial Prosthetics, American Academy of *See* American Academy of Maxillofacial Prosthetics.

Maxillofacial Radiology, American Academy of Oral and *See* American Academy of Oral and Maxillofacial Radiology.

Maxillofacial Surgeons, American Association of Oral and *See* American Association of Oral and Maxillofacial Surgeons.

Maxillofacial Surgeons, American College of Oral and *See* American College of Oral and Maxillofacial Surgeons.

Maxillofacial Surgeons, American Society of *See* American Society of Maxillofacial Surgeons.

maxillofacial surgery *See* oral and maxillofacial surgery.

Maxillofacial Surgery, American Board of Oral and *See* American Board of Oral and Maxillofacial Surgery.

maxim A succinct formulation of a fundamental principle, general truth, or rule of conduct.

maximum The greatest possible quantity or degree; the upper limit of variation, as is maximum temperature. *Compare* minimum.

maximum charge *See* fee maximum.

maximum, fee *See* fee maximum.

maximum security unit A unit in a penal or mental health facility that provides a fully secured environment for residents considered dangerous to other persons in the facility's population. *See also* unit.

may A term used in standards and scoring guidelines of the Joint Commission on Accreditation of Healthcare Organizations describing an acceptable method of standards compliance but not one that is necessarily preferred or required. *See also* Joint Commission on Accreditation of Healthcare Organizations; scoring guideline; standard.

MB *See* megabyte.

MBA *See* Master of Business Administration.

McCarran-Ferguson Act An act of Congress (1945) stating that federal laws regulating or affecting business and commerce are not applicable to the insurance business except by specific legislative action. The Act leaves regulation of insurance to individual states, unless it is specifically undertaken in federal law. *See also* insurance.

MCA *See* Maternity Center Association.

MCAT *See* Medical College Admission Test.

McBurney's point The usual point of maximum abdominal tenderness in acute appendicitis, situated between 35 and 50 millimeters from the right anterior superior iliac spine on a line between the spine and the umbilicus. *See also* appendicitis.

MCF *See* Medical Cybernetics Foundation.

MCH *See* maternal and child health services.

MCPI *See* medical consumer price index.

MD *See* Doctor of Medicine.

MDA *See* Mission Doctors Association.

MDC *See* major diagnostic category.

MDHBA *See* Medical-Dental-Hospital Bureaus of America.

MDiv *See* Master of Divinity.

ME *See* medical examiner.

Meal Programs, National Association of *See* National Association of Meal Programs.

meals on wheels A system for providing and transporting meals to the elderly and disabled at home through local authority or voluntary agencies. *See also* aged person; disabled; food; nutrition.

mean A measure of central tendency of a collection of data specifying the arithmetic average. A mean consists of the sum of all the measurements of the data set divided by the total number of measurements in the data set. The mean is best used when the distribution of data is balanced and unimodal. In a normal distribution, the mean coincides with the median and mode. *Synonym:* average. *Compare* median; mode. *See also* center line; distribution; geometric mean; measures of central tendency; regression to the mean.

mean, arithmetic *See* mean.

mean, geometric *See* geometric mean.

meaning The sense or significance of something that is conveyed, especially by language.

meaningful Having meaning, function, or purpose, as in meaningful data to improve a hospital's performance. Meaningful does not say whether the meaning is good or bad, positive or negative. *See also* significant.

meaningless Lacking meaning or significance, as in a huge quantity of meaningless data.

mean, regression to the *See* regression to the mean.

means Money, property, or other wealth, as in living within one's means. *See also* means testing.

means testing An investigation into the financial well-being of a person to determine the person's eligibility for financial assistance, as for government programs, such as Medicaid. Income tests are means tests based on income. Assets tests are means test based on personal assets. *See also* means; testing.

measles An acute infectious viral disease conferring lifelong immunity to further attacks, characterized by rash, high temperature, headache, photophobia, inflammation of the respiratory tract, and conjunctivitis. The rash usually begins inside the mouth, manifested as small white spots (Koplik's spots). Complications are usually due to secondary bacterial infection (for example, pneumonia, middle ear infection). *See also* infectious diseases; inflammation; virus.

measles, German *See* rubella.

measurable Possible to be quantified, as in measurable temperature or measurable performance. *See* *also* measure; mensurable.

measure **1.** A quantitative tool or instrument used to make measurements, as in an indicator is one kind of measure. **2.** A unit, such as an inch, specified by a measurement scale. **3.** The act or process of measuring. *See also* benchmark; measurement; performance measure; scale; standard.

measure of association A quantity that expresses the strength of association between variables. Commonly used measures of association are differences between means, proportions, or rates; the rate ratio; the odds ratio; and correlation and regression coefficients. *See also* association; correlation coefficient; mean; proportion; rate; variable.

measure of damages The extent of loss or injury for which the law allows recovery. *See also* damages.

measure, input *See* input measure.

measurement **1.** The process of quantification, that is, determining that attribute of a person, an activity, or a thing (for example, an object, an event, or a phenomenon) by which it is greater or less than some other person, activity, or thing. *See also* accuracy of a measurement; biometrics; calibration; econometrics; metrology; performance measurement; precision. **2.** The number resulting from a quantification process. *See also* mensuration. **3.** Pertaining to the process of measurement, as in measurement data or measurement error. *See also* measurement data; measurement error.

measurement, accuracy of a *See* accuracy of a measurement.

measurement data Data resulting from quantifying attributes or characteristics, as in measurement data forming an important basis for performance assessment and improvement activities. *See also* data; measurement.

measurement error Variation in measurements due to causes, such as sampling error or random error, other than real differences in the attribute being measured. *See also* error; random error; sampling error; systematic error.

measurement instrument *See* instrument.

measurement, performance *See* performance measurement.

Measurements Association, Precision *See* Precision Measurements Association.

measurement scale *See* scale.

Measurements, Conference on Precision Electromagnetic *See* Conference on Precision Electromagnetic Measurements.

Measurements, National Council on Radiation Protection and *See* National Council on Radiation Protection and Measurements.

measurement system, indicator *See* indicator measurement system.

measurement tool *See* tool.

measure, outcome *See* outcome measure.

measure, performance *See* performance measure.

measure, process *See* process measure.

measure, quality *See* quality measure.

measure of quality, structural *See* structural measure of quality.

measures of central tendency Several characteristics of the distribution of a set of measurements around a value or values at or near the middle of the set. The principal measures of central tendency are the mean, median, and mode. *See also* mean; median; mode.

measure, unit of *See* unit of measure.

mechanical airway Control and maintenance of a patient's airway by endotracheal intubation or cricothyrotomy (incision through the skin and cricothyroid membrane of the throat area to open an airway). *See also* airway; artificial respiration; endotracheal intubation.

mechanical ventilation Breathing accomplished by extrinsic means, as with a ventilator for a patient who is intubated. *See also* adult respiratory distress syndrome; artificial respiration; ventilation; ventilator.

mechanism **1.** The system or manner of parts or processes working together to serve a common function, as in gatekeeper mechanism. *See also* gatekeeper mechanism. **2.** The working parts, or the arrangement of parts, of a machine. *See also* machine.

mechanism, gatekeeper *See* gatekeeper mechanism.

mechanization Performance of tasks with machines or mechanical equipment. Mechanization does not provide for self-correcting feedback, whereas automation does. *See also* automation.

mechatronics A technology originally from Japan that combines mechanical engineering with electronics, mainly to increase automation in manufacturing industries. *See also* automation; electronic; mechanization.

meconium The green fecal material composed of secretions from intestinal glands and amniotic fluid passed by a newborn infant. *See also* feces; neonate.

medcolator A machine typically used by podiatrists

to produce direct low-voltage current for the treatment of foot and other disorders. *See also* podiatrist.

medevac Abbreviation for medical evacuation; Air transport of persons to a place where they can receive medical care, as in medevac from the island to the mainland for medical care. *See also* ambulance.

media Channels of communication that serve many diverse purposes, such as offering entertainment with either mass or specialized appeal, communicating news and information, or displaying advertising messages. *See also* journalism; mass media; media relations; multimedia; press; press kit; press release.

Media Education, Health *See* Health Media Education.

medial Situated toward the midline of the body or the central part of an organ or tissue, as in the nose is medial to the cheeks. *Compare* bilateral; lateral; unilateral.

media, mass *See* mass media.

media, multi- *See* multimedia.

median A measure of central tendency of a collection of data, consisting of the middle number of a data set when the measurements are arranged sequentially from smallest to largest or from largest to smallest. It is the most valid measure of central tendency whenever a distribution is skewed. *Compare* mean; mode. *See also* average; distribution; measures of central tendency.

Media Psychology, Association for *See* Association for Media Psychology.

media relations Organizational interactions with the print and electronic media. Positive, ongoing relationships with the media increase the probability that timely and accurate coverage of an organization's activities will result. Medical relations is typically a subfunction of public information or public relations. *See also* press; press release; public relations.

mediation In law, an attempt to bring about a peaceful settlement or compromise between disputants through the objective intervention of a neutral party who is trained in dispute resolution. *Synonym:* conciliation. *See also* arbitration; negotiation.

Mediation, Child Abuse Listening and *See* Child Abuse Listening and Mediation.

mediator An individual who acts as a neutral third party in order to help resolve disputes. *See also* conciliator; mediation.

medic **1.** A member of a military medical corps.

2. A physician or surgeon.

Medicaid The medical assistance program originating in 1965 that is jointly funded by the states and the federal government. It reimburses hospitals and physicians for providing care to needy and low-income people who cannot finance their own medical expenses. Medicaid eligibility includes a means test. It is the main source of public assistance for nursing home costs. *See also* Health Care Financing Administration; means testing; required services.

Medicaid Directors Association, State *See* State Medicaid Directors Association.

Medicaid mill A health program that primarily serves Medicaid beneficiaries, typically on an ambulatory basis. The mills, originating in the ghettos of New York City, are still found primarily in urban slums with few other medical services. They are usually organized on a for-profit basis, characterized by their great productivity, and frequently accused of a variety of abuses. *See also* Medicaid; family ganging; ping-ponging.

Medicaid (Title XIX) *See* Medicaid.

medical Relating to the study or practice of medicine. *See also* medicine.

Medi-Cal California's Medicaid program. *See* Medicaid.

Medical Accreditation, American Federation of *See* American Federation of Medical Accreditation.

medical administrator A physician administrator. *See also* administrator.

Medical Administrators, American Academy of *See* American Academy of Medical Administrators.

medical adviser A physician who provides advice to health care-related entities ranging from health insurance plans to business corporations to government agencies. *See also* adviser.

Medical Affairs, Council for *See* Council for Medical Affairs.

Medical Affairs, Forum for *See* Forum for Medical Affairs.

Medical Airlift, Mercy *See* Mercy Medical Airlift.

Medical Anthropology, Society for *See* Society for Medical Anthropology.

medical antishock trousers (MAST) *See* MAST.

medical artist *See* medical illustrator.

Medical Assistance for Aged *See* Kerr-Mills.

medical assistant An allied health professional who assists physicians in their offices or other medical settings and who performs a broad range of administrative and clinical duties including, but not limited to: scheduling and receiving patients, preparing and maintaining medical records, performing basic secretarial skills and medical transcription, handling telephone calls and writing correspondence, serving as a liaison between the physician and other individuals, managing practice finances, asepsis and infection control, taking patient histories and vital signs, performing first aid and cardiopulmonary resuscitation, preparing patients for procedures, assisting the physician with examinations and treatments, collecting and processing specimens, performing selected diagnostic tests, and preparing and administering medications as directed by the physician. More medical assistants are employed by practicing physicians than any other type of allied health personnel. Medical assistants are one type of allied health professional for which the Committee on Allied Health Education and Accreditation has accredited education programs. *See also* allied health professional; certified medical assistant.

medical assistant, certified   *See* certified medical assistant.

Medical Assistants, American Association of   *See* American Association of Medical Assistants.

Medical Assistants of American Medical Technologists, Registered   *See* Registered Medical Assistants of American Medical Technologists.

Medical Assistants, American Registry of   *See* American Registry of Medical Assistants.

Medical Assistants, American Society of Podiatric   *See* American Society of Podiatric Medical Assistants.

medical association   A national, state, regional, or local voluntary membership organization for the advancement and control of a medical profession, as in the American Medical Association. *See also* medical society.

Medical Association, Aerospace   *See* Aerospace Medical Association.

Medical Association, Alternative   *See* Alternative Medical Association.

Medical Association of America, Korean   *See* Korean Medical Association of America.

Medical Association, American   *See* American Medical Association.

Medical Association, American Holistic   *See* American Holistic Medical Association.

Medical Association, American Podiatric   *See* American Podiatric Medical Association.

Medical Association, Civil Aviation   *See* Civil Aviation Medical Association.

Medical Association, Islamic   *See* Islamic Medical Association.

Medical Association, National   *See* National Medical Association.

Medical Association, National Podiatric   *See* National Podiatric Medical Association.

Medical Association of North America, Bangladesh   *See* Bangladesh Medical Association of North America.

Medical Association of North America, Interstate Postgraduate   *See* Interstate Postgraduate Medical Association of North America.

Medical Association of North America, Ukrainian   *See* Ukrainian Medical Association of North America.

Medical Association, Pan American   *See* Pan American Medical Association.

Medical Athletic Association, American   *See* American Medical Athletic Association.

medical audit   A detailed retrospective review and evaluation of patient records along specified dimensions of care (for example, appropriateness of a procedure) usually conducted by physicians and other medical staff members. Medical audits are used in many health care settings, such as hospitals, for measuring and assessing professional and organizational performance by comparing it with accepted standards or current professional judgment. Information obtained through the medical audit process is intended for use in performance improvement activities, such as education. *See also* audit; dental audit; nursing audit; patient care audit; retrospective review.

medical bacteriology   The branch of bacteriology that deals chiefly with bacteria causing human disease. *See also* bacteriology.

medical, bio-   *See* biomedical.

medical boards   *See* medical specialty boards; state medical boards.

medical boards' disciplinary actions, state   *See* state medical boards' disciplinary actions.

Medical Boards, Federation of Podiatric   *See* Federation of Podiatric Medical Boards.

medical boards, state   *See* state medical boards.

Medical Boards of the United States, Federation of State   *See* Federation of State Medical Boards of the United States.

medical care   The provision of health services by a physician. *See also* health care; medical services.

Medical Care Program, Kaiser-Permanente   *See* Kaiser-Permanente Medical Care Program.

medical care, technical aspects of   *See* technical aspects of medical care.

medical center   A place where medical services are provided, ranging from an academic medical center encompassing several hospitals to the office of a single physician. There is no licensure requirement before the phrase may be used. *See also* academic medical center.

medical center, academic   *See* academic medical center.

medical college   *See* medical school.

Medical College Admission Test (MCAT)   A nationally standardized test, developed by the Association of American Medical Colleges and administered by the American College Testing, which nearly all US medical schools require or strongly recommend for individuals seeking admission to medical school. *See also* American College Testing; Association of American Medical Colleges; medical school; standardized test.

Medical Colleges, Association of American   *See* Association of American Medical Colleges.

Medical Communications Associations, Council for Bio-   *See* Council for Biomedical Communications Associations.

medical computer science   The branch of computer science that deals with medical applications. *See also* medical informatics.

Medical Computing, Special Interest Group on Bio-   *See* Special Interest Group on Biomedical Computing.

medical consultant   A physician who, at the request of another physician, provides medical advice regarding a patient. *See also* consultant; medical consultation.

Medical Consultants to the Armed Forces, Society of   *See* Society of Medical Consultants to the Armed Forces.

medical consultation   Upon request by a physician, another physician's review of a patient's history, examination of the patient, and recommendations. *See also* consultation.

medical consumer price index (MCPI)   The medical component of the consumer price index, providing specific data on hospital, dental, medical, and drug prices. *See also* consumer price index.

Medical Consumers and Health Care Information, Center for   *See* Center for Medical Consumers and Health Care Information.

medical control   An entity accountable for the medical competence of an emergency medical services (EMS) system. Medical control involves, among many responsibilities, the training of physicians, nurses, and emergency medical technicians in the prehospital phase of care and measurement, assessment, and improvement of the EMS system's performance. If medical control is located at one hospital, the hospital is called a *resource hospital*; other hospitals in the system are *associate hospitals*. *See also* emergency medical services system; emergency medical technician; emergency medical technician-paramedic; emergency nurse; emergency physician.

medical cybernetics   The field of knowledge and study dealing with the relationship between machinery and medical practices and procedures. *See also* cybernetics.

Medical Cybernetics Foundation (MCF)   A national organization founded in 1985 composed of 1,000 medical and medically affiliated professionals interested in researching, developing, and marketing new medical machinery, such as monitoring equipment and robotics systems. *See also* medical cybernetics; robotics.

medical deduction   A federal income tax deduction for expenditures on health insurance and other medical expenses in excess of 3% of a person's income. The medical deduction is the only national health insurance program in the United, with a deductible of 3% of income and coinsurance of one minus the marginal tax rate. Deductible medical expenses are broadly defined and include the services of physicians, dentists, podiatrists, chiropractors, and Christian Science practitioners, as well as equipment, drugs, supplies, and special diets prescribed by such professionals. *See also* marginal tax rate; medical expenses.

Medical and Dental Association, National   *See* National Medical and Dental Association.

Medical-Dental-Hospital Bureaus of America (MDHBA)   A national organization founded in 1938 composed of 200 business bureaus providing physicians, dentists, hospitals, and clinics with management, bookkeeping, finance, tax, and collection services. It sponsors the certified professional bureau executive (CPBE) certification program. *See also* certification.

Medical and Dental Society, Christian *See* Christian Medical and Dental Society.

Medical and Dental Society, Medical Group Missions of the Christian *See* Medical Group Missions of the Christian Medical and Dental Society.

medical detoxification The process of providing medical treatment and life support services when necessary for patients critically ill from a toxic substance in the body or from acute withdrawal symptoms related to the substance. *See also* detoxification; social detoxification; withdrawal symptoms.

medical device An instrument, apparatus, implement, machine, contrivance, implant, in vitro reagent, or other similar or related article, including any component, part, or accessory that is recognized in the official *National Formulary*, the *United States Pharmacopoeia*, or any supplement to them; intended for use in the diagnosis of disease or other conditions or in the cure, mitigation, treatment, or prevention of disease in humans or other animals; or intended to affect the structure or any function of the body of humans or other animals, which does not achieve its primary intended purposes through chemical action within or on the body of humans or other animals and is not dependent on being metabolized for achievement of any of its intended principal purposes. The Medical Devices Amendments of 1976 expanded the basic definition to include devices intended for use in the diagnosis of conditions other than disease, such as pregnancy and in vitro diagnostic products, including those previously regulated as drugs. Devices are classified by the Food and Drug Administration into 19 medical specialties. *See also* device; Food and Drug Administration; ECRI; GMP; Health Industry Distributors Association; Health Industry Manufacturers Association; Safe Medical Devices Act of 1990.

Medical Devices Act of 1990, Safe *See* Safe Medical Devices Act of 1990.

Medical Devices Amendments of 1976 *See* medical device.

medical dictation *See* dictation.

medical director 1. A physician employed by an organization, such as a hospital or an insurance company, who serves as the administrative head of the medical component of the organization. In hospitals, medical director tends to be the title for the chief of staff when that person is a salaried hospital employee. *Synonyms*: chief of clinical affairs; chief of medical services; dean for clinical affairs; director of medical affairs, vice president of medical affairs; vice president of professional services. *See also* chief of staff. **2.** A physician who directs and/or provides care in a health care facility; for example, medical director of a long term care facility. *See also* physician.

Medical Directors, American Academy of *See* American Academy of Medical Directors.

Medical Directors Association, American *See* American Medical Directors Association.

Medical Distributors Association, Independent *See* Independent Medical Distributors Association.

medical doctor (MD) *See* physician.

medical education The knowledge and skill obtained and developed during medical school (undergraduate medical education); internship, residency, and fellowship (graduate medical education); and continuing medical education activities. *See also* continuing medical education; fellowship; graduate medical education; internship; medical school; residency; undergraduate medical education.

Medical Education, Academy of Osteopathic Directors of *See* Academy of Osteopathic Directors of Medical Education.

Medical Education, Accreditation Council for Continuing *See* Accreditation Council for Continuing Medical Education.

Medical Education, Accreditation Council for Graduate *See* Accreditation Council for Graduate Medical Education.

Medical Education of the American Medical Association, Council on *See* Council on Medical Education of the American Medical Association.

Medical Education, Association for Hospital *See* Association for Hospital Medical Education.

medical education, continuing *See* continuing medical education.

Medical Education, Council on Podiatric *See* Council on Podiatric Medical Education.

medical education director An individual who coordinates an organization's medical education programs; for example, an educator who coordinates a hospital's programs of graduate and continuing medical education. *See also* director; education director; medical education.

medical education, graduate *See* graduate medical education.

Medical Education, Liaison Committee on *See* Liaison Committee on Medical Education.

Medical Education, Liaison Committee on Graduate *See* Liaison Committee on Graduate Medical Education.

Medical Education, Network for Continuing *See* Network for Continuing Medical Education.

Medical Education and Research in Substance Abuse, Association of *See* Association of Medical Education and Research in Substance Abuse.

medical education, undergraduate See undergraduate medical education.

Medical Effectiveness Research, Center for *See* Center for Medical Effectiveness Research.

Medical Electroencephalographic Association, American *See* American Medical Electroencephalographic Association.

Medical Electrologists, Society of Clinical and *See* Society of Clinical and Medical Electrologists.

medical emancipation *See* emancipated minor.

medical engineer *See* bioengineer.

medical epidemiologist A physician who specializes in the field of epidemiology (study of the cause, treatment, and prevention of disease). *See also* epidemiology; physician.

medical equipment Any nondrug item or apparatus needed for a diagnostic or therapeutic medical purpose. *See also* durable medical equipment; medical supplies.

medical equipment, durable *See* durable medical equipment.

Medical Equipment Suppliers, National Association of *See* National Association of Medical Equipment Suppliers.

Medic Alert Organ Donor Program (MAODP) A program founded in 1968 that provides medical identification emblems to be worn at all times, identifying the wearers' wishes to donate either some or all of their organs. It encourages organ donors to make all legal and medical arrangements to facilitate a donation, provides only emergency information, and does not counsel individuals or assist in locating recipients of organs or medical schools who may use the donation in a medical research program. *See also* donor; organ procurement.

medical ethics The values and guidelines that govern decisions in medicine. *See also* decision; ethics.

medical evidence Evidence found in treatises on medicine or surgery or furnished by physicians, nurses, and other health professionals testifying in a professional capacity as experts. *See also* evidence; expert witness.

medical examiner (ME) **1.** A physician authorized by a governmental unit to ascertain causes of deaths, especially those not occurring under natural circumstances. *See also* coroner. **2.** A member of a board of medical examiners; for example, a state board of medical examiners or a national board of medical examiners. *See also* National Board of Medical Examiners; state board of medical examiners.

Medical Examiners, National Association of *See* National Association of Medical Examiners.

Medical Examiners, National Board of *See* National Board of Medical Examiners.

Medical Examiners, National Board of Osteopathic Medical Examiners *See* National Board of Osteopathic Medical Examiners.

Medical Examiners, National Board of Podiatric *See* National Board of Podiatric Medical Examiners.

medical examiners, state board of *See* state board of medical examiners.

medical expenses Money relating to health care, including medications and health insurance premiums, spent by an individual that is allowed as an itemized deduction to the extent that such amounts (less insurance reimbursements) exceed a certain percentage of adjusted gross income. *See also* medical deduction.

Medical Fellowships, National *See* National Medical Fellowships.

medical foundation An independent organization of physicians, generally sponsored by a state or local medical association or society, concerned with the delivery of medical services at reasonable cost. It propounds beliefs, such as free choice of a physician and hospital by patients, fee-for-service reimbursement, and local peer review. Many medical foundations operate as prepaid group practices or as an individual practice association for a health maintenance organization. Although these foundations are prepaid on a capitation basis for services to some or all of their patients, they still pay their individual members on a fee-for-service basis for the services they provide. Some foundations are organized only for peer review purposes or other specific functions. *Synonym:* foundation for medical care. *See also* foundation; health maintenance organization; individual practice association; medical society; prepaid group practice.

Medical Friends of Wine, Society of *See* Society of Medical Friends of Wine.

medical geneticist A physician or scientist who specializes in medical genetics. *See also* medical genetics.

medical genetics The branch of science and specialty of medicine dealing with biological variation as it relates to health and disease, including diagnosis and therapy for patients with genetic-linked diseases. Areas of subspecialization include clinical genetics, PhD (Doctor of Philosophy) medical genetics, clinical cytogenetics, clinical biochemical genetics, and clinical molecular genetics. *See also* clinical biochemical genetics; clinical cytogenetics; clinical molecular genetics; clinical genetics; genetics; variation.

Medical Genetics, American Board of *See* American Board of Medical Genetics.

medical graduate, foreign *See* foreign medical graduate.

Medical Graduates, Educational Commission for Foreign *See* Educational Commission for Foreign Medical Graduates.

medical graduate, United States *See* United States medical graduate.

medical graduate, US *See* United States medical graduate.

Medical Group Administrators, American College of *See* American College of Medical Group Administrators.

Medical Group Management Association (MGMA) A national organization founded in 1926 composed of 11,000 persons actively engaged in the business management of medical groups consisting of three or more physicians in medical practice with centralized laboratory, x-ray, medical records, and business functions. *See also* American College of Medical Group Administrators.

Medical Group Missions of the Christian Medical and Dental Society (MGM) A mission of the Christian Medical and Dental Society founded in 1968 that conducts 35 short-term mission outreach projects annually, which send medical and nonmedical personnel to supply medical, dental, and spiritual assistance in 12 third world countries. *See also* Christian Medical and Dental Society; mission.

medical history 1. A component of a medical record consisting of an account of the events in a patient's life that have relevance to his or her mental and physical health. More than the patient's unprompted narrative, it is a specialized literary form in which a physician or other qualified health professional composes and writes an account based on facts, supplied by a patient or other informants, offered spontaneously or obtained by probing. Items are accepted for the medical record only after evaluation by the physician or other health professional, who uses his or her knowledge of the natural history of diseases to secure pertinent details and establish the sequence of events. The components of a complete medical history typically include: identification and vital statistics (such as birth date, residence, occupation); source of information and his or her relation to the patient; chief complaint(s); details of the present illness; relevant past history (including, for instance, general health, infectious diseases, operations and injuries, previous hospitalizations, and systems review); relevant inventory by body systems; social history; and family history. *Synonyms*: health history; patient history. *See also* history; medical record. **2.** The branch of history that deals with the history of medicine.

medical hold The act of holding a patient for treatment against the will of the patient, used in situations when people are thought to be suffering from mental disease and are considered a danger to self or other persons. *See also* commitment.

medical/hospital social worker (MSW) A social worker, usually with at least a master's degree in social work, who identifies and establishes beneficial resources to help patients and their families with social and emotional difficulties associated with illnesses or that are interfering with treatment. Discharge planning is an important area of practice for this group of social workers, especially since the advent of prospective payment. *See also* discharge planning; Master of Social Work; social worker.

Medical Humanities, Association for Faculty in the *See* Association for Faculty in the Medical Humanities.

Medical Illness Severity Grouping System (Medis-Groups or MEDISGRPS) A proprietary computerized data system developed by MediQual Systems, Inc, for classifying hospital patients by severity of illness using objective data specially abstracted from patients' medical records. *See also* severity of illness.

medical illustrator An artist with professional

competence in creating visual material designed to facilitate the recording and dissemination of medical, biological, and related knowledge through communication media. Medical illustrators are one type of allied health professional for which the Committee on Allied Health Education and Accreditation has accredited education programs. *Synonym*: medical artist. *See also* allied health professional.

Medical Illustrators, Association of *See* Association of Medical Illustrators.

Medical Imaging Society, Computerized *See* Computerized Medical Imaging Society.

Medical Impairment Bureau (MIB) A clearinghouse of information on people who have applied for life insurance. Adverse medical findings on previous medical examinations are recorded in code and sent to companies subscribing to the service. *See also* impairment; life insurance.

medical indigence As defined in a statute or administrative rule, the condition of having insufficient income to pay for adequate health care without depriving oneself or one's dependents of food, clothing, shelter, and other essentials of living. Medical indigence may occur when a self-supporting individual, able under ordinary conditions to provide basic maintenance for himself or herself and his or her family, is, in times of catastrophic illness, unable to finance the total cost of medical care. *See also* medically indigent; medically needy.

medical-industrial complex Business, market, and commercial orientation of the health care system with emphasis on investor-owned health care organizations. *See also* investor-owned hospital.

medical informatics The study of the management and use of biomedical information. *Synonym*: medical information science. *See also* informatics; medical computer science.

Medical Informatics Association, American *See* American Medical Informatics Association.

medical information science *See* medical informatics.

medical injury An adverse patient occurrence that may or may not have been avoidable. *See also* adverse patient occurrence; injury; negligence; potentially compensable event; tort.

Medical Institute, Howard Hughes *See* Howard Hughes Medical Institute.

Medical Instrumentation, Association for the Advancement of *See* Association for the Advancement of Medical Instrumentation.

Medical Insurance Program (Part B), Supplemental *See* Supplemental Medical Insurance Program (Part B).

medical intensive care unit (MICU) An intensive care unit for nonsurgical inpatients. *See also* intensive care unit; special care unit.

medical intervention Any medical action that is intended to interrupt or change events in progress; for example, treating a diabetic patient with insulin. *See also* intervention; nursing intervention; surgical intervention.

medical IRA *See* health IRA.

medical jurisprudence *See* forensic medicine.

Medical Jurisprudence, Society of *See* Society of Medical Jurisprudence.

medical laboratory *See* clinical laboratory.

medical laboratory technician (associate degree) An allied health professional trained in an associate degree program (two years) who performs routine laboratory tests under the supervision or direction of pathologists and other physicians, or scientists who specialize in clinical chemistry, microbiology, or the other biological sciences. Medical laboratory technicians gather data on human blood, tissues, and fluids by using a variety of precision instruments. They can demonstrate discrimination between closely similar items; can correct errors by use of preset strategies; have knowledge of specific techniques and instruments; and are able to recognize factors that directly affect procedures and results. Medical laboratory technicians (associate) are one type of allied health professional for which the Committee on Allied Health Education and Accreditation has accredited education programs. *See also* allied health professional; medical laboratory technician (certificate); medical technologist.

medical laboratory technician (certificate) An allied health professional who, under the direction of a qualified physician and/or medical technologist, performs routine, uncomplicated procedures in the areas of hematology, serology, blood banking, urinalysis, microbiology, and clinical chemistry. The procedures involve the use of common laboratory instruments in processes in which discrimination is clear, errors are few and easily corrected, and results of the procedures can be confirmed with a reference test or source within the working area. Medical laboratory technicians (certificate) are one type of allied health professional for which the Committee on

Allied Health Education and Accreditation has accredited education programs. *See also* allied health professional; medical laboratory technician (associate degree); medical technologist.

medical laboratory technologist   *See* medical technologist.

Medical Lab Personnel, National Certification Agency for   *See* National Certification Agency for Medical Lab Personnel.

medical law   The branch of law that deals with the application of medical knowledge to legal problems. *See also* health law; hospital attorney; hospital law; law.

medical legal   *See* medicolegal.

medical-legal analysis   A field of study dealing with forensic and jurisprudential aspects of medicine and surgery. *See also* analysis; forensic medicine.

Medical-Legal Analysis, American Academy of   *See* American Academy of Medical-Legal Analysis.

Medical-Legal Analysis in Medicine and Surgery, American Board of   *See* American Board of Medical-Legal Analysis in Medicine and Surgery.

Medical Letter   An organization founded in 1959 that gathers and publishes information on the therapeutic and side effects of drugs for the benefit of physicians and other health professionals. The organization emphasizes new drugs. *See also* drug; new drug.

medical liability   *See* professional liability.

medical liability insurance   *See* professional liability insurance.

medical librarian   A library specialist who acquires, organizes, catalogs, searches, retrieves, and disseminates medical information. *See also* health sciences library; librarian.

medical library   *See* health sciences library.

Medical Library Association (MLA)   A national organization founded in 1898 composed of 5,000 librarians and other individuals engaged in professional library or bibliographical work in medical and allied scientific libraries. *See also* health sciences library; library.

medical licensing   *See* medical licensure.

medical licensure   The process by which a legal jurisdiction, such as a state, grants permission to a physician to practice medicine upon finding that she or he has met acceptable qualification standards. Medical licensure also involves ongoing state regulation of physicians, including the state's authority

to revoke or otherwise restrict a license to practice. *Synonyms:* medical licensing; physician licensing; physician licensure. *See also* licensure.

Medical Literature Analysis and Retrieval System (MEDLARS)   A computerized literature retrieval service of the National Library of Medicine containing more than 4.5 million references to medical articles found in professional journals and books published since 1966. The references are made available on request to more than 1,000 hospitals, universities, government agencies, and other interested parties throughout the world. The references are filed in 15 databases including MEDLINE, TOXLINE, and CHEMLINE. *See also* MEDLINE; National Library of Medicine.

medically futile   *See* futility.

medically indigent   An individual, as defined by the federal, state, or local government, who lacks the financial ability to pay for his or her medical expenses. Medically indigent may refer to either persons whose income is low enough that they can pay for their basic living costs but not their routine medical care or, alternatively, to persons with generally adequate income who suddenly face catastrophically large medical bills. Individuals whose income and other resources fall below the defined level may be declared medically indigent and qualify for public assistance. *See also* indigent; medical indigence; medically needy; near poor.

medically needy   In the Medicaid program, individuals who have enough income and resources to pay for their basic living expenses, and so do not require welfare, but who do not have enough income and resources to pay for their medical care. These individuals receive benefits if their income after deducting medical expenses is low enough to meet the eligibility standard. *See also* Medicaid; medical indigence; medically indigent; near poor.

medically underserved area   A geographic location, such as an urban or a rural area, that has inadequate health resources to meet the health care needs of the resident population. Physician-shortage area applies to a medically underserved area that is particularly short of physicians. *See also* health service area; physician shortage area; scarcity area.

medically underserved population   A group of people with inadequate health services who may or may not reside in a specified area that is medically underserved. Thus migrants, Native Americans, or prison inmates may constitute such a population. The term is defined and used to give such populations priority for federal assistance. *See also* medically underserved area; Native American; population.

medical malpractice   A judicial determination that there has been a negligent (or, rarely, willful) failure to adhere to current standard(s) of care, resulting in injury or loss to a patient and legal liability of the provider responsible for the negligent act. Since the judgment of malpractice is sociolegal and is made on a case-by-case rather than systematic basis, standards and processes for determining malpractice may vary by area. *See also* locality rule; malpractice; standard of care.

medical malpractice insurance   Insurance against the risk of suffering financial damage because of malpractice. *See also* insurance; medical malpractice; professional liability insurance.

Medical Management Analysis System   A proprietary system for carrying out occurrence screening. *See also* occurrence screening.

medical microbiologist   A pathologist subspecializing in medical microbiology. *See* medical microbiology; microbiologist; pathology.

medical microbiology   The field of knowledge dealing with microorganisms in medicine and the pathology subspecialty consisting of the isolation and identification of microbial agents that cause infectious disease. Viruses, bacteria, fungi, and single-cell and larger parasites are identified and, when possible, tested for susceptibility to appropriate antimicrobial agents. *See also* medical microbiologist; pathology.

Medical Milk Commissions, American Association of   *See* American Association of Medical Milk Commissions.

Medical Mission Board, Catholic   *See* Catholic Medical Mission Board.

Medical Mycological Society of the Americas (MMSA)   An organization founded in 1966 composed of 408 medical professionals interested in fungi and fungal diseases. It promotes continuing education in medical mycology in association with the American Society for Microbiology. *See also* American Society fo Microbiology; fungus; mycology.

medical neglect   Withholding medically indicated treatment from an individual, especially a child. Medical neglect is one form of child abuse and neglect. *See also* child abuse; neglect.

Medical Network for Missing Children (MNMC)   A nonmembership organization founded in 1984 that helps identify missing children by medically identifiable characteristics, such as dental patterns or scars. It conducts an educational program to alert health care professionals to the problem of missing children, provides a medical-dental questionnaire to health professionals and parents of missing children, offers medical profiles of known missing children to health care professionals, and maintains archives of medical and dental profiles of missing children.

medical nuclear physics   The branch of medical physics that deals with the therapeutic and diagnostic application of radionuclides (except those used in sealed sources for therapeutic purpose) and the equipment associated with their production and use. *See also* medical physics; physics; radiological physics; radionuclides.

Medical Nurses Association, Baro-   *See* Baromedical Nurses Association.

medical office building   An office building used by physicians and other health care personnel for providing services to their patients.

medical oncologist   An internist who subspecializes in medical oncology. *See also* medical oncology.

medical oncology   The branch of medicine and subspecialty of internal medicine dealing with the diagnosis and treatment of all types of cancer and other benign and malignant tumors. Chemotherapy for malignant diseases as well as consultation with surgeons and radiotherapists are within the scope of medical oncology. *See also* internal medicine; oncology.

Medical Peer Review Association, American   *See* American Medical Peer Review Association.

Medical Personnel, Joint Review Committee for Ophthalmic   *See* Joint Review Committee for Ophthalmic Medical Personnel.

medical photographer   A photographer with training and experience in the biological sciences who photographs medical phenomena.

medical physics   The science of matter and energy and of interactions between the two, as applied to the field of medicine. *See also* medical nuclear physics; physics; radiological physics.

Medical Political Action Committee, American   *See* American Medical Political Action Committee.

medical practice   The professional business of a physician, as in solo practice or group practice. *See also* group practice; practice; solo practice.

medical practice act A state, commonwealth, or territorial statute or law governing the practice of medicine. *See also* nurse practice act.

medical practice plan The set of policies and procedures, usually presented in a single document, that governs the manner in which patient services are rendered by medical school faculty physicians, the method of obtaining reimbursement, and the disposition of the funds obtained for such services. *Synonyms*: clinical practice plan; faculty practice plan. *See also* medical school; teaching hospital.

medical profession The profession of physicians. *See also* medicine; physician; profession.

Medical Psychotherapists, American Board of *See* American Board of Medical Psychotherapists.

Medical Publishers' Association, American *See* American Medical Publishers' Association.

Medical Quality, American College of *See* American College of Medical Quality.

medical record An account compiled by physicians and other health professionals of a patient's medical history; present illness; findings on physical examination; details of treatment; reports of diagnostic tests; findings and conclusions from special examinations; findings and diagnoses of consultants; diagnoses of the responsible physician; notes on treatment, including medication, surgical operations, radiation, and physical therapy; and progress notes by physicians, nurses and other health professionals. The medical record has medical and legal purposes. Medical purposes include assisting physicians and other health professionals in making diagnoses; assisting physicians, nurses, and other health professionals in the care and treatment of the patient; and serving as a record for teaching medicine, performing clinical research, and improving practitioner and organization performance. Legal purposes include documentation of insurance claims for the patient and serving as legal proof in cases of malpractice claims, injury or compensation, cases of poisoning, and cases of homicide and suicide. *Synonyms*: chart; clinical record; health record; patient (or patient's) chart; patient (or patient's) health record; patient (or patient's) medical record; patient (or patient's) record. *See also* case-based review; consultation report; documentation; electronic medical record; Freedom of Information Act; medical history; on-line medical record; open charting; problem-oriented medical record; quality of documentation.

medical record abstracter An individual who extracts essential clinical data from a medical record using appropriate classification systems; for example, a medical record abstracter often completes a precoded form to be used as input into a hospital discharge abstract system. *Synonym*: abstracter. *See also* hospital discharge abstract system; medical record technician.

medical record abstraction The selection and separation of essential material of a medical record or other source document in order to create a summary, called an abstract, of that record or document. *Synonyms*: abstracting; abstraction. *See also* medical record abstracter.

medical record administrator (MRA) An allied health professional who manages health information systems consistent with professional standards and the medical, administrative, ethical, and legal requirements of the health care delivery system. Specifically, medical record administrators plan and develop health information systems that meet standards of accrediting and regulating agencies; design health information systems appropriate for various sizes and types of health care facilities; manage the human, financial, and physical resources of a health information service; participate in medical staff and institutional activities, including utilization management, risk management, and quality assessment; collect and analyze patient and facility data for reimbursement, facility planning, marketing, risk management, utilization management, quality assessment, and research; serve as an advocate for privacy and confidentiality of health information; and plan and offer in-service educational programs for health care personnel. Medical record administrators are one type of allied health professional for which the Committee on Allied Health Education and Accreditation has accredited education programs. *See also* allied health professional; medical record; medical record technician; registered record administrator.

medical record analyst An individual skilled in the analysis of data from medical records, who abstracts and provides data displays and analytical findings from the medical records for use by organizational management and medical staff of a hospital or other health care organization. *Synonym*: health record analyst. *See also* analysis; management; medical record abstraction; medical staff.

medical record audit   *See* medical audit; medical record review.

medical record coder   An individual who assigns and sequences codes, such as *International Classification of Diseases, Ninth Revision, Clinical Modification (ICD-9-CM)* numbers, for terms, such as congestive heart failure, for use in research, reimbursement, performance improvement, and health care planning. *See also* certified coding specialist; coder; medical record abstracter; medical record administrator; medical record coding; medical record technician.

medical record coding   The process of substituting a symbol (code), usually a number, for a term, such as a diagnosis or procedure. *See also* coding.

medical record, complete   *See* complete medical record.

medical record department   A unit of a hospital or other health care organization that provides medical record services. *See also* medical record; medical record services.

medical record, electronic   *See* electronic medical record.

medical record entry   Notes written, dated, and signed in the medical record by physicians, nurses, respiratory therapists, physical therapists, and all other health professionals permitted to do so by the organization. *See also* medical record.

medical record index   A system of indexing medical records so that they can be located according to patient names, diagnoses, procedures, physicians, and other categories. *See also* index.

medical record legibility   The degree to which writing on a medical record can be deciphered. *See also* legible.

medical record librarian   *See* medical record administrator.

medical record, on-line   *See* on-line medical record.

medical record, problem-oriented   *See* problem-oriented medical record.

medical record professional   A medical record administrator, medical record technician, registered record administrator, or other medical record specialist. *See also* medical record administrator; medical record technician; registered record administrator.

medical record progress note   A component of the medical record consisting of a pertinent chronological report of a patient's course. The SOAP format (subjective data, objective data, assessment of status, plan for care) is typically used to organize and record progress notes. *See also* medical record; problem-oriented medical record; SOAP.

medical record review   The process of reviewing patients' medical records to measure, assess, and improve organizational and practitioner performance. *See also* medical audit.

medical record review function   The medical staff responsibility, carried out in cooperation with other relevant departments/services, to measure, assess, and improve the overall quality of medical record documentation. *See also* function; medical record review; medical staff.

medical record services   The component of an organization responsible for ensuring the accuracy, completeness, timeliness, accessibility, and safe, secure, and confidential storage of patients' medical records, as in the medical record services of a hospital. *See also* medical record.

Medical Records Institute (MRI)   A national organization founded in 1979 composed of 800 medical record and computer professionals, physicians, nurses, and other individuals involved in health care interested in conducting research and education in the fields of medical documentation and computerization of patient information. Formerly (1988) Institute for Medical Record Economics. *See also* medical record.

medical record specialist   *See* medical record professional.

medical record technician (MRT)   An allied health professional who has responsibility for maintaining components of health information systems in a manner consistent with the medical, administrative, ethical, legal, accreditation, and regulatory requirements of a health care delivery system. In all types of facilities, and in various locations within a facility, the medical record technician processes, maintains, compiles, and reports health information data for reimbursement, facility planning, marketing, risk management, utilization management, quality assessment and research; abstracts and codes clinical data using appropriate classification systems; and analyzes health records according to standards. The medical record technician may be responsible for functional supervision of the various components of a health information system. Medical record technicians are one type of allied health professional for which the Committee on Allied Health Education and Accreditation has accredited education programs. *See also* accredited record technician; allied health professional; medical record; medical record administrator.

Medical Rehabilitation Administrators, Association of *See* Association of Medical Rehabilitation Administrators.

medical representative *See* detail person.

medical representative, certified *See* certified medical representative.

Medical Representatives Institute, Certified *See* Certified Medical Representatives Institute.

Medical Rescue Service, Parachute *See* Parachute Medical Rescue Service.

Medical Research Modernization Committee (MRMC) A group founded in 1978 composed of 1,500 scientists and clinicians who evaluate the medical and/or scientific merit of research modalities in an effort to identify outdated research methods and to promote sensible, reliable, and efficient methods. *See also* research.

Medical Research, National Association for Bio- *See* National Association for Biomedical Research.

medical resident A resident physician-in-training in internal medicine. *See also* housestaff; intern; internal medicine; residency.

medical review A quality-of-care review, including the appropriateness and effectiveness of services, conducted by physicians, nurses, and other health and social service personnel to meet external (for example, government) or self-imposed requirements. *See also* external review; internal review; medical review agency; utilization review.

medical review agency An agency established under a prospective payment system to carry out certain surveillance functions with respect to hospital and physician performance and detection of fraud. *See also* fraud and abuse; medical review.

medical review criteria *See* review criteria.

medical school An educational institution offering programs leading to the Doctor of Medicine (MD) degree. *Synonym*: medical college. *See also* medical education; medical practice plan; medical student; teaching hospital.

medical school admission test *See* Medical College Admission Test.

Medical School Pediatric Department Chairmen, Association of *See* Association of Medical School Pediatric Department Chairmen.

Medical Schools, Graduates of Italian *See* Gradu-

ate of Italian Medical Schools.

Medical Sciences, American Center for Chinese *See* American Center for Chinese Medical Sciences.

medical secretary An individual who performs secretarial duties in a health care setting, such as a hospital department. *See also* secretary.

Medical Service Physicians, National Association of Emergency *See* National Association of Emergency Medical Service Physicians.

medical services The services performed by physicians, nurses, and other health professionals who work under the direction of a physician. *See also* health care; physician.

Medical Services, Association of Air *See* Association of Air Medical Services.

Medical Services Training Coordinators, National Council of State Emergency *See* National Council of State Emergency Medical Services Training Coordinators.

medical social worker *See* medical/hospital social worker.

Medical Societies, Congress of County *See* Congress of County Medical Societies.

medical society Any professional association of physicians, as in county, state, or national medical societies. *See also* medical association; physician; specialty societies.

Medical Society, Chinese American *See* Chinese American Medical Society.

Medical Society Executives, American Association of *See* American Association of Medical Society Executives.

Medical Society, People's *See* People's Medical Society.

Medical Society, Undersea and Hyperbaric *See* Undersea and Hyperbaric Medical Society.

Medical Society of the United States and Mexico (MSUSM) A national organization founded in 1954 composed of 400 physicians in the United States and in Mexico. It promotes scientific and international goodwill, sponsors research and educational programs, and fosters interchange of physicians. *See also* physician.

Medical Society, Virchow-Pirquet *See* Virchow-Pirquet Medical Society.

Medical Society, Wilderness *See* Wilderness Medical Society.

Medical Sonographers, American Registry of Diagnostic *See* American Registry of Diagnostic

Medical Sonographers.

Medical Sonographers, Society of Diagnostic *See* Society of Diagnostic Medical Sonographers.

Medical Sonography, Joint Review Committee on Education in Diagnostic *See* Joint Review Committee on Education in Diagnostic Medical Sonography.

medical specialist A physician who concentrates on body systems, age group, or procedures and techniques developed to diagnose and/or treat certain types of disorders. Definitions of each specialty and of the educational and other requirements leading to eligibility (preparation) for board certification in a specialty are developed by consensus within the medical profession. To date, the certification of a medical specialist has remained separate and distinct from licensure of professionals qualified to practice medicine by civil authorities. The basic training of a physician specialist includes four years of premedical education in a college or university, four years of medical school, and, after receiving the Doctor of Medicine (MD) degree, from three to seven years of specialty training under supervision (residency). Training in various subspecialties within the general specialties can take two to three years longer. *See also* board certified; board prepared; certification; licensure; medical specialties; medical subspecialist; specialist.

medical specialties Areas of expertise in medicine. There are, for example, 23 medical specialty areas currently recognized by the American Board of Medical Specialties. These include: allergy and immunology, anesthesiology, colon and rectal surgery, dermatology, emergency medicine, family practice, medical genetics, internal medicine, neurological surgery, nuclear medicine, obstetrics and gynecology, ophthalmology, orthopaedic surgery, otolaryngology, pathology, pediatrics, physical medicine and rehabilitation, plastic surgery, preventive medicine, psychiatry and neurology, radiology, surgery, thoracic surgery, and urology. *See also* American Board of Medical Specialties; specialty.

Medical Specialties, American Board of *See* American Board of Medical Specialties.

medical specialty *See* medical specialties.

medical specialty boards **1.** National bodies that certify physicians as diplomates of one or more specialty boards when all requirements have been met. The American Board of Medical Specialties currently recognizes 23 medical specialty, such as pediatrics,

emergency medicine, and thoracic surgery. Specialty boards influence graduate medical education through setting criteria that must be met for eligibility to take the certification examinations. Each board sets the minimum length of time for education in an accredited residency program and, in part, determines the content of the training program since they determine the content of the certifying examination. *See also* American Board of Medical Specialties; board certified; board prepared; diplomate; medical specialties. **2.** *See* specialty board examination.

medical specialty resident A resident physician-in-training in a medical or surgical specialty. *See also* resident.

medical specialty societies *See* specialty societies.

Medical Specialty Societies, Council of *See* Council of Medical Specialty Societies.

Medical and Sports Music Institute of America (MSMIA) A for-profit organization founded in 1985 that develops and manufactures audiocassettes and videocassettes for exercise, insomnia, and stress management and seeks to improve and maintain fitness levels for cardiac, drug, and physical rehabilitation. It conducts research on the relationship between target heart rate during exercise and optimum exercise pace for various forms of exercises.

medical staff An organized body that has overall responsibility for the quality of the professional services provided by individuals with clinical privileges and also the responsibility of accounting to the governing body of a health care organization, such as a hospital. The medical staff includes licensed physicians and may include other licensed individuals permitted by law and by the organization to provide patient care services independently (that is, without clinical direction or supervision) in the organization. Members have delineated clinical privileges that allow them to provide patient care services independently within the scope of their clinical privileges. Members and all other persons with individual clinical privileges are subject to medical staff and departmental bylaws and are subject to review as part of the organization's performance assessment and improvement activities. *See also* attending physician; chief of staff; clinical privileges; closed staff; credentials committee; delineation of clinical privileges; governing body; hospital staff; medical staff bylaws; open staff; physician member of the medical staff; president of the medical staff; self-governance.

medical staff bylaws A governance framework that describes the roles and responsibilities of the medical staff. The bylaws are developed, adopted, and periodically reviewed by the medical staff and approved by the governing body of the health care organization. *See also* bylaws; governing body; medical staff.

medical staff, closed *See* closed staff.

medical staff credentialing *See* physician credentialing.

medical staff executive committee A group of medical staff members, a majority of whom are licensed physician members of the medical staff practicing in the organization, selected by the medical staff or appointed in accordance with governing body bylaws, who are responsible for making specific recommendations directly to the governing body for its approval and for receiving and acting on reports and recommendations from medical staff committees, clinical departments/services, and assigned activity groups. *See also* executive committee; medical staff.

medical staff, open *See* open staff.

medical staff, organized *See* organized professional staff.

medical staff, physician member of the *See* physician member of the medical staff.

medical staff president *See* chief of staff; president of the medical staff.

medical staff privileges *See* clinical privileges.

Medical Staff Services, National Association *See* National Association Medical Staff Services.

medical statistics *See* biostatistics.

medical student An individual who is enrolled in a medical school program of study to fulfill the requirements for the doctor of medicine degree. *See also* clinical clerk; clinical clerkship; doctorate; Doctor of Medicine; medical school; philiater.

Medical Subject Headings (MeSH) A standardized list of medical terms, also called a thesaurus, created by the National Library of Medicine to index the medical articles in its MEDLINE database. An average of 10 medical subject headings is assigned to describe an article's subject content, with an average of three MeSH terms designated to the main point of the article. *See also* MEDLINE; National Library of Medicine.

medical subspecialist A physician who has com-

pleted training in a general medical specialty and then takes additional training in a more specific area of that specialty (a subspecialty area). For example, forensic pathology is a subspecialty of clinical pathology and general vascular surgery is a subspecialty of surgery. The training of a subspecialist requires an additional one or more years of full-time education in a program called a fellowship. *See also* fellowship; medical specialist; subspecialist.

medical subspecialties More specific areas of a medical specialty; for example, infectious disease is a subspecialty of internal medicine and critical care medicine is a subspecialty of anesthesiology. *See also* medical specialties.

medical supplies Medical items, usually of a disposable nature, such as bandages, suture material, and sterile drapes. Supplies differ from permanent and durable capital goods, such as an examining or operating table whose use lasts over a year. *See also* medical equipment; supplies.

medical technician, ophthalmic *See* ophthalmic medical technician.

Medical Technicians, National Association of Emergency *See* National Association of Emergency Medical Technicians.

Medical Technicians, National Registry of Emergency *See* National Registry of Emergency Medical Technicians.

medical technologist (MT) An allied health professional who, in conjunction with pathologists and other physicians or scientists who specialize in clinical chemistry, microbiology, or the other biological sciences, gather data on the blood, tissues, and fluids in the human body by using a variety of precision instruments. In addition to the skills possessed by medical laboratory technicians, medical technologists perform complex analyses, fine-line discrimination, and correction of errors. They are able to recognize interdependency of tests and have knowledge of physiological conditions affecting test results in order to confirm these results and to develop data that may be used by a physician in determining the presence, extent, and, as far as possible, the cause of disease. Tests and procedures performed or supervised by medical technologists in the clinical laboratory center on major areas of hematology, microbiology, immunohematology, immunology, clinical chemistry, and urinalysis. Medical technologists are one type of allied health professional for which the Committee on Allied Health Education and Accreditation has accredited education programs. *See also* allied health professional; hematology technologist; medical laboratory technician (associate degree); medical laboratory technician (certificate).

medical technologist, ophthalmic *See* ophthalmic medical technologist.

Medical Technologists, American *See* American Medical Technologists.

Medical Technologists, Registered Medical Assistants of American *See* Registered Medical Assistants of American Medical Technologists.

medical technology The drugs, devices, and medical and surgical procedures used in health care, and the organizational and support systems within which such care is provided.

Medical Technology, American Society for *See* American Society for Medical Technology.

medical toxicologist An emergency physician, a pediatrician, or a preventive medicine physician who subspecializes in medical toxicology. *See also* medical toxicology.

medical toxicology The branch of medicine and subspecialty of emergency medicine, pediatrics, and preventive medicine dealing with the evaluation and management of patients with accidental or intentional poisoning through exposure to prescription and nonprescription medications, drugs of abuse, household or industrial toxins, and environmental toxins. Important areas of medical toxicology include, but are not limited to, acute pediatric and adult drug ingestion; drug abuse, addiction, and withdrawal; chemical poisoning exposure and toxicity; hazardous materials exposure and toxicity; occupational toxicology; biological poisons; basic concepts of toxicology, such as kinetics, dose-response relationships, indices of toxicity, and safety standards; basic principles of toxic exposure; and preventive methodologies. *Synonym*: clinical toxicology. *See also* poison control center; toxicology.

Medical Toxicology, American Board of *See* American Board of Medical Toxicology.

medical transcription *See* transcription.

Medical Transcription, American Association for *See* American Association for Medical Transcription.

medical transcriptionist An individual who translates patients' records of medical care and treatment from oral dictation to written form. *See also* transcription.

Medical Transport Association, Professional Aero- *See* Professional Aeromedical Transport Association.

Medical Treatment Effectiveness Program (MEDTEP) A component of the Agency for Health Care Policy and Research that is charged with analysis of variations in health care practices and the impact of those variations on patient outcomes. *See also* Agency for Health Care Policy and Research.

Medical Women's Association, American *See* American Medical Women's Association.

Medical Writers Association, American *See* American Medical Writers Association.

medicament *See* medicine.

medicar A vehicle that transports patients in wheelchairs between facilities or on home-hospital transfers. It is staffed with a driver only who does not provide medical care. *See also* ambulance.

Medicare A federal program administered under the Health Care Financing Administration that reimburses hospitals and physicians for health care provided to qualifying people aged 65 years and older, persons eligible for Social Security disability payments for at least two years, and certain workers and their dependents who need kidney transplantation or dialysis. Part A is hospital insurance that covers hospital costs. Part B is supplemental medical insurance that covers physician and other services. *Synonym*: Old Age, Survivors, Disability and Health Insurance Program. *See also* assignment; end stage renal disease; entitlement program; Health Care Financing Administration; Medicare, Part A; Medicare, Part B; Old Age, Survivors, Disability and Health Insurance Program; Social Security Act; Supplementary Medical Insurance Program (Part B); trust fund.

Medicare Benefits, Explanation of *See* Explanation of Medicare Benefits.

Medicare carrier *See* carrier.

Medicare Catastrophic Coverage Act of 1988 The act in which provisions were to expand Medicare benefits for both Part A and Part B. It also contained spousal impoverishment protection benefits under Medicaid. Most of the act was repealed in 1989. *See also* Medicare; Medicare Catastrophic Coverage Repeal Act of 1989.

Medicare Catastrophic Coverage Repeal Act of 1989 The act that repealed virtually the entire

Medicare Catastrophic Coverage Act except for the spousal impoverishment provision, qualified Medicare beneficiary provision, and child wellness benefit. *See also* Medicare Catastrophic Coverage Act of 1988.

Medicare conditions of participation Requirements that institutional providers (including, for example, hospitals, skilled nursing homes, and home health agencies) must meet in order to be allowed to receive payments for Medicare patients. An example is the requirement that hospitals conduct utilization review. *See also* conditions of participation; deemed status; utilization review.

Medicare costs, base year *See* base year Medicare costs.

Medicare locality A geographic area in which a Medicare carrier obtains information about prevailing charges for the purpose of making reasonable charge determinations. *See also* carrier; catchment area; health service area; Medicare; reasonable cost.

Medicare, Part A The hospital care portion of Medicare (also called Hospital Insurance [HI] Program) that automatically covers all persons aged 65 and older who are entitled to benefits under Old Age, Survivors, Disability and Health Insurance or railroad retirement plans, persons under 65 years old who have been eligible for disability for at least two years, and insured workers and their dependents needing kidney dialysis or kidney transplantation. Part A pays for inpatient care and care in skilled nursing facilities and home health agencies following a period of hospitalization, after cost-sharing requirements are met. The Part A, HI program is financed from a separate trust fund whose monies come from a contributory tax (payroll tax) levied on employers, employees, and the self-employed. *See also* Medicare.

Medicare, Part B The portion of Medicare through which individuals entitled to Medicare, Part A, may obtain assistance with payment for physicians' services. Individuals participate voluntarily through enrollment and the payment of a monthly fee. *See also* Medicare; unbundling.

Medicare participation *See* participation.

Medicare Provider Analysis and Review *MED-PAR* A database containing hospital and physician financial claims and clinical data for Medicare beneficiaries, in which data elements are defined by Medicare billing requirements and are maintained by the Health Care Financing Administration of the Department of Health and Human Services. *See also* database; Health Care Financing Administration; Medicare.

Medicare secondary payer The Medicare role in the coordination of benefits as a secondary payer to other health insurance plans, as defined in the Tax Equity and Fiscal Responsibility Act of 1982. For example, Medicare pays only the remaining part of Medicare benefits after the benefits from other insurance have been paid for persons who are eligible for health coinsurance benefits from the Veterans Administration and the Federal Employees Program. *See also* Medicare; payer; Tax Equity and Fiscal Responsibility Act.

Medicare supplement A health insurance plan that pays all or a percentage of the deductible and coinsurance amounts not covered by Medicare. Benefits not covered by Medicare (for example, prescription drugs or nursing care) are also covered under some Medicare supplement plans. *See also* Medicare; medigap policy.

medicate To treat with medicine or drugs, as in medicating a patient prior to induction of anesthesia. *See also* overmedicate.

medicate, over- *See* overmedicate.

medication Any substance intended for use in the diagnosis, cure, mitigation, treatment, or prevention of disease. *Compare* biological. *See also* drug; medicine; pharmaceutical.

medication administration The act in which a prescribed dose of an identified medication is given to a patient. *See also* administration; medication.

medication dispensing The issuing of one or more doses of a prescribed medication by a pharmacist or other authorized person to another person responsible for administering it. *See also* medication; medication administration.

medication error A discrepancy between what a physician orders and what is reported to occur. Types of medication errors include omission, unauthorized drug, extra dose, wrong dose, wrong dosage form, wrong rate, deteriorated drug, wrong administration technique, and wrong time. An omission type of medication error is the failure to give an ordered dose; a refused dose is not counted as an error if the nurse responsible for administering the dose tried, but failed, to persuade the patient to take it. Doses withheld according to written policies, such as for x-ray procedures, are not counted as omission errors. An unauthorized medication error is the administration of a dose of medication not authorized to be given to that patient. Instances of "brand or therapeutic substitution" are counted as unauthorized medication errors only when prohibited by institutional policy. A wrong dose medication error occurs when a patient receives an amount of medicine that is greater than or less than the amount ordered; the range of allowable deviation is based on each hospital's definition. *Synonym*: drug error. *See also* error; medication.

medication order   A written order by a physician, dentist or other designated health professional for medication to be dispensed by a pharmacy for administration to a patient. *See also* medication administration; medication dispensing; medication error; order.

medication system   An important organizational function composed of a series of interlinked processes required to provide medications to patients, including, at a minimum, handling a physician's (or other health professional's) order, transcribing of the order by a nurse or a pharmacist, filling the medication order in the pharmacy, transferring the medication to the nursing unit, and administering the medication to the patient. *See also* medication; medication administration; medication dispensing; medication order.

medication system, unit-dose   *See* unit-dose medication system.

Medic-Card Systems, National   *See* National Medic-Card Systems.

***Medicinae Doctor* (MD)**   *See* Doctor of Medicine.

medicine   1. The art and science of diagnosing, treating, or preventing disease and other damage to the body or mind. *See also* iatrology. **2.** An agent, such as a drug, used to treat disease or injury. *See also* drug; medication.

medicine, academic   *See* academic medicine.

Medicine, Academy of Oral Diagnosis, Radiology, and   *See* Academy of Oral Diagnosis, Radiology, and Medicine.

Medicine, Academy of Psychosomatic   *See* Academy of Psychosomatic Medicine.

medicine, addiction   *See* addiction medicine.

medicine, adolescent   *See* adolescent medicine.

medicine, allopathic   *See* allopathy.

medicine, alternative   *See* alternative medicine.

Medicine, American Academy for Cerebral Palsy and Developmental   *See* American Academy for Cerebral Palsy and Developmental Medicine.

Medicine, American Academy of Environmental   *See* American Academy of Environmental Medicine.

Medicine, American Academy of Oral   *See* American Academy of Oral Medicine.

Medicine, American Academy of Podiatric Sports   *See* American Academy of Podiatric Sports Medicine.

Medicine, American Academy of Tropical   *See* American Academy of Tropical Medicine.

Medicine, American Association for Acupuncture and Oriental   *See* American Association for Acupuncture and Oriental Medicine.

Medicine, American Association of Ayurvedic   *See* American Association of Ayurvedic Medicine.

Medicine, American Association of Colleges of Osteopathic   *See* American Association of Colleges of Osteopathic Medicine.

Medicine, American Association of Colleges of Podiatric   *See* American Association of Colleges of Podiatric Medicine.

Medicine, American Association of Electrodiagnostic   *See* American Association of Electrodiagnostic Medicine.

Medicine, American Association for the History of   *See* American Association for the History of Medicine.

Medicine, American Association of Orthomolecular   *See* American Association of Orthomolecular Medicine.

Medicine, American Association of Orthopedic   *See* American Association of Orthopedic Medicine.

Medicine, American Association of Physicists in   *See* American Association of Physicists in Medicine.

Medicine, American Board of Emergency   *See* American Board of Emergency Medicine.

Medicine, American Board of Environmental   *See* American Board of Environmental Medicine.

Medicine, American Board of Internal   *See* American Board of Internal Medicine.

Medicine, American Board of Nuclear   *See* American Board of Nuclear Medicine.

Medicine, American Board of Preventive   *See* American Board of Preventive Medicine.

Medicine, American Board of Tropical   *See* American Board of Tropical Medicine.

Medicine, American College of   *See* American College of Medicine.

Medicine, American College of Advancement in *See* American College of Advancement in Medicine.

Medicine, American College of Laboratory Animal *See* American College of Laboratory Animal Medicine.

Medicine, American College of Legal *See* American College of Legal Medicine.

Medicine, American College of Nuclear *See* American College of Nuclear Medicine.

Medicine, American College of Occupational and Environmental *See* American College of Occupational and Environmental Medicine.

Medicine, American College of Preventive *See* American College of Preventive Medicine.

Medicine, American College of Sports *See* American College of Sports Medicine.

Medicine, American Congress of Rehabilitation *See* American Congress of Rehabilitation Medicine.

Medicine, American Institute of Ultrasound in *See* American Institute of Ultrasound in Medicine.

Medicine, American Orthopaedic Society for Sports *See* American Orthopaedic Society for Sports Medicine.

Medicine, American Osteopathic Academy of Sports *See* American Osteopathic Academy of Sports Medicine.

Medicine, American Osteopathic Board of Emergency *See* American Osteopathic Board of Emergency Medicine.

Medicine, American Osteopathic College of Preventive *See* American Osteopathic College of Preventive Medicine.

Medicine, American Osteopathic College of Rehabilitation *See* American Osteopathic College of Rehabilitation Medicine.

Medicine, American Physicians Association of Computer *See* American Physicians Association of Computer Medicine.

Medicine, American Society of Addiction *See* American Society of Addiction Medicine.

Medicine, American Society of Internal *See* American Society of Internal Medicine.

Medicine, American Society of Law and *See* American Society of Law and Medicine.

Medicine, American Society of Legal and Industrial *See* American Society of Legal and Industrial Medicine.

Medicine, American Society of Podiatric *See* American Society of Podiatric Medicine.

medicine, amuletic *See* amuletic medicine.

Medicine, Association for the Advancement of

Automotive *See* Association for the Advancement of Automotive Medicine.

Medicine Association, National Emergency *See* National Emergency Medicine Association.

Medicine, Association of Professors of *See* Association of Professors of Medicine.

Medicine, Association of Program Directors in Internal *See* Association of Program Directors in Internal Medicine.

Medicine, Association for Psychoanalytic *See* Association for Psychoanalytic Medicine.

Medicine, Association of Teachers of Preventive *See* Association of Teachers of Preventive Medicine.

medicine, baro- *See* hyperbaric medicine.

medicine, behavioral *See* behavioral medicine.

medicine, bio- *See* biomedicine.

Medicine and Biology Society, IEEE Engineering in *See* IEEE Engineering in Medicine and Biology Society.

medicine, cardiovascular *See* cardiovascular medicine.

Medicine, Center for Dance *See* Center for Dance Medicine.

medicine, clinical *See* clinical medicine.

Medicine, Committee for Freedom of Choice in *See* Committee for Freedom of Choice in Medicine.

medicine, critical care *See* critical care medicine.

medicine, defensive *See* defensive medicine.

medicine, electro- *See* electromedicine.

medicine, emergency *See* emergency medicine.

medicine, folk *See* folk medicine.

medicine, forensic *See* forensic medicine.

Medicine Foundation, Royal Society of *See* Royal Society of Medicine Foundation.

medicine, geriatric *See* geriatric medicine.

medicine, group *See* group practice.

medicine, holistic *See* holistic medicine.

Medicine and Hygiene, American Society of Tropical *See* American Society of Tropical Medicine and Hygiene.

medicine, hyperbaric *See* hyperbaric medicine.

Medicine, Indians Into *See* Indians Into Medicine.

Medicine, Institute of *See* Institute of Medicine.

Medicine, Institute for Advanced Research in Asian Science and *See* Institute for Advanced Research in Asian Science and Medicine.

medicine, internal *See* internal medicine.

medicine, irregular *See* alternative medicine.

Medicine in Israel, American Physicians Fellowship for *See* American Physicians Fellowship for

Medicine in Israel.

Medicine, Lesbian, Gay and Bisexual People In *See* Lesbian, Gay and Bisexual People in Medicine.

medicine man 1. A shaman, specially a Native American shaman. *See also* Native American; shaman. **2.** A hawker of brews, potions, and other medicines among the audience in a medicine show. *See also* medicine show.

medicine, manipulative *See* manipulative medicine.

medicine, maternal-fetal *See* maternal-fetal medicine.

Medicine, Milton Helpern Institute of Forensic *See* Milton Helpern Institute of Forensic Medicine.

Medicine, National Accreditation Commission for Schools and Colleges of Acupuncture and Oriental *See* National Accreditation Commission for Schools and Colleges of Acupuncture and Oriental Medicine.

Medicine, National Institute for Burn *See* National Institute for Burn Medicine.

Medicine, National Jewish Center for Immunology and Respiratory *See* National Jewish Center for Immunology and Respiratory Medicine.

Medicine, National Library of *See* National Library of Medicine.

medicine, natural *See* naturopathy.

medicine, naturopathic *See* naturopathy.

medicine, neonatal-perinatal *See* neonatal-perinatal medicine.

Medicine, North American Academy of Musculoskeletal *See* North American Academy of Musculoskeletal Medicine.

medicine, nuclear *See* nuclear medicine.

medicine, occupational *See* occupational medicine.

medicine, orthomolecular *See* orthomolecular medicine.

medicine, over-the-counter *See* over-the-counter drug.

medicine, patent *See* over-the-counter medicine.

medicine, pediatric critical care *See* pediatric critical care medicine.

medicine, pediatric emergency *See* pediatric emergency medicine.

medicine, pediatric sports *See* pediatric sports medicine.

Medicine, Physicians Committee for Responsible *See* Physicians Committee for Responsible Medicine.

medicine, podiatric *See* podiatric medicine.

medicine, preventive *See* preventive medicine.

medicine, psychosomatic *See* psychosomatic medicine.

Medicine in the Public Interest (MIPI) A national organization founded in 1973 composed of professionals in medicine, law, and the social sciences interested in promoting and funding research into medicine and related social, legal, and ethical issues. It disseminates research findings and proposals and encourages the development of long-range public health, welfare, and social planning at the federal, state, and local levels. *See also* public interest.

medicine, pulmonary *See* pulmonary medicine.

medicine, rehabilitation *See* physical medicine and rehabilitation.

Medicine and Rehabilitation, American Academy of Physical *See* American Academy of Physical Medicine and Rehabilitation.

Medicine and Rehabilitation, American Board of Physical *See* American Board of Physical Medicine and Rehabilitation.

medicine and rehabilitation, physical *See* physical medicine and rehabilitation.

Medicine Research, Academy of Behavioral *See* Academy of Behavioral Medicine Research.

Medicine and Research, Public Responsibility in *See* Public Responsibility in Medicine and Research.

Medicine, Residency Review Committee for Emergency *See* Residency Review Committee for Emergency Medicine.

Medicine Residents' Association, Emergency *See* Emergency Medicine Residents' Association.

Medicine and Science, Joint Commission on Sports *See* Joint Commission on Sports Medicine and Science.

medicine show A traveling show, popular especially during the nineteenth century, that offered varied entertainment; between its acts brews, potions, and other medicines were sold by a medicine man. *See also* medicine man.

medicine, socialized *See* socialized medicine.

Medicine, Society for Academic Emergency *See* Society for Academic Emergency Medicine.

Medicine, Society for Adolescent *See* Society for Adolescent Medicine.

Medicine, Society of Behavioral *See* Society of Behavioral Medicine.

Medicine, Society of Critical Care *See* Society of Critical Care Medicine.

Medicine, Society for Experimental Biology and *See* Society for Experimental Biology and Medicine.

Medicine, Society of General Internal *See* Society of General Internal Medicine.

Medicine, Society of Nuclear *See* Society of Nuclear Medicine.

Medicine, Society of Prospective *See* Society of Prospective Medicine.

Medicine, Society of Teachers of Family *See* Society of Teachers of Family Medicine.

medicine, space *See* space medicine.

medicine specialist, neonatal-perinatal *See* neonatal-perinatal medicine specialist.

medicine specialist, pediatric sports *See* pediatric sports medicine specialist.

medicine, sports *See* sports medicine.

medicine, state *See* socialized medicine.

Medicine and Surgery, American Board of Industrial *See* American Board of Industrial Medicine and Surgery.

Medicine and Surgery, American Board of Medical-Legal Analysis in *See* American Board of Medical-Legal Analysis in Medicine and Surgery.

Medicine and Surgery, American Board of Neurological and Orthopaedic *See* American Board of Neurological and Orthopaedic Medicine and Surgery.

Medicine and Surgery, American College of General Practitioners in Osteopathic *See* American College of General Practitioners in Osteopathic Medicine and Surgery.

Medicine and Surgery, American Society of Contemporary *See* American Society of Contemporary Medicine and Surgery.

Medicine and Surgery, American Society for Laser *See* American Society for Laser Medicine and Surgery.

Medicine, Technologist Section of the Society of Nuclear *See* Technologist Section of the Society of Nuclear Medicine.

Medicine Technology Certification Board, Nuclear *See* Nuclear Medicine Technology Certification Board.

medicine therapy, orthomolecular *See* orthomolecular medicine therapy.

medicochirurgic Pertaining to medicine and surgery. *See also* chirurgery; medicine; surgery.

medicolegal Pertaining to medicine and law, especially to topics, such as malpractice, patient consent for services, and patient information. *Synonym:* medical legal. *See also* consent; forensic medicine; malpractice.

Medico-Legal Consultants, American Association of *See* American Association of Medico-Legal Consultants.

medigap policy A health insurance policy sold by private insurance companies designed to supplement Medicare benefits by paying for health services that are not paid by Medicare. *See also* health insurance; Medicare supplement; policy.

MedisGroups *See* Medical Illness Severity Grouping System.

MEDISGRPS *See* Medical Illness Severity Grouping System.

meditation The exercise of the mind in deep reflection or contemplation. *See also* transcendental meditation; yoga.

meditation, transcendental *See* transcendental meditation.

medium *See* culture medium.

MEDLARS *See* Medical Literature Analysis and Retrieval System.

MEDLINE A computerized bibliographic database produced by the National Library of Medicine, containing more than seven million citations, most with abstracts, from over 3,500 biomedical journals and covering the period from 1966 to the present. MEDLINE is accessed by connecting a microcomputer to a larger computer (on-line) or by using CD-ROM. *See also Index Medicus*; Medical Literature Analysis and Retrieval System; Medical Subject Headings; National Library of Medicine.

MEDPAR *See* Medicare Provider Analysis and Review.

MEDTEP *See* Medical Treatment Effectiveness Program.

meeting A gathering of people, as for business purposes. *See also* meeting process; parliamentary procedure; town meeting.

meeting process A method for conducting meetings that includes specific roles and responsibilities for a team leader, a recorder, a timekeeper, team members, and a facilitator or advisor. The steps are: clarify the objective; review roles; review the agenda; work through agenda items; review the meeting record; plan the next agenda and methods; and evaluate. *See also* agenda; meeting; parliamentary procedure; process.

meeting, town *See* town meeting.

megabit In computer science, a unit of storage capacity equal to one million bits. *See also* bit; computer.

megabyte (MB) In computer science, a storage capacity of one million bytes of information. Hard disks of microcomputers generally store 10, 20, or 30 megabytes. *See also* byte; gigabyte.

megadeath One million deaths, a unit of measure used in reference to nuclear warfare.

megadose A very large dose of something, as of a vitamin. *See also* dose; megavitamin.

megalomania Unreasonable conviction of one's own extreme greatness, goodness, or power. The ideas of a megalomaniac are called delusions of grandeur. *See also* delusions of grandeur.

megavitamin Dose of a vitamin(s) that greatly exceeds the amount required to maintain health. *See also* megadose.

melancholia A state of mental dejection, misery, depression, apathy, or withdrawal. *See also* depression.

melanin The dark brown pigment responsible for the color of the skin, eyes, hair, nipples, and other anatomical structures. *See also* melanoma.

melanoma A tumor of melanin-containing cells. *See also* melanin.

melena Abnormal tarry black stool stained with blood pigments and usually resulting from bleeding in the upper gastrointestinal tract. *Compare* hematochezia.

Mellon Foundation, Richard King *See* Richard King Mellon Foundation.

Melpomene Institute for Women's Health Research (MIWHR) A national organization founded in 1981 composed of 1,400 individuals professionally trained in health care, physical activity, and sports for girls and women. It researches and disseminates information on issues, such as body image, osteoporosis, athletic amenorrhea (cessation of menstruation), exercise and pregnancy, and aging.

meltdown A disastrous and uncontrolled event with far-reaching repercussions, especially, in financial jargon, an uncontrolled rapid fall in share values, a crash.

member **1.** A distinct part of a whole or an element of a set. *See also* membership. **2.** A person enrolled in or eligible to receive benefits from a health maintenance organization, Blue Cross plan, or other health insurance plan. *See also* beneficiary; insured; subscriber.

membership The state of being a member, as in membership in a medical specialty society. *See also* member.

Membership Section for Health Care Systems (HCS) A section of the American Hospital Association founded in 1978 composed of 304 health care systems representing 2,572 hospitals. *See also* American Hospital Association; health care system.

membrane Any thin sheet-like layer of tissue lining or enclosing an anatomical structure, or a layer of material acting as a partition or boundary; for example, the meninges. *See also* meninges; mucous membrane.

membrane, mucous *See* mucous membrane.

Membrane Society, North American *See* North American Membrane Society.

memorandum An informal record; a brief note used for communication within an organization, often typed, as in an office memorandum.

memory **1.** The mental faculty of retaining and recalling into consciousness previously experienced ideas and sensations and learned information. *See also* confabulation. **2.** In biology, the persistent modification of behavior resulting from an animal's experience. **3.** The electronic device within a computer where information is stored while being actively worked on. The memory requirements of a computer depend on the software that is used. *See also* computer; core memory; magnetic bubble memory; mind; random access memory; read-only memory; screen memory; short-term memory.

memory, core *See* core memory.

memory, magnetic bubble *See* magnetic bubble memory.

memory, random access *See* random access memory.

memory, read-only *See* read-only memory.

memory, screen *See* screen memory.

memory, short-term *See* short-term memory.

menarche The onset of menstruation (first menstrual period) at puberty. *See also* menses; puberty.

menial Work that is lacking in interest or dignity.

meninges Three connective tissue membranes that protect and enclose the brain and spinal cord, named the dura mater, the arachnoid, and the pia mater. *See also* brain; membrane; meningitis.

meningitis Inflammation of the meninges of the brain and the spinal cord, usually caused by a bacterial or viral infection and characterized by fever, headache, nausea, and stiff neck. *Synonyms:* cerebrospinal meningitis; spinal meningitis. *See also* cerebrospinal fluid; encephalitis; inflammation; lumbar puncture; meninges.

Mennonite Health Association (MHA) A national organization founded in 1952 composed of 800 health and welfare institutions (hospitals, homes for the aging, retirement communities, child welfare homes, and psychiatric centers) and individuals interested in health among Mennonite congregations and Anabaptist denominations. Formerly (1981) Mennonite Health Assembly.

Mennonite Health Assembly *See* Mennonite Health Association.

Men in Nursing, American Assembly for *See* American Assembly for Men in Nursing.

menopausal, post- *See* postmenopausal.

menopause The cessation of ovulation and menstruation, usually between the ages of 45 and 55 years, after which time a woman is unable to become pregnant. *Compare* andropause. *See also* climacteric; hormonal replacement therapy; postmenopausal; premenopausal.

Menopause Society, North American *See* North American Menopause Society.

menses The monthly flow of blood and cellular debris from the uterus that begins at puberty in women and ends at menopause. *Synonyms*: catamenia; menstrual period. *See also* menarche; menopause; puberty.

Men's Health Crisis, Gay *See* Gay Men's Health Crisis.

Menstrual Cycle Research, Society for *See* Society for Menstrual Cycle Research.

menstrual period *See* menses.

menstruation The process of discharging the menses. *See also* amenorrhea; endometriosis; menses; premenstrual syndrome.

mensurable That can be measured, as in mensurable results. *See also* measurable.

mensuration The process of measuring. *See also* measurement.

mental Of or relating to the mind, as in mental illness. *See also* mind.

mental age (MA) The age at which a person functions intellectually, determined by standardized tests. *Compare* chronological age; developmental age. *See also* intelligence quotient; standardized test.

mental anguish A compensable injury embracing all forms of mental pain, as opposed to physical pain, including deep grief, distress, anxiety, and fright. *See also* injury; pain and suffering.

mental disease *See* mental illness.

Mental Disease, Association for Research in Nervous and *See* Association for Research in Nervous and Mental Disease.

mental disorder Any disorder of the mind, such as disturbance of perceptions, memory, emotional equilibrium, thought, or behavior. It may be congenital, genetic, physical, psychological, chemical, or social. *See also* mental illness; mental retardation; mind; psychiatric hospital; psychiatry; psychology.

mental health A state of complete mental wellbeing. *Compare* mental disorder; mental illness.

Mental Health Administration, American College of *See* American College of Mental Health Administration.

Mental Health Administrators, Association of *See* Association of Mental Health Administrators.

Mental Health Association *See* National Mental Health Association.

Mental Health Association, National *See* National Mental Health Association.

Mental Health Care Accreditation Program The survey and accreditation program of the Joint Commission on Accreditation of Healthcare Organizations for eligible mental health care organizations, including the following types: alcohol and substance abuse organizations; community mental health centers; forensic psychiatric services; organizations serving persons with mental retardation and/or other developmental disabilities; and general psychiatric/mental health centers. *See also* accreditation; *Accreditation Manual for Mental Health, Chemical Dependency, and Mental Retardation/Developmental Disabilities Services*; community mental health center; developmental disability; forensic mental health services; Joint Commission on Accreditation of Healthcare Organizations; mental retardation; substance abuse; survey.

mental health center, community *See* community mental health center.

Mental Health Centers, National Council of Community *See* National Council of Community Mental Health Centers.

Mental Health, Chemical Dependency, and Mental Retardation/ Developmental Disabilities Services, Accreditation Manual for *See Accreditation Manual for Mental Health, Chemical Dependency, and Mental Retardation/Developmental Disabilities Services.*

Mental Health Clergy, Association of *See* Association of Mental Health Clergy.

Mental Health Counselors Association, American *See* American Mental Health Counselors Association.

Mental Health Law Project (MHLP) An organization founded in 1972 to clarify, establish, and enforce the legal rights of people with mental retardation and developmental disabilities. It provides technical assistance and training to lawyers, consumers, providers of mental health and special education services, and policymakers at federal, state, and local levels. Staff attorneys have represented individual plaintiffs and leading national consumer and professional associations in landmark lawsuits that have established many rights of people with mental retardation and developmental disabilities. *See also* developmental disability; law; mental retardation.

Mental Health, National Association for *See* National Mental Health Association.

Mental Health, National Association for Rural *See* National Association for Rural Mental Health.

Mental Health, National Institute of *See* National Institute of Mental Health.

mental health nursing *See* psychiatric nursing.

mental health professional Any individual who has completed a training program, has fulfilled academic, accreditation and licensing requirements, and provides mental health services for patients; for example, psychiatrists, psychologists, psychiatric nurses, and clinical social workers. *See also* health professional; mental.

Mental Health Professionals in Corrections, American Association of *See* American Association of Mental Health Professionals in Corrections.

Mental Health Program Directors, National Association of State *See* National Association of State Mental Health Program Directors.

mental health services Diagnosis, treatment, and care of patients with mental disorders. *See also* mental disorder; mental health; forensic mental health services.

Mental Health Services Administration, Substance Abuse and *See* Substance Abuse and Mental Health Services Administration.

mental health services, forensic *See* forensic mental health services.

Mental Health Services, National Consortium for Child *See* National Consortium for Child Mental Health Services.

mental health technician An individual who works with emotionally ill and mentally retarded patients. His or her occupational functions are usually determined by the broad treatment plan designed by a mental health professional. Functions may include providing admission services for patients entering a psychiatric hospital; helping patients carry out basic skills, such as eating, dressing, and personal grooming; supervising group counseling sessions; and teaching social and vocational skills that will help clients function effectively outside the hospital setting. Mental health technicians are differentiated from psychiatric aides by more extensive training and responsibility. *See also* mental health professional; psychiatric aide; technician.

mental hospital *See* psychiatric hospital.

mental illness All forms of illness in which psychologic, intellectual, emotional, or behavioral disturbances are the dominating feature. The term is relative and variable in different cultures, schools of thought, and definitions. *Compare* organic disease. *See also* illness; somatotherapy.

Mental Illness, National Resource Center on Homelessness and *See* National Resource Center on Homelessness and Mental Illness.

mentality **1.** Mental power or capacity, as in the mentality of a toddler. **2.** A way of thought or mental set, as in a physician's mentality.

Mentally Ill, National Alliance for the *See* National Alliance for the Mentally Ill.

Mental and Physical Disability Law, Commission on *See* Commission on Mental and Physical Disability Law.

Mental Research Institute (MRI) An organization founded in 1959 composed of psychiatrists, psychologists, and other professionals skilled in the disciplines related to the behavioral sciences. It conducts research, training, and service programs in the field of human behavior, with emphasis on the family as a social unit. *See also* behavioral medicine; behavioral science.

mental retardation Decreased mental development, adaptive skills, or cognitive functioning that is the result of congenital causes, brain injury, environmental deprivation (cultural-familial retardation), or disease, and is characterized by any of various difficulties, ranging from impaired learning ability to social and vocational limitations. *See also* developmental disability.

Mental Retardation, American Academy on *See* American Academy on Mental Retardation.

Mental Retardation, American Association on *See* American Association on Mental Retardation.

Mental Retardation Association of America (MRAA) A national organization founded in 1974 whose purposes include working for the improvement of the quality of life for persons with mental retardation, promoting research aimed at preventing mental retardation in future generations, and working for adequate national appropriations, supportive legislation, and implementation of statutes and regulations to benefit persons with mental retardation. *See also* mental retardation.

Mental Retardation Program Directors, National Association of State *See* National Association of State Mental Retardation Program Directors.

mentation Any mental activity. *See also* cognition; idea; mind; thought.

mentor A wise and trusted teacher and advisor. *See also* teacher.

menu In computer science, a list of choices that appears on the screen while a particular program is being executed. The menu provides options at that particular step. *See also* computer.

Mercy Medical Airlift (MMA) A nonmembership organization founded in 1984 that provides long-distance air ambulance service to patients whose physicians prescribe recovery or special treatment at a distant location. Beneficiaries include patients in need of medical and nursing care en route to hospitals or other places of continuing care, especially low-income and medically indigent families. It operates an information clearinghouse and air transportation referral services. It conducts an educational program on medical air transportation. *See also* medevac.

mercy killing *See* active euthanasia.

merger The combination of two or more entities into a single entity so that only one of the companies survives as a legal entity. *Compare* consolidation.

merit increase An increase in salary achieved through superior performance on the job. *Synonyms:* merit pay; merit raise.

merit pay *See* merit increase.

merit raise *See* merit increase.

merit rating A system in which employees are rated through a periodic employee evaluation system. The rating is often used as the basis for pay increases and promotion. *See also* employee; merit increase; meritocracy; rating.

meritocracy A system in which advancement is based on individual ability or achievement. *See also* merit rating.

mescaline A toxic and hallucinogenic alkaloid derived from the cactus *Lophophora williamsii*. Intoxication with mescaline induces hallucinations, particularly of music and color. *See also* hallucination; hallucinogen.

MeSH *See* Medical Subject Headings.

Mesmer, Franz Anton (1734-1815) An Austrian who first demonstrated hypnotism (mesmerism) in Vienna in about 1775. *See also* hypnosis; hypnotism.

mesmerism *See* hypnosis.

meta-analysis The process of using statistical methods to combine a large collection of results from individual studies for the purpose of integrating the findings and drawing conclusions. *See also* analysis.

metabolic disease A disorder of the body's normal ability to use food and produce energy; for example, diabetes mellitus is a metabolic disease. *See also* diabetes mellitus; metabolism.

metabolic rate *See* metabolism.

metabolic rate, basal *See* basal metabolic rate.

metabolism Chemical processes in the body, including the use of energy, that are necessary to maintain life. The metabolic rate is customarily expressed in calories as the heat liberated in the course of metabolism. *See also* anabolism; basal metabolic rate; calorie; catabolism; metabolic disease.

metanoia Greek word meaning "penitence, repentance, reorientation of one's way of life, spiritual conversion."

metastasis Spread of a tumor or pathogenic microorganisms (infection) from sites of origin to distant sites, usually through the bloodstream, the lymphatic system, or across a cavity, such as that continued in the peritoneum. *See also* cancer; infection; malignant.

meteorotropism Effects of climate on biological occurrences, such as angina, joint aches and pains, or insomnia. *See also* climatology.

methadone A potent synthetic narcotic drug that is less addictive than morphine or heroin and is used as a substitute for these drugs in addiction treatment programs to alleviate withdrawal symptoms. *See also* heroin; morphine; narcotics.

method An orderly arrangement of steps to accomplish an end, or a way of doing something. *See also* black box method; critical pathway method; experimental method; manner; methodology; scientific method; technique.

method, black box   *See* black box method.

method, critical pathway   *See* critical pathway method.

method, delphi   *See* delphi method.

method, experimental   *See* experimental method.

Methodist Association of Health and Welfare Ministries, United   *See* United Methodist Association of Health and Welfare Ministries.

methodology   The collection or study of methods (practices, procedures, and rules) used by those who work in a discipline or engage in an inquiry, as in the methodology of measuring, assessing, and improving performance. *See also* method; methodology expert.

methodology expert   An individual who has knowledge and experience in a methodology or methodologies and who usually is responsible for organizing and facilitating processes, such as indicator development, in which a certain method is employed. *See also* expert; methodology.

method, scientific   *See* scientific method.

method, Socratic   *See* Socratic method.

Methods Time Measurement Association for Standards and Research   *See* MTM Association for Standards and Research.

method, targeted mortality   *See* targeted mortality method.

"me too" drug   A drug that is identical, similar to, or closely related to a drug for which a new-drug application has already been approved. Many "me too" drugs are copies of approved new drugs and are introduced onto the market by manufacturers without Food and Drug Administration approval, on the belief that the original drug has become generally recognized as safe and effective. Other "me too" products are marketed with abbreviated new-drug applications, which require the submission of manufacturing, bioavailability, and labeling information, but not data relating to safety and effectiveness, which are assumed to be established. *See also* abbreviated new-drug application; generally recognized as safe; generally recognized as effective; new-drug application.

metrics, bio-   *See* biometrics.

metrics, econo-   *See* econometrics.

metrology   The science that deals with measurement.

See also biometrics; econometrics; measurement.

Metropolitan Hospitals, Section for   *See* Section for Metropolitan Hospitals.

metropolitan statistical area   A geographical designation, usually defined as an entire county, that represents an integrated social and economic unit and that contains either: **1.** a city within the area of at least 50,000 population; or **2.** an urban area of at least 50,000 with a total metropolitan population of at least 100,000.

Mexico Border Health Association, United States -   *See* United States - Mexico Border Health Association.

Mexico, Medical Society of the United States and   *See* Medical Society of the United States and Mexico.

MFI   *See* Master Facility Inventory of Hospitals and Institutions.

MGM   *See* Medical Group Missions of the Christian Medical and Dental Society.

MGMA   *See* Medical Group Management Association.

MHA   *See* Master of Health Administration; Master of Hospital Administration; Mennonite Health Association.

MHCA   *See* Managed Health Care Association.

MHIFM   *See* Milton Helpern Institute of Forensic Medicine.

MHLP   *See* Mental Health Law Project.

MHSA   *See* Master of Health Services Administration.

MI   Abbreviation for myocardial infarction (heart attack). *See* acute myocardial infarction.

MIB   *See* Medical Impairment Bureau.

microbe   A microorganism, especially a bacterium, protozoan, or fungus, that causes disease. *See also* bacteria; disease; microorganism.

Microbiological Diagnostic Manufacturers, Association of   *See* Association of Microbiological Diagnostic Manufacturers.

microbiologist   A scientist or physician who specializes in the study of bacteria, viruses, fungi, protozoa, and other microorganisms. *See also* bacteriologist; medical microbiologist; microbiology.

microbiologist, medical   *See* medical microbiologist.

microbiology   The branch of biology dealing with microorganisms, including bacteria, viruses, rickettsiae, fungi, and protozoa, and their effects on other living organisms. *See also* bacteriology; fungus; medical microbiology; virology.

Microbiology, American Academy of   *See* American Academy of Microbiology.

Microbiology, American Society for   *See* American

Society for Microbiology.

microbiology, medical *See* medical microbiology; pathology.

microbiology technologist A medical technologist specializing in performing bacteriological, viral, parasitological, immunologic, and serologic procedures in a clinical laboratory under the supervision of a pathologist or other physician or laboratory director. *See also* medical technologist.

microchip In electronics, a minute slice of a semiconducting material, such as silicon or germanium, processed to have specified electrical characteristics. A computer's microchip (or chip) contains the circuitry and components that perform the computer's functions and serve as its memory. *Synonym:* chip. *See also* computer.

microcircuit An electric circuit consisting of miniaturized components. *See also* circuit.

microcomputer In computer science, a very small computer built around a single integrated circuit (central processing unit) known as a microprocessor and designed to be used by one person at a time. All home and personal computers are microcomputers. *Synonym:* laptop computer. *See also* central processing unit; mainframe computer; microprocessor; pocket computer; portable computer.

microeconomics The study of the behavior of basic economic units, such as companies, industries, or households. Research on hospitals in the health care industry would be a microeconomic concern. *Compare* macroeconomics. *See also* economics.

microfilm A film on which printed materials are photographed at greatly reduced size for ease of storage, as in microfilming x-rays.

Microfilm Associates, Radiological Systems *See* Radiological Systems Microfilm Associates.

microfloppy disk A 3 1/2-inch disk encased in a hard protective envelope. Even though these disks are smaller than standard 5 1/4-inch floppy disk (also called diskette), they have equivalent or greater storage capacity. *See also* diskette.

Micrographic Surgery and Cutaneous Oncology, American College of Mohs *See* American College of Mohs Micrographic Surgery and Cutaneous Oncology.

microorganism A very small organism, usually visible only with a microscope; included among microorganisms are bacteria, viruses, rickettsiae, fungi, and protozoa. *See also* bacteria; fungus;

microbe; organism; protozoa; rickettsiae; virus.

microprocessor In computer science, an integrated circuit that contains the entire central processing unit of a computer on a single chip. *See also* central processing unit; integrated circuit; microchip.

microscope An instrument for producing a magnified image of an object that may be invisible to the unaided eye. *See also* electron microscope; lens; light microscope; objective; operating microscope.

microscope, electron *See* electron microscope.

microscope, light *See* light microscope.

microscope, operating *See* operating microscope.

microscopic Very small and visible only when magnified and illuminated by a microscope. *See also* microscope.

Microscopical Society, American *See* American Microscopical Society.

microscopic anatomy The study of the microscopic structure of tissues and organs, including histology (tissues) and cytology (cells). *Compare* gross anatomy. *See also* anatomy; cytology; histology.

microscopy Use of a microscope to view objects. *See also* electron microscopy; microscope.

microscopy, electron *See* electron microscopy.

Microscopy Society of America (EMSA) A national organization founded in 1942 composed of 4,500 persons interested in the electron microscope, including medical, biological, metallurgical, and polymer research scientists and technicians, and physicists interested in instrument design and improvement. It seeks to increase and disseminate information concerning electron microscopes and related instruments and results obtained through their use. Formerly (1993) Electron Microscopy Society of America. *See also* electron microscopy.

Microsoft disk operating system *See* MS-DOS.

microsurgery Surgery performed using special operating microscopes and miniaturized precision instruments to perform delicate procedures on very small structures, such as parts of the eye. *See also* operating microscope; surgery.

Microsurgery, American Board of Neurological *See* American Board of Neurological Microsurgery.

microtome An instrument for cutting very thin sections of objects for microscopic examination. *See also* paraffin bath; pathology.

micturition *See* urination.

MICU *See* medical intensive care unit; mobile intensive care unit.

midcareer plateau A time in a middle manager's career when opportunities for advancement appear to be blocked by obstacles and the current position provides insufficient challenge. A midcareer plateau is sometimes surmounted by midcareer advancement programs of education and training. *See also* middle manager.

middle age The time of human life between youth and old age, usually the years between ages 40 and 60. *Synonym:* midlife. *See also* age; andropause; climacteric; menopause; midlife crisis.

middle management A group of persons occupying managerial positions between lower and higher executives. *See also* executive; management; middle manager.

middle manager An individual with administrative responsibilities who reports to higher level managers; for example, departmental managers, assistant managers. *See also* manager; midcareer plateau; middle management.

middle-of-the-road Following a course of action between extremes, as in the politician chose the middle-of-the-road approach to the health care reform.

midget A very small person (three standard deviations below mean height for age in a child) who is otherwise normally proportioned. *Compare* giant; gigantism. *See also* dwarf; height.

midlevel The middle stage or level, as in midlevel in performance or at midlevel in a career. *See also* level.

midlife *See* middle age.

midlife crisis A period of psychological doubt and anxiety that some people experience in middle age. *See also* crisis; middle age.

midrange The middle part of a series, a progress, or a data set, as in the values in the midrange. *See also* range.

midwife *See* nurse-midwife.

midwife, certified nurse- *See* certified nurse-midwife.

midwifery The practice of a midwife. *See also* nurse-midwife.

Midwives Alliance of North America (MANA) A group founded in 1982 composed of 900 midwives, student/apprentice midwives, and persons supportive of midwifery. *See also* nurse-midwife.

Midwives, American College of Nurse- *See* American College of Nurse-Midwives.

mifepristone *See* RU-486.

migraine A severe recurring vascular headache of unknown cause, characterized by one-sided, sharp pain and often accompanied by nausea, vomiting, and visual disturbances, such as sensitivity to light. *See also* headache; hemicrania.

Migrant Health Project, East Coast *See* East Coast Migrant Health Project.

milestone A meaningful event that marks completion of some aspect of a project or course of events, as in a milestone in an organization's history or a milestone in the advancement of medicine. *See also* goal; objective; target.

military antishock trousers *See* MAST.

Military Ophthalmologists, Society of *See* Society of Military Ophthalmologists.

Military Orthopaedic Surgeons, Society of *See* Society of Military Orthopaedic Surgeons.

Military Otolaryngologists - Head and Neck Surgeons, Society of *See* Society of Military Otolaryngologists - Head and Neck Surgeons.

Military Surgeons of the United States, Association of *See* Association of Military Surgeons of the United States.

milk The mammary gland's secretion, which is the natural food of very young animals. Human milk has approximately the same fat content as cow's milk, but it contains twice as much carbohydrate and half as much protein. *See also* lactation; mammary gland; raw milk.

Milk Commissions, American Association of Medical *See* American Association of Medical Milk Commissions.

milk, evaporated *See* evaporated milk.

milk of magnesia A white suspension of magnesium hydroxide in water, used as an antacid and a laxative. *See also* antacid; laxative.

milk, raw *See* raw milk.

milk teeth *See* permanent tooth.

Milton Helpern Institute of Forensic Medicine (MHIFM) An organization founded in 1968 composed of 405 individuals who strengthen teaching and research in forensic medicine and forensic pathology. Operated by New York University and the city of New York, it trains postgraduate students, sponsors symposia, and conducts research. *See also* forensic medicine.

mind The human consciousness that originates in the brain and is manifested especially in thought, perception, emotion, will, memory, and imagination. *Synonym*: psyche. *Compare* somatic. *See also* dream; emotion; imagination; memory; perception; presence of mind; thought; will.

MIND *See* Multidisciplinary Institute for Neuropsychological Development.

minded, tough- *See* tough-minded.

mind, presence of *See* presence of mind.

mindset **1.** A mental attitude or frame of mind. **2.** An unthinking assumption or opinion. *See also* mind.

Mineral Research, American Society for Bone and *See* American Society for Bone and Mineral Research.

minicomputer A medium-sized computer processor, between a mainframe and personal computer in both size and processing capability. *See also* computer; mainframe computer; microcomputer.

minimal care unit A unit for treatment of inpatients who are ambulatory and able to meet many of their own daily living needs and require only minimal nursing care. *Synonym*: self-care unit. *See also* unit.

minimal compliance *See* compliance level.

minimax principle A strategy in game theory that is based on reducing to the lowest level the difference between the possible outcomes and the best possible outcome resulting from a decision. The minimax principle is used to select result(s) with the least amount of regret in case of failure. *See also* principle.

minimum The least possible quantity or degree; barely adequate, as in minimum standards. *Compare* maximum. *See also* minimum data set; minimum standard.

minimum data set In health care, a widely agreed-upon set of terms and definitions constituting a core of data acquired for medical records and used for developing statistics suitable for diverse types of analyses and users. Such sets have been developed for ambulatory care, hospital care, and long term care. *Synonym*: uniform basic data set. *See also* data set; hospital discharge abstract system; Uniform Clinical Data Set; Uniform Hospital Discharge Data Set.

minimum standard A statement of acceptable expectations relating to a structure, a process, or an outcome; for example, the US Food and Drug Administration has minimum standards of quality pertaining to the color, tenderness, and allowable freedom from defects permissible for many canned fruits and vegetables. *See also* minimum; standard.

Minimum Standard for Hospitals A one-page document developed in 1917 by the American College of Surgeons in response to the need for a hospital standardization program. *See also* American College of Surgeons; Joint Commission on Accreditation of Healthcare Organizations; minimum standard.

minimum wage The lowest allowable hourly wage permitted by the government or a union contract for an employee performing a particular job. *See also* minimum; wage.

minion **1.** A subordinate. *See also* peon. **2.** An obsequious follower.

Ministries, United Methodist Association of Health and Welfare *See* United Methodist Association of Health and Welfare Ministries.

ministroke *See* transient ischemic attack.

minor **1.** A person who has not yet attained an age required by law (usually between 18 and 21 years, depending on the state) for a particular purpose. For example, a minor is usually legally incompetent to give consent for medical treatment. *See also* emancipated minor; incompetent; legal age; legal guardian; mature minor. **2.** Of lesser importance, as in a minor injury, minor crossmatching, minor surgery. *See also* minor crossmatching; minor surgery.

minor crossmatching The process or act of placing red blood cells of a recipient in a donor's serum. Antiglobulin is added to increase reactivity. The presence of hemolysis or agglutination (clumping together) indicates incompatibility between donor and recipient blood. *Compare* major crossmatching. *See also* blood transfusion; crossmatching.

minor, emancipated *See* emancipated minor.

minority **1.** The smaller in number of two groups forming a whole. **2.** A racial, religious, political, national, or other group regarded as different from the larger group of which it is part.

Minority AIDS Council, National *See* National Minority AIDS Council.

Minority Health Association, National *See* National Minority Health Association.

Minority Health Professions Schools, Association of *See* Association of Minority Health Professions Schools.

minor, mature *See* mature minor.

minor surgery Surgery in which the operative procedure is neither extensive nor hazardous; for example, suturing lacerations and biopsies. *Compare* major surgery. *See also* local anesthesia; operation; surgery.

minutes An official record of what is said and done during a committee or other group meeting. *See also* committee; meeting; paper trail.

miosis Contraction of the pupil. *Compare* mydriasis. *See also* miotic; ophthalmology.

miotic An agent that contracts the pupil. *Compare* mydriatic. *See also* miosis; ophthalmology.

MIPI *See* Medicine in the Public Interest.

miracle **1.** An event, such as an act of healing, that is inexplicable by the laws of nature or science and so is thought to be supernatural in origin or an act of God. **2.** Something that excites admiring awe, as in a miracle drug. *See also* miracle drug.

miracle drug A usually new drug that proves extraordinarily effective, as in penicillin was one of the first miracle drugs. *Synonym:* wonder drug. *See also* drug; miracle.

MIS *See* management information system.

misadventure An unfortunate accident, as in a surgical misadventure. *Synonym:* mishap. *See also* accident; adverse event.

misanthrope A person who hates or mistrusts humankind.

miscarriage **1.** Premature expulsion of a nonviable fetus from the uterus. *Synonym:* spontaneous abortion. *See also* spontaneous abortion. **2.** Mismanagement, as in a miscarriage of justice.

miscommunication Lack of clear or adequate communication, as in the failure to achieve the goal was related to repeated miscommunication between the two parties. *See also* communication.

misconceive To interpret incorrectly or to misunderstand, as in misconceiving the intent of the standard. *See also* misconception.

misconception A mistaken thought, idea, or notion, as in misconceptions about the data. *Synonym:* misunderstanding. *See also* misconceive; mistake.

misdiagnose To assess incorrectly, as in the groin mass was misdiagnosed as a hernia. *See also* diagnosis.

misdiagnosis An incorrect assessment, as in the misdiagnosis resulted in a lawsuit. *See also* diagnosis.

misery index An index combining the costs of taxes, medical care, Social Security, and interest payments. It has been rising for 30 years, from about 24% of personal income in 1963 to its current level just below 40%. *See also* index.

misfile To file in the wrong place or the wrong order, as in misfiling an important document.

mishap *See* misadventure.

misidentify To specify or denote incorrectly, as in the plaintiff misidentified the physician as the one who cared for him. *Compare* identify.

misinform To provide with incorrect data or knowledge, as in the hospital did not intentionally misinform the public. *Compare* inform.

misjudge To estimate wrongly or inaccurately, as misjudging a patient's intentions to commit suicide. *Compare* judge; judgment.

mislead To direct into error of thought or action, especially by intentionally deceiving, as in deliberately misleading the jury. *Compare* lead.

mismanagement Poorly supervised activities in, for example, an organization resulting in failure of the organization to achieve its goals and a considerable waste of resources. *Compare* management.

misnomer An error in naming a person or an object. *See also* name.

misogamy Aversion to, or hatred of, marriage.

misogyny Aversion to, or hatred of, women.

misology Aversion to, or hatred of, reason, argument, or enlightenment.

misperceive To understand or comprehend incorrectly, as in misperceived intentions. *Compare* perceive.

missed abortion Retention in the uterus of an fetus that has been dead for at least eight weeks, indicated by cessation of growth and hardening of the uterus, decreasing uterine size, absence of fetal heart tones after they have been heard, and other finds of fetal death obtained by ultrasonography and other means. *See also* abortion; fetus.

Missing Children, Medical Network for *See* Medical Network for Missing Children.

mission **1.** The stated purpose of an organization, as in mission statement. *See also* mission statement. **2.** A body of persons sent to a foreign land by a religious organization, especially a Christian organization, to spread its faith or provide educational, medical, and other assistance.

Mission Board, Catholic Medical *See* Catholic Medical Mission Board.

Mission Doctors Association (MDA) An organization founded in 1957 that recruits, trains, and supports volunteer Catholic physicians and sends them to serve in third world hospitals or clinics for two to three years. *See also* mission.

Missions, American Leprosy *See* American Leprosy Missions.

Missions of the Christian Medical and Dental Society, Medical Group See Medical Group Missions of the Christian Medical and Dental Society.

mission statement A written expression that sets forth the purpose of an organization (or its component), as in a hospital's mission statement. A mission statement usually precedes the formation of goals and objectives of the organization (or its component). *See also* goal; objective; organization.

mistake **1.** An error or fault resulting from defective judgment, deficient knowledge, or carelessness. **2.** In law, an act or omission arising from ignorance or misconception, which may, depending on its character or the circumstances, justify rescission (vacating, annulling) of a contract or exoneration of a defendant from tort or criminal liability. *See also* misconception; rescission.

mistake of law Ignorance of the legal consequences of one's conduct, though one may be aware of the facts and substance of that conduct. *See also* law; mistake.

mistrial A trial terminated and declared void prior to the return of a verdict, most commonly arising from a deadlock in a jury's deliberations (hung jury), but it may also be due to some extraordinary circumstance, such as death or illness of a necessary juror or of a lawyer. *See also* jury; trial.

misunderstanding *See* misconception.

mittelschmerz Pain in the area of an ovary occurring at the time of ovulation, usually midway in the menstrual cycle. *See also* menses; ovary; ovulation.

MIWHR *See* Melpomene Institute for Women's Health Research.

mix, case *See* case mix.

mixed economy An economic system in which both market forces and government intervention and direction are used to determine resource allocation and prices. The US economy is a mixed economy; although it relies to a great extent upon markets, government also regulates some of the private economy. *See also* economy; laissez faire; mature economy.

mix index, case- *See* case-mix index.

mix management information system, case- *See* case-mix management information system.

mix, patient *See* patient mix.

mix severity, case- *See* case-mix severity.

mixed signals An unclear and confusing message, usually involving two contradicting statements.

MLA *See* Medical Library Association.

MMA *See* Mercy Medical Airlift.

MMSA *See* Medical Mycological Society of the Americas.

MNMC *See* Medical Network for Missing Children.

MO *See* modus operandi.

mobile health unit A mobile facility in which preventive, diagnostic, and therapeutic ambulatory services are provided to a community. *See also* ambulatory health care.

mobile intensive care unit (MICU) An emergency vehicle that is staffed by emergency medical technicians-paramedics and stocked with resuscitation equipment and extensive trauma supplies. *See also* advanced cardiac life support; advanced trauma life support; ambulance; ALS unit; emergency medical technician-paramedic; intensive care unit.

modality A therapeutic method or agent, such as surgery or chemotherapy, that involves the treatment of a disorder. *See also* disorder; therapeutic; therapy.

mode **1.** A measure of central tendency of a collection of data consisting of the measurement of the data set that occurs most often. *Compare* mean; median. *See also* frequency; measures of central tendency. **2.** A way or method of existing or acting, as in the hospital has a specific mode of operation that staff are expected to follow. *See also* modus operandi.

model A copy of something, such as an architectural model, or a person or thing worthy of emulating, such as a model of success. *See also* health belief model; paradigm; paragon.

model, health belief *See* health belief model.

model HMO, network *See* network model HMO.

model HMO, staff *See* staff model HMO.

Model Rules of Professional Conduct Rules adopted by the American Bar Association in 1983, with technical amendments adopted in 1987, which provide terms for resolving ethical problems that arise from "conflict between a lawyer's responsibility to clients, to the legal system and to the lawyer's own interest in remaining an upright person while earning a satisfactory living" (Preamble to the Rules). The adoption of the rules recognizes that the legal profession is largely self-governing, a status that can be maintained only as long as the profession can ensure that its regulations are conceived in the public interest and not in furtherance of self-interested concerns of the bar. These rules replace the former American Bar Association's Code of Professional Responsibility. *See also* American Bar Association.

modem (Modulator-Demodulator) In computer science, a device that links computer systems via telephone lines enabling computers in different locations to exchange information. Modems convert telephone impulses to computer-interpretable impulses. There must be a modem at each end of the communications link to either send or receive converted impulses. *See also* acoustic coupler; computer; on-line searching.

Modernization Committee, Medical Research *See* Medical Research Modernization Committee.

modified radical mastectomy A breast cancer procedure involving removal in a single block, if possible, of the entire breast and often some of the lymph glands under the arm. The chest muscles are left intact. The breast can later be reconstructed with the aid of an implant, utilizing a portion of the skin and underlying fat from a site elsewhere in the body. *Compare* lumpectomy; quadrantectomy. *See also* cancer; implant; mammary gland; mastectomy.

modified survey process An option offered by the Joint Commission on Accreditation of Healthcare Organizations to multihospital systems that own or lease at least two hospitals. The survey includes four components: a corporate orientation, the same survey team, a consecutive survey of participating organizations, and a corporate summation. *See also* accreditation survey; Joint Commission on Accreditation of Healthcare Organizations; multihospital system.

modus operandi (MO) Method of operating or means of accomplishing an end. *See also* mode.

Mohs Micrographic Surgery and Cutaneous Oncology, American College of *See* American College of Mohs Micrographic Surgery and Cutaneous Oncology.

moist gangrene Gangrene following a crushing injury or an obstruction of blood flow by an embolism (clot), tight bandages, or a tourniquet. This form of gangrene has a putrid odor, spreads rapidly, and may, if untreated, result in death in a few days. *See also* dry gangrene; embolism; gangrene.

molecular biology The study of chemical structures and events underlying biological processes, including the relation between genes and the functional characteristics they determine. *See also* biology; molecule.

Molecular Biology, American Society for Biochemistry and *See* American Society for Biochemistry and Molecular Biology.

molecular genetics The branch of genetics dealing with the chemical structure, functions, and replications of the molecules, deoxyribonucleic acid (DNA) and ribonucleic acid (RNA), involved in the transmission of hereditary information. *See also* clinical molecular genetics; deoxyribonucleic acid; genetics; ribonucleic acid.

molecular genetics, clinical *See* clinical molecular genetics.

molecule The smallest portion of a substance that can exist without losing its chemical identity. *See also* molecular genetics.

mom and pop store **1.** A small business that is typically owned and run by members of a family, such as a mom and pop restaurant. **2.** Resembling the small-scale or informal atmosphere of a mom and pop store, as in a large hospital cannot be run like a mom and pop store.

moment of truth A critical or decisive time on which much depends. *See also* truth.

momentum Impetus of a process, such as an idea or a course of events.

monetary Pertaining to money itself, the coins and currency in use, as in a monetary standard. *See also* fiscal; monetary standard.

monetary standard The manner in which a government creates faith in the value and reliability of its currency. *See also* monetary; standard.

money Coined metal, currency, and other commodities recognized by members of an economy as being reliable stores of value and a medium of exchange.

money illusion The illusion that an increase in money income increases purchasing power when, in fact, price increases of similar proportion result in the purchasing power actually remaining the same. *See also* illusion; money.

money income Income measured only in money. It contrasts with real income, which takes into account changes in the purchasing power of money due to inflation or deflation. *See also* income; real income.

moniliasis *See* candidiasis.

monitor **1.** To keep track of systematically with a view to collecting information and keeping a close watch over something, as in monitoring quality of care or admission pattern monitoring. *See also* admission pattern monitoring; monitoring and evaluation. **2.** A tool used to monitor something or someone, as in a quality assurance monitor. *See also* quality assurance monitor; tool. **3.** A video display unit of a computer workstation. A *patient monitor* can be designed for continuous measurement and/or display of particular parameters of physiological function, such as heart rate, arterial blood pressure, arterial oxygen tension, and electrocardiogram. A patient monitor is used for constant surveillance of patients under intensive care, general anesthesia, and other relevant circumstances. *See also* fetal monitor.

monitor, fetal *See* fetal monitor.

monitoring, admission pattern *See* admission pattern monitoring.

monitoring and evaluation A process designed to help health care organizations effectively use their performance measurement, assessment, and improvement resources by focusing on high-priority performance issues. The process includes identifying the most important aspects of the care the organization or its component provides; using indicators to systematically monitor these aspects of care; evaluating of the care when thresholds are approached or reached to identify opportunities for improvement or problems; taking action(s) to improve care or solve problems; evaluating the effectiveness of the action(s); and communicating findings through established channels. *See also* evaluation; monitor.

monitoring, implementation *See* implementation monitoring.

monitoring system, indicator *See* indicator measurement system.

monitoring, transcutaneous oxygen/carbon dioxide *See* transcutaneous oxygen/carbon dioxide monitoring.

monitor, quality assurance *See* quality assurance monitor.

monograph, drug *See* drug monograph.

monopolization Willful acquisition or maintenance of monopoly power is a relevant market. *See also* market; monopoly; monopoly power.

monopolize, attempt to *See* attempt to monopolize.

monopoly Exclusive control of the production and distribution of a product or service by one organization or a group of organizations acting together.

Monopoly is characterized by an absence of competition and often leads to high prices and a general lack of responsiveness to the needs and desires of consumers. The most flagrant monopolistic practices in the United States were outlawed by antitrust laws. *See also* antitrust laws; attempt to monopolize; Clayton Act; monopoly power; perfect monopoly; restraint of trade; Sherman Antitrust Act; trade.

monopoly, perfect *See* perfect monopoly.

monopoly power The ability of a single seller to fix or control prices, or to exclude competition (actual or potential) in a relevant market. *See also* market; monopolization; power.

monopoly, pure *See* perfect monopoly.

monopsony A market situation in which there is only a single consumer of the good produced. *See also* market.

monotonous Tediously repetitious or lacking in variety, as in a monotonous task or monotonous voice.

monozygotic twins *See* identical twins.

mood A pervasive and sustained emotion that, when extreme, can color one's whole view of life. *See also* affect; emotion.

moonlighting Working a second job for additional income. The word derives from the fact that many of these jobs are night jobs.

moot **1.** Subject to debate, arguable, as in a moot point. **2.** Irrelevant or of no practical importance, as in a moot question.

moral *See* morals.

moral hazard A risk to an insurance company resulting from uncertainty about the honesty of the insured, as in the tendency of the insured to spend the insurer's money more readily than he or she would spend his or her own money. For example, extra insurance provided by an employer decreases an employee's motivation to seek out lower cost health care providers. Similarly, supplemental insurance plans defeat the incentives of deductibles and coinsurance for lower utilization. *See also* hazard.

moralistic **1.** Concerned with ideas of right and wrong conduct. **2.** Characterized by a narrow-minded morality. *See also* morality.

morality A system of ideas of right and wrong conduct and how people ought to behave towards one another in order to live in peace and harmony. *See also* moralistic; morals.

moral law The law of behavior underpinning the

morality of a civilization. *See also* law; morality.

moral philosophy   Ethics. *See also* ethics.

morals   A general set of norms or mores from which people derive a sense of right and wrong. *See also* benevolence; morality.

morbid   Diseased, pathologic, or unwholesome, as in morbid thoughts or a morbid condition. *See also* moribund.

morbid anatomist   A pathologist expert in diseased tissues. *See also* pathology.

morbidity   Any subjective or objective departure from a state of physiological or psychological well-being. *Synonyms:* illness; morbid condition; sickness. *See also* comorbidity; complication; expected morbidity; morbidity rate.

morbidity, co-   *See* comorbidity.

morbidity, expected   *See* expected morbidity.

morbidity and mortality conference   In health care organizations, a medical staff conference or meeting, often department-based, in which one or more cases are presented and reviewed because they are unusual or complex, forced difficult management choices, or resulted in unexpected outcomes. Discussions typically cover many topics, such as the value of new technologies, approaches to care that might have been used, or an ethical dilemma presented by the case. Case conferences tend to be highly valued by clinicians as an effective method of learning and are typically conducted in a nonjudgmental atmosphere. They agree with medical training in that they often focus on individual cases. *See also* conference; grand rounds.

morbidity rate   The number of cases of a morbidity or illness in a population divided by the total population at risk for that specific morbidity or illness. *See also* incidence; prevalence; morbidity; rate; risk.

morbidity survey   A method for estimating the prevalence or incidence of disease or diseases in a population. A morbidity survey is usually designed simply to ascertain the facts as to disease distribution, and not to test a hypothesis. *See also* incidence; morbidity; prevalence.

morbid obesity   The condition of weighing two, three, or more, times the ideal weight; so called because it is associated with many serious and life-threatening disorders, such as diabetes mellitus, hypertension, and atherosclerosis. *See also* atherosclerosis; diabetes mellitus; hypertension; obesity.

mores   The accepted traditional customs and usages of a particular social group.

morgue   A place where the bodies of dead persons are temporarily kept for storage (until identified and claimed or until funeral arrangements have been made) and autopsy. *See also* autopsy; diener; mortuary.

moria   An abnormal tendency to joke.

moribund   Approaching death or extinction, as in the patient's moribund condition prompted the physician to call the family to the hospital. *See also* morbid.

morning-after pill   A drug, such as diethylstilbestrol (synthetic estrogen), given after sexual intercourse to prevent implantation of a fertilized ovum. *See also* contraceptive; pill.

morning sickness   Nausea and, sometimes, vomiting in the morning, especially during the first trimester of pregnancy. *See also* sickness.

moron   **1.** An obsolete term for a person with below-average mental functioning. **2.** A person regarded as very stupid.

morphine   A bitter, crystalline alkaloid extracted from opium and used in medicine as an analgesic, a light anesthetic, or a sedative. *See also* endorphin; methadone; morphinism; narcotics; opiate.

morphinism   Addiction to morphine. *See also* addiction; morphine.

morphology   The branch of biology dealing with the form, shape, and structure of organisms without consideration of function. *Compare* function; physiology. *See also* anatomy; biology; structure.

mortality   Death, as in expected mortality or neonatal mortality.

mortality, expected   *See* expected mortality.

mortality method, targeted   *See* targeted mortality method.

mortality, neonatal   *See* neonatal mortality.

mortality rate   The proportion of a population that dies during a specified period. The numerator is the number of persons dying during the period; the denominator is the size of the population, usually estimated as the midyear population. The mortality rate may be expressed as a *crude death rate* (for example total deaths in relation to total population during a year) or as rates specific for diseases and/or conditions, and, sometimes, for age, sex, place of death, and other attributes (for example, number of in-hospital deaths from acute myocardial infarction in relation to all in-hospital deaths, subcategorized by intrahospital location of death). *See also* fatality rate;

hospital mortality rate; infant mortality rate; maternal mortality rate; perinatal mortality.

mortality rate, hospital *See* hospital mortality rate.

mortality rate, infant *See* infant mortality rate.

mortality rate, maternal *See* maternal mortality rate.

mortality rate, neonatal *See* neonatal death rate.

mortality statistics Statistics (numbers) compiled from the information contained in death certificates. The statistics are usually published at regular intervals and may be stratified by age, sex, cause of death, and other variables. *See also* mortality table; statistics; variable.

mortality table A chart showing the rate of death at each age in terms of number of deaths per thousand people. *See also* mortality statistics.

mortician *See* funeral director.

mortuary A place, such as a funeral parlor or a county morgue, where dead bodies are kept awaiting burial. *See also* morgue.

mother, birth *See* birth mother.

mother board The main board of a computer, typically containing the circuitry for the central processing unit, keyboard, and monitor; it may also contain slots for accepting additional circuitry. *See also* computer.

motherhood, surrogate *See* surrogate motherhood.

mother, surrogate *See* surrogate mother.

Motility Society, American *See* American Motility Society.

motion, range of *See* range of motion.

motion sickness Nausea and vomiting caused by movement, as in travel by boat or airplane. *See also* kinesia.

motion study The process of analyzing work in order to determine the cost-efficient motions for performing tasks, developed by Frederick W. Taylor and Frank and Lillian Gilbreth. *Synonyms:* stopwatch study; time and motion study; time-motion study.

motion study, time- *See* time-motion study.

motion study, time and *See* time-motion study.

motivate To provide with an incentive or move to action. *See also* motivation.

motivation 1. The state of being incited or impelled. 2. Something or someone that incites or impels, as in there was little motivation for physicians and hospitals to discharge patients in a timely manner. *See also* field theory of motivation; motivate; motivational research; motivation psychology.

motivational research In advertising and marketing, studies conducted to determine the factors influencing consumer purchases and to assess attitudes toward products and services. *Synonym:* motivation research. *See also* advertise; motivation.

motivation, field theory of *See* field theory of motivation.

motivation psychology The branch of psychology dealing with what conscious and unconscious forces cause human beings and other animals to behave as they do. Motivational psychologists focus on bodily needs, sexual drives, aggression, and emotion. *See also* motivation; motivational research; psychology.

motivation research *See* motivational research.

motive Something that acts as an incitement to action, as in no one questioned her motive for terminating the relationship.

motor aphasia A condition in which an individual, while retaining intelligence and understanding and with the organs of speech unimpaired, is unable to utter articulate words or vocalize the particular word in his or her mind that he or she wishes to use, or utters words different from those he or she intended to speak. *Synonym:* expressive aphasia. *See also* aphasia; cerebrovascular accident; sensory aphasia.

Motorcoach Therapy, National Coalition of Psychiatrists Against *See* National Coalition of Psychiatrists Against Motorcoach Therapy.

mountain sickness Altitude sickness brought on by the diminished oxygen pressure at high elevations resulting in symptoms that include fatigue, dizziness, nausea, shortness of breath, headache, and impaired judgment. *See also* sickness.

mountebank A hawker of quack medicines who attracts customers with stories, jokes, or tricks. *See also* charlatan; quack.

mourn To feel grief or sorrow, as in the family members mourned the death of their loved one. *Synonym:* grieve.

mouse In computer science, a hand-held computer input device, connected by wire to a computer and designed to be moved about on a desk to control the position of the cursor on a monitor and to enter commands. *See also* computer; cursor; input device.

mouth-to-mouth resuscitation A technique used to revive a person who has stopped breathing, in which the rescuer presses his or her mouth against the mouth of the victim and, allowing for passive exhalation, forces air into the lungs at intervals of several seconds. *See also* cardiopulmonary resuscitation; resuscitation.

move According to the Health Security Act recently (1993) introduced to Congress, a change of residence of an individual from one alliance area to another alliance area. *See also* alliance area; Health Security Act; regional alliance.

mover and shaker A person who has a dramatic impact on an organization or a series of events; for example, an individual may be known as a mover and shaker because of her ability to get things done and achieve desired results.

MPA *See* Master of Public Administration.

MPH *See* Master of Public Health.

MRA *See* medical record administrator.

MRAA *See* Mental Retardation Association of America.

MRI *See* magnetic resonance imaging; Medical Records Institute; Mental Research Institute.

MRI scanner *See* magnetic resonance imaging scanner.

MRMC *See* Medical Research Modernization Committee.

MRT *See* medical record technician.

MS-DOS Acronym for Microsoft disk operating system; an operating system used for computers that use central processing units, such as the 8086, 8088, or 80386 microprocessor chip. *See also* disk operating system.

MSMIA *See* Medical and Sports Music Institute of America.

MSN *See* Master of Science in Nursing.

MSO *See* management services organization.

MSUSM *See* Medical Society of the United States and Mexico.

MSW *See* Master of Social Work; medical/hospital social worker.

MT *See* medical technologist.

MTM Association for Standards and Research An organization founded in 1951 composed of 1,000 persons interested in the fields of industrial engineering, industrial psychology, and human engineering. It conducts research on human motion, with emphasis on examining internal velocity, acceleration, tension, and control characteristics of a given motion under several conditions. It also studies external regularities of given groups of motion as they vary under several conditions of performance, and the proper use of motion information in measur-

ing, controlling, and improving manual activities. It conducts research on ergonomics and the effects of workplace environment on productivity. It provides information on fatigue, optimum methods of performance, the effect of practice on motion performance, and the use of motion information for determining allowances and predicting total performance time. Also known as Methods Time Measurement Association for Standards and Research. *See also* engineering psychology; ergonomics; standard.

muckraker An individual who consciously searches for corruption among public officials and other persons and then exposes it to the public. Members of the American Progressive movement of political activists during between 1890 and 1912 were muckrakers who sought to expose graft and corruption. *See also* whistleblower.

mucosa *See* mucous membrane.

mucous Containing or secreting mucus, as in dry mucous membranes showed he was dehydrated. *See also* mucus.

mucous membrane Any of the epithelial linings of the body containing mucus-secreting glands. *Synonym:* mucosa. *See also* membrane; mucous; mucus.

mucus The slippery, viscous substance secreted as a protective lubricant coating by cells and glands of the mucous membranes. *See also* mucous membrane.

multidimensional Having several facets or scopes, as in performance is multidimensional. *See also* dimensions of performance.

multidisciplinary Making use of several branches of knowledge at once, as in a multidisciplinary task force for indicator development. *See also* discipline; interdisciplinary.

Multidisciplinary Institute for Neuropsychological Development (MIND) A national organization founded in 1970 composed of 115 professionals from the fields of education, psychology, law, biomedical engineering, medicine, theology, and human services. It provides a forum for the cooperation of the arts, sciences, and technologies with the professions of law, medicine, and education in the study of human development; promotes the research, diagnosis, and remedy of learning and other disabilities; and encourages the dissemination of knowledge in human perception, communication, and behavior. *See also* disability; neuropsychology.

multifactorial Involving or dependent on several circumstances or elements, as in a multifactorial etiology of a disease. *See also* factor; multiple causation.

multifactorial etiology *See* multiple causation.

multihospital system A central association that owns, leases, or controls, by contract, two or more hospitals. Some of the benefits of such a system are improved availability of capital markets; mutual purchasing for greater economies of scale; and mutual use of technical and management personnel. There are two types of multihospital systems: not-for-profit (which includes church affiliated) and investor-owned (for profit). *Synonym*: hospital chain. *See also* economies of scale; health system; modified survey process; network.

multi-infarct dementia A dementia with a step-wise deteriorating course caused by a series of small strokes. These strokes lead to a patchy distribution of neurologic defects that affect some, and not other, functions. Multi-infarct dementia is caused by cerebrovascular disease. *See also* cerebrovascular accident; dementia.

multimedia The use of several means of communication, such as television, radio, and print, especially for the purpose of advertising or publicity, as in the hospital launched a multimedia advertising campaign to promote its services to the metropolitan community. *See also* media.

multiorganization system survey A survey option of the Joint Commission on Accreditation of Healthcare Organizations that is available to a single corporation or governmental agency that operates or governs two or more health care organizations. The survey includes: a corporate orientation; the use of a single survey team, if feasible; sequential surveys of all organizations within the system; a separate survey, accreditation decision and certificate for each member organization; and a corporate summation conference. *See also* accreditation survey; Joint Commission on Accreditation of Healthcare Organizations.

multiple causation The concept that a given disease or condition or an outcome may have more than one basis or explanation. *Synonym*: multifactorial etiology. *See also* causation; multifactorial.

multiple personality A psychological disorder in which a person exhibits two or more personalities, each functioning as a unique entity with its own memories, behaviors, and relationships. *Synonym*: split personality. *See also* personality.

multiple regression analysis *See* regression analysis.

multiple sclerosis A chronic degenerative disease of the central nervous system in which myelin is gradually destroyed in patches throughout the brain and spinal cord, interfering with the nerve pathways and causing muscular weakness, loss of coordination, and speech and visual disturbances. It occurs mainly in young adults and is thought to be caused by a defect in the immune system that may be of genetic or viral origin. *See also* central nervous system; dementia; myelin.

multiple voting A group decision-making technique designed to reduce a long list to a shorter one. *Synonym*: multivoting.

multispecialty group A medical professional group that includes a minimum of three or more physicians specializing in two or more areas of medicine. *See also* group practice.

multispecialty group practice A group practice in which the practitioners practice different specialties. *Compare* single specialty group practice. *See also* group practice.

multivariate analysis Techniques used when the variation in several variables must be studied simultaneously. In statistics, any analytic method that allows the simultaneous study of two or more dependent variables. *See also* analysis; variable.

multivisceral transplant A transplant in which a recipient receive more than one organ, as in the multivisceral transplant patient received a new stomach, pancreas, liver, small intestine, and large intestine. *See also* transplant; transplantation; viscera.

multivoting *See* multiple voting.

mumps An acute infectious viral disease, mainly of childhood, affecting predominantly the salivary glands (pain and swelling). Occasional complications include orchitis in postpubertal males, pancreatitis, thyroiditis, meningitis, and encephalitis. An attack of mumps usually confers lifelong immunity. *See also* encephalitis; immunity; infectious diseases; inflammation; orchitis; virus.

Munchausen's syndrome A condition in which a person presents himself or herself repeatedly, often to multiple physicians and hospitals, with what appears to be an acute illness, such as crushing chest pain consistent with acute myocardial infarction. The complaints are often realistic and somewhat dramatic in nature, but no clinical evidence of disease is ever found. Named after Hieronymus Karl Friedrich Frieherr Von Munchausen (1720-1797), a German swashbuckler renowned for his mendacious fables of his prowess as a soldier and sportsman. *See also* syndrome.

municipal hospital A hospital that is controlled by an agency of municipal government, for example, Bellevue Hospital in New York City. *Synonym*: city hospital. *See also* hospital.

murder The act of killing a human being intentionally and unlawfully. *See also* forensic medicine.

Murphy's law An administrative aphorism stating that whatever can go wrong, will. The law originated with developmental engineer Ed Murphy in 1949, who was allegedly frustrated by a laboratory technician's error. *See also* law.

muscle The main contractile tissue of the body, consisting of elongated muscle fibers, which on stimulation become shorter and thicker. There are three types of muscle: voluntary (striated) muscle, largely under conscious control; cardiac muscle, which is responsible for the autonomous rhythmic contraction of the heart; and involuntary (smooth) muscle, which causes contractions on the walls of blood vessels and hollow organs, such as the intestines, and which is under control of the autonomic nervous system. *See also* electromyography; myoma; rheumatology; tendon.

Musculoskeletal Medicine, North American Academy of *See* North American Academy of Musculoskeletal Medicine.

Musculoskeletal and Skin Diseases Information Clearinghouse, National Arthritis and *See* National Arthritis and Musculoskeletal and Skin Diseases Information Clearinghouse.

Music Institute of America, Medical and Sports *See* Medical and Sports Music Institute of America.

music therapist An individual who specializes in music therapy. *See also* music therapy; recreational therapy.

Music Therapists, Certification Board for *See* Certification Board for Music Therapists.

music therapy The use of music to achieve the therapeutic goals of symptom relief, emotional integration, and recovery from or adjustment to illness or disability. *See also* art therapy; dance therapy; drama therapy; manual arts therapy; poetry therapy; recreational therapy.

Music Therapy, American Association for *See* American Association for Music Therapy.

Music Therapy, National Association for *See* National Association for Music Therapy.

mutagen An agent, such as ultraviolet light or a radioactive element, that can induce or increase the frequency of mutation in an organism by causing changes in DNA (deoxyribonucleic acid). *See also* deoxyribonucleic acid; mutagenesis; mutation.

mutagenesis The formation or development of a mutation. *See also* mutation.

Mutagen Society, Environmental *See* Environmental Mutagen Society.

mutation An abrupt change in chromosomal deoxyribonucleic acid (DNA). A mutation restricted to a single gene will, by altering its DNA sequence, produce a corresponding alteration in the amino acid sequence of the protein depending on that gene. Most mutations are of this single gene type, but structural alterations in whole chromosomes can also occur. Significant mutations are those that occur in the gametes (sex cells) or their precursor cells, since these mutations will be inherited by offspring. In nature, mutations are rare, random events, which provide the basis for evolution by natural selection. Environmental mutagens can greatly increase the frequency of mutations. *See also* deoxyribonucleic acid; gene; genetics; mutagen; mutagenesis; natural selection.

mute Unable or unwilling to speak. *Synonym*: dumb. *See also* deaf-mute; mutism.

mutism Inability or refusal to speak; dumbness. *See also* deaf-mute; mute.

mutual insurance company An insurance company owned by its policyowners, who elect a board of directors that is responsible for its operation. Profits take the form of policy dividends, or refunds of part of premiums paid, which are distributed to policyowners. *Compare* stock insurance company. *See also* insurance company.

myalgia Pain affecting the muscles. *Compare* arthralgia. *See also* muscle; pain.

Mycological Society of the Americas, Medical *See* Medical Mycological Society of the Americas.

mycology The science and study of fungi. *See also* fungus; mycosis.

mycoplasma A group of the smallest free-living microorganisms known, some of which produce disease in humans, such as mycoplasma pneumonia. *See also* microorganism.

mycosis Any disease caused by a fungus. *See also* fungus; mycology.

mydriasis Dilatation of the pupil. *Compare* miosis.

See also mydriatic; ophthalmology.

mydriatic An agent that dilates the pupil. *Compare* miotic. *See also* mydriasis; ophthalmology.

myelin A fatty substance, consisting of various lipids in combination with protein, that forms the sheath enveloping all larger axons of nerve cells in the nervous system of humans. In demyelinating diseases, such as multiple sclerosis, there is patchy loss of myelin with consequent impairment of neural function. *See also* multiple sclerosis.

myelogram An x-ray of the spinal cord, spinal nerve roots, and subarachnoid space. *See also* meninges; myelography; spinal cord.

myelography A diagnostic imaging procedure in which the spinal cord and subarachnoid space are photographed after injection of a contrast medium. The resulting image is called a myelogram. *See also* myelogram.

myiasis Infestation of living tissues by maggots (larvae). *See also* maggot.

myocardial Pertaining to the heart muscle, as in acute myocardial infarction. *See also* acute myocardial infarction.

myocardial infarction *See* acute myocardial infarction.

myocardium The middle and thickest layer of muscular tissue of the heart. *See also* muscle.

myoma A tumor arising from muscle tissue. *See also* adenoma; lipoma; muscle; neurinoma.

myopia *See* nearsighted.

mysophobia An abnormal fear of dirt or contamination. *See also* phobia.

myth **1.** An ancient story dealing with supernatural beings, ancestors, or heroes that serves as an archetype in the world view of a people, explaining aspects of the natural world or delineating the psychology, customs, or ideals of society, as in the creation myth. **2.** A fiction or half-truth, especially one that forms part of an ideology, as in the administrator acted quickly to dispel the myth. *See also* belief.

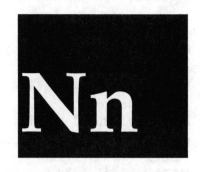

Nn

NAAAA *See* National Association of Area Agencies on Aging.

NAACLS *See* National Accrediting Agency for Clinical Laboratory Sciences.

NAACOG: The Organization For Obstetric, Gynecologic, and Neonatal Nurses *See* Association of Women's Health, Obstetric, and Neonatal Nurses.

NAADAC *See* National Association of Alcoholism and Drug Abuse Counselors.

NAAHP *See* National Association of Advisors for the Health Professions.

NAAMM *See* North American Academy of Musculoskeletal Medicine.

NAANGHT *See* National Association of Air National Guard Health Technicians.

NAAP National Association of Activity Professionals; National Association of Apnea Professionals.

NAAPABAC *See* National Association for the Advancement of Psychoanalysis and the American Boards for Accreditation and Certification.

NAATP *See* National Association of Addiction Treatment Providers.

NAB *See* National Association of Boards of Examiners for Nursing Home Administrators.

NABCO *See* National Alliance of Breast Cancer Organizations.

NABP *See* National Association of Boards of Pharmacy.

NABR *See* National Association for Biomedical Research.

NABSW *See* National Association of Black Social Workers.

NABWA *See* National Association of Black Women Attorneys.

NAC *See* CDC National AIDS Clearinghouse.

NACA *See* National Association of Childbirth Assistants.

NACC *See* National Association of Childbearing Centers; National Association of Counsel for Children.

NACDS *See* National Association of Chain Drug Stores.

NACEHSP *See* National Accreditation Council for Environmental Health Science and Protection.

NACFT *See* National Academy of Counselors and Family Therapists.

NACHC *See* National Association of Community Health Centers.

NACHFA *See* National Association of County Health Facility Administrators.

NACHO *See* National Association of County Health Officials.

NACHRI *See* National Association of Children's Hospitals and Related Institutions.

NAD *See* National Association of the Deaf.

NADA *See* National Association of Dental Assistants.

NADAP *See* National Association on Drug Abuse Problems.

NADDC *See* National Association of Developmental Disabilities Councils.

NADE *See* National Association of Disability Examiners.

NADEP *See* National Association of Disability Evaluating Professionals.

NADL *See* National Association of Dental Laboratories.

NADONA/LTC *See* National Association of Directors of Nursing Administration in Long Term Care.

NADT *See* National Association for Drama Therapy.

NAEHCA *See* National Association of Employers on Health Care Action.

NAEMSP *See* National Association of Emergency

Medical Service Physicians.

NAEMT *See* National Association of Emergency Medical Technicians.

NAER *See* National Association of Executive Recruiters.

NAF *See* National Abortion Federation.

NAFAC *See* National Association for Ambulatory Care.

NAFAR *See* National Association of First Responders.

NAHAM *See* National Association of Healthcare Access Management.

NAHC *See* National Association for Home Care.

NAHCR *See* National Association for Healthcare Recruitment.

NAHCS *See* National Association of Health Career Schools.

NAHDO *See* National Association of Health Data Organizations.

NAHHH *See* National Association of Hospital Hospitality Houses.

NAHN *See* National Association of Hispanic Nurses.

NAHQ *See* National Association for Healthcare Quality.

NAHSC *See* National Association of Homes and Services for Children.

NAHSE *See* National Association of Health Services Executives.

NAHU *See* National Association of Health Underwriters.

NAHUC *See* National Association of Health Unit Coordinators.

NALGAP *See* National Association of Lesbian/Gay Alcoholism Professionals.

NAMCP *See* National Association of Managed Care Physicians.

name A word or words used to designate a unique entity and distinguish it from other entities, as in generic name. *See also* brand name; chemical name; established name; generic name; misnomer; proprietary name; trademark.

NAME *See* National Association of Medical Examiners.

name, brand *See* brand name.

name, chemical *See* chemical name.

named insured A holder of an insurance policy whose name appears on the insurance policy. *See also* insured.

name, established *See* established name.

name, generic *See* generic name.

name, proprietary *See* proprietary name.

NAMES *See* National Association of Medical Equipment Suppliers.

Names, United States Adopted *See* United States Adopted Names.

NAMI *See* National Alliance for the Mentally Ill.

NAMO *See* National Association of Manufacturing Opticians.

NAMP *See* National Association of Meal Programs.

NAMS *See* North American Membrane Society; North American Menopause Society.

NAMSIC *See* National Arthritis and Musculoskeletal and Skin Diseases Information Clearinghouse.

NAMSS *See* National Association Medical Staff Services.

NAMT *See* National Association for Music Therapy.

NAN *See* National Academy of Neuropsychology.

NANASP *See* National Association of Nutrition and Aging Services Programs.

NANDA *See* North American Nursing Diagnosis Association.

NANN *See* National Association of Neonatal Nurses.

NANPRH *See* National Association of Nurse Practitioners in Reproductive Health.

NANR *See* National Association for Nursing Research.

NAO *See* National Academy of Opticianry.

NAON *See* National Association of Orthopaedic Nurses.

NAOO *See* National Association of Optometrists and Opticians.

NAOSW *See* National Association of Oncology Social Workers.

NAOT *See* National Association of Orthopaedic Technologists.

NAPARE *See* National Association for Perinatal Addiction Research and Education.

NAPC *See* National Assault Prevention Center.

NAPCRG *See* North American Primary Care Research Group.

NAPCWA *See* National Association of Public Child Welfare Administrators.

NAPGCM *See* National Association of Private Geriatric Care Managers.

NAPH *See* National Association of Public Hospitals.

NAPM *See* National Association of Pharmaceutical Manufacturers.

NAPN *See* National Association of Physician Nurses.

NAPNAP *See* National Association of Pediatric Nurse Associates and Practitioners.

NAPNES *See* National Association for Practical Nurse Education and Service.

NAPPH *See* National Association of Private Psychiatric Hospitals.

NAPR *See* National Association of Physician Recruiters.

Naprapathic Association, American *See* American Naprapathic Association.

naprapathy A system of medicine based on the theory that many diseases result from the displacement of connective tissues, such as tendons and ligaments, and that manipulation of these tissues, as well as dietary measures, will bring relief. *Compare* allopathy; homeopathy; naturopathy; osteopathic medicine.

NAPRR *See* National Association of Private Residential Resources.

NAPT *See* National Association for Poetry Therapy.

NAPTCC *See* National Association of Psychiatric Treatment Centers for Children.

narcissism An abnormal interest in and love of oneself, especially one's body. In psychoanalytic theory, sexual self-interest that is normal in young children but abnormal in adults. *See also* hedonism; narcissistic personality disorder; Narcissus.

narcissistic personality disorder A mental disorder characterized by excessive self-love and self-absorption, unrealistic views about one's own attributes, and little regard for other people. In some cases there is an exaggerated need for attention, preoccupation with grooming, and self-consciousness. *See also* narcissism; personality disorder.

Narcissus In Greek mythology, a youth who pined away in love for his own image in a pool of water and was transformed into the flower that bears his name. *See also* narcissism.

narcoanalysis Psychoanalysis assisted by the administration of a drug (usually a short-acting barbiturate), which causes mental disinhibition and facilitates expression of thoughts, ideas, and memories. *See also* analysis.

narcolepsy A syndrome characterized by an uncontrollable desire to sleep, sudden sleep attacks lasting from a few minutes to a few hours, episodes of momentary loss of muscle tone, and occasionally visual hallucinations before sleep. The lifelong condition usually begins in adolescence. *See also* syndrome.

narcosis A state of stupor or insensibility produced by drugs or other agents that depress the central nervous system. *See also* central nervous system; narcotics; nitrogen narcosis.

narcosis, nitrogen *See* nitrogen narcosis.

Narcotic Act, Harrison Anti- *See* Harrison Antinarcotic Act.

narcotics Any drug, as set out in the Comprehensive Drug Abuse Prevention and Control Act of 1970, produced directly or indirectly by extraction from substances of vegetable origin, or independently by means of chemical synthesis, or by a combination of extraction and chemical synthesis. The opiates are narcotics derived from the opium poppy plant and include opium, heroin, morphine, and codeine. The non-opiate synthetic narcotics include demerol and methadone. Narcotics are used clinically as painkillers and, outside of medicine, to produce euphoria. All narcotics are physically and psychologically addicting, with the likelihood of addiction depending on the drug, the frequency and duration of its use, and its dosage. *See also* controlled substances; heroin; junkie; methadone; morphine; narcosis; opiate; opium.

narcotism Addiction to narcotics, such as opium, heroin, or morphine. *See also* narcosis; narcotics.

NARD A national organization founded in 1898 composed of 30,000 owners and managers of independent drugstores and pharmacists employed in retail drugstores offering pharmacy services. It provides support for undergraduate pharmacy education through the National Association of Retail Druggists Foundation. Formerly (1988) National Association of Retail Druggists. *See also* druggist; drugstore; pharmacy.

NARF *See* National Association of Rehabilitation Facilities.

NARI *See* National Association of Rehabilitation Instructors; National Association of Residents and Interns.

NARIC *See* National Rehabilitation Information Center.

NARMH *See* National Association for Rural Mental Health.

NARN *See* National Association of Registered Nurses.

NARO *See* National Association of Reimbursement Officers.

NARPPS *See* National Association of Rehabilitation Professionals in the Private Sector.

NARS *See* National Association of Rehabilitation

Secretaries.

NAS *See* National Academy of Sciences.

NASADAD *See* National Association of State Alcohol and Drug Abuse Directors.

NASAHOE *See* National Association of Supervisors and Administrators of Health Occupations Education.

NASAR *See* National Association for Search and Rescue.

NASCD *See* National Association for Sickle Cell Disease.

NASDAD *See* National Association of Seventh Day Adventist Dentists.

NASDT *See* North American Society for Dialysis and Transplantation.

NASEMSD *See* National Association of State EMS Directors.

NASLI *See* National Association for Senior Living Industries.

NASMHPD *See* National Association of State Mental Health Program Directors.

NASMRPD *See* National Association of State Mental Retardation Program Directors.

NASN *See* National Association of School Nurses.

nasogastric Within or through the nasal passages and the stomach, as in nasogastric intubation. *See also* nasogastric feeding; nasogastric intubation.

nasogastric tube *See* nutritional support.

nasogastric feeding The process of delivering nutrients in liquid form through a tube passed into the stomach through the nose; used when a person can digest food but cannot eat. *See also* enteral formula; nutritional support.

nasogastric intubation The process of inserting a tube through the nose into the esophagus and stomach to provide a passageway to the stomach for feeding, suction, or other needs. *See also* intubation; nasogastric.

nasotracheal Within or through the nasal passages and the trachea, as in nasotracheal intubation. *See also* nasotracheal intubation.

nasotracheal intubation The process of inserting a tube through the nose into the trachea to provide an airway or to administer anesthetics. *See also* endotracheal intubation; intubation.

NASP *See* National Association of School Psychologists.

NASPE *See* North American Society of Pacing and Electrophysiology.

NASPGN *See* North American Society for Pediatric Gastroenterology and Nutrition.

NASPSPA *See* North American Society for the Psychology of Sport and Physical Activity.

NASS *See* North American Spine Society.

NASUA *See* National Association of State Units on Aging.

NASW *See* National Association of Social Workers.

NATA *See* National Athletic Trainers Association.

natal Pertaining to birth, as in prenatal, perinatal, neonatal. *See also* neonatal; perinatal; prenatal.

natal, ante- *See* prenatal.

natal, peri- *See* perinatal.

natal, post- *See* postnatal.

natal, pre- *See* prenatal.

NATCO *See* North American Transplant Coordinators Organization.

National Abortion Federation (NAF) A national organization founded in 1977 composed of 300 abortion service providers, including physician offices, clinics, feminist health centers, planned parenthood affiliates, and other individuals committed to making safe, legal abortions accessible to all women. It offers information on medical, legal, and social aspects of abortion and sets standards for abortion care. *See also* abortion.

National Academy of Counselors and Family Therapists (NACFT) A national organization founded in 1972 composed of psychologists, physicians, lawyers, counselors, psychiatrists, teachers, clergy, and social workers interested in strengthening family life through competent family counseling, family life education, and legislative activity for the good of the family unit. It accredits, among other activities, clinicians and family life educators. *See also* counseling; counselor; family life education; family therapy.

National Academy of Neuropsychology (NAN) A national organization founded in 1978 composed of 1,500 clinical neuropsychologists interested in preserving and advancing knowledge about the assessment and treatment of neuropsychological disorders. *See also* neuropsychology; psychology.

National Academy of Opticianry (NAO) A national organization founded in 1973 composed of 6,000 opticians. It offers review courses for national certification and state licensure examinations to members. *See also* certification; licensure; opticianry.

National Academy of Sciences (NAS) A private, honorary organization founded in 1863 composed of

1,540 members elected in recognition of their contributions to either science or engineering. NAS was founded by an act of Congress to serve as official adviser to the federal government on scientific and technical matters. *See also* Food and Nutrition Board; Institute of Medicine; science.

National Academy of Social Insurance An organization founded in 1986 composed of 314 experts on social insurance, including Social Security, health care financing, disability, workers' compensation, and unemployment. It furthers research and education in social security and related programs and offers seminars and workshops. *See also* disability insurance; social insurance; Social Security; unemployment insurance; workers' compensation.

national account In insurance, a group of insured persons or organizations having members in localities in more than one state who are all served by the same insurance or prepayment plan. *See also* account; Blue Cross and Blue Shield Association.

National Accreditation Association and the American Examining Board of Psychoanalysis *See* National Association for the Advancement of Psychoanalysis and the American Boards for Accreditation and Certification.

National Accreditation Commission for Schools and Colleges of Acupuncture and Oriental Medicine A national organization founded in 1982 by the National Council of Acupuncture Schools and Colleges composed of 14 members of the acupuncture community and other individuals representing the public interest. It evaluates schools and colleges of acupuncture and Oriental medicine to establish and maintain high educational standards and ethical business practices. *See also* acupuncture.

National Accreditation Council for Environmental Health Curricula *See* National Accreditation Council for Environmental Health Science and Protection.

National Accreditation Council for Environmental Health Science and Protection (NACEHSP) A national accrediting body founded in 1969 to establish a system for accreditation of environmental health curricula and related procedures and to carry out other responsibilities essential to the accreditation of academic programs leading to associate degrees, baccalaureate degrees, and graduate degrees in environmental health. Formerly (1993) National Accreditation Council for Environmental Health Curricula. *See also* accreditation; environmental health.

National Accrediting Agency for Clinical Laboratory Sciences (NAACLS) A national accrediting body founded in 1973 that accredits 734 hospitals, colleges, and universities in the allied health professions of medical technologist, medical laboratory technician, and histologic technologist in cooperation with the Committee on Allied Health Education and Accreditation. The organization establishes standards and determines which programs meet standards through self evaluation and on-site surveys. *See also* allied health professional; Committee on Allied Health Education and Accreditation; histologic technologist; medical laboratory technician; medical technologist.

National Advisory Council for Health Care Policy, Research, and Evaluation A component of the Agency for Health Care Policy and Research that acts as a policy-making, priority-setting body for the agency in conjunction with the Department of Health and Human Services Secretary. *See also* Agency for Health Care Policy and Research; Department of Health and Human Services.

National Affairs, Bureau of *See* Bureau of National Affairs.

National AIDS Clearinghouse, CDC *See* CDC National AIDS Clearinghouse.

National AIDS Information Clearinghouse *See* CDC National AIDS Clearinghouse.

National Alliance of Breast Cancer Organizations (NABCO) A national organization founded in 1986 composed of 250 breast centers, hospitals, government health offices, and support and research organizations providing information about breast cancer and breast diseases from early detection through continuing care. *See also* cancer; mammary gland.

National Alliance for the Mentally Ill (NAMI) A national organization founded in 1979 composed of 130,000 individuals and 1,000 self-help/advocacy groups interested in severe and chronic mentally ill persons. Its objectives are to provide emotional support and practical guidance to families and to educate and inform the public about mental illness. *See also* mental illness.

National Arthritis and Musculoskeletal and Skin Diseases Information Clearinghouse (NAMSIC) A national clearinghouse that collects, publishes, and disseminates professional and public educational materials for persons interested in arthritis and musculoskeletal and skin diseases. *See also* arthritis; clearinghouse.

National Assault Prevention Center (NAPC) A national organization founded in 1985 interested in preventing interpersonal violence against vulnerable populations through education, prevention training, and research. It provides services to children and adults with mental retardation and developmental disabilities, and conducts research on the causes, consequences, and prevention of interpersonal violence. *See also* violence.

National Assembly of National Voluntary Health and Social Welfare Organizations A national organization founded in 1923 composed of 36 national voluntary health and social welfare agencies interested in increasing the impact of the individual agencies and of voluntarism on human needs.

National Association of Activity Professionals (NAAP) A national organization founded in 1981 composed of 2,500 therapists, activity directors, and activity consultants in nursing homes, senior centers, retirement housing, or adult day care programs. It has set standards and established a certification process. *See also* activity professional; certification.

National Association of Addiction Treatment Providers (NAATP) A national organization founded in 1978 composed of 660 corporate and private institutional alcohol and/or drug dependency treatment facilities. It promotes awareness of chemical dependency as a treatable disease. Formerly (1987) National Association of Alcoholism Treatment Programs. *See also* addiction; chemical dependency.

National Association for the Advancement of Psychoanalysis and the American Boards for Accreditation and Certification (NAAPABAC) An organization founded in 1972 composed of 1,466 psychoanalytic training institutes and individual psychoanalysts from many schools of psychoanalytic thought interested in the advancement of psychoanalysis as a profession. It establishes standards for training and accredits psychoanalytic training institutes that may train physicians, psychologists, social workers, counselors, and other persons. It sets standards for certification of psychoanalysts and psychoanalytic psychotherapists and certifies those who have met its standards. Formerly (1981) National Accreditation Association and the Ameri-

can Examining Board of Psychoanalysis. *See also* accreditation; certification; psychoanalysis.

National Association of Advisors for the Health Professions (NAAHP) A national organization founded in 1974 composed of 1,275 college and university faculty who advise and counsel students on health careers. *See also* health professional.

National Association of Air National Guard Health Technicians (NAANGHT) A national organization founded in 1974 composed of 350 members interested in providing more effective medical services in Federal Air National Guard health facilities through interchange of ideas and dissemination of information.

National Association for Alcoholism Counselors *See* National Association of Alcoholism and Drug Abuse Counselors.

National Association of Alcoholism and Drug Abuse Counselors (NAADAC) A national organization founded in 1972 composed of 13,000 counselors in alcoholism and drug abuse treatment. It provides national representation, education, and promotion of accreditation and standards. Formerly (1982) National Association for Alcoholism Counselors. *See also* alcoholism; counselor; drug abuse.

National Association of Alcoholism Treatment Programs *See* National Association of Addiction Treatment Providers.

National Association for Ambulatory Care (NAFAC) A national organization founded in 1981 composed of 600 representatives of hospital, corporate, and independently owned ambulatory care centers. Formerly (1981) National Association of Centers for Urgent Treatment; (1984) National Association of Freestanding Emergency Centers. *See also* ambulatory health care.

National Association of Apnea Professionals (NAAP) A national organization founded in 1987 composed of 250 physicians, nurses, respiratory therapists, social workers, polysomnographers, and manufacturers and suppliers of apnea equipment. It gathers scientific and clinical information about causes and treatments of apnea and related sleep disorders and compiles statistics. *See also* apnea.

National Association of Area Agencies on Aging (NAAAA) A national organization founded in 1975 composed of 665 Area Agencies on Aging, established under the provision of the Older Americans Act of 1965. It seeks to promote and achieve a reasonable and realistic national policy on aging and acts as an advocate for the needs of older persons at the national level. *See also* aging.

National Association for Biomedical Research (NABR) A national organization founded in 1985 composed of 400 universities, research institutes, professional societies, voluntary health agencies, animal breeders and suppliers, and pharmaceutical, chemical, and testing companies that use laboratory animals for biomedical research and testing. It monitors and, when appropriate, attempts to influence legislation and regulations on behalf of members who are dependent on animals for biomedical research and testing. Formerly (1981) Research Animal Alliance. *See also* biomedical; research.

National Association of Black Social Workers (NABSW) A national organization founded in 1968 composed of 10,000 social workers and other concerned individuals who support community welfare projects and programs that will serve the interests of the black community and aid it in controlling its social institutions. *See also* social worker.

National Association of Black Women Attorneys (NABWA) A national organization founded in 1972 composed of black women who are members of the bar of any US state or territory, and associate members who include law school graduates, paralegals, and law students. It seeks to advance jurisprudence and the administration of justice by increasing the opportunities of black and nonblack women at all levels and to aid in protecting the civil and human rights of all citizens and residents of the United States. *See also* attorney; bar; lawyer.

National Association of Blue Shield Plans *See* Blue Cross and Blue Shield Association.

National Association of Boards of Examiners for Nursing Home Administrators (NAB) A national organization founded in 1972 composed of 51 state boards responsible for licensing nursing homes. It produces an examination to test the competence of nursing home administrators. *See also* nursing home; nursing home administrator.

National Association of Boards of Pharmacy (NABP) A national organization founded in 1904 composed of the pharmacy boards of US 50 states; the District of Columbia; Puerto Rico; Virgin Islands; the Canadian provinces of Alberta, Ontario, and British Columbia; and the state of Victoria, Australia. Its activities include sponsoring a uniform licensure examination, providing for interstate reci-

procity in pharmaceutic licensure based upon a uniform minimum standard of pharmaceutic education and uniform legislation, and providing legislative information and education. *See also* licensure; minimum standard; pharmacy; reciprocity; specialty boards.

National Association of Chain Drug Stores (NACDS) A national organization founded in 1933 composed of 1,055 chain drug retailers and associate members including manufacturers, suppliers, manufacturers' representatives, publishers, and advertising agencies. It interprets actions by government agencies in such areas as drugs, public health, federal trade, labor, and excise taxes. Its programs include NACDS/Merck, Sharp, Dohme; Cornell Executive Management; NACDS/Johnson & Johnson Performance Analysis Report; and Phocust (Pharmacists' Opportunities in Compliance Using Skills Training). *See also* drugstore; pharmacy.

National Association of Childbearing Centers (NACC) A national organization founded in 1983 composed of 400 birth centers and individuals and businesses interested in childbirth centers. It acts as a national information service of freestanding birth centers for state health departments, insurance companies, government agencies, consultants, hospitals, physicians, certified nurse-midwives, nurses, and families. It promotes quality care in freestanding birth centers through state licensure and national standard-setting mechanisms, educational workshops, and support of professional education for midwives. It provides standards for certification of birth centers. *See also* certification; childbirth center; nurse-midwife.

National Association of Childbirth Assistants (NACA) A national organization founded in 1985 composed of childbirth assistants. It provides information, resources, and referrals to childbearing families; conducts training workshops; and awards childbirth assistant certification. *See also* certification; childbirth.

National Association of Children's Hospitals and Related Institutions (NACHRI) A national organization founded in 1968 composed of 110 children's hospitals and related institutions whose programs are clinical, as opposed to social or custodial. Its purposes include promoting the quality of child health care through the dissemination of information, the promotion of research and education programs, and participating in charitable, scientific, and educational endeavors. *See also* children's hospital.

National Association of Community Health Centers (NACHC)   A national organization founded in 1970 composed of 950 ambulatory health care centers, administrators, clinicians, and consumers interested in continuing the growth and development of community-based health care delivery programs for medically underserved populations. *See also* community health center; medically underserved area; medically underserved population.

National Association of Counsel for Children (NACC)   A national organization founded in 1977 composed of 1,500 lawyers, judges, physicians, mental health professionals, social workers, court-appointed advocates, volunteers, and other individuals interested in improving legal representation of children. *See also* counsel.

National Association of County Health Facility Administrators (NACHFA)   A national organization founded in 1977 composed of 250 elected local officials and administrators of freestanding and hospital-based long term care facilities owned and operated by county governments or city-county consolidations. *See also* administrator; long term care facility.

National Association of County Health Officials (NACHO)   A national organization founded in 1965 composed of 2,000 county health officials interested in stimulating and contributing to the improvement of county health programs and public health practices throughout the United States. It operates a Primary Care Project, which helps to strengthen the link between local health departments and community health centers. *See also* official; public health.

National Association of the Deaf (NAD)   A national organization founded in 1880 composed of 20,000 adult deaf persons, parents of deaf children, professionals and students in the field of deafness, and organizations of and for deaf people. It protects the civil rights of the deaf in the areas of employment, elimination of communication barriers, and full citizenship benefits and obligations. Another activity is screening films and recommending which films should be captioned for hearing-impaired viewers. *See also* deafness; hearing impaired.

National Association of Dental Assistants (NADA)   A national organization founded in 1974 composed

of 4,000 dental auxiliaries. *See also* dental assistant; dental assisting.

National Association of Dental Laboratories (NADL)   A national organization founded in 1951 composed of 3,100 commercial dental laboratories, industry manufacturers and suppliers, and schools of dental technology. The association provides management seminars and a basic laboratory technician's training program. *See also* dental laboratory technician.

National Association of Dental Service Plans   *See* Delta Dental Plans Association.

National Association of Developmental Disabilities Councils (NADDC)   A national organization founded in 1975 composed of 54 state and territorial councils interested in improving the lives of developmentally disabled people. It promotes cooperation and communication among federal agencies, state governments, volunteer groups and other organizations, and individual state and territorial councils. It educates and informs the public about the needs of developmentally disabled people. *See also* developmental disability.

National Association of Directors of Nursing Administration in Long Term Care (NADONA/ LTC)   A national organization founded in 1986 composed of 1,700 directors, assistant directors, and former directors of nursing in long term care. Its goals include creating and establishing an acceptable ethical standard for practices in long term care nursing administration; developing and providing programs of education and certification for the positions of director, associate director, and assistant director; and promoting a positive image of the long term health care industry. *See also* administration; certification; long term care; nursing.

National Association of Disability Evaluating Professionals (NADEP)   A national organization founded in 1984 composed of 1,000 lawyers, doctors, psychologists, employers, and other individuals interested or involved in disability claims process, evaluation, and case management. It provides a forum for the exchange of information and functions as the membership division of the American Disability Evaluation Research Institute. *See also* disability.

National Association of Disability Examiners (NADE)   A national organization founded in 1963 composed of 2,373 disability claims examiners, attorneys, and physicians involved in determining the eligibility of applicants for social security benefits based on disability. *See also* disability.

National Association for Drama Therapy (NADT) A national association founded in 1979 composed of 325 individuals trained in the therapeutic applications of creative drama and theater and other persons trained in psychotherapy, rehabilitation, and education. *See also* drama therapy.

National Association on Drug Abuse Problems (NADAP) A national organization founded in 1971 sponsored by business and labor organizations. It serves as an information clearinghouse and referral bureau for corporations and local communities interested in prevention of substance abuse and treatment of substance abusers. *See also* drug abuse; substance abuse.

National Association of Emergency Medical Service Physicians (NAEMSP) A national organization founded in 1983 composed of 700 physicians, medical students, and other persons in the health care profession involved in emergency medical services. It acts as a forum for debate and discussion of issues relating to emergency medical services as an important facet of medical care and of the problems and responsibilities of emergency medical services physicians and related personnel. It supports research and development in the area of prehospital emergency care. *Synonym:* National Association of EMS Physicians. *See also* emergency medical services system; emergency physician.

National Association of Emergency Medical Technicians (NAEMT) A national organization founded in 1975 composed of 4,000 nationally registered or state certified emergency medical technicians (EMTs). It promotes the professional status of emergency medical technicians and national acceptance of a uniform standard of recognition for their skills. It encourages constant upgrading of these skills and qualifications and educational requirements. *See also* emergency medical technician; emergency medical technician-paramedic.

National Association of Employers on Health Care Action (NAEHCA) A national organization founded in 1976 composed of corporations and public and private organizations concerned with health care management, delivery, and cost and quality assurance. Formerly (1980) National Association of Employers on Health Maintenance Organizations;

(1987) National Association of Employers on Health Care Alternatives.

National Association of Employers on Health Care Alternatives *See* National Association of Employers on Health Care Action.

National Association of Employers on Health Maintenance Organizations *See* National Association of Employers on Health Care Action.

National Association of EMS Physicians *See* National Association of Emergency Medical Service Physicians.

National Association of Executive Recruiters (NAER) A national organization founded in 1984 composed of 125 executive recruitment and search specialist firms providing counsel and assistance in identifying and hiring candidates for middle-level and senior-level management positions. *See also* executive; recruitment.

National Association of First Responders (NAFAR) A national organization founded in 1984 composed of 864 emergency medical responders who have had 40 hours of training. It offers a national certification program for first responders and educational and research programs. Formerly (1989) American Association of First Responders. *See also* certification; emergency medical responder.

National Association of Freestanding Emergency Centers *See* National Association for Ambulatory Care.

National Association of Healthcare Access Management (NAHAM) A national organization founded in 1974 composed of 1,500 hospital admitting managers that provides educational resources for the hospital admitting field and serves as a central source of information on changes and trends in health care that affect patient access services. Formerly (1990) National Association of Hospital Admitting Managers. *See also* accessibility; admission; management.

National Association of Health Career Schools (NAHCS) A national organization founded in 1980 composed of private, vocational, technical, and junior colleges training allied health personnel. *See also* allied health professional.

National Association for Healthcare Quality (NAHQ) A national organization founded in 1976 composed of 6,500 nurses, medical records personnel, hospital administrators, physicians, risk managers, discharge planners, medical audit coordinators, and other persons engaged in the development of quality assurance programs and activities. Formerly National Association of Quality Assurance Professionals. *See also* quality; quality assurance professional.

National Association of Healthcare Recruiters *See* National Association for Healthcare Recruitment.

National Association for Healthcare Recruitment (NAHCR) A national organization founded in 1975 composed of 1,850 individuals employed directly by hospitals and other health care organizations in recruitment of allied health professionals, home health professionals, long term care professionals, nurses, and physicians. It promotes sound principles of professional health care recruitment and conducts regional seminars, symposia, and workshops. Formerly National Association of Nurse Recruiters; (1987) National Association of Healthcare Recruiters. *See also* recruitment.

National Association of Health Data Organizations (NAHDO) A national organization founded in 1986 composed of 200 state and federal health data organizations; associate and supporting members are private sector organizations, including data analysis companies, commercial insurers, health services consultants, health care researchers, third-party payers, hospital associations, and managed health care plans. It seeks to improve health care through the collection, dissemination, and application of health care data. It promotes public availability of and access to health care data, and supports use of health care data to guide formulating of health policy, purchasing, and establishing of needed health services. It encourages uniformity and accuracy in data collection to support the development of a national health care database. *See also* data; database; data collection.

National Association of Health Services Executives (NAHSE) A national organization founded in 1968 composed of 500 black health care executive managers, planners, educators, advocates, providers, organizers, researchers, and consumers. *See also* administrator; executive.

National Association of Health Underwriters (NAHU) A national organization founded in 1930 composed of 8,600 insurance agencies and individuals engaged in the promotion, sale, and administration of disability income and health insurance. *See also* disability; Disability Insurance Training Council;

health insurance; underwriting.

National Association of Health Unit Clerks-Coordinators *See* National Association of Health Unit Coordinators.

National Association of Health and Welfare Ministries of the United Methodist Church *See* United Methodist Association of Health and Welfare Ministries.

National Association of Health Unit Coordinators (NAHUC) A national organization founded in 1980 composed of 3,000 coordinators of nonclinical nursing unit activities and other persons interested in health unit coordinating. It promotes the professional practice of unit coordinating and has established standards of practice defining the role and responsibilities of health unit coordinators. It works to establish certification guidelines with a goal of national certification. Formerly (1990) National Association of Health Unit Clerks-Coordinators. *See also* certification; clerk; health unit coordinator.

National Association of Hispanic Nurses (NAHN) A national organization founded in 1976 composed of 450 Hispanic and non-Hispanic nurses concerned about the health delivery needs of the Hispanic community. *See also* nurse.

National Association for Home Care (NAHC) A national organization founded in 1982 composed of 5,000 providers of home health care, hospice, and homemaker/home health aide services. It seeks to affect legislative and regulatory processes concerning home care services; gathers and disseminates home care industry data; develops public relations strategies; and works to increase political visibility of home care services. It interprets home care services to governmental and private sector bodies affecting the delivery and financing of such services. *See also* home health care; home care program.

National Association of Homes for Children *See* National Association of Homes and Services for Children.

National Association of Homes and Services for Children (NAHSC) A national organization founded in 1975 composed of 500 residential child care homes, residential boarding home agencies, placement agencies, adoption agencies, and agencies seeking to improve group residential care and related services for children and their families. Formerly (1990) National Association of Homes for Children. *See also* residential care; residential care facility.

National Association of Hospital Admitting Managers *See* National Association of Healthcare Access Management.

National Association of Hospital Hospitality Houses (NAHHH) A national organization founded in 1985 composed of 60 hospitals, hospitality houses, and charitable foundations interested in hospital hospitality houses. *See also* hospital hospitality house.

National Association of Lesbian/Gay Alcoholism Professionals (NALGAP) A national organization founded in 1979 composed of doctors, nurses, social workers, psychologists, certified counselors, and other health professionals who work with gay and lesbian alcoholics, and drug, alcohol, and gay agencies, organizations, and institutes. Its objective is to form a network for support and communication among professionals working with chemically dependent gay and lesbian people. *See also* alcoholism; gay; lesbianism; substance abuse.

National Association of Licensed Practical Nurses. *See* National Association for Practical Nurse Education and Service.

National Association of Mail Service Pharmacies *See* American Managed Care Pharmacy Association.

National Association of Managed Care Physicians (NAMCP) A national organization founded in 1991 composed of licensed physicians and allied health professionals working in managed health care programs, such as health maintenance organizations and preferred provider organizations, medical residents and students interested in managed health care, and corporations or agencies providing services or goods to the industry. It emphasizes physician autonomy to treat patients in a manner consistent with quality health care, stronger physician-patient relationships, patient education, and public awareness of costs and benefits of services in managed health care. *See also* managed care; physician.

National Association of Manufacturing Opticians (NAMO) A national organization founded in 1975 composed of full-service optical laboratories. It initiated the development of bar coding of optical products to facilitate the ordering and processing of eyeware within the industry. *See also* bar code; optician.

National Association of Meal Programs (NAMP) A national organization founded in 1973 composed of 600 agencies that provide home-delivered meals and/or meals in a congregate setting and other health and social services, such as transportation, recreation, nutrition education, information, referral, and case management. It delivers nutritionally balanced meals to disabled and homebound elderly persons, thereby reducing or eliminating the need for institutionalization and promoting independent and community-based living arrangements. *See also* home health care; meals on wheels.

National Association of Medical Equipment Suppliers (NAMES) A national organization founded in 1982 composed of 2,100 durable medical equipment and oxygen suppliers, manufacturers, and state associations. It promotes legislative and regulatory policies that improve access to home medical equipment. *See also* durable medical equipment; medical equipment.

National Association of Medical Examiners (NAME) A national organization founded in 1966 composed of medical examiners, pathologists, and other licensed physicians who have responsibilities in connection with the official investigation of sudden, suspicious, and violent deaths. *See also* forensic medicine; medical examiner.

National Association Medical Staff Services (NAMSS) A national organization founded in 1971 composed of 2,300 individuals involved in the management and administration of medical staff services. *See also* medical staff.

National Association for Mental Health *See* National Mental Health Association.

National Association for Music Therapy (NAMT) A national organization founded in 1950 composed of 3,800 music therapists, physicians, psychologists, administrators, and educators supporting the use of music in therapy. *See also* music therapy.

National Association of Neonatal Nurses (NANN) A national organization founded in 1984 composed of 13,050 nurses currently working in neonatal intensive care units. It provides educational and networking opportunities. *See also* neonatal; neonatal intensive care unit; networking; nurse.

National Association of Nurse Practitioners in Reproductive Health (NANPRH) A national organization founded in 1980 composed of 1,400 nurse practitioners involved in reproductive health care. It advocates quality reproductive health services and reproductive freedom, and supports the rights of nurse practitioners to administer reproductive health services to patients. *See also* nurse practitioner.

National Association of Nurse Recruiters *See* National Association for Healthcare Recruitment.

National Association of Nutrition and Aging Services Programs (NANASP) A national organization founded in 1977 composed of 1,000 directors and staff of congregate and home-delivered nutrition services programs for the elderly. Its objectives include promoting professional growth and raising the standards of the profession among members and encouraging communication between aging services programs and federal agencies and governmental bodies. It has developed national standards for congregate and home-delivered services programs. *See also* meals on wheels; nutrition.

National Association of Oncology Social Workers (NAOSW) A national organization founded in 1984 composed of 750 accredited oncology social workers; associate members are professionals functioning as social workers without the professional degree and students in an accredited social work degree program. It seeks to enable social workers in oncology to better serve the needs of clients, practitioners, managers, educators, and researchers. *See also* oncology; social worker.

National Association of Optometrists and Opticians (NAOO) A national organization founded in 1960 composed of 13,225 licensed optometrists, opticians, and related corporations. It conducts public affairs programs of mutual importance to members and serves as an organizational center for special purpose programs. It also acts as a clearinghouse for information affecting the retail optical industry. *See also* clearinghouse; optometrist; optician.

National Association of Orthopaedic Nurses (NAON) A national organization founded in 1980 composed of 8,500 registered, licensed practical, or licensed vocational nurses interested in orthopaedic nursing. It stresses continuing education and the development of patient care plans and maintains liaison with and serves as a resource to hospitals, universities, industries, and government agencies. *See also* licensed practical nurse; licensed vocational nurse; orthopaedic/orthopedic surgery; registered nurse.

National Association of Orthopaedic Technologists (NAOT) A national organization founded in 1981 composed of 1,000 allied health assistants

working with orthopedic patients. It promotes continuing professional education of members and other orthopedic health care providers and administers a certification examination. *See also* certification; orthopaedic/orthopedic surgery.

National Association of Pediatric Nurse Associates and Practitioners (NAPNAP) A national organization founded in 1973 composed of 3,200 pediatric, school, and family nurse practitioners and other persons interested in the implementation and maintenance of certification of practitioners and associates, in cooperation with the National Certification Board of Pediatric Nurse Practitioners and Nurses, and other activities. *See also* certification; pediatric nurse practitioner.

National Association for Perinatal Addiction Research and Education (NAPARE) A national organization founded in 1987 composed of 750 members interested in conducting educational and research programs on substance abuse during pregnancy and the effects of substance abuse on the fetus. *See also* addiction; perinatal; substance abuse.

National Association of Pharmaceutical Manufacturers (NAPM) A national organization founded in 1954 composed of 100 pharmaceutical manufacturers, distributors, and repackagers concerned with problems arising from laws and regulations and the need to establish rapport with federal and state agencies. *See also* pharmaceutical.

National Association of Physician Nurses (NAPN) A national organization founded in 1973 composed of 3,000 physician nurses interested in bringing added stature and purpose to their profession. *See also* nurse.

National Association of Physician Recruiters (NAPR) A national organization founded in 1983 composed of 100 physician search firms. *See also* physician search firm; recruitment.

National Association for Poetry Therapy (NAPT) A national organization founded in 1969 composed of 200 psychiatrists, psychologists, social workers, teachers, nurses, librarians, paraprofessionals, counselors, recreation and rehabilitation specialists, and poets and professors of English and psychology supporting the use of poetry therapy for healing and personal growth. *See also* poetry therapy.

National Association for Practical Nurse Education and Service (NAPNES) A national organization founded in 1941 composed of 30,000 licensed practical/vocational nurses, registered nurses, physicians, hospitals, and nursing home administrators. It provides consultation services to advise schools wishing to develop a practical/vocational nursing program on required facilities, equipment, policies, curriculum, and staffing. It provides continuing education and holds national certification courses in pharmacology and other areas. Absorbed (1985) National Association of Licensed Practical Nurses. *See also* certification; licensed practical nurse; licensed vocational nurse.

National Association of Private Geriatric Care Managers (NAPGCM) A national organization founded in 1985 composed of 400 individuals interested in promoting care for elderly citizens. It provides a referral service and distributes information to individuals interested in geriatric care centers. *See also* geriatric medicine; gerontology.

National Association of Private Psychiatric Hospitals (NAPPH) A national association founded in 1933 composed of 320 private psychiatric hospitals. It safeguards and represents the private psychiatric hospital and the patients it serves in legislation, federal programs, health insurance industry, and state programs. *See also* psychiatric hospital.

National Association of Private Residential Facilities for the Mentally Retarded *See* National Association of Private Residential Resources.

National Association of Private Residential Resources (NAPRR) A national organization founded in 1970 composed of 620 agencies that serve persons with mental retardation and other developmental disabilities and other persons interested in the field of private residential services. Formerly (1987) National Association of Private Residential Facilities for the Mentally Retarded. *See also* developmental disability; mental retardation; residential care.

National Association of Psychiatric Treatment Centers for Children (NAPTCC) A national organization founded in 1983 composed of 80 residential centers for emotionally and mentally disturbed children. These residential centers are accredited by the Joint Commission on Accreditation of Healthcare Organizations. *See also* Joint Commission on Accreditation of Healthcare Organizations; psychiatry; residential care facility.

National Association of Public Child Welfare Administrators (NAPCWA) A national organiza-
tion founded in 1983 composed of 400 state and local child welfare administrators who belong to the American Public Welfare Association. It seeks to enhance the administration of services promoting the well-being of children and supports the development of public policies to prevent or alleviate family disruptions, such as child abuse and juvenile delinquency. *See also* child abuse; child welfare caseworker.

National Association of Public Hospitals (NAPH) A national organization founded in 1980 composed of 70 urban public hospitals. It promotes the development of federal, state, and local legislative and policy agendas for members. *See also* public hospital.

National Association of Quality Assurance Professionals *See* National Association for Healthcare Quality.

National Association of Registered Nurses (NARN) A national organization founded in 1979 composed of 111 nurses' associations. It offers nurses financial management programs and provides financial products, consultation, and services, including individual retirement accounts, investment services, and group life insurance. *See also* registered nurse.

National Association of Registered Nursing Homes *See* American Health Care Association.

National Association of Rehabilitation Facilities (NARF) A national organization founded in 1969 composed of 812 rehabilitation facilities in the United States and Canada that, among other services, promotes the expansion and improvement of rehabilitation services and provides educational seminars and workshops. *See also* rehabilitation hospital; rehabilitation service.

National Association of Rehabilitation Instructors (NARI) A national organization composed of 325 rehabilitation instructors interested in promoting rehabilitation of all persons with disabilities. It acts as a medium through which rehabilitation instructors can coordinate their efforts with other instructors, facilities, workshops, individuals, and organizations serving the handicapped. *See also* physical medicine and rehabilitation.

National Association of Rehabilitation Professionals in the Private Sector (NARPPS) A national organization founded in 1977 composed of 3,500 members, including private rehabilitation companies, insurance companies, rehabilitation nurses, and rehabilitation professionals in the private sector. It seeks to promote the field of private rehabilitation and to provide for information exchange on rehabilitation issues and techniques. *See also* rehabilitation.

National Association of Rehabilitation Secretaries (NARS) A national organization founded in 1971 composed of 1,349 rehabilitation secretaries. It promotes recruitment of qualified persons for secretarial and clerical positions in the rehabilitation field; determines and analyzes the skills and knowledge needed by secretaries, stenographers, and clerical workers; and devises appropriate training. *See also* rehabilitation; secretary.

National Association of Reimbursement Officers (NARO) A national organization founded in 1955 composed of 250 state and local mental health and mental retardation officials seeking to recover the cost of care, treatment, and maintenance for health care services rendered in any government hospital, institution, treatment center, school, or special medical facility. *See also* reimbursement.

National Association of Residents and Interns (NARI) A national organization founded in 1959 composed of 121,000 medical and dental students, interns, residents, and fellows. It provides secured loan plans, low-cost group insurance, group purchase discounts, and other services. *See also* fellow; intern; resident.

National Association of Retail Druggists *See* NARD.

National Association for Rural Mental Health (NARMH) A national organization founded in 1977 composed of 300 mental health practitioners and administrators and other persons interested in improving mental health services in rural areas. It promotes effective rural mental health services by acquiring funds and training professionals. It promotes the use of services by rural community dwellers. *See also* mental health; mental health services; rural.

National Association of School Nurses (NASN) A national organization founded in 1969 composed of 6,000 school nurses who conduct comprehensive school health programs in public and private schools. It provides national leadership in the promotion of health services for school children; promotes school health interests to the nursing and health community and the public; and monitors leg-

islation pertaining to school nursing. It operates the National Board for Certification of School Nurses and certifies school nurses. *See also* certification; school nurse.

National Association of School Psychologists (NASP) A national organization founded in 1969 composed of 15,520 school psychologists. It serves the mental health and educational needs of children and youth; encourages and provides opportunities for professional growth of members; informs the public on the services and practice of school psychology; and advances the standards of the profession. It operates a national school psychologist certification system. *See also* certification; school psychology.

National Association for Search and Rescue (NASAR) A national organization founded in 1970 composed of 2,900 directors or coordinators of state and regional emergency rescue services; medical rescue, fire, and emergency personnel; organizations involved in search, rescue, or survival activities; and state rescue-related agencies. It provides for liaison of state, federal, local, and private search and rescue groups; conducts training programs for search and rescue professionals; promotes the standardization of procedures; and sponsors survival education programs designed to help the public cope with disaster and emergency situations. *See also* emergency medical services system.

National Association for Senior Living Industries (NASLI) A national organization founded in 1985 composed of 1,000 businesses, associations, governmental agencies, and other groups and organizations interested in improving the quality of life for senior citizens through education and developmental programs.

National Association of Seventh Day Adventist Dentists (NASDAD) A national organization founded in 1944 composed of 600 dentists who are Seventh Day Adventists. *See also* dentist; Seventh Day Adventist.

National Association for Sickle Cell Disease (NASCD) A national organization founded in 1971 composed of community groups involved in sickle cell anemia programs throughout the United States. It provides leadership on a national level to create awareness of the negative impact of sickle cell anemia on the health, economic, social, and educational well-being of individuals and families of individuals with sickle cell disease. Its resources include counselor training, workshops and seminars, blood banks, screening and testing, and camps for children with sickle cell disease. *See also* sickle cell anemia.

National Association of Social Workers (NASW) A national organization founded in 1955 composed of 134,000 social workers who hold a minimum of a baccalaureate degree in social work; associate members are individuals engaged in social work who have a baccalaureate degree in another field. Its purposes include creating professional standards for social work practice; advocating sound public social work policies through political and legislative action; providing a wide range of membership services, including continuing education opportunities and professional programs. *See also* Academy of Certified Social Workers; social worker.

National Association of Social Workers Committee on Lesbian and Gay Issues A committee of the National Association of Social Workers (NASW) that seeks to ensure equal employment opportunities for lesbian and gay social workers and other individuals. It informs the NASW about issues, such as domestic, racial, and antigay violence, and civil rights. *See also* gay; lesbianism; National Association of Social Workers; social worker.

National Association for State Administrators of Health Occupations Education *See* National Association of Supervisors and Administrators of Health Occupations Education.

National Association of State Alcohol and Drug Abuse Directors (NASADAD) A national organization founded in 1971 composed of 67 state alcohol and drug abuse directors and their agencies. Its purposes include representing the interests of state alcohol and drug abuse directors and their agencies before Congress and federal agencies and fostering development of comprehensive alcohol and drug abuse programs on state resources. *See also* alcoholism; drug abuse.

National Association of State Directors for Disaster Preparedness *See* National Emergency Management Association.

National Association of State EMS Directors (NASEMSD) A national organization founded in 1981 composed of 55 state emergency medical services (EMS) directors interested in refining EMS activities, coordinating activities between states, and serving as a liaison with other national medical organizations. *See also* emergency medical services system.

National Association of State Mental Health Program Directors (NASMHPD) A national organization founded in 1963 composed of 55 state commissioners in charge of state mental disability programs; associate members are assistant commissioners for children and youth, research, aged, legal services, forensic services, human resource development, and community programs. It promotes cooperation of state government agencies in delivery of services to persons with mental disabilities and fosters the exchange of scientific and programmatic information in the administration of public mental health programs. It monitors state and federal and congressional activities. *See also* mental health services; mental illness.

National Association of State Mental Retardation Program Directors (NASMRPD) A national organization founded in 1963 composed of 53 state administrative personnel working with programs in the field of mental retardation. It monitors and reports on administrative, legislative, and judicial activities and other events affecting mental retardation programs. *See also* mental retardation.

National Association of State Units on Aging (NASUA) A public interest organization founded in 1964 that provides information, technical assistance, and professional development support to state units on aging. *See also* aging; geriatric medicine; gerontology; state unit on aging.

National Association of Supervisors and Administrators of Health Occupations Education (NASAHOE) A national organization composed of 35 state administrators and local supervisors of health occupations education interested in sharing resources, particularly in the area of curriculum development. Formerly (1988) National Association for State Administrators of Health Occupations Education.

National Association of VA Physicians and Dentists (NAVAP) A national organization founded in 1975 composed of 12,000 physicians and dentists employed in Veterans Administration hospitals. It works through legal means and Congress to ensure that veterans receive quality health care. Formerly (1992) National Association of VA Physicians. *See also* Veterans Administration; Veterans Administration hospital.

National Association of Vision Professionals (NAVP) A national organization founded in 1976 composed of 200 individuals responsible for or connected with vision conservation and eye health programs in public or private agencies and institutions. It serves as a forum for ideas and programs and promotes professional standards. It certifies vision screening personnel. Formerly (1986) National Association of Vision Program Consultants.

National Association of Vision Program Consultants *See* National Association of Vision Professionals.

National Association of Women Lawyers (NAWL) A national organization founded in 1911 composed of 1,200 women lawyers who have been admitted to practice in any state or territory of the United States. *See also* attorney; bar; lawyer.

National Athletic Trainers Association (NATA) A national organization founded in 1950 composed of 16,500 athletic trainers from universities, colleges, and junior colleges; professional football, baseball, basketball, and ice hockey; it also includes high schools, preparatory schools, military establishments, sports medicine clinics, and business/industrial health programs. It maintains biographical archives, a hall of fame, and a placement service. *See also* athletic trainer; sports medicine.

National Bar Association (NBA) A national organization founded in 1925 composed of 12,500 minority (predominantly black) attorneys, members of the judiciary, law students, and law faculty. *See also* attorney; bar; lawyer.

National Black Alcoholism Council (NBAC) A national organization founded in 1978 composed of 1,050 individuals concerned about alcoholism among black Americans. It works to support and initiate activities that will improve alcoholism treatment services and lead to the prevention of alcoholism in the black community. *See also* addiction; alcoholism.

National Black Nurses Association (NBNA) A national organization founded in 1976 composed of 5,000 black registered nurses, licensed practical nurses, licensed vocational nurses, and student nurses interested in providing improved health care for the black community and support for professional advancement of its members. *See also* licensed practical nurse; licensed vocational nurse; registered nurse.

National Black Women's Health Project (NBWHP) A national organization founded in 1981 composed of 2,000 individuals interested in encouraging mutual and self-help advocacy among women to bring about a reduction in health care problems prevalent among black women. It urges women to communicate with health care providers, seek out available health care resources, and communicate with other black women to minimize feelings of powerlessness and isolation. Formerly (1984) Black Women's Health Project.

National Board for Cardiopulmonary Credentialing *See* Cardiovascular Credentialing International.

National Board for Cardiovascular and Pulmonary Credentialing *See* Cardiovascular Credentialing International.

National Board for Certification of Dental Laboratories (CDL) A national board founded in 1979 composed of 600 certified dental laboratories, including commercial and private dental laboratories and dental or dental technology schools. *See also* board; certification; dental laboratory technician; dentistry.

National Board for Certification in Dental Technology (NBC) A national board founded in 1958 that establishes standards and develops and conducts examinations; it has certified 10,400 dental technicians with formal education in dental technology and a minimum of three years' experience. *See also* board; certification; dental laboratory technician.

National Board for Certification of Orthopaedic Technologists (NBCOT) A national board that determines educational standards for certification of orthopaedic technologists. *See also* board; certification; orthopaedic/orthopedic surgery.

National Board for Certified Counselors (NBCC) A national board founded in 1982 that establishes and monitors professional credentialing standards for counselors and identifies individuals who have obtained voluntary certification as a national certified counselor. *See also* board; certified counselor; counselor; credentialing; specialty boards.

national board examination A standardized national examination for medical students and physicians developed and administered by the National Board of Medical Examiners. It is given in three parts, which are generally taken during the second and fourth years of medical school and the internship year or first postgraduate year (PGY-1). Successful completion of the national board examination is a requirement for licensure as a physician in a number of states and an acceptable alternative to a state's own medical examinations in other states. *Synonym*: national boards. *See also* Federation Licensing Examination (FLEX); licensure; National Board of Medical Examiners; standardized test.

National Board of Examiners in Optometry (NBEO) A national board founded in 1951 that administers entry-level criterion-referenced credentialing examinations to students and graduates of accredited schools and colleges of optometry for use by individual state licensing boards. *See also* board; credentialing; optometry; specialty boards.

National Board of Examiners for Osteopathic Physicians and Surgeons *See* National Board of Osteopathic Medical Examiners.

National Board of Medical Examiners (NBME) An independent, nonprofit board founded in 1915 that prepares and administers qualifying examinations that, when successfully passed, certify students and graduates of United States and Canadian medical schools. *See also* board; certification; national board examination; state medical boards.

National Board of Osteopathic Medical Examiners (NBOME) A national board founded in 1935 composed of 12 osteopathic physicians elected for three-year terms, who function as the examining and evaluating board to investigate the qualifications of, and administer examinations and grant diplomate status to, osteopathic physicians. Formerly (1986) National Board of Examiners for Osteopathic Physicians and Surgeons. *See also* board; osteopathic medicine; specialty boards.

National Board of Pediatric Nurse Practitioners and Associates *See* National Certification Board of Pediatric Nurse Practitioners and Nurses.

National Board of Podiatric Medical Examiners (NBPME) A national board founded in 1956 composed of 12 podiatrists whose purpose is to prepare and administer examinations for podiatry students seeking state licensure. *See also* board; licensure; podiatric medicine; specialty boards.

National Board for Respiratory Care (NBRC) A national board founded in 1960 composed of 90,000 certified respiratory therapists, respiratory therapy technicians, and pulmonary technologists. Formerly (1982) National Board for Respiratory Therapy. *See also* board; registered respiratory therapist; respiratory therapist; respiratory therapy technician; spe-

cialty boards.

national boards *See* national board examination.

National Board of Trial Advocacy (NBTA) A national board composed of 1,500 lawyers, judges, and educators interested in improving the quality of trial advocacy, and improving public access to trial advocates of demonstrated competence. It conducts the National Certification of Criminal and Civil Trial Advocates Program and awards certification to lawyers who successfully complete all requirements, one of which is a written examination. Recertification is required every five years. *See also* American Board of Professional Liability Attorneys; board; certification; lawyer; recertification; trial.

National Bureau of Standards *See* National Institute of Standards and Technology.

National Burn Information Exchange (NBIE) A national data registry founded in 1964 composed of 137 physicians specializing in burn patient care. Its objectives include establishing standards of burn patient care and monitoring changes in standards; providing etiologic information to prevent burn accidents; and improving patient care by exchanging information on successful methods used in burn centers, units, and programs. It collects and analyzes uniform patient data on burn problems including etiology, mortality, morbidity, acute treatment, reconstruction, and cost. The database includes over 100,000 cases. *See also* burn; physician.

National Cancer Institute (NCI) *See* National Institutes of Health.

National Catholic Council on Alcoholism and Related Drug Problems (NCCA) A national organization founded in 1949 composed of 2,500 members interested in promoting adequate treatment for all clergy and religious men and women suffering from alcoholism and drug dependency through consultation and supportive services. Formerly (1988) National Clergy Council on Alcoholism and Related Drug Problems. *See also* alcoholism; alcoholism and other drug dependence.

National Catholic Pharmacists Guild of the United States (NCPG) A national organization founded in 1962 composed of 400 Catholic pharmacists, pharmacy graduates, pharmacy technicians, and students interested in upholding the principles of the Catholic faith and all laws of church and country, especially those pertaining to the practice of pharmacy. It assists ecclesiastical authorities in the diffusion of Catholic pharmacy ethics and promotes donations of funds and supplies to the needy. It opposes the sale of pornographic literature, especially that which is sold in pharmacies. *See also* pharmacist; pharmacy.

National Center for the Advancement of Blacks in the Health Professions (NCABHP) A national organization founded in 1988 composed of members of the American Public Health Association, National Black Nurses Association, the American Hospital Association, and other organizations interested in advancing blacks in the health professions. It publicizes the disparity between the health of black and white Americans and the underrepresentation of blacks in the health professions. *See also* health professional.

National Center for Clinical Infant Programs *See* Zero to Three/NCCIP.

National Center for Education in Maternal and Child Health (NCEMCH) A nonmembership organization founded in 1981 that provides information services to professionals and the public on maternal and child health. It collects and disseminates information on available materials, programs, and research and offers summer internships for graduate students in public health schools. Formerly (1982) National Clearinghouse for Human Genetic Diseases. *See also* maternal and child health services.

National Center for Health Education (NCHE) A national organization founded in 1975 composed of professionals promoting health education in schools, communities, and family settings. It manages *Growing Healthy*, a comprehensive health education curriculum. *See also* education.

National Center for Health Promotion and Aging *See* Health Promotion Institute.

National Center for Health Services Research and Health Care Technology Assessment A research center within the US Public Health Service. *See also* Health and Nutrition Examination Survey; Public Health Service.

National Center for Health Statistics (NCHS) A research center within the US Public Health Service. *See also* Cooperative Health Statistics System; Health Interview Survey; health statistics; Hospital Discharge Survey; Master Facility Inventory of Hospitals and Institutions; Public Health Service.

National Center for Homeopathy (NCH) A national organization founded in 1974 composed of 3,500 members interested in promoting the art of homeopathic healing according to the natural laws of cure. *See also* homeopathy.

National Center for Nursing Research (NANR) A research center within the National Institutes of Health, US Public Health Service, with the purpose of better integrating nursing research with other biomedical and health care research at the National Institutes of Health and across the nation. The center was authorized in 1985 and includes the research activities formerly conducted by the Division of Nursing in the Health Resources and Services Administration of the Department of Health and Human Services. *See also* National Institutes of Health; nursing; research.

National Center on Rural Aging (NCRA) A national organization founded in 1978 composed of 500 planners and providers of services for the aging, academicians and students, and other persons interested in issues related to older persons living in rural areas. *See also* aging; geriatric medicine; gerontology; rural.

National Center for Toxicological Research *See* Food and Drug Administration.

National Certification Agency for Medical Lab Personnel (NCA) A national certifying body founded in 1977 composed of 65,000 individuals employed as directors, educators, supervisors, or workers in clinical laboratory science. It develops and administers competency-based examinations for certification of clinical laboratory personnel and provides for periodic recertification by examination or through documentation of continuing education. It is affiliated with the American Society for Medical Technology and the Association of Cytogenetic Technologists. *See also* certification; clinical laboratory; recertification.

National Certification Board of Pediatric Nurse Practitioners and Nurses (NCBPNP/N) A national organization founded in 1976 composed of physician and nurse representatives from the American Academy of Pediatrics, National Association of Pediatric Nurse Associates and Practitioners, and Association of Faculties of Pediatric Nurse Associate/Practitioner Programs. It administers certification, recertification, continuing education, and self-assessment programs for general and advanced practice pediatric nursing. Formerly (1989) National Board of Pediatric Nurse Practitioners and Associates. *See also* certification; nurse practitioner; pediatric nurse.

National Certification Reciprocity Consortium/ Alcoholism and Other Drug Abuse (NCRC/ AODA) A national credentialing body founded in 1979 for drug and alcohol counselors in 39 US states, the District of Columbia, the US Air Force, Navy and Marines, and Canada. It negotiates reciprocity agreements for alcohol and drug abuse counselors with other certification bodies throughout the United States and Canada so that counselors may practice in more than one state without reapplying for certification. Formerly (1989) Certification Reciprocity Consortium/Alcoholism and Other Drug Abuse. *See also* alcoholism and other drug dependence; certification; counselor; reciprocity.

National Child Safety Council (NCSC) A national organization founded in 1949 that furnishes complete child safety education programs through local law enforcement agencies and schools. *See also* safety.

National Chronic Pain Outreach Association (NCPOA) A national organization founded in 1976 composed of 1,000 members interested in disseminating information about chronic pain and its management in an effort to lessen the suffering caused by chronic pain. It operates an information clearinghouse for pain sufferers, family members, and health professionals. *See also* clearinghouse; pain.

National Citizens Coalition for Nursing Home Reform (NCCNHR) A national organization founded in 1975 composed of 700 local consumer/citizen action groups and individuals seeking nursing home reform. It seeks to provide a consumer voice at the national, state, and local levels in the development and implementation of the long term care system. *See also* consumer; long term care.

National Clearinghouse for Human Genetic Diseases *See* National Center for Education in Maternal and Child Health.

National Clearinghouse on Licensure, Enforcement, and Regulation *See* Council on Licensure, Enforcement and Regulation.

National Clearinghouse on Marital and Date Rape (NCOMDR) A national speaking/consulting firm founded in 1980 composed of 500 students, attorneys, legislators, faculty members, rape crisis centers, shelters, and other social service groups interested in educating the public about marital, cohabi-

tant, and date rape. *See also* date rape; rape.

National Clergy Council on Alcoholism and Related Drug Problems *See* National Catholic Council on Alcoholism and Related Drug Problems.

National Coalition Against Domestic Violence (NCADV) A national organization founded in 1978 composed of 1,200 battered women's service organizations and shelters. It supplies technical assistance and makes referrals on issues of domestic violence. *See also* violence.

National Coalition Against Sexual Assault (NCASA) A national organization founded in 1978 composed of 500 members interested in building a network through which individuals and organizations working against sexual assault can share expertise, experience, and information. It acts as an advocate for and on behalf of rape victims and disseminates information on sexual assault. It sponsors Sexual Assault Awareness Month in April. *See also* networking; rape; sexual assault.

National Coalition of Arts Therapy Associations (NCATA) A national organization founded in 1979 composed of 12,000 creative arts therapists representing the American Art Therapy Association, American Association for Music Therapy, American Dance Therapy Association, American Society for Group Psychotherapy and Psychodrama, National Association for Drama Therapy, National Association for Music Therapy, and National Association for Poetry Therapy. It promotes the therapeutic and rehabilitative use of the arts in medicine, mental health, special education, and forensic and social services. *See also* art therapy.

National Coalition of Black Lung and Respiratory Disease Clinics (NCBLRDC) A national organization founded in 1981 composed of 120 clinics receiving federal aid for research or clinic operations; allied health organizations working in conjunction with black lung clinics; and interested individuals. It develops pulmonary rehabilitation programs and provides a forum for continuing education, training, facilitation of meetings, and technical assistance. It promotes networking of federally funded projects that treat miners who have been diagnosed with black lung disease. *See also* black lung disease; clinic; networking.

National Coalition for Cancer Research (NCCR) A national coalition founded in 1984 composed of cancer research and cancer care organizations and facilities. It works to educate the public and interested parties of the legislative and executive branches on the importance of cancer research and care. *See also* cancer; research.

National Coalition of Hispanic Health and Human Services Organizations (COSSMHO) A national organization founded in 1973 composed of 700 health, mental health, and human service agencies and organizations and professional individuals serving Hispanics. Its activities include health promotion and education; mental health, drug abuse, and alcohol abuse treatment and prevention; community health services; health careers development; and services to the elderly.

National Coalition on Immune System Disorders (NCISD) A national organization founded in 1983 composed of 13 professional and lay organizations with a primary interest in the immune system and its diseases. It promotes education of health professionals, policymakers, and the public on subjects related to the immune system. *See also* immune system.

National Coalition of Psychiatrists Against Motorcoach Therapy (NCPAMT) A national organization founded in 1985 composed of 430 psychiatrists, psychologists, social workers, counselors, and mental health officials who want to stop the practice of "Motorcoach Therapy," described as the "escalating and unethical practice of procuring one-way bus fares for habitual and undesirable mental health patients" upon their release from local mental health facilities. It has launched an awareness campaign targeted primarily at mental health officials. *See also* psychiatry.

National Coalition for Research in Neurological Disorders (NCR) A national organization founded in 1952 composed of 57 voluntary health agencies and professional societies interested in obtaining funds for neurological research. It stimulates public information regarding the field of neurology and neurosurgery and lobbies for increased funding for training and research in neurological disorders. Formerly (1989) National Coalition for Research in Neurological and Communicative Disorders. *See also* neurological surgery; neurology.

National Coalition for Research in Neurological and Communicative Disorders *See* National Coalition for Research in Neurological Disorders.

National College of Foot Surgeons (NCFS) A national organization founded in 1960 composed of doctors of surgical podiatry. It certifies foot surgeons as fellows and associates of the college. *See also* podiatric medicine.

National Commission on Accreditation of Alcoholism and Drug Abuse Counselor Credentialing Bodies A national organization founded in 1974 composed of 70 alcoholism and drug abuse credentialing agencies and organizations whose members are credentialed or are eligible for credentialing, and public and private corporations and governmental bodies that employ the services of substance abuse counselors. It works as an advisory agent to state credentialing organizations in developing credentialing standards for counselors and acts as an accrediting body for state certification boards. *See also* accreditation; alcoholism; counselor; credentialing; drug abuse.

National Commission for Certification of Acupuncturists (NCCA) A national certifying body founded in 1982 composed of representatives of the National Council of Acupuncture Schools and Colleges and the Association of Acupuncture and Oriental Medicine. Its purposes are to establish entry level standards of competency for the safe and effective practice of acupuncture, evaluate an applicant's qualifications by administering national board examinations in acupuncture, and certify practitioners of acupuncture who meet standards. It acts as a consultant to state agencies in development of licensure regulations and evaluation of certification mechanisms. *See also* acupuncture; certification; licensure.

National Commission on Certification of Physician Assistants (NCCPA) A national certifying body founded in 1975 that certifies physician assistants at the entry level and for continued competence. It has certified 19,000 physician assistants. Formerly (1987) National Commission on Certification of Physician's Assistants. *See also* certification; physician assistant.

National Commission on Certification of Physician's Assistants *See* National Commission on Certification of Physicians Assistants.

National Commission on Correctional Health Care (NCCHC) A national organization founded in 1983 composed of 31 professional organizations in the fields of medical and health care working to improve the quality of and set standards for medical care in correctional institutions in the United States, including prisons, jails, and detention and juvenile facilities. It acts as an accrediting body for these facilities.

National Commission for Electrologist Certification (NCEC) A certifying body for individuals interested in practicing electrolysis. It establishes and promotes safety and proficiency in the practice of permanent hair removal, and conducts research in occupational credentialing. It develops and administers credentialing examinations and seeks to enhance public confidence in electrolysis and electrolysis practitioners. *See also* certification; credentialing; electrology; electrolysis.

National Commission for Health Certifying Agencies *See* National Organization for Competency Assurance.

National Committee for Clinical Laboratory Standards (NCCLS) A national organization founded in 1968 composed of 1,300 government agencies, professional societies, clinical laboratories, and industrial firms with interests in clinical laboratory testing. Its purposes are to promote the development of national standards for clinical laboratory testing and to provide a consensus mechanism for defining and resolving problems that influence the quality and cost of laboratory work performed. *See also* clinical laboratory; standard.

National Committee for Prevention of Child Abuse (NCPCA) A national organization founded in 1972 that seeks to stimulate greater public awareness of the incidence, origins, nature, and effects of child abuse. It serves as a national advocate to prevent the neglect and physical, sexual, and emotional abuse of children. It operates the National Center on Child Abuse Prevention Research and conducts annual national media campaigns and child abuse prevention programs. *See also* child abuse; sexual assault; violence.

National Committee for Quality Assurance (NCQA) A national organization founded in 1979 composed of 14 directors representing consumers, purchasers, and providers of managed health care. It accredits quality assurance programs in prepaid managed health care organizations and develops and coordinates programs for assessing the quality of care and service in the managed health care industry. *See also* managed care; quality assurance.

National Committee for Quality Health Care (NCQHC) A national organization founded in 1978 composed of 151 health care professionals and organizations principally involved in the health care industry, including hospitals, physicians, health maintenance organizations, nursing homes, manufacturers of health care equipment, investment bankers, architects, contractors, and accountants. It works to maintain and strengthen quality health care in the United States. *See also* health care; quality.

National Committee for Radiation Victims (NCRV) A national organization founded in 1979 that serves the needs of Americans affected by exposure to human-made ionizing radiation. It offers public service information on the effects of ionizing radiation, coordinates and encourages national action on radiation health and safety issues, and serves as a clearinghouse for information and materials on radiation exposure, existing radiation standards and practices, radiation victims' organizations, and legislation affecting radiation victims. *See also* clearinghouse; radiation.

National Committee on the Treatment of Intractable Pain (NCTIP) A national organization founded in 1977 composed of 3,500 individuals promoting education and research into more effective methods of pain prevention and control with the coordinated help of professionals in the medical, legal, bioethical, psychological, and religious fields. It endorses the hospice concept of care of the dying, which allows a dying person to remain among family, friends, community, and skilled professionals and provides constant, effective medical and psychological support for pain control. It advocates legalization of heroin for medical purposes. *See also* hospice; pain; pain management.

National Conference of Black Lawyers (NCBL) A national organization founded in 1968 composed of 1,000 attorneys interested in using legal skills in the service of black and poor communities. It maintains projects in legal services to community organizations, voting rights, and international affairs and provides public education on legal issues affecting blacks and poor people. It researches racism in law schools and bar admissions. *See also* attorney; lawyer.

National Conference of Local Environmental Health Administrators (NCLEHA) A national organization founded in 1939 composed of 220 environmental health personnel engaged in or officially concerned with municipal (city, county, or district) environmental health administration or teaching of environmental health. It promotes improvement and greater use of science and practice of environmental health in community life. *See also* environmental health; public health.

National Conference of Standards Laboratories (NCSL) A national organization founded in 1961 composed of 1,200 representatives of measurements standards and calibration laboratories. It seeks cost reduction or solution of problems, both technical and administrative, that besiege all measurement activities in the physical sciences, engineering, and technology. Its committees include Biomedical and Pharmaceutical Metrology, Measurement Assurance, and Recommended Practices. *See also* laboratory; measurement; standard.

National Conference of States on Building Codes and Standards (NCSBCS) A national organization founded in 1967 composed of 250 building code officials, building-related manufacturers, associations, educators, and consumer groups seeking a cooperative solution to the multiple problems in the entire building regulatory system. *See also* building codes; standard.

National Consortium of Chemical Dependency Nurses (NCCDN) A national organization founded in 1987 composed of 3,296 nurses specializing in chemical dependency treatment. It offers a certification examination for nurses with 4,000 hours of experience in the previous five years and 30 hours of chemical dependency coursework. *See also* certification; chemical dependency; chemical dependency services; nurse.

National Consortium for Child Mental Health Services (NCCMHS) A national organization founded in 1971 composed of 20 national psychiatric, psychologic, educational, social welfare, medical, parent and teacher, and consumer organizations interested in exchanging information on child mental health services and bringing concerns regarding child mental health services to appropriate local, state, and federal agencies. *See also* child and adolescent psychiatry; mental health.

National Consumers League (NCL) A national organization founded in 1899 composed of 8,000 members interested in increasing citizen participation in governmental and industry decision making. It conducts research, educational, and advocacy programs on consumer and worker issues, such as health, insurance, privacy, communication, and

product safety and standards. *See also* consumer; consumerism.

National Contact Lens Examiners (NCLE) A national certifying body founded in 1976 that promotes continued development of opticians and technicians as contact lens fitters by formulating standards and procedures for determination of entry-level competency. It assists in the development, administration, and monitoring of a national contact lens registry examination (CLRE), which verifies entry-level competency of contact lens fitters, and it issues certificates. *See also* certification; contact lens.

National Coordinating Council on Emergency Management (NCCEM) A national organization founded in 1952 composed of 1,500 individuals responsible for preparation of emergency and civil defense plans on the city and county levels. It acts as liaison among local units of government and state and federal emergency and civil defense agencies. Formerly (1983) United States Civil Defense Council.

National Council of Acupuncture Schools and Colleges (NCASC) A national organization founded in 1982 composed of 14 schools and colleges of acupuncture that offer a minimum two-year accredited training program. Its purposes are to advance the status of acupuncture and Oriental medicine through a certification program, to provide high-quality classroom and clinical instruction, and to promote the improvement of research and teaching methods. *See also* acupuncture.

National Council Against Health Fraud (NCAHF) A national organization founded in 1977 composed of 1,500 health and legal professionals and other interested individuals interested in educating the public on fraud and quackery in health care. Its task forces include AIDS Quackery, Broadcast Media Abuse, Nutrition Diploma Mills, and Questionable Methods of Cancer Management. *See also* fraud and abuse.

National Council on the Aging (NCOA) A national organization founded in 1950 composed of 6,700 individuals in business and industry, organized labor, and the health professions; social workers, librarians, the clergy, and educators; housing, research, and government agencies; and state and local agencies on the aging. It maintains the National Association of Older Worker Employment Services, National Center on Arts and the Aging, Health Promotion Institute, National Center on

Rural Aging, National Institute on Adult Daycare, National Institute of Community-Based Long-Term Care, National Institute of Senior Centers, National Institute of Senior Housing, National Interfaith Coalition on Aging, and National Voluntary Organizations for Independent Living for the Aging. *See also* aging; geriatric medicine; gerontology; Health Promotion Institute.

National Council on Alcoholism and Drug Dependence (NCADD) A national organization founded in 1944 composed of 186 local groups working for the prevention and control of alcoholism through programs of public and professional education, medical and scientific information, and public policy advocacy. It sponsors National Alcohol Awareness Month each April and National Fetal Alcohol Syndrome Awareness Week. *See also* alcoholism; alcoholism and other drug dependence; fetal alcohol syndrome.

National Council on Alternative Health Care Policy (NCAHCP) A national organization founded in 1976 that offers technical assistance to organizations interested in developing alternative health care models, policies, and programs directed toward low-income individuals.

National Council on Child Abuse and Family Violence (NCCAFV) A national organization founded in 1984 that supports community-based prevention and treatment programs that provide assistance to children, women, the elderly, and families who are victims of abuse and violence. It is interested in the cyclical and intergenerational nature of family violence and abuse and works to increase public awareness of family violence and promote private sector financial support for prevention and treatment programs. *See also* child abuse; violence.

National Council of Community Hospitals (NCCH) A national organization founded in 1974 composed of 126 community hospitals, hospital consultant groups, and individual health delivery representatives. It acts as a lobbyist for legislation and federal issues affecting hospitals, physicians, and health care beneficiaries. *See also* community hospital.

National Council of Community Mental Health Centers (NCCMHC) A national association founded in 1969 composed of 600 community mental health centers, state provider organizations, agencies, and interested individuals. Its purpose is to improve the quality and accessibility of mental health services. It

develops state and national legislative policy issues, works for full mental health care coverage by insurance companies and federal programs, and conducts workshops relating to significant issues and changes in community mental health. *See also* community mental health center; mental health services.

National Council on Family Relations (NCFR) A national organization founded in 1938 composed of 3,900 family life professionals, including clergy, counselors, educators, home economists, lawyers, nurses, librarians, physicians, psychologists, social workers, sociologists, and researchers. It seeks to provide opportunities for members to plan and act together to advance marriage and family life through consultation, conferences, and the dissemination of information and research. *See also* family.

National Council on Family Relations Family Therapy Section *See* Family Therapy Section of the National Council on Family Relations.

National Council on the Handicapped (NCH) An independent council affiliated with the US Department of Education and interested in research, programs, services, and resources for handicapped individuals. *See also* disability; handicap; handicapped person.

National Council of Health Care Services *See* American Health Care Association.

National Council of Health Centers *See* American Health Care Association.

National Council on Health Laboratory Services (NCHLS) A national organization founded in 1952 composed of 22 representatives and alternates of national organizations and US government agencies interested in improving laboratory services. *See also* laboratory.

National Council Licensure Examination (NCLEX) An examination, developed and administered by the National Council of State Boards of Nursing, designed to test basic competency for nursing practice. The NCLEX-RN (registered nurse) test plan has three components, including nursing behaviors grouped under nursing process categories, the process of decision making that defines the role of nursing, and levels of cognitive ability. *See also* licensure; National Council of State Boards of Nursing; nursing; registered nurse.

National Council on Patient Information and Education (NCPIE) A national organization founded in 1982 composed of 240 health care organizations, pharmaceutical manufacturing organizations, federal agencies, voluntary health agencies, and consumer groups interested in increasing the availability of information and improving the dialogue between consumers and health care providers about prescription medicines. It communicates, for example, with health care providers on the importance of giving consumers oral and written information on prescription medicines and encourages consumers to ask questions about medicines and explain factors that may affect their ability to follow prescriptions. *See also* patient; pharmacy; prescription drug.

National Council for Prescription Drug Programs (NCPDP) A national organization founded in 1977 composed of 576 companies, organizations, agencies, and individuals with an active interest in third-party prescription drug programs. Its goal is to advance standardization of third-party prescription drug programs. *See also* prescription drug.

National Council on Radiation Protection and Measurements (NCRPM) A national organization founded in 1929 composed of 75 nationally recognized scientists who share the belief that significant advances in radiation protection and measurement can be achieved through cooperative effort. It conducts research focusing on safe occupational exposure levels and disseminates information. *See also* measurement; occupational safety; radiation.

National Council on Rehabilitation Education (NCRE) A national organization founded in 1961 composed of 540 academic organizations, professional educators, researchers, and students interested in improving services to persons with disabilities, determining the skills and training necessary for effective rehabilitation services, and developing standards and uniform licensure and certification requirements for rehabilitation personnel. *See also* certification; licensure; rehabilitation.

National Council of State Boards of Nursing (NCSBN) A national organization founded in 1978 composed of 61 state boards of nursing, which assists member boards in maintaining and administering the National Council Licensure Examinations for registered and practical nurses and works to ensure relevancy of the examinations to current nursing practice. It aids the boards in the collection and analysis of information pertaining to the licensure and discipline of nurses. *See also* licensed practical nurse; licensed vocational nurse; licensure;

National Council Licensure Examination; nursing; registered nurse.

National Council of State Emergency Medical Services Training Coordinators (NCSEMSTC) A national organization founded in 1977 composed of 159 individuals employed by state-level emergency medical services agencies who are responsible for coordination or supervision of emergency medical services (EMS) training programs. It promotes the responsible movement of emergency medical technicians (EMTs) throughout the nation through standardization of policies related, but not limited to, curriculum, certification, recertification, revocation, and reciprocity. It also seeks to further develop the public recognition and trust of the emergency medical technician as a health professional. *See also* certification; emergency medical services; emergency medical technician; recertification.

National Council of State Pharmaceutical Association Executives *See* National Council of State Pharmacy Association Executives.

National Council of State Pharmacy Association Executives (NCSPAE) A national organization founded in 1927 composed of 51 executive officers of state pharmaceutical associations. Formerly (1992) National Council of State Pharmaceutical Association Executives. *See also* pharmacy.

National Council for Therapeutic Recreation Certification (NCTRC) A national organization founded in 1981 that establishes national standards for certification and recertification of individuals who work in the therapeutic recreation field, grants recognition to individuals who voluntarily apply and meet established standards, and monitors adherence to standards by certified personnel. *See also* certification; recertification; recreation therapy.

National Council for Therapy and Rehabilitation Through Horticulture *See* American Horticultural Therapy Association.

national debt The debt owed by the federal government. The debt is made up of obligations, such as Treasury bills, Treasury notes, and Treasury bonds. The interest due on the national debt is one of the major annual expenses of the federal government. *See also* gross national debt.

national debt, gross *See* gross national debt.

National Demonstration Project on Quality Improvement in Health Care One of the earliest efforts at moving total quality management into the health care field, organized jointly by the Harvard Community Health Plan and the Juran Institute. The study paired 21 health care organizations with industrial total quality management experts to determine if the principles of total quality management were transferrable from industry to health care. *See also* quality improvement; total quality management.

National Dental Assistants Association (NDAA) A national association founded in 1964 composed of 500 dental assistants. It is an auxiliary of the National Dental Association. *See also* dental assistant.

National Dental Association (NDA) A national organization founded in 1913 composed of 2,500 dentists interested in providing quality dental care to the unserved and underserved public and to promote knowledge of the art and science of dentistry. It fosters the integration of minority dental health care providers in the profession and promotes dentistry as a viable career for minorities through scholarship and support programs. *See also* dentist.

National Denturist Association (NDA) A national organization founded in 1975 composed of 37 state groups of dental laboratory technicians, denturists, and dentists interested in development and advancement of standards and certification of denturists. *See also* certification; denturist.

National Digestive Diseases Education and Information Clearinghouse *See* National Digestive Diseases Information Clearinghouse.

National Digestive Diseases Information Clearinghouse (NDDIC) A national clearinghouse founded in 1980 as a national resource to inform and educate physicians, health professionals, patients and their families, and the public on digestive health and diseases. Formerly (1985) National Digestive Diseases Education and Information Clearinghouse. *See also* clearinghouse; digestive system; disease; gastroenterology.

National Drug Trade Conference (NDTC) A national federation founded in 1913 composed of 8 associations of manufacturers, wholesalers, and boards and colleges of pharmacy. *See also* board; pharmacy.

National Easter Seal Society (NESS) A national federation of state and local societies founded in 1919 that operates over 400 service centers that serve over one million people with disabilities. Also known as Easter Seal Society. Formerly (1980) National Easter Seal Society for Crippled Children and Adults. *See also* disability.

National Easter Seal Society for Crippled Children and Adults *See* National Easter Seal Society.

National Emergency Management Association (NEMA) A national organization founded in 1950 composed of 212 state emergency management directors, local emergency management representatives, and individuals, associations, and corporations with an interest in emergency management. It seeks to improve relations within the public safety community to provide a cohesive infrastructure for the protection of the public against natural and human-created hazards. It represents the local emergency management community before the federal government and produces position papers and resolutions on emergency management issues. Formerly (1980) National Association of State Directors for Disaster Preparedness. *See also* disaster; disaster preparedness plan; emergency preparedness plan/program.

National Emergency Medicine Association (NEMA) A national organization founded in 1982 composed of 5,000 individuals interested in preventing trauma and improving emergency medical care nationwide. *See also* emergency medicine.

National EMS Pilots Association (NEMSPA) A national organization founded in 1985 composed of 500 aeromedical helicopter pilots; organizations providing goods and services to the emergency medical service (EMS) industry; and medical professionals interested in improving the professionalism of EMS pilots and increasing safety in EMS operations. *See also* emergency medical services system.

National Environmental Health Association (NEHA) A national organization founded in 1930 composed of 5,600 persons engaged in environmental health and protection for governmental agencies, public health and environmental protection agencies, industry, and colleges and universities. *See also* environmental health.

National Episcopal Coalition on Alcohol *See* National Episcopal Coalition on Alcohol and Drugs.

National Episcopal Coalition on Alcohol and Drugs (NECAD) A national organization founded in 1982 composed of 800 individuals, parishes, and Episcopal church diocesan committees addressing the issue of alcohol and drug use and addiction. Formerly (1986) National Episcopal Coalition on Alcohol. *See also* addiction; alcoholism and other drug dependence.

National Eye Institute (NEI) *See* National Institutes of Health.

National Family Planning and Reproductive Health Association (NFPRHA) A national organization founded in 1971 composed of hospitals, state and city departments of health, health care providers, private nonprofit clinics, and consumers interested in the maintenance and improvement of family planning and reproductive health services. *See also* family planning.

National Federation of Catholic Physicians Guilds (NFCPG) A national organization founded in 1932 composed of 3,500 Catholic physicians and dentists and 90 local groups with a priest-moderator for each local group. *See also* physician.

National Federation of Housestaff Organizations (NFHO) A national federation founded in 1984 composed of 11 housestaff physicians' unions that assists members in collective bargaining, lobbying state and local governments, and promoting unionization among housestaff physicians. *See also* housestaff; intern; resident.

National Federation of Licensed Practical Nurses (NFLPN) A national organization founded in 1949 composed of 8,000 licensed practical and vocational nurses. *See also* licensed practical nurse; licensed vocation nurse.

National Federation of Societies for Clinical Social Work (NFSCSW) A national federation founded in 1971 composed of state societies of clinical social work united to provide a vehicle for state and regional societies to share concerns common to clinical social work, develop solutions to problems beyond the jurisdiction of any single society, and carry out appropriate courses of action. *See also* clinical social worker.

National Federation for Specialty Nursing Organizations (NFSNO) A national organization founded in 1972 composed of 29 nursing specialty organizations representing approximately 370,000 individuals. The organization provides a medium for discussion and consensus-building on common issues and problems in nursing. *See also* nursing; nursing specialties; specialty.

National Fire Protection Association (NFPA) The organization that issues the *Life Safety Code* with which the Joint Commission on Accreditation of Healthcare Organizations expects health care organizations to comply. *See also* Joint Commission on Accreditation of Healthcare Organizations; *Life Safety Code*.

National Flight Nurses Association (NFNA) A national organization founded in 1981 composed of 1,300 flight nurses. *See also* nurse.

National Flight Paramedics Association (NFPA) A national organization founded in 1986 composed of 400 flight paramedics. *See also* paramedic.

National Formulary (NF) A compendium of official standards for the preparation of various pharmaceutics not listed in the *United States Pharmacopeia*. The *National Formulary* is one of three official compendia of drugs and medications in the United States recognized by the Federal Food, Drug, and Cosmetic Act. The other two are the *Homeopathic Pharmacopeia of the United States* and the *United States Pharmacopeia*. The *National Formulary* is a publication of the United States Pharmacopeia Convention. *See also* formulary; *Homeopathic Pharmacopeia of the United States*; *United States Pharmacopeia*; United States Pharmacopeia Convention.

National Foundation for Non-Invasive Diagnostics (NFNID) A national organization founded in 1977 to provide continuing education for physicians and technologists in the field of echocardiography. It awards the designation of professional ultrasound technologist to seminar participants who meet certification standards. *See also* certification; continuing education; echocardiography.

National Geriatrics Society (NGS) A national organization founded in 1952 composed of 118 public, voluntary, and proprietary institutions providing long term care and treatment of the chronically ill aged. It promotes maintenance of standards and qualified administration of facilities caring for the aged. *See also* geriatric medicine; long term care; nursing home.

National Guard Technicians, National Association of Air *See* National Association of Air National Guard Technicians.

National Health Agencies Committee for the Combined Federal Program *See* National Voluntary Health Agencies.

National Health Board According to the Health Security Act introduced to Congress, a body created in the executive branch composed of seven members appointed by the president, by and with the advice and consent of the Senate. Its general duties and responsibilities include, but are not limited to, interpretation of a comprehensive benefit package, administration of cost-containment provisions, responsibility for a performance-based system of quality management and improvement, and development and implementation of standards to establish a national health information system to measure quality. *See also* comprehensive benefit package; Health Security Act.

National Health Care Anti-Fraud Association (NHCAA) A national organization founded in 1985 composed of 350 private insurance companies and public and private agencies that work against health insurance fraud and share information on claims. *See also* fraud and abuse.

National Health Club Association (NHCA) A national organization founded in 1988 composed of 3,000 fitness centers and health clubs. Formerly (1987) National Fitness Association. *See also* fitness.

National Health Corps *See* National Health Service Corps.

National Health Council (NHC) A national organization founded in 1920 composed of 113 voluntary and professional societies in the health field, federal government agencies concerned with health matters, and national organizations and business groups with strong health interests. It conducts research on health issues, serves as an information clearinghouse on health careers, and monitors legislation and regulations.

National Health Federation (NHF) A national watchdog organization founded in 1955 composed of 20,000 persons interested in individual freedom of choice in matters relating to health. The organization represents the belief that organized medicine, the pharmaceutical industry, and other special interests have been responsible for many laws, rules, and regulations which have served the interests of these groups rather than the interests of the American public.

national health insurance (NHI) A federal government-regulated health insurance program for financing health services for all or most citizens. The United States does not have national health insurance, but such insurance is common in many developed countries in the world. *Compare* national health service. *See also* Medicare; Medicaid; social insurance; socialized medicine; Wagner-Murray-Dingell Bill.

National Health Insurance, Committee for *See* Committee for National Health Insurance.

National Health Law Program (NHeLP) A national organization founded in 1969 composed of attorneys and health services program attorneys and their clients in matters involving health problems of the poor. It offers, among other activities, information, referral, and consultation on litigation strategy and coordinates testimony for particular hearings. *See also* attorney; health law.

National Health Lawyers Association (NHLA) A national organization founded in 1971 composed of 7,000 private, corporate, institutional, and governmental lawyers, and health professionals. It serves as an information clearinghouse on health law and sponsors health law educational programs and seminars. *See also* clearinghouse; health law; lawyer.

National Health Planning and Resources Development Act of 1974 The federal law that established health systems agencies to conduct health system planning and resource development activities in state or substate geographic areas. Federal funding of health planning ended on September 30, 1986, although many states continue planning through their health systems agencies under state funding. *See also* health planning; health system agency; statewide health coordinating council.

National Health Policy Forum (NHPF) A national nonpartisan organization founded in 1971 composed of 1,200 senior-level health policymakers from Congress and the executive branch of the federal government. Subscribers to issue papers are health policy professionals from academia and industry. The organization's primary goal is to improve the process of federal decision making in health policy. It provides continuing education for health policymakers in small, "off the record" settings to encourage the free and candid exchange of ideas. It does not lobby for or against legislative proposals, but emphasizes the discussion of underlying issues and concepts in such areas as health finance, manpower, child health and development, access to health care, aging, and preventive health care. *See also* health policy.

national health service A health program in which a national government directly operates a health system that serves some or all of its citizens. National health service and national health insurance are not synonymous; national health insurance usually refers to programs in which the government insures or otherwise arranges financing for health care without directly arranging for, owning, or operating a health care program. *Compare* national health insurance. *See also* social insurance; socialized medicine.

National Health Service Corps (NHSC) A program of the US Public Health Service, established by the Emergency Health Personnel Act of 1970, which places nurses, physicians, and dentists in underserved rural and urban areas. *Synonyms*: the Corps; National Health Corps. *See also* medically underserved population; Public Health Service.

National Health System, Coalition for a *See* Coalition for a National Health System.

National Hearing Aid Society (NHAS) A national organization founded in 1951 composed of 4,000 hearing aid specialists who test hearing for the selection, adaptation, fitting, adjusting, servicing, and sale of hearing aids. Members counsel the hearing impaired and instruct them in the care and use of hearing aids. It administers a qualification program for screening persons designated as Hearing Instrument Specialists, administers a consumer protection program, and establishes standards of education, equipment, and techniques in the fitting of hearing aids. *See also* hearing aid; hearing impaired.

National Hearing Conservation Association (NHCA) A national organization founded in 1977 composed of 450 individuals holding advanced academic degrees in a discipline involving hearing and hearing loss; professional service organizations engaged in industrial hearing conservation programs; and companies that manufacture or sell occupational noise or hearing loss products. It encourages education and standards development among members and industrial groups, and monitors legislation and regulatory activities relating to hearing conservation. *See also* hearing; hearing impaired.

National Heart, Lung and Blood Institute *See* National Institutes of Health.

National Heart Research (NHR) A project of the National Emergency Medicine Association concerned with furthering advances in the area of traumatic medicine, particularly cardiac disorders. *See also* National Emergency Medicine Association.

National Heart Savers Association (NHSA) A national organization founded in 1985 that promotes cardiac health by informing the public of the dangers of a high-cholesterol diet. It conducts public cholesterol screening programs and has been successful in persuading major food processing and fast food restaurant companies to stop using palm and coconut oil, lard, and beef tallow, which are high in saturated fats, as ingredients in prepared foods. It promotes nutrition education in public schools and lobbies for more healthful school lunches. *See also* cholesterol.

National Hormone and Pituitary Program (NHPP) A national organization founded in 1963 that collects human pituitary glands obtained through autopsies and extracts from them human growth hormone, human follicle stimulating hormone, human luteinizing hormone, human adrenocorticotrophic hormone, human thyroid stimulating hormone, human prolactin, and beta-lipotropin. These are distributed to doctors in research centers for research in endocrinology. *See also* autopsy; endocrinology; hormone; pituitary gland.

National Hospice Organization (NHO) A national organization founded in 1978 composed of 2,750 hospice organizations and individuals interested in the advancement of the hospice concept and program of care. *See also* hospice.

National Hypertension Association (NHA) A national organization founded in 1977 composed of physicians, medical researchers, and business professionals interested in prevention of the complications of hypertension. It seeks to combat hypertension by developing, directing, and implementing effective programs to educate physicians and the public about hypertension. *See also* hypertension.

National Indian Health Board (NIHB) A national organization founded in 1969 composed of Indians of all tribes and natives of Alaskan villages. It advocates the improvement of health conditions that directly or indirectly affect American Indians and Alaskan Natives and informs the public of the health conditions of Native Americans. *See also* Native American.

National Information Center for Children and Youth with Disabilities (NICHCY) A national organization founded in 1970 that provides information concerning educational rights and special services to parents and educators of children with physical, mental, and emotional handicaps. *See also* disability; handicap.

National Information Center on Deafness (NICD)
A nonmembership resource and information clearinghouse founded in 1986 that provides information on all aspects of deafness. It makes referrals and identifies other resources for persons seeking information on deafness and hearing loss. *See also* clearinghouse; deafness; hearing loss.

national information infrastructure A communications network consisting of computers and work stations, software applications and databases, and technical standards for linking users. *See also* health information infrastructure; infrastructure.

National Institute on Adult Daycare (NIAD) A national institute founded in 1979 composed of 1,300 adult daycare practitioners; health and social service planners; and individuals involved in planning and providing services for older persons. *See also* adult day care; daycare center.

National Institute on Aging *See* National Institutes of Health.

National Institute of Allergy and Infectious Diseases *See* National Institutes of Health.

National Institute of Arthritis and Musculoskeletal and Skin Diseases *See* National Institutes of Health.

National Institute for Burn Medicine (NIBM) A nonmembership organization founded in 1968 that provides consultation for development of specialized burn care facilities; prevention programs and materials; and education, information, and statistics in burn treatment and care. *See also* burn; medicine.

National Institute of Child Health and Human Development (NICHHD) A component of the National Institutes of Health that supports biomedical research on reproductive processes influencing human fertility and infertility. It develops methods for regulating fertility, evaluates the safety and effectiveness of contraceptive methods, and conducts research on the reproductive motivation of individuals and the causes and consequences of population change. *See also* National Institutes of Health.

National Institute on Community-Based Long-Term Care (NICLC) A unit of the National Council on the Aging founded in 1984 composed of 1,500 members. It promotes and develops a comprehensive long term care system that will integrate home-based and community-based services enabling older adults to live in their own homes as long as possible. It serves as information clearinghouse for long term care professionals. *See also* long term care.

National Institute of Dental Research *See* National Institutes of Health.

National Institute of Diabetes and Digestive and Kidney Diseases *See* National Institutes of Health.

National Institute on Disability and Rehabilitation Research A federal research institute administering research programs in disabilities and rehabilitation. *See also* disability; rehabilitation.

National Institute of Electromedical Information (NIEI) A national organization founded in 1984 composed of individuals interested in electromedicine. *See also* electromedicine.

National Institute of Environmental Health Sciences *See* National Institutes of Health.

National Institute for the Family (NIF) A national organization founded in 1980 that seeks to strengthen families in the United States by providing educational programs to adults. It sponsors training and assessment programs, organizes workshops and seminars and disseminates information on family education and ministries. *See also* family.

National Institute of General Medical Sciences *See* National Institutes of Health.

National Institute for Jewish Hospice (NIJH) A national organization founded in 1985 composed of individuals and organizations concerned about terminally ill Jewish people. It serves as a resource center that seeks to help terminal patients and their families deal with their grief by providing information on traditional Jewish views on death, dying, and managing the loss of a loved one. *See also* hospice care.

National Institute of Mental Health (NIMH) A branch of the National Institutes of Health responsible for sponsoring and directing research on the cause, diagnosis, treatment, and prevention of mental disorders. *See also* mental disorder; National Institutes of Health.

National Institute of Neurological and Communicative Disorders and Stroke *See* National Institutes of Health.

National Institute for Occupational Safety and Health (NIOSH) An entity within the Centers for Disease Control and Prevention that supports and conducts research on occupational safety and health issues; provides technical assistance and training; and develops recommendations for the Labor Department. *See also* Association of University Programs in Occupational Health and Safety; Centers for Disease Control and Prevention; occupational health and safety.

National Institute for Rehabilitation Engineering (NIRE) A multidisciplinary research, training, and service organization founded in 1967 to provide custom-designed and custom-made tools and devices and intensive personal task-performance and driver training to handicapped persons. It is often the organization of last resort for permanently, severely, or multihandicapped persons. It is staffed by 400 electronics engineers, physicists, psychologists, optometrists, and other individuals who work as a team for the handicapped person. *See also* handicap; rehabilitation.

National Institutes of Health (NIH) A federal agency within the US Department of Health and Human Services that is the principal biomedical research arm of the federal government. It comprises many research institutes, including the National Cancer Institute; National Eye Institute; National Heart, Lung and Blood Institute; National Institute of Allergy and Infectious Diseases; National Institute of Arthritis and Musculoskeletal and Skin Diseases; National Institutes of Diabetes and Digestive and Kidney Diseases; National Institute of Child Health and Human Development; National Institute of Dental Research; National Institute of Environmental Health Sciences; National Institute of General Medical Sciences; National Institute of Mental Health; National Institute of Neurological and Communicative Disorders and Stroke; and National Institute on Aging. The NIH is also comprised of eight components, including the National Library of Medicine, the Warren Grant Magnuson Clinical Center, the National Center for Nursing Research, the National Center for Research Resources, the John E. Fogarty International Center, the National Center for Human Genome Research, the Division of Research Grants, and the Division of Computer Research and Technology.

National Institute of Standards and Technology (NIST) A federal agency whose mission is to assist industry in developing technology to improve product quality; modernize manufacturing processes; ensure product reliability; and to facilitate rapid commercialization of products based on scientific discoveries. It is a part of the Department of Com-

merce. Formerly (1988) National Bureau of Standards. *See also* standard; technology.

National Institute for Trial Advocacy (NITA) A national organization founded in 1971 composed of lawyers and judges interested in improving the trial bar in the United States. It trains lawyers in trial advocacy skills and develops methods for teaching and learning such skills in law schools and in continuing education programs. It sponsors regional training programs featuring student performances in a courtroom atmosphere augmented by team teaching, videotape review of the students' performances, demonstrations, and lectures. *See also* judge; lawyer; trial.

National Insurance Consumer Organization (NICO) A national public interest organization founded in 1980 that educates consumers on all aspects of buying insurance and encourages people to become aware of their insurance needs and to buy insurance only as those needs dictate. It serves as a consumer advocate on public policy matters and works for reform of unfair industry practices and marketplace abuses. *See also* consumer; health insurance; insurance; public interest.

nationalization The takeover of a private company's assets or operations by a government. The company may or may not be compensated for the loss of assets. *See also* asset.

National Jewish Center for Immunology and Respiratory Medicine A national organization founded in 1978 devoted to treatment, research, and education in chronic respiratory diseases and immunological disorders, such as asthma, tuberculosis, cystic fibrosis, chronic bronchitis, emphysema, interstitial lung disease, and systemic lupus erythematosus. Formerly (1984) National Jewish Hospital/National Asthma Center. *See also* asthma; cystic fibrosis; immunology; tuberculosis.

National Jewish Hospital/National Asthma Center *See* National Jewish Center for Immunology and Respiratory Medicine.

National Kidney and Urologic Diseases Information Clearinghouse (NKUDIC) A national networking, referral, and resource center founded in 1987 that disseminates educational information on kidney and urologic diseases and their causes and treatments. It was established by the National Institutes of Health. *See also* kidney; nephrology; networking; urology.

National Leadership Coalition on AIDS (NLCOA)
A national organization founded in 1987 composed of 180 major corporations; labor, trade, and professional associations; and civic, voluntary, religious, gay, and ethnic groups. It strives to provide timely and pertinent information about AIDS to the business and labor community. *See also* acquired immunodeficiency syndrome.

National League for Nursing (NLN) A national organization founded in 1952 composed of 19,800 individuals and agencies concerned with nursing education and delivery of nursing services. It provides tests used in selecting of applicants to schools of nursing, and for evaluating nursing student progress and nursing service. It nationally accredits nursing education programs, home health agencies, and other types of home care services. *See also* American Nurses Association; Community Health Accreditation Program; nursing.

National Library of Medicine (NLM) A component of the National Institutes of Health that offers medical library services and computer-based reference services to the public, health professionals, libraries in medical schools and hospitals, and research institutions. *See also* Medical Literature Analysis and Retrieval System (MEDLARS); Medical Subject Headings (MeSH); MEDLINE; National Institutes of Health.

National Male Nurse Association *See* American Assembly for Men in Nursing.

National Marrow Donor Program (NMDP) A national organization founded in 1986 composed of 75 donor and bone marrow transplant centers. It acts as a central registry of US bone marrow donors; seeks to develop a large pool of potential donors; facilitates searches and matching of donors and recipients; and tests the effectiveness of unrelated donor transplants. *See also* bone marrow transplant; donor.

National Maternal and Child Health Clearinghouse (NMCHC) A national clearinghouse founded in 1983 that collects and disseminates information on maternal and child health, human genetics, nutrition, and pregnancy care, primarily from materials developed by the US Department of Health and Human Services. *See also* clearinghouse; maternal and child health services.

National Medical Association (NMA) A national organization founded in 1895 composed of 14,500 black physicians. *See also* medical association; physician.

National Medical and Dental Association (NMDA)
A national organization founded in 1910 composed of 600 physicians and dentists of Polish extraction. It offers specialized education and maintains a speakers' bureau and a hall of fame. *See also* dentist; physician.

National Medical Fellowships (NMF) A nonmembership organization founded in 1946 that promotes education of minority students in medicine. It conducts a financial assistance program for first-year and second-year minority medical students and conducts workshops in financial planning and management for medical and premedical students, administrators, and parents. *See also* medicine; minority.

National Medic-Card Society *See* National Medic-Card Systems.

National Medic-Card Systems (NMCS) A for-profit organization founded in 1978 that produces wallet-size medical cards that have five sections, fold into the size of a credit card, and describe individuals' medical conditions in detail. Formerly (1986) National Medic-Card Society.

National Mental Health Association (NMHA) A national consumer advocacy organization founded in 1909 composed of 550 state groups that is devoted to fighting mental illness and promoting mental health. Formerly National Association for Mental Health; (1980) Mental Health Association. *See also* mental illness.

National Minority AIDS Council (NMAC) A national organization founded in 1986 composed of 200 public health departments and AIDS service organizations. It serves as a clearinghouse of information on AIDS as it affects minority communities in the United States. *See also* acquired immunodeficiency syndrome; clearinghouse; minority.

National Minority Health Association (NMHA) A national organization founded in 1987 composed of 30,000 health care providers and associations, consumers, executives and administrators, educators, pharmaceutical and health insurance companies, and other corporations with an interest in health care. It seeks to identify and focus attention on the health needs of minorities. *See also* minority.

National Network for Social Work Managers A national organization founded in 1985 composed of 44 individuals with degrees in social work who are engaged or interested in management within the human services field. It seeks to enhance social work managers' careers in such areas as administration, management, planning, budgeting, economics, and legislative work. *See also* manager; social work; social worker.

National New Professional Health Workers *See* New Professionals Section of the American Public Health Association.

National Nurses in Business Association (NNBA) A national organization founded in 1988 composed of 650 nurses in all types of business, including medical and legal consulting and quality assurance. It promotes the growth of health-related businesses owned and operated by nurses. *See also* business; nurse.

National Nurses Society on Addictions (NNSA) A national organization founded in 1975 composed of 1,100 nurses caring for persons addicted to alcohol and other drugs, and their families. Formerly (1983) National Nurses Society on Alcoholism. *See also* addiction; alcoholism and other drug dependence.

National Nurses Society on Alcoholism *See* National Nurses Society on Addictions.

National Optometric Association (NOA) A national organization founded in 1969 composed of 350 optometrists dedicated to increasing minority optometric personnel. *See also* optometry.

National Organization of Adolescent Pregnancy and Parenting (NOAPP) A national organization founded in 1979 composed of 2,000 professionals, policymakers, community and state leaders, and other concerned individuals and organizations promoting comprehensive and coordinated services designed for the prevention and resolution of problems associated with adolescent pregnancy and parenthood. *See also* adolescence; pregnancy.

National Organization for Associate Degree Nursing (NOADN) A national organization founded in 1986 composed of 4,000 individuals interested in retaining current competency level examinations and endorsement of registered nurse licensure from state to state for associate degree nursing graduates. It represents and advances the status of associated degree nursing education and practice. *See also* associate degree; licensure; nursing; registered nurse.

National Organization of Circumcision Information Resource Centers (NOCIRC) A national umbrella organization for circumcision information centers nationwide. It seeks to educate professionals and the public about routine infant circumcision, a surgical procedure that may not be medically indicated, and end the practice of routine infant circumcision. *See also* circumcision.

National Organization for Competency Assurance (NOCA) A national organization founded in 1977 composed of 63 nonprofit organizations conducting certification programs for occupations and professionals and for trade associations representing these professionals. It seeks to increase public awareness and acceptance of private-sector credentialing as an alternative to licensure. It promotes nonlicensed but certified practitioners as a means to achieving high quality and cost containment. Formerly (1989) National Commission for Health Certifying Agencies. *See also* certification; competence; credentialing; licensure.

National Organization on Disability (NOD) A national organization founded in 1982 composed of 50 state groups concerned with promoting the full participation in all aspects of life of persons with mental and physical disabilities. It promotes for disabled persons greater educational and employment opportunities, improved access to buildings, polling places, and transportation, and increased participation in recreational, social, religious, electoral, and cultural activities. *See also* disability.

National Organization of Gay and Lesbian Scientists and Technical Professionals (NOGLSTP) A national organization founded in 1983 composed of 450 gay and lesbian individuals, and interested organizations, employed or interested in high-technology or scientific fields. Its activities include educating the public, especially the gay and scientific communities; improving members' employment and professional environment; and opposing anti-gay discrimination and stereotypes. *See also* gay; lesbianism.

National Organ Transplant Act of 1984 A federal law that prohibits the sale of human organs, provides grant assistance in organ procurement activities, established a task force for organ transplantation, and provides for a demonstration bone-marrow registry and research study to ensure public equity in the availability and appropriate use of organ transplantation. It prohibits organ purchases in interstate commerce. *See also* organ procurement; transplantation.

National Osteopathic Women Physician's Association (NOWPA) A national organization founded in 1904 composed of osteopathic women physicians. *See also* osteopathic medicine.

National Pediculosis Association (NPA) A national organization founded in 1982 composed of 3,000 physicians, school nurses, individuals representing hospitals and county health departments, and parents interested in eliminating the incidence, particularly among children, of pediculosis (head lice). It conducts public education campaigns to make pediculosis control a public health priority and acts as a consumer advocate to ensure the quality and safety of products for treating pediculosis. It encourages scientific research to discover methods of treatment that minimize the use of pesticides. It sponsors National Pediculosis Prevention Month in September. *See also* body louse; head louse; pediculosis.

National Perinatal Association (NPA) A national organization founded in 1976 composed of 5,000 organizations and individuals interested in perinatal health care. *See also* neonatal-perinatal medicine; perinatal.

National Pharmaceutical Association (NPhA) A national organization founded in 1947 composed of state and local associations of professional minority pharmacists. It provides a means whereby members may contribute to their common improvement, share their experiences, and contribute to the public good. *See also* pharmacist.

National Pharmaceutical Council (NPC) A national organization founded in 1953 composed of 30 pharmaceutical manufacturers that research and produce trade-name prescription medications and other pharmaceutical products. *See also* pharmaceutical.

National Phlebotomy Association (NPA) A national organization founded in 1978 composed of 6,000 phlebotomists and other individuals with an interest in phlebotomy. The NPA accredits phlebotomy programs and gives national certification examinations in phlebotomy at the request of approved programs, among other activities. *See also* certification; phlebotomy.

National Podiatric Medical Association (NPMA) A national organization founded in 1971 composed of 200 black podiatrists. Its activities include improvement in public health, raising standards of the podiatric profession and education, and eliminating religious and racial discrimination and segregation in American medical institutions. Formerly (1987) National Podiatry Association. *See also* podi-

atric medicine.

National Podiatry Association *See* National Podiatric Medical Association.

National Practitioner Data Bank (NPDB) A data bank established by the Health Care Quality Improvement Act of 1986 to be the sole and central repository of the following mandatory information: medical malpractice payments, whether settlement or judgment, including those made by practitioners; licensure actions taken by boards, including revocations, suspensions, censures, reprimands, probations, and license surrenders relating to professional competence or conduct; clinical privilege actions, including limitation, reduction, suspension, or revocation of longer than 30 days, when based on professional competence or conduct, or resignation from staff membership or surrender of privileges while under or to avoid investigation; and society membership activities including denial or revocation, if based on professional review action conducted through peer review process and based on assessment of practitioner's professional competence, which affected or could affect health and welfare of patients. Hospitals *must* request information from the NPDB when a physician or dentist applies for medical staff membership or clinical privileges, and every two years while the practitioner is on the staff or has privileges. A practitioner may request information concerning himself or herself at any time. A state licensing authority and nonhospital health care facilities and professional societies with formal peer review processes may also request data. Attorneys may request data only when representing a plaintiff in a professional liability claim against a hospital and specific practitioners and only when the hospital involved failed to make a mandatory NPDB request regarding the practitioner named in the action. *See also* clinical privileges; Health Care Quality Improvement Act of 1986; licensure.

National Prevention Network (NPN) A nonmembership organization founded in 1982 composed of 61 officials of state alcohol and drug agencies who work to enhance national, state, and local programs for drug and alcohol abuse prevention. It serves as a network among state agency personnel and other prevention professionals to assist in the development of effective and innovative substance abuse prevention strategies. Its parent organization is National Association of State Alcohol and Drug

Abuse Directors. *See also* alcoholism; National Association of State Alcohol and Drug Abuse Directors; prevention; substance abuse.

National Psychological Association for Psychoanalysis (NPAP) A national organization founded in 1946 composed of 342 practicing psychoanalysts. It conducts training programs leading to certification in psychoanalysis. *See also* certification; psychoanalysis.

National Rare Blood Club (NRBC) A national organization founded in 1978 composed of 16,000 persons aged 18 years to 65 years who have rare blood types and are physically able to donate blood. Formerly (1993) National Rare Blood Club/New York Blood Center. *See also* blood; blood bank; donor.

National Rare Blood Club/New York Blood Center
See National Rare Blood Club.

National Registry in Clinical Chemistry (NRCC) A national certifying body founded in 1967 that evaluates the credentials of clinical chemistry practitioners and issues certificates to those who are qualified. It provides an annual evaluation of clinical laboratory specialists in the chemical field who voluntarily present their credentials to the registry. *See also* certification; clinical chemistry.

National Registry of Emergency Medical Technicians (NREMT) A national organization founded in 1970 composed of approximately 100,000 members. It assists in the development and evaluation of educational programs to train emergency medical technicians, establishes qualifications for eligibility to apply for registration, prepares and conducts examinations designed to ensure the competence of emergency medical technicians and paramedics, establishes a system for biennial registration, establishes procedures for revocation of certificates of registration for cause, and maintains a directory of registered emergency medical technicians. *See also* emergency medical services system; emergency medical technician; paramedic.

National Rehabilitation Association (NRA) A national organization founded in 1925 composed of 17,000 physicians, counselors, therapists, disability examiners, vocational evaluators, and other persons interested in rehabilitation of persons with disabilities. *See also* disability; rehabilitation.

National Rehabilitation Counseling Association (NRCA) A division of the National Rehabilitation Association founded in 1958 composed of 4,400 professional and student rehabilitation counselors. The organization works to expand the role of counselors in the rehabilitation process. *See also* rehabilitation; rehabilitation counselor.

National Rehabilitation Information Center (NARIC) A nonmembership organization founded in 1977 whose purpose is to improve delivery of information to the rehabilitation community; for example, it disseminates the findings of programs funded by the National Institute on Disability and Rehabilitation Research. *See also* rehabilitation.

National Renal Administrators Association (NRAA) A national organization founded in 1977 composed of 475 administrative personnel involved with dialysis programs for patients with kidney failure. It provides a vehicle for the development of educational and information services for members and maintains contact with health care facilities and government agencies. *See also* administrator; hemodialysis; kidney; renal.

National Research Council (NRC) A national organization founded in 1916 composed of 9,500 volunteer scientists, engineers, and other professionals serving on approximately 1,000 study committees annually. It serves as an independent adviser to the federal government on scientific and technical questions. It is jointly administered by the National Academy of Sciences, National Academy of Engineering, and Institute of Medicine. *See also* Institute of Medicine; research.

National Resident Matching Program (NRMP) A national clearinghouse founded in 1951 for matching the preferences of medical student and intern applicants for residencies with the hospitals' choice of their applicants, in order to assist students and interns in obtaining, to the extent possible, their choices of residencies. Medical students are advised by their medical schools on the procedures of the match, how to arrange for letters of recommendation and interviews, and how to complete applications for residency training programs. They can obtain information about training programs from their faculty and from the *Directory of Graduate Medical Education Programs*, published by the American Medical Association. *See also* clearinghouse; *Directory of Graduate Medical Education*; intern; matching; resident.

National Resource Center on Homelessness and Mental Illness (NRCHMI) A nonmembership organization founded in 1988 that serves as a center for information and technical assistance on the housing and service needs of the mentally ill homeless. *See also* mental illness.

National Rural Health Association (NRHA) A national organization founded in 1987 composed of 1,650 administrators, physicians, nurses, physician assistants, health planners, academicians, and other persons interested in understanding health care problems unique to rural areas. It absorbed (1986) the American Small and Rural Hospital Association and was formed by merger of the American Rural Health Association (founded 1977) and the National Rural Health Care Association (founded 1978 and formerly [1984] National Rural Primary Care Association). *See also* rural.

National Rural Health Care Association *See* National Rural Health Association.

National Safety Council (NSC) A national nongovernmental organization founded in 1913 composed of 12,000 individuals interested in promoting accident reduction by gathering and distributing information to the public about the causes of accidents and ways to prevent them. *See also* accident; safety.

National Safety Management Society (NSMS) A national organization founded in 1968 composed of 750 individuals with managerial responsibilities related to safety/loss control management, including medical, legal, and computer technology professionals. It advances new concepts of accident prevention and loss control and promotes the role of safety management in the total management effort. It advises concentration in areas where a favorable cost-benefit return can be achieved with these new concepts, while being cognizant of humanitarian considerations. *See also* management; safety management; safety.

National Sanitation Foundation (NSF) A national foundation founded in 1944 composed of 1,800 representatives of the public, health professions, business, and industry. It cooperates in research and educational programs and develops standards in the field of environmental sanitation and health. *See also* environmental health; public health; sanitation.

National Society of Biomedical Equipment Technicians *See* Society of Biomedical Equipment Technicians.

National Society for Cardiovascular Technology/

National Society for Pulmonary Technology (NSCT/NSPT) A national organization founded in 1966 composed of 2,500 health professionals involved in cardiology technology and pulmonary technology who are employed under the direction of a physician. Formerly (1980) National Society of Cardiopulmonary Technologists; (1986) National Society for Cardiopulmonary Technology; (1988) National Alliance of Cardiovascular Technologists; (1989) American Cardiology Technologists Association. *See also* cardiovascular technologist.

National Society of Genetic Counselors (NSGC) A national organization founded in 1979 composed of 925 genetic counselors with a master's or doctorate degree in human genetics, nursing, social work, or public health; physicians, dentists, and other persons with an interest in genetic counseling; and students in an undergraduate or master's program. *See also* genetic counseling; genetic counselor.

National Society for Histotechnology (NSH) A national organization founded in 1973 composed of 3,000 histology laboratory technicians, pathologists, laboratory equipment manufacturers' representatives, and interested individuals. *See also* histologic technician; histologic technologist.

National Society of Patient Representation and Consumer Affairs of the American Hospital Association (NSPRCA) A national organization founded in 1972 in response to a 1971 recommendation by the Commission on Medical Malpractice of the Department of Health, Education and Welfare. NSPRCA is composed of 1,031 members interested in advancing the development of effective patient representative programs in health care organizations. *See also* American Hospital Association; patient representative.

National Society of Pharmaceutical Sales Trainers (NSPST) A national organization founded in 1971 composed of 360 sales training directors and sales training personnel of pharmaceutical companies interested in improving professionalism within the field by raising standards of development and training programs. It encourages members' self-development by facilitating information exchange. *See also* detail person.

National Society of Professional Sanitarians (NSPS) A national organization founded in 1956 composed of 500 publicly and privately employed sanitarians. *See also* sanitarian.

national standard rule A test used for measuring the required level of care for a patient. It is based on the level of care provided by similar practitioners throughout the country. *Compare* locality rule. *See also* rule; standard of care.

National Standards Educators Association (NSEA) A national organization founded in 1987 composed of 100 industrial executives and managers, engineers, technicians, educators, and students interested in the significance and teaching of standards within American industry. It advances the concept of management by accountability that imposes the use of detailed certifications, accreditations, registrations, and licensures to combat standards illiteracy. It seeks to institute testing of the American industrial workforce based on standards common to various fields and maintains that testing can effect a positive cultural change to bring the United States into a true state of economic competitiveness. *See also* accreditation; certification; licensure; standard.

National Sudden Infant Death Syndrome Clearinghouse (NSIDSC) A project founded in 1980 of the US Department of Health and Human Services that provides health professionals, community service workers, health educators, parents, and the public with information and educational materials on sudden infant death syndrome and related issues. It develops materials concerning the syndrome, grief, apnea, and apnea monitoring. *See also* apnea; sleep apnea; sudden infant death syndrome.

National Therapeutic Recreation Society (NTRS) A national organization founded in 1966 composed of 3,200 personnel whose full-time employment is to provide therapeutic recreation services for persons with disabilities in clinical facilities and in the community. *See also* recreation therapy.

National Tumor Registrars Association (NTRA) A national organization founded in 1974 composed of 1,700 individuals involved in central, state, regional, and hospital-based tumor registries including physicians, hospital administrators, and health care planners who maintain ongoing records of the cancer patient's history, diagnosis, therapy, and outcome. *See also* tumor registry.

National Uniform Billing System *See* UB-92.

National Voluntary Health Agencies (NVHA) A nonprofit corporation of 63 national voluntary health agencies. Its purpose is to receive funds gen-

erated by the Combined Federal Campaign and to distribute them to member agencies. Formerly (1985) National Health Agencies Committee for the Combined Federal Program. *See also* voluntary health agency.

National Wellness Association (NWA) A national organization founded in 1985 composed of 1,700 health and wellness promotion professionals from corporations, universities, hospitals, community organizations, consulting firms, government organizations, and fitness clubs. *See also* preventive medicine; wellness.

National Wellness Institute (NWI) A nonmembership organization founded in 1977 that provides national leadership in the wellness movement. It assists organizations with planning, development, implementation, and evaluation of wellness programs and assists in the development of high-quality wellness products and services. Formerly (1985) Institute for Lifestyle Improvement. *See also* preventive medicine; wellness.

National Wholesale Druggists' Association (NWDA) A national organization founded in 1876 composed of 675 wholesalers and manufacturers of drug, toiletry, and sundry products; advertising agencies; and other groups interested in improving the flow of merchandise from manufacturer to consumer. It sponsors research and specialized education programs. *See also* druggist.

National Women's Health Network (NWHN) A national organization founded in 1976 composed of 15,000 consumers, organizations, and health centers. It monitors federal health policy as it affects women, testifies before Congress and federal agencies, and supports feminist health projects. It also sponsors the Women's Health Clearinghouse, a national resource file on all aspects of women's health care.

National Women's Health Resource Center (NWHRC) A national organization founded in 1988 composed of health professionals and consumers interested in public education and research that focuses on diseases or conditions that are unique, more prevalent, or more serious in women. It develops and provides models for clinical services, especially those that will meet the needs of underserved women.

Native American A person whose ancestry originates on the North American continent, usually an American Indian. *Synonym:* American Indian. *See* *also* medicine man.

natural Neither artificial nor pathologic, as in natural childbirth or natural cardiac pacemaker. *Compare* artificial.

natural cardiac pacemaker The group of cells in the heart that rhythmically initiate the heart beat, characterized physiologically by a slow loss of membrane potential during diastole. The usual site of the pacemaker is the sinoatrial node (an area of the heart at the junction of the superior vena cava and the right atrium). *See also* artificial cardiac pacemaker; pacemaker.

natural childbirth Labor and delivery accomplished by a mother with little or no medical intervention to relieve pain or aid in the birthing process. Some advocates of natural childbirth feel that the mother should be allowed to choose her own posture during labor. *See also* labor.

natural death acts Statutes enacted in many states that establish procedures by which a competent individual can make provision for the withholding or withdrawing of medical therapy at the time when he or she loses the capacity to make such medical decisions. National death acts were enacted, in large part, to codify the increasingly popular living wills. *See also* death; durable powers of attorney for health care; living will.

natural family planning Family-planning methods that do not use contraceptive devices of any kind, using instead the natural phases of fertility. *See also* family planning.

Natural Family Planning, American Academy of *See* American Academy of Natural Family Planning.

natural food Food that does not contain any additives, such as preservatives or artificial coloring. *See also* food.

Natural Food Associates (NFA) A national organization founded in 1952 composed of 5,000 professionals and consumers interested in organic farming, natural foods, and human health. It seeks to inform the public of the values of natural, chemical-free food grown in rich, fertile soil; to expose the dangers of chemical contamination of food, water, and land; and to offer preventive measures for metabolic disease. *See also* food; natural food.

Natural Foods Association, African-American *See* African-American Natural Foods Association.

natural history of disease The ordinary course of a disease from its inception to resolution. Detection and intervention can alter the natural history of a disease. *See also* disease.

Natural Hygiene Society, American *See* American Natural Hygiene Society.

natural immunity State of being innately resistant or insusceptible to a particular disease. *Synonym:* innate immunity. *See also* immunity.

natural language A human written or spoken language as opposed to a computer language. *See also* language; natural language processing.

natural language processing (NLP) A process by which medical records produced on a word processor are converted into a relational database, allowing sophisticated queries of medical records based on complicated word searches and syntactical analysis. This technologic capability has implications for quality improvement, risk management, and automated billing. For example, a computer can automatically and instantly audit all medical records in an emergency department or other setting according to practice guidelines to answer questions, such as: "Was an adequate abdominal examination documented in the medical record?" *See also* American Association for Artificial Intelligence; artificial intelligence; Intelligence Industries Association; medical record; natural language.

natural law A law or body of laws that derives from nature and is believed to be binding upon human actions apart from or in conjunction with laws established by human authority. *See also* law.

natural medicine *See* naturopathy.

Natural Resources, Committee on Energy and *See* Committee on Energy and Natural Resources.

natural selection The process in nature by which, according to Darwin's theory of evolution, only the organisms best suited to a particular environment because of their adaptations (genotypes) tend to survive and propagate offspring with their characteristics, while those less well adapted have less chance for survival and propagation, tending to be eliminated. *Compare* artificial selection. *See also* evolution; genotype; selection; survival of the fittest.

naturopath A doctor of naturopathy who diagnoses, treats, and cares for patients, using a system of practice that bases its treatment of all physiological functions and abnormal conditions on natural and mechanical methods. These methods include air, water, heat, earth, phytotherapy (treatment by use of plants), electrotherapy, physiotherapy, minor surgery, mechanotherapy, naturopathic corrections and manipulation, and all natural methods or modalities, together with natural medicines, natural processed foods, and herbs, and natural remedies. Naturopaths exclude major surgery, therapeutic use of x-ray and radium, and use of drugs, except those assimilable substances containing elements or compounds that are compounds of bodily tissues and are physiologically compatible to body processes for maintenance of life. *Synonyms:* Doctor of Naturopathy; naturopathic physician. *See also* naturopathy.

naturopathic physician *See* naturopath.

Naturopathic Physicians, American Association of *See* American Association of Naturopathic Physicians.

naturopathy A drugless system of therapy that relies on natural remedies, such as sunlight, air, and water, supplemented with diet and massage, to treat illness. *Synonyms:* natural medicine; naturopathic medicine. *Compare* allopathy; homeopathy; naprapathy; osteopathic medicine. *See also* naturopath.

Naturopathy, Doctor of (ND) *See* naturopath.

nausea An unpleasant feeling of being about to vomit, sometimes culminating in the act of vomiting. *See also* indigestion; vomit.

NAWL *See* National Association of Women Lawyers.

NAVAP *See* National Association of VA Physicians and Dentists.

NAVP *See* National Association of Vision Professionals.

naysayer A person who is assertively negative in attitude. *See also* negativism.

NBA *See* National Bar Association.

NBAC *See* National Black Alcoholism Council.

NBC *See* National Board for Certification in Dental Technology.

NBCC *See* National Board for Certified Counselors.

NBCOT *See* National Board for Certification of Orthopaedic Technologists.

NBEO *See* National Board of Examiners in Optometry.

NBIE *See* National Burn Information Exchange.

NBME *See* National Board of Medical Examiners.

NBNA *See* National Black Nurses Association.

NBOME *See* National Board of Osteopathic Medical Examiners.

NBPME *See* National Board of Podiatric Medical Examiners.

NBRC *See* National Board for Respiratory Care.

NBTA *See* National Board of Trial Advocacy.

NBWHP *See* National Black Women's Health Project.

NCA *See* National Certification Agency for Medical Lab Personnel; Nurse Consultants Association.

NCABHP *See* National Center for the Advancement of Blacks in the Health Professions.

NCADD *See* National Council on Alcoholism and Drug Dependence.

NCADV *See* National Coalition Against Domestic Violence.

NCAHCP *See* National Council on Alternative Health Care Policy.

NCAHF *See* National Council Against Health Fraud.

NCASA *See* National Coalition Against Sexual Assault.

NCASC *See* National Council of Acupuncture Schools and Colleges.

NCATA *See* National Coalition of Arts Therapy Associations.

NCBL *See* National Conference of Black Lawyers.

NCBLRDC *See* National Coalition of Black Lung and Respiratory Disease Clinics.

NCBPNP/N *See* National Certification Board of Pediatric Nurse Practitioners and Nurses.

NCCA *See* National Catholic Council on Alcoholism and Related Drug Problems; National Commission for the Certification of Acupuncturists.

NCCAFV *See* National Council on Child Abuse and Family Violence.

NCCDN *See* National Consortium of Chemical Dependency Nurses.

NCCEM *See* National Coordinating Council on Emergency Management.

NCCH *See* National Council of Community Hospitals.

NCCHC *See* National Commission on Correctional Health Care.

NCCIP, Zero to Three/ *See* Zero to Three/NCCIP.

NCCLS *See* National Committee for Clinical Laboratory Standards.

NCCMHC *See* National Council of Community Mental Health Centers.

NCCMHS *See* National Consortium for Child Mental Health Services.

NCCNHR *See* National Citizens Coalition for Nursing Home Reform.

NCCPA *See* National Commission on Certification of Physician Assistants.

NCCR *See* National Coalition for Cancer Research.

NCEC *See* National Commission for Electrologist Certification.

NCEMCH *See* National Center for Education in Maternal and Child Health.

NCFR *See* National Council on Family Relations.

NCFS *See* National College of Foot Surgeons.

NCH *See* National Center for Homeopathy; National Council on the Handicapped.

NCHE *See* National Center for Health Education.

NCHLS *See* National Council on Health Laboratory Services.

NCHS *See* National Center for Health Statistics.

NCI National Cancer Institute. *See* National Institutes of Health.

NCIC *See* Non-Circumcision Information Center.

NCISD *See* National Coalition on Immune System Disorders.

NCL *See* National Consumers League.

NCLE *See* National Contact Lens Examiners.

NCLEHA *See* National Conference of Local Environmental Health Administrators.

NCLEX *See* National Council Licensure Examination.

NCME *See* Network for Continuing Medical Education.

NCOA *See* National Council on the Aging.

NCOMDR *See* National Clearinghouse on Marital and Date Rape.

NCPAMT *See* National Coalition of Psychiatrists Against Motorcoach Therapy.

NCPCA *See* National Committee for Prevention of Child Abuse.

NCPDP *See* National Council for Prescription Drug Programs.

NCPG *See* National Catholic Pharmacists Guild of the United States.

NCPIE *See* National Council on Patient Information and Education.

NCPOA *See* National Chronic Pain Outreach Association.

NCQA *See* National Committee for Quality Assurance.

NCQHC *See* National Committee for Quality Health Care.

NCR *See* National Coalition for Research in Neurological Disorders.

NCRA *See* National Center on Rural Aging.

NCRC/AODA *See* National Certification Reciprocity Consortium/Alcoholism and Other Drug Abuse.

NCRE *See* National Council on Rehabilitation Education.

NCRPM *See* National Council on Radiation Protection and Measurements.

NCRV *See* National Committee for Radiation Victims.

NCSBCS *See* National Conference of States on Building Codes and Standards.

NCSBN *See* National Council of State Boards of Nursing.

NCSC *See* National Child Safety Council.

NCSEMSTC *See* National Council of State Emergency Medical Services Training Coordinators.

NCSL *See* National Conference of Standards Laboratories.

NCSPAE *See* National Council of State Pharmacy Association Executives.

NCTIP *See* National Committee on the Treatment of Intractable Pain.

NCTRC *See* National Council for Therapeutic Recreation Certification.

ND Abbreviation for Doctor of Naturopathy. *See* naturopath.

NDA *See* National Dental Association; National Denturist Association; new-drug application.

NDAA *See* National Dental Assistants Association.

NDDIC *See* National Digestive Diseases Information Clearinghouse.

NDMA *See* Nonprescription Drug Manufacturers Association.

NDTA *See* Neurodevelopmental Treatment Association.

NDTC *See* National Drug Trade Conference.

NEA *See* Nutrition Education Association.

near-poor Individuals and families who earn enough money to just meet their daily needs and do not qualify for governmental assistance. Typically, they do not have health insurance. The near-poor do not qualify as medically indigent unless a severe illness or injury creates a major economic hardship that would result in the loss of basic necessities of life. *See also* medically indigent; medically needy; poor.

nearsighted Pertaining to an individual who can see well at close range but has difficulty seeing objects at a distance. *Synonym*: myopia. *See also* ophthalmology; refractive error.

NECAD *See* National Episcopal Coalition on Alcohol and Drugs.

necessary Absolutely essential, as in an operation that is medically necessary to save a patient's life. *See also* necessary cause; need.

necessary cause A cause that must exist if a given event is to occur, but may not itself result in the event. *See also* cause; necessary.

necessity, pharmaceutical *See* pharmaceutical necessity.

Neck Nurses, Society of Otorhinolaryngology and Head/ *See* Society of Otorhinolaryngology and Head/Neck Nurses.

Neck Pain and TMJ Orthopedics, American Academy of Head, Facial and *See* American Academy of Head, Facial and Neck Pain and TMJ Orthopedics.

Neck Surgeons, Society of Head and *See* Society of Head and Neck Surgeons.

Neck Surgeons, Society of Military Otolaryngologists - Head and *See* Society of Military Otolaryngologists - Head and Neck Surgeons.

Neck Surgeons, Society of University Otolaryngologists - Head and *See* Society of University Otolaryngologists - Head and Neck Surgeons.

Neck Surgery, American Academy of Otolaryngology - Head and *See* American Academy of Otolaryngology - Head and Neck Surgery.

Neck Surgery, American Society for Head and *See* American Society for Head and Neck Surgery.

necrology A death roll, an obituary notice, or a history of the dead.

necromancy The prophesying of future events by supposed communication with the spirits of the dead.

necrophilia A pathological liking for dead bodies, especially the desire to have sexual intercourse with a dead body. *Compare* necrophobia.

necrophobia An irrational fear of death or corpses. *See also* phobia. *Compare* necrophilia. *See also* corpse; death; phobia.

necropsy *See* autopsy.

necrosis Death of tissue, usually caused by disease, inadequate blood supply to the tissue, or injury. *See also* death; tissue.

need 1. Some thing or action that is essential, indispensable, required, or cannot be done or lived without. 2. A condition marked by the lack or want of some such thing or action. Needs may or may not be perceived or expressed by a person in need and must be distinguished from demands, which are expressed desires that may or may not be needed. *See also* medically needy; needs assessment; perceived need.

needle A slender, sharp, metal instrument for suturing or puncturing. *See also* aspirating needle; hypodermic needle; needle biopsy; syringe; trocar.

needle, aspirating *See* aspirating needle.

needle biopsy Removal of a segment of tissue or fluid for microscopic analysis by inserting a hollow needle through the skin or external surface of an organ and twisting the needle to obtain a sample of cells. *See also* biopsy; needle.

needle, hypodermic *See* hypodermic needle.

need, perceived *See* perceived need.

needs assessment 1. An evaluation of a population's health status. 2. An evaluation of the productivity and performance of a health care organization, department, program, or plan. A needs assessment is performed prior to establishing or redefining the goals, priorities, and tasks of a program or organization. *See also* assessment; need.

needy, categorically *See* categorically needy.

needy, medically *See* medically needy.

negative binomial distribution *See* probability distribution.

negative correlation In statistics, an inverse association between two variables, meaning that as one variable becomes large, the other becomes small. Negative correlation is represented by correlation coefficients of less than zero. *See also* correlation; correlation coefficient; positive correlation; statistics; variable.

negative, false *See* false negative.

negative feedback 1. Feedback that reduces the output of a system. *See also* feedback; output. 2. An expression of resistance or objection.

negative incentive *See* incentive.

negative predictive value of a test *See* predictive value of a negative test.

negative test, predictive value of a *See* predictive value of a negative test.

negative, true *See* true negative.

negativism A pattern of behavior characterized by opposition, resistance to suggestion, unwillingness to cooperate, and a tendency to act in a contrary way. *Compare* optimism. *See also* naysayer.

neglect To pay little or no attention to, as in child

neglect. *See also* medical neglect.

neglect, medical *See* medical neglect.

negligence **1.** The act or state of being neglectful of, for example, dress or cleanliness. **2.** In health care, failure to exercise that degree of care expected of a reasonably prudent person under similar circumstances. Active negligence occurs when one engages in conduct that causes injury. The tort of negligence requires a *duty* to exercise reasonable care; a *breach* in exercising such care; and an injury or *damage* that was proximately *caused* by that breach of duty. *See also* contributory negligence; duty; gross negligence; negligence per se; professional negligence; tort.

negligence, contributory *See* contributory negligence.

negligence, gross *See* gross negligence.

negligence per se **1.** Negligence that is recognized as such without proof as to the particular circumstances because it is so obviously contrary to accepted standards of prudence that no reasonable person would have engaged in it. *See also* negligence. **2.** Conduct that is a violation of a specific statute.

negligence, professional *See* professional negligence.

negotiate To confer with another or other persons in order to come to terms or reach an agreement. *See also* negotiated settlement.

negotiated settlement The resolution of a malpractice claim before a judicial determination. *See also* negotiate; settlement.

negotiation The process of bargaining that precedes an agreement. Successful negotiation generally results in a contract between the parties. *See also* arbitration; mediation; negotiate.

NEHA *See* National Environmental Health Association.

NEI National Eye Institute. *See* National Institutes of Health.

neighborhood health center *See* community health center.

NEJM *See New England Journal of Medicine.*

NEMA *See* National Emergency Management Association; National Emergency Medicine Association.

NEMSPA *See* National EMS Pilots Association.

neoclassical economics A school of economic theory that flourished from about 1890 until the advent of Keynesian economics. Neoclassical economics asserted that market forces always would lead to efficient allocation of resources and full employment. *See also* economics; Keynesian economics.

neohippocratism A school of medicine that tends toward a humanistic view of disease focused on the individual patient and scientific observation by the physician, representing a return to the hippocratic theory and practice, with emphasis on observation and bedside medicine. *See also* Hippocrates of Cos; Hippocratic oath.

neologism In psychiatry, invention of a new word that has meaning only to the person who coined it. It is normal in early childhood, but usually is a sign of mental illness, such as schizophrenia, in an adult. *See also* mental illness; psychiatry; schizophrenia.

neonatal Pertaining to a neonate or to the first four weeks (or month) of life after birth.

neonatal death rate The number of neonatal deaths in relation to all infants born in a given population over a given period, usually expressed as the number of neonatal deaths per 100 or 1,000 live births. *Synonym:* neonatal mortality rate. *See also* infant; live birth; neonatal mortality; rate.

neonatal ICU *See* neonatal intensive care unit.

neonatal intensive care unit (NICU) A unit of a hospital for the treatment and continuous monitoring of infants with life-threatening conditions who are generally less than 23 days old on admission to the unit. *Synonyms:* neonatal ICU; newborn intensive care unit; premature nursery. *See also* intensive care unit; special care unit; unit.

neonatal mortality Death of live-born children who have not reached four weeks or one month of age; calculated as the number of infant deaths, during the first 28 days of life, per unit of population (for example, per 1,000 live births) in a defined health care organization, geographic area, or period of time. *See also* infant mortality; mortality; neonatal death rate; perinatal mortality.

Neonatal Nurses, Association of Women's Health, Obstetric, and *See* Association of Women's Health, Obstetric, and Neonatal Nurses.

Neonatal Nurses, National Association of *See* National Association of Neonatal Nurses.

neonatal-perinatal medicine The branch of medicine and subspecialty of pediatrics dealing with the care of sick newborn infants. *Synonyms:* neonatology; perinatalogy. *See also* neonatal; pediatrics.

neonatal-perinatal medicine specialist A pediatrician who subspecializes in neonatal-perinatal medicine. *Synonyms:* neonatologist; perinatologist. *See also* neonatal-perinatal medicine.

neonatal period The first 28 days of life.

neonatal unit *See* newborn nursery.

neonate An infant from birth to four weeks (28 days) of life. *See also* Apgar scale; infant; meconium.

neonatologist *See* neonatal-perinatal medicine specialist.

neonatology *See* neonatal-perinatal medicine.

neoplasia The formation of a tumor. *See also* tumor.

neoplasm *See* tumor.

nepenthic Inducing peace and forgetfulness and freedom from sorrow.

nephrectomy Surgical removal of a kidney. *See also* kidney; nephrology.

nephritis Inflammation of the kidney. *See also* inflammation; kidney; nephrology.

nephrography Radiographic visualization of the kidneys, on plain x-ray films or with the assistance of pyelography, angiography, or computerized axial tomography. *See also* angiography; computerized axial tomography; kidney; x-ray; nephrology.

nephrolithiasis The presence of calculi (stones) within the kidney and upper urinary tract. *See also* kidney; nephrology; renal colic.

nephrologist An internist who subspecializes in nephrology. *See also* internist; nephrology; pediatric nephrologist.

nephrologist, pediatric *See* pediatric nephrologist.

nephrology A subspecialty of internal medicine and pediatrics dealing with disorders of the kidney, high blood pressure, fluid and mineral balance, dialysis of body wastes when the kidneys do not function, and consultation with surgeons about kidney transplantation. *See also* end stage renal disease; internal medicine; pediatric nephrology; renal.

Nephrology, American Society of *See* American Society of Nephrology.

Nephrology Examiners - Nursing and Technology, Board of *See* Board of Nephrology Examiners - Nursing and Technology.

Nephrology Nurses' Association, American *See* American Nephrology Nurses' Association.

nephrology, pediatric *See* pediatric nephrology.

nephrology technician *See* dialysis technician.

nephropathy Disease of the kidney. *See also* disease; kidney.

nepotism Favoritism shown or patronage granted to relatives, as in business.

nerve A bundle of sensory and/or motor nerve fibers with connective tissue and blood vessels, run-ning in a common sheath of connective tissue. Within a nerve, each nerve fiber conducts impulses independently of its fellow fibers. *See also* nerve block; nerve gas; tract.

nerve block A blocking of the passage of impulses along a nerve, especially by administration of a local anesthetic. *See also* local anesthesia; nerve.

nerve gas Any one of a group of volatile liquids that are severely toxic through their anticholinesterase action. Nerve gas inhibits the enzyme cholinesterase, which normally inactivates the neurotransmitter substance acetylcholine. Acetylcholine accumulates in excess and prevents normal neuromuscular function. *See also* gas; nerve.

nerve stimulation, transcutaneous electric *See* transcutaneous electric nerve stimulation.

nervosa, anorexia *See* anorexia nervosa.

nervosa, bulimia *See* bulimia nervosa.

nervous breakdown A severe or incapacitating emotional disorder, especially when occurring suddenly and marked by depression. *See also* depression.

Nervous and Mental Disease, Association for Research in *See* Association for Research in Nervous and Mental Disease.

nervousness A state of excitability, irritability, or restlessness.

nervous system In anatomy, the system that regulates the body's responses to internal and external stimuli. In humans, it consists of the brain, spinal cord, nerves, ganglia, and parts of the receptor and effector organs. *See also* anatomy; central nervous system; neurotransmitters; peripheral nervous system.

nervous system, central *See* central nervous system.

nervous system, peripheral *See* peripheral nervous system.

NESS *See* National Easter Seal Society.

nest egg Assets put away for a large purchase or an individual's retirement. *See also* asset; individual retirement account; retirement.

net 1. Ultimate or final, as in net result. 2. In business, what is remaining after all deductions have been made, as for expenses.

net autopsy rate *See also* adjusted autopsy rate.

net income Revenue and gains minus expenses and losses. *See also* income.

net social benefit The social benefits minus the social costs of a proposed program or project. *See also* benefit; net.

network 1. In health care, an organization that provides or provides for integrated health services to a defined population of individuals or to one or more entities contracting on behalf of individuals. Networks are exemplified by a centralized structure that coordinates and integrates services provided by components and by practitioners participating in the network. A network may take the form of a health maintenance organization, a preferred provider organization, or other cooperative system of provider organizations, practitioners, and/or insurers that contracts with purchasers to provide health services. *Synonyms:* health care network; health network. *See also* community health network; component; corporatization of health care; diversification; health system; multihospital system; network model HMO; practitioner site; primary care network. **2.** An extended group of organizations or people with similar interests who interact and remain in contact for mutual support. *See also* networking; system. **3.** In computer science, a system of computers interconnected by telephone wires or other means in order to communicate and share resources. *See also* local area network; wide area network.

Network Accreditation Program, Health Care *See* Health Care Network Accreditation Program.

Network, Chexchange *See* Chexchange Network.

network, community health *See* community health network.

Network for Continuing Medical Education (NCME) A national organization founded in 1965 composed of 800 hospitals that subscribe to continuing medical education services for physicians including biweekly videotapes, posters, program brochures, and workbooks covering the spectrum of medical topics. *See also* continuing medical education.

network, health *See* network.

networking **1.** Making use of contacts to acquire information or some professional advantage, often while appearing to be engaged only in social activity. *See also* network; old-boy network; old-girl network. **2.** In computer science, a process whereby software and hardware are arranged for interaction among computers in a multiuser system. In this process, the computers can share information and programs and use the same printers and other peripheral devices. *See also* local area network; wide area network.

network, local area *See* local area network.

network model HMO A health maintenance orga-

nization (HMO) that contracts with two or more independent group practices, possibly including a staff group, to provide health services. While a network model HMO may contain a few solo practices, it is predominantly organized around group practices. *See also* group practice; health maintenance organization; solo practice; staff model HMO.

network, old-boy *See* old-boy network.

network, old-girl *See* old-girl network.

Network for Organ Sharing, United *See* United Network for Organ Sharing.

network, primary care *See* primary care network.

Networks, Accreditation Manual for Health Care *See* Accreditation Manual for Health Care Networks.

Networks, Wellness and Health Activation *See* Wellness and Health Activation Networks.

network, wide area *See* wide area network.

net worth The total assets minus the liabilities of a professional practice, health care organization, or individual.

neurinoma A tumor arising from the outer nerve sheath or a peripheral nerve fiber. *See also* adenoma; lipoma; myoma; tumor.

neuritis Inflammation of nerve or nerves. *See also* nerve.

neuroanatomy Anatomy of the nervous system. *See also* anatomy; nervous system.

neurochemistry Chemical physiology of the nervous system. *See also* chemistry; nervous system.

neurodermatitis Any skin disorder thought to be due to or aggravated by emotional or mental factors. *See also* dermatitis; skin.

Neurodevelopmental Treatment Association (NDTA) A national organization founded in 1967 composed of 4,000 physical and occupational therapists, speech pathologists, special educators, physicians, parents, and other individuals interested in neurodevelopmental treatment. This treatment is a form of therapy for individuals who suffer from central nervous system disorders resulting in abnormal movement. Treatment attempts to initiate or refine normal states and processes in the development of movement.

Neurodiagnostic Technologists, American Society of Electro- *See* American Society of Electroneurodiagnostic Technologists.

Neuroimaging, American Society of *See* American Society of Neuroimaging.

neuroleptic Any drug used to modify the manifestations of psychoses. *Synonym*: antipsychotic. *See also* psychosis.

neurologic Pertaining to the nervous system, as in neurologic deficit. *See also* nervous system.

Neurological Association, American *See* American Neurological Association.

Neurological Disorders, National Coalition for Research in *See* National Coalition for Research in Neurological Disorders.

Neurological Microsurgery, American Board of *See* American Board of Neurological Microsurgery.

Neurological/Orthopaedic Laser Surgery, American Board of *See* American Board of Neurological/Orthopaedic Laser Surgery.

Neurological and Orthopaedic Medicine and Surgery, American Board of *See* American Board of Neurological and Orthopaedic Medicine and Surgery.

Neurological and Orthopaedic Surgeons, American Academy of *See* American Academy of Neurological and Orthopaedic Surgeons.

neurological surgeon A physician specializing in neurological surgery. *Synonym*: neurosurgeon. *See also* neurological surgery; surgeon.

Neurological Surgeons, American Association of *See* American Association of Neurological Surgeons.

neurological surgery The branch of medicine and medical specialty dealing with the operative and nonoperative management (that is, prevention, diagnosis, evaluation, treatment, critical care, and rehabilitation) of disorders of the central, peripheral, and autonomic nervous systems, including their supporting structures and vascular supply; the evaluation and treatment of pathological processes that modify functions or activity of the nervous system, including the hypophysis; and the operative and nonoperative management of pain. *Synonym*: neurosurgery. *See also* nervous system; surgery.

Neurological Surgery, American Academy of *See* American Academy of Neurological Surgery.

Neurological Surgery, American Board of *See* American Board of Neurological Surgery.

neurologic deficit, peripheral *See* peripheral neurologic deficit.

neurologist A physician who specializes in neurology. *See also* neurology.

neurology The branch and medical specialty dealing with the diagnosis and treatment of all categories of disease or impaired function of the brain,

spinal cord, peripheral nerves, muscles, and autonomic nervous system, as well as the blood vessels that relate to these structures. Clinical neurophysiology is a subspecialty of neurology. *See also* nervous system.

Neurology, American Academy of *See* American Academy of Neurology.

Neurology, American Board of Psychiatry and *See* American Board of Psychiatry and Neurology.

Neurology Society, Child *See* Child Neurology Society.

neuropathologist A pathologist who subspecializes in neuropathology. *See also* neuropathology; pathology.

Neuropathologists, American Association of *See* American Association of Neuropathologists.

neuropathology The branch of medicine and subspecialty of neurology dealing with structural and other aspects of disease of the nervous system. *See also* nervous system; neuropathologist; pathology.

neuropathy Any pathological condition affecting the peripheral nervous system; for example, diabetes mellitus, alcoholism, and malnutrition. *See also* alcoholism; diabetes mellitus; malnutrition; peripheral nervous system.

neuropharmacology The study of the action of drugs on the nervous system. *See also* nervous system; pharmacology.

neurophysiologist, clinical *See* clinical neurophysiologist.

neurophysiology The branch of physiology dealing with the functions of the nervous system. *See also* nervous system; physiology.

neurophysiology, clinical *See* clinical neurophysiology.

Neuropsychiatric Association, Central *See* Central Neuropsychiatric Association.

neuropsychiatrist A physician who specializes in neuropsychiatry. *See also* neuropsychiatry.

Neuropsychiatrists, American College of *See* American College of Neuropsychiatrists.

neuropsychiatry The combined medical study of neurological and psychiatric disorders. *See also* neurology; psychiatry.

Neuropsychological Development, Multidisciplinary Institute for *See* Multidisciplinary Institute for Neuropsychological Development.

neuropsychology The study of the psychological effects of organic brain disease. *See also* brain; organic disease; psychology.

Neuropsychology, National Academy of *See* National Academy of Neuropsychology.

Neuropsychology Special Interest Group, Behavioral *See* Behavioral Neuropsychology Special Interest Group.

Neuropsychopharmacology, American College of *See* American College of Neuropsychopharmacology.

neuroradiology The branch of radiology dealing with the nervous system. *See also* nervous system; radiology.

Neuroradiology, American Society of *See* American Society of Neuroradiology.

neuroscience Any of the sciences, such as neuroanatomy and neurobiology, that deal with the nervous system. *See also* nervous system.

Neuroscience Nurses, American Association of *See* American Association of Neuroscience Nurses.

Neuroscience Nursing, American Board of *See* American Board of Neuroscience Nursing.

Neuroscience, Society for *See* Society for Neuroscience.

neurosis A functional mental disorder in which reality testing is intact (as opposed to psychosis in which reality testing is impaired) and ego-dystonic symptoms, such as obsessions, anxiety attacks, phobias, insecurity, and depression, are prominent. *Synonym*: psychoneurosis. *Compare* psychosis. *See also* hyponchondriasis; hysteria; magical thinking; psychiatry.

neurosurgeon *See* neurological surgeon.

neurosurgery *See* neurological surgery.

Neurosurgery, American Society for Pediatric *See* American Society for Pediatric Neurosurgery.

Neurosurgery, American Society for Stereotactic and Functional *See* American Society for Stereotactic and Functional Neurosurgery.

Neurosurgical Anesthesia and Critical Care, Society of *See* Society of Neurosurgical Anesthesia and Critical Care.

Neurosurgical Society of America (NSA) A national organization founded in 1948 composed of 162 young specialists in neurological surgery. *See also* neurological surgery.

neurosyphilis Syphilis affecting the central nervous system, causing such clinical manifestations as tabes dorsalis (a degenerative condition with symptoms including loss of coordination, incontinence, and diminished muscle tone). *See also* syphilis.

neurotologist *See* otologist/neurotologist.

neurotology *See* otology/neurotology.

Neurotology Society, American *See* American Neurotology Society.

neurotransmitters Chemical substances released in minute amounts at the endings of nerve fibers in response to arrival of a nerve impulse, causing excitation of the adjacent nerve or effector organ. The best known neurotransmitters are epinephrine (adrenaline), norephinephrine (noradrenaline), acetylcholine, dopamine, and serotonin. *See also* nerve; nervous system; transmission.

New Age Movement Spiritual and consciousness-raising cultural movement of the 1980s characterized by rejection of modern Western-style values and culture and promotion of a more integrated or holistic approach in areas, such as religion, medicine, philosophy, and the environment. *See also* holistic medicine.

newborn A newborn baby. *See also* Apgar scale; baby; infant.

newborn bed *See* bassinet.

newborn bed count *See* bed count.

newborn admission The formal acceptance by a health care organization of a newborn by virtue of being born in the facility. *Synonym*: newborn inpatient admission. *See also* admission; inpatient admission.

newborn, defective *See* Baby Doe regulations.

newborn inpatient admission *See* newborn admission.

newborn intensive care unit *See* neonatal intensive care unit.

newborn nursery A unit of a hospital for the care and treatment of infants through the age of 28 days or longer if necessary. *See also* newborn.

New Deal The programs and policies to promote economic recovery and social reform introduced during the 1930s by President Franklin D. Roosevelt. *See also* Great Depression.

new drug A drug for which premarketing approval is required by the Federal Food, Drug, and Cosmetic Act. A new drug is any drug that is not generally recognized among experts qualified by scientific training and experience to evaluate the safety and effectiveness of drugs, as safe and effective for use under its prescribed conditions of use. Since 1962, most new prescription drugs have been subject to the new-drug application and premarket approval process for new drugs. The vast majority of drugs marketed over-the-counter, however, have not been through the new-drug approval process. *See also* drug; generally recognized as effective; generally recognized as safe; investigational new drug; not-new drug.

new-drug application (NDA) An application that must be approved by the US Food and Drug Administration before any new drug is marketed to the general public, which provides information designed to demonstrate safety and effectiveness. Once the application is approved, the drug may be prescribed by any physician or other health professional authorized to prescribe under state law. The new-drug application must include reports of animal and clinical investigations; a list of ingredients including the active drug and any vehicle, excipient, binder, filler, flavoring, and coloring; a description of manufacturing methods and quality control procedures; samples of the drug; and the proposed labeling. Approval of a new-drug application must be based on valid scientific evidence that the drug is safe and adequate and well-controlled clinical studies demonstrating that it is effective for its intended (labeled) uses. *See also* abbreviated new-drug application; drug; drug monograph; "me too" drug.

new-drug application, abbreviated *See* abbreviated new-drug application.

new drug, not- *See* not-new drug.

new economics Revisions of Keynesian economic theory, which appeared in the 1970s and attempted to deal with modern economic problems that were ineffectively addressed by Keynesian approaches. *See also* economics; Keynesian economics; neoclassical economics.

New England Journal of Medicine NEJM The weekly medical journal published by the Massachusetts Medical Society; it contains clinical, research, and other articles relevant to the practice of medicine. *See also* journal.

New Journalism Journalism that is characterized by a reporter's subjective interpretations. It often features fictional dramatized elements to emphasize personal involvement. *See also* journalism; subjective; subjectivism.

new patient A person who has not previously been seen by a particular physician, clinic, hospital, or other health professional or health care organization. A new patient generally requires new medical records and a complete medical history and physical examination. *See also* medical history; patient; physical examination.

New Professionals Section of the American Public Health Association A section of the American Public Health Association founded in 1969 composed of 300 professionals and paraprofessionals in the human services area. It offers specialized education. Formerly (1982) National New Professional Health Workers. *See also* American Public Health Association; public health.

newspeak Deliberately ambiguous and contradictory language used to mislead and manipulate the public. The term is derived from the language invented by George Orwell in his novel *1984*.

news release *See* press release.

next of kin The person or persons most closely related by blood to another person, as in a deceased person's spouse, child, mother, father, brother, sister, or other nearest relative, in genealogical order. *See also* kin.

NF *See* National Formulary.

NFA *See* Natural Food Associates.

NFCPG *See* National Federation of Catholic Physicians Guilds.

NFHO *See* National Federation of Housestaff Organizations.

NFLPN *See* National Federation of Licensed Practical Nurses.

NFNA *See* National Flight Nurses Association.

NFNID *See* National Foundation for Non-Invasive Diagnostics.

NFPA *See* National Fire Protection Association; National Flight Paramedics Association.

NFPRHA *See* National Family Planning and Reproductive Health Association.

NFSCSW *See* National Federation of Societies for Clinical Social Work.

NFSNO *See* National Federation of Specialty Nursing Organizations.

NGS *See* National Geriatrics Society.

NHA *See* National Hypertension Association.

NHAS *See* National Hearing Aid Society.

NHC *See* National Health Council.

NHCA *See* National Health Club Association; National Hearing Conservation Association.

NHCAA *See* National Health Care Anti-Fraud Association.

NHeLP *See* National Health Law Program.

NHF *See* National Health Federation.

NHI *See* national health insurance.

NHIS *See* Nursing Home Information Service.

NHLA *See* National Health Lawyers Association.

NHO *See* National Hospice Organization.

NHPF *See* National Health Policy Forum.

NHPP *See* National Hormone and Pituitary Program.

NHR *See* National Heart Research.

NHSA *See* National Heart Savers Association.

NHSC *See* National Health Service Corps.

NIAD *See* National Institute on Adult Daycare.

NIBM *See* National Institute for Burn Medicine.

NICD *See* National Information Center on Deafness.

NICHCY *See* National Information Center for Children and Youth with Disabilities.

niche **1.** A special area of demand for a product or a service, such as a special area in which an organization or an individual finds they prosper. "Niche strategy" in marketing is to market to a small but lucrative portion of the market. The small size of the niche generally ensures efficient marketing efforts and few if any direct competitors. *See also* marketing. **2.** A recess in a wall. **3.** The ecological role of an organism in a community.

NICHHD *See* National Institute of Child Health and Human Development.

NICLC *See* National Institute on Community-Based Long-Term Care.

NICO *See* National Insurance Consumer Organization.

nicotine An addictive, poisonous alkaloid found in tobacco leaves. Nicotine addiction is the force that drives smokers to smoke in order to maintain a high level of nicotine in their blood. In small doses nicotine stimulates the nervous system, causing an increase in pulse rate, a rise in blood pressure, and a decrease in appetite. In large doses, it is a depressant, slowing the heartbeat and leading to respiratory depression. *See also* addiction; nervous system; nicotine patch; sidestream smoke; smoking; snuff; tobacco; involuntary smoking.

nicotine patch A transdermal drug delivery system that provides systemic delivery of nicotine following its application to intact skin. It is used as an aid to stop smoking for the relief of nicotine withdrawal symptoms. *See also* addiction; nicotine; transcutaneous.

NICU *See* neonatal intensive care unit.

nidus In pathology, a central point or focus of bacterial growth in a living organism, as in the nidus of

infection was a small skin abscess. *See also* abscess; infection; pathology.

NIEI *See* National Institute of Electromedical Information.

NIF *See* National Institute for the Family.

night bed A bed regularly maintained by a health care organization for use during the night by patients who require partial hospitalization. *See also* bed; partial hospitalization.

night hospital A hospital that provides health and personal care services to patients only at night, often to those who no longer require continuous inpatient care but who are not yet able to live independently. *See also* day hospital; hospital.

night hospitalization *See* partial hospitalization.

Nightingale, Florence (1820-1910) Widely regarded as the founder of modern nursing, she elevated nursing to a noble profession during the Crimean War, established a training school for nurses at St Thomas' Hospital in London, and recognized the importance of statistical analysis of hospital records. *See also* nursing.

nightmare A dream that arouses feelings of fear, terror, panic, or anxiety. *Synonym:* oneirodynia. *See also* night terrors.

night terrors An episode, most often occurring in young children, in which the person awakens in terror, with a panicky scream, feelings of fear and anxiety, and total inability to recall any dream or incident provoking the feelings. *Synonym:* pavor nocturnus. *See also* nightmare.

NIH *See* National Institutes of Health.

NIHB *See* National Indian Health Board.

nihilism **1.** In philosophy, an extreme form of skepticism that denies all existence; a doctrine holding that all values are baseless and that nothing can be known or communicated. **2.** Rejection of all distinction in moral or religious value and a willingness to repudiate all previous theories of morality or religious belief. **3.** The belief that destruction of existing political or social institutions is necessary for future improvement. **4.** In psychiatry, a delusion that certain things or everything, including the self, does not exist. It is associated with some forms of schizophrenia. *See also* delusion.

NIJH *See* National Institute for Jewish Hospice.

NIMH *See* National Institute of Mental Health.

NIOSH *See* National Institute for Occupational Safety and Health.

NIRE *See* National Institute for Rehabilitation Engineering.

NIST *See* National Institute of Standards and Technology.

NIT *See* Nurses in Transition.

NITA *See* National Institute for Trial Advocacy.

nitrogen narcosis A condition of confusion or stupor resulting from increased levels of dissolved nitrogen in the blood, as that occurring in deep-sea divers breathing air under high pressure. *See also* hyperbaric medicine; narcosis.

nitroglycerin A thick, pale yellow substance that is used in the production of dynamite and blasting gelatin, and as a vasodilator in medicine.

nitrous oxide A gaseous anesthetic that produces light anesthesia and is used in minor surgery, childbirth, and dentistry, but not alone for major surgery. In small doses it sometimes produces exhilaration and is called laughing gas. *See also* anesthetic.

nits The ova or eggs of lice, particularly of the head louse, that firmly adhere to the hair shafts. *See also* head louse.

NKUDIC *See* National Kidney and Urologic Diseases Information Clearinghouse.

NLCOA *See* National Leadership Coalition on AIDS.

NLM *See* National Library of Medicine.

NLN *See* National League for Nursing.

NLP *See* natural language processing.

NMA *See* National Medical Association.

NMAC *See* National Minority AIDS Council.

NMCHC *See* National Maternal and Child Health Clearinghouse.

NMCS *See* National Medic-Card Systems.

NMDA *See* National Medical and Dental Association.

NMDP *See* National Marrow Donor Program.

NMF *See* National Medical Fellowships.

NMHA *See* National Mental Health Association; National Minority Health Association.

NMR Acronym for nuclear magnetic resonance. *See* magnetic resonance.

NMTCB *See* Nuclear Medicine Technology Certification Board.

NNBA *See* National Nurses in Business Association.

NNSA *See* National Nurses Society on Addictions.

NOA *See* National Optometric Association.

NOADN *See* National Organization for Associate Degree Nursing.

NOAPP *See* National Organization of Adolescent Pregnancy and Parenting.

Nobel Prize Any one of six international prizes awarded annually by the Nobel Foundation for outstanding achievements in the fields of physiology or medicine, physics, chemistry, literature, economics, and for the promotion of world peace.

NOCA *See* National Organization for Competency Assurance.

NOCIRC *See* National Organization of Circumcision Information Resource Centers.

no code *See* do-not-resuscitate order.

NOD *See* National Organization on Disability.

node In computer science, a terminal, station, communication computer, or other device in a network. *See also* computer; network.

node, lymph *See* lymph node.

no-fault medical practice liability A proposal that all people injured during medical care be automatically reimbursed, even if the care was not negligent. Patients would forfeit their right to sue and instead would be paid out of a pool funded by doctors and hospitals. No-fault liability theoretically would save money currently spent on lawsuits and distribute awards to a wider variety and number of injured people. *See also* liability; professional liability.

NOGLSTP *See* National Organization of Gay and Lesbian Scientists and Technical Professionals.

no-growth Little or no economic growth as measured by changes in the gross national product. The US economy during much of the 1970s and 1980s was characterized as no-growth since the gross national product showed only a negligible increase during much of the period. *See also* economy; gross national product.

NOHA *See* Nutrition for Optimal Health Association.

noise **1.** A sound of intensity sufficient to disturb and/or discomfort listeners. Excessive noise can cause transient or permanent deafness. *See also* deafness; noise pollution; pitch; sound. **2.** In computer science, any unwanted, spurious, or otherwise unintended data generated by a computer along with desired data. *See also* noise in data.

noise in data Irrelevant or meaningless data generated by extraneous, uncontrolled variables and/or errors on the distribution of measurements that are made in a study. Noise may render difficult or impossible the accurate determination of relationships between variables under scrutiny. *See also* data; noise; variable.

noise pollution Environmental noise that is annoying, distracting, or physically harmful. *Synonym*: sound pollution. *See also* pollution.

nomenclature A classified system of names, as of anatomical structures, organisms, or diseases. *See also International Classification of Diseases, Ninth Revision, Clinical Modification*; nosology.

Nomenclatures, Coding, and Classification, Commission on Clinical *See* Commission on Clinical Nomenclatures, Coding, and Classification.

nominal **1.** Relating to a name or names, as in nominal numbers are one, two, three, and so on. *See also* nominal data; nominalism. **2.** Insignificantly small, as in a nominal amount. *Compare* real. *See also* nominal damages.

nominal damages An award that is of insignificant value. However, it reflects the fact that there has been an invasion of a party's rights even though no real damage resulted. *See also* damages; nominal.

nominal data Qualitative data exemplified by different scores representing different *kinds* of characteristics, instead of different *amounts* of characteristics, as in 2 patients with green eyes and 34 patients with brown eyes. *Compare* ordinal data. *See also* data; nominal; nominal scale.

nominal group process *See* nominal group technique.

nominal group technique A group process technique designed to efficiently generate a large number of ideas through input from individual group members initially working independently and concurrently without fear of criticism. The technique allows a team to prioritize a large number of issues without creating "winners" and "losers." *Synonym*: nominal group process. *See also* technique.

nominalism In philosophy, a doctrine maintaining that abstract concepts, general terms, or universals have no objective reference but exist only as names. *See also* nominal.

nominal scale A scale in which classification occurs according to unordered qualitative categories, such as color of eyes, race, religion, and country of birth; hence, observations distinguished by name alone. These measurements of individual attributes are purely nominal as there is no inherent order to their categories. This is the weakest qualitative classification of samples into separate categories. *See also* interval scale; nominal; nominal data; ordinal scale; ratio scale; scale.

Non-Circumcision Information Center (NCIC) An organization founded in 1973 that seeks to provide current, accurate, and complete information to the public regarding the safety and necessity of circumcision, distribute information that discourages routine circumcision, and assist in increasing the number of uncircumcised males from 40% to 90%. *See also* circumcision.

noncoital reproduction Fertilization in which sexual intercourse is not used; for example, artificial insemination and surrogate mothering. *Synonym*: artificial reproduction. *See also* artificial insemination-donor; artificial insemination-husband; artificial reproduction; parent; gestational parent; reproduction; surrogate motherhood; test-tube baby.

noncompliance *See* compliance level.

non compos mentis Latin phrase meaning "not having control over the mind or intellect;" insane. In certain circumstances it means "not legally competent." *See also* competence; non sui juris.

nonconformities Specific occurrences of a condition that do not conform to specifications or other inspection standards; sometimes called discrepancies or defects. *See also* discrepancy.

noncontributory insurance Group health insurance in which the employer pays all of the premium. *Compare* contributory insurance. *See also* group insurance; insurance.

nondirective Pertaining to a psychotherapeutic or counseling technique in which the therapist takes an unobtrusive role in order to encourage free expression by the client or patient. *See also* counseling; psychotherapy.

nondisease factors Patient-based sources of performance variation, such as age, sex, and refusal of consent, that have an impact on care but that are not related to illness. *See also* disease; factor; patient factor.

noneconomic damages Elements of injury or loss that cannot easily and accurately be calculated in terms of money damages. For example, noneconomic losses might include pain and suffering, while economic losses would include lost wages. *See also* damages; future damages.

nonfederal government hospital A hospital that is managed by an agency or department of state or local government. *See also* federal government hospital; government hospital.

non-insulin-dependent diabetes *See* type II diabetes mellitus.

noninvasive Pertaining to a diagnostic or therapeutic technique that does not involve puncturing the skin or entering a body cavity or an organ. *Compare* invasive; invasive procedure. *See also* noninvasive vascular technology.

Non-Invasive Diagnostics, National Foundation for   *See* National Foundation for Non-Invasive Diagnostics.

noninvasive vascular technology   A specialized method of monitoring the blood flow in arms and legs in order to better diagnose disease and the presence of blood clots. *See also* noninvasive; vascular surgery.

nonjudgmental   Refraining from judgment, especially one based on personal ethical standards. *See also* judgment.

nonlinear 1. Not in a straight line. **2.** In statistics, occurring as a result of a nonadditive operation or containing a variable with an exponent other than one. *See also* nonlinear scale.

nonlinear scale   A scale in which the divisions corresponding to the steps are unequal, for example, a scale with divisions showing logarithmic or exponential change. *See also* nonlinear; scale.

nonmaleficence   A principle that guides people and organizations to refrain from causing harm. *See also* double-effect principle.

nonparticipating physician   *See* nonparticipating provider.

nonparticipating provider   A hospital or other health care organization or a health professional that has not agreed to payment schedules or charge allowances offered by a health care insurer, service plan, or prepayment plan. *See also* health care provider; participating physician; participation.

nonperformance   Failure to fulfill an obligation. *Compare* performance.

nonprescription drug   *See* over-the-counter drug.

Nonprescription Drug Manufacturers Association (NDMA)   A national organization founded in 1881 composed of 230 producers of nonprescription drugs (packaged, over-the-counter medicines) and associate members including suppliers, advertising agencies, and advertising media. It obtains and disseminates business, legislative, regulatory, and scientific information and conducts a voluntary labeling review service to assist members in complying with laws and regulations. Formerly (1989) The Proprietary Association. *See also* drug; labeling; over-the-counter drug.

non-probability sampling   A technique in which a non-representative sample is used to help define a problem or its causes when only a few cases are required for analysis and controls cannot be obtained. The technique cannot be used for drawing sweeping conclusions. Subsets are convenience sampling, purposive sampling, and quota sampling. *See also* probability; sampling.

nonproductive   Not contributing to the production of goods or services or the realization of expected results. Something that is nonproductive results in wasted effort and money. *Compare* productive.

nonprofit hospital   *See* not-for-profit hospital.

nonprofit organization   *See* not-for-profit organization.

nonrandomized control trial   An experiment in which assignment of patients to the intervention groups is at the convenience of the investigator or according to a preset plan that does not conform to the definition of random. *Compare* randomized trial. *See also* clinical trial; experiment; random; trial.

nonservice-connected disability   In the Veterans Administration health care system, a disability that was not incurred or aggravated in the line of duty during active military service. Care is available from the program for patients with such disabilities on a bed-available basis after service-connected disability patients are cared for. *Compare* service-connected disability. *See also* disability; Veterans Administration.

non sui juris   Latin phrase meaning "not by his or her own authority or legal rights." This maxim refers to legally incompetent individuals who cannot manage their own affairs. Their incompetence restricts their granting power of attorney or otherwise exercising self-judgment. *See also* non compos mentis.

nontreatment of defective newborns   *See* Baby Doe regulations.

nonurgent   Pertaining to care that does not require the resources of an emergency department. *Compare* urgent.

nonverbal communication   Communication by one person to another, consisting of facial expressions, head movements, eye contact, hand gestures, body positions and acts, tones of voice, and other unspoken demonstrations. In general, body language expresses an individual's emotions and attitudes. *Synonym:* body language. *See also* communication.

norm   1. The *average* or *usual* numerical level or pattern at which an action, event, or other measured phenomenon occurs within a defined population. For example, the norm for all surgeons in a defined geographic area in performing laparotomies for penetrating abdominal trauma. **2.** A numerical level of a *desired* action, event, or other measured phenomenon, as in the level at which several surgeons performed laparotomies for penetrating abdominal trauma was significantly below the (desired) norm. In this second sense, norm is employed as a standard against which to evaluate, for example, performance or quality. *See also* behavioral norms; normal; standard.

normal 1. Within the *usual* range of variation in a given group or population, or frequently occurring in the group or population; for example, normal body temperature or normal relations. Normal may be statistically defined as being within a range extending from two standard deviations below the mean of data set to two standard deviations above the mean. **2.** Something standard, as in a hospital's maternal mortality rate of 15% was normal for the year 1870. *See also* abnormal; norm; normal distribution; subnormal.

normal, ab- *See* abnormal.

normal delivery A baby delivered without complications. *Compare* extramural birth; premature delivery; sick baby. *See also* delivery.

normal distribution A distribution that is continuous and symmetrical with both tails of the distribution extending to infinity. The arithmetic mean, mode, and median are identical and the shape of the distribution is completely determined by the mean and standard deviation. *Synonyms:* bell-shaped curve; Gaussian distribution. *See also* distribution; mean; median; mode; probability distribution.

normalize To make normal, especially to cause to conform to a standard or norm, as in a hospital's rate for performance of primary cesarean sections began to normalize after obstetricians were provided with data showing a significantly higher hospital rate for performance of primary cesarean sections than any other hospital in the geographic area. *See also* normal.

normal limits Limits of the normal range of a test or measurement, as in the limits of normal of the hematocrit in women are 37% and 43%. *See also* limit; normal.

normal retirement age The earliest age at which one is permitted to retire and receive full benefits. *See also* retirement age.

normal saline *See* saline.

normal, sub- *See* subnormal.

normative Pertaining to the normal, usual, accepted standard or values, as in normative data and normative grammar. *See also* norm; normal; standard.

normative ethics Theories that formulate and defend basic moral principles and rules that determine what is right or wrong. *See also* ethics; normative.

normotensive Having normal blood pressure; not hypertensive or hypotensive. *See also* hypertension; hypotension.

norm, peripheral *See* behavioral norms.

norm, pivotal *See* behavioral norms.

norms, behavioral *See* behavioral norms.

North America, Arthroscopy Association of *See* Arthroscopy Association of North America.

North America, Bangladesh Medical Association of *See* Bangladesh Medical Association of North America.

North America, Interstate Postgraduate Medical Association of *See* Interstate Postgraduate Medical Association of North America.

North American Academy of Manipulative Medicine *See* North American Academy of Musculoskeletal Medicine.

North American Academy of Musculoskeletal Medicine (NAAMM) An organization founded in 1965 composed of 350 physicians interested in promoting and conducting scientific studies in manipulative and manual medicine and in promoting the use of these modalities in clinical practice. Formerly (1989) North American Academy of Manipulative Medicine. *See also* manipulative medicine.

North American ApioTherapy Society *See* American Apitherapy Society.

North American Membrane Society (NAMS) An organization founded in 1985 composed of 400 academicians, graduate students, scientists, engineers, and corporate executives interested in the advancement of membrane technology, especially synthetic membrane technology. Synthetic membranes are polymers and inorganic materials used for sterile filtration and separation processes, such as those used in gas separation, water purification, food processing, biochemistry, and the medical-pharmaceutical field. *See also* membrane.

North American Menopause Society (NAMS) An organization founded in 1989 composed of 600 physicians, scientists, research and clinical personnel, and other health professionals interested in the study of the climacteric in men and women. It offers educational programs and exchanges research plans and experience among members. *See also* andropause; climacteric; menopause.

North American Nursing Diagnosis Association (NANDA) An organization founded in 1972 composed of 1,500 registered nurses interested in developing, refining, and promoting a taxonomy of diagnostic terminology for use by nurses. *See also* diagnosis; registered nurse.

North American Primary Care Research Group (NAPCRG) An organization founded in 1972 composed of 500 physicians and other individuals interested in primary care research. It maintains 11 special interest groups including Ambulatory Sentinel Practice, Clinical Decision Making, and Health Status Group. *See also* primary care; research.

North American Society for Dialysis and Transplantation (NASDT) An organization founded in 1981 composed of 200 nephrologists, transplant surgeons and physicians, registered nurses, and transplant coordinators active in the area of teaching, manufacturing, and administration in the fields of nephrology and transplantation. *See also* dialysis; nephrology; transplantation.

North American Society of Pacing and Electrophysiology (NASPE) An organization founded in 1979 composed of 1,500 physicians, technicians, nurses, engineers, and individuals involved in pacemaker implantation and cardiac electrophysiology. It seeks to recommend standards for electrophysiologic device testing and the training of electrophysiologists and pacemaker-implanting physicians. *See also* electrophysiology; pacemaker.

North American Society for Pediatric Gastroenterology *See* North American Society for Pediatric Gastroenterology and Nutrition.

North American Society for Pediatric Gastroenterology and Nutrition (NASPGN) An organization founded in 1970 composed of 350 physicians interested and specializing in gastrointestinal, hepatobiliary (liver and bile/biliary ducts), and nutritional disorders affecting children and adolescents. It provides the public with information on gastrointestinal disorders. Formerly (1988) North American Society for Pediatric Gastroenterology. *See also* gastroenterology; nutrition; pediatric gastroenterology.

North American Society for the Psychology of Sport and Physical Activity (NASPSPA) An

organization founded in 1966 composed of 650 kinesiologists, psychologists, and physical educators interested in promoting scientific research and relations within the behavioral sciences with an application to sports psychology and motor learning, control, and development. *See also* kinesiology; psychology; sports medicine.

North American Spine Society (NASS) An educational organization founded in 1985 composed of 700 physicians, osteopathic physicians, and individuals in allied medical or surgical specialties interested in neurological and orthopaedic medicine and surgery. It maintains the American Board of Neurological and Orthopaedic Medicine and Surgery and the American Board for Medical-Legal Analysis in Medicine and Surgery. *See also* neurological surgery; orthopaedic/orthopedic surgery.

North American Transplant Coordinators Organization (NATCO) An organization founded in 1979 composed of 1,300 nurses and allied health professionals working with organ recipients and those working to obtain and distribute human organs and tissues to waiting victims of end-stage organ failure. It seeks to influence increased procurement and use of transplantable organs and tissues under the direction of individuals and institutions responsible for the employment of members. *See also* organ procurement; transplantation.

North America, Pediatric Orthopaedic Society of *See* Pediatric Orthopaedic Society of North America.

North America, Ukrainian Medical Association of *See* Ukrainian Medical Association of North America.

Nose, and Throat Advances in Children, Society for Ear, *See* Society for Ear, Nose, and Throat Advances in Children.

nosocomial Pertaining to or originating in a hospital; sometimes said of an infection not present or incubating before admission to a hospital, but generally occurring 72 hours after admission. *See also* iatrogenic; nosocomial infection.

nosocomial infection An infection acquired by a patient in a health care organization, especially a hospital. The most common nosocomial infections are urinary tract infections, followed by surgical wound infections, pneumonia, and bloodstream infections. *Synonyms:* hospital-acquired infection; postoperative infection. *Compare* community-acquired infection. *See also* infection; nosocomial; nosocomial infection rate.

nosocomial infection rate The ratio describing the number of patients with nosocomial infection divided by the number of patients at risk of developing nosocomial infection. Rates may be stratified by taking into account certain patient factors that may predispose a specified group of patients to an increased risk of acquiring a nosocomial infection (also called rate stratification by infection risk). *See also* infection; nosocomial; nosocomial infection; rate.

nosology The nomenclature and classification of diseases. *Synonyms*: nosonomy; nosotaxy. *See also* classification of diseases; classification system; nomenclature; taxonomy.

nosonomy *See* nosology.

nosotaxy *See* nosology.

not accredited An accreditation decision that results when a health care organization has been denied accreditation by the Joint Commission on Accreditation of Healthcare Organizations, when its accreditation is withdrawn by the Joint Commission, or when it withdraws from the accreditation process. This designation also describes any health care organization that has never applied for accreditation. *See also* accreditation; accreditation decision; accredited; Joint Commission on Accreditation of Healthcare Organizations; unaccredited; special analysis unit.

notarize To attest to the genuineness of a signature. A notary public performs this function. *See also* notary public.

notary public A public officer under civil and commercial law, authorized to administer oaths, to attest to and certify certain types of documents, to take depositions, and to perform certain acts in commercial matters. The seal of a notary public authenticates a document. *See also* notarize.

notch A sharp discontinuity in health or financial benefits for individuals with slightly different incomes. For example, in Medicaid, a family just below the income eligibility standard receives full subsidized coverage, while families with only slightly more income who are just above the eligibility standard receive no benefits. Spend-down provisions, governing the expenditure of assets until income eligibility levels are met, are used to compensate for notches. *See also* Medicaid.

not-for-profit carrier A health insurance, service, or prepayment organization that falls under state not-for-profit statutes; for example, Delta Dental plans and many Blue Cross and Blue Shield plans are not-for-profit carriers. *See also* Blue Cross/Blue Shield plan; carrier; Delta Dental plan.

not-for-profit hospital A general acute care, nontaxable hospital that operates on a not-for-profit basis under the ownership and control of a private corporation. Profits are turned back into maintenance and improvement of the hospital's facilities and services. Not-for-profit hospitals are usually owned by a community, a church, or another organization concerned with community services and resources. *Synonym*: nonprofit hospital. *Compare* investor-owned hospital. *See also* hospital.

Not-For-Profit Hospitals, Volunteer Trustees of *See* Volunteer Trustees of Not-For-Profit Hospitals.

not-for-profit organization An association that is allowed to exist without paying income taxes. Most not-for-profit organizations are in a socially desirable business, such as a hospital, an educational institution, or a charity. Some not-for-profit organizations are qualified by the Internal Revenue Service to receive contributions that are tax-deductible to the donor. *See also* organization.

notifiable Pertaining to certain conditions, diseases, and events that must, by law, be reported to a governmental agency, such as birth, death, smallpox, and certain violations of public health regulations. *See also* notifiable disease; public health.

notifiable disease A disease that, by statutory requirements, must be reported to the public health authority in the pertinent jurisdiction when the diagnosis is made by a provider. A notifiable disease is deemed of sufficient importance to the public health as to require that its occurrence be reported to health authorities. Examples include hepatitis, influenza, measles, and sexually transmitted diseases. *Synonym*: reportable disease. *See also* disease; notifiable; quarantine.

not-new drug A drug for which premarketing approval by the US Food and Drug Administration is not, or no longer, required. *See also* new drug.

noumenon In philosophy, an object that can be intuited only by the intellect and not perceived by the senses, as in the soul.

NOVA *See* Nurses Organization of Veterans Affairs.

NOWPA *See* National Osteopathic Women Physician's Association.

noxa An injurious agent, act, or influence.

noxious Hurtful; not wholesome.

NP *See* nurse practitioner.

NPA *See* National Pediculosis Association; National Perinatal Association; National Phlebotomy Association.

NPAP *See* National Psychological Association for Psychoanalysis.

NPC *See* National Pharmaceutical Council.

NPDB *See* National Practitioner Data Bank.

NPhA *See* National Pharmaceutical Association.

NPMA *See* National Podiatric Medical Association.

NPN *See* National Prevention Network.

NPO Abbreviation for Latin phrase *nil per os*, meaning "nothing by mouth," as in the patient remained NPO after abdominal surgery.

NRA *See* National Rehabilitation Association.

NRAA *See* National Renal Administrators Association.

NRBC *See* National Rare Blood Club.

NRC *See* National Research Council.

NRCA *See* National Rehabilitation Counseling Association.

NRCC *See* National Registry of Clinical Chemistry.

NRCHMI *See* National Resource Center on Homelessness and Mental Illness.

NREMT *See* National Registry of Emergency Medical Technicians.

NRHA *See* National Rural Health Association.

NRMP *See* National Residency Matching Program.

NSA *See* Neurosurgical Society of America.

NSC *See* National Safety Council.

NSCT/NSPT *See* National Society for Cardiovascular Technology/National Society for Pulmonary Technology.

NSEA *See* National Standards Educators Association.

NSF *See* National Sanitation Foundation.

NSGC *See* National Society of Genetic Counselors.

NSH *See* National Society for Histotechnology.

NSIDSC *See* National Sudden Infant Death Syndrome Clearinghouse.

NSMS *See* National Safety Management Society.

NSPRCA *See* National Society of Patient Representation and Consumer Affairs of the American Hospital Association.

NSPS *See* National Society of Professional Sanitarians.

NSPST *See* National Society of Pharmaceutical Sales Trainers.

NTRA *See* National Tumor Registrars Association.

NTRS *See* National Therapeutic Recreation Society.

nuclear family The immediate members of a family, including the parents and children and usually those members living under one roof. *Compare* extended family. *See also* family.

nuclear magnetic resonance (NMR) *See* magnetic resonance.

nuclear magnetic resonance imaging *See* magnetic resonance imaging.

nuclear medicine The branch and specialty of medicine dealing with the scientific and clinical delivery of diagnostic, therapeutic (exclusive of sealed radium sources), and investigative use of radionuclides for patients. The field of nuclear medicine includes radioimmunoassay; therapy with radioisotopically labelled antibodies; positron emission tomography (PET); single-proton emission computerized tomography (SPECT); the biologic effects of radiation exposure; the principles of radiation safety and protection; the management of patients who have been exposed to ionizing radiation; special knowledge in the physical sciences encompassing the fundamentals of nuclear physics and nuclear magnetic resonance; the principles and operation of radiation detection and nuclear imaging instrumentation systems; statistics; and the fundamentals of the computer sciences. *See also* nuclear radiology; radioisotope; radionuclide.

Nuclear Medicine, American Board of *See* American Board of Nuclear Medicine.

Nuclear Medicine, American College of *See* American College of Nuclear Medicine.

nuclear medicine physician A physician who specializes in nuclear medicine. *Synonym:* nuclear physician. *See also* nuclear medicine.

Nuclear Medicine, Society of *See* Society of Nuclear Medicine.

nuclear medicine technologist An allied health professional who, along with nuclear medicine physicians and other professionals in the field, applies knowledge of radiation physics and safety regulations to limit radiation exposure; prepares and administers radiopharmaceuticals; uses radiation detection devices and other kinds of laboratory equipment that measure the quantity and distribution of radionuclides deposited in the patient or in a patient specimen; performs in vivo and in vitro diagnostic procedures; and uses quality control techniques as part of a quality assurance program covering all procedures and products in the laboratory. Administrative functions may include, among other

Nuclear Medicine,
Technologist Section of the Society of   547   Nurse Anesthesia Educational Programs/
Schools, Council on Accreditation of

activities, participating in procuring supplies and equipment; documenting laboratory operations; participating in departmental inspections conducted by various licensing, regulatory, and accrediting agencies; and participating in scheduling patient examinations. Nuclear medicine technologists are one type of allied health professional for which the Committee on Allied Health Education and Accreditation has accredited education programs. *See also* accreditation; allied health professional; nuclear medicine; technologist.

Nuclear Medicine, Technologist Section of the Society of *See* Technologist Section of the Society of Nuclear Medicine.

Nuclear Medicine Technology Certification Board (NMTCB) A national board founded in 1977 composed of 12,000 nuclear medical technologists who have successfully met certification requirements. *See also* board; certification; nuclear medicine technologist.

nuclear physician *See* nuclear medicine physician.

Nuclear Physicians, American College of *See* American College of Nuclear Physicians.

nuclear physics, medical *See* medical nuclear physics.

nuclear radiology The branch of radiology that involves the analysis and imaging of radionuclides and radiolabeled substances in vitro and in vivo for diagnosis and the administration of radionuclides and radiolabeled substances for the treatment of disease. *See also* nuclear medicine; radioisotope; radiology; radionuclide.

nuclear sexing The determination of genetic sex by examining the nuclei of cells, usually in a stained smear from the buccal mucosa (inside the mouth). In normal females a large proportion of nuclei show a small stainable body (Barr body).

nuclide, radioactive *See* radioisotope.

null Amounting to nothing; absent or nonexistent.

null hypothesis The hypothesis or prediction that there is no relationship between two or more variables, as opposed to the experimental hypothesis, which predicts that there is a relationship between two or more variables. The null hypothesis states that the results observed in a study, experiment, or test are no different from what might have occurred as a result of the operation of chance alone. *Synonym:* test hypothesis. *See also* alternative hypothesis; hypothesis; level of significance; statistically significant; test statistic; variable.

nullipara A woman who has never given birth to a viable infant. *See also* pregnancy.

number One of a series of symbols of unique meaning in a fixed order that can be derived by counting. *See also* cardinal number; googol; ordinal number; statistic.

number, BNDD *See* BNDD number.

number, cardinal *See* cardinal number.

number cruncher 1. An individual who spends much time calculating and manipulating numbers. 2. A computer that performs lengthy and complex calculations. *See also* computer; statistics.

number, DEA *See* DEA number.

number generator, random *See* random number generator.

number, identification *See* identification number.

number, internal control *See* internal control number.

number, ordinal *See* ordinal number.

numerator The upper portion of a common fraction to indicate the number of parts of the whole; for instance, the numerator of an indicator might be the number of women receiving cesarean sections, while the denominator might be the number of women giving birth during a given period of time. *Compare* denominator. *See also* indicator.

numeric keypad On a computer keyboard, a separate set of keys beside the main alphabetic keypad that contains the digits 0 to 9 and a decimal point key. The digits are arranged in the same way as they are on an adding machine. A numeric keypad is easier and quicker to use than the number keys on the regular keyboard row. *See also* computer.

nurse 1. An individual qualified by education and authorized by law to practice nursing. There are many different types and specialties of nurses whose names are generally descriptive of their special responsibilities, such as nurse anesthetist, charge nurse, licensed practical nurse, public health nurse, and nurse executive. *See also* certified nurse; licensed practical nurse; licensed vocational nurse; nursing; nursing care; registered nurse. 2. To feed at the breast; suckle. *Synonym:* breastfeed. *See also* wet nurse.

nurse, advanced practice *See* advanced practice nurse.

nurse, agency *See* pool nurse.

nurse aide *See* nursing assistant.

Nurse Anesthesia Educational Programs/ Schools, Council on Accreditation of *See* Council on Accreditation of Nurse Anesthesia Educational Programs/Schools.

nurse anesthetist A registered nurse who is qualified by special training to administer anesthesia in collaboration with a physician or dentist and who can assist in the care of patients who are in critical condition. *See also* advanced practice nurse; certified registered nurse anesthetist.

nurse anesthetist, certified registered *See* certified registered nurse anesthetist.

Nurse Anesthetists, American Association of *See* American Association of Nurse Anesthetists.

Nurse Anesthetists, Council on Certification of *See* Council on Certification of Nurse Anesthetists.

Nurse Associates and Practitioners, National Association of Pediatric *See* National Association of Pediatric Nurse Associates and Practitioners.

nurse association, visiting *See* visiting nurse association.

Nurse Associations of America, Visiting *See* Visiting Nurse Associations of America.

Nurse Attorneys, The American Association of *See* The American Association of Nurse Attorneys.

nurse, cardiac care *See* cardiac care nurse.

nurse, certified *See* certified nurse.

nurse, certified critical care *See* certified critical care nurse.

nurse, charge *See* charge nurse.

nurse, circulating *See* circulating nurse.

nurse clinical instructor A registered nurse who teaches and supervises nursing students in a clinical area, such as pediatrics or surgery. *See also* registered nurse; student nurse.

nurse clinician *See* nurse practitioner.

Nurse Consultants, American Association of Legal *See* American Association of Legal Nurse Consultants.

Nurse Consultants Association (NCA) A national organization founded in 1979 composed of 150 registered nurses working in consulting roles in industry and business. It aids members in educating health care personnel in the use of current technologies and in encouraging greater understanding between manufacturers and health care personnel regarding product and service promotion. *See also* consultant; registered nurse.

nurse coordinator A registered nurse who coordinates and manages the activities of nursing personnel for two or more nursing units. *Synonyms:* patient care coordinator; supervisory nurse. *See also* registered nurse; supervising nurse.

Nurse Corps The branch within each of the armed services comprised of registered nurses within that service; for example, Army Nurse Corps. The members of the Nurse Corps have the rank, title, responsibilities, and status of officers. *See also* corps; nurse.

Nurse Corps Association, Retired Army *See* Retired Army Nurse Corps Association.

nurse, critical care *See* critical care nurse.

nurse, degree *See* degree nurse.

nurse, diploma *See* diploma nurse.

Nurse Education and Service, National Association for Practical *See* National Association for Practical Nurse Education and Service.

nurse, emergency *See* emergency nurse.

nurse epidemiologist A registered nurse, usually with postgraduate training in epidemiology. *See also* epidemiologist; medical epidemiologist; registered nurse.

nurse executive A registered nurse on the hospital executive management team who is responsible for the management of the nursing organization (that is, nursing department, nursing division, nursing service) and for the clinical practice of nursing throughout a health care organization. *Synonyms:* director of nursing; nursing service administrator; nursing service director; vice president for nursing. *See also* chief of nursing; registered nurse.

Nurse Executives, American Organization of *See* American Organization of Nurse Executives.

nurse, float *See* float nurse.

nurse, floor *See* floor nurse.

nurse, general duty *See* staff nurse.

nurse, geriatric *See* geriatric nurse.

nurse, head *See* charge nurse.

nurse, industrial *See* occupational health nurse.

nurse, infection control *See* infection control practitioner/specialist.

nurse, intensive care *See* critical care nurse; certified critical care nurse.

nurse intern An individual who has completed educational preparation in nursing who undergoes practical clinical experience, usually under the supervision of a head nurse or other qualified person in the clinical area in accordance with state nurse practice laws or statutes. *See also* head nurse; intern; nurse practice act; student nurse.

nurse, licensed practical *See* licensed practical

nurse.

nurse, licensed vocational   *See* licensed vocational nurse.

nurse manager   A registered nurse holding 24-hour accountability for the management of a unit(s) or area(s) where nursing care is delivered within a health care institution. *See also* head nurse; manager; registered nurse.

nurse-midwife   A registered nurse who has received special training to examine expectant mothers and perform or assist in routine labor and delivery of normal infants. After a baby's birth, nurse-midwives care for newborns, assist new mothers in learning to care for their infants, and provide interconceptual care (between pregnancies) or family-planning approaches. *Synonym:* midwife. *See also* advanced practice nurse; nurse.

nurse-midwife, certified   *See* certified nurse-midwife.

Nurse-Midwives, American College of   *See* American College of Nurse-Midwives.

nurse, obstetric   *See* obstetric nurse.

nurse, occupational health   *See* occupational health nurse.

nurse, office   *See* office nurse.

nurse, operating room   *See* operating room nurse.

nurse, pediatric   *See* pediatric nurse.

nurse, pool   *See* pool nurse.

nurse, practical   *See* licensed practical nurse.

nurse practice act   A state, commonwealth, or territorial statute or law delineating the legal scope of the practice of nursing within the geographic boundaries of the jurisdiction. *See also* dental practice act; medical practice act.

nurse practitioner (NP)   A registered nurse who has completed additional training beyond basic nursing education and who provides primary health care services in accordance with state nurse practice laws or statutes. Tasks performed by nurse practitioners vary with practice requirements mandated by geographic, political, economic, and social factors. Nurse practitioner specialists include, but are not limited to, family nurse practitioners, gerontological nurse practitioners, pediatric nurse practitioners, obstetric-gynecologic nurse practitioners, and school nurse practitioners. *See also* advanced practice nurse; registered nurse.

nurse practitioner, obstetric-gynecologic   *See* obstetric-gynecologic nurse practitioner.

nurse practitioner, pediatric   *See* pediatric nurse practitioner.

Nurse Practitioners, American Academy of   *See* American Academy of Nurse Practitioners.

Nurse Practitioners and Nurses, National Certification Board of Pediatric   *See* National Certification Board of Pediatric Nurse Practitioners and Nurses.

nurse practitioner specialist   *See* nurse practitioner.

Nurse Practitioners in Reproductive Health, National Association of   *See* National Association of Nurse Practitioners in Reproductive Health.

nurse, primary   *See* primary nurse.

nurse, private   *See* private-duty nurse.

nurse, private-duty   *See* private-duty nurse.

nurse, psychiatric   *See* psychiatric nurse.

nurse, public health   *See* public health nurse.

nurse, registered   *See* registered nurse.

nursery   *See* newborn nursery.

nursery, newborn   *See* newborn nursery.

nursery, premature   *See* neonatal intensive care unit.

nurse's aide   *See* nursing assistant.

Nurses in AIDS Care, Association of   *See* Association of Nurses in AIDS Care.

Nurses, American Association of Critical-Care   *See* American Association of Critical-Care Nurses.

Nurses, American Association of Neuroscience   *See* American Association of Neuroscience Nurses.

Nurses, American Association of Occupational Health   *See* American Association of Occupational Health Nurses.

Nurses, American Association of Office   *See* American Association of Office Nurses.

Nurses, American Association of Spinal Cord Injury   *See* American Association of Spinal Cord Injury Nurses.

Nurses, American Board for Occupational Health   *See* American Board for Occupational Health Nurses.

Nurses, American Society of Ophthalmic Registered   *See* American Society of Ophthalmic Registered Nurses.

Nurses, American Society of Plastic and Reconstructive Surgical   *See* American Society of Plastic and Reconstructive Surgical Nurses.

Nurses, American Society of Post Anesthesia   *See* American Society of Post Anesthesia Nurses.

Nurses and Associates, Society of Gastroenterology   *See* Society of Gastroenterology Nurses and

Associates.

Nurses Association, American *See* American Nurses Association.

Nurses Association, American Holistic *See* American Holistic Nurses Association.

Nurses Association, American Licensed Practical *See* American Licensed Practical Nurses Association.

Nurses' Association, American Nephrology *See* American Nephrology Nurses' Association.

Nurses Association, American Psychiatric *See* American Psychiatric Nurses Association.

Nurses Association, American Radiological *See* American Radiological Nurses Association.

Nurses Association, Baromedical *See* Baromedical Nurses Association.

Nurses' Association, Dermatology *See* Dermatology Nurses' Association.

Nurses Association, Emergency *See* Emergency Nurses Association.

Nurses Association, Hospice *See* Hospice Nurses Association.

Nurses Association, National Black *See* National Black Nurses Association.

Nurses Association, National Flight *See* National Flight Nurses Association.

Nurses, Association of Operating Room *See* Association of Operating Room Nurses.

Nurses, Association of Pediatric Oncology *See* Association of Pediatric Oncology Nurses.

Nurses, Association of Rehabilitation *See* Association of Rehabilitation Nurses.

Nurses, Association of Women's Health, Obstetric, and Neonatal *See* Association of Women's Health, Obstetric, and Neonatal Nurses.

Nurses in Business Association, National *See* National Nurses in Business Association.

nurse, school *See* school nurse.

nurse, scrub *See* scrub nurse.

nurse service, visiting *See* visiting nurse association.

Nurses and Health Professionals, Federation of *See* Federation of Nurses and Health Professionals.

Nurses' House An organization founded in 1925 composed of 900 registered nurses and other individuals interested in assisting registered nurses in financial and other crises by providing short-term financial aid for shelter, food, and utilities until the nurses obtain entitlements or jobs; offering counseling on emotional problems, such as drug and alcohol dependency, and referral to those needing psy-

chological care; and encouraging homebound or retired nurses through a volunteer corps. *See also* registered nurse.

Nurses, National Association of Hispanic *See* National Association of Hispanic Nurses.

Nurses, National Association of Orthopaedic *See* National Association of Orthopaedic Nurses.

Nurses, National Association of Neonatal *See* National Association of Neonatal Nurses.

Nurses, National Association of Physician *See* National Association of Physician Nurses.

Nurses, National Association of Registered *See* National Association of Registered Nurses.

Nurses, National Association of School *See* National Association of School Nurses.

Nurses, National Certification Board of Pediatric Nurse Practitioners and *See* National Certification Board of Pediatric Nurse Practitioners and Nurses.

Nurses, National Consortium of Chemical Dependency *See* National Consortium of Chemical Dependency Nurses.

Nurses, National Federation of Licensed Practical *See* National Federation of Licensed Practical Nurses.

Nurses Organization of the Veterans Administration *See* Nurses Organization of Veterans Affairs.

Nurses Organization of Veterans Affairs (NOVA) A national organization founded in 1980 composed of 2,400 registered nurses of the Department of Veterans Affairs. Formerly (1989) Nurses Organization of the Veterans Administration. *See also* registered nurse; Department of Veterans Affairs.

nurse specialist *See* clinical nurse specialist.

nurse specialist, clinical *See* clinical nurse specialist.

Nurses Society on Addictions, National *See* National Nurses Society on Addictions.

Nurses Society, Intravenous *See* Intravenous Nurses Society.

Nurses, Society of Otorhinolaryngology and Head/Neck *See* Society of Otorhinolaryngology and Head/Neck Nurses.

Nurses Support Network *See* Nurses in Transition.

nurse, staff *See* staff nurse.

Nurses in Transition (NIT) An organization founded in 1978 composed of 200 nurses seeking to expand their role and their autonomy in health care and to incorporate holistic health practices into nursing. Formerly (1985) Nurses Support Network. *See also* holistic health; nurse; transition.

nurse, student *See* student nurse.

nurse, supervising *See* nursing supervisor.

nurse, supervisory *See* nurse coordinator.

nurse, surgical *See* surgical nurse.

nurse, team *See* team nurse.

nurse, visiting *See* public health nurse.

nurse, vocational *See* licensed vocational nurse.

nurse, wet *See* wet nurse.

nursing **1.** The health profession dealing with nursing care as defined in relevant state, commonwealth, or territory nurse practice acts and other applicable laws and regulations, and as permitted by a health care organization in accordance with these definitions. *Synonym*: nursing practice. *See also* home nursing; nurse; nursing care; nursing home. **2.** *See also* lactation; nurse.

Nursing Administration, American Academy of Ambulatory *See* American Academy of Ambulatory Nursing Administration.

Nursing Administration in Long Term Care, National Association of Directors of *See* National Association of Directors of Nursing Administration in Long Term Care.

nursing aide *See* nursing assistant.

Nursing, American Academy of *See* American Academy of Nursing.

Nursing, American Assembly for Men in *See* American Assembly for Men in Nursing.

Nursing, American Association of Colleges of *See* American Association of Colleges of Nursing.

Nursing, American Association for the History of *See* American Association for the History of Nursing.

Nursing, American Board of Neuroscience *See* American Board of Neuroscience Nursing.

nursing assistant An individual who performs routine patient-care-related tasks under the supervision of a nurse. Duties may include, but are not limited to, aiding patients in getting out of bed and walking; giving back rubs and bathing and shaving patients; taking temperatures; serving food and assisting in feeding; and cleaning rooms and changing bed linens. Specialties of nursing assistants include psychiatric aides and home health aides. *Synonyms*: nurse aide; nursing aide. *See also* aide; home health aide; orderly; psychiatric aide.

Nursing Assistant's Association, American *See* American Nursing Assistant's Association.

Nursing Association, Drug and Alcohol *See* Drug and Alcohol Nursing Association.

Nursing, Association of State and Territorial Directors of *See* Association of State and Territorial Directors of Nursing.

nursing audit A patient-chart review conducted by one or more peer nurses to assess documentation of nursing care provided in a health care organization. *See also* dental audit; medical audit.

nursing care Services intended to assist an individual in the performance of those activities contributing to health or its recovery (or to peaceful death) that he or she would perform unaided if he or she had the necessary strength, will, or knowledge. This includes, but is not limited to, assisting patients in carrying out therapeutic plans and understanding the health needs of patients. The special content of nursing care varies in different countries and situations, and, as defined, it is not given solely by nurses, but also by many other health professionals. *See also* nurse; nursing.

nursing care facility *See* nursing home.

nursing care institution *See* nursing home.

nursing care plan A formal plan of the nursing care activities to be conducted in behalf of a given patient and used to coordinate the activities of all nursing personnel involved in that patient's care. *See also* care plan.

nursing care, skilled *See* skilled nursing care.

nursing care unit An organized entity within the nursing service of a hospital or long term care facility (nursing home) in which continuous nursing care is provided. *See also* nursing; nursing care; unit.

Nursing Certification, American Board of Post Anesthesia *See* American Board of Post Anesthesia Nursing Certification.

nursing, chief of *See* chief of nursing.

Nursing Diagnosis Association, North American *See* North American Nursing Diagnosis Association.

Nursing Education, Institute for Hospital Clinical *See* Institute for Hospital Clinical Nursing Education.

Nursing Education and Licensure, Federation for Accessible *See* Federation for Accessible Nursing Education and Licensure.

nursing facility, skilled *See* skilled nursing facility.

Nursing Faculty in Higher Education, Association of Black *See* Association of Black Nursing Faculty in Higher Education.

nursing home A nonhospital health care organization with inpatient beds and an organized professional staff that provides continuous nursing and other health-related, psychosocial, and personal services to patients who are not in an acute phase of illness, but who require continued care on an inpatient basis. Nursing homes provide a broad range of services and levels of care, ranging from skilled nursing care to custodial care. *Synonym:* nursing care facility; nursing care institution. *See also* intermediate care facility; long term care; skilled nursing facility.

nursing, home *See* home nursing.

nursing home administration Management of the operations of a nursing home. *See also* administration; nursing home; nursing home administrator.

nursing home administrator An individual, often licensed by the state, who is responsible for the management of a nursing home. *See also* administrator; nursing home.

Nursing Home Administrators, American College of *See* American College of Health Care Administrators.

Nursing Home Administrators, National Association of Boards of Examiners for *See* National Association of Boards of Examiners for Nursing Home Administrators.

Nursing Home Association, American *See* American Health Care Association.

Nursing Home Information Service (NHIS) A project of the National Senior Citizens Research and Education Center that provides information on nursing home standards and regulations, alternative community and health services, criteria for choosing a nursing home, and guidelines for obtaining medigap insurance (insurance covering medical expenses after Medicare's percentage is paid). It encourages consumer advocacy by persons desiring long term care for themselves or for family or friends. It promotes compliance with the Nursing Home Patients Bill of Rights, a document listing some of the requirements for a federally certified nursing home. *See also* bill of patient rights; certified; Medicare; medigap policy; nursing home.

Nursing Home Reform, National Citizens Coalition for *See* National Citizens Coalition for Nursing Home Reform.

Nursing, Interagency Council on Library Resources for *See* Interagency Council on Library Resources for Nursing.

nursing intervention Any nursing action that is intended to interrupt or change events in progress; for example, turning a comatose patient to avoid

development of decubitus ulcers (bed sores), or teaching insulin injection technique to a newly diagnosed diabetic patient. *See also* health intervention; intervention; medical intervention; surgical intervention.

nursing journal *See* journal.

Nursing, Master of Science in *See* Master of Science in Nursing.

nursing, mental health *See* psychiatric nursing.

Nursing, National Council of State Boards of *See* National Council of State Boards of Nursing.

Nursing, National League for *See* National League for Nursing.

Nursing, National Organization for Associate Degree *See* National Association for Associate Degree Nursing.

nursing orders Instructions for implementing the nursing care plan based on the assessment of patient needs that includes, but is not limited to, timing of activities, patient and family education, and discharge preparation. *See also* nursing; order.

Nursing Organizations, National Federation for Specialty *See* National Federation for Specialty Nursing Organizations.

nursing practice *See* nursing.

nursing, primary *See* primary nursing.

nursing, psychiatric *See* psychiatric nursing.

nursing record The portion of the medical record completed by nurses, containing the care plan, nursing orders, and nursing notes about all nursing activities in behalf of the patient. *See also* care plan; medical record.

Nursing Research, National Center for *See* National Center for Nursing Research.

Nursing Schools, Commission on Graduates of Foreign (CGFNS) *See* Commission on Graduates of Foreign Nursing Schools.

Nursing Society, Oncology *See* Oncology Nursing Society.

Nursing, Society for Vascular *See* Society for Vascular Nursing.

nursing staff Registered nurses, licensed practical/vocational nurses, nursing assistants, and other nursing personnel who perform nursing services in a health care organization. *See also* staff; staff nurse.

nursing service administrator *See* nurse executive.

nursing service director *See* nurse executive.

nursing specialties Areas of specialized nursing including, for example, surgical, school, or psychiatric nursing. *See also* nurse practitioner; specialty.

nursing supervisor   A nurse whose function is the administrative and clinical leadership of the nursing service of a division of a health care organization, such as a nursing supervisor of emergency department nurses. *Compare* floor nurse. *See also* nurse manager; unit manager.

nursing, team   *See* team nursing.

nursing unit, skilled   *See* skilled nursing unit.

nutrient   A substance that must be supplied by the diet to provide for normal health of the body, energy supplies, and materials for growth. Nutrients include proteins, fats, carbohydrates, vitamins, and minerals. *See also* essential nutrient; malabsorption; nutritional support; trace elements.

nutrient, essential   *See* essential nutrient.

nutrition   **1.** Nourishment. *See also* malnutrition; meals on wheels; pica; trace elements; vitamin. **2.** All of the physical processes involved in the ingestion, digestion, absorption, assimilation, and excretion of nutrients. *See also* nutrient. **3.** The study of food and drink as related to the needs of the body. *See also* nutritional support; total parenteral nutrition.

Nutrition and Aging Services Programs, National Association of   *See* National Association of Nutrition and Aging Services Programs.

Nutritional Consultants, American Association of   *See* American Association of Nutritional Consultants.

nutritional support   Methods of delivering food and water by artificial methods when a patient is unable to consume adequate amounts by eating, drinking, and swallowing. Tube feedings are most frequently accomplished with intravenous, nasogastric, and gastrostomy tubes. An intravenous tube is placed in a neck or arm vein; a nasogastric tube is passed through the nose and throat ending in the stomach; and a gastrostomy tube is passed through an artificial opening of the abdominal wall into the stomach. *See also* gastrostomy; nasogastric feeding; nutrient; total parenteral nutrition.

Nutrition, American Board of   *See* American Board of Nutrition.

Nutrition, American College of   *See* American College of Nutrition.

Nutrition, American Council of Applied Clinical   *See* American Council of Applied Clinical Nutrition.

Nutrition, American Institute of   *See* American Institute of Nutrition.

Nutrition, American Society for Clinical   *See* American Society for Clinical Nutrition.

Nutrition, American Society for Parenteral and Enteral   *See* American Society for Parenteral and Enteral Nutrition.

Nutrition Board, Food and   *See* Food and Nutrition Board.

Nutrition Council, Enteral   *See* Enteral Nutrition Council.

Nutrition, Council for Responsible   *See* Council for Responsible Nutrition.

Nutrition Education Association (NEA)   A national organization founded in 1977 composed of 25,000 health professionals and other individuals interested in educating the public on good nutrition as a means of acquiring and maintaining good health. *See also* nutrition.

Nutrition Education, Society for   *See* Society for Nutrition Education.

Nutrition Forum, Child   *See* Child Nutrition Forum.

nutrition and infusion therapy services, enteral and parenteral   *See* enteral and parenteral nutrition and infusion therapy services.

Nutrition Institute, Community   *See* Community Nutrition Institute.

nutritionist   A person who is trained in or expert in the field of nutrition. *See also* nutrition.

nutritionist, clinical   *See* dietitian.

Nutritionists Association, American   *See* American Nutritionists Association.

nutrition, mal-   *See* malnutrition.

Nutrition, North American Society for Pediatric Gastroenterology and   *See* North American Society for Pediatric Gastroenterology and Nutrition.

Nutrition for Optimal Health Association (NOHA)   A national organization founded in 1972 composed of 500 persons interested in promoting good nutrition as a means of achieving and maintaining optimal health. Its activities include conducting nutrition programs and seminars. *See also* nutrition.

nutrition, parenteral   *See* parenteral nutrition.

nutrition, public health   *See* public health nutrition.

NVHA   *See* National Voluntary Health Agencies.

NWA   *See* National Wellness Association.

NWDA   *See* National Wholesale Druggists' Association.

NWHN   *See* National Women's Health Network.

NWHRC   *See* National Women's Health Resource Center.

NWI   *See* National Wellness Institute.

nyctophilia   Abnormal preference for night over day.

nyctophobia Irrational fear of the night. *See also* phobia.

nymphomania Intense sexual excitement in the female, indiscriminately directed at any male (or female) and unrelieved by orgasm. Nymphomania is a rare episodic state that may have an organic basis. *See also* mania; orgasm.

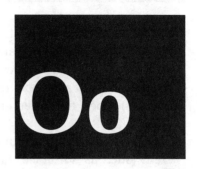

Oo

OAA *See* Opticians Association of America.

OASDHI *See* Old Age, Survivors, Disability and Health Insurance Program.

OASDI *See* Old Age, Survivors, and Disability Insurance.

oath A formal declaration or promise to fulfill a pledge. *See also* affidavit; Hippocratic oath; testify; testimony.

oath of Hippocrates *See* Hippocratic oath.

oath, Hippocratic *See* Hippocratic oath.

OB *See* obstetrician.

obesity An abnormal increase in body weight beyond the limitation of skeletal and physical requirements as the result of an excessive accumulation of fat in the body. *Synonym:* adiposity. *See also* bariatrics; endogenous obesity; exogenous obesity; morbid obesity; overweight; sedentary.

obesity, endogenous *See* endogenous obesity.

obesity, exogenous *See* exogenous obesity.

obesity, morbid *See* morbid obesity.

obfuscation The act of rendering, or process of becoming, obscure.

OB-GYN *See* obstetrics and gynecology.

object Something perceptible by one or more of the senses, especially by vision or touch. *See also* objective; sensation; sense.

objective **1.** Pertaining to reality as it can be determined by observations and the external senses, made by individuals who are not experiencing the event. *See also* object; observation. **2.** Free of personal bias and opinion, as in an objective evaluation. *Compare* subjective. *See also* objectivism. **3.** A quantifiable statement of a desired future state or condition with a stated deadline for achieving the objective, which must have a relationship to the attainment of a goal. *See also* goal; management by objec-

tives; mission statement; target. **4.** In an optical system, such as microscope, a lens or complex of lenses, that is nearest the object being examined. *See also* microscope.

objectives, management by *See* management by objectives.

objectivism In philosophy, one of several doctrines holding that all reality is objective and external to the mind and that knowledge is reliably based on observed objects and events. Subjectivism, by contrast, is the doctrine that all knowledge is restricted to the conscious self and its sensory states. *Compare* subjectivism. *See also* objective.

objectivity The state of being uninfluenced by emotions or personal prejudices. *Compare* subjectivity. *See also* objective.

obligation The act of binding oneself by a social, legal, or moral tie, such as a duty, contract, or promise. An obligation compels an individual to follow or avoid a particular course of action, as in the Hippocratic oath describes a physician's obligation to do no harm. *See also* duty; responsibility.

oblivion The condition of being completely forgotten, as in the hard lessons learned being consigned to posterity and oblivion.

oblivious Lacking all memory; lacking conscious awareness, as in the psychiatric patient was oblivious to her surroundings.

OBRA '89 Acronym for Omnibus Budget Reconciliation Act of 1989. *See* Agency for Health Care Policy and Research; Physician Payment Reform.

observant Quick to perceive or apprehend; alert, as in an observant patient.

observation The act or process of watching carefully and attentively. *See also* observation period; scientific method.

observational study A study in which nature is allowed to take its course and observed changes are studied in relation to changes in others, as in an observational study of a baboon troop in Kenya. The investigator(s) does not intervene in an observational study.

observation period A time period following an event (such as administration of a penicillin injection) during which a patient is watched closely for evidence that the care provided does no harm (for example, an allergic reaction to penicillin). *See also* observation.

observer One who observes. *See also* observation.

obsession An abnormally persistent focus on a single thought, image, or impulse that is unwanted and distressing and involuntarily comes to mind despite attempts to ignore or suppress it. Common obsessions involve thoughts of violence, contamination, and self-doubt. *See also* compulsion; obsessive-compulsive.

obsessive-compulsive Characterized by a compulsive tendency to repeat certain acts or rituals, such as brushing teeth more than is necessary, usually to relieve anxiety. *See also* obsessive-compulsive personality disorder.

obsessive-compulsive personality disorder A mental disorder characterized by an uncontrollable need to repeat certain acts or rituals, such as washing hands more than is necessary. *See also* obsessive-compulsive; personality disorder.

obsolescence The process of passing out of usefulness, as in technological obsolescence. *See also* obsolete; technological obsolescence.

obsolescence, technological *See* technological obsolescence.

obsolete No longer in use, as in newer technologies have rendered obsolete many older technologies. *See also* obsolescence; technological obsolescence.

Obstetrical Society, American Gynecological and *See* American Gynecological and Obstetrical Society.

Obstetric Anesthesia and Perinatology, Society for *See* Society for Obstetric Anesthesia and Perinatology.

obstetric forceps Any of a variety of instruments designed to assist in the extraction of the fetal head during childbirth. *See also* birth; forceps; obstetrics.

obstetric-gynecologic nurse practitioner A nurse practitioner specializing in obstetrics and gynecology. *See also* nurse practitioner; obstetrics

and gynecology.

obstetrician A physician specializing in obstetrics. *See also* obstetrics.

obstetrician-gynecologist A physician specializing in obstetrics and gynecology. *See also* obstetrics; obstetrics and gynecology.

Obstetricians and Gynecologists, American College of *See* American College of Obstetricians and Gynecologists.

Obstetricians and Gynecologists, American College of Osteopathic *See* American College of Osteopathic Obstetricians and Gynecologists.

Obstetric, and Neonatal Nurses, Association of Women's Health, *See* Association of Women's Health, Obstetric, and Neonatal Nurses.

obstetric nurse A registered nurse who specializes in obstetrics. *See also* obstetrics; registered nurse.

obstetrics The branch of medicine dealing with the management of pregnancy, labor, and the post labor recovery period. *See also* labor; obstetrics and gynecology; pregnancy; puerperium.

Obstetrics, American Society for Psychoprophylaxis in *See* American Society for Psychoprophylaxis in Obstetrics.

Obstetrics, Association of Professors of Gynecology and *See* Association of Professors of Gynecology and Obstetrics.

obstetrics and gynecology (OB-GYN) The branch and specialty of medicine that deals with the management of pregnancy, labor, and the postlabor recovery period (obstetrics) and diseases of the female genital tract (gynecology). Subspecialty areas of obstetrics and gynecology include critical care medicine, gynecologic oncology, maternal-fetal medicine, and reproductive endocrinology. *See also* critical care medicine; gynecologic oncology; maternal-fetal medicine; reproductive endocrinology.

Obstetrics and Gynecology, American Board of *See* American Board of Obstetrics and Gynecology.

Obstetrics and Gynecology, Council on Resident Education in *See* Council on Resident Education in Obstetrics and Gynecology.

obstipation Profound constipation. *See also* constipation.

obstruction Blockage; interruption of a process or progress, as in intestinal obstruction. *See also* ileus; intestine.

obstructive pulmonary disease, chronic *See* chronic obstructive pulmonary disease.

obvious Easily perceived or understood.

Occam's razor *See* Ockham's razor.

occasional Occurring now and then, at random. *See also* continuous; frequent; intermittent; periodic; sporadic.

occasion of service A specific identifiable act of service provided a patient, such as performance of a test, medical examination, treatment, or procedure. *See also* service.

occlusion **1.** A blockage or closing off of a vessel or passageway in the body, as in a clot occluding a blood vessel. *See also* coronary occlusion. **2.** The manner in which the teeth in the opposing jaws meet in biting, as in malocclusion. *See also* malocclusion; orthodontics.

occult Hidden or difficult to observe directly, as in occult blood in stool. *See also* occult blood.

occult blood A very small or hidden amount of blood, not observable and usually detected only by chemical test or microscopic analysis. *See also* blood; occult.

occupancy In a health care organization, such as a hospital, the ratio of average daily census to the average number of beds maintained during the reporting period. *See also* bed; census; occupancy rate.

occupancy factor (T) The level of occupancy of an area adjacent to a source of radiation, used to determine the amount of shielding required in the walls. *T* is rated as full, for an office or laboratory next to an x-ray facility; partial, for corridors and restrooms; and occasional, for stairways, elevators, closets, and outside areas. *See also* radiation; x-ray.

occupancy permit, beneficial *See* beneficial occupancy permit.

occupancy rate A measure of inpatient health facility use, determined by dividing available bed days by patient days. It measures the average percentage of a hospital's beds occupied and may be institutionwide or specific for one department or service. *See also* occupancy; patient days; rate.

occupation An activity that serves as one's regular source of livelihood. *See also* job; occupational; profession; vocation; work.

occupational Pertaining to engagement in a particular occupation. *See also* occupation.

occupational accident An accidental injury that occurs in the workplace. *See also* occupational hazard.

occupational certification A practice that permits practitioners in a particular occupation to claim at least a minimum level of competence for that occupation. As a means of regulation, however, certification does not prevent uncertified persons from supplying the same services as certified ones. *See also* certification; occupation.

occupational disability A condition in which an employee is unable to perform the functions required to complete a job satisfactorily because of an occupational disease or an occupational accident; for example, a mail-sorter developing carpal tunnel syndrome or a baseball pitcher developing elbow problems. *See also* disability; occupational accident; occupational disease.

occupational disease A disease resulting from the conditions of a person's employment, usually from long-term exposure to a noxious substance or from continuous repetition of certain acts. *Synonym:* industrial disease. *See also* disease; occupational.

Occupational and Environmental Health, Society for *See* Society for Occupational and Environmental Health.

Occupational and Environmental Medicine, American College of *See* American College of Occupational and Environmental Medicine.

occupational hazard Any condition of a job, such as exposure to radiation or chemicals, that can result in injury or illness. *See also* hazard; occupational.

occupational health The degree to which an employee is able to function at an optimum level of well-being at work as reflected by productivity, work attendance, disability compensation claims, and employment longevity. *See also* environmental health; occupational; health.

occupational health nurse A registered nurse who works in the field of occupational health. Many occupational health nurses have advanced training in occupational health or public health. *Synonym:* industrial nurse. *See also* nurse; occupational; occupational health services; registered nurse.

Occupational Health Nurses, American Association of *See* American Association of Occupational Health Nurses.

Occupational Health Nurses, American Board for *See* American Board of Occupational Health Nurses.

occupational health and safety The recognition, control, and prevention of health hazards and illnesses associated with occupations and the work environment. This includes promotion of the mental and physical health of employed persons. *See also* occupational health; occupational hazard.

Occupational Health and Safety, Association of University Programs in *See* Association of University Programs in Occupational Health and Safety.

occupational health services Health services involving the physical, mental, and social well being of individuals in relation to their work and working environment. *Synonym*: industrial health services. *See also* employee health service.

Occupational Hearing Conservation, Council for Accreditation in *See* Council for Accreditation in Occupational Hearing Conservation.

occupational medicine The branch of medicine dealing with the prevention and treatment of disease and injuries occurring at work or in specific occupations. *See also* medicine; occupation.

occupational nurse *See* occupational health nurse.

Occupational Safety and Health Act of 1970 The principal federal statute providing for the health and safety of employees on the job, administered by the Occupational Safety and Health Administration and the National Institute for Occupational Safety and Health. The act created the Occupational Safety and Health Review Commission, the Occupational Safety and Health Administration, and the National Institute for Occupational Safety and Health. *Synonym*: Williams-Steiger Act. *See also* Occupational Safety and Health Administration; Occupational Safety and Health Review Commission.

Occupational Safety and Health Administration (OSHA) A component of the Department of Labor established by the Occupational Safety and Health Act of 1970, that develops and promulgates standards relating to occupational safety and health, develops and issues regulations in this area, conducts investigations and inspections to determine the status of compliance with safety and health standards and regulations, and issues citations and proposes penalties for noncompliance with safety and health standards and regulations. *See also* Department of Labor; occupational safety and health standard.

Occupational Safety and Health, National Institute for *See* National Institute for Occupational Safety and Health.

Occupational Safety and Health Review Commission (OSHRC) An independent federal agency established by the Occupational Safety and Health Act of 1970 to adjudicate enforcement actions initiat-ed under the act when they are contested by employers, employees, or representatives of employees. The Occupational Safety and Health Act, covering virtually every employer in the United States requires employers to provide a place of employment free from hazards recognized to cause or likely to cause death or serious physical harm, and to comply with occupational safety and health standards set forth under the act. The OSHRC adjudicates when a citation is issued against an employer as a result of an inspection and the citation is contested within 15 working days thereafter. *See also* Occupational Safety and Health Act of 1970.

occupational safety and health standard A standard that requires conditions or the adoption of one or more practices, means, methods, operations, or processes reasonably necessary or appropriate to provide safe or healthful employment and places of employment. Safety standards may be adopted by national consensus or established by federal regulation. *See also* Occupational Safety and Health Act of 1970; Occupational Safety and Health Administration; standard.

occupational social worker *See* industrial social worker.

occupational therapist (OT) An allied health professional who provides occupational therapy services including, but not limited to, education and training in activities of daily living; the design, fabrication, and application of orthoses (splints); guidance in the selection and use of adaptive equipment; therapeutic activities to enhance functional performance, work readiness, and skills; and consultation concerning the adaptation of physical environments for the handicapped. These services are provided to individuals or groups, to both inpatients and outpatients, and to employers in business and industry. Occupational therapists are one type of allied health professional for which the Committee on Health Education and Accreditation has accredited education programs. *See also* accreditation; allied health professional; occupational therapy; occupational therapy assistant.

occupational therapy (OT) The use of productive or creative activity in the treatment or rehabilitation of physically or emotionally disabled people. OT focuses on the active involvement of a patient in specially designed therapeutic tasks and activities to improve function, performance capacity, and the ability to cope with demands of daily living. *See also* adult day care; disability; occupational medicine; occupational therapy services; therapy.

occupational therapy assistant An allied health professional who, under the direction of an occupational therapist, directs an individual's participation in selected tasks to restore, reinforce, and enhance performance; to facilitate learning of those skills and functions essential for adaptation and productivity; to diminish or correct pathology; and to promote and maintain health. Occupational therapy assistants are one type of allied health professional for which the Committee on Allied Health Education and Accreditation has accredited education programs. *See also* accreditation; allied health professional; occupational therapist; occupational therapy.

Occupational Therapy Association, American *See* American Occupational Therapy Association.

Occupational Therapy Certification Board, American *See* American Occupational Therapy Certification Board.

occupational therapy services Services that provide goal-directed purposeful activity to aid in the development of adaptive skills and performance capacities by individuals of all ages who have physical disabilities and related psychological impairment(s). Such therapy is designed to maximize independence, prevent further disability, and maintain health. *See also* disability; occupational therapy; service.

occurrence **1.** A happening, event, incident, or episode, as in an adverse occurrence. **2.** In epidemiology, the frequency of a disease or other attribute or event in a population or group without distinguishing between incidence and prevalence. *See also* adverse patient occurrence; episode; frequency; incident.

occurrence, adverse patient *See* adverse patient occurrence.

occurrence-based coverage Insurance that covers claims only when the event that gives rise to the claim happens during the period of time that the policy is in effect, regardless of when the claim is made. *See also* claims-made coverage; coverage; occurrence policy.

occurrence criteria Criteria used in occurrence reporting and occurrence screening systems to screen for and identify adverse patient occurrences. Examples of occurrence criteria include unplanned return to operating room or delivery room on same admission, transfer from a general care to a special care unit, and nosocomial infection. *Synonyms*: occurrence screening; occurrence screening criteria. *See also* adverse patient outcome; criteria; occurrence reporting; occurrence screening.

occurrence policy A professional liability insurance policy that covers the holder during the period an alleged act of malpractice occurred. Occurrence policies are said to have a "long tail," because the statute of limitations on malpractice allegations is unlimited. Thus an individual could be sued years after an event had taken place yet, if the individual held an occurrence type of malpractice policy, there would be protection under that policy. *Compare* claims-made coverage. *See also* malpractice; occurrence-based coverage; professional liability.

occurrence reporting A system for identifying adverse patient occurrences (APOs) through relying on individuals to report events that correspond to objective occurrence criteria. Occurrence reporting can be hospitalwide, although typically it focuses on high-risk areas within a hospital. Occurrence reporting provides data concurrently and generally outperforms incident reporting in its yield of APOs (40% to 60%). However, occurrence reporting systems are event-oriented and seldom identify misdiagnoses or inappropriate treatment patterns that would be found in a criterion-based review of a patient's chart. Occurrence reporting is also subject to personal interpretations and other impediments to individuals' filing reports. *See also* adverse patient occurrence; HCFA generic quality screens; incident reporting; occurrence; occurrence criteria; occurrence screening.

occurrence screening A system for concurrent or retrospective, or concurrent and retrospective identification of adverse patient occurrences (APOs) through medical chart-based review according to objective screening criteria. Examples of criteria include admission for adverse results of outpatient management, readmission for complications or incomplete management of problems on previous hospitalization, or unplanned removal, injury, or repair of an organ or structure during surgery, an invasive procedure, or vaginal delivery. Criteria are used hospitalwide or adapted for departmental or topic-specific screening. Occurrence screening identifies about 80% to 85% of APOs. It will miss APOs that are not identifiable from the medical record. *See also* adverse patient occurrence; HCFA generic quality screens; incident reporting; occurrence; occurrence criteria; occurrence reporting; screening; surprise rate.

occurrence screening criteria   *See* occurrence criteria.

occurrence screens   *See* occurrence criteria.

Ockham's razor   William of Ockham's fourteenth-century dictum stating that entities should not be multiplied needlessly. This rule has been interpreted in science and philosophy to mean that the simplest of two or more competing theories is preferable and that an explanation for unknown phenomena should first be attempted in terms of what is already known. *Synonyms*: law of parsimony; Occam's razor; scientific parsimony. *See also* parsimony.

OCOO   *See* Osteopathic College of Ophthalmology and Otorhinolaryngology.

oculist   *See* ophthalmologist.

OD   *See* Doctor of Optometry.

odontalgia   A toothache. *See also* dentistry; pain.

odontology   The study of the structure, development, and abnormalities of the teeth. *See also* tooth.

Odontology, American Society of Forensic   *See* American Society of Forensic Odontology.

odontology, forensic   *See* forensic dentistry.

odor   A volatile emanation that is perceived by the sense of smell. *See also* sense; sense organ; smell.

ODPHP National Health Information Center (ONHIC)   A national organization founded in 1979 and funded by the Office of Disease Prevention and Health Promotion (ODPHP), Public Health Service, US Department of Health and Human Services, that operates the National Information Center for Orphan Drugs and Rare Diseases. It aids consumers and health professionals in locating health information. *See also* drug; orphan drug.

OEA   *See* Optometric Editors Association.

Oedipus   In Greek mythology, a son of Laius and Jocasta, who was abandoned at birth and unwittingly killed his father and then married his mother. *See also* Oedipus complex.

Oedipus complex   In psychoanalysis, repressed sexual feelings of a child toward the parent of the opposite sex and feelings of competition with the parent of the same sex. If unresolved, this complex may result in neurosis and an inability to form normal sexual relationships in adulthood. *See also* Oedipus; psychoanalysis.

OEPF   *See* Optometric Extension Program Foundation.

office   **1.** A place in which business, clerical, or professional activities are conducted, as in physician's office. *See also* receptionist; secretary. **2.** A duty or function assigned to or assumed by someone, as in office of chief operating officer.

office, admitting   *See* admitting department.

office, admissions   *See* admitting department.

office building, medical   *See* medical office building.

office, business   *See* business office.

office diagnosis   *See* bedside diagnosis.

Office of Disease Prevention and Health Promotion   An organizational unit within the office of the Assistant Secretary for Health of the Department of Health and Human Services, established by the Health Promotion and Disease Prevention Amendments of 1984. It coordinates activities with the Department of Health and Human Services relating to disease prevention, prevention services, health promotion, and health information and education concerning the appropriate use of health care services; coordinates the previous activities with similar private-sector activities; provides a national information clearinghouse on these activities; and conducts research and supports projects. *See also* health promotion; preventive medicine.

Office of the Forum for Quality and Effectiveness in Health Care   A component of the Agency for Health Care Policy and Research (AHCPR) that is developing multidisciplinary clinical practice guidelines based on medical appropriateness and effectiveness research and expert consensus. In setting priorities for clinical guideline development, AHCPR has targeted conditions or procedures that meet one or more of the following criteria: affecting a large number of individuals, amenable to prevention or early intervention, associated with high variation in clinical practice, of particular relevance to the Medicare population, likely to incur high costs, and having an existing base of scientific knowledge. To date, initial guideline development is being focused on prediction, prevention, and early treatment of pressure sores; management of chronic pain; diagnosis and treatment of depressed outpatients in primary care settings; treatment of urinary incontinence in adults; treatment of visual impairment in adults; delivery of comprehensive care in sickle cell disease; treatment of human immunodeficiency virus infections in the outpatient setting; and diagnosis and treatment of benign prostatic hypertrophy. *See also* Agency for Health Care Policy and Research;

practice guideline.

Office of Health Planning and Evaluation An organization within the US Public Health Service that monitors and assists state-funded and state-directed programs in health planning and directs selected health evaluation programs and projects. *See also* evaluation; health planning; Public Health Service.

Office of Health Technology Assessment A component of the Agency for Health Care Policy and Research that concentrates its review on those technologies being considered for Medicare reimbursement. *See also* Agency for Health Care Policy and Research; Medicare; technology assessment.

Office of Human Development Services A federal agency within the Department of Health and Human Services that includes the Administration on Aging; Administration for Children, Youth and Families; Administration on Developmental Disabilities; and Administration for Native Americans.

Office Laboratory Assessment, Commission on *See* Commission on Office Laboratory Assessment.

office management The process of organizing and administering the activities that normally occur in any day-to-day business office environment. *See also* management; office.

Office of Management and Budget (OMB) An organization within the executive office of the president of the United States which develops the president's proposed federal budget for submission to Congress each year, monitors the established budget and its execution by the Departments and Offices, and provides executive oversight in areas, such as procurement policy and regulation. *See also* budget; management.

office manager An individual who has the administrative responsibilities of office management. *See also* business office manager; manager; office management.

office manager, business *See* business office manager.

office nurse An individual employed by a physician in his or her office to perform or to assist in the performance of certain procedures. This person may be a registered nurse, licensed practical nurse, licensed vocational nurse, or nursing assistant who provides services according to education and as authorized by state laws or statutes. *See also* licensed practical nurse; licensed vocational nurse; nursing assistant; office; registered nurse.

Office Nurses, American Association of *See* American Association of Office Nurses.

Office of Personnel Management The federal agency responsible, among other activities, for administering the Federal Employees Health Benefits Program. *See also* Federal Employees Health Benefits Program; personnel management.

Office of Population Affairs The office within the US Public Health Service concerned with adolescent pregnancy and family planning programs. *See also* family planning; public health.

officer A person holding a position of authority, either by election or appointment, in an organization; for example admitting officer, chief executive officer, chief financial officer.

officer, admitting *See* admitting officer.

officer, chief executive *See* chief executive officer.

officer, chief financial *See* chief financial officer.

officer, chief information *See* chief information officer.

officer, chief operating *See* chief operating officer.

Office of Science and Data Development A component of the Agency for Health Care Policy and Research that is responsible for database development for the agency. *See also* Agency for Health Care Policy and Research.

Officers, National Association of Reimbursement *See* National Association of Reimbursement Officers.

Office of the Surgeon General The office of the chief medical officer of the United States within the US Public Health Service. *See also* Public Health Service; surgeon general; surgeon general of the United States.

Office of Technology Assessment (OTA) An organization of the US Congress established by the Technology Assessment Act of 1972 as a nonpartisan support agency to help Congress deal with issues of advanced technology and to anticipate and plan for the consequences of the use of technology. Health care related technology issues are handled by the OTA's Health and Life Science Division. *See also* Prospective Payment Assessment Commission.

office visit A visit by a patient for care at a physician's office. *See also* visit.

official **1.** Relating to an office, as in official duties. **2.** Authorized by proper authority, as in official permission. **3.** Pertaining to drugs authorized by or contained in the *United States Pharmacopoeia* or *National Formulary*. *See also National Formulary; United States*

Pharmacopoeia.

official accreditation decision report *See* survey report.

officialese Language characteristic of official documents or statements, especially when obscure, pretentiously wordy, or excessively formal. *See also* bureaucratese; language; legalese; official.

officialism Rigid adherence to official regulations, forms, and procedures.

Officials, National Association of County Health *See* National Association of County Health Officials.

off-line A computer system that does not allow the user direct access to the mainframe or stored files. Typically, information is stored on magnetic tape and must be loaded onto the mainframe before information can be retrieved. New data entered to the system accumulates in temporary storage until a file update can be run that merges the new data into the existing file. *Compare* on-line. *See also* computer; mainframe computer.

off-load In computer science, to transfer data to a peripheral device. *See also* computer.

off-the-record Not for publication or attribution. *Compare* on-the-record.

off time A period of time when not in service, as in off time for a computer or machine is when it is not scheduled for use or needs maintenance, alterations, or repairs. *See also* time.

OHS *See* Optometric Historical Society.

oil Any greasy liquid that is insoluble in water and soluble in alcohol and ether. Mineral oils are mixtures of various hydrocarbons, but animal and vegetable oils are simple lipids, mixtures of fatty acid glycerides distinguished from fats only by their liquidity. *See also* lipid.

ointment Any greasy, water-insoluble preparation for external application to the body, usually containing a medicinal substance, as in cortisone ointment or calomine ointment. *Synonyms:* salve; unction; unguent. *See also* paste.

OJT *See* on-the-job training.

OLA *See* Optical Laboratories Association.

Old Age, Survivors, and Disability Insurance Program (OASDI) A federal program created by the Social Security Act, which taxes both workers and employers to pay benefits to retired and disabled persons, their dependents, widows or widowers, and the children of deceased workers. *Synonym:* Social Security. *See also* Old Age, Survivors, Disabili-

ty and Health Insurance Program; Social Security.

Old Age, Survivors, Disability and Health Insurance Program (OASDHI) A program administered by the Social Security Administration that provides monthly cash benefits to retired and disabled workers and their dependents, and to survivors of insured workers. The OASDHI also provides health insurance benefits for persons aged 65 years and older, and for disabled persons younger than age 65. The legislative authority for the OASDHI is in the Social Security Act, originally enacted in 1935. The health insurance component of OASDHI, known as Medicare, was initiated in 1965. *See also* Medicare; Old Age, Survivors, and Disability Insurance Program.

old-boy network An informal, exclusively male system of mutual assistance and friendship through which men belonging to a particular group exchange favors and connections, as in politics or business. *See also* network; networking.

Older Americans Act of 1965 A federal statute that, as amended, attempts to provide a national policy for assisting older Americans in securing equal opportunity and an enhanced quality of life.

old-girl network An informal, exclusively female system of mutual assistance and friendship through which women belonging to a particular group exchange favors and connections, as in politics or business. *See also* network; networking.

old guard Individuals with long tenure in a group or an organization, who tend to be conservative, defensive of established programs and procedures, reactionary, and resistant to change.

old school A group committed to traditional ideas or practices, as in a physician or nurse of the old school.

olfaction The sense of smell. *See also* smell.

OMA *See* Optical Industry Association.

OMB *See* Office of Management and Budget.

ombudsman *See* ombudsperson.

ombudsperson A person who investigates complaints and reports findings, especially between aggrieved parties, such as patients, and an organization, such as a hospital or a component of a hospital. *See also* patient representative.

omission The act of withholding treatment. *See also* withdrawing treatment; withholding treatment.

Omnibus Budget Reconciliation Act of 1989 *See* Agency for Health Care Policy and Research; Physician Payment Reform.

omniprecipience The quality of being "all feeling" and able to understand how other people feel. *See also* ideal ethical observer.

omniscience **1.** The quality of knowing everything; having unlimited knowledge. **2.** The quality of knowing all the relevant facts. *See also* ideal ethical observer.

OMT *See* osteopathic manipulative treatment.

onanism The extravaginal depositing of semen, as in masturbation or coitus interruptus. *See also* coitus interruptus; masturbation; semen.

oncogene A viral gene, that is, segments of deoxyribonucleic acid (DNA) thought to be capable of inducing malignant transformation in cells. *See also* cancer; deoxyribonucleic acid; gene; malignant; virus.

oncologist A physician who specializes in oncology. *See also* gynecologic oncologist; medical oncologist; oncology; pediatric hematologist-oncologist.

oncologist, gynecologic *See* gynecologic oncologist.

oncologist, medical *See* medical oncologist.

oncologist, pediatric *See* pediatric hematologist-oncologist.

oncologist, pediatric hematologist- *See* pediatric hematologist-oncologist.

Oncologists, Society of Gynecologic *See* Society of Gynecologic Oncologists.

oncology The branch of medicine and subspecialty of gynecology, internal medicine, and pediatrics, dealing with the diagnosis and treatment of patients with cancer. *See also* gynecologic oncology; medical oncology; pediatric hematology-oncology; radiation oncology.

Oncology Administrators, Society for Radiation *See* Society for Radiation Oncology Administrators.

Oncology, American College of Mohs Micrographic Surgery and Cutaneous *See* American College of Mohs Micrographic Surgery and Cutaneous Oncology.

Oncology, American Society of Clinical *See* American Society of Clinical Oncology.

Oncology, American Society of Pediatric Hematology/ *See* American Society of Pediatric Hematology/Oncology.

Oncology, American Society of Preventive *See* American Society of Preventive Oncology.

Oncology, American Society for Therapeutic Radiology and *See* American Society for Therapeutic

Radiology and Oncology.

Oncology Centers, Association of Freestanding Radiation *See* Association of Freestanding Radiation Oncology Centers.

Oncology Group, Gynecologic *See* Gynecologic Oncology Group.

Oncology Group, Radiation Therapy *See* Radiation Therapy Oncology Group.

oncology, gynecologic *See* gynecologic oncology.

oncology, medical *See* medical oncology.

Oncology Nurses, Association of Pediatric *See* Association of Pediatric Oncology Nurses.

Oncology Nursing Society (ONS) A national organization founded in 1975 composed of 19,000 registered nurses interested in oncology. It seeks to promote high professional standards in oncology nursing, provide a network for the exchange of information, encourage nurses to specialize in oncology, and promote and develop educational programs in oncology nursing. *See also* network; nursing; oncology; registered nurse.

oncology, pediatric *See* pediatric hematology-oncology.

oncology, pediatric hematology- *See* pediatric hematology-oncology.

oncology, radiation *See* radiation oncology.

Oncology Social Workers, Association of Pediatric *See* Association of Pediatric Oncology Social Workers.

Oncology Social Workers, National Association of *See* National Association of Oncology Social Workers.

Oncology, Society of Surgical *See* Society of Surgical Oncology.

on demand When asked for; for example, a hospital emergency department generally provides health services to patients on demand (when the patient shows up to the emergency department).

oneirism An abnormal dreamlike state of consciousness. *See also* dream; oneirology.

oneirodynia *See* nightmare.

oneirology The science of dreams. *See also* dream.

one-to-one service A method of organizing nursing services in an inpatient care unit by which one registered nurse assumes responsibility for all nursing care provided one patient for the duration of one shift. *See also* registered nurse; service.

ongoing In progress or evolving, as in the ongoing measurement of important outcomes and processes.

See also continuous.

ONHIC *See* ODPHP National Health Information Center.

on-line Connected to and communicating directly with a computer's central processing unit. It is the type of computer system in which information entered into the system is immediately reflected in the database so that inquiries will always reflect up-to-the-minute transaction status. *Compare* off-line. *See also* central processing unit; computer; computer terminal; mainframe computer.

on-line database A database stored on a main-frame computer, which is transmitted by telephone, microwaves, or other means and can be accessed with a decoding device (modem) and displayed on a monitor or as a printout. *See also* database; modem; on-line.

on-line medical record A medical record stored in a computer, with constant instantaneous access via a computer terminal. *See also* electronic medical record; medical record.

on-line searching The process of connecting a microcomputer to a remote computer through a telecommunications network, requiring a personal computer, a modem, and communications software. A *modem* converts information on a microcomputer from digital to analog signals for transmission to the remote computer, and vice versa. The modem most commonly transmits across telephone lines; however, dedicated cables can be installed on local computer networks. *Communications software* translates the transmissions to and from the modem into information that may be printed or stored on disk. In order to gain access or log onto an on-line database, the searcher must have a subscription and password from a *database service. See also* database services; modem; on-line database.

on-line system In computer science, a system in which data are entered into a device, such as a terminal, that is connected directly to a computer. The user interacts with the computer through a terminal. *See also* computer; system.

ONS *See* Oncology Nursing Society.

on-the-job training (OJT) Work-related training that occurs on the actual work site while engaged in the occupation or profession; hands-on instruction.

on-the-record Intended for publication or attribution. *Compare* off-the-record.

oophorectomy Surgical removal of one or both ovaries. *Compare* orchiectomy. *See also* gynecology; hysterectomy; ovary.

OOSS *See* Outpatient Ophthalmic Surgery Society.

OPA *See* organ procurement agency.

OPD Abbreviation for outpatient department. *See* outpatient service.

open access In health care, describes a health plan member's ability to self-refer for specialty care with a participating provider without first obtaining referral from another physician. *Compare* gatekeeper mechanism.

open charting A system of medical record keeping in which the patient has access to his or her chart. Open charting in varying degrees is authorized in some mental health institutions. *See also* medical record.

open date A date stamped on a product so that the consumer can determine its freshness. Open dating is a relatively recent consumer marketing practice. *See also* best-before date; pack date.

open-door policy A management policy of encouraging a relaxed environment with employees by leaving the manager's door open to encourage informal employee interaction. *See also* management; policy.

open-ended programs Entitlement programs, such as Medicaid, in the federal budget for which eligibility requirements are determined by law. Actual obligations and outlays are only limited by the number of eligible persons who apply for benefits and the actual benefits received. *See also* entitlement; entitlement authority; Medicaid.

open enrollment A period of time when new subscribers may enroll in a group or individual health insurance plan or prepaid group practice. Individuals perceived as high-risk (for example, because of a preexisting illness) may be subjected to high premiums or exclusion during open enrollment periods. *See also* enrollment; exclusions; preexisting condition; premium.

open heart surgery Surgery on a dry, nonbeating heart; cardiopulmonary function is temporarily taken over by a heart-lung machine. *See also* cardiac rehabilitation program; heart-lung machine; perfusionist; surgery; thoracic surgery.

opening statement In litigation, a statement made by the attorney for each party after the jury has been selected and before any evidence has been presented. It outlines for the jury the evidence that each party intends to present and informs the jury of the party's theory of the case. *See also* closing statement.

open medical staff *See* open staff.

open panel group practice A medical or dental group practice that invites all physicians or dentists who meet its membership requirements to participate in marketing, delivery, and business administration of the group's health or dental care services. *Synonym*: open panel practice. *Compare* closed panel group practice. *See also* group practice; practice.

open panel practice *See* open panel group practice.

open staff An arrangement in which a medical staff of a hospital accepts new physician applicants to the medical staff, if the physicians are qualified and approved by the governing body of the organization. The term is also applied to hospital-physician contracts in which physicians provide administrative and clinical services to a hospital on a nonexclusive basis. *Synonym*: open medical staff. *Compare* closed staff; exclusive contract. *See also* medical staff.

operant conditioning In behavior therapy, a form of learning in which an individual is rewarded for the desired response and punished for the undesired responses. It is used to break harmful habits and reinforce desirable behavior. *See also* behavior modification; behavior therapy; conditioning; shaping.

operating environment In computer science, the shell surrounding the disk operating system (DOS) of a personal computer. It turns the display into a desktop that is basically a menu from which one selects and runs personal computer applications. *See also* disk operating system.

operating expense The amount of money paid to maintain property, such as insurance and utilities. It excludes financing expenses, depreciation, and income taxes.

operating microscope A binocular microscope used in surgery to enable the surgeon to clearly view small and inaccessible parts of the body, such as parts of the eye or ear. *See also* microscope; microsurgery.

operating officer, chief *See* chief operating officer.

operating room (OR) A unit of a hospital or other health care facility in which surgical procedures requiring anesthesia are performed. *Synonym*: operating theater. *See also* surgical suite.

operating room nurse (OR nurse) A registered nurse qualified by education and training to work in an operating room. An operating room supervisor, a circulating nurse, and a scrub nurse are three types

of OR nurses. *See also* circulating nurse; registered nurse; scrub nurse.

Operating Room Nurses, Association of *See* Association of Operating Room Nurses.

operating room supervisor *See* operating room nurse.

operating room technician A person who performs certain functions relating to the cleanliness, safety, and efficiency of an operating room. An operating room technician works under the supervision of an operating room nurse and the medical staff of a hospital or other surgical facility. *See also* operating room; technician.

operating statement A financial statement showing an organization's revenues and expenses and, usually, the budgeted monies, actual monies, and any discrepancy or variance between the two, in dollars and percentages. *See also* financial statement.

operating surgeon The surgeon responsible for a given surgical operation and the care directly associated with the operation. *See also* operation; surgeon.

operating system In computer science, a program that controls a computer and makes it possible for users to enter and run other programs. Most computers are set up so that, when first turned on, they automatically begin running a small program supplied in read-only memory (ROM) or occasionally in another form. This program enables the computer to load its operating system from disk or tape. *See also* boot; disk operating system; read-only memory.

operation Any surgical procedure performed on the body with instruments or by the hands of a surgeon, in order to remedy an injury, an ailment, a defect, or a dysfunction. Examples of operations include hysterectomy, appendectomy, and tooth extraction. *See also* major surgery; minor surgery; surgery; wound infection.

operational control The power of management over the daily activities of a business. *See also* management.

operational data A form of secondary data that are collected and maintained by an organization to meet its ongoing information needs; for example, hospital medical records and hospital billing records. *See also* data; data source; primary data; secondary data.

operational definition A description in quantifiable terms of what to measure and the steps to follow to consistently measure it. A desirable operational definition includes a criterion to be applied, a way to determine whether the criterion is satisfied, and a way to interpret the results of the test. An operational definition is developed for each key quality characteristic or key process variable before data are collected. *See also* key process variable; key quality characteristic.

operative   Pertaining to a surgical operation. *See also* perioperative; postoperative; preoperative.

operative care, post-   *See* postoperative care.

operative care, pre-   *See* preoperative care.

Operative Dentistry, Academy of   *See* Academy of Operative Dentistry.

operative, peri-   *See* perioperative.

operative, post-   *See* postoperative.

operative, pre-   *See* preoperative.

Ophthalmic Administrators, American Society of   *See* American Society of Ophthalmic Administrators.

ophthalmic assistant   *See* ophthalmic medical technician; ophthalmic medical technologist.

ophthalmic laboratory technician   An individual trained in the operation and maintenance of machines that grind lenses and make eyeware as prescribed by an optometrist or ophthalmologist. *See also* laboratory; ophthalmology; optometry; technician.

Ophthalmic Medical Personnel, Joint Review Committee for   *See* Joint Review Committee for Ophthalmic Medical Personnel.

ophthalmic medical technician   An allied health professional who assists ophthalmologists by performing tasks delegated to him or her by ophthalmologists. Ophthalmic medical technicians are qualified to take a medical history, administer diagnostic tests, take anatomical and functional ocular measurements, test ocular functions (including visual acuity, visual fields, and sensorimotor functions), administer topical ophthalmic medications, and instruct the patient (as in home care and use of contact lenses). Other tasks include caring for and maintaining ophthalmic instruments, sterilizing surgical instruments, assisting in ophthalmic surgery in the office or hospital, assisting in the fitting of contact lenses, and adjusting and making minor repairs on spectacles. Ophthalmic medical technicians are one type of allied health professional for which the Committee on Allied Health Education and Accreditation has accredited education programs. *Synonym:* paraophthalmic. *See also* allied health professional; ophthalmic medical technologist; ophthalmology;

technician.

ophthalmic medical technologist   An allied health professional who performs all duties carried out by ophthalmic medical technicians but is expected to do so at a higher level of expertise and to exercise considerable clinical technical judgment. Additionally, technologists may be expected to perform ophthalmic clinical photography and fluorescence angiography, ocular motility and binocular function tests, and electrophysiological and microbiological procedures, as well as to provide instruction and supervision of other ophthalmic personnel and patients. Ophthalmic medical technologists are one type of allied health professional for which the Committee on Allied Health Education and Accreditation has accredited education programs. *Synonym:* paraophthalmic. *See also* allied health professional; ophthalmic medical technician; ophthalmology.

Ophthalmic Photographers' Society (OPS)   A national organization founded in 1969 composed of 1,200 ophthalmologists, pathologists, medical and ophthalmic photographers, nurses, and other persons actively involved with ophthalmology or ophthalmic photography. *See also* ophthalmic photography; ophthalmology.

ophthalmic photography   Photography of the eye for documentation and diagnostic purposes.

Ophthalmic Practice, Pharmacists in   *See* Pharmacists in Ophthalmic Practice.

Ophthalmic Registered Nurses, American Society of   *See* American Society of Ophthalmic Registered Nurses.

Ophthalmic Research Institute (ORI)   An organization founded in 1972 that conducts coordinated vision research and instrumentation and procedure evaluation needed by the ophthalmic industry. Its research programs include new examination and treatment methods. Formerly (1988) Optometric Research Institute. *See also* ophthalmology; optometry; research.

Ophthalmic Surgery Society, Outpatient   *See* Outpatient Ophthalmic Surgery Society.

Ophthalmological Society, American   *See* American Ophthalmological Society.

ophthalmologist   A physician who specializes in ophthalmology. *Synonym:* oculist. *Compare* optician; optometrist. *See also* ophthalmology.

Ophthalmologists, Contact Lens Association of   *See* Contact Lens Association of Ophthalmologists.

Ophthalmologists, Society of Military   *See* Society of Military Ophthalmologists.

ophthalmology   The branch and specialty of medicine dealing with comprehensive eye and vision care, including diagnosis, monitoring, and medically or surgically treating all eyelid and orbital problems affecting the eye and visual pathways. Vision services, such as prescribing glasses and contact lenses, are included in the area of ophthalmology. *See also* glaucoma; ophthalmologist; opticianry; optometry; orthoptics; spectacles.

Ophthalmology, American Academy of   *See* American Academy of Ophthalmology.

Ophthalmology, American Board of   *See* American Board of Ophthalmology.

Ophthalmology, American Society of Contemporary   *See* American Society of Contemporary Ophthalmology.

Ophthalmology, Association for Research in Vision and   *See* Association for Research in Vision and Ophthalmology.

Ophthalmology, Association of Technical Personnel in   *See* Association of Technical Personnel in Ophthalmology.

Ophthalmology, Association of University Professors of   *See* Association of University Professors of Ophthalmology.

Ophthalmology, Joint Commission on Allied Health Personnel in   *See* Joint Commission on Allied Health Personnel in Ophthalmology.

Ophthalmology and Otorhinolaryngology, Osteopathic College of   *See* Osteopathic College of Ophthalmology and Otorhinolaryngology.

Ophthalmology, Pan-American Association of   *See* Pan-American Association of Ophthalmology.

Ophthalmology and Strabismus, American Association for Pediatric   *See also* American Association for Pediatric Ophthalmology and Strabismus.

ophthalmoscope   An instrument containing a perforated mirror and lenses used to examine the interior of the eye. *Synonym:* fundoscope. *See also* ophthalmology; ophthalmoscopy.

ophthalmoscopy   The process of examining the interior of the eye with an ophthalmoscope, as in performing ophthalmoscopy to diagnose for signs of diabetic retinopathy or hypertensive vascular changes. *Synonym:* fundoscopy. *See also* ophthalmology.

opiate   A drug that contains opium, is derived from opium (a substance derived from poppy plants), or

is produced synthetically and has opiatelike characteristics. Examples of opiates include morphine, codeine, and heroin. *See also* enkephalin; heroin; morphine; narcotics; opium.

opinion   **1.** A belief or conclusion held with confidence but not substantiated by positive knowledge or proof. *See also* assumption; judgment; opinionated; public opinion; public opinion poll; tenet. **2.** A judgment based on special knowledge and given by a expert, as in a medical opinion or a legal opinion.

opinionated   Holding stubbornly and often unreasonably to one's own opinions. *See also* opinion.

opinion leader   An individual whose ideas and behavior serve as a model to other persons. Opinion leaders communicate messages to a primary group, influencing the attitudes and behavior change of people in the group. *See also* leader.

opinion poll   *See* public opinion poll.

opinion poll, public   *See* public opinion poll.

opinion program, second-   *See* second-opinion program.

opinion, public   *See* public opinion.

Opinion Research, American Association for Public   *See* American Association for Public Opinion Research.

opinion, second   *See* second opinion.

opium   An extract of the capsules of the opium poppy (*Papaver somniferum*). It is the source of the narcotic, analgesic, and addictive opium alkaloids, which include morphine, codeine, and papaverine. *See also* morphine; opiate; paregoric; poppy.

opportunist   An individual who takes advantage of any opportunity to achieve an end, often with no regard for principles or consequences.

opportunistic infection   An infection by microorganisms whose normally low pathogenicity is enhanced by depression of the host's humoral or cellular immune defenses, such as occurs in immune deficiency syndromes and the administration of immunosuppressive drugs (for example, for transplantation patients). The systemic fungal infections, such as aspergillosis, and systemic candidiasis, toxoplasmosis, cytomegalovirus infection, and pneumocystic pneumonia, are examples. *See also* acquired immunodeficiency syndrome; candidasis; infection; organ transplantation; *Pneumocystis*; transplantation.

opportunity   A favorable or advantageous circumstance or combination of circumstances.

opportunity cost   The value that resources, used in

a particular way, would have if used in the best possible or another specified alternative way. When opportunity costs exceed the value the resources have in the way they are being used, they represent lost opportunities to get value from the resources. For example, the opportunity cost of attending medical school is wages that would have been earned from working four years instead of attending medical school for those four years. The opportunity cost of devoting physician time to tertiary care is the lost value of devoting the same time to primary care. *See also* cost; opportunity.

opportunity statement A concise description of a process or an outcome in need of improvement, its boundaries, the general area of concern where a quality improvement team should begin its efforts, and why work on the improvement is a priority. *See also* problem statement.

OPS *See* Ophthalmic Photographers' Society.

opt To decide or make a choice, as in a medical student opting for a residency in a high-paying specialty area.

optical character recognition Any of various systems whereby graphic information is input directly into a computer by means of an optic device. *See also* Automatic Identification Manufacturers; optical character reader.

optical character reader An input device that reads characters on printed documents by their shapes, translating them into computer machine language for further manipulation. *See also* computer; input device; machine language; optical character recognition.

optical disk *See* compact disk.

Optical Industry Association (OMA) A national organization founded in 1916 composed of 100 manufacturers of ophthalmic frames, lenses, cases, and optical machinery; associate members are suppliers of materials and parts. Formerly (1992) Optical Manufacturers Association. *See also* ophthalmology; opticianry; optometry.

Optical Laboratories Association (OLA) A national organization founded in 1962 composed of 350 independent, wholesale ophthalmic laboratories and suppliers serving the ophthalmic field. *See also* laboratory; ophthalmology; opticianry; optometry.

Optical Manufacturers Association *See* Optical Industry Association.

optical-stripe card A smart card that uses the same

technology as a compact disk for music or data and can hold about two megabytes (two million bytes) of data. This may translate to approximately 2,000 pages of data and adequate space to also hold a number of digital images, such as ultrasound pictures of a fetus, electrocardiograms, or even a low-resolution chest x-ray. The device that reads from the card and writes information to the card must operate with a great deal of precision. *See also* smart card in health care.

optician A person who makes and dispenses lenses and frames (spectacles) prescribed by optometrists and ophthalmologists. Although some opticians grind lenses themselves, this work is usually done by optical laboratory technicians. *Synonym*: dispensing optician. *Compare* ophthalmologist; optometrist. *See also* opticianry.

optician, dispensing *See* dispensing optician.

opticianry The discipline of making and dispensing lenses and frames prescribed by optometrists and ophthalmologists. *See also* optician; spectacles.

Opticianry Accreditation, Commission on *See* Commission on Opticianry Accreditation.

Opticianry, American Board of *See* American Board of Opticianry.

Opticianry, National Academy of *See* National Academy of Opticianry.

Opticians Association of America (OAA) A national organization founded in 1926 composed of 700 retail dispensing opticians who fill prescriptions for glasses or contact lenses written by a vision care specialist. *See also* optician.

Opticians, National Association of Manufacturing *See* National Association of Manufacturing Opticians.

Opticians, National Association of Optometrists and *See* National Association of Optometrists and Opticians.

optics The study of light. *See also* fiberoptics.

optics, fiber- *See* fiberoptics.

Optics Manufacturers' Association, Laser and Electro- *See* Laser and Electro-Optics Manufacturers' Association.

Optics Society of America (OSA) A national organization founded in 1916 composed of 11,000 persons interested in any branch of optics, including research, instruction, optical applications, manufacture, distribution of optical equipment, and physiological optics. Its technical groups focus on areas, such as lasers, medical optics, optical design, and vision. *See also* laser; optics.

Optics Society, IEEE Lasers and Electro- *See* IEEE Lasers and Electro-Optics Society.

optimal Most favorable or desirable, as in optimal health.

Optimal Health Association, Nutrition for *See* Nutrition for Optimal Health Association.

optimism A tendency to expect the best possible outcome or dwell on the most hopeful aspects of a situation. *Compare* negativism; pessimism.

optimist A person who usually expects a favorable outcome.

optimum The point at which the condition, degree, or amount of something is the most favorable, as in optimum achievable. *See also* optimum achievable standard.

optimum achievable standard A statement of expectation about the highest level of performance that is practically attainable. *See also* optimum; standard.

optimum capacity The level of output that produces the lowest cost per unit. *See also* capacity.

optional services Services that may be provided or covered by a health program or provider and, if provided, will be paid for in addition to any required services that must be offered. Examples of optional services under Medicaid in many states are prescribed drugs, dental services, and skilled nursing facility services for individuals younger than 21 years. *Compare* basic health services.

options Alternative courses of action, as in options that face a decision maker.

optometric assistant *See* optometric assistant and technician.

optometric assistant and technician An individual who assists an optometrist in providing vision care. He or she may, for example, perform preliminary vision capability tests; determine the power of old and new lenses; take facial and frame measurements and assist patients in frame selection; order lenses prescribed by the optometrist; and assist the fitting of contact lenses and teach the patient how to wear and care for them. An optometric technician is a person who has received training beyond that of an optometric assistant and who performs more advanced duties, such as examining the curvature of the cornea and recording eye pressures or tensions. *Synonym:* paraoptometrics. *See also* optometry.

Optometric Association, American *See* American Optometric Association.

Optometric Association, National *See* National Optometric Association.

Optometric Care, Council on Clinical *See* Council on Clinical Optometric Care.

Optometric Editors Association (OEA) A national organization founded in 1965 composed of 45 present or past editors or assistant editors of serial optometric publications; associate members include editors of ophthalmic publications. It promotes standards of excellence in optometric communications. *See also* optometry.

Optometric Education, Council on *See* Council on Optometric Education.

Optometric Educators, Association of *See* Association of Optometric Educators.

Optometric Extension Program Foundation (OEPF) A national organization founded in 1928 composed of 4,000 registered optometrists and optometric assistants enrolled for continuing education courses. It conducts training seminars and graduate clinical seminars in topics related to vision. *See also* optometry.

Optometric Historical Society (OHS) A national organization founded in 1969 composed of optometrists and other individuals or groups interested in optometry, optics, and related disciplines. Its purposes are to encourage the collection and preservation of materials relating to the history of optometry and to assist in the care of archives of optometric interest. *See also* history; optometry.

Optometric Research Institute *See* Ophthalmic Research Institute.

Optometric Society, Armed Forces *See* Armed Forces Optometric Society.

optometric technician *See* optometric assistant and technician.

optometrist An individual qualified by education and authorized by law to practice optometry. He or she may examine the eyes and vision system for visual defects, diagnose impairments, prescribe corrective lenses, and provide other types of treatment. An optometrist can use drugs for diagnostic purpose and (in most states) prescribe them for therapeutic purposes. *Compare* optician; ophthalmologist. *See also* optometry.

Optometrists and Opticians, National Association of *See* National Association of Optometrists and Opticians.

Optometrists in Vision Development, College of
See College of Optometrists in Vision Development.

optometry   The profession dealing with problems of human vision and their correction through the prescription and adaptation of visual training (orthoptics), lenses, or other optical aids. Optometry is not a branch of medicine. *See also* ophthalmology; opticianry; optometrist; orthoptics; spectacles.

Optometry, American Academy of   *See* American Academy of Optometry.

Optometry, Association of Schools and Colleges of   *See* Association of Schools and Colleges of Optometry.

Optometry, National Board of Examiners in   *See* National Board of Examiners in Optometry.

OR   *See* operating room.

Oral Biology, American Institute of   *See* American Institute of Oral Biology.

oral contraceptive   A pill, usually containing estrogen or progesterone, that inhibits ovulation and thereby prevents conception. *Synonym*: birth control pill. *See also* birth control; contraception.

Oral Diagnosis, Organization of Teachers of   *See* Organization of Teachers of Oral Diagnosis.

Oral Diagnosis, Radiology, and Medicine, Academy of   *See* Academy of Oral Diagnosis, Radiology, and Medicine.

oral hygiene   *See* dental hygiene.

oral and maxillofacial surgeon   A dentist who specializes in oral and maxillofacial surgery. *Synonym*: oral surgeon. *See also* oral and maxillofacial surgery.

Oral and Maxillofacial Radiology, American Academy of   *See* American Academy of Oral and Maxillofacial Radiology.

Oral and Maxillofacial Surgeons, American Association of   *See* American Association of Oral and Maxillofacial Surgeons.

Oral and Maxillofacial Surgeons, American College of   *See* American College of Oral and Maxillofacial Surgeons.

oral and maxillofacial surgery   A branch and specialty of dentistry that includes a broad scope of diagnostic, operative, and related services dealing with diseases, injuries, and defects in the jaw and associated structures. *Synonym*: oral surgery. *See also* dental specialties; oral and maxillofacial surgeon; surgery.

Oral and Maxillofacial Surgery, American Board of   *See* American Board of Oral and Maxillofacial Surgery.

Oral Medicine, American Academy of   *See* American Academy of Oral Medicine.

oral pathologist   A dentist who specializes in oral pathology. As a diagnostician, an oral pathologist does not necessarily treat the diseases directly but may provide counsel and guidance to other specialists who do provide treatment. *See also* dental specialties; dentist; oral pathology.

oral pathology   A dental specialty dealing with the nature of mouth diseases through study of their causes, processes, and effects. *See also* dental specialties; oral pathologist; pathology.

Oral Pathology, American Academy of   *See* American Academy of Oral Pathology.

Oral Pathology, American Board of   *See* American Board of Oral Pathology.

oral poliovirus vaccine   *See* Sabin vaccine.

oral surgeon   *See* oral and maxillofacial surgeon.

oral surgery   *See* oral and maxillofacial surgery.

orchidectomy   *See* orchiectomy.

orchiectomy   Surgical removal of one or both testes. *Synonym*: orchidectomy. *Compare* oophorectomy. *See also* testis; urology.

orchitis   Inflammation of the testes. *See also* inflammation; mumps; testis.

order   **1.** A condition of comprehensible arrangement among the elements of a group. *See also* ordered data set. **2.** A directive, for example, about treatment, examination, drugs, and other care to be given to a patient, as in a physician's order. *See also* back order; medication order; nursing orders; prescribe; standing orders.

order, back   *See* back order.

order, do-not-resuscitate   *See* do-not-resuscitate order.

ordered data set   A data set that has been arranged to show the observations from the smallest to the largest value. *See also* data set.

orderly   An attendant in a hospital who performs routine, nonmedical work in a hospital or other health care facility. *See also* nursing assistant.

order, medication   *See* medication order.

order not to resuscitate   *See* do-not-resuscitate order.

order, pecking   *See* pecking order.

orders, nursing   *See* nursing orders.

orders, standing   *See* standing orders.

order, temporary restraining   *See* temporary

restraining order.

ordinal Being of a specified position in a numbered series, as in an ordinal rank of fifth. *See also* ordinal data; ordinal number; ordinal scale.

ordinal data Data resulting from use of an ordinal scale. *Compare* nominal data. *See also* ordinal scale.

ordinal number A number indicating position in a series of order, as in first (1st), second (2nd), third (3rd), and so on. *Compare* cardinal number. *See also* number; ordinal scale.

ordinal scale A scale in which classification occurs along ordered qualitative categories where the values have a distinct order, but their categories are qualitative in that there is no natural numerical distance between the possible values. Only the relative sizes of numbers (larger than, smaller than) are important. Examples of ordinal scales are American Society of Anesthesiologists - Physical Status categories, as in P1, P2, and so forth, or a classification of level of compliance for standards published by the Joint Commission on Accreditation of Healthcare Organizations, as in a score of 1 [substantial compliance], 2 [significant compliance], and so forth). *See also* compliance level; ordinal number; scale.

ordinary care Care that will offer reasonable hope of benefit to a patient with less chance of creating the burdens that may be associated with extraordinary care. *Compare* extraordinary care.

organ A structural part of a system of the body that is composed of tissues and cells that enable it to perform a particular function or functions, as in the liver, spleen, and kidney. *See also* organ bank; organ donor; tissue; viscera.

organ bank A repository and registry service, within a major hospital or network of hospitals, for human tissues and organs for use or implantation in patients. *See also* bank; implantation; organ; organ donor; tissue bank.

organ donor An individual who permits an organ to be removed from his or her body for transplantation to another person. *See also* donor.

Organ Donor Program, Medic Alert *See* Medic Alert Organ Donor Program.

organic Pertaining to organs or an organ of the body, as in organic disease. *See also* organ; organic disease.

organic disease Disease caused by damage or change to organs or tissues. *Compare* mental illness. *See also* disease; organic.

organic psychosis A psychosis caused by physical causes such as infection; for example, general paresis (a condition characterized by dementia and paralysis) caused by syphilis. *See also* psychosis; toxic psychosis.

organism Any living animal, plant, fungus, bacterium, or virus. *See also* bacteria; fungus; microorganism; virus.

organism, micro- *See* microorganism.

organization **1.** An orderly, systematic structure of roles and responsibilities that function to accomplish predetermined objectives; an entity that is made up of elements with varied functions that contribute to the whole and to collective functions; for example, a hospital or a health maintenance organization. *See also* corporate structure; corporation; functional organization; health care organization; management services organization; physician-hospital organization. **2.** The manner of being orderly and systematic, as in a high degree of organization. **3.** The act or process of putting into an order or a system, as in departmental reorganization was efficiently performed. *See also* reorganization; shakeup.

organization, action *See* action organization.

organizational behavior An academic field of study, primarily taught in business schools and psychology departments, dealing with human behavior in organizations. The field deals with subject matter such as motivation, group dynamics, leadership, organization structure, decision making, careers, conflict resolution, and organizational development. *Synonym*: organizational psychology. *See also* behavior; organization.

organizational chart A diagram showing all the interrelationships of positions within an organization in terms of authority and responsibility. *See also* chart.

organizational culture The fundamental beliefs and attitudes that powerfully affect the behavior of people in and around an organization over time. The organizational culture is transmitted to new members through socialization processes; is maintained and transmitted through a network of rituals, rites, myths, communication, and interaction patterns; and is enforced and reinforced by group norms and the organization's system of rewards and controls. Sources of organizational culture include the attitudes and behaviors of dominant, early organization "shapers" and "heroes"; the organization's nature of work, including its functions and interactions with the external environment; and new members' attitudes, values, and willingness to act. Organizational culture provides a framework for the shared understanding of events, defines behavioral expectations, provides a source of and focus for members' commitment, and functions as an organizational control system. *See also* culture; organization.

organizational development Planned, systematic processes in which behavioral science principles and practices are used to improve an organization's functioning. *See also* development; organization; organizational planning.

organizational performance The way in which an organization, such as a hospital, carries out or accomplishes its important functions so as to increase the probability that desired outcomes will be achieved. *See also* organization; outcome; performance.

organizational planning The process of transforming organizational objectives into specific management strategies and tactics designed to achieve objectives. Organizational planning is one of the most important management responsibilities. *See also* management; organization; planning.

organizational psychology *See* organizational behavior.

organization, articles of *See* articles of organization.

organization-based factor *See* organization factor.

organization, charitable *See* charitable organization.

organization, exclusive provider *See* exclusive provider organization.

organization, experimental medical care review *See* experimental medical care review organization.

organization factor An organization-related variable that may contribute to variation in organizational performance. An organization factor is usually controllable by the organization and is the object of performance measurement and improvement processes. *Synonym:* organization-based factor. *Compare* external environmental factor; patient factor; practitioner factor. *See also* factor; variable.

organization, functional *See* functional organization.

organization, health care *See* health care organization.

organization, health maintenance *See* health maintenance organization.

organization leaders In health care organizations, the group of individuals that set expectations, develop plans, and implement procedures to assess and improve the quality of the organization's governance, management, clinical, and support processes. For example, leaders in hospitals include at least the leaders of the governing body; the chief executive officer and other senior managers; the elected and/or appointed leaders of the medical staff and the clinical departments and other medical staff members in an organization's administrative positions; and the nursing executive and other senior nursing leaders. *See also* leader; organization; organization planning.

organization, learning *See* learning organization.

organization man/organization woman A person whose identity, behavior, and lifestyle slavishly conform to the social mores of an organization; derived from William F. Whyte's book *The Organization Man*.

organization, management services *See* management services organization.

organization, matrix *See* matrix organization.

organization, not-for-profit *See* not-for-profit organization.

Organization, Pan American Health *See* Pan American Health Organization.

organization, peer review *See* peer review organization.

organization, physician-hospital *See* physician-hospital organization.

organization, preferred provider *See* preferred provider organization.

organization, professional *See* professional organization.

organization, professional standards review *See* professional standards review organization.

organization, re- *See* reorganization.

Organizations, American Association of Preferred Provider *See* American Association of Preferred Provider Organizations.

organization, shared service *See* shared service organization.

Organizations, Leadership Council on Aging *See* Leadership Council on Aging Organizations.

Organizations, National Association of Health Data *See* National Association of Health Data Organizations.

Organizations, National Coalition of Hispanic Health and Human Services *See* National Coalition of Hispanic Health and Human Services Organizations.

Organizations, National Federation of Housestaff *See* National Federation of Housestaff Organizations.

Organizations, National Federation for Specialty Nursing *See* National Federation for Specialty Nursing Organizations.

organization structure The manner in which responsibility and authority is apportioned among the members of an organization, as in a line and staff organization. *See also* organization; structure.

Organization of Teachers of Oral Diagnosis A national organization founded in 1963 composed of 200 teachers and university departments of oral diagnosis (oral medicine and oral pathology). *See also* Academy of Oral Diagnosis, Radiology, and Medicine; oral pathology.

organization unit A functional division of an organization, as in an intensive care unit. *See also* organization; unit.

organization, voluntary *See* voluntary health agency.

organizationwide Throughout an organization; across multiple structural and staffing components, as in organizationwide quality improvement. *See also* organization.

organization worker, community *See* community organization worker.

Organization, World Health *See* World Health Organization.

organize To put together into an orderly, functional, structured whole. *See also* organized; organized professional staff.

organized As used in accreditation reviews of hospitals and other health care organizations, administratively and functionally structured; for example, organized medical or professional staff. *See also* organize; organized professional staff.

organized medical staff *See* organized professional staff.

organized professional staff A formal organization of the professional personnel of a hospital that includes one or more physicians and to whom is delegated the responsibility for maintaining standards of medical care and/or health-related care. *Synonyms:* organized medical staff; organized staff. *See also* medical staff; staff.

organotherapy The treatment of disease by administration of extracts of animal organs, usually endocrine glands, now replaced by the use of pure hormones. *See also* endocrine; gland; hormone.

organ procurement The process of obtaining vital human organs, such as livers, hearts, and kidneys, for implantation in other humans who need them. Organs can be procured from live donors or cadavers, such as patients on life-support systems who are proclaimed dead. There are many ethical issues involved with organ procurement. For example, informed consent must be obtained without coercion prior to removal of an organ from a live donor, yet coercion is difficult to avoid when one family member is being asked to donate an organ for another family member. *See also* anatomical gift; informed consent; organ; organ procurement agency; presumed consent; procurement; required request law; transplantation.

organ procurement agency (OPA) An organization set up to keep records of persons needing organ transplants and of donor organs available, and to match the two with such speed that the surgery can be performed successfully. *See also* organ procurement.

Organs, American Society for Artificial Internal *See* American Society for Artificial Internal Organs.

organ, sense *See* sense organ.

Organ Sharing, United Network for *See* United Network for Organ Sharing.

Organ Transplant Act of 1984, National *See* National Organ Transplant Act of 1984.

organ transplantation To transfer an organ from one body to another. Solid organs, such as the heart, kidney, and liver, are viable only from patients in whom an intact circulatory system can be maintained despite brain death. *Compare* tissue transplantation. *See also* opportunistic infection; organ procurement; transplantation.

orgasm The culmination or climax of sexual intercourse, arousing an intensely pleasurable sensation in both sexes, and accompanied in the male by ejaculation of semen. *Synonym:* climax. *See also* nymphomania; reproduction; sexual intercourse.

ORI *See* Ophthalmic Research Institute.

Oriental Bodywork Therapy Association, American *See* American Oriental Bodywork Therapy Association.

Oriental Medicine, American Association for Acupuncture and *See* American Association for Acupuncture and Oriental Medicine.

Oriental Medicine, National Accreditation Commission for Schools and Colleges of Acupuncture and *See* National Accreditation Commission for Schools and Colleges of Acupuncture and

Oriental Medicine.

orientation **1.** A person's awareness of self with regard to position, time, place, and personal relationships, as in sexual orientation. *See also* sexual orientation. **2.** Introductory instructions concerning a new situation, as in orientation of new medical staff members.

orientation, sexual *See* sexual orientation.

OR nurse *See* operating room nurse.

orphan drug Any pharmaceutical product that may be available to physicians and patients in countries other than the United States but that has not been "adopted" by a domestic pharmaceutical manufacturer or distributor. An orphan drug may not be available in the United States for several reasons, including total sales would not justify the expense of research and development, the product may not have been approved by the Bureau of Drugs of the Food and Drug Administration, or the medication may be a natural substance that cannot be effectively protected by patent laws against competition from a similar form of the product. The US Orphan Drug Act of 1982 offers federal financial incentives to commercial and nonprofit organizations to develop and market drugs previously unavailable in the United States. *See also* drug; Food and Drug Administration.

Orphan Drug Act of 1982 A federal law providing tax incentives and developmental grants for the testing of drugs designated by the Secretary of Health and Human Services as possibly effective for the treatment of many diseases and conditions that affect only small numbers of persons. *See also* orphan drug.

ORS *See* Orthopedic Research Society.

orthesis *See* orthosis.

ORTHO *See* American Orthopsychiatric Association.

orthodontia *See* orthodontics.

orthodontic appliance A device that is fixed to the teeth or removable that applies force to the teeth and their supporting structures to modify tooth position. *Synonym*: dental appliance. *See also* appliance; brace; retainer.

orthodontics A dental specialty involving treatment of problems relating to irregular dental development, missing teeth, and other abnormalities in order to establish normal function and appearance. *Synonyms*: orthodontia; orthodonture. *See also* dental specialties; dentist; malocclusion; orthodontist.

Orthodontics, American Association for Functional *See* American Association for Functional Orthodontics.

Orthodontics, American Board of *See* American Board of Orthodontics.

Orthodontics, American Society for the Study of *See* American Society for the Study of Orthodontics.

Orthodontics, College of Diplomates of the American Board of *See* College of Diplomates of the American Board of Orthodontics.

Orthodontics for the General Practitioner, American Academy of *See* American Academy of Orthodontics for the General Practitioner.

Orthodontic Society, American *See* American Orthodontic Society.

orthodontist A dentist who specializes in orthodontics. The orthodontist is skilled in straightening teeth and correcting the position of jaws by using braces and/or other appliances that affect oral growth and development. *See also* dental specialties; dentist; orthodontics.

Orthodontists, American Association of *See* American Association of Orthodontists.

orthodonture *See* orthodontics.

orthomolecular medicine The study of the concentrations of substances, such as vitamins, normally found in the body but appearing disproportionately in schizophrenics, alcoholics, children with learning disabilities, and older people suffering memory loss, depression, and other senile illnesses. *See also* medicine; orthomolecular medicine therapy.

Orthomolecular Medicine, American Association of *See* American Association of Orthomolecular Medicine.

orthomolecular medicine therapy The treatment of mental disorders by the provision of the optimum molecular environment for the mind, especially the optimum concentrations of substances, such as vitamins, normally present in the body. *See also* orthomolecular medicine.

Orthopaedic Association, American *See* American Orthopaedic Association.

Orthopaedic Foot and Ankle Society, American *See* American Orthopaedic Foot and Ankle Society.

Orthopaedic Laser Surgery, American Board of Neurological/ *See* American Board of Neurological/Orthopaedic Laser Surgery.

Orthopaedic Medicine and Surgery, American Board of Neurological and *See* American Board of Neurological and Orthopaedic Medicine and Surgery.

Orthopaedic Nurses, National Association of *See* National Association of Orthopaedic Nurses.

Orthopaedic Section, American Physical Therapy Association A national association founded in 1974 composed of 10,758 orthopaedic physical therapists who belong to the American Physical Therapy Association, physical therapy educators, and students. *See also* American Physical Therapy Association; physical therapy.

Orthopaedic Society, Academie *See* Academie Orthopaedic Society.

Orthopaedic Society, Clinical *See* Clinical Orthopaedic Society.

Orthopaedic Society of North America, Pediatric *See* Pediatric Orthopaedic Society of North America.

Orthopaedic Society, Ruth Jackson *See* Ruth Jackson Orthopaedic Society.

Orthopaedic Society for Sports Medicine, American *See* American Orthopaedic Society for Sports Medicine.

orthopaedic/orthopedic surgeon A physician who specializes in orthopaedic surgery. *See* orthopaedic/orthopedic surgery; surgeon.

Orthopaedic Surgeons, American Academy of *See* American Academy of Orthopaedic Surgeons.

Orthopaedic Surgeons, American Academy of Neurological and *See* American Academy of Neurological and Orthopaedic Surgeons.

Orthopaedic Surgeons, Society of Military *See* Society of Military Orthopaedic Surgeons.

orthopaedic/orthopedic surgery The branch and specialty of medicine dealing with the preservation, investigation, and restoration of the form and function of the extremities, spine, and associated structures by medical, surgical, and physical means. Orthopaedic surgery involves the care of patients whose musculoskeletal problems are present at birth or develop at any time during their lifetime. It also involves diagnosis and treatment of congenital deformities, trauma, infections, tumors, and metabolic disturbances of the musculoskeletal system. Hand surgery is a subspecialty of orthopaedic surgery. *See also* arthroscopy; bone; cast; fracture; hand surgery; hip replacement; joint; orthopedics; splint; traction.

Orthopaedic Technologists, National Association of *See* National Association of Orthopaedic Technologists.

Orthopaedic Technologists, National Board for Certification of *See* National Board for Certification of Orthopaedic Technologists.

orthopaedist/orthopedist *See* orthopaedic/orthopedic surgeon.

Orthopedic Medicine, American Association of *See* American Association of Orthopedic Medicine.

Orthopedic Research Society (ORS) A national organization founded in 1954 composed of 1,500 orthopedic surgeons and other investigators who are elected as active members on the basis of previous scientific activity, continued participation in the field of research, and accomplishments in orthopedic surgery. It promotes orthopedic research and provides a place for presentation and discussion of orthopedic research activities. *See also* orthopaedic/orthopedic surgery; research.

Orthopedic Resident Education, Advisory Council for *See* Advisory Council for Orthopedic Resident Education.

orthopedics The branch of medicine that deals with the prevention or correction of injuries or disorders of the skeletal system and associated muscles, joints, and ligaments. *See also* orthopaedic/orthopedic surgery.

Orthopedics, American Academy of Gnathologic *See* American Academy of Gnathologic Orthopedics.

Orthopedics, American Academy of Head, Facial and Neck and TMJ *See* American Academy of Head, Facial and Neck and TMJ Orthopedics.

Orthopedics, American Osteopathic Academy of *See* American Osteopathic Academy of Orthopedics.

Orthopedics, American Board of Podiatric *See* American Board of Podiatric Orthopedics.

Orthopedics, American College of Chiropractic *See* American College of Chiropractic Orthopedics.

Orthopedics, Council on Chiropractic *See* Council on Chiropractic Orthopedics.

orthopedics, pediatric *See* pediatric orthopedics.

orthopedics, podiatric *See* podiatric orthopedics.

Orthopedic Surgery, American Board of *See* American Board of Orthopedic Surgery.

Orthopedic Surgical Manufacturers Association (OSMA) A national organization founded in 1955 composed of 24 manufacturers of orthopedic surgical items. *See also* orthopaedic/orthopedic surgery.

orthopedist/orthopaedist *See* orthopaedic/orthopedic surgeon.

Orthopedists, American College of Foot *See* American College of Foot Orthopedists.

Orthopsychiatric Association, American *See* American Orthopsychiatric Association.

orthopsychiatry The psychiatric study, treatment, and prevention of emotional and behavioral problems, especially those that arise during early development. *See also* psychiatry.

Orthoptic Council, American *See* American Orthoptic Council.

orthoptics Practice of using nonsurgical measures, especially eye exercises, to treat abnormalities of vision and uncoordinated eye movement, such as strabismus (muscular disorder, such as "cross eye") and amblyopia (decrease in sharpness of vision). Orthoptics means "straight eyes." *See also* orthoptist; optometry; strabismus.

orthoptist A health professional who specializes in the treatment of eye coordination defects. *See also* orthoptics.

Orthoptists, American Association of Certified *See* American Association of Certified Orthoptists.

orthosis An orthopedic appliance or apparatus used to support, align, prevent, or correct deformities or to improve the function of movable parts of the body. *Synonym*: orthesis. *See also* appliance; orthotics.

Orthotic Clinics, Association of Children's Prosthetic- *See* Association of Children's Prosthetic-Orthotic Clinics.

Orthotic and Prosthetic Association, American *See* American Orthotic and Prosthetic Association.

orthotic/prosthetic technician An individual who, under the direction of a orthotist/prosthetist, follows prescriptions and specifications to determine a device, such as a brace, to be made and the materials and tools needed to make the device. The technician then develops the devices. *See also* orthosis; orthotics; prosthetics; technician.

orthotics The science dealing with the use of specialized mechanical devices to support or supplement weakened or abnormal joints or limbs. *See also* joint; orthosis; pedorthics; prosthetics.

Orthotics and Prosthetics, American Board for Certification in *See* American Board for Certification in Orthotics and Prosthetics.

orthotist/prosthetist A person who makes, fits, and teaches individuals how to use braces, artificial limbs (prostheses), and other orthotic/prosthetic

appliances. The most common prosthetic replacements are artificial legs, feet, arms, and hands. *See also* appliance; brace; orthosis; prosthesis.

Orthotists and Prosthetists, American Academy of *See* American Academy of Orthotists and Prosthetists.

orotracheal intubation The process of inserting a tube through the mouth into the trachea to serve as an airway. *See also* intubation; nasotracheal intubation.

OSA *See* Optical Society of America.

oscilloscope A cathode ray tube that displays electrical variations. *See also* cathode ray tube.

OSHA *See* Occupational Safety and Health Administration.

OSHRC *See* Occupational Safety and Health Review Commission.

OSMA *See* Orthopedic Surgical Manufacturers Association.

osteoarthritis The most common form of degenerative joint disease, in which a breakdown of the joint cartilage occurs, causing joint pain and stiffness. It has no relation to nutrition, except that obesity worsens it because of excess weight on the joints. *See also* arthritis; joint; orthopaedic/orthopedic surgery; rheumatology.

osteology The study and knowledge of the bones. *See also* bone.

osteomalacia The adult form of rickets, a disease in which low levels of calcium and phosphate in the blood prevent bone calcification. It is caused by a deficiency of vitamin D in the diet, lack of skin exposure to sunlight, or by conditions inhibiting vitamin D absorption or use. *See also* bone; rickets; vitamin.

osteomyelitis Infection of the bone. *See also* bone.

osteopath *See* osteopathic physician.

Osteopathic Academy of Orthopedics, American *See* American Osteopathic Academy of Orthopedics.

Osteopathic Academy of Sclerotherapy, American *See* American Osteopathic Academy of Sclerotherapy.

Osteopathic Academy of Sports Medicine, American *See* American Osteopathic Academy of Sports Medicine.

Osteopathic Association, American *See* American Osteopathic Association.

Osteopathic Association, Bureau of Professional Education of the American *See* Bureau of Professional Education of the American Osteopathic Association.

Osteopathic Board of Emergency Medicine, American *See* American Osteopathic Board of Emergency Medicine.

Osteopathic Board of General Practice, American *See* American Osteopathic Board of General Practice.

Osteopathic Board of Pediatrics, American *See* American Osteopathic Board of Pediatrics.

Osteopathic College of Allergy and Immunology, American *See* American Osteopathic College of Allergy and Immunology.

Osteopathic College of Anesthesiologists, American *See* American Osteopathic College of Anesthesiologists.

Osteopathic College of Dermatology, American *See* American Osteopathic College of Dermatology.

Osteopathic College of Ophthalmology and Otorhinolaryngology (OCOO) A national organization founded in 1916 composed of 385 osteopathic physicians who have completed formal specialty training or are acquiring such training in ophthalmology, otorhinolaryngology, and orofacial plastic surgery and those who are certified specialists in one or more of these areas. It develops application of osteopathic concepts in this specialty and determines minimum standards of education at undergraduate and postgraduate levels. *See also* ophthalmology; osteopathic medicine; otolaryngology.

Osteopathic College of Pathologists, American *See* American Osteopathic College of Pathologists.

Osteopathic College of Preventive Medicine, American *See* American Osteopathic College of Preventive Medicine.

Osteopathic College of Proctology, American *See* American Osteopathic College of Proctology.

Osteopathic College of Radiology, American *See* American Osteopathic College of Radiology.

Osteopathic College of Rehabilitation Medicine, American *See* American Osteopathic College of Rehabilitation Medicine.

Osteopathic Directors of Medical Education, Academy of *See* Academy of Directors of Osteopathic Education.

Osteopathic Emergency Physicians, American College of *See* American College of Osteopathic Emergency Physicians.

Osteopathic Examiners, American Association of *See* American Association of Osteopathic Examiners.

Osteopathic Healthcare Executives, College of *See* College of Osteopathic Healthcare Executives.

Osteopathic Hospital Association, American *See* American Osteopathic Hospital Association.

Osteopathic Internists, American College of *See* American College of Osteopathic Internists.

osteopathic manipulative treatment (OMT) The use of osteopathic physicians' hands to diagnose injury and illness and to encourage the body's natural tendency toward good health. OMT is employed in combination with all other medical procedures to provide care. *See also* manipulative medicine; osteopathic medicine.

Osteopathic Medical Examiners, National Board of *See* National Board of Osteopathic Medical Examiners.

osteopathic medicine A system of medicine based on the theory, originally propounded in 1874 by Dr Andrew Taylor Still (1828-1917), that the normal body, when in correct adjustment, is a vital mechanical organism naturally capable of making its own responses to and defenses against diseases. The physician of this school searches for and, if possible, corrects any peculiar position of the joints or tissue or peculiarity of diet or environment that is a factor in destroying the natural resistance. The measures used are physical, hygienic, medicinal, and surgical. Today osteopathic medicine is distinguished from allopathy mainly, if at all, by its greater reliance on manipulation. Osteopathic physicians are licensed to perform medicine and surgery in all states, eligible for graduate medical education in either osteopathic or allopathic programs, reimbursed by Medicare and Medicaid for their services, supported under health personnel legislation, and generally treated identically with allopathic physicians. *Synonym*: osteopathy. *Compare* allopathy; homeopathy; naprapathy; naturopathy.

Osteopathic Medicine, American Association of Colleges of *See* American Association of Colleges of Osteopathic Medicine.

Osteopathic Medicine and Surgery, American College of General Practitioners in *See* American College of General Practitioners in Osteopathic Medicine and Surgery.

Osteopathic Obstetricians and Gynecologists, American College of *See* American College of Osteopathic Obstetricians and Gynecologists.

Osteopathic Pediatricians, American College of *See* American College of Osteopathic Pediatricians.

osteopathic physician A practitioner of osteopathic medicine. *Synonyms*: doctor; doctor of osteopathy;

osteopath; physician. *See also* osteopathic medicine.

Osteopathic Specialists, American Association of *See* American Association of Osteopathic Specialists.

Osteopathic State Executive Directors, Association of *See* Association of Osteopathic State Executive Directors.

Osteopathic Surgeons, American College of *See* American College of Osteopathic Surgeons.

Osteopathic Women Physician's Association, National *See* National Osteopathic Women Physician's Association.

osteopathy *See* osteopathic medicine.

Osteopathy, American Academy of *See* American Academy of Osteopathy.

osteoporosis A condition in which bones lose mass and become porous and fragile, markedly increasing susceptibility to fractures; results over a period of years from a complex interplay of genetic, hormonal, nutritional, and other factors. Adequate dietary calcium while bone is being laid down (birth to age 35 years) delays onset. *See also* bone; calcitonin; geriatric medicine; orthopaedic/orthopedic surgery; rheumatology.

osteotripsy Bone surgery performed by the use of bone burrs and bone files. *See also* bone.

ostomy A surgical procedure in which an opening is made to allow the passage of urine from the bladder or feces from the intestines. *See also* colostomy; ileostomy; stoma.

OT *See* occupational therapist; occupational therapy.

OTA *See* Office of Technology Assessment.

otalgia Earache. *See also* otitis; pain.

OTC drug *See* over-the-counter drug.

other diagnosis Any medical condition of a patient other than the principal diagnosis, which exists at the time of patient admission or develops subsequently and affects the treatment received and/or the length of stay in a health care organization. The other diagnosis is coded using the *International Classification of Diseases, Ninth Revision, Clinical Modification*. *Synonym:* secondary diagnosis. *See also* comorbidity; diagnosis; principal diagnosis.

otitis Inflammation of a part(s) of the ear, as in otitis media (inflammation of the middle ear). *See also* inflammation; otalgia.

Otolaryngic Allergy, American Academy of *See* American Academy of Otolaryngic Allergy.

otolaryngologist *See* otolaryngologist-head and neck surgeon; pediatric otolaryngologist.

otolaryngologist-head and neck surgeon A physician specializing in otolarnygology - head and neck surgery. *Synonyms:* ear, nose, and throat physician/specialist/surgeon. *See also* otolaryngology; surgeon.

Otolaryngologist-Head and Neck Surgeons, Society of Military *See* Society of Military Otolaryngologist - Head and Neck Surgeons.

otolaryngologist, pediatric *See* pediatric otolaryngologist.

Otolaryngologists-Head and Neck Surgeons, Society of University *See* Society of University Otolaryngologists-Head and Neck Surgeons.

otolaryngology The branch and specialty of medicine dealing with medical and surgical treatment of the head and neck, including the ears, nose, and throat. Head and neck oncology and facial plastic and reconstructive surgery are areas of expertise. Otology/neurotology and pediatric otolaryngology are two subspecialties of otolaryngology. *Synonym:* otorhinolaryngology. *See also* laryngology; otology/neurotology; pediatric otolaryngology; rhinology; tonsillectomy.

Otolaryngology Administrators, Association of *See* Association of Otolaryngology Administrators.

Otolaryngology, American Board of *See* American Board of Otolaryngology.

Otolaryngology-Head and Neck Surgery, American Academy of *See* American Academy of Otolaryngology-Head and Neck Surgery.

otolaryngology, pediatric *See* pediatric otolaryngology-head and neck surgery.

Otological Society, American *See* American Otological Society.

Otological Society, American Laryngological, Rhinological and *See* American Laryngological, Rhinological and Otological Society.

otologist *See* otologist/neurotologist.

otologist/neurotologist An otolaryngologist who subspecializes in otology/neurotology. *See also* otolaryngology; otology/neurotology.

otology/neurotology The branch of medicine and subspecialty of otolaryngology concerned with diagnosis, management, prevention, cure, and care of patients with diseases of the ear and temporal bone, including disorders of hearing and balance. The subspecialty deals specifically with care for patients in need of cochlear implants, implantable hearing aids, and extensive reconstruction of the tympanum (eardrum) and ossicular chains (small bones of the middle ear).

otorhinolaryngology *See* otolaryngology.

Otorhinolaryngology and Head/Neck Nurses, Society of *See* Society of Otorhinolaryngology and Head/Neck Nurses.

Otorhinolaryngology, Osteopathic College of Ophthalmology and *See* Osteopathic College of Ophthalmology and Otorhinolaryngology.

otoscope An endoscope used to examine the external ear, the tympanic membrane (eardrum) and, through the eardrum, the small bones of the middle ear. It consists of a light, a magnifying lens, and a device for insufflation (blowing air into the ear). *See also* endoscope.

out-of-area coverage Benefits that a health plan will provide to its members who are outside the plan's coverage area. With rare exceptions, out-of-area coverage is limited to emergency services only. *See also* coverage; emergency services; health plan.

outbreak *See* epidemic.

outcome In health care, the cumulative effect at a defined point in time of performing one or more processes in the care of a patient; for example, patient survival (or death) following a health intervention is an outcome. *See also* health intervention; patient health outcome; product.

outcome assessment Evaluation based on the premise that care is delivered in order to bring about certain results; criteria are developed to measure the actual outcomes of patient care and service against the predetermined criteria. *See also* assessment; outcome; outcome criteria.

outcome of care *See* patient health outcome.

outcome criteria Criteria against which the level of outcomes achieved may be compared. *See also* criteria; outcome; outcome assessment.

outcome data Data collected to evaluate a specified outcome, such as changes in a patient's health status attributable to care processes received by the patient. *See also* data; outcome; process data.

outcome following suicide attempt A completed or incomplete suicide attempt, that is, a suicide attempt that does or does not result in death. *See also* suicide; suicide attempt.

outcome indicator An indicator that measures what happens or does not happen after a process(es), service(s), or activity(ies) is performed or not performed. *See also* indicator; outcome measure; process indicator.

outcome measure A measure of what happens or does not happen after a process(es), service(s), or activity(ies) is performed or not performed, or a structural component (such as a technology or a medical specialist) exists or does not exist. Outcome measures quantify an organization's, a practitioner's, or a community's actual results in providing services the organization is capable of providing. *Compare* input measure; process measure. *See also* measure; outcome indicator.

outcome, patient health *See* patient health outcome.

outcomes management A philosophy of making health care-related choices based on better insight and understanding into the effect of these choices on a patient's life. *See also* management; outcome.

outcomes research Health services research that attempts to identify the clinical outcomes of the delivery of health care services. *See also* outcome; research.

outcome standard A statement of expectation set by competent authority concerning a degree or level of acceptable outcome achieved by an individual, group, organization, community, or nation, according to preestablished requirements and/or specifications. *See also* outcome; process standard; standard.

outdated blood Donated whole blood that has been stored under refrigeration for more than 21 days and consequently is unusable for transfusion. *See also* blood; blood transfusion.

outlier **1.** Observations differing so widely from the rest of a set of data as to lead one to suspect that a gross error may have been committed or suggest that these values come from a different population; for example, health care providers with performance or outcomes rates that are outside the range of expected rates after adjustment for patient or other characteristics are called outliers. **2.** A patient having either an extremely long length of stay or incurring an extraordinarily high cost when compared with most patient discharges classified in the same diagnosis-related group (DRG). *Compare* inlier. *See also* cost outlier; diagnosis-related groups; high-mortality outlier; low-mortality outlier.

outlier, cost *See* cost outlier.

outlier, high-mortality *See* high-mortality outlier.

outlier, low-mortality *See* low-mortality outlier.

out-of-body experience An experience in which a person perceives himself or herself from an external perspective, as though the mind or soul has left the physical body and is acting of its own volition.

out-of-pocket costs *See* out-of-pocket payments.

out-of-pocket payments Payments or costs borne directly by a patient without benefit of insurance. *See also* insurance.

outpatient An individual who receives health care services in a clinic, emergency department, or other health care facility without being admitted to (lodged overnight in) a health care facility as an inpatient. *Compare* inpatient. *See also* outpatient bed; patient.

outpatient admission, clinic *See* clinic outpatient admission.

outpatient admission, emergency *See* emergency department admission.

outpatient admission, referred *See* referred outpatient admission.

outpatient bed A bed regularly maintained by a health care organization for patients who require medical services for less than 24 hours. *See also* bed; outpatient.

outpatient care Care that is provided to patients who are not confined to an institutional bed as inpatients during the time services are rendered, such as an emergency department visit that does not result in hospitalization overnight. *Synonym:* ambulatory care; ambulatory health care. *See also* ambulatory health care; clinic outpatient admission.

outpatient clinic *See* outpatient service.

outpatient department (OPD) *See* outpatient service.

Outpatient Ophthalmic Surgery Society (OOSS) A national organization founded in 1981 composed of ophthalmic surgeons interested in gathering and sharing information about outpatient eye surgery in order to promote high-quality, low-cost patient care. *See also* ophthalmology; surgery.

outpatient service Service providing diagnosis and treatment to patients who do not require admission as inpatients. *Synonyms:* outpatient clinic; outpatient department. *See also* clinic; inpatient; outpatient; service.

Outpatient Surgeons, American Society of *See* American Society of Outpatient Surgeons.

outpatient surgery *See* ambulatory surgery.

outpatient visit All services provided an outpatient in the course of a single appearance in an outpatient or inpatient unit. *See also* outpatient; visit.

outplacement Assistance in finding a new job,

given by an employer to an employee who has been laid off or whose employment has been terminated. *See also* employee; layoff.

output 1. The process or act of producing, or the yield, or the total of anything produced; for example, cardiac output (the effective volume of blood expelled by either ventricle of the heart per unit of time), or units of service output (for example, number of cardiac catheterizations performed by a hospital per unit time). The output of a process can be the input to a succeeding process. *See also* feedback; health services research; input; task. **2.** The information produced by a computer from a specified input. *See also* computer; electronic data processing.

outreach program A hospital-sponsored and hospital-administered program whose purpose is to bring a specified type of health service, such as primary care or home care, into the community the hospital serves. *See also* community health care.

outside director A member of an organization's governing body who is not an employee of or otherwise associated with an organization. Outside directors are considered important because they can bring unbiased opinion to major corporate decisions and they also can contribute diverse experience to the decision-making process. *See also* director; governing body.

outsourcing The process of having components of a project or endeavor supplied by individuals or companies outside of an organization, in order to cut costs, improve quality, or both. *See also* consultant.

ova Plural of ovum. *See* ovum.

ova banking Storing ova (eggs) for future use in producing a human baby. *See also* bank; ovum; sperm banking; zygote banking.

ovary In humans, the paired female reproductive organ that produces ova (eggs), estrogen, and progesterone. *Compare* testis. *See also* genitalia; ovulation; ovum.

overage Too much; the opposite of shortage. For example, the legislation resulted in an overage of health professionals in urban as compared to suburban and rural areas.

overcharge Retail price charged that is greater than the actual retail price of an item; excessive price. In health care, an excessive fee or charge.

overcompensation A conscious or unconscious exaggerated attempt to overcome or neutralize a real or imagined defect or unwanted characteristic. *See* *also* compensation.

overcorrect To remedy beyond what is needed, appropriate, or usual, especially when the overcorrection results in a mistake. *See also* correct.

overcrowd To cause to be excessively crowded, as in emergency department overcrowding.

overdose An excessive amount, as in an overdose of heroin. *See also* dose; megadose.

overhead Indirect expenses of running a business not directly associated with a particular item or service sold; for example, electricity, insurance, and benefits paid to hospital employees are overhead expenses.

overhead projector A projector capable of projecting enlarged images of written or pictorial material onto a screen or wall from a transparency placed horizontally below the projector and lighted from underneath.

overheating Pertaining to an economy that is expanding so rapidly that economists fear a rise in inflation. In an overheated economy, too much money is chasing too few goods, leading to price rises, and the productive capacity of a nation is usually nearing its limit. *See also* economy.

overhype To promote or publicize to excess. *See also* overkill; promotion.

overkill An excess of something beyond what is required or suitable for a particular purpose; for example, an expensive promotional effort that produces diminishing returns because it repels rather than attracts customer interest. *See also* marketing.

overlay A later addition superimposed on an already existing condition, mass, or state; for example, an emotional overlay. *See also* emotional overlay; psychosomatic illness.

overlay, emotional *See* emotional overlay.

overlay, psychogenic *See* emotional overlay.

overmedicate To medicate a patient excessively. *See also* medicate.

overpay To pay too much, as in the officer or the hospital was overpaid. *See also* pay.

overpopulation Excessive population of an area to the point of overcrowding, depletion of natural resources, or environmental deterioration. *See also* population.

overprescribe To prescribe an excessive amount of a medication. *See also* prescribe.

overproduction Excessive production; supply beyond market demand at remunerative prices;

glut.

overqualified Educated or skilled beyond what is necessary or desired for a particular job. *See also* qualified.

overresponse An abnormally intense response to a stimulus. *See also* response.

oversight Watchful care or management. *See also* executive oversight.

oversight, executive *See* executive oversight.

over-the-counter (OTC) drug A nonprescription medication that is legally sold over the counter in a retail store. Over-the-counter medicines can be purchased in any quantity without restrictions at the retail store level. *Synonyms*: nonprescription drug; over-the-counter medicine; patent medicine. *Compare* prescription drug. *See also* drug.

over-the-counter medicine *See* over-the-counter drug.

overtime Time worked in excess of an agreed upon time for normal working hours by an employee. For example, hourly employees must be compensated at the rate of one and one-half their normal hourly rate for overtime work beyond 40 hours in a workweek.

overtransfusion Overloading of the circulation by excessive transfusion of blood or other fluid. *See also* blood transfusion.

overtriage The process of transporting patients to trauma centers when the patients could have received appropriate care in a nontrauma center. The use of trauma scoring instruments, such as the Glasgow coma scale, are intended to increase the probability of matching trauma patients with the appropriate level of trauma care. *See also* Glasgow coma scale; trauma score; triage; undertriage.

overview 1. A broad comprehensive perspective; a survey. 2. A summary or review; for example, a type of medical literature review in which primary research relevant to a clinical topic or question is examined and summarized, and an effort is made to identify all available published and unpublished literature that pertains to the topic or question, as in an overview of penicillin allergy.

overweight Excessive increase in adipose tissue (obesity) or muscle and skeletal tissues (muscular overweight). *See also* obesity.

ovolactovegetarian A vegetarian who abstains from meat, poultry, and fish, but eats dairy products and eggs. *See also* vegetarian.

ovulation The release of an egg (ovum) from a

Graafian follicle on the surface of the ovary; then it passes via the fallopian tube into the uterus. Ovulation occurs once a month on about the 15th day of the menstrual cycle throughout the female reproductive period (from menarche to menopause). It is marked by slight fever and in some women by mittelschmerz (pain in the area of the ovary). *See also* fertility drug; mittelschmerz; ovary; ovum.

ovum The female reproductive cell or gamete; egg. *See also* ova banking; ovary; ovulation; spermatozoa.

owner In quality improvement, a person(s) who has or is given the responsibility and authority to lead the continuing improvement of a process. Process ownership is a designation made by leaders of organizations and depends on the boundaries of a process. *See also* boundary.

oximeter An instrument for measuring the oxygen saturation of hemoglobin in arterial blood. *See also* oximetry; transcutaneous oxygen/carbon dioxide monitoring.

oximetry A technique of measurement to noninvasively monitor patient oxygenation through either spectrophotometric evaluations of arterial blood flow or simple diffusion measurements of oxygen through capillary membranes. *See also* pulse oximetry.

oximetry, pulse *See* pulse oximetry.

ozone An unstable gas with a pungent smell and powerful oxidizing properties, formed when oxygen is exposed to the silent discharge of electricity. It makes up the naturally occurring ozone layer in the earth's upper atmosphere, which absorbs most of the sun's harmful ultraviolet radiation. *See also* ozone depletion.

ozone depletion A reduction of ozone concentration in the ozone layer caused by atmospheric pollution and the build-up in the atmosphere of ozone-depleting chemicals. *See also* ozone; ozone hole.

ozone hole An area of the ozone layer in which serious ozone depletion has occurred. *See also* ozone; ozone depletion.

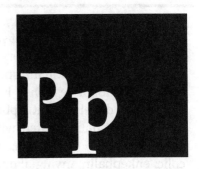

PA *See* physician assistant; Parapsychological Association.

PA Abbreviation for professional association. *See* professional corporation.

PAAO *See* Pan-American Association of Ophthalmology.

PAAS *See* Pan American Allergy Society.

pabulum Food of any kind. *See also* food.

PAC *See* Pediatric AIDS Coalition; political action committee.

pacemaker An object that influences the rate at which the heart beats, that is, either a natural cardiac (heart) pacemaker or an artificial cardiac pacemaker. *See also* artificial cardiac pacemaker; demand pacemaker; fixed rate pacemaker; natural cardiac pacemaker.

pacemaker, artificial cardiac *See* artificial cardiac pacemaker.

pacemaker, demand *See* demand pacemaker.

pacemaker, fixed-rate *See* fixed-rate pacemaker.

pacemaker, natural cardiac *See* natural cardiac pacemaker.

pacesetter One that takes the lead or sets an example for other persons to follow. *See also* trendsetter; vanguard.

pacing Maintaining the heartbeat by repetitive stimulation of the heart muscle with a pacemaker. *See also* artificial cardiac pacemaker; natural cardiac pacemaker.

Pacing and Electrophysiology, North American Society of *See* North American Society of Pacing and Electrophysiology.

package A container in which something is packed for storage or transport, as in medication package. *See also* labeling; package insert.

package, comprehensive benefit *See* comprehen-sive benefit package.

package insert The labeling approved by the US Food and Drug Administration for a prescription drug product, which accompanies a product when it is shipped by a manufacturer to a pharmacist. The package insert is used by prescribing professionals, principally physicians. It states indications and contraindications of a drug, mode(s) of administration, dosage information, and warnings. *See also* contraindication; Food and Drug Administration; labeling; package; *Physicians' Desk Reference*; prescription drug.

packaging laws *See* labeling.

Packard Foundation, The David and Lucile *See* The David and Lucile Packard Foundation.

pack date A date stamped on frozen or canned items to indicate when the food was processed, manufactured, or packaged. *See also* best-before date; open date.

packed cells A preparation of blood cells separated from the liquid blood plasma used to restore adequate levels of red blood cells without overloading the circulatory system with too much fluid. *See also* blood transfusion; overtransfusion.

padding Adding unnecessary material or expenses for the purpose of increasing size or volume, as in padding an expense account to increase reimbursement from an organization.

pagination The process of dividing a document into pages. Many computer word processors offer a "paginate" command that shows where page breaks will occur in the printed text. *See also* computer.

PAHO *See* Pan American Health Organization.

PAI *See* Human Resource Certification Institute.

pain An unpleasant sensory or emotional experience connected with actual or potential tissue damage, or described in terms of such damage. Pain has two components: the sensory input and feeling of injury and the emotional response to the injury. Part of the emotional response is shaped by previous experience, development, upbringing, and personality. Pain is usually treated with analgesics. *See also* ache; analgesic; anesthesia; anesthetic; arthralgia; colic; enkephalin; myalgia; odontalgia; otalgia; pain threshold; sciatica; suggestion.

pain management A subspecialty of anesthesiology dealing with patients experiencing problems with acute or chronic pain in both hospital and ambulatory settings. *See also* anesthesiology; management; pain; physical medicine and rehabilitation; transcutaneous electric nerve stimulation.

pain management program A specialized program for the management of chronic and acute pain, using a multidisciplinary approach with medical, nursing, and allied health professionals. *See also* pain; pain management.

Pain, National Committee on the Treatment of Intractable *See* National Committee on the Treatment of Intractable Pain.

Pain Outreach Association, National Chronic *See* National Chronic Pain Outreach Association.

pain, referred *See* referred pain.

Pain Society, American *See* American Pain Society.

pain and suffering In law, an element of damages that one may recover for physical or mental pain and suffering that result from a wrong done or suffered. The loss of ability or capacity to work because of physical pain or emotional or mental suffering is a type of pain and suffering. Recovery for pain and suffering is restricted by statute in certain states. *See also* cap; mental anguish.

pain threshold A point at which a stimulus activates pain receptors to produce a feeling of pain. Individuals differ in pain threshold, some experiencing pain earlier than other individuals with a higher pain threshold. *See also* pain; threshold.

Pain and TMJ Orthopedics, American Academy of Head, Facial and Neck *See* American Academy of Head, Facial and Neck Pain and TMJ Orthopedics.

palate The partition separating the oral and nasal cavities; it comprises a bony portion in front (the hard palate) and a fleshy portion behind (the soft palate). The latter is drawn up during swallowing to block off the back of the nose. *See also* cleft palate.

palate, cleft *See* cleft palate.

paleopathology The study of disease in ancient peoples, as deduced from examination of bony remains, mummies, and other evidence, such as ancient writings. *See also* pathology.

palliative Relieving pain or other symptoms without effecting a cure, as in palliative care for a terminally ill patient. *See also* palliative care.

palliative care A range of treatments intended to relieve or alleviate pain and suffering without attempting to cure their source. *Synonym:* palliative treatment. *See also* pain; palliative; terminal illness.

palliative treatment *See* palliative care.

palmistry Fortune-telling from inspection of the pattern of creases in the palm of the hand. *See also* inspection; table.

palpable Perceivable by touch.

palpation In physical diagnosis, the act of feeling by the sense of touch. Palpation is used on all parts of the human body accessible to the examining fingers, such as palpating the abdomen for tenderness or palpating the size, shape, consistency, motility, and/or pulsation of masses. Special methods of palpation include light and deep palpation, ballottement, fluctuation, and fluid wave. *See also* physical examination; pulse.

palpitation A subjective awareness of the beat of the heart, usually as an unpleasant thumping sensation in the chest or at the root of the neck. It occurs in normal subjects when the force of the beat is abruptly increased, as by emotion or on lying down in bed. Disturbances of cardiac rhythm may also cause palpitations. *Synonym:* heart palpitation. *See also* anxiety; heart.

palsy Paralysis, as in cerebral palsy, Bell's palsy, or crossed-leg palsy. *See also* cerebral palsy.

Palsy Associations, United Cerebral *See* United Cerebral Palsy Associations.

palsy, cerebral *See* cerebral palsy.

Palsy and Developmental Medicine, American Academy for Cerebral *See* American Academy for Cerebral Palsy and Developmental Medicine.

PAMA *See* Pan American Medical Association.

panacea A universal remedy for all diseases, evils, or difficulties; a cure-all. *See also* Panacea.

Panacea One of two sisters, the other being Hygeia, who were the daughters of Aesculapius. *See also* Aesculapius; Hippocratic oath; panacea.

Pan American Allergy Society (PAAS) An international organization founded in 1956 composed of

695 physicians throughout the Western Hemisphere who include allergy diagnosis and management in their practices. Its purpose is to serve as a forum by improving social communication among members. *See also* allergy and immunology.

Pan-American Association of Ophthalmology (PAAO) An international organization founded in 1939 composed of 8,000 ophthalmologists throughout the Western Hemisphere who are interested in improving the treatment of eye disease and prevention of blindness in the Americas through the exchange of ideas and treatments. *See also* ophthalmology.

Pan American Health Organization (PAHO) An international organization founded in 1902 composed of 38 governments of Western Hemisphere nations concerned with improving physical and mental health in the Americas. It coordinates regional activities combatting disease, including exchange of statistical and epidemiological information, development of local health services, and organization of disease control and eradication programs. *See also* World Health Organization.

Pan American League Against Rheumatism (PANLAR) An international organization founded in 1942 composed of 5,500 physicians and other professionals interested in the prevention and treatment of rheumatic diseases. It conducts biomedical and epidemiological research, offers assistance in the coordination of national, professional, and social agencies, and seeks to educate health professionals. *See also* rheumatism; rheumatology.

Pan American Medical Association (PAMA) An international organization founded in 1925 composed of 6,000 physicians and other individuals interested in fostering the exchange of medical information and research results among physicians in Western Hemisphere countries. It has a large number of allied sections (for example, alcoholism, fundamental sciences), specialty sections (for example, anesthesiology, pathology, psychiatry, transplantation of organs), and subspecialty sections (for example, vascular surgery). Also known as Associacion Medica Pan Americana. *See also* medical association.

pan, bed *See* bed pan.

pancreas A large, elongated digestive and endocrine gland lying behind the stomach, which secretes pancreatic juice for protein digestion into the duodenum and insulin, glucagon, and somato-

statin into the bloodstream. *See also* diabetes mellitus; endocrine; gland; glucagon; insulin; type I diabetes mellitus; type II diabetes mellitus.

Pancreatic Society, American *See* American Pancreatic Society.

pancreatitis Inflammation of the pancreas. *See also* inflammation; pancreas.

pandemic An epidemic of intercontinental or worldwide proportions, as in the malaria pandemic among early settlers until the introduction of quinine, or the pandemic fear that gripped Europe during Hitler's reign. *Compare* endemic; epidemic. *See also* epidemiology; influenza.

panel 1. A group of people gathered to plan or discuss an issue, judge a contest, or act as a team. *See also* arbitration panel; closed panel group practice; expert panel; open panel group practice. **2.** The list of persons who have been summoned for jury duty and from whom a jury may be chosen. *See also* impanel; screening panel.

panel, arbitration *See* arbitration panel.

panel, defense *See* screening panel.

panel, expert *See* expert panel.

panel, exploratory *See* screening panel.

panel group practice, closed *See* closed panel group practice.

panel group practice, open *See* open panel group practice.

panel practice, closed *See* closed panel group practice.

panel practice, open *See* open panel group practice.

panel, screening *See* screening panel.

panic Intense, overwhelming fear, producing terror, physiological changes, and often immobility or hysterical behavior, as in a panic disorder.

PANLAR *See* Pan American League Against Rheumatism.

Papanicolaou smear *See* Pap smear.

paper trail Documentary evidence of an individual's or group's actions. *See also* minutes.

paperwork Work involving the handling of reports, letters, and forms, as in burdensome paperwork.

Pap smear A test for cervical and uterine cancer developed by George Papanicolaou, a Greek anatomist in the United States (1883-1962). *Synonyms*: Papanicolaou smear; Pap test. *See also* gynecology.

parachute, golden *See* golden parachute.

Parachute Medical Rescue Service (PMRS) A

national organization founded in 1975 composed of 100 parachute volunteer teams of physicians, paramedics, and other specialists. It provides medical services and supplies in remote and otherwise inaccessible areas that have been devastated by hurricanes, earthquakes, or other natural disasters. It performs damage assessment and reporting and conducts periodic training assemblies to improve teamwork and individual qualifications. It holds annual parachute jump schools.

paradigm A model, example, or pattern that is effective in explaining or demonstrating a complex process, as in Pavlov's dogs were a paradigm of the conditioned-response theory. *See also* model; paradigm shift.

paradigm shift A time when the model, example, or pattern that underlies a science or discipline changes in such a fundamental way that the beliefs and behavior of the people involved in the science or discipline are changed. Many people feel that a major paradigm shift is currently underway in health care. *See also* paradigm; shift.

paraffin bath **1.** A form of physical therapy used by podiatrists and other professionals consisting of applying wet heat to a patient's feet by dipping them in melted wax. *See also* bath; physical therapy. **2.** The process of preparing tissues for microscopic examination by use of a microtome to slice the blocks of fixed tissue. *See also* microtome; pathology.

paragon A model of excellence or perfection of a kind, as in a paragon of virtue. *See also* model.

paralegal A person other than a licensed attorney who is employed, usually by a law office, to perform a variety of legal-assistance tasks, including document and exhibit preparation for trials and legal research using an on-line database, such as Lexis. *See also* attorney; law; paraprofession; trial.

parallel interface In computer science, the printer or other computer peripheral device connected to a computer in such a way as to simultaneously transmit all of the bits in a byte of information. This contrasts to a serial interface in which a printer or other peripheral device connected to a computer transmits the bits of a byte of information sequentially, or one after another. *See also* interface; serial interface.

parallel processing In computer science, the simultaneous performance of two or more tasks by a computer.

paralysis Loss or impairment of the ability to move

a body part, usually as a result of damage to its nerve supply. *See also* paraplegia.

paramedic A person who is certified by a state agency to perform advanced cardiac life support procedures and other emergency medical treatment under the direction of a physician. *See also* allied health professional; advanced cardiac life support; emergency medical technician-paramedic.

paramedical personnel Health professionals who are not physicians or nurses. Examples include medical technicians, aides, nutritionists, and physician assistants. The preferred term for these occupations is allied health professional. *See also* allied health professional; paraprofession; personnel.

Paramedic, Joint Review Committee on Educational Programs for the EMT- *See* Joint Review Committee on Educational Programs for the EMT-Paramedic.

Paramedics Association, National Flight *See* National Flight Paramedics Association.

parameter **1.** In mathematics, a constant in an equation or a model; in statistics and epidemiology, one of a set of measurable characteristics, such as temperature and pulse, of a group or population. **2.** In medicine, statements that delineate the ways in which it is acceptable for physicians and other health professionals to treat patients. *See also* boundary; estimate; limit; practice guideline; practice parameter.

parameter, practice *See* practice parameter.

parametric test A statistical test that depends on assumption(s) about the distribution of the data; for example, the assumption that the data will be normally vs bimodally distributed. *See also* data; distribution; probability distribution; statistics; test.

paranoia A mental disorder characterized by delusions of persecution (and, sometimes, of grandeur), which are often organized into an elaborate and logical system of thinking and often centered on a specific theme, such as job persecution. Suspiciousness, hostility, and resistance to therapy are often characteristic of a paranoic person. Paranoia is classically associated with schizophrenia but may also occur in depression, alcoholism, and senile dementia. *See also* alcoholism; depression; schizophrenia.

paranormal Beyond the range of normal experience or scientific explanation, as in telepathy is considered a paranormal experience and phenomenon. *See also* parapsychology.

Paranormal, Committee for the Scientific Investigation of Claims of the *See* Committee for the Scientific Investigation of Claims of the Paranormal.

paraophthalmic *See* ophthalmic technician; ophthalmic technologist.

paraoptometric *See* optometric assistant and technician.

paraplegia Paralysis of the lower half of the body including both legs, usually caused by damage to the spinal cord. *See also* paralysis; quadriplegia.

Paraplegia Society, American *See* American Paraplegia Society.

paraprofession Occupations requiring successful completion of a training program at or above the college level or its equivalent, typically lasting one to two years; the program resembles that of the profession's to which it corresponds, except that the paraprofessional program is shorter and more limited in content. Members of the occupation work under the direction and supervision of the professionals whose service capabilities they extend and to whom they are responsible. Paraprofessionals work in many fields, including law, medicine, library science, teaching, and social services. Examples of paraprofessionals in health care include physician assistants and dental hygienists. *See also* allied health professional; paralegal; profession.

paraprofessional *See* allied health professional.

Parapsychological Association (PA) A national organization founded in 1957 composed of 280 persons who hold a doctorate degree or its equivalent and other individuals who are actively engaged in advancing parapsychology as a branch of science. It encourages parapsychological research and disseminates information on scientific findings. It is affiliated with the American Association for the Advancement of Science. *See also* parapsychology.

Parapsychological Services Institute (PSI) A counseling, educational, and research center for individuals who are experiencing psychical or spiritual events (including dreams that foretell the future, visitations by deceased persons, poltergeist manifestations, and hauntings) or who wish to explore the meaning and transformative value such experiences may have on their lives. *See also* parapsychology.

parapsychology The study of extrasensory perception and allied phenomena (for example, clairvoyance and telepathy) that appear to transcend natural laws. *See also* clairvoyance; sixth sense; telepathy.

Parapsychology, American Association for *See* American Association for Parapsychology.

parasite **1.** An organism living in or on another and obtaining food from it. A parasite may or may not harm its host, but confers no benefit upon it. Parasites of humans include bacteria, viruses, fungi, and protozoa. *See also* body louse; head louse; parasitology; pediculosis; scabies; virus; worm. **2.** One who habitually takes advantage of the generosity of other people without making any useful return.

Parasitologists, American Society of *See* American Society of Parasitologists.

parasitology The scientific discipline dealing with the study of parasites. *See also* helminth; parasite; protozoa.

paregoric An opium derivative used to treat diarrhea and to relieve pain. Its adverse effects include constipation. *See also* opium.

parens patriae The power of the government to protect an individual for his or her own good.

parent **1.** A father or mother of a child. The advent of noncoital reproduction has made distinction among genetic parents, gestational mother, and rearing parents important. *See also* genetic parent; gestational parent; noncoital reproduction; rearing parent. **2.** To act as a parent, to raise and nurture, as in adolescent parenting. **3.** Pertaining to parenting, as in parent company. *See also* parent company.

parent company A company that owns or controls subsidiaries through the ownership of voting stock. A parent company is often an operating company in its own right. A parent company that has no business of its own is often called a holding company. *See also* company; holding company.

parenteral Not through the alimentary tract, but rather by injection through another route, such as subcutaneous, intramuscular, intraorbital, intracapsular, intraspinal, intrasternal, and intravenous. *See also* alimentary tract; intramuscular; intravenous; subcutaneous.

parenteral alimentation, total *See* total parenteral nutrition.

Parenteral Drug Association (PDA) A national association founded in 1946 composed of 3,500 individuals working in the research, development, or manufacture of parenteral (injectable) drugs and sterile products. It serves as a liaison with pharmaceutical manufacturers, suppliers, users, academics, and government regulatory officials. *See also* drug; parenteral.

Parenteral and Enteral Nutrition, American Society for *See* American Society for Parenteral and Enteral Nutrition.

parenteral nutrition The intravenous (directly into the bloodstream) administration (via tubing) of nutrient fluids, amino acids, carbohydrates, fats, vitamins, and/or minerals. *See also* nutrition; parenteral; total parenteral nutrition.

parenteral nutrition, total *See* total parenteral nutrition.

parenteral nutrition and infusion therapy services, enteral and *See* enteral and parenteral nutrition and infusion therapy services.

parenteral product A sterile pharmaceutical preparation taken into the body through a route other than the alimentary canal. *See also* parenteral; product.

parent, genetic *See* genetic parent.

parent, gestational *See* gestational parent.

Parenthood Federation of America, Planned *See* Planned Parenthood Federation of America.

Parenting Fitness, Positive Pregnancy and *See* Positive Pregnancy and Parenting Fitness.

Parenting, National Association of Adolescent Pregnancy and *See* National Association of Adolescent Pregnancy and Parenting.

parent, rearing *See* rearing parent.

Pareto analysis The application of the principle of determining which few steps in a process are vital or most important and taking action to alter or reinforce these steps rather than the many other incidental steps in the process. *See also* analysis; Pareto, Vilfredo; useful many; vital few.

Pareto chart A special form of vertical bar graph that displays information in such a way that priorities for process improvement can be established. It displays the relative importance of all the data and is used to direct efforts to the largest improvement opportunity by highlighting the vital few in contrast to the many others. *See also* chart; check sheet; Pareto analysis; Pareto, Vilfredo.

Pareto principle A principle that is employed to identify the "vital few" (for example, customers, customer needs, product features, process features, or inputs) to help direct resources and attention to areas where they do the most good. For example, the Pareto principle states that a *few* contributors to the cost of poor quality are responsible for *the bulk* of the cost. These vital few contributors need to be identified so that improvement resources can be concentrated in the few contributors. *See also* awkward zone; Pareto analysis; Pareto chart; Pareto, Vilfredo.

Pareto, Vilfredo An Italian economist and sociologist (1848-1923) after whom the Pareto principle is named. *See also* Pareto analysis; Pareto chart; Pareto principle.

parity **1.** The condition of having given birth to children. **2.** In obstetrics, the classification of women by their number of live-born children and stillbirths delivered at more than 28 weeks of gestation; or the total number of times a woman has been pregnant minus the number of abortions and/or miscarriages occurring up to 28 weeks of gestation. A para 4 (P4) gravida 5 (G5) means four deliveries after 28 weeks and one abortion or miscarriage before 28 weeks. **3.** In computer science, the characteristic of a number being odd or even. When groups of bits (1's and 0's) are being transmitted or stored by a computer, an extra bit is often added so that the total number of 1's is always odd (or, alternatively, always even). This is called *parity of the data*. *See also* bit; byte; parity check.

parity check A test performed by checking a unit of data for even or odd parity to determine whether a mistake has taken place in reading, writing, or transmitting information. For example, if data are written, the computed parity bit is compared to the parity bit already appended to the data. If these match, it indicates that the data are correct. If they do not agree, a *parity error* exists. *See also* parity.

parity of data *See* parity.

parity error *See* parity check.

Parkinson's disease A progressive neurological disorder characterized by resting tremors, shuffling gait, stooped posture, rolling motions of the fingers, and muscle weakness and rigidity. Named after the English physician James Parkinson (1755-1824). *Synonym*: parkinsonism. *See also* dementia.

Parkinson's Law Any of several satirical observations propounded as economic laws, especially "Work expands to fill the time allotted to it." Named after Cyril Northcote Parkinson, a British historian born in 1909, noted for his humorous works that ridicule the inefficiency of bureaucracies.

Park Ridge Center (PRC) An organization founded in 1985 composed of 2,000 physicians and other health professionals, theologians, ethicists, clergy, and pastoral counselors interested in the interreligious, multidisciplinary study of health, faith, and ethics. *See also* ethics; Lutheran General Health Care System.

parliamentary procedure Formal procedure followed in the conduct of any meeting, usually following Roberts' Rules of Order. Parliamentary procedure is followed to expedite the orderly conduct of a meeting's agenda. *See also* agenda; meeting; meeting process.

paronychia Infection of the tissue around the nails. *Synonym*: whitlow. *See also* hangnail.

paroxysm A sudden, but temporary, violent attack; for example, a paroxysm of coughing.

parsimony Adoption of the simplest assumption in the formulation of a theory or in the interpretation of data, especially in accordance with the rule of Ockham's razor. *See* Ockham's razor.

parsimony, law of *See* Ockham's razor.

parsimony, scientific *See* Ockham's razor.

Part A, Medicare *See* Medicare, Part A.

Part B, Medicare *See* Medicare, Part B.

partial Being or affecting only a part, as in partial disability.

partial care program Mental health services provided to individuals who spend only part of a 24-hour period in a facility. These mental health services are provided in an environment that is more structured than that of an outpatient program, but less structured than that of either a residential treatment program or an inpatient treatment program. *See also* mental health services; residential care facility.

partial compliance *See* compliance level.

partial disability An illness or injury that prevents a person from performing one or more functions of his or her occupation or profession. *See also* disability.

partial hospitalization Formal programs of care in a hospital or other health care organization for periods of less than 24 hours a day, typically involving services usually provided to inpatients. There are two principal types: *night hospitalization*, for patients who need hospitalization but can work or attend school outside the hospital during the day, and *day hospitalization*, for people who require in-hospital diagnostic or treatment services but can safely spend nights and weekends at home. *See also* day bed; hospitalization; night bed; partial hospitalization ser-

vices; weekend hospitalization.

Partial Hospitalization, American Association for *See* American Association for Partial Hospitalization.

partial hospitalization services Psychiatric treatment and/or the treatment of alcohol and other drug dependencies for patients not in an acute phase of illness requiring 24 hour inpatient care. *See also* alcoholism and other drug dependence; partial care program; partial hospitalization; psychiatry.

partial hysterectomy A hysterectomy in which the cervix is left in place. *Synonyms*: subtotal hysterectomy; supracervical hysterectomy; supravaginal hysterectomy. *See also* hysterectomy.

participate To take part or share in something. *See also* participation.

participating *See* participation.

participating insurance An insurance policy that pays a dividend to its owner. *See also* insurance; participating policy.

participating physician Under Medicare, a physician who has signed a contract agreeing to refrain from charging a Medicare patient the difference between the physician's usual charge and Medicare payment allowance. *Compare* nonparticipating provider. *See also* Medicare; participation; physician.

participating plan A Blue Cross and Blue Shield plan that agrees to process national account claims in its jurisdiction on behalf of another plan that serves as the control plan for that national account. *See also* Blue Cross plan; Blue Shield plan; control plan.

participating policy Insurance coverage under which the insured receives dividends on company earnings that may be applied to reduce the amount of premium that must be paid by the insured. *See also* participating insurance.

participating provider *See* participation.

participation The act of taking part or sharing in something, as in a physician participates in an insurance plan when he or she agrees to accept the plan's preestablished fee or reasonable charge as the maximum amount that can be collected for services rendered. A nonparticipating physician may charge more than the insurance program's maximum allowable amount for a particular service. The patient is then liable for the excess above the allowed amount. This system was developed in the private sector as a method of providing the insured with specific health care services at no out-of-pocket costs. Participation is used more loosely in Medicare and Medicaid to mean any physician who accepts reimbursement from either program. Any physician accepting Medicaid payments must accept them as payment in full. A hospital or other health program is called a *participating provider* when it meets the various requirements of, and accepts reimbursement from, a public or private health insurance program. *See also* conditions of participation; Medicaid; Medicare; patient participation; penetration.

Participation, Association for Quality and *See* Association for Quality and Participation.

participation, conditions of *See* conditions of participation.

participation, patient *See* patient participation.

participative leadership Consultative management method that encourages other individuals to participate. Leadership decisions are achieved as the end result of group participation. *See also* leadership.

particle A minute mass of matter, such as a proton or electron.

parting shot An act of aggression or retaliation, such as a threat, that is made upon one's departure or at the end of a heated argument.

partisan Devoted to a cause, person, group, or idea, as in partisan politics.

partner An individual who is associated with another or other persons in an organization, activity, or endeavor. *See also* general partner; junior partner; limited partner; partnership; silent partner.

partner, general *See* general partner.

partner, junior *See* junior partner.

partner, limited *See* limited partner.

partners *See* governing body.

partnership A legal relationship between two or more competent persons (parties) who have contracted to place their money, effects, and labor in commerce or business with a proportionate sharing of profits and losses. *Compare* joint venture; limited partnership. *See also* partner.

partnership, brokered *See* brokered partnership.

partnership, limited *See* limited partnership.

partner, silent *See* silent partner.

part-time For less than the customary time, as in a part-time employee. Part-time employees usually do not receive the same health insurance, retirement, and other benefits full-time employees receive. *Compare* full-time. *See also* employment; job sharing.

part-time worker According to the Bureau of Labor Statistics, a person employed less than 35 hours per week. *Compare* full-time worker.

parturient Pertaining to giving birth. *See also* parturition.

parturition The process of childbirth. *See also* delivery; labor.

party payer, third- *See* third-party payer.

party, responsible *See* responsible party.

PAS *See* Professional Activity Study.

PASG Abbreviation for pneumatic antishock garment. *See* MAST.

passive Not active; not initiated by the self, as in passive exercise or passive immunity.

passive aggressive personality disorder A personality disorder characterized by an indirect resistance to demands for adequate social and occupational performance; anger and opposition to authority and the expectations of other people that is expressed covertly by obstructionism, procrastination, stubbornness, dawdling, forgetfulness, and intentional inefficiency. *See also* passive; personality disorder.

passive euthanasia Allowing death to occur by withholding or withdrawing treatment from a patient who is hopelessly ill. *Synonym:* "letting die." *Compare* active euthanasia. *See also* euthanasia.

passive exercise A therapeutic exercise in which movement is provided by a therapist or a machine instead of the patient. *See also* physical therapy.

passive immunization The conferring of specific immune reactivity on previously nonimmune individuals by the administration of sensitized lymphoid cells or serum from immune individuals, as in administering hepatitis B immunoglobulin. *Compare* active immunization. *See also* immunization.

passive negligence *See* vicarious liability.

passive smoking *See* involuntary smoking.

pass-through cost A hospital cost, such as undergraduate and graduate medical education, which is not incorporated in diagnosis-related group (DRG) prices. Medicare funds are provided to the hospital directly, that is, the costs are "passed through" (around) the DRG mechanism. *See also* cost; diagnosis-related groups; Medicare.

password In computer science, a sequence of characters required to gain access to a computer system. *See also* computer; log on.

paste A semiliquid medicinal preparation intended for external application. Pastes usually contain a high proportion of finely powdered solids, such as starch and zinc oxide, and are fairly stiff. They are used for circumscribed skin lesions, such as those that may occur in psoriasis. *See also* ointment.

pasteurization Process of heating milk and other fluids (to temperatures of 140° F or 60° C) for a specified time (for example, 60 minutes) to destroy or retard the development of disease-transmitting microorganisms, especially bacteria. *See also* microorganism; raw milk.

pastor A Christian minister or priest or layperson having spiritual charge over a person or a congregation or other group. *See also* pastoral.

pastoral Pertaining to the duties of a pastor, as in pastoral counseling for hospitalized patients. *See also* chaplaincy service.

pastoral care *See* chaplaincy service.

Pastoral Counseling, American Board of Examiners in *See* American Board of Examiners in Pastoral Counseling.

pastoral counseling department *See* chaplaincy service.

pastoral counselor, clinical *See* clinical pastoral counselor.

Pastoral Counselors, American Association of *See* American Association of Pastoral Counselors.

Pastoral Education, Association for Clinical *See* Association for Clinical Pastoral Education.

Pastoral Research, Commission on *See* Commission on Pastoral Research.

PATA *See* Professional Aeromedical Transport Association.

patch, nicotine *See* nicotine patch.

patent medicine *See* over-the-counter drug.

paternalism 1. A policy or practice of treating or governing people in a fatherly manner, especially by providing for their needs without giving them rights or responsibilities. *See also* beneficence. 2. In organizational management, the setting of limits on individual autonomy in an effort to benefit, or prevent harm to, the person whose autonomy is limited. The term is sometimes used pejoratively in the sense that management assumes inferior status for employees. Paternalistic behavior may be ethically justifiable if a person has some defect or encumbrance in understanding or deciding, if serious harm is likely unless there is intervention, and if the probable benefit from the intervention will outweigh the probable harm of nonintervention. *See also* autonomy.

paternity The state of being a father. *Compare* maternity.

paternity leave The leave of absence from work granted to a father to care for his infant. *See also* maternity leave.

paternity test A comparison of blood types among mother, child, and a man suspected of fathering the child in an effort to determine the father. If the child's blood group could not have resulted from the combination of the man's blood group with that of the woman, then the man is definitely not the father of the child. However, other results are not conclusive, since a finding that the man could be the father does not prove that he is the father. Thus, blood group analysis is used to disprove putative paternity; it cannot prove paternity. *See also* blood groups; hematology; paternity; test.

path A course of action or conduct, as in critical pathway. *See also* clinical pathway; critical pathway.

path, clinical *See* clinical pathway.

pathogen Any agent capable of producing disease, especially a living microorganism, such as a bacterium or fungus. *See also* disease; microorganism; pathogenesis; pathogenicity.

pathogenesis The mechanisms by which an etiologic agent, such as a microorganism, produces disease. *See also* disease; etiology; microorganism; pathogen.

pathogenic Producing disease, as in pathogenic bacteria. *See also* disease; pathogen; pathogenicity.

pathogenicity 1. The property of an agent, such as a microorganism or a toxic chemical, that determines the degree to which overt disease is produced in an infected or affected population. 2. The power of an agent to produce disease. *See also* disease; pathogen; virulence.

pathognomonic Describing a sign or symptom that is specific to or characteristic of a particular disease; for example, Koplik's spots are pathognomonic of measles. *See also* disease; sign; symptom.

pathologic stage classification system, American Joint Committee on Cancer *See* American Joint Committee on Cancer pathologic stage classification system.

pathologist A physician who specializes in pathology. *See also* pathology.

pathologist, anatomical *See* anatomical pathologist.

pathologist, blood banking *See* blood banking specialist.

pathologist, chemical *See* chemical pathologist.

pathologist, clinical *See* clinical pathologist.

pathologist, forensic *See* forensic pathologist.

pathologist, immuno- *See* immunopathologist.

pathologist, oral *See* oral pathologist.

pathologist, pediatric *See* pediatric pathologist.

Pathologists, American Association of *See* American Association of Pathologists.

Pathologists, American Association of Neuro- *See* American Association of Neuropathologists.

Pathologists, American Osteopathic College of *See* American Osteopathic College of Pathologists.

Pathologists, American Society of Clinical *See* American Society of Clinical Pathologists.

pathologist's assistant An individual who assists a pathologist in the preparation, dissection, and completion of work with autopsy and operating room specimens. *See also* autopsy; pathologist; prosector.

Pathologists' Assistants, American Association of *See* American Association of Pathologists' Assistants.

Pathologists, College of American *See* College of American Pathologists.

Pathologists, Society of Toxicologic *See* Society of Toxicologic Pathologists.

pathologist, speech *See* speech pathologist.

pathology The branch and specialty of medicine dealing with the essential nature of disease, especially the structural and functional changes in tissues and organs of the body that cause or are caused by disease. These changes are detected by means of information gathered from the microscopic examination of tissue specimens, cells, and body fluids and from clinical laboratory tests on body fluids and secretions. Ten subspecialties of pathology are blood banking, chemical pathology, cytopathology, dermatopathology, forensic pathology, hematology, immunopathology, medical microbiology, neuropathology, and pediatric pathology. *See also* blood banking; chemical pathology; cytopathology; dermatopathology; forensic pathology; hematology; immunopathology; medical microbiology; neuropathology; pediatric pathology.

Pathology, American Academy of Oral *See* American Academy of Oral Pathology.

Pathology, American Board of *See* American Board of Pathology.

Pathology, American Board of Oral *See* American Board of Oral Pathology.

Pathology, American Registry of *See* American Registry of Pathology.

Pathology, American Society for Colposcopy and Cervical *See* American Society for Colposcopy and Cervical Pathology.

Pathology, American Society for Dermato- *See* American Society for Dermatopathology.

Pathology, Armed Forces Institute of *See* Armed Forces Institute of Pathology.

Pathology and Audiology, Council on Professional Standards in Speech-Language *See* Council on Professional Standards in Speech-Language Pathology and Audiology.

Pathology Chairmen, Association of *See* Association of Pathology Chairmen.

pathology, chemical *See* chemical pathology.

pathology, clinical *See* clinical pathology.

pathology and clinical laboratory services Services of a health care organization that provide information on diagnosis, prevention, or treatment of disease through the examination of the structural and functional changes in tissues and organs of the body that cause or are caused by disease. *See also* clinical laboratory; disease; pathology.

Pathology and Clinical Laboratory Services, Accreditation Manual for *See Accreditation Manual for Pathology and Clinical Laboratory Services.*

Pathology, Department of Environmental and Toxicologic *See* Department of Environmental and Toxicologic Pathology.

pathology, forensic *See* forensic pathology.

Pathology Foundation, American *See* American Pathology Foundation.

pathology, immuno- *See* immunopathology.

Pathology Information, Intersociety Committee on *See* Intersociety Committee on Pathology Information.

Pathology, Institute for Gravitational Strain *See* Institute for Gravitational Strain Pathology.

pathology, oral *See* oral pathology.

pathology, paleo- *See* paleopathology.

pathology, pediatric *See* pediatric pathology.

Pathology Practice Association (PPA) A national organization founded in 1980 composed of 500 pathologists interested in having their views represented on legislative issues. *See also* pathology.

Pathology Society, Gastrointestinal *See* Gastrointestinal Pathology Society.

Pathology, Society for Hemato- *See* Society for Hematopathology.

pathology, speech *See* speech pathology.

Pathology, Universities Associated for Research and Education in *See* Universities Associated for Research and Education in Pathology.

pathophysiology The physiology of disordered function. *See also* physiology.

pathway, clinical *See* clinical pathway.

pathway, critical *See* critical pathway.

pathway, fifth *See* fifth pathway.

pathway method, critical *See* critical pathway method.

patient **1.** A person who receives health services from a health care provider and who gives consent for the provider to provide those services. Persons receiving mental health services provided by health care personnel other than psychiatrists are often called *clients*, but physicians and many allied health professionals typically treat *patients*. *See also* client; health care provider; health services; inpatient; outpatient; patient-centered; patient-centered care; patient-centered standards. **2.** Bearing or enduring pain, difficulty, provocation, or annoyance with calmness.

patient abandonment Improper withdrawal from the care of a patient after the creation of a physician-patient relationship. Generally, a duty of care continues until a physician's services are no longer required; there is a mutual consent to termination; the patient dismisses the physician; or the physician elects to discontinue care. To avoid abandonment, the physician should provide adequate notice and an adequate opportunity for a patient to obtain substitute care. *See also* abandonment; patient.

patient account manager An individual who manages personnel engaged in credit and collection functions for hospitals, clinics, and other health care organizations. *See also* American Guild of Patient Account Management; certified patient account manager.

patient account manager, certified *See* certified patient account manager.

patient advocate *See* patient representative.

patient assessment The systematic collection and analysis of patient-specific data necessary to determine patient care and treatment needs. *See also* assessment; needs assessment; patient.

patient-based factor *See* patient factor.

patient bill of rights *See* bill of patient rights.

patient care audit A retrospective review of selected hospital medical records, performed by a multi-disciplinary professional committee for the purpose of comparing the quality of care provided with accepted standards. *See also* audit; dental audit; medical audit; nursing audit.

patient care committee A hospital committee composed of medical, nursing, and other professional staff members whose purpose is to monitor patient care practices to increase the probability that predetermined standards are met. *See also* patient care audit.

patient care continuity *See* continuity of care.

patient care coordinator *See* nurse coordinator.

patient care function, invisible *See* invisible patient care function.

patient care function, visible *See* visible patient care function.

patient care plan *See* care plan.

patient care plan, interdisciplinary *See* interdisciplinary patient care plan.

patient care, progressive *See* progressive patient care.

patient care unit *See* inpatient care unit.

patient-centered **1.** Organized around what is done with, for, or to a patient. **2.** Adopting a patient's perspective. *See also* patient; patient-centered care; patient-centered standards.

patient-centered care An approach to care that consciously adopts a patient's perspective; this perspective can be characterized around dimensions, such as respect for patient's values, preferences, and expressed needs; coordination and integration of care; information, communication, and education; physical comfort; emotional support and alleviation of fear and anxiety; involvement of family and friends; and transition and continuity. *See also* patient; patient-centered; patient-centered standards.

patient-centered standards Standards that are organized around what is done with, for, or to patients, such as assessment, treatment, and education. *See also* patient; patient-centered; patient-centered care; standard.

patient chart *See* medical record.

patient, clinic *See* clinic patient.

patient collection Pertaining to methods of obtaining payment of overdue accounts receivable and bad debts in individual patient accounts. *See also* collection agency.

patient compensation fund A fund established by state law, most commonly financed by a surcharge on malpractice premiums of all professional liability policyholders in a state and used to pay malpractice claims. *See also* malpractice; professional liability insurance.

patient complaint **1.** An expression of dissatisfaction issued by a patient. **2.** A system for identifying adverse patient occurrences (APOs) through information from dissatisfied patients and/or representatives of these patients. *See also* adverse patient outcomes; occurrence screening.

patient compliance *See* compliance.

patient consent *See* informed consent.

patient days A measure of institutional use, usually measured as the number of inpatients at a specified time (for example, at midnight). *See also* occupancy rate.

patient discharge Formal release or dismissal of a patient from a health care organization or program. *See also* discharge; dismissal; disposition.

patient dropout *See* against medical advice.

patient dumping The denial or limitation of the provision of medical care to, or the transfer to other institutions of, patients who are not able to pay or for whom payment methods do not pay the hospital enough to cover its costs. The Consolidated Omnibus Budget Reconciliation Act (COBRA) of 1985 was passed in 1986 to protect patients against dumping because of suspicion that hospitals with emergency services were limiting access to conserve money. *See also* Consolidated Omnibus Budget Reconciliation Act; transfer agreement.

patient education Teaching and learning directed toward increasing a patient's ability to manage personal health, as in patient education for newly diagnosed diabetics. *See also* health education.

patient education department A department in a health care organization providing patients and their families with instructions relating to health maintenance and the management of illness and disability. *See also* patient education.

patient, emergency *See* emergency patient.

patient empowerment *See* shared decision making.

patient escort service A service often provided by hospital volunteers to accompany patients who need help in moving about a hospital. *See also* service.

patient, established *See* established patient.

patient factor An individual patient-related variable that may influence performance data; includes severity of illness (factors related to the degree or stage of disease before treatment), comorbid conditions (disease factors, not intrinsic to the primary disease, which may have an impact on patient suitability for, or tolerance of, diagnostic or therapeutic care), and nondisease factors (such as female or male sex and refusal of consent). Patient factors usually are not within practitioners' or organizations' control. *Synonym:* patient-based factor. *See also* external environmental factor; factor; nondisease factors; organization factor; practitioner factor.

patient health outcome The result that happens to a patient from performance (or nonperformance) of one or more processes, services, or activities carried out by health care providers. A patient health outcome represents the cumulative effect of one or more processes at a defined time, as in survival to discharge following a gunshot wound to the chest or an acute myocardial infarction. *Synonym:* outcome of care. *See also* efficiency; outcome; quality of care.

patient history *See* medical history.

patient identification system An organized procedure for establishing accurate and complete patient identity. *See also* system.

patient, in- *See* inpatient.

Patient Information and Education, National Council on *See* National Council on Patient Information and Education.

patient isolation *See* isolation.

patient medical record *See* medical record.

patient mix The numbers and types of patients served by a hospital or other health care organization or program. Patients may be classified according to socioeconomic characteristics, diagnoses, or severity of illness. Knowledge of an organization's patient mix is important for planning and comparison. *See also* case mix; scope of services.

patient, new *See* new patient.

patient occurrence, adverse *See* adverse patient occurrence.

patient origin study A study to determine the geographic distribution of the homes of patients served by hospitals or health programs, used to define catchment areas and to plan the development of health services and facilities. *See also* catchment area.

patient, out- *See* outpatient.

patient participation Patient involvement in the decision-making process in matters pertaining to his or her health. *See also* informed consent; participation; respect and caring.

patient perspectives on care *See* respect and caring.

patient-physician relationship A relationship initiated and sustained by a patient who has legal and moral authority over the relationship. An agreement is established in a relationship in which the physician will respond to the patient's preferences and the patient will accept the physician's recommendations. *Synonym:* doctor-patient relationship. *See also* patient; physician.

patient, private *See* private patient.

patient profile A list of all health care services provided to a particular patient during a specified period of time, for example, during a hospitalization. *See also* patient; profile; profiling.

patient record *See* medical record.

patient record, computer-based *See* computer-based patient record.

Patient Record Institute, Computer-Based *See* Computer-Based Patient Record Institute.

patient record system, computer-based *See* computer-based patient record system.

Patient Representation and Consumer Affairs of the American Hospital Association, National Society of *See* National Society of Patient Representation and Consumer Affairs of the American Hospital Association.

patient representative A person who investigates and mediates patients' problems and complaints in relation to a hospital's (or other type of health care organization's) services. *Synonyms*: ombudsman; ombudsperson; patient advocate. *See also* ombudsperson.

patient right, confidentiality as a *See* confidentiality as a patient right.

patient rights Liberties and privileges that individuals retain during their status as patients, to the extent permitted by law. *See also* bill of patient rights; confidentiality as a patient right; patient's right of autonomy.

patients' assessments *See* patients' ratings; patients' reports.

patient's chart *See* medical record.

patients' compensation *See* patient compensation fund.

Patient Self-Determination Act (PSDA) Legislation signed by President George Bush in 1990 stating that hospitals, skilled nursing facilities, hospices, home health care agencies, and health maintenance organizations are responsible for developing patient information for distribution. The information must include patients' rights, advance directives (living wills), ethics committees' consultation and education functions, limited medical treatment (supportive/comfort care only), mental health treatment, resuscitation, restraints, surrogate decision making, and transfer of care. The purpose of the act is to assure that individuals receiving health care services will be given an opportunity to participate in and direct health care decisions affecting themselves. *See also* advance directives; durable power of attorney for health care; living will.

patient, self-pay *See* self-pay patient.

patient, self-responsible *See* self-pay patient.

patient service representative An individual trained to complete health insurance claim forms and to assist health care providers, such as physicians and hospitals, in collecting payments for services from patients and insurers. *See also* health insurance.

patient's family The person(s) who plays a meaningful role in a patient's life. This definition includes an individual(s) who may or may not be legally related to the patient. *See also* family; patient.

patient's medical record *See* medical record.

patients' ratings Personal evaluations of aspects of health care providers and services. Ratings are inherently subjective because they reflect personal experiences, expectations, and preferences, as well as the standards patients apply when evaluating the care they have received. *See also* patients' reports.

patients' reports Information from patients about things that did or did not happen during their health care. Patients' reports are inherently more objective than patients' ratings and can be more readily confirmed by an outside observer. *See also* patients' ratings.

patient's record *See* medical record.

patient's right of autonomy The patient's right to determine what shall be done with his or her own body. A patient, for example, has a right to refuse treatment by withholding consent. A physician or other health professional may believe that an operation or other form of treatment is desirable or necessary, but the law does not permit the physician or other health professional to substitute his or her own judgment for that of the patient by any form of artifice or deception except as ordered by the court (for example, if a fetus is threatened by its mother's refusal of treatment). *See also* autonomy; consent;

informed consent; patient rights.

Patients, The Information Exchange on Young Adult Chronic *See* The Information Exchange on Young Adult Chronic Patients.

patient transfer *See* intrahospital transfer; transfer.

patient treatment plan *See* care plan.

patient, ward *See* ward patient.

patriarchy A social system in which the father is the head of the family and descent is traced through the father's side of the family. *Compare* matriarchy.

patricide The killing of one's father. *Compare* matricide. *See also* murder.

pattern A particular design or arrangement of natural or accidental origin, as in a pattern in the data was readily identified. *See also* data pattern; practice pattern analysis; trend; data trend.

pattern analysis, practice *See* practice pattern analysis.

pattern of care The distribution of rates of performance among members of a group of practitioners, health care organizations, or communities. *See also* pattern; performance.

pattern, data *See* data pattern.

pattern monitoring, admission *See* admission pattern monitoring.

pauper An individual who is destitute and dependent on other persons for support.

Pavlov, Ivan A Russian physiologist (1849-1936) who is best known for describing the conditioned response. *See also* conditioned reflex; conditioning.

pavor nocturnus *See* night terrors.

pawn A person or organization at the mercy of another's will.

pay Compensation to personnel for services performed. *See also* overpay; payer; payment; severance pay; third-party payer.

payback period The time necessary for a new item of equipment to produce revenues or result in savings equal to its cost.

payer An organization (such as the federal government or a commercial insurance company) or a person who furnishes the money to pay for the provision of health care services. *See also* all-payer system; primary payer; single-payer system; third-party payer.

payer, Medicare secondary *See* Medicare secondary payer.

payer, primary *See* primary payer.

payer system, all- *See* all-payer system.

payer system, single- *See* single-payer system.

payer, third-party *See* third-party payer.

payment An amount paid, as in full payment for services rendered. *See also* cost-based payment; prospective payment; prospective payment system; third-party payment; unified payment.

Payment Assessment Commission, Prospective *See* Prospective Payment Assessment Commission.

payment, cost-based *See* cost-based reimbursement.

payment, fee-for-service *See* fee for service.

payment, prospective *See* prospective payment.

Payment Reform, Physician *See* Physician Payment Reform (OBRA '89).

payment, retroactive *See* retrospective reimbursement.

payments, out-of-pocket *See* out-of-pocket payments.

payment system, prospective *See* prospective payment system.

payment, third-party *See* third-party payment.

payment, unified *See* unified payment.

pay, over- *See* overpay.

pay plan, incentive *See* incentive pay plan.

pay or play A proposal for restructuring the health care system in the United States so that all employers would be required to either provide health insurance for their workers or pay a tax to finance a government plan to cover them and everyone else. *See also* employer; health insurance.

payroll deduction A specified amount taken out of a person's pay to finance a benefit. Payroll deductions may be either a set payroll tax, as the social security tax, or a required payment for a benefit, for example, a group health insurance premium or pension contributions. *See also* deduction; payroll tax.

payroll premium *See* payroll tax.

payroll tax A tax levied on wages and salaries, such as for social security and unemployment insurance. A government requirement that an employer pay a set portion of the premium on group health insurance benefits for his or her employees is a payroll tax on the employer. *Synonym*: payroll premium. *See also* payroll deduction; tax; unemployment insurance.

pay, severance *See* severance pay.

pay, take-home *See* take-home pay.

pay, under- *See* underpay.

PC *See* personal computer; professional corporation.

PCB 1. Polychlorinated biphenyl, any of a number

of chemical compounds that are obtained by adding chlorine atoms to biphenyl, which cause persistent environmental pollution. *See also* pollution. **2.** Abbreviation for printed circuit board, a flat sheet carrying the printed circuits and microchips in a microcomputer or other microelectronic device. *See also* microchip; microcomputer.

PC clone A computer copy of International Business Machines' (IBM's) personal computer (PC) first marketed in 1982. *Synonyms*: IBM compatible; IBM look-alike. *See also* clone; personal computer.

PC compatibility In computer science, compatible with an IBM personal computer, that is, able to run the same computer software. There are many levels of compatibility. *See also* computer software; personal computer.

PCE *See* potentially compensable event.

PCHRG *See* Public Citizen Health Research Group.

PCLG *See* Public Citizen Litigation Group.

PCP **1.** Abbreviation for phencyclidine hydrochloride, an illegal drug taken for its hallucinogenic effects. The drug was introduced as an anesthetic in the late 1950s but was soon limited therapeutically to veterinary use. PCP has over 150 street names, such as angel dust. **2.** Abbreviation for *Pneumocystis carinii* pneumonia. *See Pneumocystis.*

PCRM *See* Physicians Committee for Responsible Medicine.

PCRS *See* Precision Chiropractic Research Society.

PDA *See* Parenteral Drug Association.

PDCA cycle *See* Plan-Do-Check-Act cycle.

PDR *See Physicians' Desk Reference.*

PDR for Nonprescription Drugs A compendium of information on over-the-counter drugs, published annually by Medical Economics Data. *See also* over-the-counter drug; *Physicians' Desk Reference.*

PE *See* probable error.

peak flow meter A portable instrument used by and for people with asthma to monitor small changes in breathing capacity. *See also* asthma; spirometer.

pecking order **1.** A hierarchy among a group of people, classes, or nations. **2.** The social hierarchy in a flock of domestic fowl, such as chickens, in which each bird pecks subordinate birds and submits to being pecked by dominant birds.

pedal Pertaining to the foot, as in pedal pulses. *See also* pedal illness.

pedal illness In podiatry, foot ailments. *See also*

podiatric medicine.

pederast A man who has a sexual relationship with a boy. *See also* pederasty.

pederasty Homosexual anal intercourse, especially that between a man and a young boy who is the passive partner. *See also* homosexuality; pederast; pedophilia; sexual intercourse.

Pediatric AIDS Coalition (PAC) An organization of child advocacy and health groups interested in advancing AIDS research, treatment, and education. It seeks financial assistance from government and private sources. *See also* acquired immunodeficiency syndrome; pediatrics.

Pediatric Association, Ambulatory *See* Ambulatory Pediatric Association.

pediatric basic life support *See* basic life support.

pediatric cardiologist A pediatrician who specializes in pediatric cardiology. *See also* pediatric cardiology.

pediatric cardiology The branch of medicine and subspecialty of pediatrics dealing with the heart and blood vessels and the assessment of cardiovascular disease in children from fetal life to young adulthood. *See also* cardiology; pediatrics.

pediatric critical care medicine The branch of medicine and subspecialty of pediatrics dealing with all aspects of the management of critically ill pediatric patients in the intensive care unit setting. *See also* pediatric critical care specialist; pediatric intensive care unit; pediatrics.

pediatric critical care specialist A pediatrician who subspecializes in pediatric critical care medicine. *See also* critical care physician; pediatric critical care medicine; pediatric intensive care unit.

pediatric dentist A dentist specializing in pediatric dentistry. *Synonym:* pedodontist. *See also* pediatric dentistry.

pediatric dentistry A dental specialty dealing with the diagnosis and treatment of children, adolescents, and young adults whose dental development is not complete. *Synonyms:* pedodontia; pedodontics. *See also* dental specialities; pediatric dentist.

Pediatric Dentistry, American Academy of *See* American Academy of Pediatric Dentistry.

Pediatric Dentistry, American Board of *See* American Board of Pediatric Dentistry.

Pediatric Department Chairmen, Association of Medical School *See* Association of Medical School Pediatric Department Chairmen.

Pediatric Dermatology, Society for *See* Society for

Pediatric Dermatology.

pediatric endocrinologist A pediatrician who subspecializes in pediatric endocrinology. *See also* pediatric endocrinology.

pediatric endocrinology The branch of medicine and subspecialty of pediatrics dealing with infants, children, and adolescents who have diseases that result from an abnormality in the endocrine glands. These diseases include, but are not limited to, diabetes mellitus, growth failure, unusual size for age, early or late puberty development, birth defects, the genital region, and disorders of the thyroid, adrenal, and pituitary glands. *See also* diabetes mellitus; endocrinology; pediatrics; pituitary gland; thyroid gland.

pediatric emergency medicine The branch of medicine and subspecialty of emergency medicine and pediatrics dealing with the management of emergencies in infants and children. *See also* emergency medicine; emergency physician; pediatrics.

pediatric emergency physician A pediatrician who subspecializes in pediatric emergency medicine. *See also* pediatric emergency medicine.

pediatric gastroenterologist A pediatrician who subspecializes in pediatric gastroenterology. *See also* pediatric gastroenterology.

pediatric gastroenterology The branch of medicine and subspecialty of pediatrics dealing with management of disorders of the digestive systems of infants, children, and adolescents. *See also* digestive system; gastroenterology; pediatrics.

Pediatric Gastroenterology and Nutrition, North American Society for *See* North American Society for Pediatric Gastroenterology and Nutrition.

pediatric hematologist-oncologist A pediatrician who subspecializes in pediatric hematology-oncology. *See also* pediatric hematology-oncology.

pediatric hematology-oncology The branch of medicine and subspecialty of pediatrics dealing with blood disorders and cancerous diseases in pediatric patients. *See also* hematology; oncology; pediatrics.

Pediatric Hematology/Oncology, American Society of *See* American Society of Pediatric Hematology/Oncology.

pediatrician A physician who specializes in pediatrics. *See also* pediatrics.

Pediatricians, American College of Osteopathic *See* American College of Osteopathic Pediatricians.

pediatric infectious disease The branch of medicine and subspecialty of pediatrics dealing with the prevention and treatment of infectious diseases in children. *See also* infectious diseases; pediatrics.

pediatric infectious disease specialist A pediatrician who subspecializes in pediatric infectious disease. *See also* pediatric infectious disease; pediatrics.

pediatric inpatient An inpatient who is under a certain age as determined by a hospital. *See also* adult inpatient; inpatient.

pediatric inpatient bed A bed regularly maintained by a hospital for pediatric inpatients, other than newborns, who are receiving continuing hospital services. *See also* bed; newborn; pediatric inpatient.

pediatric inpatient bed count *See* bed count.

pediatric intensive care unit An intensive care unit for pediatric inpatients. *See also* intensive care unit; pediatric critical care medicine; pediatric critical care specialist; special care unit; unit.

pediatric medical toxicologist *See* medical toxicologist.

pediatric medical toxicology *See* medical toxicology.

pediatric nephrologist A pediatrician who subspecializes in pediatric nephrology. *See also* pediatric nephrology.

pediatric nephrology The branch of medicine and subspecialty of pediatrics dealing with the normal and abnormal development and maturation of the kidneys and the urinary tract, the mechanisms by which the kidneys can be damaged, the evaluation and treatment of renal diseases, fluid and electrolyte abnormalities, hypertension, and renal replacement therapy in children from fetal life to young adulthood. *See also* hypertension; nephrology; pediatrics.

Pediatric Neurosurgery, American Society for *See* American Society for Pediatric Neurosurgery.

pediatric nurse A registered nurse who specializes in providing nursing care to children from birth to adolescence. *See also* registered nurse.

Pediatric Nurse Associates and Practitioners, National Association of *See* National Association of Pediatric Nurse Associates and Practitioners.

pediatric nurse practitioner (PNP) A nurse practitioner specializing in pediatrics. *See also* nurse practitioner; pediatrics; registered nurse.

Pediatric Nurse Practitioners and Nurses, National Certification Board of *See* National Certification Board of Pediatric Nurse Practitioners and Nurses.

pediatric oncologist *See* pediatric hematologist-oncologist.

pediatric oncology *See* pediatric hematology-oncology.

Pediatric Oncology Nurses, Association of *See* Association of Pediatric Oncology Nurses.

Pediatric Oncology Social Workers, Association of *See* Association of Pediatric Oncology Social Workers.

Pediatric Ophthalmology and Strabismus, American Association for *See* American Association for Pediatric Ophthalmology and Strabismus.

Pediatric Orthopaedic Society of North America (POSNA) An organization founded in 1983 composed of 500 orthopedic surgeons interested in continuing education in the field of pediatric orthopedics. It conducts tutorial programs. *See also* orthopaedic/orthopedic surgery; pediatric orthopedics.

pediatric orthopedics Orthopedic surgery applied to infants and children. *See also* orthopaedic/orthopedic surgery.

pediatric otolaryngologist An otolaryngologist who subspecializes in pediatric otolaryngology-head and neck surgery. *See also* pediatric otolaryngology-head and neck surgery.

pediatric otolaryngology-head and neck surgery The branch of medicine and subspecialty of otolaryngology dealing with management of infants and children with disorders that include congenital and acquired conditions involving the aerodigestive tract, nose, paranasal sinuses, ear, and other areas of the head and neck. *See also* otolaryngology; pediatric otolaryngologist; pediatrics; surgery.

pediatric pathologist A pathologist who subspecializes in pediatric pathology. *See also* pediatric pathology.

pediatric pathology The branch of medicine and subspecialty of pathology dealing with the essential nature of disease, especially of the structural and functional changes in tissues and organs of the body that cause or are caused by disease in the fetus, infant, and child. *See also* pathology; pediatrics.

Pediatric Psychology, Society for *See* Society for Pediatric Psychology.

pediatric pulmonologist A pediatrician who subspecializes in pediatric pulmonology. *See also* pediatric pulmonology.

pediatric pulmonology The branch of medicine and subspecialty of pediatrics dealing with the pre-

vention and treatment of all respiratory diseases affecting infants, children, and young adults. *See also* pediatrics; pulmonary medicine.

Pediatric Radiology, Society for *See* Society for Pediatric Radiology.

Pediatric Research, Society for *See* Society for Pediatric Research.

pediatric rheumatologist A pediatrician who subspecializes in pediatric rheumatology. *See also* pediatric rheumatology.

pediatric rheumatology The branch of medicine and subspecialty of pediatrics dealing with the prevention, diagnosis, and treatment of the various rheumatic disorders in infants, children, and adolescents. *See also* pediatrics; rheumatology.

pediatrics The branch and specialty of medicine dealing with the physical, emotional, and social health of children from birth to young adulthood. Fourteen subspecialties of pediatrics are adolescent medicine, pediatric cardiology, pediatric critical care medicine, pediatric endocrinology, pediatric emergency medicine, pediatric gastroenterology, pediatric hematology-oncology, pediatric infectious disease, neonatal-perinatal medicine, pediatric nephrology, pediatric pulmonology, pediatric rheumatology, pediatric sports medicine, and medical toxicology. *See also* adolescent medicine; pediatric cardiology; pediatric critical care medicine; pediatric endocrinology; pediatric emergency medicine; pediatric gastroenterology; pediatric hematology-oncology; pediatric infectious disease; neonatal-perinatal medicine; pediatric nephrology; pediatric pulmonology; pediatric rheumatology; pediatric sports medicine; medical toxicology.

Pediatrics, American Academy of *See* American Academy of Pediatrics.

Pediatrics, American Board of *See* American Board of Pediatrics.

Pediatrics, American College of Podo- *See* American College of Podopediatrics.

Pediatrics, American Osteopathic Board of *See* American Osteopathic Board of Pediatrics.

pediatrics, podo- *See* podopediatrics.

pediatric sports medicine The branch of medicine and pediatric subspecialty dealing with the physiology and biomechanics of exercise; basic nutrition and its application to exercise; psychological aspects of exercise, performance, and competition; guidelines for evaluation prior to participation in exercise;

physical conditioning requirements for various activities; effects of disease on exercise and the use of exercise in the care of medical problems; prevention, evaluation, management, and rehabilitation of injuries; understanding effects of therapeutic, performance-enhancing, and recreational drugs; and promotion of healthy life-styles in the pediatric population. *See also* exercise; nutrition; pediatrics; sports medicine.

Pediatric Society, American *See* American Pediatric Society.

pediatric sports medicine specialist A pediatrician who subspecializes in pediatric sports medicine. *See also* pediatric sports medicine.

Pediatrics, Society for Behavioral *See* Society for Behavioral Pediatrics.

pediatric surgeon A general surgeon who specializes in pediatric surgery. *See also* pediatric surgery; surgeon.

pediatric surgery The branch of medicine and subspecialty of general surgery dealing with management of surgical conditions in premature and newborn infants, children, and adolescents. *See also* general surgery; pediatrics; surgery.

Pediatric Surgical Association, American *See* American Pediatric Surgical Association.

Pediatric Urology, Society for *See* Society for Pediatric Urology.

pediculosis Infestation with lice. *See also* body louse; head louse; pesticide; public health.

Pediculosis Association, National *See* National Pediculosis Association.

pedodontia *See* pediatric dentistry.

pedodontics *See* pediatric dentistry.

pedodontist *See* pediatric dentist.

pedophilia Sexual orientation, either homosexual or heterosexual, of an adult towards children. *See also* pederasty.

pedorthics The area of health care concerned with fitting and providing prescription footwear to clients referred by physicians and assisting in the design of pedorthic devices. *See also* orthotics.

Pedorthics, Board of Certification in *See* Board of Certification in Pedorthics.

peer **1.** A person who has equal standing with another person or other persons, as in education, age, training, rank, or status. **2.** In utilization and quality-of-care reviews of health care organizations, peers are defined as professionals in the same spe-

cialty of professional practice or a related specialty as the professionals whose services are being reviewed. *See also* peer review.

peer review **1.** In health care, concurrent or retrospective review of a health professional's performance (for example, a physician's performance) of clinical professional activities by peer(s) through formally adopted written procedures that provide for adequate notice and an opportunity for a hearing of the professional under review. Immunity from civil damage actions attaches to a hospital and hospital medical staff members if certain rights are afforded the physician as part of the disciplinary hearing process. *See also* concurrent review; peer review committee; retrospective review; second opinion. **2.** Review of research proposals, manuscripts submitted for publication, and abstracts submitted for presentation at scientific meetings; whereby these are judged for scientific and technical merit by other scientists in the same field.

Peer Review Association, American Medical *See* American Medical Peer Review Association.

peer review committee A committee composed of individuals (such as physicians) appointed or elected by a body (such as a medical staff of a hospital or medical society) to evaluate the performance of peers. *See also* committee; peer review.

peer review organization (PRO) A medical review organization established by the Tax Equity and Fiscal Responsibility Act of 1982 as a part of the prospective payment system to review the appropriateness of settings of care and the quality of care provided to Medicare beneficiaries. A PRO is under contract with the US Department of Health and Human Services. It replaces the professional standards review organization. *Synonym*: Utilization and Quality Control Peer Review Organization. *See also* experimental medical care review organization; Health Standards and Quality Bureau; Medicare; professional standards review organization; Tax Equity and Fiscal Responsibility Act of 1982.

pelvic Pertaining to the pelvis. *See also* pelvic examination; pelvic inflammatory disease; pelvis.

pelvic examination A physical examination of the female pelvic organs by a physician or other qualified health professional. *See also* bimanual; pelvis; physical examination.

pelvic inflammatory disease (PID) Inflammatory condition of the female pelvic organs, often associated with bacterial infection, characterized by lower abdominal pain, fever, and vaginal discharge. It is treated by antibiotics. It may lead to scarring of the fallopian tubes, sometimes leading to infertility. *See also* chlamydia; gonorrhea; inflammation; pelvis.

pelvis The lower part of the trunk of the body, comprising the region bounded by the two hip bones and the sacral and coccygeal portion of the spine. *See also* pelvic inflammatory disease.

PEN *See* Physicians Education Network.

pending claim A delayed health insurance claim held by an insurer because of omissions or errors in the claims information used for determining the eligibility of the patient, provider, or services for payment. *See also* claim.

penetrating trauma Trauma due to penetrating force that may occur as a result of, for example, a stab wound or a gunshot wound. *See also* blunt trauma; trauma.

penetration In marketing, the percentage of possible subscribers who have contracted for benefits with a specific health insurance or prepayment organization or plan, or a percentage of the total possible patient population that is actually served by a health care organization in a given geographic area. *See also* market penetration; marketing; saturation.

penetration, market *See* market penetration.

penicillin Any of a group of broad-spectrum antibiotics obtained from penicillium molds or produced synthetically. *See also* antibiotic.

penis The male external organ of urination and copulation, developmentally homologous with the female clitoris. *Compare* clitoris. *See also* circumcision; genitalia; phallus.

Pennsylvania Health Care Cost Containment Council *See* state data initiatives.

peon A person who works in a servile capacity. *See also* minion.

people intensive A process requiring many people to complete; not easily automated. For example, medication usage in a hospital is a people-intensive process requiring numerous interlinked steps. *See also* labor intensive.

People's Medical Society (PMS) A national public affairs organization founded in 1982 composed of 80,000 people interested in cost, quality, and management of the American health care system. It seeks to train and encourage individuals to study local health care systems, practitioners, and institutions

and promote preventive health care and medical cost control by these groups; address major policy issues and control health costs; encourage more preventive practice and research; promote self-care and alternative health care procedures; launch an information campaign to assist individuals in maintaining personal health and to prepare them for appointments with health professionals. *See also* medical society; preventive health services.

peptic ulcer An open sore in the lining of the stomach or duodenum related to acidic gastric secretions penetrating the protective mucous membrane of the gastrointestinal wall, thereby reaching the underlying muscular layers. Recent research suggests the possible involvement of a microorganism. *See also* antacid; duodenum; gastric ulcer; microorganism; ulcer.

per capita By or for each individual. Anything figured per capita is calculated by the number of individuals involved and is divided equally among all. *See also* capitation.

perceive **1.** To become aware of directly through any of the senses, especially sight or hearing, as in to perceive the approach of a storm. **2.** To achieve an understanding of, as in perceiving the importance of an event. *See also* mind; misperceive; perception.

perceived need A felt need, meaning that the need is felt by an individual or group, but the need may not be perceived by other individuals or groups. *See also* need.

perceive, mis- *See* misperceive.

percentile The set of divisions that produce exactly 100 equal parts in a series of continuous values, used to indicate the ranking or to establish a maximum of some amount, item, occurrence, or other entity distributed along the equal scale. *See also* quantile; scale.

perception The process by which information received by the senses is recognized, interpreted, and analyzed to become meaningful. Recognition and interpretation of sensory stimuli is based chiefly on memory. *See also* clairvoyance; cognition; mind; perceive; sixth sense; telepathy; wit.

perception psychology The branch of psychology that studies how an organism becomes aware of objects, events, and relationships in the outside world through its senses. Psychologists in the field of perception analyze vision, hearing, taste, smell, touch, movement, and other topics. *See also* perception; psychology.

percussion In physical diagnosis, the method of examination in which the surface of the body is struck to emit sounds that vary in quality according to the density of the underlying tissues, as in hyperresonance, dullness, tympany, or flatness on percussion of a patient's abdomen. *See also* physical examination.

percutaneous Through the skin, as in percutaneous transluminal angioplasty. *See also* percutaneous transluminal angioplasty.

percutaneous transluminal angioplasty A procedure in which a narrowing blood vessel is dilated by means of a balloon catheter inserted through the skin and through the lumen of the vessel to the site of the narrowing. There the balloon is inflated to flatten plaque against the vessel wall. *Synonym*: balloon angioplasty. *See also* angioplasty; percutaneous; percutaneous transluminal coronary angioplasty; plaque.

percutaneous transluminal coronary angioplasty (PTCA) Dilatation of a coronary (heart) blood vessel by means of a balloon catheter inserted through the skin and through the lumen of the vessel to the site of the narrowing, where the balloon is inflated to flatten plaque against the artery wall. *See also* angioplasty; percutaneous; percutaneous transluminal angioplasty; plaque.

per diem cost The cost per day; for example, the inpatient institutional costs per day or for a day of care. Hospitals occasionally charge for their services on the basis of a *per diem rate* derived by dividing their total costs by the number of inpatient days of care given. Per diem costs are an average and do not reflect the true cost for each patient. *See also* cost.

per diem rate *See* per diem cost.

perfect competition A market condition in which no buyer or seller has the power to alter the market price of a good or service. A perfectly competitive market has a large number of buyers and sellers, a homogeneous (similar) good or service, an equal awareness of prices and volume, an absence of discrimination in buying and selling, total mobility of productive resources, and complete freedom of entry. Perfect competition exists only as a theoretical ideal. *Synonym*: pure competition. *See also* competition.

perfected Complete beyond practical or theoretical improvement; practical application of technological development that cannot be improved substantially.

perfect monopoly A market dominated by a single producer, in which no competition of any kind can arise. *See also* monopoly.

perform **1.** To begin and carry through to completion, as in a surgeon performing an operation. **2.** To take action in accordance with the requirements of; fulfill, as in performing one's obligations to patients. *See also* accomplish; performance.

performance **1.** In health care, the way in which an individual, group, or organization carries out or accomplishes its important functions and processes; for example, measuring the performance of a hospital in providing obstetrical care of high quality. *Compare* nonperformance. *See also* organizational performance; performance assessment; performance data; performance improvement; performance measurement; performance area; performance standard; track record. **2.** In law, the degree to which an obligation or promise is fulfilled, especially completion of one's duty under a contract. *See also* contract. **3.** In marketing, the level of capability in a product, such as a high-performance car. *See also* marketing.

performance area An element of an accreditation decision grid used by the Joint Commission on Accreditation of Healthcare Organizations that summarizes a standard or group of standards. For example, education and communication, or continuum of care, are two performance areas on the accreditation decision grid. The performance areas identified on the accreditation decision grid are most critical to the final accreditation decision. *See also* accreditation decision; accreditation decision grid; aggregate survey data; Joint Commission on Accreditation of Healthcare Organizations; performance.

performance assessment An analysis and interpretation of performance measurement data to transform them into useful information; the second segment of a performance measurement, assessment, and improvement system. The product of assessment is information. *See also* assessment; indicator; indicator measurement system; information; measurement data; performance; performance improvement; performance measurement; track record.

performance-based quality-of-care evaluation A system of evaluation using three distinct, but interlinked, tools: performance measures, such as indicators; guidelines and standards; and a performance database. *See also* evaluation; indicator; performance database; practice guideline; quality of care; standard.

performance data Data that provide information about performance, as in organizational performance data. *See also* economic credentialing; data; performance; performance database.

performance database In health care, an organized collection of data designed primarily to provide information concerning organizational and/or practitioner performance. *See also* database; indicator measurement system; performance.

performance dimensions *See* dimensions of performance.

performance improvement The study and adaptation of functions and processes to increase the probability of achieving desired outcomes; the third segment of a performance measurement, assessment, and improvement system. *See also* function; improvement; outcome; performance; performance assessment; performance measurement; process.

performance index A measurement approach in which several different measures of performance are weighted as to their relative importance and then displayed simultaneously against a 100% attainment goal. *See also* index; performance.

performance indicator An instrument that measures performance. *See also* indicator; performance.

performance measure Any instrument (such as an indicator) for quantifying levels of performance. *See also* measure; performance; performance measurement.

performance measurement The quantification of processes and outcomes using one or more dimensions of performance, such as timeliness or availability. *See also* dimensions of performance; indicator measurement system; measurement; performance; performance measure; reliability testing.

performance, organizational *See* organizational performance.

performance rate A measurement produced by using a performance measure, providing a quantitative evaluation of patient care events being monitored. *See also* measurement; performance; rate.

performance standard A statement of expectation set by competent authority concerning a degree or level of requirement, excellence, or attainment in performance of a task achieved by an individual, group, organization, community, or nation, according to preestablished requirements and/or specifications. *See also* outcome standard; performance;

process standard; standard.

perfusion **1.** To pour or diffuse a liquid over or through something. **2.** The blood flow through an organ, tissue, or part, as in organ perfusion. *See also* perfusionist.

Perfusion, American Board of Cardiovascular *See* American Board of Cardiovascular Perfusion.

perfusionist An allied health professional who specializes in operating extracorporeal circulation equipment during any medical situation in which it is necessary to support or temporarily replace a patient's cardiopulmonary-circulatory function. A perfusionist selects equipment and techniques used during cardiopulmonary bypass, is responsible for the induction of hypothermia, and may administer blood products, anesthetic agents, or drugs through the extracorporeal circuit on prescription. Final medical responsibility for extracorporeal perfusion rests with the surgeon in charge. Perfusionists are one type of allied health professional for which the Committee on Allied Health Education and Accreditation has accredited education programs. *Synonyms:* circulation technologist; perfusion technologist. *See also* accreditation; allied health professional; American Society of Extra-Corporeal Technology; heart-lung machine; hypothermia; open-heart surgery; perfusion.

perfusion technologist *See* perfusionist.

peril **1.** Exposure to the risk of harm or loss. **2.** A risk or accident covered by an insurance policy. *See also* hazard; insurance; risk.

perinatal Pertaining to or occurring in the period shortly before to shortly after birth, for instance, the time between the completion of the 28th week of gestation and seven days after birth or, alternatively, a few months before and after birth. *See also* natal; postnatal; prenatal.

Perinatal Addiction Research and Education, National Association for *See* National Association for Perinatal Addiction Research and Education.

Perinatal Association, National *See* National Perinatal Association.

perinatal medicine, neonatal- *See* neonatal-perinatal medicine.

perinatal medicine specialist, neonatal- *See* neonatal-perinatal medicine specialist.

perinatal mortality Mortality during the perinatal period. *See also* perinatal; stillbirth.

perinatologist *See* neonatal-perinatal medicine

specialist.

perinatology   *See* neonatal-perinatal medicine.

Perinatology, Society for Obstetric Anesthesia and   *See* Society for Obstetric Anesthesia and Perinatology.

period   **1.** Any interval of time. **2.** The constant time interval between recurrences of a periodic (regularly repetitive) function. **3.** *See* menstrual period.

period, accounting   *See* accounting period.

period, base   *See* base period.

periodic   Occurring at regular, predictable intervals. *See also* continuous; frequent; intermittent; occasional; sporadic.

period, incubation   *See* incubation period.

period, menstrual   *See* menstrual period.

period, neonatal   *See* neonatal period.

period, observation   *See* observation period.

periodontal   Pertaining to the area around a tooth.

periodontal disease   Disease of the tissues around a tooth, often leading to damage to the bony sockets of the teeth. *See also* periodontal; periodontitis.

periodontia   *See* periodontics.

periodontics   A dental specialty concerned with diseases that affect the oral mucous membranes and tissues that surround and support the teeth. *Synonyms*: periodontia; periodontology. *See also* dental specialties.

periodontist   A dentist who specializes in periodontics. *Synonym*: periodontologist. *See also* dental specialties; dentist; periodontics.

periodontitis   Inflammation and destruction of the periodontal membrane, the tissue that surrounds the roots of the teeth and holds them to the jaw. *See also* inflammation; periodontal disease.

periodontologist   *See* periodontist.

periodontology   *See* periodontics.

Periodontology, American Academy of   *See* American Academy of Periodontology.

Periodontology, American Board of   *See* American Board of Periodontology.

period, payback   *See* payback period.

period, safe   *See* safe period.

period, transition   *See* transition period.

period, waiting   *See* waiting period.

perioperative   Pertaining to the time before, during, and after surgery; for example, perioperative indicators. *See also* intraoperative; operation; preoperative; postoperative.

peripheral   Pertaining to the outside, surface, or area away from the center of an organ or of the body; for example, peripheral nervous system. *See also* peripheral neurologic deficit; peripheral nervous system; peripheral vascular disease.

peripheral nervous system   The nerves of the body and their supporting tissues considered collectively, excluding those contained in the brain and spinal cord and also excluding the autonomic nervous system. *See also* autonomic nervous system; central nervous system; nervous system; peripheral; peripheral neurologic deficit.

peripheral neurologic deficit   Functional defect, such as wrist drop, involving one or more peripheral nerves. *See also* deficit; neurologic; peripheral.

peripheral norm   *See* behavioral norms.

peripherals   Computer equipment other than the main processor used in printing, storing, communicating, and related functions. *See also* computer; peripheral.

peripheral vascular disease   Abnormal narrowing of vessels that carry blood outside the heart, especially to the arms and legs. *See also* disease; peripheral; vascular.

peristalsis   The wavelike contractions of the intestines that propel nutrients and intestinal contents forward toward the anus. *See also* intestine; nutrient.

peritoneal   Pertaining to the peritoneum. *See also* peritoneum.

peritoneal cavity   The abdominal and pelvic space between the two layers of peritoneum (parietal and visceral). *See also* cavity; peritoneum.

peritoneal dialysis   Dialysis through the peritoneum often used by patients with renal impairment. The dialyzing solution is introduced into and removed from the peritoneal cavity as either a continuous or an intermittent procedure. *See also* dialysis; hemodialysis; peritoneum.

peritoneoscope   *See* laparoscope.

peritoneoscopy   *See* laparoscopy.

peritoneum   The strong, two-layered membrane lining the abdomen and pelvis and encapsulating the abdominal organs. *See also* peritoneal cavity; peritoneal dialysis; peritonitis.

peritonitis   Inflammation of the peritoneum, caused by bacteria or irritating substances and characterized by abdominal pain, nausea, vomiting, rebound tenderness, chills, and fever. A ruptured appendix is the most frequent cause of peritonitis. *See also* appendicitis; inflammation; peritoneum.

peritonsillar abscess *See* quinsy.

perjury The criminal offense of making false statements under oath or affirmation. *See also* suborn.

perk *See* perquisite.

permanent Remaining or lasting without essential change, as in permanent tooth. *See also* permanent disability; permanent injunction; permanent tooth.

permanent disability A continuous condition resulting from illness or injury that prevents an individual from performing some or all of the functions of his or her occupation. *See also* disability; permanent.

Permanente Medical Groups *See* Kaiser-Permanente Medical Care Program.

permanent injunction A court order to do or refrain from doing some act that is issued as part of the final judgment by the court in a lawsuit. *See also* injunction; permanent.

permanent teeth *See* permanent tooth.

permanent tooth Any of the set of 32 teeth that appear during and after childhood and, in the optimal case, last until old age. In each jaw, there are four incisors, two canines, four premolars, and six molars. They replace the 20 deciduous (milk, primary) teeth of early childhood, usually starting to erupt in the sixth year and continuing to erupt until the 18th to 25th year (eruption of the third molars or wisdom teeth). *See also* tooth; permanent; wisdom teeth.

permit A document, issued by a government regulatory authority, that allows the bearer to take some specific action, as in a building permit, driver's permit, or license to sell alcoholic beverages. *See also* beneficial occupancy permit.

permit, beneficial occupancy *See* beneficial occupancy permit.

perquisite Any special privilege, service, or benefit made in conjunction with employment in addition to basic wages and salaries; for example, health insurance, pensions, automobiles, and vacation areas. Executive perks may include limousines, club memberships, and corporate aircraft use. *Synonyms:* fringe benefit; perk.

perseveration The persistent repetition of words or actions despite a patient's efforts to say or do something else. *See also* language.

per se violation A term of antitrust law regarding violations, such as price fixing, that are so plainly anticompetitive that no elaborate study of the industry is necessary to establish their illegality and no justification is permitted on the basis of special circumstances in the particular market. *See also* antitrust laws; price fixing; violation.

persistency In insurance, the rate at which policies written in a given line of insurance or for members of a given group are maintained in force until the completion of the terms of the policies. *See also* insurance.

persistent generalized lymphadenopathy A clinical condition characterized by a positive test for human immunodeficiency virus (HIV) and diffuse lymph node enlargement for longer than three months but no other signs or symptoms of human immunodeficiency virus. *See also* HIV infection; lymph node.

persistent vegetative state *See* vegetative state.

person **1.** A living human being, as in an aged person. *See also* aged person. **2.** In law, an individual or incorporated group having certain legal rights and responsibilities.

persona In psychology, the personality role that a person assumes and presents to the world. *Compare* anima. *See also* psychology.

person, aged *See* aged person.

personal Pertaining to a person; private.

personal care Assistance with activities of daily living, such as bathing, dressing, and eating, that are typically provided by home health aides or other personnel. *Synonym:* personal care services. *See also* activities of daily living; adult day care; home health aide; maintenance home health care.

personal care institution *See* residential care facility.

personal care services *See* personal care.

personal computer (PC) A small computer built around a microprocessor and designed to be used by one person at a time. *See also* computer; microcomputer; personal.

personal effects Tangible property privately owned by a person and regularly worn or carried on one's person; for example, keys, jewelry, wallet, and clothing. *See also* personal.

personal health care *See* personal health services.

personal health services Health services provided to individuals, in contrast to health services directed at populations, such as environmental health, community health, public health, consultation, and education services, and health education. *Synonym:* personal health care. *See also* health services; personal.

personal influence The power of an individual to sway or control the decisions and actions of one or more other individuals. *See also* influence; personal; persuasion.

personal injury In law, wrongful conduct causing false arrest, invasion of privacy, libel, slander, defamation of character, or bodily injury. The injury is against a person in contrast to property damage or destruction. In workers' compensation acts, "personal injury" means any harm or damage to the health of an employee, however caused, whether by accident, disease, or otherwise, which arises in the course of and out of his or her employment, and incapacitates him or her in whole or in part. *See also* American Board of Professional Disability Consultants; injury; personal; workers' compensation acts.

personality The totality of behavioral, attitudinal, intellectual, and emotional characteristics of an individual, as in personality disorder or personality psychology. *See also* personality disorder; personality psychology.

personality, addictive *See* addictive personality.

Personality Assessment, Society for *See* Society for Personality Assessment.

personality disorder A mental disorder, such as obsessive compulsive disorder or passive aggressive disorder, characterized by maladaptive and usually rigid patterns of behavior that greatly affects social functioning. *See also* disorder; personality.

personality disorder, narcissistic *See* narcissistic personality disorder.

personality disorder, obsessive-compulsive *See* obsessive-compulsive personality disorder.

personality disorder, passive aggressive *See* passive aggressive personality disorder.

personality disorder, sadistic *See* sadistic personality disorder.

personality, multiple *See* multiple personality.

personality psychology The branch of psychology referring to the characteristics that make individuals different from one another and account for the way they behave. Personality psychologists investigate how an individual's personality develops, the chief personality types, and the measurement of personality traits. *See also* personality; psychology.

personality, sadistic *See* sadistic personality disorder.

personality, sociopathic *See* psychopath.

personality, split *See* multiple personality.

personal physician **1.** A physician who assumes responsibility for the care of an individual on a continuing basis. **2.** A physician whom a patient designates as his or her principal physician. *See also* personal; physician.

personkind A nonsexist substitute for "mankind." *Synonyms:* humanity; humankind.

personnel People who actually compose an organization's work force; an organization's human resources. *See also* human resources.

personnel administration *See* personnel management.

Personnel, American Society for Healthcare Central Service *See* American Society for Healthcare Central Service Personnel.

personnel costs Total costs to an organization of its employees' salaries, fringe benefits, and other direct and indirect components of its total employee compensation package. *See also* cost; organization; personnel.

personnel department An organizational unit providing for the planning and management of an organization's human resources, including recruiting, interviewing, and screening job applicants; providing benefits and maintaining salary scales; providing orientation for new employees; maintaining a control system over positions of employment; handling labor relations; and performing risk appraisal. *Synonym:* human resources department. *See also* department; human resources; personnel.

Personnel, Joint Review Committee for Ophthalmic Medical *See* Joint Review Committee for Ophthalmic Medical Personnel.

personnel management Management that deals with the planning and management of an organization's human resources. *Synonym:* personnel administration. *See also* human resources management; personnel department.

Personnel Management, Office of *See* Office of Personnel Management.

Personnel in Ophthalmology, Association of Technical *See* Association of Technical Personnel in Ophthalmology.

Personnel in Ophthalmology, Joint Commission on Allied Health *See* Joint Commission on Allied Health Personnel in Ophthalmology.

personnel, paramedical *See* paramedical personnel.

personnel psychology The branch of psychology

dealing with the study and improvement of personnel practices in industry and government. *See also* industrial psychology; psychology.

personnel files *See* personnel record.

personnel record Recorded information about employees kept by an employer. *Synonym:* personnel files. *See also* employee; personnel.

person, reasonable *See* reasonable person.

perspective **1.** A view or mental outlook. **2.** The ability to perceive things in their actual interrelations or comparative importance.

perspiration The colorless saline moisture excreted by the sweat glands. *Synonym:* sweat.

persuasion The act or process of inducing another or other persons to undertake a course of action or embrace a point of view by means of reasoning or emotion. In advertising, persuasion is a primary objective that can be achieved by creating advertisements with some combination of the following elements: effective attention-getting devices, a strong appeal to self-interest, a stimulation of desire for a product or service, and a powerful call-to-action response. *See also* brainwashing; personal influence.

PERT *See* Program Evaluation and Review Technique.

PERT chart *See* Program Evaluation and Review Technique.

PERT diagram *See* Program Evaluation and Review Technique.

Peruvian Heart Association (PHA) An organization founded in 1967 composed of 400 Peruvian physicians, nurses, and other health professionals specializing in cardiology. It offers continuing education courses for Peruvian physicians, enabling them to fulfill the coursework required by Peruvian law for continuance of medical practice. It provides information to residents of Lima, Peru, concerning heart attacks, high blood pressure, cholesterol, and other diseases, and conducts programs in conjunction with the American College of Cardiology and the American Heart Association. *See also* cardiology.

perversion Action considered abnormal or unnatural, especially a sexual activity deviating from what is considered normal. *Synonym:* sexual deviance.

pessary A vaginal suppository, or a mechanical device inserted into the vagina to provide tissue support or to prevent insemination of the uterus. *See also* uterus; vagina.

pessimism A tendency to stress the negative or unfavorable or to take the gloomiest possible view. *Compare* optimism. *See also* negativism.

pesticide Chemicals, such as insecticides and rodenticides, used to destroy or control pests, such as insects and rats. *See also* pediculosis.

PET *See* positron emission tomography.

PET scan A cross-sectional image produced by a PET scanner. *See also* positron emission tomography.

PET scanner A machine that produces cross-sectional x-rays of metabolic processes by means of positron emission tomography. *See also* positron emission tomography.

Peter principle A theory that people rise in their career in every hierarchy to the level of their own incompetence. It is based on the book *The Peter Principle and Why Things Always Go Wrong* by Lawrence J. Peter. Work in organizations, according to the Peter principle, is accomplished by employees who have not yet reached their level of incompetence. *See also* incompetent.

petit jury An ordinary trial jury, as opposed to a grand jury. Petit juries, traditionally composed of 12 members, determine issues of fact in civil and criminal cases and reach a verdict in conjunction with those findings. *See also* grand jury; jury; jury trial.

Petri dish A circular, flat-bottomed, vertical-sided shallow glass dish with a slightly larger glass cover of similar shape, in which microorganisms are cultured on a nutrient medium. *See also* bacteriology; culture; microorganism.

petty Of small importance or trivial, as in petty cash. *See also* petty cash.

petty cash A small money fund commonly kept in a cash box, as in a physician's office, and maintained by a secretary or receptionist. Petty cash is used to pay for small, unexpected items without prior authorization and without the necessity for writing a check. *See also* petty.

Pew Charitable Trusts, The *See* The Pew Charitable Trusts.

PF *See* Physicians Forum.

PGY-1 Abbreviation for postgraduate year 1, the first year of a physician residency program that is sponsored by a single medical specialty department. Subsequent years are called PGY-2, PGY-3, and so on, depending on the length of the residency program which varies according to specialty and is usually from three to seven years. *See also* medical specialties; residency.

PH *See* public health.

PHA *See* Peruvian Heart Association.

phallus An erect penis. *Synonym:* priapus. *See also* penis.

phantom limb An illusion of the presence of an amputated limb, which may be associated with pain, numbness, and tingling referred to the absent part. *See also* illusion; sense.

PharD *See* PharmD.

pharmaceutic *See* pharmaceutical.

pharmaceutical **1.** Relating to drugs or to a pharmacy or pharmacist. *See also* decentralized pharmaceutical services; pharmaceutical services. **2.** A medicinal drug. *Synonym:* pharmaceutic. *See also* drug; pharmacist; pharmacy.

pharmaceutical aid *See* pharmaceutical necessity.

Pharmaceutical Association, American *See* American Pharmaceutical Association.

Pharmaceutical Association, National *See* National Pharmaceutical Association.

Pharmaceutical Council, National *See* National Pharmaceutical Council.

Pharmaceutical Education, American Council on *See* American Council on Pharmaceutical Education.

pharmaceutical equivalence The degree to which two formulations of the same medication are identical in strength, concentration, and dosage form. *See also* bioequivalence; chemical equivalence; pharmaceutical.

Pharmaceutical Industry Association, Generic *See* Generic Pharmaceutical Industry Association.

Pharmaceutical Manufacturers Association (PMA) A national organization founded in 1958 composed of 93 manufacturers of ethical pharmaceutical and biological products that are distributed under their own labels. It encourages high standards for quality control and good manufacturing practices; research toward development of new medical products; and enactment of uniform and reasonable drug legislation. It disseminates information on governmental regulations and policies, but does not maintain or supply information on specific products, prices, distribution, promotion, or sales policies of its individual members. *See also* drug; pharmaceutical; pharmacy.

Pharmaceutical Manufacturers, National Association of *See* National Association of Pharmaceutical Manufacturers.

pharmaceutical necessity A substance having slight or no value therapeutically, but is used in the preparation of various pharmaceuticals, including preservatives, solvents, ointment bases, and flavoring, coloring, diluting, emulsifying, and suspending agents. *Synonym:* pharmaceutical aid. *See also* excipient; pharmaceutical.

pharmaceutical representative *See* detail person.

Pharmaceutical Research and Science, Academy of *See* Academy of Pharmaceutical Research and Science.

Pharmaceutical Sales Trainers, National Society of *See* National Society of Pharmaceutical Sales Trainers.

Pharmaceutical Scientists, American Association of *See* American Association of Pharmaceutical Scientists.

pharmaceutical services The activities pertaining to the appropriate, safe, and effective storage, preparation, dispensing, and administration of drugs in hospitals and other health care organizations. *See also* decentralized pharmaceutical services; home pharmaceutical services.

pharmaceutical services, decentralized *See* decentralized pharmaceutical services.

pharmaceutical services, home *See* home pharmaceutical services.

Pharmaceutical Society of America, Jewish *See* Jewish Pharmaceutical Society of America.

pharmaceutist *See* pharmacist.

pharmacist An individual qualified by education and authorized by law to practice pharmacy. *Synonym:* pharmaceutist. *See also* apothecary; druggist; pharmacy.

Pharmacists, American Association of Homeopathic *See* American Association of Homeopathic Pharmacists.

Pharmacists, American Society of Consultant *See* American Society of Consultant Pharmacists.

Pharmacists, American Society of Hospital *See* American Society of Hospital Pharmacists.

Pharmacists Guild of the United States, National Catholic *See* National Catholic Pharmacists Guild of the United States.

Pharmacists in Ophthalmic Practice (PIOP) A national organization founded in 1984 composed of 26 pharmacists who serve as directors or chief pharmacists of institutions that specialize in ophthalmology or otolaryngology. It exchanges information and determines standards relating to ophthalmological pharmacy, pharmacology, and formulations. *See also* ophthalmology; pharmacology; pharmacy.

pharmacodynamics The study of the biochemical and physiological effects of drugs and the mechanisms of their actions, including the correlation of actions and effects of drugs with their chemical structure. *See also* drug; pharmacokinetics; pharmacology.

pharmacognosy The study of drugs of natural origin.

Pharmacognosy, American Society of *See* American Society of Pharmacognosy.

pharmacokinetics The study of the action of drugs in the human body over a period of time, including the method and rate of absorption and excretion and the duration of effect. *See also* cell kinetics; drug; kinetics; pharmacodynamics; pharmacology.

pharmacologist A person with a graduate degree in pharmacology who studies the actions of drugs, including conducting drug research relating to the development of new drugs. *See also* pharmacist; pharmacology.

pharmacology The science of drugs, including their composition, uses, and effects. *See also* clinical pharmacology; pharmacologist; psychopharmacology.

Pharmacology, American College of Clinical *See* American College of Clinical Pharmacology.

Pharmacology, American College of Neuropsycho- *See* American College of Neuropsychopharmacology.

Pharmacology, Associates of Clinical *See* Associates of Clinical Pharmacology.

pharmacology, clinical *See* clinical pharmacology.

Pharmacology and Experimental Therapeutics, American Society for *See* American Society for Pharmacology and Experimental Therapeutics.

pharmacology, neuro- *See* neuropharmacology.

pharmacology, psycho- *See* psychopharmacology.

Pharmacology Society, Behavioral *See* Behavioral Pharmacology Society.

Pharmacology and Therapeutics, American Society for Clinical *See* American Society for Clinical Pharmacology and Therapeutics.

pharmacomania An uncontrollable desire to take or to administer medicines. *Compare* pharmacophobia. *See also* drug; mania; medication.

pharmacopoeia An authoritative treatise on recognized drugs used in medicine and including their preparations, formulas, doses, and standards of purity. *See also* United States Pharmacopeia.

Pharmacopeial Convention, United States *See* United States Pharmacopeial Convention.

Pharmacopeia, United States *See United States Pharmacopeia.*

pharmacophobia An irrational fear of drugs or medicines. *Compare* pharmacomania. *See also* pharmaceutical; phobia.

pharmacotherapeutics The study of drugs used in the treatment of disease. *See also* pharmacology; therapeutics.

pharmacy **1.** The branch of health sciences dealing with the preparation, preserving, compounding, dispensing, and proper use of drugs. *See also* drug; polypharmacy. **2.** A place where pharmacy is practiced. *See also* apothecary; druggist; pharmacist.

Pharmacy, American Association of Colleges of *See* American Association of Colleges of Pharmacy.

Pharmacy, American College of Clinical *See* American College of Clinical Pharmacy.

Pharmacy, American Institute of the History of *See* American Institute of the History of Pharmacy.

pharmacy assistant An individual who assists a pharmacist in technical tasks, such as reviewing the past medication histories of patients for drug interactions, packaging prescriptions, conducting inventory control, and managing purchase records. *Synonym*: pharmacy technician. *See also* pharmacy.

Pharmacy Association, American Managed Care *See* American Managed Care Pharmacy Association.

Pharmacy Association Executives, National Council of State *See* National Council of State Pharmacy Association Executives.

pharmacy department A unit of an organization, such as a hospital, that controls the preparation, preservation, compounding, dispensing, storage, and control of drugs. *See also* department; pharmacy.

Pharmacy, Doctor of *See* Doctor of Pharmacy.

Pharmacy Graduate Examination Committee, Foreign *See* Foreign Pharmacy Graduate Examination Committee.

Pharmacy Law, American Society for *See* American Society for Pharmacy Law.

Pharmacy, National Association of Boards of *See* National Association of Boards of Pharmacy.

pharmacy, poly- *See* polypharmacy.

Pharmacy Practice and Management, Academy of *See* Academy of Pharmacy Practice and Management.

pharmacy, satellite *See* decentralized pharmaceutical services.

pharmacy technician *See* pharmacy assistant.

pharmacy and therapeutics A medical staff responsibility, carried out in cooperation with the pharmaceutical department/service, the nursing department/service, management and administrative services, and other services and individuals of a health care organization to measure, assess, and improve the policies and procedures relating to drug and diagnostic testing material and investigational or experimental drug usage; develop and maintain a drug formulary; and review all significant untoward drug reactions. *See also* drug adverse reaction; formulary; medical staff; pharmacy; pharmacy and therapeutics committee; therapeutics.

pharmacy and therapeutics committee The medical staff committee that performs the pharmacy and therapeutics function. *See also* pharmacy and therapeutics.

Pharmacy and Therapeutics for the Elderly, Center for the Study of *See* Center for the Study of Pharmacy and Therapeutics for the Elderly.

PharmB Abbreviation for the Latin phrase *Pharmaciae Baccalaureus*, meaning "Bachelor of Pharmacy." *See* bachelor's degree; pharmacy.

PharmD Abbreviation for the Latin phrase *Pharmaciae Doctor*, meaning "Doctor of Pharmacy." *See* Doctor of Pharmacy.

PharM Abbreviation for the Latin phrase *Pharmaciae Magister*, meaning "Master of Pharmacy." *See* Master of Pharmacy.

pharyngitis Inflammation of the pharynx (throat). *See also* inflammation; tonsils.

phase A distinct stage of development through which an individual, organization, process, disease, or other entity may pass.

PhD Abbreviation for the Latin phrase *Philosophiae Doctor*, meaning Doctor of Philosophy. *See* Doctor of Philosophy.

phencyclidine hydrochloride *See* PCP.

phenome A group of organisms related by phenotype. *See also* phenotype.

phenomena, threshold *See* threshold phenomena.

phenomenology **1.** In philosophy, the study of all possible appearances in human experience, during which considerations of objective reality or purely subjective responses are left out of account. *See also* phenomenon. **2.** In psychiatry, the theory that behavior is determined by the way an individual

perceives reality rather than by external reality in objective terms. *See also* psychiatry.

phenomenon **1.** An observable event or sign that is perceptible by the senses. **2.** In medicine, a phenomenon may be relatively specific to a particular disease and therefore of diagnostic significance; for example, Duckworth's phenomenon (arrest of breathing before stoppage of the heart's action in certain fatal brain conditions) and dawn phenomenon (the early-morning increase in plasma glucose concentration, and thus insulin requirement, in a patient with insulin-dependent diabetes). **3.** An unusual or unaccountable fact or occurrence, such as a marvel. *See also* phenomenology; threshold phenomena.

phenotype The characteristics of an organism that can be observed (for example, eye color, height) and are the result of genetic makeup (genotype) and environmental factors. *Compare* genotype. *See also* phenome.

PHEWA *See* Presbyterian Health, Education and Welfare Association.

PHHSA *See* Protestant Health and Human Services Assembly.

philanthropy The effort to provide humanitarian or charitable assistance. Philanthropy, in contrast to charity, implies that some form of improvement in public welfare or general benefit is expected from the donation. *Compare* charity. *See also* humanitarian.

Philanthropy, Association for Healthcare *See* Association for Healthcare Philanthropy.

-philia Having a tendency toward, as in hemophilia.

-philiac One that has a tendency toward, as in hemophiliac.

philiater An individual interested in medical science, particularly a medical student. *See also* medical student.

Phillips curve An economic proposition stating that there is a negative relationship between unemployment and the level of inflation, meaning that as inflation increases, unemployment decreases and vice versa. *See also* inflation.

phleb- Pertaining to a vein, as in phlebitis.

phlebitis Inflammation of a vein. *See also* inflammation; vein.

phlebotomist An individual who practices phlebotomy. *See also* phlebotomy.

phlebotomize To take blood from an individual by phlebotomy. *See also* intravenous team; phlebotomy.

Phlebotomus A genus of very small, bloodsucking sandflies, many species of which are vectors of disease-causing organisms. *Synonym:* sandfly. *See also* phlebotomy; vector.

phlebotomy Incision or puncture of a vein for removing blood, as in collecting blood from a blood donor or collecting a blood specimen for laboratory analysis. *See also* blood letting; intravenous team.

Phlebotomy Association, National *See* National Phlebotomy Association.

phlegm **1.** Thick, viscid mucous secretion produced by the mucous membranes of the respiratory passages. *See also* mucous membrane. **2.** In humoralism, one of the four humors of the body. *See also* humoralism; phlegmatic.

phlegmatic Characterized by an excess of the humor called phlegm; hence heavy, dull, and apathetic. *See also* humoralism; phlegm.

PHN *See* public health nurse.

PHO *See* physician-hospital organization.

phobia An exaggerated and illogical fear which may be insistent and intense, giving rise to panic and a compelling need to flee whatever causes the fear. When a phobia is a source of marked distress or interferes with social functioning, it is considered a mental disorder. Treatment includes desensitization therapy and other techniques of behavior therapy. *See also* behavior therapy.

phobia, agora- *See* agoraphobia.

phobia, anthropo- *See* anthropophobia.

phobia, cancero- *See* cancerophobia.

phobia, claustro- *See* claustrophobia.

phobia, geronto- *See* gerontophobia.

phobia, homo- *See* homophobia.

phobia, hydro- *See* hydrophobia.

phobia, necro- *See* necrophobia.

phobia, nycto- *See* nyctophobia.

phobia, pharmaco- *See* pharmacophobia.

phobia, xeno- *See* xenophobia.

phobia, zoo- *See* zoophobia.

phobophobia Irrational fear of one's own fears or of acquiring a phobia. *See also* phobia.

phocomelia A severe congenital anomaly in which the limbs fail to develop normally, so that the hands and feet may be directly attached to the body. *See also* thalidomide.

phonation The production of voice sounds. *See also* speech.

phonetics The study of voice, vocal sounds, spoken language, and pronunciation. *See also* phonation; speech.

Photographers' Society, Ophthalmic *See* Ophthalmic Photographers' Society.

Photographic Association, Biological *See* Biological Photographic Association.

photography, ophthalmic *See* ophthalmic photography.

phototherapy The treatment of disease, such as acne and hyperbilirubinemia (high levels of bilirubin in the blood) in the newborn, with exposure to light, such as ultraviolet and infrared radiation. *See also* infrared radiation therapy; ultraviolet.

PHR *See* Physicians for Human Rights.

phrenology The set of beliefs purporting that mental development and mental faculties are related to the external configuration of the skull. *See also* physiognomy.

PHS *See* Public Health Service.

PHSA *See* Public Health Service Act.

physiatrician *See* physiatrist.

physiatrics *See* physical medicine and rehabilitation.

physiatrist **1.** A physician who specializes in physical medicine. **2.** A health professional who administers physical therapy. *Synonym:* physical medicine specialist. *See also* physical medicine and rehabilitation; physical therapy.

Physiatrists, Association of Academic *See* Association of Academic Physiatrists.

physiatry *See* physical medicine and rehabilitation.

physical Pertaining to the body, to material things, or to physics. *See also* physics.

Physical Activity, North American Society for the Psychology of Sport and *See* North American Society for the Psychology of Sport and Physical Activity.

physical dependence A physiologic state that occurs due to the administration of habit-forming substances, such as opiates. It will occur in most adults and children if, for example, they receive narcotics for seven days or more. Such patients require a gradual tapering of the narcotic to avoid withdrawal symptoms. *See also* addiction; dependence; narcotics.

physical diagnosis Diagnostication by physical examination including the processes of inspection, palpation, percussion, and auscultation. *See also* auscultation; diagnosis; inspection; palpation; percussion; physical examination.

Physical Disability Law, Commission on Mental and *See* Commission on Mental and Physical Disability Law.

physical examination An examination in which a clinician brings the five senses of sight, hearing, touch, smell, and taste to bear on the patient through inspection, palpation, percussion, and auscultation. The experienced clinician assigns special meanings to his or her perceptions as the result of practice and knowledge of normal and abnormal anatomy and physiology. When the clinician recognizes the abnormal in the physical examination, he or she uses the facts of pathology to make a diagnosis. The major effort in becoming a diagnostician consists of acquiring the intellectual background to make perceptions meaningful. *See also* auscultation; examination; inspection; medical history; medical record; palpation; percussion.

Physical Fitness Centers, Association of *See* Association of Physical Fitness Centers.

physical fitness program A health promotion program designed to improve body performance with emphasis on cardiovascular fitness, strength, and flexibility and other motor fitness elements, such as agility and balance. *See also* fitness; wellness; wellness program.

physical medicine and rehabilitation The branch and specialty of medicine concerned with diagnosing and treating patients with impairments or disabilities that involve musculoskeletal, neurologic, cardiovascular, or other body systems. The primary focus is on maximal restoration of physical, psychological, social, and vocational function and on alleviation of pain. For diagnosis and evaluation, a physiatrist (a specialist in physical medicine) may use the techniques of electromyography and electrodiagnosis as supplements to the medical history, physical examination, x-ray examination, and laboratory examination. In addition to traditional treatment modes a physiatrist may use therapeutic exercise, prosthetics, orthotics, and mechanical and electrical devices. *Synonyms*: physiatrics; physiatry. *See also* electromyography; electrodiagnosis; orthotics; pain management; physical medicine service; physical therapy; prosthetics.

Physical Medicine and Rehabilitation, American Academy of *See* American Academy of Physical Medicine and Rehabilitation.

Physical Medicine and Rehabilitation, American Board of *See* American Board of Physical Medicine and Rehabilitation.

physical medicine specialist *See* physiatrist.

physical medicine service Service that provides physical therapy and other physical restorative and maintenance programs. *See also* physical medicine and rehabilitation; physical therapy; rehabilitation service.

physical plant and maintenance department *See* maintenance department.

physical rehabilitation services The professional and technical care that assists physically disabled persons to increase, attain, and/or maintain functional capacity. *See also* physical medicine and rehabilitation.

physical restraint *See* restraint.

physical science Sciences, such as physics, chemistry, astronomy, and geology, that analyze the nature and properties of energy and nonliving matter. *See also* chemistry; physics; science.

physical therapist (PT) A health professional who specializes in physical therapy. *Synonym*: physiotherapist. *See also* physical therapy; physical therapy services.

physical therapy (PT) The health care field concerned primarily with the treatment of disorders with physical agents and methods, such as massage, manipulation, therapeutic exercises, cold, heat (including shortwave, microwave, and ultrasonic diathermy), hydrotherapy, electric stimulation, and light to assist in rehabilitating patients and in restoring normal function after an illness or injury. *Synonym*: physiotherapy. *See also* activities of daily living; hand massage; hand vibrator; hydrotherapy; infrared radiation therapy; massage; passive exercise; range of motion; ultrasound physical therapy.

physical therapy assistant An individual who works under the supervision of a physical therapist to assist him or her in providing physical therapy services. A physical therapy assistant may, for instance, help patients follow an appropriate exercise program that will increase their strength, endurance, coordination, and range of motion and train patients to perform activities of daily life. *See also* activities of daily living; physical therapy; range of motion.

Physical Therapy Association, American *See* American Physical Therapy Association.

Physical Therapy Association, Orthopaedic Section, American *See* American Physical Therapy Association, Orthopaedic Section.

Physical Therapy Association, Private Practice Section, American *See* American Physical Therapy Association, Private Practice Section.

Physical Therapy Association, US *See* US Physical Therapy Association.

physical therapy services Services that provide identification, prevention, remediation, and rehabilitation of acute or prolonged physical dysfunction or pain, with emphasis on movement dysfunction. Such therapy encompasses examination and analysis of patients and the therapeutic application of physical and chemical agents, exercise, and other procedures to maximize functional independence. *See also* physical therapy.

physical therapy, ultrasound *See* ultrasound physical therapy.

physician 1. An individual qualified by education and authorized by law to practice medicine. *See also* iatros; medical practice act; medicine. 2. A person who practices medicine as distinct from surgery. Thus, a surgeon is also a physician (meaning 1), but a physician is not necessarily a surgeon (meaning 2). *See also* surgeon.

physician - administrative, public health *See* public health physician - administrative.

physician, admitting *See* admitting physician.

physician, allopathic *See* allopathic physician.

Physician Art Association, American *See* American Physician Art Association.

physician assistant (PA) An allied health professional who provides health care services with the direction and supervision of a doctor of medicine or an osteopathic physician, who is ultimately responsible for the decision making required to initiate and sustain therapy. Tasks performed by PAs vary with practice requirements mandated by geographic, political, economic, and social factors. Functions of the PA include performing diagnostic, therapeutic, preventive, and health maintenance services in any setting in which the physician renders care, to allow more effective and focused application of the physician's particular knowledge and skills. Physician assistants are one type of allied health professional for which the Committee on Allied Health Education and Accreditation has accredited education programs. *Synonym*: physician extender. *See also* physician.

Physician Assistant Programs, Association of *See* Association of Physician Assistant Programs.

Physician Assistants, Accreditation Review Committee on Education for *See* Accreditation Review Committee on Education for Physician Assistants.

Physician Assistants, American Academy of *See* American Academy of Physician Assistants.

Physician Assistants, National Commission on Certification of *See* National Commission on Certification of Physician Assistants.

physician, attending *See* attending physician.

physician, board-certified *See* board-certified physician.

physician, board-eligible *See* board-eligible.

physician, chiropractic *See* chiropractor.

physician - clinical, public health *See* public health physician - clinical.

physician compliance *See* compliance.

physician, contract *See* contract physician.

physician credentialing A process of evaluating a physician's competence, which includes assessing his or her education, licensure, and specialty certification and conferring hospital privileges with the goal of protecting public safety. *See also* certification; credentialing; licensure; physician.

physician, critical care *See* critical care physician.

physician director of quality assurance A full-time or part-time physician who directs or advises medical staff concerning issues of clinical quality and performance and oversees and gives clinical credibility to the organization's quality assurance or related program. The physician usually works closely with a quality assurance manager or coordinator to form a clinical/administrative team and typically assists the coordinator and other staff with clinical judgments and day-to-day communications with department chiefs or other medical staff members. Other functions include chairing the hospitalwide or medical staff quality assurance committee and, with department chiefs, following up problems or potential problems referred to their departments for study and action. A physician quality assurance director generally reports to the medical director or medical staff executive committee. *See also* medical staff; quality assurance; quality assurance program.

physician, emergency *See* emergency physician.

physician, emergency department *See* emergency physician.

physician, emergency medicine *See* emergency

physician.

physician, emergency room *See* emergency physician.

physician epidemiologist *See* medical epidemiologist.

physician executive A physician whose primary professional responsibility is management of a health care organization. *See also* executive; health care organization; physician.

Physician Executives, American College of *See* American College of Physician Executives.

physician extender *See* physician assistant.

physician, hospital-based *See* hospital-based physician.

physician-hospital organization (PHO) A legal entity formed by a hospital and a group of physicians to further mutual interests and to achieve market objectives. A PHO generally combines physicians and a hospital into a single organization for the purpose of obtaining payer contracts. Doctors maintain ownership of their practices. They agree to accept managed care patients according to the terms of a professional services agreement with the PHO. The PHO serves as a collective negotiating and contracting unit. The PHO typically is owned and governed jointly by a hospital and shareholder physicians. *See also* group practice without walls; integrated provider; management services organization; medical foundation; organization.

physician, impaired *See* physician impairment.

physician impairment The inability of a physician to practice medicine with reasonable skill and with safety to patients due to a disability, such as alcohol or drug abuse, mental illness, handicap, or senility. *See also* impaired health care provider; impairment.

physician licensing *See* medical licensure.

physician licensure *See* medical licensure.

physician member of the medical staff A doctor of medicine or osteopathic physician who, by virtue of education, training, and demonstrated competence, is granted medical staff membership and clinical privileges by a health care organization to perform specified diagnostic or therapeutic procedures. *See also* medical staff; physician; physician credentialing.

physician, nonparticipating *See* nonparticipating provider.

physician, nuclear *See* nuclear medicine physician.

physician, nuclear medicine *See* nuclear medicine physician.

Physician Nurses, National Association of *See* National Association of Physician Nurses.

physician, osteopathic *See* osteopathic physician.

physician, participating *See* participating physician.

physician-patient privilege In law, a privilege protecting communications between a physician and a patient in the course of their professional relationship from disclosure unless consent is given by the patient. This privilege is statutory and did not exist under common law. Its purpose is to allow persons to secure medical service without the fear of betrayal or humiliation. This privilege, however, does not hold if a physician examines a patient for a purpose other than treatment, such as by court order (determining sanity or obtaining a blood sample to determine intoxication). The privilege does not preclude a physician from giving expert opinion testimony in response to a hypothetical question involving the physical or mental condition of the patient when such testimony is not dependent on information protected by the privilege. In general, the privilege does not apply to a nurse, unless acting as the doctor's assistant, medical students, dentists, pharmacists, or chiropractors. It does not extend after the death of the patient. *Synonym*: doctor-patient privilege. *See also* patient; physician; privileged communication; psychotherapist-patient privilege.

Physician Payment Reform (OBRA '89) Legislation enacted that provides for a major change in the Medicare physician payment rules enacted in 1992 and stronger enforcement of restricting "antitrust" and financial relationships with clinical laboratories and equipment providers. *See also* antitrust acts; clinical laboratory; Medicare; physician.

Physician Payment Review Commission (PPRC) (PhysPRC) A federal advisory body created in 1986 by Congress to design reasonable and rational payments to physicians by Medicare. After three years of study and consultation, the commission recommended that the work of William Hsiao and his colleagues at Harvard University in developing the resource-based relative-value scale be adopted as the method used to revamp the Medicare fee schedule. *See also* Medicare; resource-based relative-value scale.

physician, pediatric emergency *See* pediatric emergency physician.

physician, personal *See* personal physician.

physician, primary care *See* primary care

physician.

physician profile A longitudinal or cross-sectional statistical summary of physician-specific objective health care data used to assess and improve health care delivery. *See also* physician; physician profiling; profile.

physician profiling A process of aggregation and analysis of physician-related health care data, often in the form of tables or graphs, representing distinctive features or characteristics of a physician or group of physicians. *See also* physician profile; profile; profiling.

Physician Program, Impaired *See* Impaired Physician Program.

physician, provider-based *See* provider-based physician.

Physician Recruiters, National Association of *See* National Association of Physician Recruiters.

physician recruitment Locating, soliciting, and attracting physicians to a hospital or area. *See also* physician; recruitment.

physician, resident *See* medical resident.

Physicians Abroad, Association of Haitian *See* Association of Haitian Physicians Abroad.

physician, salaried *See* salaried physician.

Physicians in America, Association of Philippine *See* Association of Philippine Physicians in America.

Physicians, American Academy of Disability Evaluating *See* American Academy of Disability Evaluating Physicians.

Physicians, American Academy of Family *See* American Academy of Family Physicians.

Physicians, American Academy of Sports *See* American Academy of Sports Physicians.

Physicians, American Association of Naturopathic *See* American Association of Naturopathic Physicians.

Physicians, American Association of Public Health *See* American Association of Public Health Physicians.

Physicians, American Association of Senior *See* American Association of Senior Physicians.

Physicians, American Association of Testifying *See* American Association of Testifying Physicians.

Physicians, American Board of Quality Assurance and Utilization Review *See* American Board of Quality Assurance and Utilization Review Physicians.

Physicians, American College of *See* American College of Physicians.

Physicians, American College of Chest *See* American College of Chest Physicians.

Physicians, American College of Emergency *See* American College of Emergency Physicians.

Physicians, American College of Nuclear *See* American College of Nuclear Physicians.

Physicians, American College of Osteopathic Emergency *See* American College of Osteopathic Emergency Physicians.

Physicians, American Society of Bariatric *See* American Society of Bariatric Physicians.

Physicians, American Society of Handicapped *See* American Society of Handicapped Physicians.

Physicians, American Society of Psychoanalytic *See* American Society of Psychoanalytic Physicians.

physician's assistant *See* physician assistant.

Physician's Assistants in Cardio-Vascular Surgery, Association of *See* Association of Physician's Assistants in Cardio-Vascular Surgery.

physician's associate *See* physician assistant.

Physicians, Association of American *See* Association of American Physicians.

Physicians, Association of American Indian *See* Association of American Indian Physicians.

Physicians Association of Computer Medicine, American *See* American Physicians Association of Computer Medicine.

Physicians Association, Federal *See* Federal Physicians Association.

Physician's Association, National Osteopathic Women *See* National Osteopathic Women Physician's Association.

Physicians, Association of Pakistani *See* Association of Pakistani Physicians.

Physicians, Association of Professional Baseball *See* Association of Professional Baseball Physicians.

Physicians Association, Renal *See* Renal Physicians Association.

Physicians Association, Turkish American *See* Turkish American Physicians Association.

Physicians Committee for Responsible Medicine (PCRM) A national organization founded in 1985 composed of 30,000 physicians, scientists, health professionals, and other persons interested in increasing public awareness about the importance of preventive medicine and nutrition. It also raises scientific and ethical questions about the use of animals in medical research. It supports research in US agricultural policies and develops programs to encourage a shift in agricultural subsidies toward healthful crops. *See also* nutrition; preventive medicine.

Physicians' Current Procedural Terminology (CPT) A systematic listing and coding of procedures and services performed by physicians that is widely used for coding in billing and payment for physician services. The book is divided into five sections: medicine (except anesthesiology), anesthesiology, surgery, radiology, and pathology and laboratory. Each procedure or service is identified with a five-digit code, such as a radiologic examination of the skull (complete, minimum of four views, with or without stereo) has the code 70260. *CPT* is published by the American Medical Association. *See also* American Medical Association; coding.

Physicians and Dentists, National Association of VA *See* National Association of VA Physicians and Dentists.

Physicians and Dentists, Union of American *See* Union of American Physicians and Dentists.

Physicians' Desk Reference (PDR) A compendium of labeling information on pharmaceutical and diagnostic products, published annually by Medical Economics Data. Sections include full product information (information found in package inserts required by law) for most pharmaceuticals, both prescription and over the counter, product overviews for selected drugs and accurate photographs of many products for identification. Information is also provided on active and inactive ingredients, educational materials, pregnancy categories used in drug labeling, poison control centers, and procedures for reporting drug and vaccine adverse events. *See also* compendium; package insert; *PDR for Nonprescription Drugs.*

physician search firm A company that recruits physicians to fill positions nationwide. *See also* physician; recruitment.

Physicians Education Network (PEN) A national organization founded in 1977 composed of ophthalmologists and other individuals interested in promoting consumer safety legislation; opposing legislation that could allow lower medical standards; and promoting required referral legislation in each state, which would require optometrists to refer patients to ophthalmologists for any medical treatment or prescription. It campaigns against optometric drug use legislation. *See also* network; ophthalmology; optometry.

Physicians Fellowship for Medicine in Israel, American *See* American Physicians Fellowship for Medicine in Israel.

Physicians Forum (PF) A national organization founded in 1939 composed of physicians, particularly those holding salaried positions, who work for health care as a human right. It promotes development of a national health service with a single class of medical care for all, financed by a progressive income tax surcharge for health. *See also* national health service.

Physicians Guilds, National Federation of Catholic *See* National Federation of Catholic Physicians Guilds.

physician shortage area A geographic area with an inadequate supply of physicians, usually defined as an area having a physician-to-population ratio of less than some defined standard, such as 1 to 4,000. *See also* medically underserved area; physician.

Physicians for Human Rights (PHR) A national organization founded in 1986 composed of 2,000 health professionals who bring the skills of the medical profession to the protection of human rights. It specifically works to prevent the participation of doctors in torture, defend imprisoned health professionals, prevent physical and psychological abuse of citizens by governments, and provide medical and humanitarian aid to victims of repression. *See also* humanitarian; human rights.

Physicians for Human Rights, American Association of *See* American Association of Physicians for Human Rights.

Physicians for Human Rights, Bay Area *See* Bay Area Physicians for Human Rights.

Physicians, National Association of Emergency Medical Service *See* National Association of Emergency Medical Physicians.

Physicians, National Association of Managed Care *See* National Association of Managed Care Physicians.

physician specialist *See* medical specialist.

Physicians Poetry Association, American *See* American Physicians Poetry Association.

physician, sports medicine *See* sports medicine physician.

physicians, reappointment of *See* reappointment of physicians.

Physicians for Research in Cost-Effectiveness (PRICE) A national organization founded in 1989 composed of 1,500 physicians interested in sharing information and learning about cost-effective medical care. It acts as an educational forum and sponsors specialty committees. *See also* cost-effective; cost-effectiveness analysis.

Physicians for Social Responsibility (PSR) A national organization founded in 1961 composed of 55,000 medical professionals with doctoral degrees, medical students, and other persons concerned with the threat of nuclear war. It educates the public on the medical effects of nuclear war and nuclear weapons and on the implications of national policy and legislative actions on arms control issues.

Physicians, Society of Air Force *See* Society of Air Force Physicians.

Physicians and Surgeons, American Association of Podiatric *See* American Association of Podiatric Physicians and Surgeons.

Physicians and Surgeons, Association of American *See* Association of American Physicians and Surgeons.

Physicians and Surgeons, Interamerican College of *See* Interamerican College of Physicians and Surgeons.

physicians' and surgeons' professional liability insurance Malpractice insurance. *See* medical malpractice insurance.

Physicians and Surgeons (of United States of America), Royal College of *See* Royal College of Physicians and Surgeons (of United States of America).

Physicians, Uniformed Services Academy of Family *See* Uniformed Services Academy of Family Physicians.

Physicians, United States Association of *See* American Association of Ayurvedic Medicine.

Physicians Who Care (PWC) A national organization founded in 1985 composed of 2,800 independent physicians who are interested in educating patients about making wise choices in health care between health maintenance organizations and the more traditional independent physician's practice. *See also* health maintenance organization.

physician, teaching *See* teaching physician.

physician volume The number of a procedure performed (such as an endoscopy) or a condition (such as acute myocardial infarction) treated by individual physicians. *See also* physician; volume.

Physicists in Medicine, American Association of *See* American Association of Physicists in Medicine.

physics The science of matter and energy and of interactions between the two, grouped in fields, such as electromagnetism, atomic and nuclear physics, and solid-state physics. *See also* biophysics; diagnostic radiological physics; health physics; magnetism; medical nuclear physics; medical physics; physical science; radiological physics.

Physics, American Board of Health *See* American Board of Health Physics.

physics, bio- *See* biophysics.

physics, diagnostic radiological *See* diagnostic radiological physics.

physics, health *See* health physics.

physics, medical *See* medical physics.

physics, medical nuclear *See* medical nuclear physics.

physics, radiological *See* radiological physics.

Physics Society, Health *See* Health Physics Society.

physics, therapeutic radiological *See* therapeutic radiological physics.

physiognomy The determination of temperament and character from facial features. *See also* phrenology; temperament.

physiological Normal, as in a physiological, not pathological, heart murmur. *See also* physiology.

physiological chemist *See* biochemist.

physiological psychology The branch of psychology that examines the relationship between behavior and body structures or functions, particularly the workings of the nervous system. Physiological psychologists explore the functions of the brain, how hormones affect behavior, and the physical processes involved in learning and emotions. *See also* behavior; nervous system; physiology; psychology.

Physiological Research, Society for Psycho- *See* Society for Psychophysiological Research.

physiological saline A sterile solution of sodium chloride that is isotonic to body fluids in humans, used to temporarily maintain living tissue and as a solvent for parenterally administered drugs. *See also* Ringer's solution; saline.

Physiological Society, American *See* American Physiological Society.

Physiological Therapeutics, Council on Chiropractic *See* Council on Chiropractic Physiological Therapeutics.

physiologist An individual who specializes in physiology. *See also* physiology.

physiology The branch of biology that deals with

the functions of the living organism and its parts and of the physical and chemical factors and processes involved, as in renal (kidney) physiology or gastrointestinal physiology. *Compare* anatomy; structure. *See also* biology; electrophysiology; neurophysiology.

Physiology and Chronic Health Evaluation (APACHE), Acute   *See* Acute Physiology and Chronic Health Evaluation.

physiology, electro-   *See* electrophysiology.

physiology, neuro-   *See* neurophysiology.

Physiology, North American Society of Pacing and Electro-   *See* North American Society of Pacing and Electrophysiology.

physiology, patho-   *See* pathophysiology.

Physiology, Society for the Study of Male Psychology and   *See* Society for the Study of Male Psychology and Physiology.

physiotherapist   *See* physical therapist.

physiotherapy   *See* physical therapy.

physique   The body's proportions, muscular development, and appearance, as in a long-distance runner's physique. *See also* habitus.

PhysPRC   *See* Physician Payment Review Commission.

pica   The craving and ingestion of particular, often bizarre, substances, such as earth, clay, cornstarch, ice, baking soda, ashes, paint, paraffin, and coffee grounds. It occurs in pregnancy, some mental disorders, and some cases of nutritional deficiency. *See also* malnutrition; nutrition.

PID   *See* pelvic inflammatory disease.

piece of work   A remarkable person, achievement, or product.

piecework   Work performed by outside contractors who are paid by the piece. Pieceworkers typically agree to perform certain production services on an individual basis; they often do piecework in their homes.

pie chart   A circle representing a whole amount, with wedge-shaped sectors indicating the fraction in each category. *See also* chart.

pig   A lead container used to ship and store radioactive materials. *See also* radiation.

pile   *See* hemorrhoid.

pill   **1.** A small pellet or tablet containing pharmaceutical agents, taken by swallowing whole or by chewing. The active substance (or substances) is mixed with a vehicle (excipient), to confer cohesion and firmness. *See also* excipient; tablet. **2.** An oral contraceptive. *See also* oral contraceptive; morning-after pill.

pill, birth control   *See* oral contraceptive.

pill, morning-after   *See* morning-after pill.

Pilots Association, National EMS   *See* National EMS Pilots Association.

pilot study   A study designed to prove or test methods that may be used in full-scale plans. A pilot study reduces the investment risk in unproven methods. *See also* feasibility study.

ping-ponging   The process of passing a patient from one physician to another in a health program for unnecessary cursory examinations so that the program can charge the patient's third-party payer for a physician visit to each physician. The practice and term originated and is most common in Medicaid mills. *See also* family ganging; Medicaid; Medicaid mills.

pink eye   Acute conjunctivitis (inflammation of the delicate membrane that covers the exposed part of the eyeball). *See also* inflammation; membrane.

PIOP   *See* Pharmacists in Ophthalmic Practice.

pitch   The quality of a sound, which is determined by the frequency of vibration of a sound source; a high frequency produces a sound of high pitch. *See also* noise; sound.

pitfall   An unapparent or unexpected source of trouble or danger, as in diagnostic pitfalls in clinical medicine.

pituitary gland   A small endocrine gland attached to the base of the brain that secretes substances which control the other endocrine glands and influence growth, metabolism, and maturation. *Synonym:* pituitary body. *See also* endocrine; endocrinology; giant; gland; growth hormone; hormone; pediatric endocrinology.

Pituitary Program, National Hormone and   *See* National Hormone and Pituitary Program.

pivotal norm   *See* behavioral norms.

PL   Abbreviation for Public Law (or federal statute). The term is always followed by a number identifying the session number of the Congress that enacted the statute and the sequential number of the statute passed by that Congress.

PLA   Abbreviation for "person living with AIDS." *See also* PLWA; PWA.

placebo   Any therapeutic procedure or chemically inert substance, such as sugar or distilled water, or less-than-effective dose of a harmless substance prescribed and administered as if it were an effective dose of a needed drug. Originally, a placebo was given solely for the psychophysiological effects of the treatment. More recently, placebos have been administered to a control group in a controlled clinical trial so that the specific and nonspecific effects of the experimental treatment can be distinguished. In such trials, the experimental treatment must produce better results than the placebo to be considered effective. A physician may deceptively, but ethically, prescribe a placebo to a patient if the condition being treated has a high response rate to placebo, if the alternative to placebo is continued illness or a drug with known toxicity, and if the patient demands a prescription to improve his or her condition. *See also* ethics; placebo effect; suggestion.

placebo effect A usually beneficial change in a patient following a particular treatment that arises from the patient's expectations concerning the treatment and the power of suggestion, rather than from the treatment itself. *See also* halo effect; placebo.

placenta An organ that develops within the pregnant uterus about the third month of pregnancy, through which the fetus receives nourishment and oxygen and the mother's body removes fetal waste products. *See also* abruptio placenta; placenta previa.

placenta, abruptio *See* abruptio placenta.

placenta previa A placenta that develops in the lower uterine segment, in the zone of dilatation, so that it covers or adjoins the internal cervical opening. Painless hemorrhage in the last trimester, particularly during the eighth month, is the most common symptom. Placenta previa is an important cause of maternal death and stillbirth (fetal death). *See also* abruptio placenta; maternal death; stillbirth.

plaintiff The party that initially institutes a lawsuit in a court. In a personal action, he or she seeks a remedy in a court of justice for an injury to, or a withholding of, his or her rights. *Compare* defendant. *See also* lawsuit; malicious prosecution.

plan **1.** A scheme, program, or method worked out beforehand for the accomplishment of an objective, as in a retirement plan. *See also* retirement plan. **2.** In organizations, a sequence of predetermined actions management has chosen to complete future organizational objectives. Planning is one of the primary responsibilities of organizational managers. *See also* care plan; control plan; health plan; home plan; host

plan; nursing care plan; participating plan; quality plan.

plan, Blue Cross *See* Blue Cross plan.

plan, Blue Cross/Blue Shield *See* Blue Cross/Blue Shield plan.

plan, Blue Shield *See* Blue Shield plan.

plan, care *See* care plan.

plan, clinical practice *See* medical practice plan.

plan, control *See* control plan.

plan of correction, conditional accreditation A health care organization's written plan, approved by staff of the Joint Commission on Accreditation of Healthcare Organizations, that outlines the actions that the organization will take to address compliance issues that caused the Accreditation Committee to make a decision of conditional accreditation. The plan is the basis for the follow-up survey at a specified time, once the plan is approved. *See also* Accreditation Committee; conditional accreditation; follow-up survey; Joint Commission on Accreditation of Healthcare Organizations.

plan of correction, plant, technology, and safety management A health care organization's written plan that must be approved by staff of the Joint Commission on Accreditation of Healthcare Organizations, detailing the procedures to be taken to correct existing life safety deficiencies and lists the extraordinary life safety measures to be implemented to temporarily reduce the hazards associated with the deficiencies. *See also* Joint Commission on Accreditation of Healthcare Organizations; life safety management program; plant, technology, and safety management.

plan, Delta Dental *See* Delta Dental plan.

plan, dental *See* dental insurance.

plan, disaster preparedness *See* disaster preparedness plan.

Plan-Do-Check-Act (PDCA) cycle A planning and improvement methodology in which improvements are planned and tested for feasibility. *Synonyms:* Deming cycle; Shewhart cycle. *See also* continuous quality improvement; FADE process; FOCUS-PDCA.

plan, employee health benefit *See* employee health benefit plan.

Planes, The Angel *See* The Angel Planes.

plan, faculty practice *See* medical practice plan.

plan, fee-for-service *See* fee-for-service.

plan, health *See* health plan.

plan, home   *See* home plan.

plan, host   *See* host plan.

plan, incentive benefit   *See* incentive benefit plan.

plan, incentive pay   *See* incentive pay plan.

plan, individual practice   *See* individual practice plan.

plan, Keogh   *See* Keogh plan.

plan, managed care   *See* managed care.

plan, managed indemnity   *See* managed indemnity plan.

plan, marketing   *See* marketing plan.

plan, medical practice   *See* medical practice plan.

Planned Parenthood Federation of America   An educational, research, and medical services organization concerned with fertility-related health topics, including abortion, contraception, family planning, and international population control. *See also* abortion; contraception.

planner, health   *See* health planner.

planning   The conscious design of desired future states. *See also* plan; contingency planning; strategic planning.

Planning Association, American Health   *See* American Health Planning Association.

planning, contingency   *See* contingency planning.

planning, corporate   *See* corporate planning.

planning and development agency, state health   *See* state health planning and development agency.

planning, discharge   *See* discharge planning.

Planning and Evaluation, Office of Health   *See* Office of Health Planning and Evaluation.

planning, family   *See* family planning.

planning, health   *See* health planning.

planning, Hoshin   *See* Hoshin planning.

planning, long-term   *See* strategic planning.

Planning and Marketing of the American Hospital Association, Society for Healthcare   *See* Society for Healthcare Planning and Marketing of the American Hospital Association.

planning, natural family   *See* natural family planning.

planning, organizational   *See* organizational planning.

planning, quality   *See* quality planning.

planning, social work discharge   *See* social work discharge planning.

planning, strategic   *See* strategic planning.

plan, nursing care   *See* nursing care plan.

plan, participating   *See* participating plan.

plan, patient care   *See* care plan.

plan, patient treatment   *See* care plan.

plan, prepayment   *See* prepayment plan.

plan, point-of-service   *See* point-of-service plan.

plan, quality   *See* quality plan.

plan, retirement   *See* retirement plan.

plan, state health   *See* state health plan.

plant   Assets comprising land, buildings, machinery, natural resources, furniture and fixtures, and all other equipment permanently used. In a more narrow sense, "plant" refers to only buildings or only land and buildings. *See also* fixed asset; maintenance department.

plantar verrucae   *See* verrucae.

plant engineer   *See* administrative engineer.

plant, technology, and safety management (PTSM)   An organizational management program designed to provide a physical environment free of hazards and to manage staff activities to reduce the risk of human injury. *See also* equipment management; plan of correction, plant, technology, and safety management; plant; *PTSM*; safety management.

plaque   **1.** A fatty deposit of material on the inner lining of an arterial wall, characteristic of atherosclerosis. *See also* atherosclerosis; percutaneous transluminal angiography; transient ischemic attack. **2.** A film of mucus and bacteria on a tooth surface. *See also* dentistry; tooth.

plasma   *See* blood plasma.

plasmapheresis   A process in which plasma is taken from donated blood and the remaining components, mostly red blood cells, are returned to the donor. *See also* blood plasma.

plasmid   An extrachromosomal genetic element existing and replicating autonomously in the cytoplasm of a cell. Bacterial plasmids are closed loops of deoxyribonucleic acid (DNA) consisting of only a few genes, capable, for example, of conferring antibiotic resistance on the host cell. Plasmids are used in genetic engineering. *See also* cell; chromosome; deoxyribonucleic acid; genetic engineering.

plaster   Fabric coated with an adhesive substance and applied to the skin for protective and medicinal purposes. *See also* cast; plaster of Paris.

plaster of Paris   Powdered calcium sulphate, obtained by heating gypsum (hydrated calcium sulphate) so that it loses three-quarters of its water of crystallization. On mixing with water, plaster of Paris sets and rapidly hardens. It is particularly useful for making casts and bandages for purposes of immobilization. *See also* cast; emergency medicine; orthopaedic/orthopedic surgery; plaster.

Plastic and Reconstructive Surgeons, American Society of *See* American Society of Plastic and Reconstructive Surgeons.

Plastic and Reconstructive Surgery, American Academy of Facial *See* American Academy of Facial Plastic and Reconstructive Surgery.

Plastic and Reconstructive Surgical Nurses, American Society of *See* American Society of Plastic and Reconstructive Surgical Nurses.

plastic surgeon A physician who specializes in plastic surgery. *See also* plastic surgery; surgeon.

Plastic Surgeons, American Association of *See* American Association of Plastic Surgeons.

plastic surgery The branch and specialty of medicine dealing with the repair and reconstruction of defects of form and function of the skin and its underlying musculoskeletal system, with emphasis on the craniofacial structures, the oropharynx, the upper and lower limbs, the breast, and the external genitalia. It also includes aesthetic surgery of structures with undesirable form, the design and transfer of flaps, the transplantation of tissues, the replantation of structures, excisional surgery, the management of complex wounds, and the use of alloplastic materials. Surgery of the hand is a subspecialty of plastic surgery. *Synonym*: reconstructive surgery. *See also* alloplastic; cosmetic surgery; mammaplasty; rhinoplasty; surgery.

Plastic Surgery, American Board of *See* American Board of Plastic Surgery.

Plastic Surgery, American Society for Aesthetic *See* American Society for Aesthetic Plastic Surgery.

Plastic Surgery Facilities, American Association for Accreditation of Ambulatory *See* American Association for Accreditation of Ambulatory Plastic Surgery Facilities.

Plastic Surgery Research Council (PSRC) A national organization founded in 1955 composed of 232 members interested in fostering fundamental research in the fields of plastic and reconstructive surgery. *See also* plastic surgery.

platelet A small disk-shaped cellular element of blood that contains no hemoglobin and is essential for blood clotting (coagulation). A normal platelet count is between 200,000 and 300,000 platelets per one cubic milliliter of blood. *See also* apheresis; blood cell.

plausible Apparently valid, likely, or acceptable; credible, as in a plausible assertion.

play therapy A form of psychotherapy for children in which play with games and toys is used to gain insight into the child's feelings and thoughts and to help treat conflicts and psychological problems. *See also* child and adolescent psychiatry; psychotherapy; therapy.

pleading, responsive *See* responsive pleading.

pleadings The formal written documents, in legal format, filed with the court by the parties that set out the plaintiff's allegations (cause of action) and the defendant's answer to those allegations. Pleadings generally include the complaint, answer, response to affirmative defenses raised in the answer, third-party claims, counterclaims, and the answer to each. *See also* affirmative defense; allegation; answer; complaint; responsive pleading.

pleasure principle In psychoanalytic theory, the tendency to pursue actions or objects that provide immediate gratification of instinctual drives and to avoid discomfort and pain. *Compare* reality principle.

pleonasm The use of more words than are required to express an idea.

plethora **1.** Congestion with blood. **2.** An overabundance or excess.

pleurisy Inflammation of the lining of the lungs causing chest pain (pleurodynia), fever, and dry cough. *See also* inflammation; lung.

plexor A small, rubberheaded hammer used in examination or diagnosis by percussion, as in elicitation of a knee jerk reflex.

plexus Any network of vessels or nerves, as in brachial plexus. *See also* network.

plot To locate points on a graph or to draw a graph; a graph so produced. *See also* graph.

plotter In computer science, a computer output device that draws graphs or pictures, usually by moving a pen. *Synonyms*: plotting board; plotting table. *See also* computer.

plotting board *See* plotter.

plotting table *See* plotter.

plumbism Lead poisoning. *See also* lead; poison.

pluralism **1.** In ethics, identifying more than one intrinsic good. *See also* ethics. **2.** A concept that advocates that people of diverse ethnic, racial, religious, or social groups retain their culture or beliefs while living elsewhere. *See also* culture; religion.

PLWA   Abbreviation for "person living with AIDS." *See also* PLA; PWA.

PMA   *See* Pharmaceutical Manufacturers Association; Precision Measurements Association.

PMRS   *See* Parachute Medical Rescue Service.

PMS   *See* People's Medical Society; premenstrual syndrome.

PN   Abbreviation for "pneumonia" or "practical nurse." *See* licensed practical nurse; licensed vocational nurse; pneumonia.

pneumatic antishock garment (PASG)   *See* MAST.

pneumococcus   A gram-positive bacterium called *Streptococcus pneumoniae* that is the most common cause of bacterial pneumonia. It also causes meningitis and other infectious diseases. *See also* bacteria; meningitis; pneumonia.

pneumoconiosis   A lung disease produced by the inhalation and pulmonary deposition of dusts of occupational or other environmental origin. Examples of pneumoconioses are anthracosis or black lung disease, siderosis, silicosis, and asbestosis. *See also* black lung disease; brown lung.

Pneumocystis   A genus of microorganism thought to be protozoa but its life-cycle has not been established with certainty. *Pneumocystis carinii* is the causative agent of a life-threatening form of pneumonia that characteristically occurs as an opportunistic infection. *See also* opportunistic infection; pneumonia; protozoa.

pneumonia (PN)   Inflammation of the lungs with solidification of its air spaces, usually caused by infection with bacteria, viruses, fungi, or rickettsiae. Symptoms include fever, chills, cough, chest pain, and shortness of breath. *See also* inflammation; pneumococcus; *Pneumocystis*; pneumonitis; rales.

pneumonic   **1.** Pertaining to the lungs, as in pneumonic infiltrate. **2.** Pertaining to pneumonia or pneumonitis. *See also* pneumonia; pneumonitis.

pneumonitis   Inflammation of the lung tissues from any cause, including chemical and physical agents. *See also* inflammation; pneumonia.

pneumothorax   Collection of air or gas in the pleural cavity of the chest, causing the lung to collapse. Symptoms include sharp chest pain and difficulty in breathing. *See also* emergency medicine; thoracic surgery.

PNP   *See* pediatric nurse practitioner.

pocket computer   A computer small enough to be carried in one hand. Programmable calculators, which are capable of storing instructions and are therefore on the verge of being true computers, were introduced in the 1970s. Laptop computers and portable computers are much larger than pocket computers. *See also* computer; microcomputer; portable computer.

podagra   *See* gout.

Podiatric Administration, American Academy of   *See* American Academy of Podiatric Administration.

podiatric assistant   An individual who assists a podiatrist in tasks, such as exposing and developing x-rays; taking and recording patient histories; assisting in biomechanical evaluations and negative castings; preparing and sterilizing instruments and equipment; providing the patient with postoperative instructions; applying surgical dressings; preparing the patient for treatment, padding, and strapping; and performing routine office procedures. *Synonym:* podiatric medical assistant. *See also* podiatric medicine.

Podiatric Circulatory Society, American   *See* American Podiatric Circulatory Society.

Podiatric Dermatology, American Society of   *See* American Society of Podiatric Dermatology.

podiatric medical assistant   *See* podiatric assistant.

Podiatric Medical Assistants, American Society of   *See* American Society of Podiatric Medical Assistants.

Podiatric Medical Association, American   *See* American Podiatric Medical Association.

Podiatric Medical Association, National   *See* National Podiatric Medical Association.

Podiatric Medical Boards, Federation of   *See* Federation of Podiatric Medical Boards.

Podiatric Medical Education, Council on   *See* Council on Podiatric Medical Education.

Podiatric Medical Examiners, National Board of   *See* National Board of Podiatric Medical Examiners.

podiatric medicine   The profession of the health sciences dealing with the examination, diagnosis, treatment, and prevention of diseases, conditions, and malfunctions affecting the human foot and its related or governing structures, by use of medical, surgical, or other means. Formerly called chiropody. *See also* bunion.

Podiatric Medicine, American Association of Colleges of   *See* American Association of Colleges of Podiatric Medicine.

Podiatric Medicine, American Society of *See* American Society of Podiatric Medicine.

podiatric orthopedics One of three specialty areas of podiatric medicine currently recognized by the American Podiatric Medical Association in which the podiatric practitioner can become certified as a specialist by meeting criteria, including written and oral examinations, and demonstrating knowledge and experience in the specialty. *See also* American Podiatric Medical Association; podiatric public health; podiatric surgery.

Podiatric Orthopedics, American Board of *See* American Board of Podiatric Orthopedics.

Podiatric Physicians and Surgeons, American Association of *See* American Association of Podiatric Physicians and Surgeons.

podiatric practitioner *See* podiatrist.

podiatric public health One of three specialty areas of podiatric medicine currently recognized by the American Podiatric Medical Association in which the podiatric practitioner can become certified as a specialist by meeting criteria including written and oral examinations, and demonstrating knowledge and experience in the specialty. *See also* American Podiatric Medical Association; podiatric orthopedics; podiatric surgery; public health.

Podiatric Radiologists, American College of *See* American College of Podiatric Radiologists.

podiatric specialist A podiatrist who specializes in an area of podiatric medicine including podiatric orthopedics, podiatric public health, or podiatric surgery. *See also* podiatric medicine; podiatric specialties; specialist.

podiatric specialties Specialty areas of podiatric medicine, including podiatric orthopedics, podiatric public health, and podiatric surgery. *See also* podiatric medicine; podiatric orthopedics; podiatric public health; podiatric surgery; specialty.

Podiatric Sports Medicine, American Academy of *See* American Academy of Podiatric Sports Medicine.

podiatric surgery One of three specialty areas of podiatric medicine currently recognized by the American Podiatric Medical Association in which a podiatric practitioner can become certified as a specialist by meeting criteria, including written and oral examinations, and demonstrating knowledge and experience in the specialty. *See also* American Podiatric Medical Association; podiatric medicine; surgery.

Podiatric Surgery, American Board of *See* American Board of Podiatric Surgery.

podiatrist A health professional qualified by education and authorized by law to practice podiatric medicine. Formerly called chiropodist. *Synonyms:* doctor of podiatric medicine; foot surgeon; podiatric practitioner. *See also* podiatric medicine.

Podiatrists, American Association of Hospital *See* American Association of Hospital Podiatrists.

podiatry *See* podiatric medicine.

Podiatry Executives, Conference of *See* Conference of Podiatry Executives.

podopediatrics The study of children's foot ailments. *See also* pediatrics; podiatric medicine.

Podopediatrics, American College of *See* American College of Podopediatrics.

poetic justice An outcome in which virtue is rewarded and vice punished, often in an especially appropriate or ironic manner. *See also* justice.

Poetry Association, American Physicians *See* American Physicians Poetry Association.

Poetry, Association for Applied *See* Association for Applied Poetry.

poetry therapist An individual who specializes in poetry therapy. *See also* poetry therapy.

poetry therapy The use of poetry for healing and personal growth in patients with mental states ranging from neurosis to acute psychosis, as well as in people with physical or learning disabilities. Methods of using poetry for therapy include reading poems and encouraging clients to write their own poetry. The purpose is to lead a person into talking or writing about himself or herself and bringing out emotions not previously shown or discussed. *See also* art therapy; dance therapy; drama therapy; manual arts therapy; music therapy; recreational therapy.

Poetry Therapy, National Association for *See* National Association for Poetry Therapy.

point-of-service plan A type of health plan allowing the covered person to choose to receive a service from a participating or a nonparticipating provider, with different benefit levels associated with the use of participating providers. Point-of-service can be provided in several ways, including, for example, a health maintenance organization allowing its members to obtain limited services from nonparticipating providers, or a preferred provider organization being used to provide both participating and non-participating levels of coverage and access. *See also* health care provider; health maintenance organization; health plan; preferred provider organization.

poison A substance that when inhaled, ingested, or absorbed impairs health or causes death. *See also* antidote; carbon monoxide; cyanide; lead; poison control center.

poison control center A facility that provides information concerning poisons and the management of poisoning in emergency situations. *See also* medical toxicology; poison.

Poison Control Centers, American Association of *See* American Association of Poison Control Centers.

Poisoning, Alliance to End Childhood Lead *See* Alliance to End Childhood Lead Poisoning.

poisoning, blood *See* septicemia.

poisoning, food *See* food poisoning.

Poisson distribution A type of probability distribution typically applied to distributions that are not continuous. Named after Simeon Denis Poisson (1781-1840), French mathematician. *See also* probability distribution.

polemic **1.** An argument that refutes or attacks a specific opinion or doctrine. **2.** An individual engaged in or inclined to polemics. *See also* polemics.

polemics The art or practice of controversy, argumentation, or refutation. *See also* polemic.

policies and procedures *See* policy; procedure.

policies and procedures manual A compendium of an organization's (or a component thereof) current and formally adopted policies and the methodological procedures supporting them, as in a hospital's policy and procedures manual. *See also* policy.

policy **1.** The act, method, or manner of proceeding in some process or course of action adopted and pursued by an individual or a organization. **2.** Any course of action or way of doing something adopted as proper, advantageous, or expedient. The US Congress, for example, makes policy principally by writing legislation and conducting oversight activities. In insurance, a policy is the written contract of insurance between an insurer and the insured. In the executive branch of the federal government, policies are documents that interpret or enlarge upon rules, sometimes referred to as guidelines. Policies bear the same relationship to rules (regulations) as rules do to law, except that unlike regulations, they do not have the force of law. *See also* confidentiality and dis-

closure policy; fiscal policy; health policy; participating policy.

Policy Advisory Center, Health *See* Health Policy Advisory Center.

Policy, Americans for a Sound AIDS *See* Americans for a Sound AIDS Policy.

policy analysis A set of techniques used to determine the effects of a policy before they actually occur. *See also* analysis; policy.

policy analyst An individual who studies the effects of a proposed or actual policy. *See also* policy analysis.

policy, confidentiality and disclosure *See* confidentiality and disclosure policy.

Policy Council, Economic *See* Economic Policy Council.

policy, fiscal *See* fiscal policy.

Policy Forum, National Health *See* National Health Policy Forum.

policy, health *See* health policy.

policyholder An individual or other entity who owns an insurance policy. *Synonym*: policyowner. *See also* insurance policy.

policy, insurance *See* insurance policy.

policy, medigap *See* medigap policy.

Policy, National Council on Alternative Health Care *See* National Council on Alternative Health Care Policy.

policy, occurrence *See* occurrence policy.

policy, open-door *See* open-door policy.

policyowner *See* policyholder.

policy, participating *See* participating policy.

policy, public *See* public policy.

Policy, Public Voice for Food and Health *See* Public Voice for Food and Health Policy.

policy, quality *See* quality policy.

Policy, Research, and Evaluation, National Advisory Council for *See* National Advisory Council for Policy, Research, and Evaluation.

policy, trolley car *See* trolley car policy.

polio *See* poliomyelitis.

poliomyelitis An acute viral infection, with a worldwide distribution confined to primates. It is spread from person to person, the portal of entry being the gastrointestinal tract. In the vast majority of instances, infection produces either no symptoms at all or only those of an influenza-like illness. A proportion of patients, however, manifest signs of meningitis and a proportion of these develop the motor paralysis that was the much-feared complication of the epidemic disease in communities with good sanitation (and hence a low level of naturally acquired immunity) before the advent of active immunization programs. *Synonyms:* infantile paralysis; polio. *See also* poliovirus; Sabin vaccine; Salk vaccine; vaccine.

poliovirus The causative agent of poliomyelitis, consisting of a small non-enveloped ribonucleic acid virus belonging to the enterovirus genus. *See also* poliomyelitis; ribonucleic acid; virus.

political action committee (PAC) An organization formed by business, labor, or other special-interest groups to raise money and make contributions to the campaigns of political candidates whom they support. *See also* action organization.

Political Action Committee, American Medical *See* American Medical Political Action Committee.

political science The study of the processes, principles, and structure of government and of political institutions. *See also* politics; social science.

politics The art or science of government or governing, especially the governing of a political entity and the management of its internal and external affairs. *See also* government; ideology; political science.

Politics and the Life Sciences, Association for *See* Association for Politics and the Life Sciences.

pollen Microspores of seed plants containing male gametophytes, carried by wind or insects to plants for germination. Many pollens are potent allergens. *See also* allergy.

poll, public-opinion *See* public-opinion poll.

pollster An individual who takes public-opinion surveys. *Synonym:* polltaker. *See also* public opinion poll.

polltaker *See* pollster.

pollutant Something that pollutes, especially a waste material that contaminates air, soil, or water. *See also* pollution.

pollution Disposal of waste products into air, water, and soil, leading to harmful or undesirable effects on health or offensive, though not necessarily harmful, effects on health. *See also* Environmental Protection Agency; noise pollution; PCB; pollutant.

pollution, noise *See* noise pollution.

pollution, sound *See* noise pollution.

polyandry Multiple husbands. *Compare* polygyny. *See also* polygamy.

polygamy The practice of having more than one spouse concurrently, subdivided into polyandry and polygyny. *See also* polyandry; polygyny.

polygyny Multiple wives. *Compare* polyandry. *See also* polygamy.

polypharmacy The act of prescribing or administering more than one drug to a patient. The possibility of drug interaction must be considered in these cases. *See also* pharmacy.

Polysomnographic Technologists, Association of *See* Association of Polysomnographic Technologists.

polysomnographic technology The field dealing with the measurement and recording of multiple physiological activity, such as eye movement and heart rate, during sleep. *See also* sleep; sleep apnea; somnology; technology.

POMR *See* problem-oriented medical record.

pool, high-risk *See* high-risk pool.

pool nurse A registered nurse, licensed practical nurse, or licensed vocational nurse, who is not a member of the nursing staff of a health care organization but who is hired through an agency to provide patient care on a temporary basis when inadequate numbers of regular nursing staff are available to provide care. *Synonym:* agency nurse. *See also* licensed practical nurse; licensed vocational nurse; registered nurse.

pool, risk *See* risk pool.

poor Having little or no wealth and few or no possessions; needy; medically needy. *See also* medically needy; near poor; poverty; working poor.

poor, near *See* near poor.

poor, working *See* working poor.

poppy Any plant of the genus *Papaver* which includes the opium poppy, or of related genera *Meconopsis* and *Glaucium*. *See also* opium.

population 1. The inhabitants of a geographic area considered together. 2. The number of inhabitants of an area. *See also* overpopulation. 3. In statistics, a set of objects or individuals from which a sample is drawn. *See also* epidemiology; statistics.

Population Affairs, Office of *See* Office of Population Affairs.

population, indicator *See* indicator population.

population, medically underserved *See* medically underserved population.

population, over- *See* overpopulation.

population profile A longitudinal or cross-sectional statistical summary of population-specific objective health care data used to assess and improve health care delivery. *See also* population; population profiling; profile; profiling.

population profiling A process of aggregation and analysis of population-specific health care data, often in the form of tables or graphs, representing distinctive features or characteristics of a population. *See also* population profile; profile; profiling.

population, reference *See* reference population.

pornography The depicting of events calculated to arouse sexual excitement in the reader, listener, or beholder.

port In computers, a connection point for a peripheral device. *See also* peripherals.

portability The circumstance in which an individual is guaranteed health insurance coverage with a new employer, without a waiting period or having to meet additional deductible requirements, when the individual changes jobs or residence. *See also* health insurance.

portable computer A light microcomputer that can be carried easily. *See also* computer; microcomputer.

portable equipment *See* medical equipment.

position 1. A place or location. 2. A point of view or attitude on a certain question or issue. *See also* positioning; position paper.

positioning A marketing and public relations term used to describe the process and activities undertaken to change or solidify an organization's share of the market, or to change or solidify the image of the organization in the marketplace. *See also* marketing; position.

position, lithotomy *See* lithotomy position.

position paper A detailed report explaining, justifying, or recommending a particular course of action. *See also* position.

positive 1. Having a value greater than zero, as in positive correlation. *See also* positive correlation. 2. Indicating existence or presence of something; for example, presence of pregnancy indicated by a positive blood test. 3. Characterized by affirmation or cooperation, as in a positive approach to the assignment. *Compare* negativism.

positive, antibody *See* antibody positive.

positive correlation A direct association between two variables meaning that as one variable becomes large, the other also becomes large, and vice versa. Positive correlation is represented by a correlation coefficient greater than zero. *See also* correlation; correlation coefficient; negative correlation; positive; variable.

positive, false *See* false positive.

positive incentive *See* incentive.

positive predictive value (of a test) *See* predictive value of a positive test.

Positive Pregnancy and Parenting Fitness (PPPF) A national organization founded in 1982 composed of 350 nurses, childbirth educators, certified midwives and lay midwives, yoga instructors, physical therapists, psychologists, health care providers, and other persons interested in pregnancy and parenting education. It promotes a holistic approach to pregnancy and parenting and works to improve parent-child relationships in order to foster the development of strong family units. It supports increased availability of prenatal and neonatal health care. *See also* fitness; holistic health; pregnancy.

positive test, predictive value of a *See* predictive value of a positive test.

positive, true *See* true positive.

positron A positive electron, a particle having the mass of the electron but with a positive electric charge. *See also* positron emission tomography.

positron emission tomography (PET) An x-ray technique (photographing a single plane of a structure) in which a computer-generated image of a biological activity within the body is produced through the detection of gamma rays that are emitted when introduced radionuclides decay and release positrons. It is used to localize abnormalities in the brain and other organs by imaging a radioactive substance injected into the body that collects in the cells of these organs. *Synonym*: positron tomography. *See also* imaging; positron; tomography.

positron tomography *See* positron emission tomography.

POSNA *See* Pediatric Orthopaedic Society of North America.

posology The medical or pharmacological study of the dosages of medicines and drugs. *See also* dosage; drug.

Post Anesthesia Nurses, American Society of *See* American Society of Post Anesthesia Nurses.

Post Anesthesia Nursing Certification, American Board of *See* American Board of Post Anesthesia Nursing Certification.

postdoctoral Pertaining to academic study beyond the level of a doctoral degree. *See also* doctorate.

Postdoctoral and Internship Centers, Association of Psychology *See* Association of Psychology Postdoctoral and Internship Centers.

posterior Pertaining to, situated in, or toward the back of a structure. *Compare* anterior.

Postgraduate Medical Association of North America, Interstate *See* Interstate Postgraduate Medical Association of North America.

postgraduate year 1 *See* PGY-1.

posthumous birth **1.** Delivery of a child by cesarean section after the death of the mother. **2.** Birth of a child after the father's death. *See also* birth.

postindustrial Pertaining to a period in the development of an economy or a nation in which the relative importance of manufacturing lessens and that of services, information, and research grows. *See also* industrial; industrialism.

postmature infant Infant born after 42 weeks' gestation and usually showing signs of placental insufficiency. *Compare* premature infant. *See also* infant.

postmenopausal Pertaining to the time after menopause. *See also* menopause.

postmortem After death. *See also* autopsy.

postmortem examination *See* autopsy.

postnatal Existing or occurring immediately following the infant's birth; applies to mother and infant. *See also* perinatal; prenatal.

postoperative Pertaining to the period after surgery, including the emergence from anesthesia and the abatement of the acute signs of anesthesia and surgery. *See also* intraoperative; operation; preoperative; postoperative care.

postoperative autotransfusion The collection, processing, and reinfusion of a patient's blood shed from the mediastinum following open heart or chest surgery or from the chest following traumatic hemothorax (collection of blood in the chest cavity). *See also* autotransfusion; intraoperative autotransfusion.

postoperative care Provision of medical, nursing, and other health services for patients following surgery. *Synonym*: postsurgical care. *See also* postoperative; preoperative care; recovery room; wound infection.

postoperative recovery room *See* recovery room.

postpartum Pertaining to the first few days after birth, as in postpartum care. *See also* birth; postpartum care.

postpartum care Provision of medical, nursing, and other health-related services to patients following childbirth. *See also* postpartum; wound infection.

postsurgical care *See* postoperative care.

posttraumatic Occurring as a result of, or after, mental or physical injury. *See also* posttraumatic stress disorder; trauma.

posttraumatic stress disorder (PTSD) A psychological disorder affecting individuals who have experienced profound emotional trauma, such as torture or rape, characterized by recurrent flashbacks of the traumatic event, nightmares, eating disorders, anxiety, fatigue, forgetfulness, and social withdrawal. *Synonym*: posttraumatic stress syndrome. *See also* disorder; stress; trauma.

postulate **1.** Something assumed without proof as being self-evident or generally accepted, especially when used as a basis for an argument. **2.** A requirement, as in Koch's postulates. *See also* Koch's postulates.

postulates, Koch's *See* Koch's postulates.

posture General attitude, position, and deportment of the body, normally maintained by unconscious reflex activity.

pot *See* cannabis.

potable Drinkable, as in potable water.

potency **1.** The strength or power of a drug, toxin, or hazard. **2.** Ability of a male to achieve and maintain an erection and thus engage in coitus. *See also* impotence.

potential **1.** Existing and ready for action but not yet active. **2.** Possible as opposed to actual, as in a potential improvement opportunity or a potential problem. **3.** The inherent ability or capacity for growth, development, or coming into being, as in a potential for greatness or a potential for disaster.

potential demand (for health services) *See* demand (for health services).

potentially compensable event (PCE) An adverse patient care event that ultimately may be involved in a liability claim. The event involves a disability (temporary or permanent) caused by health care management (including acts of commission and omission by health care providers). This term was originally coined by researchers in the California Medical Insurance Feasibility Study (1976) sponsored by the California Medical Association and the California Hospital Association. In this study, over 20,000 patient charts from 23 hospitals were reviewed for the presence of adverse events that might result in litigation for malpractice compensation. These adverse events were called potentially compensable events (PCEs). The 20 PCEs developed by physicians and medical audit experts during this study later became the basis for occurrence screening criteria, adapted and modified for use by individual institutions. A PCE is not the same as an adverse patient occurrence (APO) or negligence. *See also* adverse patient occurrence; negligence; occurrence criteria; occurrence screening.

Potentials, American Society for Clinical Evoked *See* American Society for Clinical Evoked Potentials.

potomania An abnormal craving for alcoholic drink. *Synonym*: dipsomania. *See also* alcohol; alcoholism; mania; thirst.

poultice A hot dressing for application to the skin, either for the purpose of counter-irritation or in order to increase local blood flow.

poverty **1.** The condition of having an inadequate supply of money, resources, goods, or means to maintain life and health at a subsistence level. **2.** A relative measure within a society, being the state of having income and/or wealth so low as to be unable to maintain what is considered a minimum standard of living. *See also* poor; poverty area; poverty level; standard of living; subsistence.

poverty area An urban or rural geographic area with a high proportion of families with low income and/or other indications of poverty, such as poor housing conditions, high illegitimate birth rates, and high incidence of juvenile delinquency. *See also* poverty.

poverty level An income level judged inadequate to provide a family or individual with the essentials of life. The figure for the United States is adjusted regularly to reflect changes in the Consumer Price Index. *See also* Consumer Price Index; level; poverty.

power **1.** The ability or capacity to perform or act effectively. **2.** Strength of force exerted or capable of being exerted. *See also* monopoly power. **3.** The ability or official capacity to exercise control; authority. **4.** In statistics, a characteristic of a statistical hypothesis test, denoting the probability that the null hypothesis will be rejected if it is false. *See also* null hypothesis; statistics.

power of attorney A legal instrument by which a person, as principal, grants authority to another to act as his or her attorney or agent. The primary purpose of a power of attorney is to evidence the authority of the agent to third parties with whom the agent deals. A person need not be an attorney-at-law to have the power of attorney to act for another. *See also* attorney; durable power of attorney for health care.

power of attorney for health care, durable *See* durable power of attorney for health care.

power, market *See* market power.

power, monopoly *See* monopoly power.

power, purchasing *See* purchasing power.

power, statistical *See* statistical power.

power surge A sudden increase in voltage that enters a computer or word processor through a power line; potentially damaging to electrical equipment, especially computers. *See also* computer.

pox Diseases, such as smallpox, cowpox, and chickenpox, that are characterized by pocks or eruptive blisters containing pus on the skin. *See also* chickenpox; infectious diseases; smallpox.

pox, chicken- *See* chickenpox.

pox, small- *See* smallpox.

PPA *See* Pathology Practice Association.

PPO *See* preferred provider organization.

PPPF *See* Positive Pregnancy and Parenting Fitness.

PPRC *See* Physician Payment Review Commission.

***p* (probability) value** The probability of concluding that a statistical association exists between, for instance, a risk factor and a health endpoint, when in fact, there is no real association; the likelihood that an observed association in a study is due to chance alone. The letter p, followed by the abbreviation n.s. (not significant) or by the symbol < (less than) and a decimal notation, such as 0.01, 0.05, is a statement of the probability that the difference observed could have occurred by chance, if the groups are really alike as required under the null hypothesis. Most biomedical work sets significance levels at a p value of less than 5% (p less than 0.05) or 1% (p less than 0.01), meaning that the test result is sufficiently unlikely to have occurred by chance to justify the designation "statistically significant." *See also* level of significance; statistical significance type I error.

PPS *See* Private Practice Section/American Physical Therapy Association; prospective payment system; prospective pricing system.

PR *See* public relations.

practical **1.** Acquired through practice or action, rather than study, theory, or ideas, as in practical experience. **2.** Intended to serve a purpose without elaboration. **3.** Level-headed, efficient. *See also* pragmatic.

practical nurse (PN) *See* licensed practical nurse; licensed vocational nurse.

Practical Nurse Education and Service, National Association for *See* National Association for Practical Nurse Education and Service.

practical nurse, licensed *See* licensed practical nurse.

Practical Nurses Association, American Licensed *See* American Licensed Practical Nurses Association.

Practical Nurses, National Federation of Licensed *See* National Federation of Licensed Practical Nurses.

practical nurse, vocational *See* licensed vocational nurse.

practice **1.** Use of one's knowledge in a particular profession, as in the practice of medicine. **2.** The business of a professional person, as in an obstetrician's medical practice. *See also* family practice; general practice; group practice; medical practice; unauthorized practice.

practice act, dental *See* dental practice act.

practice act, medical *See* medical practice act.

practice act, nurse *See* nurse practice act.

Practice, American Board of Family *See* American Board of Family Practice.

Practice, American Osteopathic Board of General *See* American Osteopathic Board of General Practice.

Practice Association, American Group *See* American Group Practice Association.

Practice Association, American Professional *See* American Professional Practice Association.

practice association, individual *See* individual practice association.

practice association model HMO, independent *See* independent practice association model HMO.

Practice Association, Pathology *See* Pathology Practice Association.

practice, contract *See* contract practice.

practice, family *See* family practice.

practice, general *See* general practice.

practice, group *See* group practice.

practice guideline Descriptive tool(s) or standardized specification(s) for care of the typical patient in the typical situation, developed through a formal process that incorporates the best scientific evidence of effectiveness with expert opinion. *Synonyms or near-synonyms*: algorithm; clinical criteria; clinical practice guideline; clinical protocol; guideline; parameter; practice parameter; preferred practice pattern; protocol; review criteria. *See also* acceptable

alternative; algorithm; guideline; parameter; practice parameter; protocol.

practice, medical *See* medical practice.

practice nurse, advanced *See* advanced practice nurse.

practice, open panel *See* open panel group practice.

practice parameter Strategies for patient management developed to assist practitioners in clinical decision making. *Synonyms and near-synonyms*: clinical policy; clinical standard; critical pathway; guideline; patient management strategy; practice guideline. *See also* clinical pathway; critical pathway; parameter; practice guideline.

practice pattern analysis A method of aggregating data by practitioner, diagnosis, diagnosis-related group (DRG), or other defined category to show patterns of care and/or variations in care. *Synonym*: practice profiling. *See also* analysis; diagnosis; diagnosis-related groups; economic credentialing; pattern; practitioner profile; variation.

Practice, Pharmacists in Ophthalmic *See* Pharmacists in Ophthalmic Practice.

practice plan, individual *See* individual practice plan.

practice plan, medical *See* medical practice plan.

practice policy A flexible strategy for management of patient care.

practice, prepaid group *See* prepaid group practice.

practice, private *See* private practice.

practice privileges *See* admitting privileges.

practice profiling *See* practice pattern analysis.

practice, single specialty group *See* single specialty group practice.

practice, solo *See* solo practice.

practice, unauthorized *See* unauthorized practice.

practitioner Any individual who is qualified to practice a profession; for example, a physician or nurse. Practitioners are often required to be licensed as defined by law. *See also* licensed independent practitioner; licensure; medical practice act; nurse practice act.

Practitioner Data Bank, National *See* National Practitioner Data Bank.

practitioner factor Individual practitioner-related variable that may contribute to variation in performance data; usually controllable and the object of a thorough monitoring process. *See also* external environmental factor; factor; organization factor; patient factor.

practitioner, licensed independent *See* licensed independent practitioner.

practitioner, nurse *See* nurse practitioner.

practitioner, obstetric-gynecologic nurse *See* obstetric-gynecologic nurse practitioner.

practitioner, pediatric nurse *See* pediatric nurse practitioner.

practitioner, primary care *See* primary care provider.

practitioner profile A longitudinal or cross-sectional aggregation of objective health care data used to assess and improve practitioner performance in health care delivery; for example, a practitioner profile may be used to evaluate physician members of a clinical department in a hospital, who are up for reappointment and renewal or expansion of clinical privileges. The data that appear on a practitioner's profile are not "grades" and cannot be automatically translated into reappoint/don't reappoint decisions. However, the use of practitioner profiles acknowledges that the clinical department chief may not be intimately familiar with all department members, and that quantitative and qualitative peer review data can be helpful in making an objective performance evaluation. *See also* peer review; practitioner; profile; profiling.

practitioner profiling A process of aggregation and analysis of practitioner-specific health care data, often in the form of tables or graphs, representing distinctive features or characteristics of a practitioner or group of practitioners. *See also* practitioner; practitioner profile; profile; profiling.

Practitioners, American Academy of Nurse *See* American Academy of Nurse Practitioners.

Practitioners in Infection Control, Association for *See* Association for Practitioners in Infection Control.

practitioner site The office of a licensed practitioner who is a member of the practitioner panel of a health care network. *See also* licensed; network; practitioner.

Practitioners, National Association of Pediatric Nurse Associates and *See* National Association of Pediatric Nurse Associates and Practitioners.

Practitioners and Nurses, National Certification Board of Pediatric Nurse *See* National Certification Board of Pediatric Nurse Practitioners and Nurses.

Practitioners in Osteopathic Medicine and Surgery, American College of General *See* American College of General Practitioners in Osteopathic Medicine and Surgery.

practitioner, specialty care *See* specialist.

pragmatic Dealing or concerned with facts or actual occurrences. *See also* practical; pragmatism.

pragmatism A practical, matter-of-fact way of approaching or assessing situations or of solving problems. It holds that the whole meaning of a conception lies in its practical consequences. *See also* common sense.

praise Expression of approval or admiration, as in praise for reaching a milestone.

prandial Pertaining to a meal, as in postprandial chest discomfort.

PRC *See* Park Ridge Center.

PRCLR *See* PR Committee for Licensing and Registration.

PR Committee for Licensing and Registration (PRCLR) A nonmembership organization founded in 1985 composed of members of the Public Relations Society of America who are interested in professionalizing the field of public relations through licensing and certification of qualified public relations counselors, with legal sanctions. It furnishes model standards for public relations professionals and lobbies US state governments regarding licensing laws and sanctions. *See also* certification; licensure; public relations; Public Relations Society of America; sanction; standard.

preadmission certification *See* admissions review.

preadmission process for admission The formal acceptance by a hospital or other health care organization of a patient for preliminary tests on an outpatient basis before admission as an inpatient. *See also* admissions review; inpatient; outpatient.

preadmission review *See* admissions review.

precancerous Pertaining to a pathologic process or lesion that tends to become malignant. *See also* cancer; malignant.

precision 1. Sharply defined through exact detail; for example, in mathematics, a measurement with three significant figures is more precise than a measurement with two. 2. In statistics, the extent to which a measurement procedure gives the same results when repeated under identical conditions, the inverse of the variance. Under certain conditions, this may also be called reliability. Precision is not the same as accuracy. For example, a faulty measurement may be expressed precisely, but may not be accurate. Measurements should possess an acceptable degree of both accuracy and precision. *Compare* accuracy of a measurement. *See also* measurement; reliability; variance.

Precision Chiropractic Research Society (PCRS) A national organization founded in 1976 composed of 200 doctors of chiropractic specializing in spinal stress. It conducts research into spinal problems and treatments, such as investigating the relationship between headaches and spinal adjustments. It documents research by x-raying patients before treatment and again after treatments to determine change (if any) of spinal position. Also known as Spinal Stress Research Society. *See also* chiropractic; research.

Precision Electromagnetic Measurements, Conference on *See* Conference on Precision Electromagnetic Measurements.

Precision Measurements Association (PMA) A national organization founded in 1959 composed of 600 engineers, scientists, and technically skilled persons interested in measurement science. It sponsors one-day courses in pressure measurement instruments; linear, optical, and electronic measurement; and basic metrology. *See also* measurement; metrology; precision.

precocity Premature development.

preconception An opinion or a conception formed in advance of full or adequate knowledge or experience, thus a prejudice or bias. *See also* concept; conception.

precondition A condition that must exist or be established before something can occur or be considered, as in demonstrating acceptable reliability of a test as a precondition to accepting resulting data as credible.

precordial Pertaining to the area of the chest directly over the heart, as in precordial chest pain.

precursor Something that precedes something else; in clinical medicine, for example, a sign or symptom that heralds another.

prediction Foretelling of a future event. Predictions are probability estimates of future occurrences based on many different estimation methods, including past patterns of occurrence and statical projections of current data. *See also* forecasting; projection.

predictive validity The ability of an indicator or other measure to predict future events. *See also* external validity; indicator; validity.

predictive value of a negative test In medicine, the probability that an individual with a negative

test does not have the condition being tested for. *See also* test.

predictive value of a positive test In medicine, the probability that an individual with a positive test is a true positive (does have the condition being tested for). *See also* test.

predictive value of a screening test A probability determined by the sensitivity and specificity of a test, and by the prevalence of the condition for which the test is used. When the prevalence of a given condition is low in a tested population, a test with a high sensitivity functions fairly well at both ruling in the correct diagnosis and ruling out the incorrect one. But as the prevalence increases, the sensitivity of the test must also increase to maintain the same number of false negatives. *See also* prevalence; sensitivity; specificity; test.

predisposition A tendency to be affected by a particular disease or to develop or react in a certain way. It may be genetic or result from environmental factors.

preeclampsia A condition of late pregnancy characterized by hypertension, swelling of the extremities, and protein in the blood; when convulsions and coma are associated, it is called eclampsia. *Synonyms*: toxemia; toxemia of pregnancy. *See also* eclampsia; pregnancy.

preembryo An organism formed two to three days after fertilization. *See also* embryo; fertilization; preembryo transfer.

preembryo transfer A technique of fertilization in which a husband's sperm is used to fertilize a donor's or wife's egg in vitro and the resultant preembryo is transferred to his wife or the couple's preembryo is transferred to a surrogate mother. *See also* fertilization; preembryo; surrogate motherhood; transfer.

preexisting condition In the field of health insurance, an injury occurring, a disease contracted, or a physical condition that exists prior to the issuance of a health insurance policy. It usually results in an exclusion from coverage under the policy for costs resulting from the condition. *See also* exclusions; job lock.

preference A choice of one alternative over another; for example, some people show a preference for certain physicians over other physicians because of bedside manner.

preferred practice pattern *See* practice guideline.

preferred provider *See* preferred provider organization.

preferred provider organization (PPO) A prenegotiated arrangement between purchasers and providers to furnish specified health services to a group of employees/patients. An insurance company or employer negotiates discounted fees with networks of health care providers in return for guaranteeing a certain volume of patients. Providers under contract in such arrangements are called preferred providers. Enrollees in a PPO can receive treatment outside the network but must pay higher copayments or deductibles for it. PPO contracts usually have three distinguishing features: discounts from standard charges, monetary incentives for single subscribers to utilize contracting providers, and broad utilization management programs. *See also* health maintenance organization; network.

Preferred Provider Organizations, American Association of *See* American Association of Preferred Provider Organizations.

prefrontal lobotomy A surgical procedure in which the white fibers that connect the thalamus to the prefrontal and frontal lobes of the brain are severed. It is performed as a treatment for intense anxiety or violent behavior. *Synonym:* frontal lobotomy. *See also* neurological surgery; psychiatry; psychosurgery.

pregnancy The condition in which a woman carries a developing fetus in the uterus from the time of conception to birth of the child. Pregnancy lasts 266 days from the day of fertilization but is usually calculated as 280 days from the first day of the last menstrual period. *See also* amenorrhea; amniocentesis; artificial reproduction; gestation; gestational diabetes; gravity; noncoital reproduction; obstetrics; preeclampsia; pseudocyesis; quickening; uterus.

pregnancy counseling Help and counseling for unmarried parents and their families, consisting of assisting with decision making, foster care for the infant, the legal freeing of a child for adoption, and teaching parenting skills. *See also* counseling; pregnancy.

Pregnancy Discrimination Act of 1978 An amendment to Title VII of the Civil Rights Act of 1964, which holds that discrimination on the basis of pregnancy, childbirth, or related medical conditions constitutes unlawful sex discrimination.

pregnancy, ectopic *See* ectopic pregnancy.

Pregnancy and Parenting Fitness, Positive *See* Positive Pregnancy and Parenting Fitness.

Pregnancy and Parenting, National Organization of Adolescent *See* National Organization of Adolescent Pregnancy and Parenting.

pregnancy, pseudo- *See* pseudopregnancy.

pregnancy test A test for the detection of pregnancy, which uses chemical, bioassay, or radioimmunoassay techniques for the estimation of hormone levels in urine or blood plasma. *See also* bioassay; hormone; pregnancy; radioimmunoassay; test.

pregnancy, toxemia of *See* preeclampsia.

pregnant Carrying developing offspring within the body. *See also* pregnancy.

prejudice, dismissal with *See* dismissal with prejudice.

prejudice, dismissal without *See* dismissal without prejudice.

preliminary injunction A court order to do or refrain from doing some act that is issued during the course of a lawsuit and remains effective until the dispute is settled or judgment is reached. *See also* injunction; permanent injunction.

premature Occurring before the expected time; therefore, not fully developed, especially a premature infant.

premature baby *See* premature infant.

premature birth A birth that occurs after an infant is generally capable of independent life and before the end of the term. *Compare* abortus. *See also* birth; premature; premature infant; term.

premature delivery A baby delivered with time and/or weight factors qualifying it for premature status. *See also* delivery; premature; premature infant.

premature infant An infant born before full term, that is, after a gestation period of less than 38 weeks. A premature infant is usually of low birth weight. The prognosis depends on the maturity of the organ systems of the infant's body and on the postnatal care provided, optimally in a neonatal intensive care unit. Prematurity is also defined as a birth weight less than 2.5 kilograms (5.5 pounds). *Synonym:* premature baby. *Compare* postmature infant. *See also* infant; premature.

premature nursery *See also* neonatal intensive care unit.

premedical Preceding and preparing for the study of medicine, as in premedical studies required for admission to medical school.

premenopausal Pertaining to the years or stage of life before menopause. *See also* menopause.

premenstrual Occurring before menstruation, as in premenstrual syndrome. *See also* menstruation; premenstrual syndrome.

premenstrual syndrome (PMS) A set of physical and emotional symptoms that occur before each menstrual period in some women. The symptoms are related to hormonal changes and water retention and may include bloating, headache, irritation, appetite changes, and breast tenderness. *See also* hormone; menses; menstruation; premenstrual.

premise A basis for reasoning; a proposition upon which an argument is based or from which a conclusion is drawn.

premium The amount paid or payable, often in installments, by an insured person or policyholder to an insurer or third-party payer for insurance coverage under an insurance policy. Premium amounts are related to the actuarial value of the benefits provided by the policy, plus a loading to cover administrative costs and profit. Premiums are paid for coverage whether benefits are actually used or not. Premiums should not be confused with cost sharing (copayments, coinsurance, and deductives), which are paid only if benefits are actually used. Premiums can be established by either an experience rating or a community rating method. *See also* community rating; cost sharing; experience rating; loading.

prenatal Existing before or occurring before birth. *Synonym:* antenatal. *See also* natal; perinatal; postnatal.

preoperative Pertaining to the period before surgery, when a patient is prepared for surgery by limitations on intake of food and fluids, premedication, and other procedures. *See also* operation; perioperative; postoperative; preoperative care.

preoperative care Physiological and psychological preparation of a patient for surgery. *See also* preoperative; postoperative care.

prepaid group practice A contractual arrangement in which an association of three or more physicians provides a defined set of services to persons over a specified time period in return for a fixed periodic prepayment made in advance of the use of service. *Compare* closed panel group practice. *See also* group practice; health maintenance organization; medical foundation.

prepaid health plan A contract between an insurer and a subscriber or group of subscribers whereby the prepaid health plan provides a specified set of health benefits in return for a period premium. *See also* health plan; Kaiser Foundation Health Plan; point-of-service plan.

preparation The act of making ready, as in drug preparation or patient preparation for surgery.

prepayment In health care, any payment ahead of time to a health care provider for anticipated services. A prepayment system, for instance, involves a fee paid to a third-party payer, such as a health maintenance organization or a Blue Cross/Blue Shield plan, which then agrees to pay for stipulated services when they are provided. *See also* health care provider; prepayment plan.

prepayment plan A contractual arrangement for health services in which a prenegotiated payment is made in advance, covering a certain time period, and the health care provider agrees, for this payment, to furnish certain services to the beneficiary. *See also* health care provider; health plan; prepayment.

preprocedure review Evaluation conducted after admission but before a procedure is performed to ensure that the procedure is medically reasonable and necessary and could not be performed safely and effectively in an alternative setting. *See also* procedure.

preponderance of the evidence A test used by a fact finder (judge or jury) to determine which side has prevailed on a point under contention. Alternatively described as the greater weight of the evidence, it generally requires that one side prove that the fact at issue is more likely than not. It is in contrast to "clear and convincing evidence" and "proof beyond a reasonable doubt," which are progressively higher standards of proof. *See also* evidence; fact finder.

preretirement counseling Counseling that involves attention to Social Security benefits, private pension plans, medical and life insurance plans, educational and training opportunities, and employment opportunities that might be available if clients desire full-time, part-time, or volunteer employment as a second career. *See also* counseling; retirement.

prerogative An exclusive or peculiar right, or a distinctly superior advantage belonging to a person or group. *See also* privilege.

Presbyterian Health, Education and Welfare Association (PHEWA) A national organization founded in 1955 composed of 1,800 health, education, and welfare agencies and programs related to the United Presbyterian Church, USA; and individuals interested in issues in the health, education, and welfare fields. Its member agencies include children's homes and services, hospitals and health services, homes and services for the aging, community centers, and neighborhood houses. It establishes standards for the effectiveness of services and organizes social action and research.

prescribe To direct the selection, preparation, and administration of a medication or other treatment. *See also* order; overprescribe; prescription.

prescribe, over- *See* overprescribe.

prescription A written direction by a physician, dentist, or other authorized health care provider for the preparation and administration of a medication, therapy, or device. A prescription consists of a heading or *superscription* (the symbol *Rx* or the word *Recipe*, meaning "take"); the *inscription* (the names and quantities of ingredients); the *subscription* (directions for compounding); and the *signature* (directions for the patient that are to be marked on the receptacle). *See also* ancillary charge; over-the-counter drug; prescription drug.

prescription drug A drug that can only be provided to a person on the prescription of a physician, dentist, or other authorized health professional. The prescription specifies the drug to be given, the amount of the drug to be dispensed, and the directions necessary for the patient to use the drug. *Synonym*: prescription medicine. *Compare* over-the-counter drug. *See also* drug; legend drug; package insert.

prescription drug, non- *See* over-the-counter drug.

Prescription Drug Manufacturers Association, Non- *See* Nonprescription Drug Manufacturers Association.

Prescription Drug Programs, National Council for *See* National Council for Prescription Drug Programs.

prescription medicine *See* prescription drug.

presence of mind The ability to think and act calmly and efficiently, especially in an emergency. *See also* mind.

present To appear or to show, as a patient presenting to the emergency department with a complaint of chest pain.

presentation **1.** The complex of symptoms and signs that first manifest the presence of a disease process. *See also* disease. **2.** In obstetrics, the particular part of a fetus presented to the birth canal at the onset of labor. *See also* labor. **3.** A setting forth in words and visuals to enlighten an audience and persuade them to commit themselves to a course of action or thought. An effective presentation is usually planned, organized, and tailored to a specific audience to help facilitate a behavior change desired by the presenter.

present state In force-field analysis, the description of an organization as it currently exists. It includes both formal and informal happenings within the organization. *See also* force-field analysis.

preservative Something added to preserve, as in a chemical added to foods to inhibit spoilage. Synonym: food preservative. *See also* additive; sulfites.

president *See* chief executive officer.

president of the medical staff A member of a hospital medical staff who is elected or appointed by the medical staff to serve as its administrative head for a designated time. *See also* chief of staff; medical staff.

president's budget In the federal budget, the budget for a particular fiscal year specifying proposed budget authority, obligations, and outlays transmitted to Congress by the president in accordance with the Budget and Accounting Act of 1921, as amended. Some elements of the budget, such as the estimates for the legislative branch and the judiciary, are included without review by the Office of Management and Budget or approval by the president. *See also* budget; Congressional budget.

press **1.** The entirety of media and agencies that collect, publish, transmit, or broadcast the news. **2.** The people involved in the media, such as news reporters, photographers, publishers, and broadcasters. *See also* journalism; mass media; media; press kit; press release.

press kit A set of prepared press releases and related materials given to the press for general dissemination. Press kits are prepared by an organization, typically by its public relations or press department, to give an official statement or view regarding a particular newsworthy event or to give background or supplementary information on the organization. *See also* press; press release.

press release An announcement made by an organization of an event or other newsworthy item that is issued to the press. *Synonym*: news release. *See also* mass media; media relations; press; press kit; public relations.

pressure group An interest group or lobbying organization that endeavors to influence public policy and especially governmental legislation, regarding its special concerns and priorities. *See also* group; public interest group; special interest.

pressure sore A lesion caused by prolonged pressure in a person allowed to lie too still in bed for a long period of time. *Synonyms*: bed sore; decubitus; decubitus ulcer; pressure ulcer. *See also* sore; ulcer.

pressure ulcer *See* pressure sore.

prestige pricing Pricing reflecting the assumption that customers will not pay less than a predetermined price floor for services or merchandise since it is believed that otherwise the services or merchandise will be of inferior quality. *See also* pricey; tailgate pricing.

presume To take for granted as being true in the absence of proof to the contrary, as in presumed consent. *See also* presumed consent; presumption.

presumed consent A policy advocated by some people that would presume that an individual would allow his or her organs to be retrieved for transplantation after death unless he or she specifically issues a directive that forbids organ harvesting or retrieval. Currently, the practice allows for cadaver donation when there is consent from living relatives of a deceased donor or when the donor has issued a directive prior to death permitting organ retrieval. *See also* consent; organ procurement.

presumption A legal concept by which an assumption is made that a fact exists based on the existence of another or other facts. *See also* fact; irrebuttable presumption; rebuttable presumption.

presumption, irrebuttable *See* irrebuttable presumption.

presumption, rebuttable *See* rebuttable presumption.

prevailing charge A charge that falls within the range of charges most frequently used in a locality for a particular medical service or procedure. The top of this range establishes an overall limitation on the charges that a carrier, which considers prevailing charges in reimbursement, will accept as reasonable for a given service, without adequate special justification. *See also* charge.

prevalence The existing number of individuals (or cases) with an attribute, a condition, or a disease in a given population at a specific time, as in the number of individuals with acquired immunodeficiency syndrome (AIDS) in a city as of the first day of the year. There is no distinction between new and old cases. *Compare* incidence. *See also* prevalence rate.

prevalence rate The total number of individuals who have an attribute, a condition, or a disease at a particular time or during a particular period, divided by the population at risk of having the attribute, condition, or disease at a specified time or midway through a period of time, multiplied by 100. *Compare* incidence rate. *See also* prevalence; rate.

prevention A future-oriented strategy that improves quality and performance by directing analysis and action toward correcting the production process, rather than identifying and removing defects at the end of the production process. *Compare* detection; inspection. *See also* preventive.

Prevention Center, National Assault *See* National Assault Prevention Center.

Prevention, Centers for Disease Control and *See* Centers for Disease Control and Prevention.

Prevention of Child Abuse, National Committee for *See* National Committee for Prevention of Child Abuse.

prevention cost The cost of all activities undertaken to prevent defects in design and development, purchasing, labor, and other aspects of beginning and creating a product or service, for example, process capability studies, operation training, quality audits, preventive maintenance. *See also* appraisal cost; cost; cost of quality; failure cost; prevention.

Prevention and Health Promotion, Office of Disease *See* Office of Disease Prevention and Health Promotion.

Prevention Movement, Cesarean *See* Cesarean Prevention Movement.

Prevention Network, National *See* National Prevention Network.

preventive 1. Seeking to avert the occurrence of. 2. In health care, having the goal or effect of decreasing the probability of occurrence of diseases or accidents, or the consequences thereof; for example, immunizations and education are preventive measures.

preventive health services Services designed to promote health and prevent disease. *See also* health services; preventive medicine.

preventive maintenance *See* maintenance.

preventive medicine The branch and specialty of medicine that focuses on the health of individuals and defined populations in order to protect, promote, and maintain health and well-being, and to prevent disease, disability, and premature death. It includes biostatistics, epidemiology, health services administration, environmental and occupational influences on health, social and behavioral influences on health, and measures which prevent the occurrence, progression, and disabling effects of disease or injury. Medical toxicology is a subspecialty of preventive medicine. *See also* biostatistics; epidemiology; medical toxicology; wellness.

Preventive Medicine, American Board of *See* American Board of Preventive Medicine.

Preventive Medicine, American College of *See* American College of Preventive Medicine.

Preventive Medicine, American Osteopathic College of *See* American Osteopathic College of Preventive Medicine.

Preventive Medicine, Association of Teachers of *See* Association of Teachers of Preventive Medicine.

Preventive Oncology, American Society of *See* American Society of Preventive Oncology.

priapus *See* phallus.

price The amount of money or goods asked for or given in exchange for something else, as in price discrimination or pricey. *See also* price blending; price discrimination; price fixing.

PRICE *See* Physicians for Research in Cost-Effectiveness.

price blending Under the prospective pricing system in health care, a method for the equitable determination of prices for diagnosis-related groups (DRGs) by the comparison of an individual hospital's range of cost per case for any given DRG to the national average for that DRG. *See also* diagnosis-related groups; price.

price discrimination The act of selling goods or services at different prices to different purchasers. *See also* discrimination; price.

price fixing Under the federal antitrust laws, combination or conspiracy for the purpose of and with the effect of raising, depressing, fixing, pegging, or stabilizing the price of a commodity in interstate commerce. The test is not what the actual effect is on prices, but whether such agreements interfere with the freedom of traders and thereby restrain their ability to sell in accordance with their own judg-

ment. *See also* Sherman Antitrust Act.

price index, consumer *See* consumer price index.

price, market *See* market price.

price, unit *See* unit price.

pricey A product or service offered at a price at or near the top of what the market will bear. *See also* market; price.

pricing, prestige *See* prestige pricing.

pricing system, prospective *See* prospective pricing system.

pricing, tailgate *See* tailgate pricing.

prickly heat An itchy rash due to obstruction of the sweat gland ducts and escape of sweat into the skin. It is associated with prolonged excessive heat load. *See also* hyperpyrexia.

prima facie case A case that appears to have enough evidence to prevail in a lawsuit if it is not contradicted by evidence proving otherwise. *See also* case; lawsuit.

primary care Basic health care and a branch of medicine that emphasizes the point when a patient first seeks assistance in a health care system and the care of the simpler and more common illnesses and injuries. Primary care can be provided by primary care physicians and health professionals other than physicians, notably nurse practitioners or physician assistants. Thus, primary care is typically characterized by the nature of the contact (first contact in the health care system) rather than the qualifications of the practitioners providing that care. *See also* care; primary care center; primary care network; primary care physician; secondary care; tertiary care.

primary care center A facility that provides primary care on a scheduled basis and is open approximately eight hours per day, that is staffed by a physician or other qualified practitioner (such as a physician assistant), that is supported by basic laboratory and sometimes radiology services, and that provides continuity of care. A primary care center typically offers first contact health care only and patients requiring specialized medical care are referred elsewhere. *See also* continuity of care; freestanding ambulatory care center; primary care.

primary care network A group of primary care physicians who have joined together to share the financial risk of providing prepaid care to those of their patients who are members of a given health plan. *See also* health plan; network; primary care.

primary care physician A general practitioner,

family practitioner, primary care internist, or primary care pediatrician who usually provides only primary care services. A person with specialty qualifications may also provide primary care, alone or in combination with referral services. *See also* gatekeeper mechanism; physician; primary care; primary care provider.

primary care practitioner *See* primary care provider.

primary care provider An individual, such as a physician or other qualified practitioner (for example, nurse practitioner, physician assistant), who provides primary care services and manages routine health care needs. Care requiring more specialized knowledge or skill is obtained by referral from the primary care provider to a specialist for consultation or continued care. *Synonym:* primary care practitioner. *See also* health care provider; primary care physician; specialist.

Primary Care Research Group, North American *See* North American Primary Care Research Group.

primary cesarean section First cesarean section. *See also* cesarean section.

primary contact A person in direct contact with a communicable disease case. *See also* contact; secondary contact.

primary data Data that do not exist prior to conducting a study. *See also* data; data source; secondary data.

primary health care *See* primary care.

primary nurse A registered nurse who provides all nursing care to an assigned group of patients throughout their hospitalization. *See also* primary nursing; registered nurse; team nurse.

primary nursing A system of nursing care in which one nurse is responsible around the clock for planning, supervising, and, when present, giving nursing care to an assigned individual or group of patients. This approach to nursing care is replacing team nursing, in which a group of individuals of different levels of skill, rather than a given individual, carries out nursing functions. *See also* team nursing.

primary payer The insurer obligated to pay losses before any liability of other, secondary insurers. Medicare, for instance, is a primary payer with respect to Medicaid. *See also* coordination of benefits; duplication; Medicaid; Medicare.

primary standards The set of Joint Commission on Accreditation of Healthcare Organizations standards, or the accreditation manual that represents the majority of standards, surveyed in an organization during a tailored survey. *See also* Joint Commission on Accreditation of Healthcare Organizations; secondary standards; standard; tailored survey.

PRIM&R *See* Public Responsibility in Medicine and Research.

primum non nocere Latin phrase meaning "above all, do no harm." *See also* double effect principle; nonmaleficence.

principal diagnosis The diagnosis that, after study, is judged to be the principal reason for hospitalization or other care. This diagnosis is coded using the *International Classification of Diseases, Ninth Revision, Clinical Modification. See also* diagnosis; other diagnosis.

principle A basic truth, law, or assumption, as in democratic principles, or a standard or rule, as in the principle of honesty. *See also* assumption; doctrine; rule of thumb; tenet.

principle, double-effect *See* double-effect principle.

principle of the least advantaged In an ethical dilemma, the weakest party receives special consideration in decision making. *See also* ethical dilemma.

principle, least-effort *See* least-effort principle.

principle, minimax *See* minimax principle.

principle, Pareto *See* Pareto principle.

principle, Peter *See* Peter principle.

principle, pleasure *See* pleasure principle.

principle, prudent buyer *See* prudent buyer principle.

principle, reality *See* reality principle.

printed circuit board *See* PCB.

printer A device for putting computer output on paper. *See also* hard copy; line printer; daisy wheel printer; dot-matrix printer; ink jet printer; laser printer.

printer, daisy wheel *See* daisy wheel printer.

printer, dot-matrix *See* dot-matrix printer.

printer, ink jet *See* ink jet printer.

printer, laser *See* laser printer.

printer, line *See* line printer.

printout Hard-copy output from a computer, such as selected information from a computer file or a printout of the information currently on the computer screen. *See also* computer; hard copy.

prior authorization A requirement imposed by a third-party payer, under many systems of utilization review, that a provider must justify before a peer review committee, insurance company representative, or state agent the need for delivering a particular service to a patient before actually providing the service in order to receive reimbursement. This generally applies to expensive nonemergency services or services that are overused or abused. *See also* preadmission certification.

priorities Objectives ordered by level of importance or urgency, those with the greatest importance having the highest priority. *See also* prioritize.

prioritize To arrange in order of importance or urgency. *See also* priorities.

priority *See* priorities.

prison hospital *See* security hospital.

privacy **1.** The condition of being secluded from the presence or view of other persons. **2.** The state of being free from unwanted intrusion. *See also* confidentiality; private; right of privacy.

Privacy Act of 1974 A federal statute that reasserts the fundamental right to privacy as derived from the Constitution of the United States. It provides a series of basic safeguards for individuals so as to prevent the misuse of personal information by the federal government. Safeguards include, for example, making known to the public the existence and characteristics of all personal information systems kept by federal agencies, permitting individuals access to records containing personal information about that individual, and providing for civil remedies for individuals whose records are kept or used in contravention of the requirements of the act. *See also* privacy; right of privacy.

privacy, right of *See* right of privacy.

private Confined to the individual, as in a private opinion, private research, or private patient. *See also* privacy.

private-duty nurse A nurse who, as an independent contractor employed by a patient, provides direct nursing care to the patient. *See also* nurse.

private foundation A corporation or trust, whose endowments are dedicated to philanthropy and whose proceeds are directed to the public good. Private foundations are controlled and usually financially supported by a single source, such as an individual, family, or corporation. *See also* foundation.

Private Geriatric Care Managers, National Association of *See* National Association of Private Geriatric Care Managers.

private health agency *See* voluntary health agency.

private hospital Investor-owned or not-for-profit hospital that is controlled by a legal entity other than

a government agency. *See also* hospital.

private nurse *See* private-duty nurse.

private patient A patient whose care is the responsibility of an individual physician and whose care is paid for directly by the patient or a third-party payer, as opposed to a public, service, or ward patient, whose care is the financial responsibility of a health program or institution. *Compare* ward patient. *See also* patient; third-party payer.

private practice A medical or other type of practice in which the practitioner and his or her practice are independent of any external policy control. It usually requires that the practitioner be self-employed, except when he or she is salaried by a partnership in which he or she is a partner with similar practitioners. It is not synonymous with fee-for-service practice, in which the practitioner may sell his services by another method, such as capitation; or solo practice because group practices may be private. Regulation, which does exert external control, is not generally thought to make all practice public. *See also* clinical social worker, private practice; fee for service; practice; practitioner.

private practice, clinical social worker *See* clinical social worker, private practice.

Private Practice Section/American Physical Therapy Association (PPS) A national group founded in 1955 composed of 4,500 physical therapists who are members of the American Physical Therapy Association and who are in private practice. One main purpose of the group is to provide physical therapists with information on establishing and managing a private practice. *See also* American Physical Therapy Association; physical therapy; private practice.

Private Psychiatric Hospitals, National Association of *See* National Association of Private Psychiatric Hospitals.

Private Residential Resources, National Association of *See* National Association of Private Residential Resources.

private review Utilization review performed by or on behalf of private payers of health services. *See also* utilization review.

private room A hospital room designed and equipped to house one inpatient. *See also* inpatient; room accommodations; semiprivate room; ward.

Private Sector, National Association of Rehabilitation Professionals in the *See* National Association of Rehabilitation Professionals in the Private Sector.

privilege   An advantage not enjoyed by all; a special benefit enjoyed by a person, company, or class beyond the common advantages of other citizens. *See also* prerogative.

privilege, attorney-client   *See* attorney-client privilege.

privilege, doctor-patient   *See* physician-patient privilege.

privileged communication   A confidential communication that is legally protected from discovery in a lawsuit or use as evidence in a trial. Communications, for example, between a physician and patient are privileged communications and cannot be revealed without the permission of the patient or a court order. Most of the contents of a medical record are also protected by this privilege. A patient can waive the privilege but the privilege cannot be waived by a physician or hospital, nor can the physician invoke the privilege if the patient waives it. *See also* admissible evidence; attorney-client privilege; communication; physician-patient privilege; psychotherapist-patient privilege.

privilege, physician-patient   *See* physician-patient privilege.

privilege, psychotherapist-patient   *See* psychotherapist-patient privilege.

privilege, therapeutic   *See* therapeutic privilege.

privileges, admitting   *See* admitting privileges.

privileges, clinical   *See* clinical privileges.

privileges, emergency   *See* emergency privileges.

privileges, hospital   *See* admitting privileges.

privileges, practice   *See* admitting privileges.

privileges, temporary   *See* temporary privileges.

privileging   *See* clinical privileges.

Prize, Nobel   *See* Nobel Prize.

prn   Abbreviation for the Latin phrase *pro re na'ta* meaning "according as circumstances may require," for example, taking a medication *prn*.

PRO   *See* peer review organization.

probability   **1.** The chance or likelihood that something will happen or has happened. *See also* actuarial science; stochastic. **2.** The limit of the relative frequency of an event in a sequence of *N* random trails as *N* approaches infinity. *See also* statistics. **3.** A measure, ranging from zero to one, of the degree of belief in a hypothesis or statement. *See also* hypothesis.

probability distribution   A mathematical formula that relates the values of a characteristic being measured with their probability of occurrence in a population. When the characteristic being measured can take on any value (subject to the fineness of the measuring process), its probability distribution is called a *continuous probability distribution*. The probability distribution for time spent by emergency medicine technicians at a trauma scene is an example of a continuous probability distribution because the characteristic being measured (time) could have any value, limited only by the fineness of the measuring instrument. Experience has shown that most continuous characteristics follow one of several common probability distributions: the normal distribution, the exponential distribution, and the Weibull distribution. When the characteristic being measured can take on only certain specific values, such as greater than 20 minutes *or* less than or equal to 20 minutes spent by emergency medical technician-paramedics at a trauma scene, its probability distribution is called a *discrete probability distribution*. The common discrete distributions are the Poisson, binomial, negative binomial, and hypergeometric. *See also* binomial distribution; continuous data; continuous variable indicator; discrete data; discrete variable; distribution; joint probability; normal distribution; rate-based indicator.

probability distribution, continuous   *See* probability distribution.

probability distribution, discrete   *See* probability distribution.

probability, joint   *See* joint probability.

probability theory   The branch of mathematics dealing with the purely logical properties of probability. Its theorems underlie most statistical methods. *See also* probability; theory.

probability value   *See* p (probability) value.

probable error (PE)   In statistics, the amount by which the arithmetic mean of a sample is expected to vary because of chance alone. *See also* chance; error.

probe   **1.** Any surgical instrument used primarily for exploratory purposes. **2.** Any instrument or method used for exploration, for example, in biology or genetics. **3.** *See* key items, probes, and scoring guidelines.

probes, and scoring guidelines, key items,   *See* key items, probes, and scoring guidelines.

problem   **1.** A question to be answered. **2.** A situation, matter, or person that presents perplexity or difficulty. *See also* project; systemic problem; trouble; troubleshooter.

problem-oriented medical record (POMR) A type of medical record in which a patient's history, physical findings, laboratory results, and other data and information are organized according to problems, such as chest pain or vomiting blood, instead of according to diseases, such as pneumonia or peptic ulcer, or no organization at all. The problem-oriented record includes subjective, objective, assessment(s), and diagnostic and treatment plan(s) (SOAP) for each problem. This contrasts with a medical record in which information is recorded in a less organized manner without regard for careful documentation of subjective, objective, assessment, and planning information about individual problems. *See also* medical record; SOAP.

problem prone Refers to a function, process, activity, or service that has historically caused problems for an organization, practitioners, patients, and/or a community. *See also* problem.

Problems, National Association on Drug Abuse *See* National Association on Drug Abuse Problems.

problem solving A structured process for acquiring and analyzing data in a way that will identify the root causes of problems and remove or reduce those causes. *See also* problem.

problem statement A description in specific and measurable terms of how a perplexing or difficult question or issue affects the performance of an organization. *See also* opportunity statement; problem.

problem, systemic *See* systemic problem.

procedural due process *See* due process of law.

procedure **1.** A series of steps taken to accomplish a desired end, as in a therapeutic, cosmetic, or surgical procedure. *See also* appendectomy; method; surgery; technique. **2.** A unit of health care, as in services and procedures. *See also* operation; policy; surgery.

procedure-coding manual A book used by claims examiners and issued by health insurers to health care providers to assist them in coding and describing services provided and claimed. *See also* coding; procedure.

procedure, death-delaying *See* death-prolonging procedure.

procedure, death-prolonging *See* death-prolonging procedure.

procedure, life-prolonging *See* life-prolonging procedure.

procedure, parliamentary *See* parliamentary procedure.

procedure review, pre- *See* preprocedure review.

procedures manual *See* policies and procedures manual.

process **1.** An interrelated series of activities, actions, events, mechanisms, or steps that transform inputs into outputs for a particular beneficiary or customer, as in the hospital admission process. *See also* health services research; high-risk process; high-volume process; important process. **2.** A projection, prominence, protuberance, outgrowth, or extension of or from the main body of an anatomical structure, such as the xiphoid process at the bottom of the sternum.

process, abuse of *See* abuse of process.

process, administrative *See* administrative process.

process for admission, preadmission *See* preadmission process for admission.

process assessment Evaluation procedure that focuses on how care is delivered. It is based on the premise that there are standards of performance for activities or services undertaken in delivering patient care; the specific actions taken, events occurring, and human interactions can be compared with the accepted standards. The degree to which specific actions taken compare favorably with standards of performance yields an assessment of performance. *See also* assessment; process.

process capability The measured, built-in reproducibility or consistency of a product turned out by a process. Such a determination is made using statistical methods, not wishful thinking. The statistically determined pattern or distribution can only then be compared to specification limits to decide if a process can consistently deliver a product within those parameters. *See also* analysis; capability; parameter; process.

process capability analysis An analysis that quantifies the inherent ability of a process to meet the demands of performance objectives. *See also* analysis; process capability.

Process Control Society, Statistical *See* Statistical Process Control Society.

process control, statistical *See* statistical process control.

process data Data describing what is done to, for,

or by patients, as in performance of a procedure. *See also* data; outcome data.

process, data verification *See* data verification process.

process, high-risk *See* high-risk process.

process, high-volume *See* high-volume process.

process, important *See* important process.

process improvement The continuous endeavor to learn about all aspects of a process and to use this knowledge to change the process to reduce variation and complexity and to improve the level of its performance. Process improvement begins by understanding how customers define quality, how processes work, and how understanding the variation in those processes can lead to wise management action. *See also* boundary; improvement; process.

process indicator An indicator that measures a discrete process, service, or activity. The best process indicators focus on processes that are closely linked to outcomes, meaning that a scientific basis exists for believing that the process, when executed well, will increase the probability of achieving a desired outcome. *See also* indicator; outcome indicator.

process, indicator testing *See* indicator testing process.

processing, accreditation decision *See* accreditation decision processing.

processing, batch *See* batch processing.

processing, blood *See* blood processing.

processing, data *See* data processing.

processing, natural language *See* natural language processing.

processing, parallel *See* parallel processing.

processing, word *See* word processing.

process measure A measure of a discrete process, service, or activity. *See also* input measure; measure; output measure; process indicator.

process, meeting *See* meeting process.

process, modified survey *See* modified survey process.

processor, word *See* word processor.

process owner *See* owner.

process quality audit An analysis of elements of a process and appraisal of completeness, correctness of conditions, and probable effectiveness. *See also* audit; process.

process standard A statement of expectation set by competent authority concerning a degree or level of acceptable performance of a process achieved by an individual, group, organization, community, or nation, according to preestablished requirements and/or specifications. *See also* outcome standard; process; standard.

process variable, key *See* key process variable.

process variation The spread of process output over time. There is variation in every process, and all variation is caused. The causes are of two types: special or common. A process can have both types of variation at the same time or only common-cause variation. The management action necessary to improve the process is different depending on the type of variation being addressed. *See also* common-cause variation; special-cause variation; variation.

pro-choice In favor of a woman's right to choose whether or not to have an abortion. *Compare* pro-family; pro-life; right-to-life. *See also* abortion.

procidentia A severe degree of prolapse of the uterus or rectum, with most or all of the organ outside the body. *See also* prolapse; uterus.

proctology The study of disorders of the anus and rectum. *See also* colon and rectal surgery.

Proctology, American Osteopathic College of *See* American Osteopathic College of Proctology.

proctoscope An endoscope with illumination for inspecting the rectum. *See also* endoscope.

proctoscopy Inspection of the rectum with a proctoscope. *See also* proctoscope.

proctosigmoidoscope An endoscope for illuminating and viewing the rectum and sigmoid colon. *See also* endoscope.

proctosigmoidoscopy Inspection of the rectum and sigmoid colon with a proctosigmoidoscope.

procure To get by special effort, as in procuring an organ for transplantation. *See also* procurement.

procurement Acquisition of items required to carry on an enterprise, as in organ procurement for transplantation. *See also* organ procurement.

procurement agency, organ *See* organ procurement agency.

procurement, organ *See* organ procurement.

prodrome Premonitory symptoms or signs heralding the onset of some disease, such as migraine headache. *See also* disease; sign; symptom.

produce To make, fabricate, or bring forth something, as in to produce an agenda. *See also* product; productive.

producers, database *See* database producers.

product Something produced; the output or end

result of any process. Products are either goods or services. *See also* goods; parenteral product; service.

product evaluation committee In health care, an organizational committee composed of medical, nursing, purchasing, and administrative staff members whose purpose is to evaluate products and advise on their procurement. *See also* evaluation; product.

productive **1.** Producing or capable of producing. *See also* produce. **2.** Producing abundantly. **3.** Yielding favorable or useful results. *Compare* nonproductive. *See also* productivity.

productivity **1.** The quality of being productive. *See also* productive. **2.** In economics, the relationship between the number of units of service provided or products produced per unit of labor required, per unit of time. For example, an increase in productivity is achieved through an increase in production per unit of labor over time.

Productivity Management Association, Quality and *See* Quality and Productivity Management Association.

Productivity and Quality Center, American *See* American Productivity and Quality Center.

product liability The onus on a producer or others to make restitution for loss related to personal injury, property damage, or other harm caused by a product. *See also* liability; service liability.

Product Liability Alliance, The *See* The Product Liability Alliance.

product, parenteral *See* parenteral product.

product quality audit A quantitative assessment of conformance to required product characteristics. *See also* audit; product.

products of conception *See* conceptus.

pro-family Promoting family life and return to a moral code based on the family unit; opposed to the legalizing of abortion. *Compare* pro-choice. *See also* family; pro-life; right-to-life.

profession Any field, occupation, or career requiring considerable training and specialized study and adhering to a high standard of ethical behavior; for example, professions of law, medicine, engineering, public accountancy, architecture, and teaching. *See also* job; occupation; paraprofession; professional; work.

profession, para- *See* paraprofession.

professional **1.** One who is a specialist in a particular field or occupation, as a physician and a lawyer

are professionals. *See also* health professional. **2.** Pertaining to one's profession or occupation, as in professional liability. **3.** Conforming to the standards of a profession. *Compare* unprofessional. **4.** Engaging in a given activity as a source of livelihood or as a career, as in a professional blood donor. *See also* professional blood donor. **5.** Having or showing great skill.

professional, activity *See* activity professional.

Professional Activity Study (PAS) The oldest hospital automated discharge abstract system, developed and sold by the Commission on Professional and Hospital Activities and used by many acute short-stay hospitals in the United States. *See also* Commission on Professional and Hospital Activities; hospital discharge abstract system; quality assurance monitor.

Professional Aeromedical Transport Association (PATA) A national organization founded in 1986 composed of 200 firms that provide air ambulance services, primarily by means of fixed-wing aircraft, and suppliers to the industry. *See also* ambulance.

professional, allied health *See* allied health professional.

Professional Baseball Physicians, Association of *See* Association of Professional Baseball Physicians.

professional blood donor A blood donor who is paid for the blood he or she donates to a blood bank. *Compare* voluntary blood donor. *See also* blood donor; donor; professional.

Professional Business Consultants, Institute of Certified *See* Institute of Certified Professional Business Consultants.

Professional Business Consultants, Society of *See* Society of Professional Business Consultants.

professional code of ethics *See* code of ethics.

Professional Conduct, Model Rules of *See* Model Rules of Professional Conduct.

professional corporation (PC) A legal entity whose shareholders must be licensed members of the same profession, such as medicine or dentistry. A PC has certain advantages, such as limited liability for its professional stockholder(s) and corporate ownership of equipment including vehicles. *Synonym*: professional association (PA). *See also* professional.

Professional Disability Consultants, American Board of *See* American Board of Professional Disability Consultants.

**Professional Education of the American
Osteopathic Association, Bureau of**   643   **Professionals, National Association of
Lesbian/Gay Alcoholism**

Professional Education of the American Osteopathic Association, Bureau of   See Bureau of Professional Education of the American Osteopathic Association.

professional, health   See health professional.

Professional and Hospital Activities, Commission on   See Commission on Professional and Hospital Activities.

Professional Hypnotherapists, American Association of   See American Association of Professional Hypnotherapists.

professionalization   The process by which occupations acquire professional status. See also profession.

professional liability   In health care, the legal obligation of a health professional or health care organization resulting from a breach (performing or failing to perform something that was done or should have been done), for which the law provides a remedy. A physician, for example, who fails to make a diagnosis resulting in patient injury is professionally liable for the injury. Professional liability is not the same as professional negligence. Synonym: medical liability. See also liability; malpractice; occurrence policy; professional; professional liability insurance; professional negligence.

Professional Liability Attorneys, American Board of   See American Board of Professional Liability Attorneys.

professional liability insurance   Insurance covering the risk of loss from patient injury or illness resulting from professional negligence or other professional liability. Professional liability insurance pays malpractice claims. Often, a hospital's professional liability policy will not cover the actions of physicians on the medical staff, in which case those physicians need to obtain their own individual policies. See also insurance; medical malpractice insurance; professional.

professional library   The resource center in a health care organization that provides for the informational, educational, and, when appropriate, research-related needs of professional staff and others. See also library.

professional, medical record   See medical record professional.

professional, mental health   See mental health professional.

professional negligence   In health care, failure of a professional, such as a physician, to exercise the degree of care considered reasonable under the circumstances, resulting in an unintended injury to another party. Negligence is one kind of tort that results in legal liability. The tort of negligence requires a duty to exercise reasonable care; a failure to exercise such care; and an injury that was proximately caused by that failure. A careless act may be committed, but if no one is injured as a result, there is no "negligence" as far as legal liability is concerned. Professional negligence is not synonymous with professional liability. See also negligence; professional liability; tort.

professional organization   An organization that promotes a particular profession, as in a medical society or a legal society. See also organization; profession.

Professional Practice Association, American   See American Professional Practice Association.

Professional Psychology, American Board of   See American Board of Professional Psychology.

professional, quality assurance   See quality assurance professional.

professional in quality assurance, certified   See certified professional in quality assurance.

Professional Responsibility, American Bar Association Center for   See American Bar Association Center for Professional Responsibility.

Professional Sanitarians, National Society of   See National Society of Professional Sanitarians.

Professionals, Associated Bodywork and Massage   See Associated Bodywork and Massage Professionals.

Professionals, Association of Reproductive Health   See Association of Reproductive Health Professionals.

Professionals, Federation of Nurses and Health   See Federation of Nurses and Health Professionals.

Professional Sleep Societies, Association of   See Association of Professional Sleep Societies.

Professionals, National Association of Activity   See National Association of Activity Professionals.

Professionals, National Association of Apnea   See National Association of Apnea Professionals.

Professionals, National Association of Disability Evaluating   See National Association of Disability Evaluating Professionals.

Professionals, National Association of Lesbian/Gay Alcoholism   See National Association of Lesbian/Gay Alcoholism Professionals.

Professionals, National Association of Quality Assurance *See* National Association of Quality Assurance Professionals.

Professionals, National Association of Vision *See* National Association of Vision Professionals.

Professionals, National Organization of Gay and Lesbian Scientists and Technical *See* National Organization of Gay and Lesbian Scientists and Technical Professionals.

Professionals in the Private Sector, National Association of Rehabilitation *See* National Association of Rehabilitation Professionals in the Private Sector.

Professionals Section of the American Public Health Association, New *See* New Professionals Section of the American Public Health Association.

Professionals Society, Regulatory Affairs *See* Regulatory Affairs Professionals Society.

professional staff, organized *See* organized professional staff.

Professional Standards Review Council of America (PSRCA) A national organization founded in 1977 composed of physicians, nurses, health care administrators, and consumers concerned with monitoring the quality, appropriateness, and cost of health care given to patients in hospitals, ambulatory clinics, nursing facilities, and physicians' offices. *See also* standard.

professional standards review organization (PSRO) A now defunct organization of physicians in a designated area, state, or community established to monitor health care services paid for through Medicare, Medicaid, and Maternal and Child Health programs to ensure that services provided are medically necessary, meet professional standards, and are provided in the most economic medically appropriate health care agency or institution. The requirement for the establishment of PSROs was added to the Social Security Act via the Social Security Amendments of 1972. PSROs were preceded by experimental medical care review organizations (EMCROs). PSROs have since 1982 been replaced in function by utilization and quality control peer review organizations (PROs). *See also* experimental medical care review organization; Medicaid; Medicare; peer review organization; Social Security Act.

Professional and Technical Advisory Committee (PTAC) A group of public and health care professional organization representatives who provide staff of the Joint Commission on Accreditation of Healthcare Organizations, for each accreditation program, with knowledge and experience and who help to establish and refine standards and strengthen the accreditation process. *See also* Joint Commission on Accreditation of Healthcare Organizations.

profession, para- *See* paraprofession.

Professions, American Society of Allied Health *See* American Society of Allied Health Professions.

Professions Association, Arthritis Health *See* Arthritis Health Professions Association.

Professions, National Association of Advisors for the Health *See* National Association of Advisors for the Health Professions.

Professions, National Center for the Advancement of Blacks in the Health *See* National Center for the Advancement of Blacks in the Health Professions.

professor A teacher or an instructor, as in a university or medical school professor. *See also* academic medicine; faculty; tenure.

Professors, Association of Environmental Engineering *See* Association of Environmental Engineering Professors.

Professors of Child and Adolescent Psychiatry, Society of *See* Society of Professors of Child and Adolescent Psychiatry.

Professors of Gynecology and Obstetrics, Association of *See* Association of Professors of Gynecology and Obstetrics.

Professors of Medicine, Association of *See* Association of Professors of Medicine.

Professors of Ophthalmology, Association of University *See* Association of University Professors of Ophthalmology.

proficiency Having an advanced degree of competence, as in an art, vocation, profession, or branch of learning. *See also* ability; proficiency testing; skill.

proficiency testing The assessment of technical knowledge and skills relating to certain occupations. The Secretary of the Department of Health and Human Services was required by the Social Security Amendments of 1972 to develop and conduct a program to determine the proficiency of individuals in performing the tasks of practical nurses, therapists, medical technologists, cytotechnologists, radiologic technologists, psychiatric technicians, and other health care technicians and technologists. This program was finally repealed by Section 608(b) (technical corrections section) of the Family Support Act of 1988. *See also* proficiency; testing.

profile   In health care, a longitudinal or cross-sectional aggregation of health care data used to assess and improve some aspect of health care delivery. *See also* diagnostic profile; hospital profile; patient profile; physician profile; population profile; practitioner profile; profiling.

profile analysis   Use of aggregate statistical data at the level of a practitioner, a region, or the nation to compare and assess various characteristics of practice patterns. *See also* analysis; profile.

profile, diagnostic   *See* diagnostic profile.

profile, hospital   *See* hospital profile.

profile, patient   *See* patient profile.

profile, physician   *See* physician profile.

profile, population   *See* population profile.

profile, practitioner   *See* practitioner profile.

profiling   An aggregation and analysis of health care data, often in the form of a table or graph, representing distinctive features or characteristics of the object of the data, as in profiling patients, physicians, hospitals, or populations. *See also* patient profile; physician profiling; practice pattern analysis; profile.

profiling, diagnostic   *See* diagnostic profiling.

profiling, hospital   *See* hospital profiling.

profiling, physician   *See* physician profiling.

profiling, population   *See* population profiling.

profiling, practice   *See* practice pattern analysis.

profiling, practitioner   *See* practitioner profiling.

profit   The gain made by the sale of a good or service after deducting expenses, such as the value of labor, materials, and interest on capital involved in its production. Economists define profit as return to (or on) capital investment and distinguish normal (competitive) and excessive (more than competitive) profit. *See also* product; profit center; profiteer; profit motive; underwriting profit.

profit center   A segment of a business organization that is responsible for producing profits on its own. *See also* profit.

profiteer   One who makes excessive profits, often to the detriment of others. *See also* profit.

profit motive   A desire to earn a favorable financial return on a business venture. The profit motive underlies the free enterprise system. *See also* capitalism; profit.

profit, underwriting   *See* underwriting profit.

progeny   Offspring.

prognosis   **1.** In health care, the forecasting or foretelling of the outcome of a disease or condition. **2.** The forecast so produced.

program   An outline of work to be done or a prearranged plan or procedure to conduct an activity, as in a cost-containment program or an accreditation program. *See also* computer program.

Program, Ambulatory Care Accreditation   *See* Ambulatory Care Accreditation Program.

program, cardiac rehabilitation   *See* cardiac rehabilitation program.

program, categorical   *See* categorical program.

program, computer   *See* computer program.

program, degree   *See* degree program.

Program, Diagnostic and Therapeutic Technology Assessment   *See* Diagnostic and Therapeutic Technology Assessment Program.

Program Directors in Internal Medicine, Association of   *See* Association of Program Directors in Internal Medicine.

Program Directors, National Association of State Mental Retardation   *See* National Association of State Mental Retardation Program Directors.

program, employee assistance   *See* employee assistance program.

program, employee benefit   *See* employee benefit program.

program, entitlement   *See* entitlement program.

Program Evaluation and Review Technique (PERT)   A planning and control technique that minimizes interruptions and/or delays in a process with interrelated functions. PERT is used to assist in reducing the time required for completion of a project. A *PERT chart* (also called PERT diagram) shows the sequence and interrelationships of activities from the beginning of a project to the end and uses probabilities for activity start and completion dates. *See also* evaluation; program; review; technique.

Program Foundation, Optometric Extension   *See* Optometric Extension Program Foundation.

program, health aide   *See* health aide program.

Program, HIV/AIDS   *See* HIV/AIDS Program.

program, home care   *See* home care program.

Program, Home Care Accreditation   *See* Home Care Accreditation Program.

Program, Health Care Network Accreditation   *See* Health Care Network Accreditation Program.

Program, Hospital Accreditation   *See* Hospital

Accreditation Program.

Program, Impaired Physician *See* Impaired Physician Program.

Program, Kaiser-Permanente Medical Care *See* Kaiser-Permanente Medical Care Program.

Program, Long Term Care Accreditation *See* Long Term Care Accreditation Program.

Program, Medic Alert Organ Donor *See* Medic Alert Organ Donor Program.

Program, Mental Health Care Accreditation *See* Mental Health Care Accreditation Program.

programmer *See* computer programmer.

programmer, computer *See* computer programmer.

programmer, systems *See* systems programmer.

programming language In computer science, a series of rules for writing instructions in terms and in a format that the computer can understand. *See also* computer; language.

programming, structured *See* structured programming.

Program, National Hormone and Pituitary *See* National Hormone and Pituitary Program.

Program, National Marrow Donor *See* National Marrow Donor Program.

Program, National Resident Matching *See* National Resident Matching Program.

program, outreach *See* outreach program.

program, pain management *See* pain management program.

program, partial care *See* partial care program.

program, physical fitness *See* physical fitness program.

program, quality assurance *See* quality assurance program.

program, rehabilitation *See* rehabilitation program.

program, residential *See* residential program.

program, residential treatment *See* residential treatment program.

program review An assessment of a health program operating in a specific setting, performed to provide a basis for decisions concerning the operation of the program. *See also* program; review.

Programs, Association of Maternal and Child Health *See* Association of Maternal and Child Health Programs.

Programs, Association of Physician Assistant *See* Association of Physician Assistant Programs.

program, second-opinion *See* second-opinion program.

programs, federal assistance *See* federal assistance programs.

programs, maternal and child health *See* maternal and child health services.

Programs, National Association of Meal *See* National Association of Meal Programs.

Programs, National Association of Nutrition and Aging Services *See* National Association of Nutrition and Aging Services Programs.

Programs, National Council for Prescription Drug *See* National Council for Prescription Drug Programs.

Programs of North America, Association of Halfway House Alcoholism *See* Association of Halfway House Alcoholism Programs of North America.

Programs in Occupational Health and Safety, Association of University *See* Association of University Programs in Occupational Health and Safety.

programs, open-ended *See* open-ended programs.

program, staff development *See* staff development program.

program, wellness *See* wellness program.

progressive **1.** Advancing, going forward, as in progressive ideas or progressive change. *See also* progressive patient care. **2.** Going from bad to worse, as in progressive illness.

progressive patient care A common method of organizing nursing services within a health care organization by which patients are grouped into levels of inpatient care units (intensive, intermediate, and self-care) according to their degree of illness. Patients are moved from one unit to another as their illness advances or their condition improves. *See also* inpatient.

progressive tax A tax in which the rate increases as the amount subject to tax increases, as in the federal personal income tax, which taxes the wealthy at a higher rate than the poor or middle class. *See also* regressive tax; proportional tax; tax.

progress note, medical record *See* medical record progress note.

progress report, written *See* written progress report.

project A unique endeavor with a beginning and an end to be completed by one or more people within the constraints of time, budget, and quality; a problem scheduled for solution. *See also* project grant; project management; project team.

project grant A grant that directs funding to a specific project. *Compare* general support grant. *See also* grant; project.

projection Estimate of future performance made, for example, by corporate planners, economists, and credit and securities analysts. Economists use econometric models to project gross national product, inflation, unemployment, and many other economic factors. *See also* econometrics; forecasting.

project management A set of principles, methods, and techniques for effective planning of objective-oriented work, thereby establishing a sound basis for effective scheduling, controlling, and replanning in the management of projects. *See also* management; project.

projector, overhead *See* overhead projector.

project, quality improvement *See* quality improvement project.

project team A cross-functional team of workers throughout an organization assigned the responsibility of diagnosing and improving a problem. *See also* project; team.

prolapse A falling or slipping down of an organ, as in prolapse of the uterus. *See also* procidentia.

pro-life In favor of upholding the right to life of the developing fetus; opposed to abortion. *Compare* pro-choice; RU-486. *See also* anti-choice; pro-family; right-to-life.

PROM Acronym for programmable read-only memory; in computer science, a memory that can be programmed only once. *See also* computer.

promotion 1. The act of raising to a more important or responsible job or rank. 2. To contribute to the progress or growth of, as in health promotion. 3. In external relations, the presentation of a product for consumer or public acceptance, through a program of direct contact methods and media relations. *See also* overhype; research and development.

promotion, health *See* health promotion.

Promotion Institute, Health *See* Health Promotion Institute.

Promotion, Office of Disease Prevention and Health *See* Office of Disease Prevention and Health Promotion.

prompt 1. Carried out or performed in a timely manner, without delay, as in prompt service. 2. A symbol that appears on a computer terminal screen to signal to the user that the computer is ready to receive input.

promulgate To make known by public declaration.

proof 1. The evidence or argument that compels the mind to accept an assertion as true. *See also* burden of proof; prove. 2. The concentration of alcohol in an alcoholic beverage. In the United States, proof is two times the alcohol content; for example, 20 percent alcohol is 40-proof alcohol.

proof, burden of *See* burden of proof.

proof of the pudding The ultimate evidence or proof attesting the true nature of something.

proofread To review written material in order to find errors and make corrections.

ProPaC *See* Prospective Payment Assessment Commission.

property 1. A characteristic quality, ability, capability, or function, as in the properties of catgut make it well-suited for suture material. 2. Something owned or possessed.

property insurance Insurance that pays for damage to the insured's own property. *See also* insurance; property.

prophecy 1. A prediction. *See also* self-fulfilling prophecy. 2. An inspired utterance of a prophet, viewed as a revelation of divine will.

prophecy, self-fulfilling *See* self-fulfilling prophecy.

prophylaxis The prevention of disease; preventive treatment, as in prophylaxis for bacterial endocarditis. *See also* chemoprophylaxis.

prophylaxis, chemo- *See* chemoprophylaxis.

Prophylaxis in Obstetrics, American Society for Psycho- *See* American Society for Psychoprophylaxis in Obstetrics.

proportion 1. The relation of one part to another or to the whole. 2. A type of ratio in which the numerator is expressed as a subset of the denominator; for example, the number of patients with primary cesarean section divided by the number of all patients with cesarean section. *See also* denominator; numerator; rate; ratio.

proportional tax A tax imposed at a fixed and uniform rate in proportion to the property subject to the tax. The social security payroll tax is proportional up to a specified limit on income to which it applies. *See also* progressive tax; regressive tax; tax.

proposition 1. A plan suggested for acceptance; a proposal. 2. An expression in language or signs of something that can be believed, doubted, or denied or is either true or false. *See also* theory.

proprietary Owned by a private individual or corporation and operated for the purpose of making a profit for its owners, as in a proprietary hospital or proprietary medicine. *See also* proprietary drug; proprietary name.

proprietary blood bank *See* commercial blood bank.

proprietary drug A drug manufactured and sold only by the owner of the patent, formula, brand name, or trademark associated with the drug. *See also* drug; proprietary.

proprietary hospital *See* investor-owned hospital.

proprietary name A brand name or trademark under which a proprietary product is marketed. *See also* name; proprietary.

PRO scope of work (PRO-SOW) A contract which details the specific obligations of a peer review organization (PRO). It defines the duties and functions of the Medicare review for a specific contract cycle. The first SOW, for instance, was used during the first contract cycle (1984-1986) and emphasized the detection of inappropriate utilization and payments under the new Medicare hospital prospective payment system after October 1983. Contract activities, which concentrated on inpatient hospital care, included reducing unnecessary admissions, ensuring that payment rates matched diagnostic and procedural information contained in the patient records, and reviewing patients who were transferred or readmitted to an acute care hospital within seven days of discharge. *See also* Medicare; peer review organization.

PRO-SOW *See* PRO scope of work.

prosector An individual who performs anatomical dissections and prepares autopsy specimens for pathological examination or demonstration. *See also* autopsy; pathologist's assistant.

prosecute In law, to initiate civil or criminal court action against. *See also* prosecution.

prosecution **1.** In law, the institution and conduct of a legal proceeding. **2.** *See* prosecuting attorney.

prosecution, malicious *See* malicious prosecution.

prosecuting attorney A lawyer empowered to prosecute cases on behalf of a government and its people. *Synonyms*: prosecution; prosecutor. *See also* attorney; prosecution.

prosecutor *See* prosecuting attorney.

prospective Likely or expected to happen in the future, as in prospective payment.

prospective data collection The process of data collection in anticipation of an event or occurrence, as compared with retrospective data collection, which is the process of data collection for events that have already occurred. *See also* data; data collection; prospective.

Prospective Medicine, Society of *See* Society of Prospective Medicine.

prospective payment Payment for services in which the payment is set before the services are actually provided (that is, prospectively), and this payment is issued regardless of the cost incurred providing the services. This contrasts to retrospective payment in which payment for services is based on actual costs determined after the services have been provided. *Synonym*: prospective reimbursement. *Compare* retrospective reimbursement. *See also* cost outlier; payment; prospective pricing system; prospective payment system.

Prospective Payment Assessment Commission (ProPaC) An advisory body established by the Social Security Act Amendments of 1983 to advise the Secretary of Health and Human Services on recommended adjustments in the weights and classification of diagnosis-related groups under Medicare, and to review and recommend any percentage or amount needed to reflect increases in the cost or mix of goods and services. The commission is comprised of 15 experts selected by the director of the Congressional Office of Technology Assessment. *See also* assessment; Medicare; Office of Technology Assessment; payment; prospective.

prospective payment system (PPS) The prospective pricing system for paying for services for Medicare patients by diagnosis-related groups (DRGs). *Compare* cost-based reimbursement. *See also* Medicare; prospective payment; prospective pricing system; uniform capital factor.

prospective pricing system (PPS) The method of third-party payment by which rates of payment to health care providers for services to patients are established in advance (prospectively) for the coming fiscal year. Providers are paid these rates for services delivered regardless of the cost actually incurred in providing these services. Prospective pricing is best exemplified by the prospective payment system for Medicare patients established by the Tax Equity and Fiscal Responsibility Act of 1981. *See also* cost-based reimbursement; Medicare; retrospective reimbursement.

prospective reimbursement *See* prospective payment.

prospective review Review of a proposed scheduled of treatment, which could include patient care or discharge plans, and any policies or procedures that specify how care is or will be provided. *Compare* retrospective review.

prospective study An inquiry planned to observe and gather data for events that have not yet occurred, as compared with a retrospective study, which is planned to examine events that have already occurred. *Compare* retrospective study.

prostaglandin A family of hormonelike compounds that have a wide range of actions in the body, which may be desirable or undesirable depending on the situation. For example, prostaglandins stimulate uterine contractions during childbirth, help lower blood pressure and open airways, regulate body temperature, and regulate acid secretion in the stomach. Aspirin and other nonsteroidal anti-inflammatory drugs inhibit prostaglandin production.

prostate A gland in the male reproductive system that surrounds the neck of the bladder and the urethra. The prostate contributes to the seminal fluid a secretion containing acid phosphatase, citric acid, and proteolytic enzymes, which account for the liquefaction of the coagulated semen. *See also* benign prostatic hypertrophy; prostatectomy; prostatitis.

prostatectomy Surgical removal of the prostate or a part of it. There are many ways to accomplish removal, including perineal prostatectomy, transurethral resection of the prostate (TUR, TURP) (performed by means of a cystocope passed through the urethra), retropubic prevesical prostatectomy, and suprapubic transvesical prostatectomy. *See also* prostate; prostatitis.

prostatic hypertrophy, benign *See* benign prostatic hypertrophy.

prostatitis Inflammation of the prostate. *See also* prostate.

prosthesis An artificial substitute for a missing body part, such as an artificial arm, leg, eye, tooth, hearing aid, and implanted pacemakers. Prostheses are used for functional or cosmetic reasons, or both.

Prosthetic Association, American Orthotic and *See* American Orthotic and Prosthetic Association.

Prosthetic-Orthotic Clinics, Association of Children's *See* Association of Children's Prosthetic-Orthotic Clinics.

prosthetics The field of knowledge relating to the design and use of prostheses, appliances used to correct extremity ailments. *See also* orthotics; orthotist/prosthetist.

Prosthetics, American Academy of Maxillofacial *See* American Academy of Maxillofacial Prosthetics.

Prosthetics, American Board for Certification in Orthotics and *See* American Board for Certification in Orthotics and Prosthetics.

prosthetist *See* orthotist/prosthetist.

Prosthetists, American Academy of Orthotists and *See* American Academy of Orthotists and Prosthetists.

Prosthodontic Organizations, Federation of *See* Federation of Prosthodontic Organizations.

prosthodontics A dental specialty dealing with the restoration and maintenance of oral function, comfort, appearance, and health by the replacement of missing natural teeth and associated structures with fixed or removable substitutes, such as dentures and bridgework. *See also* bridge; crown; dental specialties; denture; implant dentistry; prosthodontist.

Prosthodontics, American Academy of Fixed *See* American Academy of Fixed Prosthodontics.

Prosthodontics, American Academy of Implant *See* American Academy of Implant Prosthodontics.

Prosthodontics, American Board of *See* American Board of Prosthodontics.

prosthodontics, implant *See* implant dentistry.

Prosthodontic Society, American *See* American Prosthodontic Society.

prosthodontist A dentist who specializes in prosthodontics. *See also* dental specialties; dentist; prosthodontics.

Prosthodontists, American College of *See* American College of Prosthodontists.

prostration A state of helplessness or total exhaustion. *See also* exhaustion.

protection for adults (adult protection) Services that determine the need for protective intervention, correct hazardous living conditions or situations in which vulnerable adults are unable to care for themselves, and investigate evidence of neglect, abuse, or exploitation. *Synonyms:* adult protection; adult protection services. *See also* protection for children.

Protection Agency, Environmental *See* Environmental Protection Agency.

Protection Association, National Fire *See* National Fire Protection Association.

protection for children (child protection) Services

that help families recognize the cause of any problems and strengthen parental ability to provide acceptable care.

Protection Engineers, Society of Fire *See* Society of Fire Protection Engineers.

Protection and Measurements, National Council on Radiation *See* National Council on Radiation Protection and Measurements.

Protection, National Accreditation Council for Environmental Health Science and *See* National Accreditation Council for Environmental Health Science and Protection.

protege/protegee One whose welfare, training, or career is promoted by an influential person.

protein Complex organic molecules that are composed of amino acids and are a fundamental component of all living cells. Types of proteins include enzymes, hormones, and antibodies. Proteins can be obtained from meat, fish, eggs, milk, and legumes. *See also* antibodies; enzyme; gluten; hormone.

protein, lipo- *See* lipoprotein.

Protestant Health Association, American *See* American Protestant Health Association.

Protestant Health and Human Services Assembly (PHHSA) A national organization founded in 1970 composed of 17 institutions and agencies involved in serving the health and welfare needs of people. It exercises influence and uses resources consistent with Christian healing and caring. Formerly (1987) Protestant Health and Welfare Assembly.

Protestant Health and Welfare Assembly *See* Protestant Health and Human Services Assembly.

protocol A plan, or set of steps, to be followed in a study, an investigation, or an intervention, as in clinical protocols used in the care of trauma patients. *See also* algorithm; practice guideline.

protoplasm The matter of which all biological cells consist, which in nucleated cells is subdivided into that composing the nucleus (nucleoplasm) and that surrounding the nucleus (cytoplasm). *See also* biology; cell.

protozoa Single-celled microorganisms, comprising the simplest phylum of the animal world. A few are parasitic in humans and therefore have medical importance; for example, protozoa are the causative agents of giardia, malaria, amoebiasis, toxoplasmosis, and trichomoniasis. *See also* microorganism; parasite.

prove To establish the truth or validity of by pre-

sentation of argument or evidence. *See also* proof.

provider One that makes something, such as a service, available; for example, health care provider. *See also* health care provider.

provider-based physician Under Medicare, a physician who performs services in a provider setting and has a financial arrangement under which he or she is compensated through or by a provider or provider-related entity. *See also* Medicare; physician.

provider, free choice of *See* free choice of provider.

provider, health care *See* health care provider.

provider, health service *See* health care provider.

provider, impaired health care *See* impaired health care provider.

provider, integrated *See* integrated provider.

provider, nonparticipating *See* nonparticipating provider.

provider organization, preferred *See* preferred provider organization.

Provider Organizations, American Association of Preferred *See* American Association of Preferred Provider Organizations.

provider, participating *See* participating provider.

provider, primary care *See* primary care provider.

provider, referral *See* referral provider.

Provider Reimbursement Review Board (PRRB) A body appointed by the Secretary of Health and Human Services to provide an appeal mechanism for health care providers to whom Medicare fiscal intermediaries deny reimbursement for services under Medicare. *See also* Medicare.

Providers, National Association of Addiction Treatment *See* National Association of Addiction Treatment Providers.

provisional accreditation An accreditation decision that results when a health care organization has demonstrated compliance with selected structural standards of the Joint Commission on Accreditation of Healthcare Organizations used in the first of two surveys conducted under the early survey policy. The second survey is conducted approximately six months later to allow the health care organization sufficient time to demonstrate a track record of performance. Provisional accreditation status remains until a health care organization completes a full survey. *See also* accreditation decision; early survey option; Joint Commission on Accreditation of Healthcare Organizations.

proximal Nearest; closer to any point of reference,

as in the elbow is proximal to the wrist (point of reference, shoulder). *Compare* distal.

proximate cause   In negligence law, an act or omission that naturally and directly produces a consequence. In some jurisdictions, for an act to be considered the proximate cause of a loss or injury, it must be proved that, but for the act or omission, the injury or loss would not have occurred. *See also* cause.

proxy   A person authorized to decide (act) for another person, particularly in some meeting or action. *See also* durable power of attorney for health care.

PRRB   *See* Provider Reimbursement Review Board.

PRSA   *See* Public Relations Society of America.

prudence   Displaying foresight and discretion in one's actions.

prudent buyer principle   The principle that Medicare or other third-party payers should not reimburse a provider for a cost that is not reasonable because it is more than the amount that a prudent and cost-conscious buyer would be expected to pay. *See also* health care provider; Medicare; principle; third-party payer.

Prudent Use of Antibiotics, Alliance for the   *See* Alliance for the Prudent Use of Antibiotics.

pruritis   Itching, as in a pruritic rash. *Compare* antipruritic. *See also* itch.

PS   *See* Psychology Society; Psychometric Society; Psychonomic Society.

PSI   *See* Parapsychological Services Institute.

pseudocyesis   A usually psychosomatic condition in which physical symptoms of pregnancy, such as weight gain and amenorrhea (absence of menstruation), are manifested without conception. *Synonym:* pseudopregnancy. *See also* amenorrhea; conception; pregnancy; psychosomatic illness.

pseudopregnancy   *See* pseudocyesis.

psoriasis   A common chronic skin condition in which the epidermal cells grow rapidly, causing the skin to become thickened, red, and scaly. *See also* dermatology; skin.

PSR   *See* Physicians for Social Responsibility.

PSRC   *See* Plastic Surgery Research Council.

PSRCA   *See* Professional Standards Review Council of America.

PSRO   *See* professional standards review organization.

PSW   *See* psychiatric social worker.

psyche   *See* mind.

psychedelic   **1.** Pertaining to a mental state with visual hallucinations, altered perceptions, and usually strong emotions, in some cases, similar to that observed in psychosis. **2.** A drug, such as LSD (lysergic acid), that produces such effects. *See also* hallucination; hallucinogen; lysergic acid; psychosis.

psychiatric aide   An individual who works with mentally ill patients performing a variety of tasks under the supervision of a nurse or other qualified professional. These tasks can involve assisting the patient in bathing, dressing, and grooming; escorting the patient inside and on the grounds; recording a patient's behavior and physical condition; and helping the patient to gain confidence and skills. A psychiatric aide is a nurse assistant specialty. *See also* aide; mental health technician; nursing assistant; psychiatry.

Psychiatric Administrators, American Association of   *See* American Association of Psychiatric Administrators.

Psychiatric Association, American   *See* American Psychiatric Association.

Psychiatric Association, American Ortho-   *See* American Orthopsychiatric Association.

Psychiatric Association, Central Neuro-   *See* Central Neuropsychiatric Association.

psychiatric care   Provision by or under the direction of a psychiatrist of services related to the diagnosis and treatment of mental or emotional disorders. *See also* psychiatry.

psychiatric emergency services   A 24-hour-per-day hospital service providing immediate initial evaluation and treatment to patients with mental or emotional disorders. *See also* emergency medicine; emergency services; psychiatry.

psychiatric hospital   A hospital that provides diagnostic and treatment services to patients with mental or emotional disorders. *See also* mental disorder; hospital.

Psychiatric Hospitals, National Association of Private   *See* National Association of Private Psychiatric Hospitals.

psychiatric inpatient unit   A unit in a hospital for treatment of patients who require psychiatric care. *See also* inpatient; psychiatry; unit.

psychiatric nurse   A registered nurse qualified by specialized education and training to provide nursing care to patients with mental or emotional disorders. *See also* psychiatry; registered nurse.

Psychiatric Nurses Association, American *See* American Psychiatric Nurses Association.

psychiatric nursing The branch of nursing dealing with the prevention and treatment of mental or emotional disorders. *Synonym:* mental health nursing. *See also* nursing; psychiatric nurse; psychiatry.

Psychiatric Residency Training, American Association of Directors of *See* American Association of Directors of Psychiatric Residency Training.

Psychiatric Services for Children, American Association of *See* American Association of Psychiatric Services for Children.

psychiatric social worker (PSW) A social worker who works in a psychiatric hospital, residential treatment center, psychiatric unit of a general hospital, or a mental health center. A PSW assists individuals and their families in dealing with social, emotional, and environmental problems resulting from mental illness or disability. A PSW serves as a link between patient, psychiatrist or clinical psychologist, family, and community. *See also* psychiatry; psychotherapist; social worker.

Psychiatric and Substance Abuse Services, Special Constituency Section for *See* Special Constituency Section for Psychiatric and Substance Abuse Services.

Psychiatric Treatment Centers for Children, National Association of *See* National Association of Psychiatric Treatment Centers for Children.

psychiatrist A physician who specializes in psychiatry. *See also* psychiatry.

psychiatrist, neuro- *See* neuropsychiatrist.

Psychiatrists Against Motorcoach Therapy, National Coalition of *See* National Coalition of Psychiatrists Against Motorcoach Therapy.

Psychiatrists in Alcoholism and Addictions, American Academy of *See* American Academy of Psychiatrists in Alcoholism and Addictions.

Psychiatrists of America, Black *See* Black Psychiatrists of America.

Psychiatrists, American Academy of Clinical *See* American Academy of Clinical Psychiatrists.

Psychiatrists, American Association of Community *See* American Association of Community Psychiatrists.

Psychiatrists, American College of *See* American College of Psychiatrists.

Psychiatrists, American College of Neuro- *See*

American College of Neuropsychiatrists.

Psychiatrists, Association of Gay and Lesbian *See* Association of Gay and Lesbian Psychiatrists.

Psychiatrists from India, American Association of *See* American Association of Psychiatrists from India.

psychiatry The branch of medicine and medical specialty dealing with the prevention, diagnosis, and treatment of mental, addictive, and emotional disorders, such as psychoses, depression, anxiety disorders, substance abuse disorders, developmental disabilities, sexual dysfunctions, and adjustment reactions. Addiction psychiatry, child and adolescent psychiatry, clinical neurophysiology, forensic psychiatry, and geriatric psychiatry are psychiatric subspecialties. *See also* addiction psychiatry; child and adolescent psychiatry; clinical neurophysiology; forensic psychiatry; geriatric psychiatry.

psychiatry, addiction *See* addiction psychiatry.

psychiatry, adolescent *See* child and adolescent psychiatry.

Psychiatry, American Academy of Child *See* American Academy of Child and Adolescent Psychiatry.

Psychiatry, American Academy of Child and Adolescent *See* American Academy of Child and Adolescent Psychiatry.

Psychiatry, American Association of Chairmen of Departments of *See* American Association of Chairmen of Departments of Psychiatry.

Psychiatry, American Association for Geriatric *See* American Association for Geriatric Psychiatry.

Psychiatry, American Association for Social *See* American Association for Social Psychiatry.

Psychiatry, American Board of Forensic *See* American Board of Forensic Psychiatry.

Psychiatry, American Society for Adolescent *See* American Society for Adolescent Psychiatry.

psychiatry, child and adolescent *See* child and adolescent psychiatry.

psychiatry, forensic *See* forensic psychiatry.

psychiatry, geriatric *See* geriatric psychiatry.

Psychiatry, Group for the Advancement of *See* Group for the Advancement of Psychiatry.

Psychiatry, Institute on Hospital and Community *See* Institute on Hospital and Community Psychiatry.

Psychiatry and the Law, American Academy of *See* American Academy of Psychiatry and the Law.

Psychiatry and Neurology, American Board of

See American Board of Psychiatry and Neurology.

psychiatry, social *See* social psychiatry.

Psychiatry, Society of Professors of Child and Adolescent *See* Society of Professors of Child and Adolescent Psychiatry.

Psychical Research, American Society for *See* American Society for Psychical Research.

psychoanalysis A method of psychiatric therapy and branch of psychiatry that originated with the Austrian physician Sigmund Freud during the late 1800s and early 1900s. According to Freud, mental disorders could be cured by uncovering a patient's unconscious wishes and fears. Freud believed that all behavior is influenced by instincts, fears, and unconscious mental processes not controlled by rational thought. He claimed that early childhood bodily experiences, especially sexual ones, shape individual behavior in later life. Psychoanalysts believe that unpleasant experiences, especially during childhood, may become buried in the unconscious mind and cause mental illness. Psychoanalytic treatment tries to bring these experiences out of a patient's unconscious mind and into the conscious mind through use of free association, dream interpretation, and analysis of resistance and transference. Psychoanalytic theory includes the following ideas: the mind is divided into the id, the ego, and the superego; there are five overlapping stages of psychosexual development (oral phase, anal phase, phallic stage, latency, and adolescence); and there is a strong attraction of children to the parent of the opposite sex, called the Oedipus complex. *See also* Oedipus; Oedipus complex; repression.

Psychoanalysis, American Academy of *See* American Academy of Psychoanalysis.

Psychoanalysis and the American Boards for Accreditation and Certification, National Association for the Advancement of *See* National Association for the Advancement of Psychoanalysis and the American Boards for Accreditation and Certification.

Psychoanalysis, Association for Applied *See* Association for Applied Psychoanalysis.

Psychoanalysis, Association for Child *See* Association for Child Psychoanalysis.

Psychoanalysis, National Psychological Association for *See* National Psychological Association for Psychoanalysis.

psychoanalyst An individual who specializes in psychoanalysis. *See also* psychoanalysis.

Psychoanalysts, American College of *See* American College of Psychoanalysts.

Psychoanalytic Association, American *See* American Psychoanalytic Association.

Psychoanalytic Medicine, Association for *See* Association for Psychoanalytic Medicine.

Psychoanalytic Physicians, American Society of *See* American Society of Psychoanalytic Physicians.

psychoanalyze To analyze and treat by psychoanalysis. *See also* psychoanalysis.

psychobabble Psychological jargon, especially that of psychotherapy. *See also* jargon; psychotherapy.

psychobabbler One who uses psychobabble. *See also* psychobabble.

psychodrama A therapeutic method developed by Dr JL Moreno (1889-1974), used to afford catharsis and social relearning. *See also* drama therapy.

Psychodrama, American Society of Group Psychotherapy and *See* American Society of Group Psychotherapy and Psychodrama.

psychogenic Originating in the mind, not in the body, as in psychogenic illness. *See also* hysteria; psychosomatic.

psychogenic overlay *See* emotional overlay.

psychohistory Application of the principles of psychology to the study of history. *See also* history; psychology.

psycholinguistics A branch of linguistics that deals with the interrelation between the acquisition, use, and comprehension of language and the processes of the mind. *See also* language; linguistics; psychology.

Psychological Association, American *See* American Psychological Association.

Psychological Association, Asian American *See* Asian American Psychological Association.

Psychological Association, Division of Psychotherapy of the American *See* Division of Psychotherapy of the American Psychological Association.

Psychological Association for Psychoanalysis, National *See* National Psychological Association for Psychoanalysis.

Psychological and Cognitive Sciences, Federation of Behavioral, *See* Federation of Behavioral, Psychological and Cognitive Sciences.

Psychological Development, Multidisciplinary Institute for Neuro- *See* Multidisciplinary Institute for Neuropsychological Development.

Psychological Hypnosis, American Board of *See*

American Board of Psychological Hypnosis.

Psychological Studies, Christian Association for *See* Christian Association for Psychological Studies.

Psychological Study of Lesbian and Gay Issues, Society for the *See* Society for the Psychological Study of Lesbian and Gay Issues.

Psychological Study of Social Issues, Society for the *See* Society for the Psychological Study of Social Issues.

psychological trauma *See* trauma.

Psychological Type, Association for *See* Association for Psychological Type.

psychologist An individual who specializes in psychological research, testing, and/or therapy. *See also* clinical psychologist; personnel psychologist; psychology; school psychologist.

psychologist, clinical *See* clinical psychologist.

psychologist, personnel *See* personnel psychologist.

Psychologists in Addictive Behaviors, Society of *See* Society of Psychologists in Addictive Behaviors.

Psychologists, Association of Aviation *See* Association of Aviation Psychologists.

Psychologists, Association of Black *See* Association of Black Psychologists.

psychologist, school *See* school psychologist.

Psychologists, Division of Applied Experimental and Engineering *See* Division of Applied Experimental and Engineering Psychologists.

Psychologists, National Association of School *See* National Association of School Psychologists.

Psychologists and Social Workers, American Association of Spinal Cord Injury *See* American Association of Spinal Cord Injury Psychologists and Social Workers.

Psychologists, Society of Experimental *See* Society of Experimental Psychologists.

psychology The branch of science that deals with mental processes and behavior, composed of the following major fields: abnormal, clinical, comparative, counseling, developmental, educational, engineering, experimental, industrial, learning, motivation, perception, personality, physiological, psychometrics, school, and social psychology. *See also* social science.

psychology, abnormal *See* abnormal psychology.

Psychology, American Academy of Forensic *See* American Academy of Forensic Psychology.

Psychology, American Association for Correctional *See* American Association for Correctional Psychology.

Psychology, American Board of Bionic Rehabilitative *See* American Board of Bionic Rehabilitative Psychology.

Psychology, American Board of Professional *See* American Board of Professional Psychology.

Psychology, Association for Advancement of *See* Association for Advancement of Psychology.

Psychology, Association for Birth *See* Association for Birth Psychology.

Psychology, Association for Humanistic *See* Association for Humanistic Psychology.

Psychology, Association for Media *See* Association for Media Psychology.

Psychology, Association for Women in *See* Association for Women in Psychology.

psychology, clinical *See* clinical psychology.

Psychology, Council for the National Register of Health Service Providers in *See* Council for the National Register of Health Service Providers in Psychology.

psychology, counseling *See* counseling psychology.

psychology, developmental *See* developmental psychology.

Psychology, Division of Family *See* Division of Family Psychology.

psychology, educational *See* educational psychology.

psychology, engineering *See* engineering psychology.

psychology, industrial *See* industrial psychology.

Psychology - Law Society, American *See* American Psychology - Law Society.

psychology, learning *See* learning psychology.

Psychology, National Academy of Neuro- *See* National Academy of Neuropsychology.

psychology, para- *See* parapsychology.

psychology, perception *See* perception psychology.

psychology, personality *See* personality psychology.

psychology, personnel *See* personnel psychology.

Psychology and Physiology, Society for the Study of Male *See* Society for the Study of Male Psychology and Physiology.

Psychology Postdoctoral and Internship Centers, Association of *See* Association of Psychology Postdoctoral and Internship Centers.

psychology, school *See* school psychology.

psychology, social *See* social psychology.

Psychology Society (PS) A national organization founded in 1960 composed of 3,200 psychologists who have a doctoral degree and are certified/licensed in the state where they practice. It seeks to further the use of psychology in therapy, family and social problems, behavior modification, and treatment of drug abusers and prisoners. *See also* psychology.

Psychology, Society for the Advancement of Social *See* Society for the Advancement of Social Psychology.

Psychology, Society for Pediatric *See* Society for Pediatric Psychology.

Psychology of Sport and Physical Activity, North American Society for the *See* North American Society for the Psychology of Sport and Physical Activity.

psychometrician A psychologist who deals with measurement of psychological phenomena. *See also* psychometrics.

psychometrics The branch of psychology that deals with the design, administration, and interpretation of quantitative tests for the measurement of psychological variables, such as intelligence, aptitude, and personality traits. *Synonym*: psychometry. *See also* measurement; psychology.

Psychometric Society (PS) A national organization founded in 1935 composed of 2,200 persons interested in development of quantitative models for psychological phenomena and quantitative methodology in the social and behavioral sciences. *See also* psychometrics.

psychometry *See* psychometrics.

psychomotor Relating to motor movement (muscle activity) associated with mental processes, as in psychomotor skills.

psychoneurosis *See* neurosis.

Psychonomic Society (PS) A national organization founded in 1959 composed of 2,400 persons qualified to conduct and supervise scientific research in psychology or allied sciences. Members hold a Doctor of Philosophy (PhD) degree or its equivalent and have published significant research other than a doctoral dissertation. *See also* psychology.

psychopath A person with an antisocial personality disorder, especially one manifested in aggressive, perverted, criminal, or amoral behavior. *Synonym*: sociopath. *See also* personality disorder.

Psychopathological Association, American *See* American Psychopathological Association.

psychopathology *See* abnormal psychology.

Psychopathology of Expression, American Society of *See* American Society of Psychopathology of Expression.

psychopharmacology The branch of pharmacology that deals with the study of the actions and effects of psychoactive drugs. *See also* drug; pharmacology.

Psychopharmacology, American College of Neuro- *See* American College of Neuropsychopharmacology.

Psychophysiological Research, Society for *See* Society for Psychophysiological Research.

Psychophysiology and Biofeedback, Association for Applied *See* Association for Applied Psychophysiology and Biofeedback.

Psychoprophylaxis in Obstetrics, American Society for *See* American Society for Psychoprophylaxis in Obstetrics.

psychosexual Pertaining to the mental and emotional aspects of sexual behavior. *See also* sex.

psychosis A severe mental disorder, with or without organic damage, characterized by derangement of personality, loss of contact with reality, and deterioration of normal social functioning. Hallucinations and delusions characterize psychoses. *Compare* neurosis. *See also* neuroleptic; organic psychosis; personality; psychedelic; toxic psychosis.

psychosis, organic *See* organic psychosis.

psychosis, toxic *See* toxic psychosis.

psychosocial Relating social conditions to mental health.

psychosomatic Pertaining to a disorder having physical symptoms but originating from mental or emotional causes, as in psychosomatic abdominal pain. *Compare* somatic. *See also* hysteria; psychogenic; psychosomatic illness; psychosomatic medicine.

psychosomatic disease *See* psychosomatic illness.

psychosomatic illness A disorder having physical symptoms but originating from mental or emotional causes. For instance, disorders that are thought to be related to or exacerbated by emotional disturbances include asthma, peptic ulcer, and neurodermatitis. *Synonym*: psychosomatic disease. *See also* asthma; illness; neurodermatitis; overlay; peptic ulcer; psychosomatic medicine.

psychosomatic medicine The use of methods and principles of psychology in the treatment of physical ailments. *See also* medicine; psychology; psychosomatic.

Psychosomatic Medicine, Academy of *See* Academy of Psychosomatic Medicine.

Psychosomatic Society, American *See* American Psychosomatic Society.

psychosurgery Brain surgery involving destruction of brain tissue to treat severe, intractable mental or behavioral disorders. *See also* neurological surgery; prefrontal lobotomy; psychiatry.

psychotherapist A mental health professional who provides psychotherapy. Psychiatrists, psychologists, and psychiatric or clinical social workers are three kinds of psychotherapists. *See also* mental health professional; psychiatric social worker; psychiatrist; psychologist; psychotherapy.

psychotherapist-patient privilege A privilege, recognized by many states, similar to the physician-patient privilege for disclosures to psychologists or other general practitioners treating mental or emotional disorders, such as drug or alcohol dependence. Such a privilege arises from the special therapeutic need to assure the patient that disclosures will not be made. *See also* patient; physician-patient privilege; psychotherapist.

Psychotherapists, American Academy of *See* American Academy of Psychotherapists.

Psychotherapists, American Board of Medical *See* American Board of Medical Psychotherapists.

psychotherapy A treatment technique of alleviating or curing certain forms of mental disorders by suggestion, persuasion, encouragement, the inspiration of hope or confidence, the discouragement of morbid memories, associations, or beliefs, and other similar means. Psychotherapy relies principally on verbal communications within the relationship between a mental health professional (psychotherapist) and a patient(s). The primary treatment modalities of psychotherapy are individual, family, and group therapies. The length of the treatment may be short-term or long-term. *See also* behavior therapy; gestalt therapy; group therapy; psychotherapist; sex therapy; therapy; transference.

Psychotherapy, American Board of Examiners of Psychodrama, Sociometry, and Group *See* American Board of Examiners of Psychodrama, Sociometry, and Group Psychotherapy.

Psychotherapy of the American Psychological Association, Division of *See* Division of Psychotherapy of the American Psychological Association.

Psychotherapy, Association for the Advancement of *See* Association for the Advancement of Psychotherapy.

Psychotherapy Association, American Group *See* American Group Psychotherapy Association.

psychotherapy, gestalt *See* gestaltism.

psychotherapy, group *See* group therapy.

Psychotherapy, Institute for Research in Hypnosis and *See* Institute for Research in Hypnosis and Psychotherapy.

Psychotherapy and Psychodrama, American Society of Group *See* American Society of Group Psychotherapy and Psychodrama.

psychotropic drug Any drug that alters perception or behavior. These include, but are not limited to, those drugs that produce drug dependence. *See also* alcoholism and other drug dependence; deinstitutionalization; drug; hallucinogen.

PT *See* physical therapist; physical therapy.

PTAC *See* Professional and Technical Advisory Committee.

PTCA *See* percutaneous transluminal coronary angioplasty.

PTSD *See* posttraumatic stress disorder.

PTSM *See* plant, technology, and safety management.

PTSM A handbook and ongoing series of monographs that provide information on the standards of the Joint Commission on Accreditation of Healthcare Organizations and issues relating to plant, technology, and safety management applicable to all types of health care organizations. *See also* Joint Commission on Accreditation of Healthcare Organizations; plant, technology, and safety management.

puberty The period during which secondary sex characteristics begin to develop and the capability of sexual reproduction is attained. *See also* adolescence; menarche; menstruation.

public The community or the people as a whole sharing a common interest, as in the aggregate of the citizens of a state, nation, or municipality.

public accountability *See* accountability.

public administration The discipline and practice of organizing and managing people and other resources to achieve the goals of government. *See also* administration; Master of Public Administration; public.

public affairs 1. Issues, questions, and responses pertaining to social, governmental, military, scientific, economic, or corporate activities that are of concern to the people at large. 2. *See* public relations.

public agency *See* administrative agency.

public assistance Aid, such as money or food, given to homeless and other financially needy people. *See also* public.

Public Child Welfare Administrators, National Association of *See* National Association of Public Child Welfare Administrators.

Public Citizen A citizens' interest group founded in 1971 by Ralph Nader to support the work of citizen advocates. Its areas of focus include consumer rights in the marketplace, safe products, a healthful environment and work place, clean and safe energy sources, corporate and government accountability, group buying to enhance marketplace clients, and citizen empowerment. In health care, its interests include hospital quality and costs, doctors' fees, physician discipline and malpractice, state administration of Medicare programs, unnecessary surgery, comprehensive health planning, dangerous drugs, carcinogens, medical devices, and overuse of medical and dental x-rays. It favors a single-payer comprehensive health care system. Its methods for change include lobbying, litigation, monitoring government agencies, research, and public education. It acquires funding primarily through direct mail and payment for publications and court awards.

Public Citizen Health Research Group (PCHRG) A citizens' interest group founded in 1971 that works on issues of health care delivery, workplace safety and health, drug regulation, food additives, medical device safety, and environmental influences on health. It petitions or sues federal agencies on consumers' behalf, testifies before Congress on health matters, and monitors the enforcement of health and safety legislation. It publicizes important health findings and makes available to the public a broad spectrum of research and consumer action materials in the form of books and reports. *See also* Public Citizen.

Public Citizen Litigation Group (PCLG) A national public interest group founded in 1972 by Ralph Nader that files consumer cases dealing with economic issues; cases involving health and safety of consumers and workers; cases compelling various federal agencies to comply with the laws they administer; cases concerning open government; and cases relating to other areas of concern to consumers and citizens. *See also* consumer; litigation; Public Citizen.

public domain In law, land and water in possession of and owned by the United States and the states individually, as distinguished from lands privately owned by individuals or corporations; in copyright law, public ownership status of writings, documents, or publications that are not protected by copyrights. *See also* domain.

public health (PH) The science and practice of protecting and improving the health of a community, as by preventive medicine, health education, control of communicable diseases, application of sanitary measures, and monitoring of environmental hazards. *See also* board of health; health planner; preventive medicine; public.

public health administrator An individual who is responsible for assisting in the formulation of departmental policies and procedures, developing budgets, assisting in development of legislation, overseeing and monitoring contracts, and other administrative duties. *See also* administrator; public health.

Public Health, American Board of Dental *See* American Board of Dental Public Health.

Public Health Association, American *See* American Public Health Association.

Public Health Association, New Professionals Section of the American *See* New Professionals Section of the American Public Health Association.

Public Health, Association of Schools of *See* Association of Schools of Public Health.

public health bacteriology The branch of bacteriology dealing with the spread and prevention of bacterial disease. *See also* bacteriology; public health.

public health consultant An individual with a master's degree in public health or a related field usually working at the state and federal levels who provides technical assistance to local health agencies by making on-site visits and helping plan, implement, and evaluate health care programs. He or she may also meet with private organizations to assist in designing health care programs and procedures. *See also* consultant; public health.

Public Health, Council on Education for *See* Council on Education for Public Health.

public health dental hygienist A dental hygienist who works in a clinical setting, such as a public health clinic, state hospital, or state correctional facility, or in a community setting, such as a school clinic where he or she may assist in the development and operation of the clinic, distribution of dental supplies, education, and other tasks. *See also* dental hygienist; public health.

public health dentist A dentist who specializes in dental public health. A public health dentist may work in state facilities, public health clinics, or state or local health departments. *See also* dental specialties; dentist; public health dentistry.

public health dentistry A dental specialty involving the control and prevention of dental disease and the promotion of oral health through organized community efforts. It is the form of dental practice that treats the community, rather than the individual, as a patient. *Synonym*: dental public health. *See also* dental specialties; dentist; public health dentist.

Public Health Dentistry, American Association of *See* American Association of Public Health Dentistry.

Public Health Education, Association of State and Territorial Directors of *See* Association of State and Territorial Directors of Public Health Education.

Public Health Education, Society for *See* Society for Public Health Education.

public health educator An individual usually based in the health department who is responsible for working with health department staff, community agencies, professional groups, schools, and the general public in organizing community health resources, disseminating health information materials, conducting promotional campaigns, and stimulating interest in the improvement of the health practices of the public. *See also* public health.

public health engineer An individual who oversees and directs the performance of a variety of environmental engineering activities to protect and improve land and water resources and their quality to maintain a clean environment. *See also* engineer; public health.

public health field investigator An individual who usually locates, prevents, and controls sexually transmitted diseases through investigation, treatment, and educational services. He or she interviews infected patients and their contacts in an effort to locate the source of disease and refers them to local clinics for treatment. The public health investigator maintains regular contact with private physicians, laboratory personnel, and state and local health department personnel to improve case reporting and remain current on treated cases and diagnostic techniques. *See also* public health; sexually transmitted disease.

Public Health Laboratorians, Conference of *See* Conference of Public Health Laboratorians.

Public Health, Master of *See* Master of Public Health.

public health nurse (PHN) A specially prepared registered nurse employed in a community agency, who generally is involved in health department programs for child health, maternity care, family planning, general communicable diseases, and sexually transmitted diseases. Much of the work of the public health nurse centers on health education and prevention of disease. *See also* public health; registered nurse.

public health nutrition An individual who provides technical and advisory services to local health departments and related community agencies about nutrition. He or she often provides services directed toward the nutrition of pregnant women, infants, and children. *See also* nutrition; public health.

public health physician - administrative A physician who deals with health administration rather than the direct delivery of medical services; for example, as the medical director of a community health department. *See also* health administration; physician; public health.

public health physician - clinical A physician who is engaged primarily in providing direct medical services in a public health clinic or, at a higher level, developing and supervising diagnostic and treatment programs for a large specialty public health clinic or for all clinic activities in a designated health district or area. *See also* physician; public health.

Public Health Physicians, American Association of *See* American Association of Public Health Physicians.

public health, podiatric *See* podiatric public health.

Public Health Service (PHS) A component of the Health and Human Services Department that promotes the protection and advancement of physical and mental health; establishes national health policy; maintains cooperative international health-related agreements and programs; administers programs to develop health resources and improve delivery of health services; works to prevent and control communicable diseases; conducts and supports research in medical and related sciences, and provides scientific information; protects against impure or unsafe foods, drugs, and cosmetics; and develops education for the health professions. Elements of the Public Health Service include Centers for Disease Control and Prevention, Food and Drug Administration, National Institutes of Health, Health Resources and Services Administration, Substance Abuse and Mental Health Services Administration, Agency for Health Care Policy and Research, Agency for Toxic Substances and Disease Registry, and the Indian Health Service. *See also* Department of Health and Human Services; Indian Health Service; Public Health Service Act; Substance Abuse and Mental Health Services Administration.

Public Health Service Act (PHSA) One of the principal acts of Congress providing legislative authority for federal health activities. Originally enacted July 1, 1944, the PHS Act was a complete codification of all the accumulated federal public health laws. Generally, the PHS Act contains authority for public health programs, biomedical research, health personnel training, family planning, emergency medical services systems, health maintenance organizations, regulation of drinking water supplies, and health planning and resources development. *See also* Clinical Laboratory Improvement Act of 1967; Public Health Service.

Public Health Service, Commissioned Officers Association of the United States *See* Commissioned Officers Association of the United States Public Health Service.

public health social worker A social worker who provides social work services to children and adults in public health agencies, through public health clinics, and in state facilities, such as hospitals and institutions for the developmentally disabled. *See also* public health; social worker.

Public Health Workers, Lesbian and Gay Caucus of *See* Lesbian and Gay Caucus of Public Health Workers.

public hospital A hospital that is owned or operated by a unit of state or local government, is a public or private nonprofit corporation that is formally granted governmental powers by a unit of state or local government, or is a private nonprofit hospital that has a contract with a state or local government to provide health services to low-income individuals who are not entitled to benefits under Title XVIII of the Social Security Act or eligible for assistance under a state's plan under this title. *See also* hospital.

Public Hospitals, National Association of *See* National Association of Public Hospitals.

public information *See* public relations.

public information interview The opportunity during an on-site accreditation survey conducted by the Joint Commission on Accreditation of Healthcare Organizations for the presentation of information by the public or other interested parties, as well as by personnel and staff of the health care organization undergoing survey. *See also* accreditation survey; interview; Joint Commission on Accreditation of Healthcare Organizations.

public interest Values generally thought to be shared by the public at large; for the common good. There is, however, no one public interest and what one person or organization claims is for the common good may not be commonly accepted as good. *See also* public interest group.

Public Interest, Center for Science in the *See* Center for Science in the Public Interest.

public interest group An organized group seeking to develop positions and support causes relating to a broader definition of the public good as opposed to any specific social or economic interest. Examples of public interest groups are Common Cause, the League of Women Voters, the Sierra Club, and the right-to-life groups. *See also* pressure group; public interest; special interest.

Public Interest, Medicine in the *See* Medicine in the Public Interest.

Public Law *See* PL.

public opinion Public consensus pertaining to an issue or a situation. *See also* opinion; public.

public-opinion poll A survey of the public to acquire information, using a statistically sampled cross-section of a targeted population. The data obtained from public-opinion polls is usually used descriptively, such as to describe public attitudes about issues or political candidates. *Synonym*: opinion poll. *See also* pollster; public opinion.

Public Opinion Research, American Association for *See* American Association for Public Opinion Research.

public patient *See* ward patient.

public policy Community common sense and common conscience, extended and applied through the state to matters of public morals, health, safety, and welfare. *See also* policy; public.

public relations (PR) **1.** The art or science of establishing and promoting a favorable relationship with the public. It often involves a form of communication that is primarily directed to image building and that tends to deal with issues rather than specifically with products or services. **2.** An organizational management function that evaluates public opinion, identifies the policies and services of an organization with the public interest, and develops and executes programs to earn public understanding and acceptance. It is also responsible for media relations. *Synonyms*: public affairs; public information. *See also* image consultant; media relations.

Public Relations, American Society for Health Care Marketing and *See* American Society for Health Care Marketing and Public Relations.

Public Relations, American Society for Hospital *See* American Society for Health Care Marketing and Public Relations.

public relations consultant An organization or individual who contracts to provide assistance in developing, implementing, and evaluating a public relations program. It is sometimes associated with an advertising agency. *See also* consultant; public relations.

public relations director An individual who plans and implements programs to communicate with an organization's audiences and to enhance the public's perception of the organization. *See also* director; public relations.

Public Relations Society of America (PRSA) A national organization founded in 1947 composed of 15,357 public relations practitioners in business and industry, counseling firms, hospitals, schools, government, and nonprofit organizations. It conducts professional development programs and maintains a job referral service. *See also* PR Committee for Licensing and Registration; public relations.

public representation The persona of an organization as presented to a public, for example, in brochures, logos, names, stationery. Public representation can address such issues as type of service provided, type of populations served, and accreditation status.

Public Responsibility in Medicine and Research (PRIM&R) A nonmembership organization founded in 1974 composed of health and legal professionals, subjects/patients, and laypersons interested in research, primarily with human subjects and animals. It was formed to question the development of procedures regulating research and the growth of increasingly hostile public sentiment towards the field. Its activities include aiding members in assembling data they might need for testimony before legislative and other hearings.

public servant A person who holds a government position by election or appointment. *See also* public; public service.

public service **1.** Employment within a governmental system, such as a nurse in the Public Health Service. **2.** A service performed for the benefit of the public, especially by a nonprofit organization, as in public service required for graduation.

Public Voice for Food and Health Policy (PVFHP) A national organization founded in 1982 composed of 300 consumers concerned about food and health issues. It promotes consumer interests in public and private decision making on food and health policy and works with congressional leaders and federal officials to strengthen food safety and labeling laws, farm subsidy programs, sugar and grain price supports, school lunch nutrition, and food programs for the rural poor. *See also* consumer; consumerism; health policy.

public welfare The prosperity, well-being, or convenience of the public at large or of a whole community, as distinguished from the advantage of an individual or particular class. It embraces the primary social interests of order, morals, safety, economic interest, and non-material and political interest. *See also* public; welfare.

Public Welfare Association, American *See* American Public Welfare Association.

Publishers' Association, American Medical *See* American Medical Publishers' Association.

puerperal fever An illness resulting from infection of the endometrium of the uterus following childbirth or abortion, marked by fever and septicemia and typically caused by unsterile technique. *Synonym*: childbed fever. *See also* fever; obstetrics; puerperium; Semmelweiss, Ignaz Philipp; uterus.

puerperium **1.** The state of a woman during childbirth or immediately thereafter. **2.** The six-week period lasting from childbirth to the return of normal uterine size. *See also* obstetrics; puerperal fever.

pull-by date *See* sell-by date.

pulmonary Relating to the lungs, as in pulmonary medicine. *See also* lung; respiration.

pulmonary disease, chronic obstructive *See* chronic obstructive pulmonary disease.

pulmonary function laboratory A laboratory for examination and evaluation of patients' respiratory functions by means of electromechanical equipment. *See also* laboratory; pulmonary medicine.

pulmonary medicine A subspecialty of internal medicine and pediatrics dealing with diseases of the lungs and airways, such as pneumonia, cancer, pleurisy, asthma, occupational diseases, bronchitis, sleep disorders, emphysema, and other disorders. Pulmonology involves testing lung functions, performing endoscopy of the bronchial airways, and prescribing and monitoring mechanical assistance to ventilation. Many pulmonary disease experts are also experts in critical care. *See also* asthma; bronchitis; emphysema; internal medicine; lung; pediatric pulmonology; pulmonary function laboratory; respiration.

Pulmonary Rehabilitation, American Association of Cardiovascular and *See* American Association of Cardiovascular and Pulmonary Rehabilitation.

Pulmonary Technology, National Society for Cardiovascular Technology/National Society for *See* National Society for Cardiovascular Technology/National Society for Pulmonary Technology.

pulmonologist An internist or pediatrician who specializes in pulmonary medicine. *See also* pediatric pulmonology; pulmonary medicine.

pulmonologist, pediatric *See* pediatric pulmonologist.

pulmonology *See* pulmonary medicine.

pulmonology, pediatric *See* pediatric pulmonology.

pulse A pressure wave in a blood vessel resulting in rhythmical throbbing produced by the regular contractions of the heart, especially as palpated at the wrist or in the neck. *See also* palpation; pulse oximetry; vital signs; wave.

pulse oximetry A noninvasive method of determining arterial oxygen saturation by interposing a fingertip or other vascular-rich appendage between a two-wavelength light source and a light detector. The apparatus requires brief warm-up and may be used continuously; results are not affected by skin pigmentation. Its use is limited in low-perfusion states, such as a patient in cardiac arrest. *See also* oximetry.

pump priming An economic policy of increasing government expenditures and/or reducing taxes in order to stimulate the economy to higher levels of output. Pump-priming measures are supposed to be temporary, existing only until the economy sponta-

neously develops and sustains growth on its own. *See also* economy.

punish To subject to a penalty for an offense, a sin, or a fault, as in a supervisor punishing an employee.

punitive damages A sum of money awarded in the courts, not to compensate the injured party, but to punish the defendant and deter him or her and other persons from similar acts. It generally requires that the act be willful, wanton, or reckless. *Synonym:* exemplary damages. *Compare* compensatory damages. *See also* damages.

purchase 1. To obtain in exchange for money or its equivalent; to buy. **2.** Something bought. **3.** The act or process of buying.

purchaser One that purchases something, as in the federal government as a purchaser of health services for the aged. *See also* network; purchase.

purchasing alliance *See* health alliance.

purchasing alliance, regional *See* regional alliance.

purchasing department An organizational unit providing for purchasing of equipment and supplies. *See also* materials management department; purchase.

purchasing, director of An individual who is responsible for the procurement of supplies and equipment. *See also* director; purchase; purchasing department.

purchasing, group *See* group purchasing.

purchasing power The value of money as measured by the goods and services it can buy. For example, consider the amount of goods and services that a dollar can buy in a particular market, as compared with prior periods. It might be reported, for instance, that one dollar in 1970 had 59 cents of purchasing power in 1985 because of erosion caused by inflation. *See also* purchase; real income.

purchasing and stores *See* materials management department.

pure Free from mixture with or contamination by other materials or ideas, as in perfect competition. *See also* perfect competition.

pure competition *See* perfect competition.

purgation Administration of a laxative (purgative) in order to induce defecation. *See also* laxative.

purgative *See* laxative.

purulent Pertaining to pus, as in a purulent discharge from the wound. *See also* pus.

pus Thick, yellowish or greenish fluid, containing

dead white blood cells, bacteria, and dead tissue, formed at an infection site. *See also* abscess.

"putting out fires" approach   *See also* Juran, Joseph M.; management by crisis.

***p* value**   *See p* (probability) value.

PVFHP   *See* Public Voice for Food and Health Policy.

PWA   Abbreviation for "person with AIDS." *See also* PLA; PLWA.

PWC   *See* Physicians Who Care.

pyogenic   Pus forming, as in pyogenic bacteria. *See also* pus.

pyrexia   *See* fever.

pyrexia, hyper-   *See* hyperpyrexia.

pyrogen   A fever-producing agent, such as bacterial endotoxin. *See also* bacteria; fever.

pyrosis   *See* heartburn.

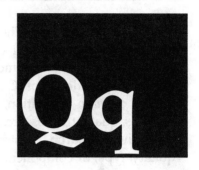

QA *See* quality assurance.

QAP *See* quality assurance program.

QC *See* quality control.

QFD *See* quality function deployment.

QHR *See* Quality Healthcare Resources.

QI *See* quality improvement.

QIC *See* quality improvement council.

QIP *See* quality improvement project.

QIT *See* quality improvement team.

QM *See* quality management.

QPMA *See* Quality and Productivity Management Association.

QRB Abbreviation for *Quality Review Bulletin*. *See The Joint Commission Journal on Quality Improvement*.

quack A person who fraudulently misrepresents his or her ability and experience in the diagnosis and treatment of disease or the effect to be achieved by the treatment offered. *See also* charlatan; mountebank.

quacksalver A person who claims special merit for treatment with his or her medications and salves.

quadrantectomy A breast cancer procedure involving removal of cancerous tissue plus a wedge of surrounding tissue, leaving the breast slightly smaller. Portions of the underarm lymph nodes may also be removed. *Compare* lumpectomy; mammary gland; mastectomy; modified radical mastectomy.

quadriplegia Paralysis affecting all four limbs and the trunk of the body below the level of spinal cord injury; usually caused by trauma. *Synonym*: tetraplegia. *See also* paralysis; paraplegia.

quadruplets Four offspring from a single gestation. *See also* fertility drug; gestation.

qualification **1.** A quality, an ability, or an accomplishment that makes an individual suitable or eligible for a particular position or task, as in qualifications necessary to make a good manager. **2.** A con-

dition or circumstance that must be met or complied with, as in physician qualifications for participation in an insurance program.

qualified Meeting the qualifications for a position or a task, as in a qualified perfusionist, qualified physician, or qualified oral surgeon. *See also* overqualified; qualified handicapped individual.

qualified handicapped individual With respect to employment, a person who with reasonable accommodation can perform the essential functions of a job. *See also* handicapped person; qualified.

qualified, over- *See* overqualified.

qualify **1.** To declare competent or capable; to certify, as in a board qualifying a podiatrist. *See also* certification. **2.** To make legally capable; to license. *See also* licensure.

qualitative Pertaining to quality or qualities, as opposed to quantitative, which pertains to expressing amounts. For example, a qualitative analysis of a substance involves determining the kinds of elements that make up the substance; determination of the amount of each element present is a quantitative assessment. *Compare* quantitative. *See also* analysis; qualitative analysis; qualitative data; qualitative evaluation; qualitative research; semiquantitative.

qualitative analysis Analysis of an object of interest to determine the nature of the elements or ingredients of which it is composed. *Compare* quantitative analysis. *See also* analysis; qualitative.

qualitative data Data characterized by measurement on a dichotomous scale or a nominal scale or, if the categories are ordered, an ordinal scale. Examples are sex, hair color, death or survival, and nationality. *Compare* quantitative data. *See also* data; dichotomous scale; nominal scale; ordinal scale; scale.

qualitative evaluation The non-numerical examination and interpretation of observations for the purpose of discovering underlying meanings and patterns of relationships. *Compare* quantitative evaluation. *See also* evaluation; qualitative; qualitative analysis; qualitative research.

qualitative research Research that deals with the quality, type, or components of a group, substance, or mixture. For example, qualitative research is often used in advertising to determine the quality of audience response to advertising. Qualitative research is exploratory in nature and uses procedures, such as in-depth interviews and focus group interviews, to gain insights and guide subsequent decision-making processes. *Compare* quantitative research. *See also* qualitative; research.

quality **1.** A character, characteristic, or property of anything that makes it good or bad, commendable or reprehensible; thus the degree of excellence that a thing possesses. **2.** The totality of features and characteristics of a product or service that bear on its ability to satisfy stated or implied needs. *See also* relative quality. **3.** Fitness for use. *See also* quality of care; value.

Quality, American College of Medical *See* American College of Medical Quality.

quality assessment In health care, measurement and analysis of the quality of care for individuals, groups, or populations. *See also* assessment; measurement; performance assessment; quality.

quality assurance (QA) **1.** All planned or systematic actions necessary to provide adequate confidence that a service or product will satisfy given requirements for quality. **2.** Designing a product or service, as well as controlling its production, so well that quality is inevitable. **3.** In health care, the activities and programs intended to provide adequate confidence that the quality of patient care will satisfy stated or implied requirements or needs. *See also* assurance; quality.

quality assurance, certified professional in *See* certified professional in quality assurance.

quality assurance coordinator *See* quality assurance professional.

quality assurance engineering The name given Joseph M. Juran's system of total quality management. *See also* Juran, Joseph M.; quality assurance; total quality management.

quality assurance monitor A part of the Profes-

sional Activity Study (PAS) program in which patient care is compared with standards established by clinical specialty societies with findings presented for hospital use in quality management. *See also* monitor; Professional Activity Study; quality assurance.

Quality Assurance, National Committee for *See* National Committee for Quality Assurance.

quality assurance, physician director of *See* physician director of quality assurance.

quality assurance professional In health care, an individual who specializes in conducting quality assurance (quality management) activities in a health care organization. Quality assurance professionals include quality assurance coordinators and directors, utilization review coordinators, risk managers, quality managers, discharge planners, and peer review coordinators. *See also* certified professional in quality assurance; National Association for Healthcare Quality.

Quality Assurance Professionals, National Association of *See* National Association for Healthcare Quality.

quality assurance program (QAP) An organized set of activities designed to demonstrate that patient care and services provided by a hospital or other health care organization or program are the best possible with available resources and consistent with achievable goals. This is accomplished through ongoing assessment of important aspects of patient care, the correction of identified problems, and follow-up activities to determine that corrected problems have not recurred. *See also* quality assurance.

Quality Assurance and Utilization Review Physicians, American Board of *See* American Board of Quality Assurance and Utilization Review Physicians.

quality audit A systematic and independent examination and evaluation to determine whether quality activities and results comply with planned arrangements and whether these arrangements are implemented effectively and are suitable to achieve objectives. *See also* audit; quality.

quality audit, process *See* process quality audit.

quality audit, product *See* product quality audit.

Quality Award, Malcolm Baldridge *See* Malcolm Baldridge Quality Award.

quality of care The degree to which health services for individuals and populations increase the likelihood of desired health outcomes and are consistent with current professional knowledge. *See also* health services; patient health outcome; quality.

quality-of-care evaluation, performance-based
See performance-based quality-of-care evaluation.

Quality Center, American Productivity and *See*
American Productivity and Quality Center.

quality characteristics Characteristics of the output of a process (service or product) that are important to a customer. The identification of quality characteristics requires knowledge of customer needs and expectations. *See also* key quality characteristic.

quality circle A small group of professionals or employees of a health care organization who perform similar work and who meet regularly to learn and apply techniques for identifying, analyzing, and solving work-related problems. Quality circles originated in Japan as a total quality management technique in which groups of workers were organized and empowered to make improvements in the areas in which they worked. *See also* quality; total quality management.

quality college A center within organizations, such as Motorola and Whirlpool, devoted to formal instruction, applied research, and pure research on quality matters. Employees typically are rotated through as students and managers as instructors. *See also* quality.

quality control (QC) **1.** The process through which actual performance is measured, the performance is compared with goals, and the difference is acted on. **2.** The use of operational techniques and statistical methods to measure and predict quality.

quality control circle *See* quality circle.

Quality Control, American Society for *See* American Society for Quality Control.

quality control, statistical *See* statistical quality control.

quality, cost of *See* cost of quality.

quality of documentation The degree to which data and information recorded in source documents, such as medical records, are accurate, complete, and recorded in a timely manner. *See also* documentation; medical record; quality.

Quality and Effectiveness in Health Care, Office of the Forum for *See* Office of the Forum for Quality and Effectiveness in Health Care.

quality engineering The branch of engineering that deals with the principles and practice of product and service quality assurance and control. *See also* engineering; quality; quality assurance; quality control.

quality function deployment (QFD) An approach to quality in which an organization is organized to assess the needs of external customers. The "house of quality," a set of seven matrixes, is the basic graphic used in QFD for showing customer requirements and means of meeting requirements. It often is used by service departments within organizations to survey customers' needs and assess the degree to which these needs are being met. *See also* customer; function; quality.

Quality Health Care, National Committee for *See* National Committee for Quality Health Care.

Quality Healthcare Resources (QHR) A not-for-profit subsidiary of the Joint Commission on Accreditation of Healthcare Organizations that makes available to the health care field consultative support and technical assistance services generally applicable to performance measurement, assessment, and improvement activities. *See also* Joint Commission on Accreditation of Healthcare Organizations; performance assessment; performance improvement; performance measurement.

quality improvement (QI) The attainment, or process of attaining, a new level of performance or quality that is superior to any previous level of quality. *See also* facilitator; improvement; quality.

quality improvement, continuous *See* continuous quality improvement.

quality improvement council (QIC) A group composed of the senior leadership of an organization that is primarily responsible for planning, strategy development, deployment, monitoring, educating, and promoting the acquisition and application of the knowledge necessary for improvement of quality. *See also* quality improvement.

Quality Improvement in Health Care, National Demonstration Project on *See* National Demonstration Project on Quality Improvement in Health Care.

quality improvement project (QIP) A discrete activity in the process of continuous quality improvement consisting of a process that has been identified as needing improvement and has been given priority. A team composed of representatives from all departments and disciplines involved in the process is assigned to measure, assess, and improve the process. To be successful, the team must be supported by management in its project. *See also* continuous quality improvement; storyboard; storybook.

quality improvement project team *See* quality improvement team.

quality improvement storyboard *See* storyboard.

quality improvement storybook *See* storybook.

quality improvement storytelling *See* storytelling.

quality improvement team (QIT) Groups of employees, often cross-departmental, who plan, direct, develop strategy, teach, train, assess, provide feedback, and praise in order to reach a solution to a system or process in need of improvement within an organization. *See also* charter statement; facilitator; quality improvement; remedial journey; team.

quality inspection A process in which organizations sample, measure, and sort to remove defective goods or services and thereby improve quality, rather than designing quality into the product or service. *See also* inspection; quality.

quality, letter *See* letter quality.

quality level, acceptable *See* acceptable quality level.

quality of life That which makes life worth living or, in a more quantitative sense, an estimate of remaining life free of impairment, disability, or handicap. *See also* life; quality.

quality management (QM) That aspect of the overall management function that determines and implements the quality policy. *See also* management; quality; quality policy.

quality management, total *See* total quality management.

quality measure A quantitative measure of the features and characteristics of a service or product. *See also* measure.

Quality, National Association for Healthcare *See* National Association for Healthcare Quality.

Quality and Participation, Association for *See* Association for Quality and Participation.

quality of patient care *See* quality of care.

quality plan A document setting out the specific quality practices, resources, and activities relevant to a particular product, process, service, contract, or project. *See also* plan; quality planning.

quality planning The activity, according to Joseph M. Juran, of developing the goods and services required to meet customer needs. This involves a series of universal steps: determining who are the customers, determining the needs of the customers, developing features of goods or services that respond to customers' needs, developing processes that are able to produce these features, and transferring the resulting plans to the operating forces. *See also* Juran, Joseph M.; planning; quality plan.

quality policy The overall intentions and direction of an organization regarding quality as formally expressed by top management. *See also* policy; quality; quality management.

Quality and Productivity Management Association (QPMA) A national organization founded in 1975 composed of 1,000 corporate employees in middle-management and senior-management positions who are interested in implementing productivity improvement programs. Formerly (1990) American Productivity Management Association. *See also* productivity; quality; quality management.

quality, relative *See* relative quality.

Quality Review Bulletin (QRB) *See The Joint Commission Journal on Quality Improvement.*

quality screens, HCFA generic *See* HCFA generic quality screens.

quality, structural measure of *See* structural measure of quality.

quality surveillance The continuing monitoring and verification of the status of procedures, methods, conditions, products, processes, and services and analysis of records in relation to stated references to ensure that requirements for quality are being met. *See also* quality; surveillance.

quality system The organizational structure, responsibilities, procedures, processes, and resources for implementing quality management. *See also* quality management; quality system audit.

quality system audit A documented activity performed to verify, by examination and evaluation of objective evidence, that applicable elements of the quality system are suitable and have been developed, documented, and effectively implemented in accordance with specified requirements. *See also* audit; quality system.

quality trilogy The processes of quality planning, quality control, and quality improvement. *See also* quality control; quality improvement; quality planning.

quantification **1.** The expression of the quantity of something. **2.** Determination of that attribute of a thing by which it is greater or less than some other thing. *See also* measurement. **3.** Assignment of numbers to objects or events to describe their properties.

quantify To determine or express (measure) the quantity of something. *See also* quantity.

quantile A division of a distribution into equal, ordered subgroups. Deciles are tenths; quartiles, quarters; quintiles, fifths; terciles, thirds; and centiles, hundredths. *See also* quartile.

quantitative Expressed or expressible as a quantity. *Compare* qualitative. *See also* quantitative analysis; quantitative evaluation; quantitative data; quantitative research.

quantitative analysis Analysis dealing with actual measurement of the amounts or proportions of the various components of an object or thing being measured. It is distinguished from qualitative analysis, which may assess, for example, the character of management or the state of employee morale. *Compare* qualitative analysis. *See also* analysis; measurement; semiquantitative.

quantitative data Data expressed in numerical quantities, such as continuous measurements or counts. *Compare* qualitative data. *See also* continuous data; data; scale.

quantitative evaluation The numerical representation and manipulation of observations for the purpose of describing and explaining the phenomena that those observations reflect. *Compare* qualitative evaluation. *See also* evaluation; quantitative; quantitative analysis; quantitative data; quantitative research.

quantitative research Research that deals with the quantities of things and that involves the measurement of quantity or amount. *Compare* qualitative research. *See also* quantitative; research.

quantitative, semi- *See* semiquantitative.

quantity 1. The property of something that can be determined by measurement. *See also* measurement; quantify. 2. That attribute of anything by which it is greater or less than some other thing.

quantum 1. A quantity or an amount. 2. Something that can be measured or counted.

quantum leap An abrupt change or step, especially in method, information, or knowledge.

quarantine 1. The limitation of freedom of movement of susceptible persons who have been exposed to a communicable disease, in order to prevent spread of the disease. *See also* communicable disease. 2. Enforced isolation. *See also* isolation; notifiable disease; public health.

quarterly Every three months (one quarter of a year), for example, performance data published quarterly.

quartile The value of the boundary at the 25th, 50th, or 75th percentiles of a frequency distribution divided into four parts, each containing one quarter of the population. The first quartile is the point below which 25% of the observations lie. The third quartile is the point below which 75% of the observations lie. *See also* distribution; quantile.

quassation The crushing of drugs, or their reduction to small pieces. *See also* drug.

question, information *See* information question.

question, leading *See* leading question.

questionnaire An instrument made up of a predetermined set of questions, used to collect data.

quick and dirty Cheaply made or done and of inferior quality.

quickening A pregnant woman's first awareness of the movement of the fetus, usually occurring about the 16th week of pregnancy but sometimes earlier. *See also* pregnancy.

quick study A person who is able to understand and deal with something easily, quickly, and successfully.

quid pro quo Something required in return for another thing of like value, as in requiring health professional schools to produce needed health personnel in return for their receiving federal capitation payments.

quiet room A room in which a patient may be involuntarily confined for clinical reasons. *See also* seclusion.

quinsy Pus-filled inflammation of the tonsils and palate, usually a complication of tonsillitis. *Synonym:* peritonsillar abscess. *See also* inflammation; palate; pus.

quintile *See* quantile.

quintuplets Five offspring from a single gestation. *See also* fertility drug; gestation.

quorum The number of members of any body who must necessarily be present in order for the body to conduct and transact business, as in at least a majority of committee members must be present to constitute a quorum.

quotient The result of the division of a numerator by a denominator. In 10 divided by 5 equals 2, 2 is the quotient.

QWERTY Pertaining to the traditional configuration of typewriter or computer keyboard keys (from the first six letters in the upper left row of the keyboard). See also console.

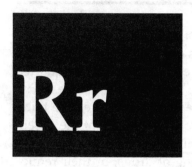

Rr

R *See* roentgen.

rabies An acute infectious viral disease of most warm-blooded animals that attacks the central nervous system. It is transmitted by the bite of infected animals, such as cats, dogs, or wolves, and is almost uniformly fatal without treatment. *Synonym:* hydrophobia. *See also* infectious diseases; virus.

rad A unit of measure for radioactivity absorbed by living organisms or present in a physical environment. One rad is equal to an energy absorption of 0.01 joule per kilogram of irradiated material. The rad has replaced the roentgen as the measure of choice for expressing exposure limitations for persons undergoing radiation treatment or working with equipment and substances that emit radiation. *See also* radiation; roentgen.

radiant energy *See* radiation.

radiation Electromagnetic energy emitted in the form of rays or particles, including gamma rays, x-rays, ultraviolet rays, visible light, and infrared radiation. Some of these types of radiation are used in health care for diagnosis (for example, x-rays) and treatment (for example, radioactive elements, such as radium, used in cancer treatment). *Synonym:* radiant energy. *See also* film badge; occupancy factor; rad; rem; x-ray.

radiation, beam *See* beam radiation.

Radiation Control Program Directors, Conference of *See* Conference of Radiation Control Program Directors.

radiation oncology The branch of radiology that deals with the therapeutic applications of radiant energy and its modifiers and the study and management of disease, especially malignant tumors. *Synonym:* therapeutic radiology. *See also* oncology; radiology.

Radiation Oncology Administrators, Society for *See* Society for Radiation Oncology Administrators.

Radiation Oncology Centers, Association of Free-standing *See* Association of Freestanding Radiation Oncology Centers.

Radiation Protection and Measurements, National Council on *See* National Council on Radiation Protection and Measurements.

Radiation Research Society (RRS) A national organization founded in 1952 composed of 2,025 biologists, physicists, chemists, and physicians contributing to knowledge of radiation and its effects. It promotes original research in the natural sciences relating to radiation and facilitates integration of different disciplines in the study of radiation effects. *See also* radiation; research.

radiation sickness An abnormal condition caused by exposure to ionizing radiation, as from exposure to nuclear bomb explosions or exposure to radioactive chemicals in the workplace. Symptoms and prognosis depend on the amount of radiation, the exposure time, and the part of the body affected. Severe exposure can cause death within hours, whereas mild or moderate exposure can cause nausea, vomiting, and headache, which may be followed by hair loss and bleeding disorders. *See also* radiation; sickness.

radiation therapy The use of beam radiation, radioactive implants, or radioisotopes for cancer-directed therapeutic intent. The radiation interferes with the division of cells and the synthesis of deoxyribonucleic acid (DNA) in the cells. Many cancer cells are destroyed by radiation; the major disadvantage is possible damage to cells and tissues in adjacent areas. *Synonym:* radiotherapy. *See also* beam radiation; cyclotron; radioactive implant; radioisotope; x-ray therapy.

radiation therapy, infrared *See* infrared radiation therapy.

Radiation Therapy Oncology Group (RTOG) A national organization founded in 1971 composed of 120 clinical radiation therapy investigative centers that conduct cooperative clinical trials and studies to improve the care of patients with cancer. *See also* radiation oncology; radiation therapy.

radiation therapy technologist An allied health professional who, under the supervision of radiation oncologists, administers radiation therapy services to patients. A radiation therapy technologist exercises judgment in the administration of prescribed courses of treatment, tumor location, and dosimetry; maintains records; and is responsible for radiation protection for the patient, self, and other persons while carrying out tasks. Radiation therapy technologists are one type of allied health professional for which the Committee on Allied Health Education and Accreditation has accredited education programs. *See also* allied health professional; radiation oncology; radiation therapy; technologist.

Radiation Victims, National Committee for *See* National Committee for Radiation Victims.

radical hysterectomy A hysterectomy with pelvic lymphadenectomy (removal of lymph nodes) and wide lateral excision of parametrial and paravaginal supporting structures. *See also* hysterectomy.

radioactive Emitting radiation. *See also* radiation.

radioactive implant A type of radiation therapy that includes all interstitial implants, molds, seeds, needles, or intracavity applications of radioactive materials, such as cesium, radium, radon, and radioactive gold. *See also* implant; radiation therapy; radioactive; radioisotope.

radioactive nuclide *See* radioisotope; radionuclide.

radioactive isotope *See* radioisotope.

radioactivity Emission of radiation in the form of particles or waves as a result of the spontaneous disintegration (decay) of the nuclei of certain naturally occurring radioactive elements (for example, radium) or of artificially produced radioisotopes, such as iodine-131. *See also* radiation; radioisotope.

radiobiology The branch of biology concerned with the effects of radiation on living organisms and the behavior of radioactive substances in biological systems. *See also* biology; radiation.

radiochemistry The chemistry of radioactive materials. *See also* chemistry; radioisotope.

radiograph An image produced on a radiosensitive surface, such as a photographic film, by radiation other than visible light, especially by x-rays passed through an object or by photographing a fluoroscopic image. *See also* roentgenogram; x-ray.

radiographer An allied health professional who provides patient services using imaging equipment, as directed by physicians qualified to order and/or perform radiologic procedures. A radiographer exercises independent judgment in the technical performance of medical imaging procedures by adapting variable technical parameters of the procedure to the condition of the patient and is responsible for radiation protection for patients, self, and other persons. Radiographers are one type of allied health professional for which the Committee on Allied Health Education and Accreditation has accredited education programs. *Synonym:* radiologic technologist. *See also* allied health professional; radiology.

radiography The process by which radiographs (film records) are made of internal structures of the body by passage of x-rays or gamma rays through the body to act on specially sensitized film. *Synonyms:* roentgenography; roentgenology; skiagraphy. *See also* mammography; radiograph; radiology.

Radiography Technologists, American Registry of Clinical *See* American Registry of Clinical Radiography Technologists.

radioimmunoassay (RIA) A method of determining the concentration of a protein, such as a hormone, in the blood serum by monitoring any reaction produced by the injection of a radioactively-labeled substance known to react in a particular way with the protein under study. *See also* assay; immunoassay; ligand assay; pregnancy test.

radioimmunology The study of immunity using radiolabeling and other radiological methods. *See also* immunology; radiolabel.

radioisotope A natural or artificially produced radioactive isotope of a chemical element, such as iodine-131 or phosphorus-32, given orally, into a cavity, or by intravenous injection, used in medicine for diagnosis or therapy. *Synonym:* radioactive isotope. *See also* half-life; iodine; isotope; nuclear radiology; radiation therapy; radioactive implant; radionuclide.

radiolabel To tag a substance, such as a hormone, an enzyme, or a protein, with a radioactive tracer. *See also* radioimmunology.

Radiological Nurses Association, American *See* American Radiological Nurses Association.

radiological physics The branch of medical physics that includes therapeutic radiological physics, diagnostic radiological physics, and medical nuclear physics. *See also* diagnostic radiological physics; medical nuclear physics; therapeutic radiological physics.

radiological physics, diagnostic *See* diagnostic radiological physics.

radiological physics, therapeutic *See* therapeutic radiological physics.

Radiological Society of North America (RSNA) An organization founded in 1915 composed of 25,000 radiologists and scientists in fields closely related to radiology. *See also* radiology.

Radiological Systems Microfilm Associates (RSMA) A national organization founded in 1979 composed of medical microfilm service bureaus and manufacturers of medical microfilming equipment. It seeks promotion of the industry image, establishment of industry quality control standards, and the use of combined purchasing power to reduce costs. *See also* microfilm.

radiologic technologist *See* radiographer.

Radiologic Technologists, American Chiropractic Registry of *See* American Chiropractic Registry of Radiologic Technologists.

Radiologic Technologists, American Registry of *See* American Registry of Radiologic Technologists.

Radiologic Technologists, American Society of *See* American Society of Radiologic Technologists.

Radiologic Technology, Joint Review Committee on Education in *See* Joint Committee on Education in Radiologic Technology.

radiologist A physician who specializes in radiology. A radiologist may have special expertise in the branches of radiology including therapeutic radiology (radiation oncology), diagnostic radiology, nuclear radiology, or radiological physics, which includes therapeutic radiological physics, diagnostic radiological physics, and medical nuclear physics. *See also* radiology.

Radiologists, American Association for Women *See* American Association for Women Radiologists.

Radiologists, American College of Podiatric *See* American College of Podiatric Radiologists.

Radiologists, American Society of Clinic *See* American Society of Clinic Radiologists.

Radiologists, Association of University *See* Association of University Radiologists.

Radiologists Business Managers Association *See* Radiology Business Management Association.

radiology The branch of health sciences and medical specialty dealing with radioactive substances and radiant energy and with the diagnosis and treatment of disease by means of both ionizing (for example, roentgen rays) and nonionizing (for example, ultrasound) radiations. Branches of radiology include therapeutic radiology (radiation oncology), diagnostic radiology, nuclear radiology, and radiological physics, which includes therapeutic radiological physics, diagnostic radiological physics, and medical nuclear physics. *See also* diagnostic radiology; medical nuclear physics; nuclear radiology; radiation oncology; radiological physics.

Radiology Administrators, American Healthcare *See* American Healthcare Radiology Administrators.

Radiology Administrators, American Hospital *See* American Healthcare Radiology Administrators.

Radiology, American Academy of Oral and Maxillofacial *See* American Academy of Oral and Maxillofacial Radiology.

Radiology, American Board of *See* American Board of Radiology.

Radiology, American College of *See* American College of Radiology.

Radiology, American Osteopathic College of *See* American Osteopathic College of Radiology.

Radiology, American Society of Neuro- *See* American Society of Neuroradiology.

Radiology Business Management Association (RBMA) A national organization founded in 1968 composed of 1,400 business managers for radiology groups and vendors of equipment, services, or supplies. Formerly (1990) Radiologists Business Managers Association. *See also* management; radiology.

radiology, diagnostic *See* diagnostic radiology.

Radiology, and Medicine, Academy of Oral Diagnosis, *See* Academy of Oral Diagnosis, Radiology, and Medicine.

radiology, nuclear *See* nuclear radiology.

Radiology and Oncology, American Society for Therapeutic *See* American Society for Therapeutic Radiology and Oncology.

radiology service Service providing diagnosis and treatment through the use of x-rays and other forms of radiant energy. *See also* radiology; service.

Radiology, Society of Cardiovascular and Interventional   *See* Society of Cardiovascular and Interventional Radiology.

Radiology, Society for Pediatric   *See* Society for Pediatric Radiology.

Radiology, Society of Thoracic   *See* Society of Thoracic Radiology.

radiology, therapeutic   *See* radiation oncology.

radiolucent   Allowing the passage of x-rays or other radiation and therefore not opaque. *Compare* radiopaque. *See also* radiation; radiology; x-ray.

radionuclide   A nuclide (a type of atom specified by its atomic number, atomic mass, and energy state, such as carbon-14) that exhibits radioactivity (emits nuclear radiation). *See also* medical nuclear physics; nuclear radiology; radioisotope.

radiopaque   Impervious (not transparent) to x-rays or other radiation; for example, a radiopaque lead shield to protect a patient's reproductive organs or radiopaque iodine isotope used as contrast media in producing x-ray images during intravenous pyelography. *Compare* radiolucent. *See also* radiation; radiology; radiopaque dye; x-ray.

radiopaque dye   A chemical that does not permit the passage of x-rays, used to outline the interior of certain organs (for example, stomach, intestines, kidneys) during x-ray and fluoroscopic procedures. *See also* contrast medium.

radiotherapy   *See* radiation therapy.

radium   A naturally occurring radioactive metallic element used in radiation therapy as a source of beta particles and gamma rays. Its half-life is 1,620 years. *See also* radiation; radiation therapy; radioactive implant; radium therapy.

Radium Society, American   *See* American Radium Society.

radium therapy   The use of radium (a highly radioactive metallic element) in treating cancer. *See also* radium; therapy.

Railway Surgeons, American Association of   *See* American Association of Railway Surgeons.

raison d'être   Reason or justification for existing.

rales   Moist bubbling sounds heard on auscultation of the lungs, indicating the presence of fluid in the air passages. *See also* lung; pneumonia.

RAM   *See* random access memory.

RANCA   *See* Retired Army Nurse Corps Association.

RAND Corporation   A research organization in Santa Monica, California, that assesses alternative reimbursement schemes for health care. Its interests include the role and changing character of academic medicine, medical human resources and technology, and care of the elderly.

random   **1.** Having no specific pattern, purpose, or objective. *Compare* deterministic. *See also* random access; random error. **2.** In statistics, relating to the same or equal chances or probability of occurrence for each member of a group; for example, in clinical research, the probability of assignment of a given subject to a specified treatment group is fixed and constant (typically 0.50) but the subject's actual assignment cannot be known until it occurs.

random access   In computer science, the method whereby data are obtained on disks by going directly to the location of the data, as contrasted with securing an item of data from a tape on which the data elements are reviewed serially. *Synonym*: direct access. *Compare* sequential access. *See also* computer; data element; random.

random access memory (RAM)   In computer science, a memory device in which information can be accessed in any order and any location in memory can be found, on average, as quickly as any other location. A computer's RAM is its main memory where it can store data, so the size of the RAM, measured in kilobytes or megabytes, is an important indicator of the capacity of the computer. *See also* read-only memory (ROM).

random allocation   *See* randomization.

random controlled trial   *See* randomized trial.

random error   The portion of variation in a measurement that has no apparent connection to any other measurement or variable and that is generally regarded as due to chance. *See also* chance; error; measurement; random; reliability.

randomize   To make random in arrangement, especially in order to control the variables in an experiment. *See also* random; variable.

randomization   Placement of individuals in groups by chance, usually with the aid of a table of random numbers. Within the limits of chance variation, randomization makes the control and experimental groups similar at the start of the inquiry, thereby reducing any investigator or observer bias that might otherwise be introduced into the inquiry. Randomization is different from systematic allocation (for example, on even and odd days of the month) or allocation at the convenience or discretion of an investigator. *Synonym*: random allocation. *See also* random; randomize.

randomized clinical trial (RCT) *See* randomized trial.

randomized control trial (RCT) *See* randomized trial.

randomized control trial, non- *See* nonrandomized control trial.

randomized controlled trial (RCT) *See* randomized trial.

randomized trial An experiment in which individuals are randomly allocated to receive or not receive an experimental preventive, therapeutic, or diagnostic procedure and then followed to determine the effect of the intervention. *Synonyms*: random control trial; randomized clinical trial; randomized controlled trial; randomized control trial. *Compare* nonrandomized control trial. *See also* randomize; trial.

random number generator A program that generates a sequence of numbers that seem to be completely random. Random numbers provide a way of selecting a sample without human bias. *See also* number; random sample.

random sample A sample derived by selecting sampling units (for example, individual patients) such that each unit has an independent and fixed (generally equal) chance of selection. Whether a given unit is selected is determined by chance (for example, by a table of randomly ordered numbers) *See also* population; random; random sampling; sample.

random sampling Obtaining a sample that has been randomly selected from a population. *See also* sampling; simple random sampling; stratified random sampling.

random sampling, simple *See* simple random sampling.

random sampling, stratified *See* stratified random sampling.

random, unannounced survey *See* unannounced survey.

random variable In statistics, a variable whose values are distributed according to a probability distribution. *See also* probability distribution; random; regression; stochastic; *t*-distribution; variable.

range In statistics, a measure of the variation in a set of data calculated by subtracting the lowest value in the data set from the highest value in that same set. *Synonym*: range of distribution. *See also* midrange; statistics.

range of distribution *See* range.

range, mid- *See* midrange.

range of motion (ROM) The extent of movement of a limb or other body part, often used as a measure of rehabilitation. *See also* physical therapy.

rank A relative position or degree of value in a graded group.

rank and file In an organization or a group, those people who form the major portion, excluding the leaders and officers.

ranking scale A scale that arranges the members of a group from high to low according to the magnitude of the observations, assigns numbers to the ranks, and neglects distances between members of the group. See also measurement; ordinal scale; rank; scale.

rape The crime of forcing another person to submit to sex acts, especially sexual intercourse. Most states have replaced the common-law rape definition with "sexual assault" statutes, which are generally gender neutral (both the actor and the victim can be either male or female) and provide that it is a crime to knowingly cause another person to engage in a sexual act by force or threat. The federal statute specifically terms the offense "aggravated sexual abuse." *See also* date rape; rape shield law; sexual assault; statutory rape.

rape, date *See* date rape.

Rape, National Clearinghouse on Marital and Date *See* National Clearinghouse on Marital and Date Rape.

rape shield law A law that prohibits the defense in a rape case from cross-examination regarding the plaintiff's prior sexual conduct. *See also* law; rape.

rape, statutory *See* statutory rape.

rapist One who commits the crime of rape. *See also* rape.

rapport Relationship of mutual trust or emotional affinity achieved through activities encouraging this result.

RAPS *See* Regulatory Affairs Professionals Society.

rash Any temporary skin eruption. *See also* dermatitis; dermatology; psoriasis; ringworm; roseola; skin.

rate A measure of a part with respect to a whole; an expression of the frequency with which an event occurs in a defined population per unit of time (for example, the heart rate is the number of beats per minute) or per number of possible occurrences (for example, one illness per 100 people exposed to the illness). The use of rates rather than raw numbers is essential for comparison of experience between populations at different times, different places, or among different categories of persons. The components of a rate are the numerator, the denominator, the specified time in which events occur, and usually a multiplier, a power of 10, which converts the rate from an awkward fraction or decimal to a whole number (for example, 1.35/1,000 is transformed to 135/100,000). Rates can be expressed either as a proportion or as a ratio. In a proportion, the numerator is expressed as a subset of the denominator (for example, the number of patients with primary cesarean section over all patients who have a cesarean section). In a ratio, the numerator and denominator measure different phenomenon (for example, the number of patients with central lines who develop infections over the number of patient days in which a central line is in place). *See also* denominator; numerator; proportion; ratio; underreporting.

rate, adjusted autopsy   *See* adjusted autopsy rate.

rate, autopsy   *See* autopsy rate.

rate, basal metabolic   *See* basal metabolic rate.

rate-based indicator   An aggregate data indicator in which the value of each measurement is expressed as a proportion or as a ratio. *Synonym:* discrete variable indicator. *See also* aggregate data indicator; indicator; probability distribution; rate.

rate, bed-turnover   *See* bed-turnover rate.

rate, birth   *See* birth rate.

rate, child death   *See* child death rate.

rate, collection   *See* collection rate.

rate, fatality   *See* fatality rate.

rate, fertility   *See* fertility rate.

rate, gross autopsy   *See* autopsy rate.

rate, incidence   *See* incidence rate.

rate, infant mortality   *See* infant mortality rate.

rate, infection   *See* nosocomial infection rate.

rate, interim   *See* interim rate.

rate, marginal tax   *See* marginal tax rate.

rate, metabolic   *See* metabolism.

rate, morbidity   *See* morbidity rate.

rate, mortality   *See* mortality rate.

rate, neonatal death   *See* neonatal death rate.

rate, neonatal mortality   *See* neonatal death rate.

rate, net autopsy   *See* adjusted autopsy rate.

rate, nosocomial infection   *See* nosocomial infec-

tion rate.

rate, occupancy   *See* occupancy rate.

rate, performance   *See* performance rate.

rate, prevalence   *See* prevalence rate.

rate, readmission   *See* readmission rate.

rate, response   *See* response rate.

rate, surprise   *See* surprise rate.

rating   **1.** A position assigned on a scale. *See also* scale. **2.** In insurance, the process of determining rates, or the cost of insurance, for individuals, groups, or classes of risks, as in community rating. *See also* bond rating; community rating; credit rating; experience rating; merit rating; scale.

rating, bond   *See* bond rating.

rating, community   *See* community rating.

rating, credit   *See* credit rating.

rating, experience   *See* experience rating.

rating, merit   *See* merit rating.

ratio   The relationship between two quantities when the numerator and denominator measure different phenomena; for example, the number of patients with bloodstream infection divided by the number of patients with central line or umbilical catheters in place, over 12 months. A ratio is an expression of the relationship between a numerator and a denominator when the two usually are separate and distinct quantities, neither being included in the other, as with a proportion. *See also* denominator; likelihood ratio; numerator; proportion; rate.

ratio, likelihood   *See* likelihood ratio.

ration   A fixed portion or allotment. *See also* rationing.

rational   Exercising the ability to reason. *Compare* irrational. *See also* reason.

rationale   The fundamental reason or basis for something, as in the rationale behind an indicator.

rationale, indicator   *See* indicator rationale.

Rational-Emotive Therapy, Institute for   *See* Institute for Rational-Emotive Therapy.

rationalism   **1.** Reliance on reason as the best guide for belief and action. *See also* reason. **2.** In philosophy, the theory that the exercise of reason, rather than the acceptance of empiricism, authority, or spiritual revelation, provides the only valid basis for action or belief; also that reason is the prime source of knowledge and of spiritual truth. *See also* empirical.

rationalization   A mental defense mechanism in which actions or attitudes are justified after the event by the finding of reasons for them. *See also* psychology; reason.

rationing A method for limiting the purchase or use of an item when the quantity demanded of the item exceeds the quantity available at a specific price. For example, health care rationing refers to restricting allotments of health care services to a fixed amount because the quantity demanded of health services exceeds the quantity available at a specific price. *See also* ration; resource allocation; triage.

ratio scale A type of interval scale with a meaningful and true zero point; thus products involving the data points demonstrate the relations between the data points. For example, one can say that one person's weight is so many times another person's weight. A ratio scale is the most powerful measurement scale because not only are the differences between observations quantifiable, but the observations can themselves be expressed as a ratio. *See also* interval scale; nominal scale; ordinal scale; scale.

ratio, staffing *See* staffing ratio.

raw data Initial data a researcher has before beginning analysis. *See also* data.

raw material Unprocessed material; for example, data as the raw material for analysis.

raw milk Milk that is not pasteurized. *See also* pasteurization.

ray The rectilinear path along which directional energy (for example, electromagnetic energy) travels from its source, as in x-ray. *See also* x-ray.

ray, x- *See* x-ray.

RBC *See* red blood cell.

RBMA *See* Radiology Business Management Association.

RBRV *See* resource-based relative value.

RBRVS *See* resource-based relative-value scale.

RCPS *See* Royal College of Physicians and Surgeons (of the United States of America).

RCT Abbreviation for randomized clinical trial; randomized control trial, and randomized controlled trial. *See* randomized trial.

RD Abbreviation for registered dietitian. *See* dietitian.

R & D *See* research and development.

RDAs *See* recommended dietary allowances.

RDIs *See* recommended dietary intakes.

reaccreditation 1. The process of renewing the accreditation of an organization, such as a hospital. 2. Renewal of accreditation status. *See also* accreditation.

reaction A response to a stimulus, especially in

medicine, as in an drug adverse reaction. *See also* drug adverse reaction; reaction formation; transfusion reaction.

reaction, drug adverse *See* drug adverse reaction.

reaction formation In psychiatry and psychology, a defense mechanism in which a person unconsciously develops attitudes and behavior that are contrary to repressed unacceptable drives and impulses and that serve to conceal them; for example, a strong moral stance that hides an impulse to lust. *See also* psychiatry; psychology.

reaction, transfusion *See* transfusion reaction.

readable 1. Interesting to read, as in a readable book. 2. Capable of being read, as in machine readable. *See also* legible; machine readable.

readable, machine *See* machine readable.

readership The readers of a publication considered as a group.

reading, lip *See* lip reading.

readmission Admission to a hospital or other health care organization within a specified period of time after a prior admission or because of complications relating to a prior admission. *See also* admission; readmission rate.

readmission rate A number showing the proportion of a hospital's patients (or a class of patients, such as asthmatics) who reenter the hospital within a specified interval after discharge with the same diagnosis (such as asthma). *See also* rate; readmission.

read-only memory (ROM) In computer science, a device containing instructions that do not need to be changed, such as the instructions for calculating arithmetic functions. The computer can read instructions out of ROM, but no data can be added to or stored in ROM. *See also* CD-ROM disk; memory; operating system; random access memory (RAM).

read-out In computer science, presentation of data, usually in digital form, from calculations or storage. *See also* computer.

Reaganomics General collection of conservative, free-market economic policies favored by President Ronald Reagan and his administration. *See also* trickle-down theory.

real 1. Actual, as opposed to nominal (existing in name only). *Compare* nominal. 2. In economics, pertains to measures, such as price and income, which are corrected for inflation over time so as to permit a comparison of actual purchasing power. *See also* purchasing power; real income.

real earnings Wages, salaries, and other earnings, corrected for inflation over time so as to produce a measure of actual changes in purchasing power. *Synonym:* real wages.

real income Income of an individual, group, or country adjusted for changes in purchasing power caused by inflation. For example, if the cost of an item increases from $100 to $120 in ten years, reflecting a 20% decline in purchasing power, salaries must rise by 20% if real income is to be maintained. *See also* income; money income; purchasing power.

realist A person who is inclined to literal truth and pragmatism. *Compare* idealist. *See also* pragmatism.

reality principle In psychoanalytic theory, the ego functions that modify the demands of the pleasure principle to meet the demands and requirements of the external world. *Compare* pleasure principle. *See also* principle.

Reality Therapy, Institute for *See* Institute for Reality Therapy.

real resources All inputs, such as money, time, and other goods and services used to produce a product or service. *See also* real; resources.

real time **1.** In computer science, the actual time in which a physical process under computer study or control occurs. **2.** The time a computer takes to solve a problem, measured from the time data are fed in to the time a solution is received. **3.** A type of computer system in which information is updated at the same rate as data are received, as with automatic pilot or automated teller machines.

real wages *See* real earnings.

reappointment of physicians The process of assessing a physician's current clinical competence and compliance with a medical staff's bylaws, rules, and regulations for the purpose of reappointment and renewal of his or her clinical privileges. Medical staff appointments and clinical privileges are usually granted for one to two years. Items that are verified at the time of reappointment include, for instance, current licensure, liability claims pending and closed since the last appointment, current professional liability insurance coverage, satisfactory physical and mental health status, and compliance with medical staff bylaws, rules, and regulations, particularly those involving completion of medical records and participation in departmental meetings and quality assurance activities. *See also* licensure; medical staff; medical staff bylaws; professional lia-

bility; recredentialing.

rearing parent A parent who actually rears a child. *See also* noncoital reproduction; parent.

reason The capacity for logical, rational, and analytic thought; intelligence, good judgment, sound sense. *See also* mind; think; thought; rationalism; rationalization.

reasonable Being within the bounds of sound sense; not excessive or extreme; fair.

reasonable charge For any specific service covered under Medicare, the lower of the customary charge by a particular physician for that service and the prevailing charge by physicians in the geographic area for that service. Generically, the term is used for any charge payable by an insurance program that is determined in a similar, but not necessarily identical, fashion. *See also* charge.

reasonable cost The amount a third-party payer using cost-related reimbursement will actually reimburse. Costs are considered reasonable if they are not unnecessary or excessive. Virtually all major purchasers of health care have already abandoned, or are planning to abandon, reasonable cost in favor of prospective payment and contracted price mechanisms, which provide greater long-term price stability for health care services. *See also* cost; prospective payment; purchaser; reasonable charge; third-party payer.

reasonable person A phrase used to denote a hypothetical person who exercises qualities of intelligence, judgment, and knowledge that society requires of its members for the protection of their own interest and the interests of other persons. *See also* reasonable person standard.

reasonable person standard In law, a test often used by a fact finder (judge or jury) to measure conduct in his or her determination of negligence; the general level of care expected of individuals under the same or similar circumstances. For physicians defending themselves in a negligence suit, this generally refers to the behavior expected of a reasonable physician, familiar with the appropriate standards of practice that should be applied in circumstances, such as those under question in a lawsuit. *See also* reasonable person; standard.

reasoning Use of reason to form conclusions or make judgments or inferences. *See also* deductive reasoning; inductive reasoning; judgment; reason.

Reasoning, Association for Automated *See* Association for Automated Reasoning.

reasoning, deductive *See* deductive reasoning.

reasoning, inductive *See* inductive reasoning.

reason, rule of *See* rule of reason.

rebuttable presumption A legal proposition that, depending on a jurisdiction, allows the party opposing a presumed fact to offer evidence to contradict that fact. *Compare* irrebuttable presumption. *See also* presumption; res ipsa loquitur.

receptionist An office worker employed chiefly to receive visitors and answer the telephone. *See also* office; secretary.

receptive aphasia *See* sensory aphasia.

recertification To renew certification, especially that given by a licensing or certification board, as in recertification of a hospital for Medicare by Health Care Financing Administration or recertification of a physician by a medical specialty board. *See also* certification.

recession An extended downturn in general business activity, typically defined as at least two consecutive quarters of decline in a country's real gross national product. *See also* economy; gross national product.

reciprocity Relationship between persons, corporations, states, or countries in which privileges granted by one are returned by the other; for example; recognition by one jurisdiction of the licenses of physicians of a second jurisdiction when the second jurisdiction extends the same recognition to physician licenses of the first jurisdiction. *See also* endorsement in professional licensure; state medical boards.

Reciprocity Consortium/Alcoholism and Other Drug Abuse, National Certification *See* National Certification Reciprocity Consortium/Alcoholism and Other Drug Abuse.

recognition **1.** Acknowledgement, as in recognition for a job well done. **2.** Known to be something that has been perceived before, as in voice recognition. *See also* voice recognition.

recognition, voice *See* voice recognition.

recombinant DNA A molecule of deoxyribonucleic acid (DNA) in which genes have been artificially rearranged and genetic material from another organism has been inserted. Recombinant DNA technology is used to produce human insulin and growth hormone. *See also* biotechnology; deoxyribonucleic acid; gene; gene splicing; recombinant human insulin.

recombinant DNA technology *See* genetic engineering.

recombinant human insulin A type of insulin made from recombinant DNA techniques and used in the treatment of diabetes mellitus. It is identical to natural human insulin and is used by diabetics who are allergic or resistant to beef and pork insulin. The trade name for recombinant human insulin is Humulin. *See also* diabetes mellitus; insulin; recombinant DNA.

recommend To advise or counsel, as in recommending a certain course of action. *See also* recommendation.

recommendation Something, such as a course of action, that is advised. *See also* recommend; supplemental recommendation; type I recommendation.

recommendation, consultative *See* supplemental recommendation.

recommendation, first generation type I *See* first generation type I recommendation.

recommendation, second generation type I *See* second generation type I recommendation.

recommendation, supplemental *See* supplemental recommendation.

recommendation, type I *See* type I recommendation.

recommendation, type II *See* supplemental recommendation.

recommended dietary allowances (RDAs) Standards created by nutrition experts and adopted by the Food and Nutrition Board of the National Research Council of the National Academy of Sciences for levels of average daily intake of essential nutrients. These levels not only encompass the nutritional needs of essentially all healthy persons, but also include a slight excess to allow the buildup of a reserve against future need. US RDAs are derived by the Food and Drug Administration and appear on food and vitamin and mineral pill labels. *See also* nutrient; recommended dietary intakes.

recommended dietary intakes (RDIs) Standards set by the World Health Organization for the level of average daily nutrient intake to encompass the nutritional needs of essentially all healthy persons, plus some extra for storage. RDIs are international RDAs. *See also* recommended dietary allowances.

Reconstructive Surgeons, American Society of Plastic and *See* American Society of Plastic and Reconstructive Surgeons.

reconstructive surgery *See* plastic surgery.

Reconstructive Surgery, American Academy of Facial Plastic and *See* American Academy of Facial Plastic and Reconstructive Surgery.

Reconstructive Surgical Nurses, American Society of Plastic and *See* American Society of Plastic and Reconstructive Surgical Nurses.

record **1.** An account of information or facts that is set down in writing as a means of preserving the information or facts; for example, medical record. *See also* medical record; track record. **2.** In data processing, a collection of related data items. A collection of records is called a file. *See also* accounting records; file; nursing record; record cycle; records management.

record administrator, registered *See* registered record administrator.

record, clinical *See* medical record.

record cycle The period during which a record is created, used, stored for retrieval, transferred to inactive status, and destroyed. *See also* cycle; record; records management.

record, health *See* medical record.

record, medical *See* medical record.

record, nursing *See* nursing record.

record, off-the- *See* off-the-record.

record, on-the- *See* on-the-record.

record, patient *See* medical record.

record, patient's health *See* medical record.

record, personnel *See* personnel record.

record, problem-oriented medical *See* problem-oriented medical record.

records, accounting *See* accounting records.

Records Institute, Medical *See* Medical Records Institute.

records management A system used to collect, record, store, and eventually discard an organization's records. *See also* management; record cycle.

records, vital *See* vital records.

record technician, accredited *See* accredited record technician.

record, track *See* track record.

recovery **1.** In health care, return to a previous state or condition of health or function that preceded the occurrence of a disease or disability, as in patient recovery. *See also* recovery room; rehabilitation. **2.** In economics, a period in a business cycle when economic activity picks up and the gross national product grows, leading into the expansion phase of the cycle. *See also* economy. **3.** In law, the money awarded by a court to the successful plaintiff in a lawsuit. *See also* damages.

recovery room An area in a hospital or other health care setting for monitoring and treating postoperative patients. *Synonym:* postoperative recovery room. *See also* postoperative care.

recreation Refreshment of the mind or body through play activities that amuse or stimulate.

recreational therapist An individual who specializes in recreational therapy. *Synonym:* activities director. *See also* recreational therapy; therapist.

recreational therapy The use of recreational activities, such as athletics, arts and crafts, movies, and camping to rehabilitate and restore patients' physical and emotional health. Recreational therapists provide services for special populations, such as the elderly, handicapped, and mentally ill in hospitals, nursing homes, recreation centers, and long term care facilities. *Synonym:* therapeutic recreation. *See also* adult day care; art therapy; dance therapy; drama therapy; manual arts therapy; music therapy; poetry therapy.

recreational therapy technician An individual who, under the direction of a recreational therapist, assists patients in performing medically approved recreational activities. *See also* recreational therapist; recreational therapy; technician.

Recreation Association, American Therapeutic *See* American Therapeutic Recreation Association.

Recreation Certification, National Council for Therapeutic *See* National Council for Therapeutic Recreation Certification.

Recreation Society, National Therapeutic *See* National Therapeutic Recreation Society.

recredentialing The process of determining and certifying the competence of a physician or other professional at some time after the initial determination of his or her qualification for licensure or hospital privileges. Recredentialing is required at periodic intervals (such as every two years) in most hospitals and other types of health care organizations. Recredentialing focuses on physicians' actual performance, rather than on physicians' capacity to perform well, as reflected, for example, in passing a written examination. *See also* credentialing; physician credentialing; reappointment of physicians.

Recruiters, National Association of Executive *See* National Association of Executive Recruiters.

Recruiters, National Association of Physician *See* National Association of Physician Recruiters.

recruitment The act of seeking prospective new employees or members for an organization. Recruitment is an important function for an organization to maintain personnel. *See also* headhunter; physician recruitment.

recruitment bonus A bonus often given by employers and employment agencies for locating potential employees, especially for employee categories in which a scarcity of qualified candidates exists.

Recruitment, National Association for Healthcare *See* National Association for Healthcare Recruitment.

recruitment, physician *See* physician recruitment.

Rectal Surgeons, American Society of Colon and *See* American Society of Colon and Rectal Surgeons.

Rectal Surgery, American Board of Colon and *See* American Board of Colon and Rectal Surgery.

rectum The terminal portion of the large intestine, extending from the sigmoid flexure to the anal canal and anus. *See also* colon; colon and rectal surgery; intestine.

recurring clause A provision in some health insurance policies that specifies a time period during which the recurrence of a condition is considered a continuation of a prior period of disability or hospital confinement rather than a separate spell of illness. *See also* health insurance.

recuperation Recovery or return to a normal or previous state of health. *See also* rehabilitation.

red bead experiment A simple exercise developed by W. Edwards Deming to model a production system. The exercise demonstrates that many managers hold workers to standards beyond workers' control, that variation is part of any process, and that workers work within a system beyond their control. The simulation also shows that some workers always will be above average, some average, and some below average; that the system, not the skills of individual workers, determines to a large extent how workers perform in carrying out repeating processes; and that only management can change the system or empower other persons to change it. *Synonyms*: red bead game; red bead parable. *See also* Deming, W. Edwards; experiment.

red bead game *See* red bead experiment.

red bead parable *See* red bead experiment.

red blood cell (RBC) A cell in human blood that contains hemoglobin and transports oxygen and carbon dioxide to and from tissues. *Synonyms*: erythrocyte; red cell. *See also* blood cell.

red cell *See* red blood cell.

red crescent In Muslim countries, a red crescent replaces a red cross as the symbol of the Red Cross. *See also* Red Cross.

Red Cross An international organization that cares for the wounded, sick, and homeless in wartime, according to the terms of the Geneva Convention of 1864, and now also during and following natural disasters. The emblem of the organization is a Geneva cross or a red Greek cross on a white background. *See also* American Red Cross National Headquarters; red crescent.

Red Cross National Headquarters, American *See* American Red Cross National Headquarters.

red herring An issue that may be important generally but which has no relevant importance to the question at hand. It tends to draw attention away from the central issue.

red tape Extensive paperwork necessary to gain approval by an entity in order to accomplish a goal, as in bureaucratic red tape.

Reduction Act of 1984, Deficit *See* Deficit Reduction Act of 1984.

reduction in force *See* RIF.

refer In health care, to direct a patient to a health care provider who has specialized qualifications or resources to diagnose or treat specific health conditions or diseases, as in to refer a patient to a specialist in rheumatology. *See also* referral.

refereed journal A professional or literary journal in which articles or papers are selected for publication by a panel of referees who are experts in the field. Their evaluation of each of the articles submitted for publication is often used to make decisions as to whether to publish or reject for publication the article or paper. *See also* journal.

reference 1. A source of information about the qualifications, credit, and character of a person or an organization. 2. A note in a publication referring the reader to another passage or source.

reference database In health care, a public or private database containing aggregate data about many patients or cases that can be used for effectiveness research, financial analyses, and other purposes. A reference database provides authoritative information against which an individual, organization, or community being studied can be evaluated and compared. *See also* database; reference.

reference population   The population to which one can refer for authoritative information and against which a population being studied can be evaluated and compared. *See also* population; reference database.

referral   The process whereby a patient is sent by one practitioner or program to another practitioner or program for services or consultation that the referring source is not prepared or qualified to provide. *See also* consultation; referral center; referral provider; selective referral.

referral center   Under Medicare prospective pricing, those rural hospitals that are paid the appropriate urban rate, adjusted by the rural wage index, because they meet the specified criteria as a referral center. *See also* Medicare; prospective pricing system.

referral provider   A provider (usually a specialty physician or other health entity) who renders a service to a patient who has been sent by a participating provider in a health plan. *See also* health care provider; provider; referral.

referral, selective   *See* selective referral.

referred care   Medical care provided to a patient when referred by one health professional to another with more specialized qualifications or interests. There are two levels of referred care: secondary and tertiary. Secondary care is usually provided by a broadly skilled specialist, such as a general surgeon, a general internist, or an obstetrician. Tertiary care is provided on referral of a patient to a subspecialist, such as a neonatologist or a pediatric pulmonologist. *See also* primary care; secondary care; tertiary care.

referred outpatient admission   The formal acceptance by a health care organization of an outpatient who, upon the referral of a physician or another hospital, is to receive only designated services. *See also* admission; outpatient.

referred pain   Pain that is felt in a part of the body at a distance from the area of pathology, as pain in the right shoulder derived from a ruptured ectopic pregnancy. *See also* pain.

reflex   Any involuntary or automatic response to a stimulus, as in gag reflex. *See also* gag reflex.

reflex, gag   *See* gag reflex.

reflux   Retrograde flow, as in reflux esophagitis. *See also* gastroesophageal reflux; reflux esophagitis.

reflux esophagitis   Inflammation of the lower part of the esophagus caused by regurgitation of gastric contents containing acid and pepsin. *See also* esophagus; gastroesophageal reflux; heartburn; indigestion; inflammation.

reflux, gastroesophageal   *See* gastroesophageal reflux.

Reform, American Council for Health Care   *See* American Council for Health Care Reform.

Reform Association, American Tort   *See* American Tort Reform Association.

Reform, National Citizens Coalition for Nursing Home   *See* National Citizens Coalition for Nursing Home Reform.

refractive error   Any impairment of the lens function of the eyes, such as myopia. *See also* nearsighted; ophthalmology.

Refractive Surgery, American Society of Cataract and   *See* American Society of Cataract and Refractive Surgery.

refusal   Preventing or stopping medical care by a patient or his or her representative. *See also* informed refusal.

refusal, informed   *See* informed refusal.

regeneration   Replacement or regrowth of a substance or a structure in its original form and by natural processes.

regimen   A planned treatment program designed to achieve a specific result, as in a therapeutic regimen consisting of bedrest, heat, and anti-inflammatory agents.

regional alliance   **1.** According to the Health Security Act introduced to Congress, a health alliance consisting of a nonprofit organization, an independent state agency, or an agency of the state that is governed by a board of directors consisting of members who represent employers whose employees purchase health coverage through the alliance and members who represent individuals who purchase such coverage, including employees. Each regional alliance contracts with any willing state-certified health plan to enter into a contract with the alliance for the enrollment of eligible individuals in the alliance area. Each regional alliance must provide to each eligible enrollee a choice of health plans among the plans that have contracts in effect with the regional alliance, including at least one fee-for-service plan. Each regional alliance is responsible for the collection of all amounts owed the alliance by individuals or employers and is responsible for providing payment to each regional alliance health plan. Each regional alliance is responsible for the issuance of health security cards (health cards) to regional alliance eligible individuals. *Synonyms:* regional health alliance; regional purchasing alliance. *See also* alliance area; corporate alliance; health alliance; health card; health plan; Health Security Act; regional alliance employer; state-certified health plan. **2.** A formal arrangement among several health care organizations and/or health systems from two or more states, for specific purposes, that functions under a set of bylaws or other written rules that each member agrees to follow. *See also* health system; multihospital system; network.

regional alliance eligible individual According to the Health Security Act introduced to Congress, an eligible individual with respect to whom a regional alliance health plan is an applicable health plan. *See also* corporate alliance eligible individual; regional alliance; regional alliance health plan.

regional alliance employer According to the Health Security Act introduced to Congress, an employer who is not a corporate alliance employer. *See also* corporate alliance employer; Health Security Act; regional alliance.

regional alliance health plan According to the Health Security Act introduced to Congress, a health plan offered by a regional alliance. *See also* corporate alliance health plan; health plan; regional alliance.

regional anesthesia Anesthesia of an area of the body through administration of a local anesthetic that blocks a group of sensory nerve fibers, as in epidural anesthesia or spinal anesthesia. *See also* anesthesia; general anesthesia; local anesthesia.

Regional Anesthesia, American Society of *See* American Society of Regional Anesthesia.

regional health alliance *See* regional alliance.

regional purchasing alliance *See* regional alliance.

register **1.** An official recording of items, names, or actions, such as vital statistics (births, deaths, and marriages). **2.** To enter in an official register.

registered Officially qualified or certified, as in a registered hospital or registered nurse. *See also* registration.

registered biological photographer *See* Biological Photographic Association.

registered dietitian (RD) A dietitian who has successfully completed an examination and maintains continuing education requirements of the Commis-

sion on Dietetic Registration. *See also* dietitian; registered; registration.

Registered Encephalographic Technicians and Technologists, American Board of Certified and *See* American Board of Certified and Registered Encephalographic Technicians and Technologists.

registered hospital A hospital recognized by the American Hospital Association as having the essential characteristics of a hospital. *See also* hospital; registered; registration.

Registered Medical Assistants *See* Registered Medical Assistants of American Medical Technologists.

Registered Medical Assistants of American Medical Technologists (RMAAMT) A program founded in 1976 of the American Medical Technologists that has certified 9,000 assistants to physicians in office practice, clinics, hospitals, and private health care facilities. Formerly (1991) Registered Medical Assistants. *See also* American Medical Technologists; medical assistant; registered; registration.

registered nurse (RN) A nurse who has passed a state registration examination and has been licensed to practice nursing. The registration license is intended to ensure minimum levels of competence and thus protect the public, not to indicate the educational background of a nurse. Registered nurses' duties vary depending on the setting in which they work, including, for example, hospitals, physicians' offices, public health clinics, industrial plants, and schools. General responsibilities may include nursing care of patients, teaching health care, counseling, patient assessment, analyzing laboratory reports, and operating equipment, such as respirators and electrocardiographic machines. Registered nurses may also oversee the work of other health care workers. *See also* associate degree; baccalaureate degree program; certified nurse; diploma nurse; diploma school; licensed practical nurse; nurse; nurse anesthetist; nurse practitioner; registered; registration.

registered nurse anesthetist, certified *See* certified registered nurse anesthetist.

Registered Nurses, American Society of Ophthalmic *See* American Society of Ophthalmic Registered Nurses.

Registered Nurses, National Association of *See* National Association of Registered Nurses.

registered record administrator (RRA) A medical

record administrator who has been certified by the American Health Information Management Association as meeting its standards in medical record science. *See also* administrator; American Health Information Management Association; medical record administrator; registered; registration.

registered respiratory therapist (RRT) A respiratory therapist who has been registered by the National Board for Respiratory Care. *See also* National Board for Respiratory Care; registered; registration; respiratory; respiratory therapist.

registered social worker A social worker who has a graduate degree from an accredited school of social work, has successfully completed the Academy of Certified Social Workers examination, and has met other requirements necessary for certification. *See also* Academy of Certified Social Workers; certification; registered; registration; social worker.

Register of Health Service Providers in Psychology, Council for the National *See* Council for the National Register of Health Service Providers in Psychology.

registrar An individual whose responsibility is to maintain records.

Registrars Association, National Tumor *See* National Tumor Registrars Association.

registration **1.** The act of making a list, catalogue, schedule, or register that has the purpose and effect of giving notice and preventing fraud and deception. **2.** A formal process by which qualified individuals are listed on an official roster or registry maintained by a government or nongovernmental agency, enabling such persons to use a particular title and attesting to employing agencies and individuals that minimum qualifications have been met and maintained. *See also* registered; registry.

Registration of Electroencephalographic and Evoked Potentials Technologists, American Board of *See* American Board of Registration of Electroencephalographic and Evoked Potentials Technologists.

Registration, PR Committee for Licensing and *See* PR Committee for Licensing and Registration.

registry A database containing data pertinent to a specified topic, as in a tumor registry or a registry of clinical chemistry practitioners or emergency medical technicians. *See also* database.

Registry in Clinical Chemistry, National *See* National Registry in Clinical Chemistry.

Registry of Clinical Radiography Technologists, American *See* American Registry of Clinical Radiography Technologists.

Registry of Emergency Medical Technicians, National *See* National Registry of Emergency Medical Technicians.

Registry of Interpreters for the Deaf (RID) A national organization founded in 1964 composed of 4,000 professional interpreters and transliterators for the deaf. It maintains a registry of certified interpreters and transliterators, works to establish certification standards, and offers a national certification evaluation. *See also* certification; deaf; deafness.

Registry of Medical Assistants, American *See* American Registry of Medical Assistants.

Registry, National Bone Marrow Donor *See* National Marrow Donor Program.

Registry of Pathology, American *See* American Registry of Pathology.

Registry of Radiologic Technologists, American *See* American Registry of Radiologic Technologists.

Registry of Radiologic Technologists, American Chiropractic *See* American Chiropractic Registry of Radiologic Technologists.

registry, trauma *See* trauma registry.

registry, tumor *See* tumor registry.

regression In statistics, the relationship between the mean value of a random variable and the corresponding values of one or more independent variables. A common form of regression is a linear regression in which the model chosen for the analysis is a linear equation. *See also* independent variable; random variable; regression analysis; statistics; variable.

regression analysis A statistical procedure for determining the best approximation of the relationship between a dependent variable, such as the revenues of a hospital, and one or more independent variables, such as gross national product or per capita income. By measuring exactly how large and significant each independent variable has historically been in its relation to the dependent variable, the future value of the dependent variable can be predicted. Regression analysis attempts to measure the degree of correlation between dependent and independent variables, thereby establishing the predictive value of the independent variable. The most common form of regression analysis is a linear regression model. Multiple regression analysis is a method for measuring the effects of several factors concurrently. *See also* dependent variable; independent variable; variable.

regression line A line calculated in regression analysis that is used to estimate the relation between two quantities, the independent variable and the dependent variable. *See also* dependent variable; independent variable; regression analysis; variable.

regression to the mean The tendency for measurements, such as scores, that are extremely unusual to revert back to more normal levels on retest. *See also* mean; regression.

regressive **1.** Decreasing proportionately as the amount taxed increases, as in regressive tax. *See also* regressive tax. **2.** Characterized by a tendency to regress or go back.

regressive tax A tax that takes a decreasing proportion of income as income rises, such as sales taxes and the social security payroll tax on earnings above the maximum to which the tax applies. A regressive tax, for example, takes a higher percentage of the earnings of a low-income family than of a high-income family. A sales tax on food is considered regressive since low-income people pay the same amount of tax to buy a dozen eggs, for example, as do high-income people. *See also* progressive tax; proportional tax; tax.

regularly maintained beds The total number of beds that a health care organization has regularly set up and staffed for use by patients. *See also* bed.

regular survey *See* triennial survey.

regulate To control; to impose standards; to govern by rules. *See also* regulation.

regulated industry An industry that is regulated by government. The utility industries are an example of regulated industry because their pricing, profits, and, sometimes, production methods are regulated by both federal and state governments. *See also* industry; regulate; regulation.

regulation Rules or other directives issued by administrative agencies that are used to carry out a law. Many government agencies prepare regulations to administer a law. Regulatory programs can be described in terms of their purpose (such as to control charges), who or what is regulated (for example, regulating hospitals), who regulates (for example, state government), and method of regulation (for instance, prospective rate review). *See also* safe harbor regulations.

Regulation, Council on Licensure, Enforcement

and *See* Council on Licensure, Enforcement and Regulation.

regulation of insurance business *See* McCarran-Ferguson Act.

regulations, safe harbor *See* safe harbor regulations.

Regulatory Affairs Professionals Society (RAPS) A national organization founded in 1976 composed of professionals in the drug, medical device, biotechnology, diagnostic, cosmetic, and food industries, and lawyers, physicians, and consultants interested in advancing the regulatory affairs profession dealing with health care products. *See also* regulation.

regulatory agency A government body responsible for control and supervision of a particular activity or area of public interest, as in regulatory affairs concerning health care products. *See also* administrative agency; public interest.

Regulatory Boards, Federation of Associations of *See* Federation of Associations of Regulatory Boards.

rehabilitation **1.** Restoration of an individual or of a part of the body to functioning after injury, disease, or other abnormal state. **2.** The combined and coordinated use of medical, social, educational, and vocational measures for training or retraining individuals disabled by disease or injury. The goal is enabling patients to achieve their highest possible level of functional ability. *See also* cardiac rehabilitation program; habilitation; recovery; recuperation; vocational rehabilitation.

Rehabilitation Act of 1973 (PL 93-112) Legislation prohibiting government agencies, certain entities contracting with the federal government, certain recipients of federal grants, and recipients of federal financial assistance from discriminating against the handicapped. Section 504 of the act provides that "no otherwise qualified handicapped individual shall, solely by reason of his handicap, be excluded from the participation in, be denied the benefits of, or be subjected to discrimination under any program or activity receiving Federal Financial Assistance (FFA) (health care programs in receipt of Medicare or Medicaid funds are deemed to be recipients of FFA). Regulations implementing this legislation define "handicapped individual" very broadly (including individuals who regard themselves as being handicapped and alcoholics and drug addicts); prohibit discrimination in employment on the basis of handicap; require FFA recipients to make reasonable accommodations so that a qualified handicapped individual may be able to perform the essential elements of a job; require FFA recipients to make their services/programs accessible to the handicapped; require that all hospitals with emergency services establish procedures for effective communication with the hearing impaired; and prohibit discrimination in the treatment and admission of patients addicted to drugs and alcohol. *See also* Americans with Disabilities Act of 1990; handicapped person; rehabilitation.

rehabilitation administrator An individual who specializes in administering medical rehabilitation programs for federal, state, and nongovernmental hospitals and centers. *See also* administrator; rehabilitation.

Rehabilitation Administrators, Association of Medical *See* Association of Medical Rehabilitation Administrators.

Rehabilitation, American Academy of Physical Medicine and *See* American Academy of Physical Medicine and Rehabilitation.

Rehabilitation, American Association of Cardiovascular and Pulmonary *See* American Association of Cardiovascular and Pulmonary Rehabilitation.

Rehabilitation, American Board of Physical Medicine and *See* American Board of Physical Medicine and Rehabilitation.

Rehabilitation Association, American Deafness and *See* American Deafness and Rehabilitation Association.

Rehabilitation Association, National *See* National Rehabilitation Association.

rehabilitation center A health care organization specializing in rehabilitation. *See also* alcoholism rehabilitation center; health care organization; rehabilitation hospital.

rehabilitation center, alcoholism *See* alcoholism rehabilitation center.

Rehabilitation, Council of State Administrators of Vocational *See* Council of State Administrators of Vocational Rehabilitation.

Rehabilitation Counseling Association, American *See* American Rehabilitation Counseling Association.

Rehabilitation Counseling Association, National *See* National Rehabilitation Counseling Association.

rehabilitation counselor An individual who counsels disabled persons toward attaining their maximum functional capacity. A rehabilitation counselor also assists patients and clients to identify and use rehabilitation services designed to facilitate employment placement, full job performance, and job satisfaction. *Synonym:* vocational rehabilitation counselor. *See also* counselor; rehabilitation; rehabilitation counselor aide.

rehabilitation counselor aide An individual who assists a rehabilitation counselor in planning and implementing rehabilitation programs and activities for patients and clients. An aide may locate employment opportunities and match clients to available jobs. *See also* aide; rehabilitation counselor.

Rehabilitation Education, National Council on *See* National Council on Rehabilitation Education.

Rehabilitation Engineering, National Institute for *See* National Institute for Rehabilitation Engineering.

Rehabilitation Facilities, Commission on Accreditation of *See* Commission on Accreditation of Rehabilitation Facilities.

Rehabilitation Facilities, National Association of *See* National Association of Rehabilitation Facilities.

rehabilitation facility *See* rehabilitation hospital.

rehabilitation hospital A hospital or facility that provides health-related, social, and/or vocational services to disabled persons to help them attain their maximum functional capacity. *Synonym:* rehabilitation facility. *See also* hospital; rehabilitation.

Rehabilitation Hospitals and Programs, Section for *See* Section for Rehabilitation Hospitals and Programs.

Rehabilitation Information Center, National *See* National Rehabilitation Information Center.

Rehabilitation Instructors, National Association of *See* National Association of Rehabilitation Instructors.

rehabilitation medicine *See* physical medicine and rehabilitation.

Rehabilitation Medicine, American Congress of *See* American Congress of Rehabilitation Medicine.

Rehabilitation Medicine, American Osteopathic College of *See* American Osteopathic College of Rehabilitation Medicine.

rehabilitation nurse A registered nurse who engages in the practice of rehabilitation nursing. *See also* registered nurse; rehabilitation.

Rehabilitation Nurses, Association of *See* Association of Rehabilitation Nurses.

Rehabilitation Professionals in the Private Sector, National Association of *See* National Association of Rehabilitation Professionals in the Private

Sector.

rehabilitation program *See* rehabilitation service.

rehabilitation program, cardiac *See* cardiac rehabilitation program.

Rehabilitation Secretaries, National Association of *See* National Association of Rehabilitation Secretaries.

rehabilitation service An organizational service providing medical, health-related, social, and vocational services for disabled persons to help them attain or retain their maximum functional capacity. *Synonym:* rehabilitation program. *See also* physical medicine and rehabilitation; physical medicine service.

rehabilitation services, physical *See* physical rehabilitation services.

Rehabilitation Specialists, Council of *See* Council of Rehabilitation Specialists.

Rehabilitation Therapy, American Association for *See* American Association for Rehabilitation Therapy.

rehabilitation unit A unit in a hospital or other health care organization for treatment of inpatients who require assistance in attaining and/or retaining their maximum functional capacity. *See also* rehabilitation hospital.

rehabilitation, vocational *See* vocational rehabilitation.

Rehabilitative Audiology, Academy of *See* Academy of Rehabilitative Audiology.

Rehabilitative Psychology, American Board of Bionic *See* American Board of Bionic Rehabilitative Psychology.

reimbursement Compensation to another party for money spent or losses incurred, as in reimbursement made by an insurance company to a hospital for services provided to patients covered by an insurance contract. *See also* cost-based reimbursement; reimbursement specialist; retroactive reimbursement; retrospective reimbursement.

reimbursement, cost-based *See* cost-based reimbursement.

Reimbursement Officers, National Association of *See* National Association of Reimbursement Officers.

reimbursement, retroactive *See* retroactive reimbursement.

reimbursement, retrospective *See* retrospective reimbursement.

Reimbursement Review Board, Provider *See* Provider Reimbursement Review Board.

reimbursement specialist An individual who pre-

pares materials to obtain third-party payment and who may also negotiate reimbursement structures with third-party payers. *Synonym:* insurance clerk. *See also* reimbursement; third-party payer.

reinforcement In psychology, strengthening of a particular response or behavioral pattern by rewarding desirable behavior and punishing undesirable behavior. *See also* behavior; psychology; shaping.

reinsurance Special insurance coverage obtained by a provider or health plan to protect against certain unanticipated and potentially crippling losses incurred on covered services for members. Such insurance may limit exposure on a per-case or an aggregate basis. In some cases, physicians can obtain reinsurance through the contracted health plan. *See also* health care provider; health plan; insurance.

rejection **1.** In medicine, immunological response whereby substances or organisms that the system recognizes as foreign are not accepted, as in rejection of a transplanted organ. *See also* immunology; transplantation. **2.** Denying attention or affection to another person.

relapse To show again the signs and symptoms of a disease or condition after partial or complete remission. *Compare* remission.

relation A logical or natural association between two or more things. *See also* relationship.

relational file In computer science, a record (such as a medical record) in which certain content has been indexed, meaning that certain words have been set apart into specially formatted fields for future queries. Thus, in a large collection of relational files, it would be possible to ask: "How many records contain the diagnosis of sprained ankle?" In a relational database, "diagnosis" is a formatted field, and this question would be easily asked and answered. *Compare* flat file. *See also* field; file; medical record.

relationship Connection or association between two or more things, as in the relationship between administration of high-dose epinephrine and improved survival after cardiac arrest could not be demonstrated. *See also* relation; scale relationship.

relationship, scale *See* scale relationship.

relations, labor *See* labor relations.

relations, media *See* media relations.

relations, public *See* public relations.

relative quality The degree of excellence of a service or product. *See also* quality.

relative value scale (RVS) A numerical scale

designed to permit comparisons of the resources needed for various units of service provided. *See also* relative value unit; resource-based relative value; resource-based relative value scale; scale.

relative value unit (RVU) A unit of measure designed to permit comparison of the amounts of resources required to perform various provider services by assigning weight to such factors as personnel time, level of skill, and sophistication of equipment required to render service. *See also* resource-based relative value.

relativism In philosophy, a theory that ideas about truth and moral values are not absolute but are relative to the persons or groups holding them.

release **1.** In medicine, a mechanism by which an individual relinquishes a health care organization or other provider from responsibility or liability resulting from the patient's refusing treatment, cooperation, or compliance with a physician's orders. **2.** In law, a mechanism by which an individual relinquishes his or her right to maintain a claim or cause of action. *See also* cause of action.

release of information A consent form signed by a patient authorizing information to be given to a third party, such as an insurance company or lawyer. *See also* release.

release, press *See* press release.

relevance An item that is capable of making a difference in decision making. There are three elements of relevance: information must be available in a timely fashion before it loses its value in decision making; data must have an acceptable level of predictive value about outcomes past, present, and future; and information must have feedback value that provides information about earlier expectations.

reliability **1.** The ability of an item to perform a required function under stated conditions. *See also* reliability engineering. **2.** In performance measurement, consistency in results of a measure, including the tendency of the measure to produce the same results twice when it measures some entity or attribute believed not to have changed in the interval between measurements. **3.** Statistically, reliability refers to the degree to which scores are free from random error. Two major types of reliability are test, retest and split-half. *See also* data reliability; indicator reliability; interobserver reliability; intrarater reliability; random error; reliability engineering; split-half reliability; test, retest reliability.

reliability assessment *See* reliability testing.

reliability coefficient, interobserver *See* interobserver reliability coefficient.

reliability, conspect *See* interobserver reliability.

reliability, data *See* data reliability.

reliability engineering The engineering function dealing with the principles and practices related to the design, specification, assessment, and achievement of product or system reliability requirements and involving aspects of prediction, evaluation, production, and demonstration. *See also* engineering; reliability.

reliability, indicator *See* indicator reliability.

reliability, interobserver *See* interobserver reliability.

reliability, interjudge *See* interobserver reliability.

reliability, interrater *See* interobserver reliability.

reliability, intrarater *See* intrarater reliability.

reliability, scorer *See* interobserver reliability.

reliability, split-half *See* split-half reliability.

reliability testing In health care performance measurement, quantification of the accuracy and completeness with which indicator occurrences are identified from among all cases at risk of being indicator occurrences; a component of an indicator testing process. *See also* indicator; indicator testing process; performance measurement; reliability; split-half reliability; testing; test, retest reliability.

reliability, test, retest *See* test, retest reliability.

religion Belief in and reverence for a supernatural power or powers regarded as creator and governor of the universe. *See also* culture; faith; religious; sacred; subculture; worldview.

religious Accepting a higher power as a controlling influence for the good in one's life. *See also* religion; sacred.

Religious Therapists, American Association of *See* American Association of Religious Therapists.

rem The standard unit of measurement of absorbed radiation in living tissue. A millirem is a thousandth of a rem. A diagnostic chest x-ray involves between 20 millirems and 30 millirems of radiation. Each American, on average, receives 100 millirems to 200 millirems of radiation each year from natural background sources, such as cosmic rays, and artificial sources, such as diagnostic x-rays. There is considerable debate among scientists over the safety of repeated low doses of radiation. *See also* rad; radiation.

remedial Pertaining to correcting a deficiency, as in remedial journey. *See also* remedial journey.

remedial journey A sequence of problem-solving steps that move a quality improvement team from the identified root cause of a problem to the implementation of a solution or remedy that will hold the gains the team has made. *See also* quality improvement; quality improvement team.

remedies, exhaustion of *See* exhaustion of remedies.

remedy **1.** In health care, a medicine or therapy that relieves pain, cures disease, or corrects a disorder or condition. *See also* iamatology; treatment. **2.** In law, relief available from a court by which the violation of a legal right is prevented or a legal wrong is redressed. *See also* exhaustion of remedies.

remission A partial or complete disappearance of, or a lessening of the severity of, the symptoms of a disease, as in breast cancer in remission. It may be spontaneous or result from therapy and may be temporary or permanent. *Compare* relapse.

remote cause In law, a cause that does not necessarily produce an event without which an injury would not occur. A cause that is not considered proximate is regarded as remote. *See also* cause; proximate cause.

renal Pertaining to the kidney or the region of the kidneys, as in end stage renal disease. *See also* end stage renal disease; kidney; nephrology.

Renal Administrators Association, National *See* National Renal Administrators Association.

renal colic Severe colic due usually to impaction of a stone in the urinary tract. *See also* colic; nephrolithiasis; nephrology; urology.

renal disease Disease of the kidney. *See also* disease; kidney; nephrology; urology.

renal disease, end stage *See* end stage renal disease.

renal dialysis *See* hemodialysis.

renal failure A situation in which the kidneys, because of disease or destruction, are no longer able to maintain physiological homeostasis, in particular the excretion of nitrogenous and other waste products and the regulation of water, electrolyte, and acid-base balance. *See also* failure; kidney; nephrology; renal.

Renal Physicians Association (RPA) A national organization founded in 1973 composed of 1,500 physicians specializing in the treatment of renal (kidney) diseases. Its activities include expressing the concerns and needs of renal physicians to congressional and governmental agencies legislating,

executing, and regulating the federal End Stage Renal Disease Program. *See also* nephrology.

reorganization A thorough alteration of the structure of an organization. *See also* organization.

repeal To abolish, annul, or rescind by legislative act.

Rephael Society (RS) A national organization founded in 1966 composed of 600 Orthodox Jewish physicians, dentists, physical therapists, nurses, and other professionals in the health care field interested in studying medical issues and problems as they relate to Orthodox Jewish law and promoting the welfare of Orthodox Jews in the health care field. *See also* religion.

replacement blood donor A blood donor whose donation replaces blood used by a specific patient, thereby cancelling charges to the patient for blood. *See also* blood donor; donor.

replacement therapy Administration of a body substance to compensate for the loss, as from disease or surgery, of a gland or tissue that would normally produce this substance. *See also* hormone replacement therapy.

replacement therapy, hormone *See* hormone replacement therapy.

replant In medicine, to reattach an organ or limbs surgically to the original site, as in finger replantation. *See also* implant; transplant.

report **1.** A detailed account or statement describing an event, occurrence, or incident, such as the proceedings or transactions of a group. *See also* incident report. **2.** A written result of a study or investigation. *See also* interim report; report card. **3.** To relate or tell about, as in investigative reporting. *See also* investigative reporting; underreporting.

reportable disease *See* notifiable disease.

report card A report of progress presented periodically, as in a report card on quality of health services designed to inform patients and health care purchasers of practitioner and organizational performance. *See also* report.

reporter **1.** A writer, an investigator, or a presenter of news stories. **2.** In law, a person authorized to write and issue official accounts of judicial or legislative proceedings.

report, incident *See* incident report.

reporting, investigative *See* investigative reporting.

reporting, occurrence *See* occurrence reporting.

reporting, under- *See* underreporting.

reporting, uniform *See* uniform reporting.

report, interim *See* interim report.

representative, certified medical *See* certified medical representative.

representative, patient *See* patient representative.

representative, patient service *See* patient service representative.

representative sample A sample that resembles the population in some way. *See also* sample.

Representatives Association, Health Industry *See* Health Industry Representatives Association.

Representatives Institute, Certified Medical *See* Certified Medical Representatives Institute.

repression In psychoanalysis, an unconscious defense mechanism whereby unacceptable thoughts, feelings, memories, and impulses are pushed from the conscious into the unconscious, where they are submerged but remain important in influencing behavior and are often the source of anxiety. *See also* psychiatry; psychoanalysis.

repressive tax A tax designed to discourage a certain activity rather than to produce revenue. High taxes on tobacco and alcohol are repressive in the sense that they discourage consumption of the taxed product by raising its price. *See also* tax.

reproduction **1.** The act of producing a counterpart, an image, or a copy. **2.** In biology, to generate offspring by sexual or asexual means. *See also* artificial reproduction; biology; noncoital reproduction; ovum; spermatozoa.

reproduction, artificial *See* artificial reproduction.

reproduction, noncoital *See* noncoital reproduction.

Reproduction, Society for the Study of *See* Society for the Study of Reproduction.

reproductive endocrinologist An obstetrician-gynecologist who subspecializes in reproductive endocrinology. *See also* endocrinology; reproduction; reproductive endocrinology.

Reproductive Endocrinologists, Society of *See* Society of Reproductive Endocrinologists.

reproductive endocrinology A subspecialty of obstetrics and gynecology concerning management of complex problems relating to reproductive endocrinology and infertility. *See also* endocrinology; obstetrics and gynecology; reproduction.

Reproductive Health Association, National Family Planning and *See* National Family Planning and Reproductive Health Association.

Reproductive Health, Institute for *See* Institute for Reproductive Health.

Reproductive Health, National Association of Nurse Practitioners in *See* National Association of Nurse Practitioners in Reproductive Health.

Reproductive Health Professionals, Association of *See* Association of Reproductive Health Professionals.

Reproductive Surgeons, Society for *See* Society for Reproductive Surgeons.

reproductive technologies A variety of ways of achieving reproduction; for example, in-vitro fertilization, preembryo transfer, and surrogate motherhood. *See also* artificial insemination; fertilization; noncoital reproduction; preembryo transfer; reproduction; surrogate motherhood.

Reproductive Technology, Society for Assisted *See* Society for Assisted Reproductive Technology.

require To impose an obligation on or compel, as in required to comply with certain standards for accreditation. *See also* requirement.

required request law A law that requires hospitals to develop programs for asking families of deceased patients to donate the organs of the deceased for transplantation. *Synonym:* routine inquiry law. *See also* organ; organ procurement; transplantation.

required services Services that must be offered by a health program in order to meet some external standard. For example, under Title XIX of the Social Security Act, each state must offer certain basic health services before it can qualify as having a Medicaid program and thus be eligible for receiving federal matching funds. Examples of required services include hospital services, skilled nursing facility services for individuals aged 21 years and over, and home health care services for all persons eligible for skilled nursing facility services. *See also* standard.

requirement Something necessary or obligatory, often as a condition; for example, a requirement to meet a standard to achieve certification or accreditation. *See also* accreditation; certification; licensure; require; resource requirements; standard.

rescission The cancellation of a contract and the return of the parties to the positions they would have occupied if the contract had not been made. *See also* contract; mistake.

Rescue, National Association for Search and *See* National Association for Search and Rescue.

Rescue Service, Parachute Medical *See* Parachute

Medical Rescue Service.

research 1. Conscious action to acquire deeper knowledge or new facts about scientific, technical and other subjects. **2.** To study something thoroughly so as to present in a detailed, accurate manner, as in researching a subject. *See also* research design; research and development.

Research, Academy of Behavioral Medicine *See* Academy of Behavioral Medicine Research.

Research, Alliance for Aging *See* Alliance for Aging Research.

Research in Ambulatory Health Care Administration, Center for *See* Center for Research in Ambulatory Health Administration.

Research, American Association for Cancer *See* American Association for Cancer Research.

Research, American Association for Dental *See* American Association for Dental Research.

Research, American Association for Public Opinion *See* American Association for Public Opinion Research.

Research, American Federation for Aging *See* American Federation for Aging Research.

Research, American Federation for Clinical *See* American Federation for Clinical Research.

Research, American Society for Bone and Mineral *See* American Society for Bone and Mineral Research.

Research, American Society for Psychical *See* American Society for Psychical Research.

Research Animal Alliance *See* National Association for Biomedical Research.

Research in Asian Science and Medicine, Institute for Advanced *See* Institute for Advanced Research in Asian Science and Medicine.

Research, Association for Health Services *See* Association for Health Services Research.

Research in the Behavioral Sciences, American Institutes for *See* American Institutes for Research in the Behavioral Sciences.

research center A facility in which research is the primary activity. Research centers may be independent or affiliated with other organizations, such as universities or hospitals. Funding for research centers may come from many sources including grants, contracts, and public appropriations. *Synonym:* research institute. *See also* research.

Research, Center for Death Education and *See* Center for Death Education and Research.

Research, Center for Hazardous Materials *See* Center for Hazardous Materials Research.

Research, Center for Medical Effectiveness *See* Center for Medical Effectiveness Research.

Research, Central Society for Clinical *See* Central Society for Clinical Research.

Research, Child Abuse Institute of *See* Child Abuse Institute of Research.

Research in Child Development, Society for *See* Society for Research in Child Development.

Research, Commission on Pastoral *See* Commission on Pastoral Research.

Research in Cost-Effectiveness, Physicians for *See* Physicians for Research in Cost-Effectiveness.

Research Council, National *See* National Research Council.

Research Council, Plastic Surgery *See* Plastic Surgery Research Council.

research design The predetermined procedures and methods used by an investigator in conducting research. *See also* research.

research and development (R & D) Activities performed by a team of professionals working to transform a product idea into a technically sound product capable of being promoted. *See also* development; idea; promotion; research.

research dietitian A registered dietitian qualified by advanced preparation in dietetics and research techniques who plans, investigates, evaluates, and applies knowledge in dietetics. *See also* dietitian; registered dietitian.

Research Dissemination and Liaison, Center for *See* Center for Research Dissemination and Liaison.

Research and Educational Trust, Hospital *See* Hospital Research and Educational Trust.

Research and Education, National Association for Perinatal Addiction *See* National Association for Perinatal Addiction Research and Education.

Research and Education in Pathology, Universities Associated for *See* Universities Associated for Research and Education in Pathology.

Research, and Evaluation, National Advisory Council for Health Care Policy, *See* National Advisory Council for Health Care Policy, Research, and Evaluation.

Research, Foundation for Health Services *See* Foundation for Health Services Research.

Research Group, North American Primary Care *See* North American Primary Care Research Group.

Research Group, Public Citizen Health *See* Public

Citizen Health Research Group.

research, health services *See* health services research.

Research, Huxley Institute for Biosocial *See* Huxley Institute for Biosocial Research.

Research in Hypnosis and Psychotherapy, Institute for *See* Institute for Research in Hypnosis and Psychotherapy.

research institute *See* research center.

Research Institute, Acupuncture *See* Acupuncture Research Institute.

Research, Institute for Aerobics *See* Institute for Aerobics Research.

Research Institute, Mental *See* Mental Research Institute.

Research Institute, Ophthalmic *See* Ophthalmic Research Institute.

research, marketing *See* marketing research.

Research Modernization Committee, Medical *See* Medical Research Modernization Committee.

research, motivation *See* motivational research.

research, motivational *See* motivational research.

Research, National Association for Biomedical *See* National Association for Biomedical Research.

Research, National Center for Nursing *See* National Center for Nursing Research.

Research, National Coalition for Cancer *See* National Coalition for Cancer Research.

Research, National Heart *See* National Heart Research.

Research, National Institute on Disability and Rehabilitation *See* National Institute on Disability and Rehabilitation Research.

Research in Nervous and Mental Disease, Association for *See* Association for Research in Nervous and Mental Disease.

Research in Neurological Disorders, National Coalition for *See* National Coalition for Research in Neurological Disorders.

research, outcomes *See* outcomes research.

Research, Public Responsibility in Medicine and *See* Public Responsibility in Medicine and Research.

research, qualitative *See* qualitative research.

research, quantitative *See* quantitative research.

Research and Science, Academy of Pharmaceutical *See* Academy of Pharmaceutical Research and Science.

Research Society on Alcoholism (RSA) A national organization founded in 1976 composed of 770

scientists holding a Doctor of Medicine (MD) or Doctor of Philosophy (PhD) degree and other individuals actively engaged in research on alcoholism and alcohol-related problems. *See also* alcoholism.

Research, Society for Epidemiologic *See* Society for Epidemiologic Research.

Research, Society for Life History *See* Society for Life History Research.

Research, Society for Menstrual Cycle *See* Society for Menstrual Cycle Research.

Research Society, Orthopedic *See* Orthopedic Research Society.

Research, Society for Pediatric *See* Society for Pediatric Research.

Research Society, Precision Chiropractic *See* Precision Chiropractic Research Society.

Research, Society for Psychophysiological *See* Society for Psychophysiological Research.

Research Society, Radiation *See* Radiation Research Society.

Research Society, Scoliosis *See* Scoliosis Research Society.

Research, Society for Sex Therapy and *See* Society for Sex Therapy and Research.

Research Society, Sleep *See* Sleep Research Society.

Research in Substance Abuse, Association of Medical Education and *See* Association of Medical Education and Research in Substance Abuse.

research trial *See* clinical trial.

Research in Vision and Ophthalmology, Association for *See* Association for Research in Vision and Ophthalmology.

resect To surgically remove a portion of a structure or organ, as in resection of the prostate gland. *See also* dissect.

reserve **1.** In insurance, the money or other negotiable instruments set aside by an insurance company to ensure the fulfillment of its commitments to pay future claims. *See also* insurance. **2.** The keeping of one's feelings, thoughts, or affairs to oneself.

reserve, lifetime *See* lifetime reserve.

residence *See* domicile.

residency A period of on-the-job training of variable length beginning after an individual graduates from a medical, dental, podiatric, or other professional school. The professional-in-training performs professional duties under supervision. Satisfactory completion of a residency is a requirement for credentialing in some professional fields and specialities. The first graduate year of training following completion of medical school and the awarding of the doctor of medicine (MD) degree is now generally called the PGY-1 (postgraduate year 1), though internship has been the more traditional term. Medical residencies for graduate physicians are approved by a formal review system. *See also* internship; medical education; medical resident; PGY-1; residency program; Residency Review Committee; transitional year.

Residency Electronic Interactive Data Access, Fellowship and *See* Fellowship and Residency Electronic Interactive Data Access.

residency program A program in graduate medical, dental, podiatric or other health professional education to train specialists. These programs are principally based in hospitals, though during a residency physicians, dentists, and other health professionals may be assigned to clinics or other ambulatory centers (especially in the primary care specialties). *See also* chief resident; residency.

Residency Review Committee (RRC) A committee sponsored by the medical specialty boards, the specialty societies, and the American Medical Association that accredits residency programs. The accrediting process involves a review of certain written information, a site visit to the training program, and consideration of the information by a Residency Review Committee. Accreditation of a residency program indicates that it is judged to be in substantial compliance with the *Essentials of Accredited Residencies*. The Accreditation Council for Graduate Medical Education oversees the accreditation of training in all specialties and must approve or disapprove the recommendations of the Residency Review Committee. *See also* accreditation; Accreditation Council for Graduate Medical Education; residency; residency; Residency Review Committee for Emergency Medicine.

Residency Review Committee for Emergency Medicine (RRCEM) An accrediting body founded in 1982 composed of 12 representatives of the American College of Emergency Physicians, the American Board of Emergency Medicine, Council on Medical Education of the American Medical Association and the Emergency Medicine Residents' Association, that accredits residency training programs in emergency medicine. *See also* American College of Emergency Physicians; American Board of Emergency

Medicine; Council on Medical Education of the American Medical Association; emergency medicine; Emergency Medicine Residents' Association; residency.

Residency Training, American Association of Directors of Psychiatric *See* American Association of Directors of Psychiatric Residency Training.

resident 1. A person who resides in a particular place permanently or for an extended period, as in a nursing home resident. *Synonym*: long-term resident. **2.** An individual (such as a physician) undergoing training by performing duties and tasks under supervision in a residency program within an organization (such as a hospital), as in a medical resident. *Synonym*: resident physician. *See also* administrative resident; chief resident; dental resident; medical resident; medical specialty resident; residency; surgical resident.

resident, administrative *See* administrative resident.

resident bed A bed regularly maintained for use by persons who require custodial care and personal service but not nursing or medical services. *See also* bed; custodial care; resident.

resident, chief *See* chief resident.

resident, dental *See* dental resident.

Resident Education, Advisory Council for Orthopedic *See* Advisory Council for Orthopedic Resident Education.

Resident Education in Obstetrics and Gynecology, Council on *See* Council on Resident Education in Obstetrics and Gynecology.

residential care Care including lodging and board provided in a protective environment, such as a residential care facility, community-based living unit, group home, apartment, or foster home, to patients, including the mentally retarded, chemically dependent, or mentally ill who are not in an acute phase of illness and would be capable of self-preservation during a disaster. *See also* custodial care; residential care facility; residential community-based care.

residential care facility A live-in facility that provides custodial care to persons who, because of their physical, mental, or emotional condition, are not able to live independently. *Synonyms*: personal care institution; residential center; residential facility; residential treatment facility. *See also* custodial care; home for the aged; residential care.

Residential Centers, American Association of

Children's *See* American Association of Children's Residential Centers.

residential community-based care   Care including board and lodging for the mentally retarded, chemically dependent, or mentally ill with minimum supervision and little or no formal program activity within a residential facility; facilities for emotionally handicapped children, involving therapeutic care in child-caring institutions and group homes; halfway houses, which are therapeutic and supportive living arrangements for the chemically dependent and the mentally ill and that bridge the gap between residential treatment and community living; and extended care, very long term care and treatment for the chemically dependent and the mentally ill with 24-hour supervision and almost all services provided in the facility. *Synonym*: board and lodging. *See also* domiciliary care; halfway house; residential care; residential care facility.

residential facility   *See* residential care facility.

residential facility, community   *See* community residential facility.

residential occupancy   A classification of living quarters defined by the *Life Safety Code*® as the presence of overnight sleeping accommodations used by a population able to take action for self-preservation in the event of a fire. *See also Life Safety Code* ®.

residential program   A system of organized services for individuals with mental illness and substance abuse who require a less restrictive environment than an inpatient facility. *See also* residential care; residential care facility; residential community-based care; residential treatment program.

Residential Resources, National Association of Private   *See* National Association of Private Residential Resources.

residential treatment facility   *See* residential care facility.

residential treatment program   A setting in which mental health services are provided to individuals who require an overnight but less structured environment than that of an inpatient program, but who also require more structure than that of either a partial care program or an outpatient program. *See also* residential program.

resident, long-term   *See* resident.

Resident Matching Program, National   *See* National Resident Matching Program.

resident, medical   *See* medical resident.

resident, medical specialty   *See* medical specialty resident.

resident physician   *See* resident.

Residents' Association, Emergency Medicine   *See* Emergency Medicine Residents' Association.

Residents, Committee of Interns and   *See* Committee of Interns and Residents.

Residents and Interns, National Association of   *See* National Association of Residents and Interns.

resident, surgical   *See* surgical resident.

resignation   A formal notice given by a departing employee that his or her relationship with the employing organization is being terminated. *See also* employee.

res ipsa loquitur   Latin phrase meaning "the thing speaks for itself"; a rule of evidence in court that allows a fact finder (judge or jury) to assume negligence when an instrument causing an injury was in the control of a defendant and when the incident does not ordinarily occur without negligence. For example, depending on the jurisdiction, pursuant to the doctrine of res ipsa loquitur, a jury may infer the existence of negligence on the part of a surgeon from the fact that a sponge was left inside a patient; no other proof would be required. A rebuttable presumption allows a defendant an opportunity to attempt to disprove his or her presumed negligence. *See also* fact finder; rebuttable presumption.

resistant, tamper   *See* tamper resistant.

resolution   **1.** Firm determination. **2.** In medicine, the subsiding or termination of an abnormal condition, such as fever resolution. *See also* resolve. **3.** Discrimination between objects or values that are close together, usually applied to optical systems. *See also* contrast resolution.

resolution, contrast   *See* contrast resolution.

resolve   **1.** To make a firm decision about. *See also* determination. **2.** To bring to a usually successful conclusion, as in resolving a conflict, or a resolving infection. *See also* resolution.

resonance imaging, magnetic   *See* magnetic resonance imaging.

Resonance Imaging, Society for Magnetic   *See* Society for Magnetic Resonance Imaging.

resource   *See* resources.

resource allocation   In health care, societal or organizational decisions about the distribution of available health care resources involving, among other scarce resources, expensive life-saving technologies, location of physician's practices, and intensive care unit access. *See also* allocation; economics; rationing; resource requirements.

resource-based relative value (RBRV) The actual figure or value arrived at in relative, nonmonetary work units (relative value units) that can later be converted into dollar amounts as a means for determining reimbursement for provider (such as physicians and hospital) services. The formula for RBRV for a given service is: RBRV = (TW) (1 + RPC) (1 + AST), in which TW represents total work input by the provider; RPC is an index of relative specialty practice cost; and AST is an index of amortized value for the opportunity cost of specialized training. Total work input is defined by four attributes: time, mental effort and judgment, technical skill and physical effort, and psychological stress. *See also* relative value scale; relative value unit; resource-based relative-value scale.

resource-based relative-value scale (RBRVS) A method of reimbursement under Medicare that attempts to base physician reimbursement on the amount of resources, including cognitive and evaluative skills, required to diagnose and treat conditions. The approach weighs what resources, such as practice costs and the cost of specialty training, have gone into the "manufacture" of a service or procedure. Since the 1930s physicians have been paid according to the "customary, prevailing and reasonable" fee for a region of the country, and fee schedules reimbursed disproportionately for procedural services. *See* Medicare; Physician Payment Review Commission; relative value scale; relative value unit; resource-based relative value; scale.

resource capacity The number, type, and distribution of providers and facilities available for the delivery of health services for a defined population, such as people within a geographic or political area. *See also* capacity; resources.

Resource Center, National Women's Health *See* National Women's Health Resource Center.

resource constraint The maximum amount of resources available to produce a product or service. *See also* resources.

Resource Group, North American Primary Care *See* North American Primary Care Resource Group.

resource hospital *See* medical control.

resource requirements The material, facilities, financing, and human resources required to achieve

an objective, such as conducting a program or rendering services. *See also* requirement; resources.

resources Money, people, time, and equipment necessary for an organization or individual to carry out objectives. *See also* economics; health resources; human resources.

Resources Administration, American Society for Healthcare Human *See* American Society for Healthcare Human Resources Administration.

Resources Association, American Blood *See* American Blood Resources Association.

Resources, Committee on Energy and Natural *See* Committee on Energy and Natural Resources.

Resources Development Act of 1974, National Health Planning and *See* National Health Planning and Resources Development Act of 1974.

resources, health *See* health resources.

resources, human *See* human resources.

Resources Institute, Hazardous Materials Control *See* Hazardous Materials Control Resources Institute.

Resources, Institute of Laboratory Animal *See* Institute of Laboratory Animal Resources.

Resources, National Association of Private Residential *See* National Association of Private Residential Resources.

Resources for Nursing, Interagency Council on Library *See* Interagency Council on Library Resources for Nursing.

Resources, Quality Healthcare *See* Quality Healthcare Resources.

resources, real *See* real resources.

respect To feel or show deferential regard for; esteem. *See also* respect and caring.

respect and caring In health care, a performance dimension addressing the degree to which a patient, or a designee, is involved in his or her own care decisions and to which those providing services do so with sensitivity and respect for the patient's needs, expectations, and individual differences. *See also* caring; dimensions of performance; patient participation; respect; sensitivity.

respiration The act or process of breathing (inhaling and exhaling). *See also* artificial respiration; lung; ventilation; vital signs.

respiration, artificial *See* artificial respiration.

respirator A device that supplies oxygen or a mixture of oxygen and carbon dioxide for breathing, used especially in artificial respiration. *See also* artificial respiration; iron lung.

respiratory Pertaining to the exchange of oxygen and carbon dioxide between the atmosphere and the cells of the body. The process includes ventilation (inspiration and expiration), the diffusion of oxygen from pulmonary alveoli to the blood and of carbon dioxide from the blood to the alveoli, and the transport of oxygen to and carbon dioxide from body cells. *See also* adult respiratory distress syndrome; lung; respiration; respiratory arrest.

respiratory arrest Cessation of breathing. *See also* adult respiratory distress syndrome; cardiac arrest.

Respiratory Care, American Association for *See* American Association for Respiratory Care.

Respiratory Care, National Board for *See* National Board for Respiratory Care.

Respiratory Disease Clinics, National Coalition of Black Lung and *See* National Coalition of Black Lung and Respiratory Disease Clinics.

respiratory diseases unit A unit of a health care organization for treatment of inpatients with respiratory diseases. *See also* asthma; bronchitis; disease; emphysema; pneumonia; respiratory.

respiratory distress syndrome A disease, especially of premature infants, characterized by distressful breathing, cyanosis (bluish discoloration due to lack of oxygen), and the formation of a membrane (hyaline membrane) over the alveoli of the lungs. *See also* adult respiratory distress syndrome; syndrome.

respiratory distress syndrome, adult *See* adult respiratory distress syndrome.

respiratory failure The circumstance in which the respiratory system is unable to maintain normal body homeostasis, particularly with respect to arterial gas tensions of oxygen and carbon dioxide, indicating extensive impairment of lung function. *See also* failure; respiratory; respiratory distress syndrome.

Respiratory Health Association (RHA) A national organization founded in 1905 composed of pulmonary physicians, nurses, and other individuals interested in promoting respiratory health and the prevention and control of respiratory disease. It conducts Better Breathing classes to teach improved breathing techniques, exercises, proper use of medications, nutrition, and practical skills for daily living. It offers anti-smoking and smoking cessation education programs for youth and adults, corporate wellness programs, and respiratory activity programs for individuals with chronic lung disease. *See also* lung; pulmonary medicine; respiration; respiratory.

respiratory isolation A category of patient isolation intended to prevent transmission of infectious diseases over short distances through the air. A private room is indicated but patients infected with the same organism may share a room. Masks are for those who come in close contact with the patient; gowns and gloves are not. *See also* infectious diseases; isolation; respiratory.

Respiratory Medicine, National Jewish Center for Immunology and *See* National Jewish Center for Immunology and Respiratory Medicine.

respiratory therapist An allied health professional who assumes primary responsibility for respiratory care processes, including the supervision of respiratory therapy technician functions. The respiratory therapist may review, collect and recommend obtaining additional data, which he or she then evaluates to determine the appropriateness of the prescribed respiratory care, and may participate in the development of the respiratory care plan; selects, assembles, and checks all equipment used in providing respiratory care; initiates and conducts therapeutic procedures, and modifies prescribed therapeutic procedures to achieve one or more specific objectives; maintains patient records and communicates relevant information to other members of the health care team; and assists the physician in performing special procedures in a clinical laboratory, procedure room, or operating room. Respiratory therapists are one type of allied health professional for which the Committee on Allied Health Education and Accreditation has accredited education programs. *Synonym:* inhalation therapist. *See also* allied health professional; registered respiratory therapist; respiratory therapy; respiratory therapy technician.

respiratory therapist, registered *See* registered respiratory therapist.

respiratory therapy (RT) The health care field dealing with treatment of diseases or disability due to respiratory illness or injury. *Synonym:* inhalation therapy. *See also* respiratory therapist.

Respiratory Therapy, American Association for *See* American Association for Respiratory Care.

Respiratory Therapy Education, Joint Review Committee for *See* Joint Review Committee for Respiratory Therapy Education.

Respiratory Therapy, National Board for *See*

National Board for Respiratory Care.

respiratory therapy technician An allied health professional who administers general respiratory care and may assume clinical responsibility for specified respiratory care processes involving the application of well-defined therapeutic techniques under the supervision of a respiratory therapist and a physician. Specifically, the respiratory therapy technician reviews clinical data, the history, and respiratory therapy orders; collects clinical data by interview and examination of the patient; recommends and/or performs and reviews additional bedside procedures, x-rays, and laboratory tests; evaluates data to determine the appropriateness of the prescribed respiratory care; assembles and maintains equipment used in respiratory care; ensures cleanliness and sterility by the selection and/or performance of appropriate disinfecting techniques and monitors their effectiveness; and initiates, conducts, and modifies prescribed therapeutic procedures. Respiratory therapy technicians are one type of allied health professional for which the Committee on Allied Health Education and Accreditation has accredited education programs. *See also* respiratory therapist; respiratory therapy; technician.

respite care Short-term care to individuals in the home or an institution in order to provide temporary relief to the family home care giver. This care may be provided during the day or overnight.

respondeat superior Latin phrase meaning "let the master answer"; a rule that holds a master liable for the acts of his or her servant, an employer for the acts of his or her employee, and a principal for the acts of his or her agent. It requires that the act for which the master, employer, or principal is held liable be done within the scope of the business. For example, a physician may be liable for the acts of his or her employed nurse in treating patients even though the employer's conduct is faultless. *See also* captain of the ship doctrine; master and servant; vicarious liability.

respondent **1.** *See* appellee. **2.** One who responds to a survey. *See also* survey.

response A reply or reaction to a stimulus, such as a patient response in a clinical research study or a response to a survey. *See also* overresponse; respondent; response rate.

response, over- *See* overresponse.

response rate In survey research, the percentage of persons given questionnaires who complete and return them. *See also* rate; response; survey.

responsibility The state, quality, or fact of being responsible. *See also* accountability; duty; obligation; responsible.

Responsibility, American Bar Association Center for Professional *See* American Bar Association Center for Professional Responsibility.

Responsibility in Medicine and Research, Public *See* Public Responsibility in Medicine and Research.

Responsibility, Physicians for Social *See* Physicians for Social Responsibility.

responsible **1.** Liable to be required to give account of one's actions, as in the hospital held responsible for the outcome. **2.** Able to make moral or rational decisions on one's own and therefore answerable for one's behavior, as in a physician being responsible for providing a service. **3.** Able to be trusted or depended upon, as in a responsible person. *See also* accountability; responsibility.

Responsible Genetics, Council for *See* Council for Responsible Genetics.

Responsible Medicine, Physicians Committee for *See* Physicians Committee for Responsible Medicine.

Responsible Nutrition, Council for *See* Council for Responsible Nutrition.

responsible party **1.** An individual or organization responsible for placing a patient in a health care facility and ensuring that adequate care is provided; for example, a parent is usually the responsible party for a child. **2.** The party responsible for payment of services. *See also* responsibility.

responsive Readily reacting to suggestions, influences, or appeals, as in a responsive hospital administration.

responsive pleading A formal written answer to allegations set out in a pleading filed by another party. *See also* pleadings; responsive.

rest home A facility providing custodial care and, sometimes, limited nursing care, as by a visiting nurse. *See also* custodial care.

Restoration, Eye-Bank for Sight *See* Eye-Bank for Sight Restoration.

restrain To hold back or keep in check. *See also* restraint; restraint of trade.

restraining order, temporary *See* temporary restraining order.

restraint **1.** In health care, use of a physical or mechanical device to involuntarily restrain the movement of the whole or a portion of a patient's body as a means of controlling his or her physical activities in order to protect him or her or other persons from injury. Restraint differs from mechanisms usually and customarily used during medical, diagnostic, or surgical procedures that are considered a regular part of such procedures. These mechanisms include, but are not limited to, body restraint during surgery, arm restraint during intravenous administration, and temporary physical restraint before administration of electroconvulsive therapy. Devices used to protect the patient, such as bed rails, tabletop chairs, protective nets, helmets, or the temporary use of halter-type or soft-chest restraints, and mechanisms, such as orthopedic appliances, braces, wheelchairs, or other appliances or devices used to posturally support the patient or assist him or her in obtaining and maintaining normative bodily functions are not considered restraint interventions. *See also* seclusion; straitjacket. **2.** Control or repression of feelings. *See also* restrain.

restraint order, temporary *See* temporary restraining order.

restraint of trade In common law and as used in antitrust laws, contracts or combinations that tend or are designed to eliminate or stifle competition, effect a monopoly, artificially maintain prices, or otherwise hamper or obstruct the course of trade and commerce as it would be carried on if left to the control of natural economic forces. *See also* antitrust laws; monopoly.

Restorative Dentistry, American Academy of *See* American Academy of Restorative Dentistry.

restricted fund Money donated to an organization that can be expended for a specified purpose only. *Compare* unrestricted fund. *See also* fund.

restricted fund, un- *See* unrestricted fund.

restructuring Reorganization of an organization, such as a hospital in order to better deal with new functions, enterprises, and demands. *See also* corporate restructuring; diversification.

restructuring, corporate *See* corporate restructuring.

resurvey The next triennial survey of a health care organization conducted by the Joint Commission on Accreditation of Healthcare Organizations. *See also* accreditation survey; Joint Commission on Accreditation of Healthcare Organizations.

resuscitation The process or act of reviving, or attempting to revive, patients from the absence of respiration or cardiac activity, as in restoration of breathing after respiratory arrest or reviving the heartbeat after cardiac arrest. *See also* cardiopulmonary resuscitation; mouth-to-mouth resuscitation; respiration.

resuscitation, cardiopulmonary *See* cardiopulmonary resuscitation.

resuscitation cart *See* crash cart.

resuscitation, mouth-to-mouth *See* mouth-to-mouth resuscitation.

retail store dentistry Dental services offered within a retail department or drug store business. Space is usually leased from a store by a separate administrative group, which, in turn, subleases to a dentist or dental group providing dental services. Appointments are usually unnecessary. *See also* dentistry.

retainer **1.** An advance fee paid to a professional to ensure the availability of her or his services at a later time. **2.** *See* orthodontic appliance.

retardation Slowness, as in mental retardation or psychomotor retardation. *See also* mental retardation.

Retardation, American Academy on Mental *See* American Academy on Mental Retardation.

Retardation, American Association on Mental *See* American Association on Mental Retardation.

Retardation Association of America, Mental *See* Mental Retardation Association of America.

retardation, mental *See* mental retardation.

Retardation Program Directors, National Association of State Mental *See* National Association of State Mental Retardation Program Directors.

Retarded, Association for Advancement of Blind and *See* Association for Advancement of Blind and Retarded.

retention *See* risk charge.

retention rate *See* risk charge.

retch To attempt unsuccessfully to vomit.

Reticuloendothelial Society *See* Society for Leukocyte Biology (A Reticuloendothelial Society).

Reticuloendothelial Society), Society for Leukocyte Biology, (A *See* Society for Leukocyte Biology (A Reticuloendothelial Society).

reticuloendothelial system The cells of the blood and body tissues, including macrophages, lymphocytes, and granulocytes, that are involved in the immune response, inflammation, and functions in host defense against such problems as malignancies, infection, and environmental pathogens. *See also* Hodgkin's disease; immune system; inflammation;

lymphocyte; reticulosis; white blood cell.

reticulosis Any proliferative disorder of the reticuloendothelial system. *See also* Kaposi's sarcoma; reticuloendothelial system.

retire To withdraw, leave, or depart from a particular activity or situation. *See also* retirement.

Retired Americans, Association of *See* Association of Retired Americans.

Retired Army Nurse Corps Association (RANCA) A national organization founded in 1977 composed of 2,190 Army Nurse Corps officers retired from either active or reserve duty; associate members are officers with 16 or more years of service still serving on active duty and former members of the Army Nurse Corps who were honorably discharged. It provides educational opportunities for members; disseminates information to the public; and seeks to preserve the history of the US Army Nurse Corps. *See also* corps; nurse; Nurse Corps; retired.

Retired Dentists, American Society of *See* American Society of Retired Dentists.

Retired Persons, American Association of *See* American Association of Retired Persons.

Retired Persons Services (RPS) A mail service pharmacy founded in 1959 for members of the American Association of Retired Persons. It provides prescription and nonprescription drugs, vitamins, and other health care items through mail service and walk-in facilities in California, Texas, Missouri, Oregon, Indiana, Connecticut, Florida, Pennsylvania, Nevada, Virginia, and Washington, DC. It encourages consumer awareness, comparison shopping, and use of generic drugs. *See also* American Association of Retired Persons; generic drug law; prescription drug.

retirement Leaving active employment because of age, disability, illness, or personal choice. *See also* disability retirement; preretirement counseling; retirement age; retirement plan.

retirement age The age at which an employee stops working; the point at which retirement benefits are payable. A 1978 amendment to the Age Discrimination in Employment Act raised the minimum mandatory retirement age to 70 years. *See also* automatic retirement age; deferred retirement age; early retirement age; normal retirement age.

retirement age, automatic *See* automatic retirement age.

retirement age, deferred *See* deferred retirement age.

retirement age, early *See* early retirement age.

retirement age, normal *See* normal retirement age.

retirement center A facility or organized program that provides social services and activities to retired persons who generally do not require ongoing health care. *See also* retirement.

retirement community, continuing care *See* continuing care retirement community.

retirement counseling, pre- *See* preretirement counseling.

retirement, disability *See* disability retirement.

Retirement Income Security Act, Employee *See* Employee Retirement Income Security Act.

retirement plan A plan provided by an employer or a self-employed individual for an employee's or self-employed individual's retirement. Because of the tax advantages, most retirement plans are designed to ensure a present deduction to the employer while the employee is permitted to avoid recognizing the income until he or she has actually or constructively received it. *See also* individual retirement account; Keogh plan.

retractor In medicine, a surgical instrument used to hold back organs or the edges of an incision during surgery so that underlying structures can be adequately exposed. *See also* surgery.

retrieval **1.** To find and bring back, as in data retrieval. **2.** In computer science, the process of accessing information from memory or other storage devices.

retroactive Applying to a period before enactment, as in a retroactive pay increase. *See also* retroactive date; retroactive reimbursement.

retroactive date The date stipulated in a claims-made insurance policy as the earliest date an event may occur and be covered under that claims-made policy. *See also* claims-made coverage.

retroactive reimbursement Additional payment by a third-party payer to an institution for services not identified at the time of initial reimbursement. *See also* reimbursement; retroactive; retrospective reimbursement.

retrospective Pertaining to events in the past, as in retrospective reimbursement. *See also* retrospective data collection; retrospective reimbursement.

retrospective data collection Collection of data for events that have already occurred. *See also* data collection.

retrospective reimbursement   A method of third-party payment in which costs incurred by a provider in providing services to covered patients are based on actual costs determined after the services have been provided, usually at the end of a fiscal period. This contrasts to prospective pricing in which rates of payments to providers for patient services are established in advance for the coming fiscal year, and providers are paid these rates for services delivered regardless of the costs actually incurred in providing these services. *See also* prospective pricing system; reimbursement; retroactive reimbursement; retrospective.

retrospective review   A method of determining medical necessity and/or appropriate billing practice for services that have already been rendered. *Compare* prospective review. *See also* audit; medical audit; retrospective; retrospective study.

retrospective study   An inquiry planned to observe and collect data for events that have already occurred, as compared with a prospective study, which is planned to observe events that have not yet occurred. A case-control study is usually retrospective. *Compare* prospective study. *See also* case-control study; retrospective; retrospective review.

retrovirus   A ribonucleic (RNA) virus characterized by the presence of an enzyme, reverse transcriptase, that enables transcription of RNA to deoxyribonucleic acid (DNA) inside an affected cell and replication within the cell. A well-known retrovirus is the human immunodeficiency virus (HIV), which makes copies of itself in host cells, such as T4 helper lymphocytes, leading to a disruption of normal immune responses. *See also* deoxyribonucleic acid; HIV; immune system; ribonucleic acid; virus.

revenue   Increase in an organization's assets or a decrease in its liabilities during an accounting period. *See also* income; general revenue; revenue sharing; uncollected revenue.

Revenue Act of 1934   An act of Congress that prohibited tax-exempt organizations from attempting to influence legislation and from engaging in propaganda activities.

revenue, general   *See* general revenue.

revenue sharing   Distribution of a portion of federal tax revenues to state and municipal governments. *See also* revenue.

revenue, uncollected   *See* uncollected revenue.

review   **1.** To study or examine with an eye to criticism or correction, or, alternatively, improvement. **2.** A written evaluation or study.

Review Accreditation Commission, Utilization   *See* Utilization Review Accreditation Commission.

review, admissions   *See* admissions review.

review agency, medical   *See* medical review agency.

Review Association, American Managed Care and   *See* American Managed Care and Review Association.

Review Association, American Medical Peer   *See* American Medical Peer Review Association.

review, blood usage   *See* blood usage review.

review board, institutional   *See* institutional review board.

Review Board, Provider Reimbursement   *See* Provider Reimbursement Review Board.

review, capital expenditure   *See* capital expenditure review.

review, case-based   *See* case-based review.

review, claims   *See* claims review.

Review Commission on Education for Physician Assistants, Accreditation   *See* Accreditation Review Commission on Education for Physician Assistants.

Review Committee for Educational Programs in Surgical Technology, Accreditation   *See* Accreditation Review Committee for Educational Programs in Surgical Technology.

review committee, peer   *See* peer review committee.

review committee, utilization   *See* utilization review committee.

review, concurrent   *See* concurrent review.

review, continued-stay   *See* continued-stay review.

review coordinator, utilization   *See* utilization review coordinator.

Review Council of America, Professional Standards   *See* Professional Standards Review Council of America.

review criteria   A guideline or standard, or a series of guidelines or standards, against which activity can be assessed for the purpose of evaluation. *See also* criteria; criteria set; practice guideline.

review, design   *See* design review.

review, drug utilization   *See* drug usage evaluation.

review, explicit   *See* explicit review.

review, external   *See* external review.

review function, medical record   *See* medical record review function.

review, implicit   *See* implicit review.

review, internal   *See* internal review.

review, medical   *See* medical review.

review, medical record   *See* medical record review.

review organization, peer   *See* peer review organization.

review, peer   *See* peer review.

Review Physicians, American Board of Quality Assurance and Utilization   *See* American Board of Quality Assurance and Utilization Review Physicians.

review, preadmission   *See* admissions review.

review, preprocedure   *See* preprocedure review.

review, private   *See* private review.

review, program   *See* program review.

review, prospective   *See* prospective review.

review, retrospective   *See* retrospective review.

review, surgical case   *See* surgical case review.

Review Technique, Program Evaluation and   *See* Program Evaluation and Review Technique.

review, utilization   *See* utilization review.

revised trauma score (RTS)   *See* trauma score.

revocation   The recall of a power or authority conferred, as in the revocation of a physician's license.

revolving door   A term used to describe an organization whose members or personnel remain only a short time before going elsewhere. *See also* organization.

rework   The act of performing a task two or more times because it was not performed correctly the first time. Rework occurs for many reasons, including insufficient planning, failure of a customer to specify the needed input, and failure of a supplier to provide a consistently high-quality output. *See also* cost of quality; customer; failure cost; squander; rework loop; supplier; waste; work.

rework loop   A sequence of steps in a process that checks work that has been completed and reworks and corrects some or all of the work that is inadequate. *See also* rework.

Rh   Pertaining to the Rh factor, as in Rh antigen or Rh incompatibility. *See also* Rh factor.

RHA   *See* Respiratory Health Association.

rheology   The science of the deformation and flow of matter. It is often used in medicine to mean the study of blood flow in the circulatory system. *See also* circulatory system.

rhesus factor   *See* Rh factor.

rhetoric   **1.** The art of using language effectively and persuasively. **2.** A style of speaking or writing that is elaborate, pretentious, insincere, or intellectually vacuous.

rheumatism   Various afflictions of the muscles, tendons, joints, bones, or nerves, leading to discomfort and disability. *See also* arthritis; rheumatology.

Rheumatism, Pan American League Against   *See* Pan American League Against Rheumatism.

rheumatologist   An internist or pediatrician who specializes in rheumatology. *See also* pediatric rheumatology; rheumatology.

rheumatologist, pediatric   *See* pediatric rheumatologist.

rheumatology   The branch of medicine and subspecialty of internal medicine and pediatrics dealing with the management of diseases of joints, muscle, bones, and tendons. *See also* bone; gout; internal medicine; joint; osteoarthritis; pediatric rheumatology.

Rheumatology, American College of   *See* American College of Rheumatology.

rheumatology, pediatric   *See* pediatric rheumatology.

Rh factor   Any of several substances on the surface of red blood cells that induce a strong response in individuals lacking the substance. It is called Rh factor because it was first identified in the blood of rhesus monkeys. Approximately 85% of people have Rh factor. Persons having the factor are designated Rh-positive; those lacking the factor, Rh-negative. If an Rh-negative person receives Rh-positive blood, hemolysis, and anemia can result. Rh is an abbreviation for rhesus. *See also* red blood cell; blood groups.

rhinitis   *See* hay fever.

Rhinolaryngology and Head/Neck Nurses, Society of Oto-   *See* Society of Otorhinolaryngology and Head/Neck Nurses.

Rhinological and Otological Society, American Laryngological,   *See* American Laryngological, Rhinological, and Otological Society.

Rhinologic Society, American   *See* American Rhinologic Society.

rhinology   The branch of medicine dealing with the anatomy, physiology, and pathology of the nose. *See also* otolaryngology.

rhinophyma   Disfiguring irregular enlargement of the nose due to an abnormal increase in the number of sebaceous glands, occurring in rosacea. *See also* rosacea; sebaceous gland; skin.

rhinoplasty   Any plastic surgical procedure on the nose. *See also* otolaryngology; plastic surgery; rhinology.

rhythm   A pattern displayed by recurrent events, as

in a regular rhythm characterized by the same event or sequence of events repeated at uniform intervals. *See also* arrhythmia; circadian rhythm.

rhythm, circadian   *See* circadian rhythm.

rhythm method of contraception   *See* safe period.

RIAL   *See* radioimmunoassay.

ribonucleic acid (RNA)   A nucleic acid that in most cells transmits genetic information from the deoxyribonucleic acid (DNA) in the nucleus to the cytoplasm and functions in the synthesis of proteins. It is the genetic material of some viruses. *See also* deoxyribonucleic acid; molecular genetics; poliovirus; retrovirus; virus.

Richard King Mellon Foundation   A private foundation established in 1947 with local grant programs emphasizing conservation, higher education, cultural and civic affairs, social services, medical research, and health care. It also provides support for conservation of natural areas and wildlife preservation. It donates money primarily in Pittsburgh and western Pennsylvania, except for nationwide conservation programs. *See also* foundation; private foundation.

rickets   Defective development and growth of bones due to inadequate absorption and use of calcium. The usual cause is vitamin D deficiency in childhood. Vitamin D promotes calcium absorption from the intestine and its incorporation into bone structure. The clinical features of rickets are soft and fragile bones, inadequate growth, deformities of the limbs, thoracic cage, pelvis, and skull, and characteristic x-ray changes. *See also* osteomalacia.

rickettsiae   Bacterialike microorganisms that live as parasites in ticks, fleas, lice, and mites and are transmitted to humans by these vectors. Rickettsia-caused diseases include Rocky Mountain spotted fever and typhus. *See also* microorganism; vector.

RID   *See* Registry of Interpreters for the Deaf.

rider   **1.** An amendment or addition attached to a document, such as an insurance policy, identifying changes in coverage. These changes may include either expanding or decreasing the policy's benefits or adding or excluding certain conditions from the policy's coverage. **2.** In the legislative process, a provision in a bill that is not germane to the main purpose of the law.

RIF   Acronym for reduction in force, meaning the elimination of specific job categories in organizations. A person who has been "riffed" has not been fired but nevertheless is without a job. *See also* voluntary demotion.

riff   To lose one's job without being fired. *See also* RIF.

right   *See* rights.

right of autonomy, patient's   *See* patient's right of autonomy.

right, confidentiality as a patient   *See* confidentiality as a patient right.

right to die   The legal right to refuse life-saving or life-sustaining (or, alternatively, death-prolonging) procedures. A competent adult has the legal right to refuse medical treatment, even if that treatment is essential to sustaining life. *See* autonomy; patient's right of autonomy.

Right to Die, Choice in Dying - The National Council for the   *See* Choice in Dying-The National Council for the Right to Die.

right-to-life   **1.** Pertaining to protecting the rights of the developing fetus. Right-to-life supporters are opposed to allowing a woman to choose whether to have an abortion. *See also* pro-life. **2.** Pertaining to protecting the rights of the terminally ill, people on life-support machines, and other groups of people in similar circumstances. *Compare* right to die.

right-to-lifer   A supporter of the right-to-life position. *See also* right-to-life.

right-to-live   *See* autonomy; patient's right of autonomy.

right of privacy   The constitutional right of privacy to prohibit unwanted invasion, especially of one's own body. This right is the basis for informed consent and restriction of governmental intrusion in areas, such as birth control, sterilization, abortion, and the right to refuse medical treatment. *See also* confidentiality; informed consent; privacy.

right to refuse treatment   *See* autonomy; patient's right of autonomy.

rights   Individual liberties either expressly provided for in state or federal constitutions, such as the right to assembly or free speech, or which have been found to exist as those constitutions have been interpreted, such as the right to refuse medical treatment or the right to an abortion. *See also* adjective law; autonomy; bill of patient rights; human rights; patient rights; patient's right of autonomy; substantive right; women's rights.

rights, bill of patient   *See* bill of patient rights.

rights, human   *See* human rights.

rights, patient   *See* patient rights.

Rights of the Terminally Ill, Center for the   *See*

Center for the Rights of the Terminally Ill.

right, substantive *See* substantive right.

rights, women's *See* women's rights.

rigor The sensation of shivering experienced when the body temperature rises sharply. *Synonyms*: chill; shake. *See also* shivering.

rigor mortis Stiffness or hardness of the muscles, which occurs shortly after death.

Ringer's solution Physiological saline solution with potassium and calcium chlorides added. *See also* physiological saline; saline.

ringworm A fungal (*Tinea*) infection in which centrifugal spread of the fungus in the skin accompanied by central healing of the lesion leads to a circular rash (*Tinea circinata*). *See also* fungus; rash.

RISC Acronym for reduced instruction set computer, a type of computer designed to perform a limited set of operations, and therefore having relatively simple circuitry and able to work at high speed. CISC (complex instruction set computing), by contrast, is the more traditional, slower approach to computing. *See also* computer.

risk **1.** Any measurable or predictable chance of loss, injury, disadvantage, hazard, danger, peril, or destruction. Risk to a health care organization may arise, for example, through general or professional liability or physical property damage. Insurance is purchased to cover such exigencies. *See also* hazard; peril. **2.** The chance of occurrence of disease, injury, or death among various groups of individuals and from different causes. An applicant for a health insurance policy whose physical condition fails to meet health status standards is referred to as an impaired risk. *See also* health risk.

risk adjustment In performance measurement in health care, the use of severity-of-illness measures, such as age, to estimate the risk (the measurable or predictable chance of loss, injury, or death) to which a patient is subject before receiving some health care intervention. For example, patients with an advanced state of a disease, such as emphysema, who receive an intervention, such as surgery requiring general anesthesia, will usually have a higher risk of morbidity and mortality than a patient with normal lung function receiving the identical intervention. Risk (or severity) adjustment is important so that performance and quality can be meaningfully compared across organizations, practitioners, and communities. *See also* adjustment; severity adjust-

ment; severity of illness.

risk analysis In health insurance, the process of evaluating the expected health care costs for a prospective group and determining what product, benefit level, and price to offer to best meet the needs of the group and carrier. *See also* analysis; carrier; risk.

risk appraisal, health *See* health risk appraisal.

risk assessment The qualitative or quantitative estimation of the likelihood of (adverse) effects that may result from exposure to specified events or processes or from the absence of beneficial influences. *See also* assessment; health risk appraisal; risk.

risk, assumption of *See* assumption of risk.

risk, at *See* at risk.

risk-benefit analysis The process of analyzing and comparing on a single scale the benefits and risks of an action or failure to act. *See also* analysis; benefit; risk.

risk capital Money invested in a business venture for which stock is issued. *See also* capital; risk.

risk charge In insurance, the fraction of a premium that goes to generate or replenish surpluses that a carrier must develop to protect against the possibility of excessive losses under its policies. Profits, if any, on the sale of insurance are also taken from the surpluses developed using risk charges. *Synonyms*: retention; retention rate. *See also* carrier; charge; premium.

risk, credit *See* credit risk.

risk factor A factor that increases one's chances of contracting a particular disease, as in risk factors for coronary artery disease. *See also* factor; risk.

risk, health *See* health risk.

risk, impaired *See* risk.

risk management In health care, the function of planning, organizing, and directing a comprehensive program of activities to identify, evaluate, and take corrective action against risks that may lead to patient injury, employee injury, and property loss or damage with resulting institutional financial loss or legal liability. Three components of many risk management programs include risk financing (determining the types of potential exposures to the institution and then ensuring that adequate insurance coverage is available in the event that a loss occurs); claims management (involves investigating and disposing of claims in such a manner as to minimize dollar loss to the organization); and loss prevention (establishing systems to identify, evaluate, and minimize or prevent potential areas of risk). *See also* incident reporting; management; risk; risk management activities; risk manager.

risk management activities   Clinical and administrative activities that health care organizations undertake to identify, evaluate, and reduce the risk of injury and loss to members, personnel, and visitors of health care organizations. *See also* risk; risk management; risk manager.

Risk Management, American Society for Healthcare   *See* American Society for Healthcare Risk Management.

Risk Management, American Society for Hospital   *See* American Society for Healthcare Risk Management.

risk management contract   A contract between a group purchaser and an insurer, service plan, medical foundation, or other third party in which the third-party organization agrees to administer, but not underwrite, the group's health care coverage plan. The third-party organization receives an administrative fee for its services but the payment of benefits comes from funds provided by the group. The group purchaser self-insures its employees or group members. *See also* contract; management; purchaser.

risk manager   An individual who specializes in risk management. Risk managers have varied backgrounds, including insurance, law, administration, nursing, and safety engineering. Their responsibilities may include claims management (such as immediate investigation of unexpected, undesirable occurrences); establishment of management information systems to encourage personnel to report occurrences of actual or potential loss; education of hospital and medical staffs because personnel and medical staffs generally need to improve their understanding of what situations may constitute loss potential; review of policies and procedures; and evaluation of insurance coverages and contracts. *See also* risk management.

risk pool   A pool of money that is large enough to meet the costs of care for a group of individuals in relation to their health care risks. *See also* high risk pool; risk.

risk pool, high-   *See* high-risk pool.

risk sharing   The distribution of financial risk among parties furnishing a service. For example, if a

hospital and a group of physicians from a corporation provide health care at a fixed price, a risk-sharing arrangement would entail both the hospital and the group being held liable if expenses exceed revenues. *See also* risk; share.

ritual   A detailed method of procedure faithfully or regularly followed; a behavior that has a cultural origin in an organization, a society, or other group. *See also* circumcision.

ritual abuse   *See* child abuse.

RJS   *See* Ruth Jackson Orthopaedic Society.

RMAAMT   *See* Registered Medical Assistants of American Medical Technologists.

RN   *See* registered nurse.

RNA   *See* ribonucleic acid.

Robert Wood Johnson Foundation, The   *See* The Robert Wood Foundation.

Robert W Woodruff Foundation, Inc   An independent foundation established in 1937. Its fields of interest include expansion and improvement of medical, nursing, and educational facilities, youth programs and child welfare, care of the aged, and cultural and civic affairs. It donates money primarily in Atlanta, Georgia. *See also* foundation; private foundation.

robot   Computerized machine that can be programmed to perform certain tasks.

robotics   The science of robots. *See also* cybernetics; medical cybernetics.

rock the boat   To upset the status quo. An individual or group that rocks the boat challenges the customary sequence of procedures or events.

roentgen (R)   A unit of radiation exposure equal to the quantity of ionizing radiation that will produce one electrostatic unit of electricity in $1cm^3$ of dry air at 0° C and standard atmospheric pressure. *See also* rad.

roentgenogram   A photograph made with x-rays. *Synonym*: roentgenograph. *See also* mammogram; radiograph; x-ray.

roentgenograph   *See* roentgenogram.

roentgenography   Photography with the use of x-rays. *See also* radiography.

roentgenology   Radiology using x-rays. *See also* radiology.

roentgenoscope   *See* fluoroscope.

roentgenotherapy   The treatment of disease with x-rays. See also x-ray.

roentgen ray   *See* x-ray.

Roentgen Ray Society, American   *See* American Roentgen Ray Society.

Roentgen, Wilhelm Konrad   German physicist (1845-1923) who discovered x-rays (roentgen rays) in 1895 and developed x-ray photography, revolutionizing medical diagnosis.

role playing   A technique designed to reduce the conflict inherent in various social situations, in which participants act out particular behavioral roles in order to achieve a better understanding of a situation by experiencing a realistic simulation. It is useful in therapeutics (psychology) and as a training exercise. *See also* psychology.

rollout   The inauguration or initial public exhibition of a new service, policy, or product.

ROM   *See* range of motion; read-only memory.

room accommodations   The types of rooms provided for patient care in a health care organization, for example, private room, semiprivate room, ward. *See also* private room.

room, birthing   *See* birthing room.

rooming-in   A method of organizing obstetric services in which mothers share accommodations with and assume the care of newborn infants with help as needed from nursing personnel. *See also* obstetrics.

room, labor   *See* labor room.

room, operating   *See* operating room.

room, postoperative recovery   *See* recovery room.

room, private   *See* private room.

room, quiet   *See* quiet room.

room, recovery   *See* recovery room.

room, semiprivate   *See* semiprivate room.

room, scrub   *See* scrub room.

root cause   The original cause for not meeting the requirements of a process. *See also* cause.

Rorschach test   A psychodiagnostic method devised by the Swiss psychiatrist Hermann Rorschach (1884-1922). A subject is shown a series of 10 cards, each of which bears a bilaterally symmetrical inkblot, five of which are in black and white, three in black and red, and two multicolored. The subject is invited to interpret what he or she sees on each card, and the responses are recorded. The test is said to aid in assessment of personality, intellect, and emotion and to assist the differential diagnosis of psychiatric disorders. Objective validation of these claims has been disappointing. *Synonym*: inkblot test. *See also* psychiatry; test; validation.

rosacea   A chronic disorder of the skin of the nose, cheeks, and forehead marked by persistent capillary dilatation causing reddening of the skin, and papule and pustule formation. In some longstanding cases, rhinophyma may result. *See also* capillary; dermatology; rhinophyma.

roseola   An infection of infancy presumed to be due to an as yet unidentified virus. It is marked by fever for 3 to 4 days, followed by appearance of a rose-colored rash. Recovery is uneventful. *See also* infection; infectious diseases; rash; virus.

rotor-wing   *See* ambulance.

round file   Wastepaper basket. *Synonym*: circular file.

rounds   Visits by a physician or other health professional, or a group of health professionals, to the bedsides of patients in a hospital or other health care organization. The purpose of rounds is to evaluate treatment, analyze and document progress, and determine whether current care should be continued or changed. *See also* grand rounds; teaching rounds.

rounds, grand   *See* grand rounds.

rounds, teaching   *See* teaching rounds.

rounds, ward   *See* teaching rounds.

routine inquiry law   *See* required request law.

routine services   **1.** Services that do not require specialized equipment, knowledge, or human resources, and which are inpatient services provided to most patients. **2.** Outpatient services which usually are included in an office visit or limited examination.

Royal College of Physicians and Surgeons (of the United States of America) (RCPS)   An organization founded in 1987 composed of physicians and allied health professionals interested in tropical medicine. It provides postgraduate continuing medical education, and confers certificates and diplomas. *See also* tropical medicine.

Royal Society of Medicine Foundation (RSMF)   An organization founded in 1967 composed of 3,500 physicians. It serves as a forum for the discussion of topics relevant to the medical community in the United States and the United Kingdom. It sponsors conferences and exchange programs in conjunction with the Royal Society of Medicine.

RPA   *See* Renal Physicians Association.

RPS   *See* Retired Persons Services.

RRA   *See* registered record administrator.

RRC   *See* Residency Review Committee.

RRCEM   *See* Residency Review Committee for Emergency Medicine.

RRS *See* Radiation Research Society.

RRT *See* registered respiratory therapist.

RS *See* Rephael Society.

RSA *See* Research Society on Alcoholism.

RSMA *See* Radiological Systems Microfilm Associates.

RSMF *See* Royal Society of Medicine Foundation.

RSNA *See* Radiological Society of North America.

RT *See* respiratory therapy.

RTOG *See* Radiation Therapy Oncology Group.

RTS Acronym for revised trauma score. *See* trauma score.

RU-486 Mifepristone, an abortifacient antiprogestin drug used clinically in the United Kingdom and France for pregnancy interruption (nonsurgical abortion) early in the first trimester. Because it is an abortifacient, not a contraceptive, it has been the object of intense political opposition by pro-life forces in the United States. *See also* abortion; abortifacient; induced abortion; pro-life.

rubella A common and mild virus infection affecting principally children and young adults. One attack usually confers lifelong immunity. It is characterized by a slight fever, inflammation of lymph nodes, and a pink spotted rash on the face, trunk, and extremities, in that order. The major importance of rubella lies in the consequences, including congenital heart disease, brain damage, eye cataracts, and deafness, it produces in the fetus when a mother becomes infected during the first three or four months of pregnancy. Active immunization with live attenuated (weakened) virus is effective. *Synonym:* German measles. *See also* infectious diseases; teratogen; teratology; vaccinate.

rule **1.** Prescribed guide for action or conduct, regulation or principle. *See also* principle. **2.** In the executive branch of the federal government, a statement of general or particular applicability and future effect designed to implement, interpret, or prescribe law or policy, or describing the organization, procedure, or practice requirements of an agency. Commonly also called a regulation. Rules are published in the *Federal Register*. A rule, once adopted in accordance with the procedures specified in the Administration Procedure Act, has the force of law. *See also Federal Register*; regulation.

rule, discovery *See* discovery rule.

rule, locality *See* locality rule.

rule, national standard *See* national standard rule.

Rules of Professional Conduct, Model *See* Model Rules of Professional Conduct.

rule of reason In antitrust law, the principle that the law is to be applied only to "unreasonable" restraints of trade. *See also* antitrust laws; monopoly; restraint of trade.

rules and regulations In health care organizations, official statements authorized by the governing body of a health care organization as to the conduct of the organization's affairs in specified areas. *See also* regulation; rule.

rule of thumb A useful principle having wide application but not intended to be strictly accurate or reliable in every situation. *See also* principle.

run A pattern in data on a run chart or control chart in which a number of points occur on only one side of the center line, when a certain number of consecutive points occur in either ascending or descending order, or when the pattern becomes predictable (such as alternative points above and below the center line). Such data runs can help differentiate between special and common-cause variation. *See also* common-cause variation; control chart; data; data pattern; run chart; special-cause variation.

run chart A display of data in which data points are plotted as they occur over time (for example, observed weights plotted over time) to detect trends or other patterns and variation occurring over time. Run charts, as opposed to tabular frequency displays, are capable of time-ordering analytic studies. *Synonym:* time plot. *See also* chart; run.

runner *See* ambulance chaser.

rupture *See* hernia.

rural Pertaining to areas outside larger and moderate-sized cities and surrounding population concentrations, generally characterized by farms, ranches, small towns, and unpopulated regions. *See also* suburban; urban.

Rural Aging, National Center on *See* National Center on Rural Aging.

Rural Health Association, National *See* National Rural Health Association.

Rural Hospital Association, American Small and *See* National Rural Health Association.

Rural Hospitals, General Constituency Section for Small or *See* General Constituency Section for Small or Rural Hospitals.

Rural Mental Health, National Association for *See* National Association for Rural Mental Health.

rurban Areas on the fringe of urban development that are in the process of being developed for urban uses. *Compare* rural; suburban; urban.

Ruth Jackson Orthopaedic Society (RJS) An organization founded in 1983 composed of 189 women orthopedic surgeons seeking to advance the science of orthopedic surgery and provide support for women orthopedic surgeons. Named after Dr Ruth Jackson (b. 1902), the first woman certified by the American Board of Orthopedic Surgery and the first female member of the American Academy of Orthopedic Surgeons. Formerly (1991) Ruth Jackson Society. *See also* orthopaedic/orthopedic surgery.

RVS *See* relative value scale.

RVU *See* relative value unit.

Rx Abbreviation for *recipe*, meaning "take," as in a prescription for medication. *See also* prescription.

SA *See* surgeon assistant.

SAAC *See* Society for the Advancement of Ambulatory Care.

Sabin vaccine An oral vaccine consisting of live attenuated (weakened) polio viruses, used to immunize individuals against poliomyelitis. Named after Albert Bruce Sabin, an American physician and bacteriologist. *Synonyms*: oral poliovirus vaccine; trivalent live oral poliomyelitis vaccine. *See also* poliomyelitis; Salk vaccine; vaccine; virus.

sabotage A direct interference with or destruction of productive capabilities of an organization by those opposed to an organization's management or to a country in time of warfare. Disgruntled employees have become an important source of saboteurs in recent years. *See also* employee; management; organization.

saccharin A white crystalline non-nutritive powder having a taste about 550 times sweeter than ordinary sugar. It is used as a calorie-free sweetener. *See also* sugar-free.

sacred Worthy of religious veneration. *See also* religion; religious; sanctity of life; taboo.

sacred cow A person or an object that is immune from criticism, often unreasonably so. *See also* sacred.

sacred disease *See* epilepsy.

sacrifice **1.** Forfeiture of something highly valued for the sake of something else considered to have a greater value or claim, as in personal sacrifice for one's family. **2.** To kill an experimental animal.

SAD *See* seasonal affective disorder.

sadism **1.** Delight in cruelty. **2.** The act or an instance of deriving sexual gratification from inflicting pain on other persons. Named after Marquis de Sade (1740-1814). *See also* masochism; sadistic per-

sonality disorder; sadomasochism.

sadistic personality disorder A personality disorder characterized by a pervasive pattern of cruel, demeaning, and aggressive behavior. Satisfaction is gained in intimidating, coercing, and humiliating other persons. There is social intolerance, broad-ranging authoritarianism, and fascination with violence. *See also* personality disorder; sadism.

sadomasochism (S & M) Deriving pleasure from simultaneous sadism and masochism. *See also* masochism; sadism.

SAEM *See* Society for Academic Emergency Medicine.

safe Secure from danger, harm, or evil, as in a safe patient care environment.

safeguard A precautionary measure that serves as a protection or guard.

safe harbor regulations Regulations that describe certain acts or behaviors that are not illegal under a specific law, even though they might otherwise be illegal. In health care, this has been applied to certain joint ventures and other arrangements between hospitals and physicians or among physicians, meaning that these activities would not violate Medicare fraud and abuse laws. *See also* fraud and abuse; joint venture; Medicare; regulation.

Safe Medical Devices Act of 1990 A federal law that imposes reporting requirements on the users and manufacturers of medical devices. The Food and Drug Administration requires medical device manufacturers, distributors, and device user facilities (such as hospitals) to report deaths, serious illnesses, and serious injuries that have been or may have been caused by medical devices. *See also* device; malfunction; medical device.

safe period The period of the menstrual cycle during which conception is least likely to occur, usually taken as the 10 days preceding menstruation and the seven days following. Sexual intercourse is avoided during the time before and after ovulation. *Synonym:* rhythm method of contraception. *See also* conception; contraception; menses; period; sexual intercourse.

safe sex   Sexual activity in which precautions are taken to reduce the risk of spreading sexually transmitted diseases, especially AIDS. This usually involves avoidance of promiscuity, abstinence from orogenital and rectal sex, and the use of condoms. *Synonym:* safer sex. *See also* acquired immunodeficiency syndrome; casual sex; sex; sexually transmitted disease.

safer sex   *See* safe sex.

safety   **1.** Freedom from danger, risk, or injury. **2.** In health care, a performance dimension addressing the degree to which the risk of an intervention (for example, use of a drug or a procedure) and risk in the care environment are reduced for a patient and other persons, including health care practitioners. *See also* risk; security.

Safety Association, Exer-   *See* Exer-Safety Association.

Safety Commission, Consumer Product   *See* Consumer Product Safety Commission.

Safety Engineers, American Society of   *See* American Society of Safety Engineers.

Safety and Health Act of 1970, Occupational   *See* Occupational Safety and Health Act of 1980.

Safety and Health Administration, Occupational   *See* Occupational Safety and Health Administration.

Safety and Health, National Institute for Occupational   *See* National Institute for Occupational Safety and Health.

Safety and Health Review Commission, Occupational   *See* Occupational Safety and Health Review Commission.

safety and health standard, occupational   *See* occupational safety and health standard.

safety management   In health care organizations, management of general safety, safety education, emergency preparedness, hazardous material and wastes, and safety devices and operational practices. *See also* emergency preparedness plan/program; hazardous materials; hazardous waste; management; safety.

safety management, plant, technology, and   *See*

plant, technology, and safety management.

safety management program, life   *See* life safety management program.

Safety Management Society, National   *See* National Safety Management Society.

Safety, National Council   *See* National Safety Council.

Safety Professionals, Board of Certified   *See* Board of Certified Safety Professionals.

safety standard, occupational   *See* occupational safety and health standard.

SAFP   *See* Society of Air Force Physicians.

SAGES   *See* Society American Gastrointestinal Endoscopic Surgeons.

salaried physician   A physician who is employed as a physician by a hospital or other health care organization on a salaried basis. *See also* physician; salary; teaching physician.

salary   A form of earnings that is usually expressed in monthly or annual terms, as in a nurse's salary. *See also* base salary; wage.

salary, base   *See* base salary.

Sales Trainers, National Society of Pharmaceutical   *See* National Society of Pharmaceutical Sales Trainers.

saline   A solution of salt (sodium chloride, NaCl). Saline containing 0.9 grams NaCl per 100 milliliters has the same electrolyte strength as blood and is referred to as normal, physiological, isotonic saline. *See also* physiological saline; Ringer's solution; tears.

saline, physiological   *See* physiological saline.

saliva   A fluid secreted by the parotid, submaxillary, and sublingual salivary glands that assists chewing by moistening the mouth. The saliva also contains an enzyme that initiates the process of digestion by hydrolyzing starch. *See also* digestion; salivary glands.

salivary glands   Specialized paired structures, including the parotid, submaxillary, and sublingual glands, that secrete saliva. *See also* saliva.

Salk vaccine   A vaccine administered by injection, consisting of inactivated polioviruses, used to immunize against poliomyelitis in individuals with deficient immune systems and in unvaccinated adults. Named after Jonas Edward Salk, an American microbiologist who developed the first effective killed-virus vaccine against polio in 1954. *See also* poliomyelitis; Sabin vaccine; vaccine.

salve   *See* ointment.

SAM *See* Society for Adolescent Medicine; Society for Advancement of Management.

Samaritan, Good *See* Good Samaritan.

Samaritan laws, Good *See* Good Samaritan laws.

same-day surgery *See* ambulatory surgery.

sample A group of items chosen from a population. In statistics, a sample is a limited number of measurements taken from a larger source (the population or universe) used to estimate the characteristics of the population or universe. *See also* consecutive sample; convenience sample; population; random sample; sampling.

sample, consecutive *See* consecutive sample.

sample, convenience *See* convenience sample.

sample, random *See* random sample.

sample, representative *See* representative sample.

sample, sequential *See* consecutive sample.

sampling A basic statistical tool consisting of drawing a limited number of measurements from a larger source (population) and then analyzing those measurements to estimate characteristics of the population from which the measurements have been drawn. *See also* non-probability sampling; random sampling; simple random sampling; stratified random sampling; systematic sampling.

sampling error The unavoidable potential for error whenever a random sample is used rather than a whole population, due to the smaller size of the sample.

sampling, non-probability *See* non-probability sampling.

sampling, random *See* random sampling.

sampling, simple random *See* simple random sampling.

sampling statistics The science of inferring the characteristics of a population from a sample. *See also* inference; sample; sampling; statistics.

sampling, stratified random *See* stratified random sampling.

sampling, systematic *See* systematic sampling.

sanatorium An institution for the treatment of chronic diseases or for medically supervised recuperation, as in a tuberculosis sanatorium. *See also* sanitarium.

sanction **1.** An authoritative permission or approval that makes a course of action valid. *See also* approved. **2.** A penalty, specified or in the form of moral pressure, that acts to ensure compliance or conformity, as in economic sanctions. *See also* economic sanctions.

sanctions, economic *See* economic sanctions.

sanctity of life Considering life as sacred or holy. *See also* sacred.

sandfly *See Phlebotomus.*

sanitarian In public health, an individual who performs a wide spectrum of services, depending on his or her level of education and experience. A beginning sanitarian may perform inspections and investigations at food service establishments, food processing plants, and food distribution facilities to determine compliance with environmental health laws and regulations. He or she also may inspect schools, motels, and recreation areas, checking food protection, water supply, waste disposal, lighting conditions, ventilation, fire safety, cleanliness, and animal or insect vectors of disease, such as mosquitoes and rats. He or she may inspect operational aspects of swimming pools, small untreated water supplies (wells), and sewage disposal facilities. A beginning sanitarian in a specialized program may participate in the inspection of larger facilities or systems, such as air pollution sources, water supply systems and plants, industrial and domestic waste treatment systems, and solid and hazardous waste management systems. In the upper levels, sanitarians may deal with the inspection of nursing homes and other facilities that are subject to complex state and federal regulations and standards and may be responsible for all of the environmental programs in a district, or be responsible for one program, such as milk sanitation. *Synonyms:* environmental health practitioner; environmental health specialist. *See also* industrial hygienist; sanitarian aide.

sanitarian aide An individual who, under the direct supervision of a sanitarian, performs routine inspections of facilities, runs tests on consumer products, and reports violations of environmental laws or regulations. *See also* aide; sanitarian.

Sanitarians, American Academy of *See* American Academy of Sanitarians.

Sanitarians, National Society of Professional *See* National Society of Professional Sanitarians.

sanitarium An institution for the promotion of health. The word was originally coined to designate the institution established by the Seventh-Day Adventists at Battle Creek, Michigan, to distinguish it from institutions providing care for mental or tuberculous patients. *See also* health promotion;

sanatorium.

sanitary Free from elements, such as filth or pathogens, that endanger health. *See also* hygiene.

sanitary engineer An engineer specializing in the maintenance of urban environmental conditions conducive to the preservation of public health. *See also* engineer; engineering; public health; sanitary.

Sanitary Engineering, American Society of *See* American Society of Sanitary Engineering.

Sanitary Engineers, American Academy of *See* American Academy of Environmental Engineers.

sanitation Formulation and application of measures designed to protect public health, particularly with respect to the provision of toilet facilities, drainage, and the disposal of sewage. *See also* public health; sanitarian; sanitary.

Sanitation Foundation, National *See* National Sanitation Foundation.

sanitation worker An individual employed to remove rubbish. *See also* sanitation; sanitary.

sanitorium *See* sanatorium.

sanity The quality or condition of being of sound mind. *Compare* insanity. *See also* mind.

sapphism *See* lesbianism.

sarcasm A cutting remark, intended to hurt.

sarcoma A malignant tumor arising from connective tissue, bone, muscle, and other tissues. Sarcomas are much less common than carcinomas (which arise from epithelial tissue) but are often highly malignant. *See also* Kaposi's sarcoma.

sarcoma, Kaposi's *See* Kaposi's sarcoma.

SART *See* Society for Assisted Reproductive Technology.

SASP *See* Society for the Advancement of Social Psychology.

satellite **1.** An associated or subsidiary enterprise, as in satellite hospital. *See also* satellite hospital. **2.** An object launched to orbit Earth or another celestial body. *See also* satellite communications.

satellite communications Use of orbital satellites to send voice, data, video, and graphics from one location to another; for example, teleconferencing and television programs for continuing medical education and education for patients. *See also* communication; satellite.

satellite hospital Part of a hospital that is geographically separated from the hospital and that offers limited services to persons in its geographical area. *See also* hospital; satellite.

satellite pharmacy *See* decentralized pharmaceutical services

satisfaction The fulfillment or gratification of a desire, a need, or an appetite, as in patient satisfaction survey. *See also* job satisfaction.

satisfaction, job *See* job satisfaction.

saturated fat A fat, usually of animal origin, whose fatty acid chains cannot incorporate additional hydrogen atoms. An excess of these fats in the diet is thought to raise the blood cholesterol level. *See also* cholesterol; fat; hydrogenation.

saturation In marketing insurance or health maintenance organizations, the point at which further penetration of a market is improbable or too costly. *See also* market; penetration.

Saturday night special A cheap handgun easily obtained and concealed.

saturnism Lead poisoning. *See also* lead; poison.

Say's Law A nineteenth century (classical) proposition in economics that supply creates its own demand, that whatever quantity is supplied will also be demanded. It is named after the nineteenth century French economist, JB Say. *See also* law of supply and demand; supply.

SBBT *See* specialist in blood bank technology.

SBET *See* Society of Biomedical Equipment Technicians.

SBM *See* Society of Behavioral Medicine.

SBP *See* Society for Behavioral Pediatrics.

SC *See* Society for Cryobiology.

SCA *See* Society of Cardiovascular Anesthesiologists.

scabies Infestation of the skin with the contagious itch mite, *Acarus scabiei*, also known as *Sarcoptes scabiei*. *See also* parasite.

SCA&I *See* Society for Cardiac Angiography and Interventions.

scale A system of ordered marks at fixed intervals representing predetermined units, used as a reference standard in measurement. *See also* abbreviated injury scale; Apgar scale; Celsius scale; centigrade scale; dichotomous scale; Fahrenheit scale; Glasgow coma scale; interval scale; Kelvin scale; nominal scale; nonlinear scale; ordinal scale; ratio scale; ranking scale; relative-value scale; resource-based relative-value scale; sliding scale.

scale, abbreviated injury *See* abbreviated injury scale.

scale, Apgar *See* Apgar scale.

scale, Celsius *See* Celsius scale.

scale, centigrade   *See* centigrade scale.

scale, dichotomous   *See* dichotomous scale.

scale, economies of   *See* economies of scale.

scale, Fahrenheit   *See* Fahrenheit scale.

scale, Glasgow coma   *See* Glasgow coma scale.

scale, interval   *See* interval scale.

scale, Kelvin   *See* Kelvin scale.

scale, measurement   *See* scale.

scale, nominal   *See* nominal scale.

scale, nonlinear   *See* nonlinear scale.

scale, ordinal   *See* ordinal scale.

scale, ranking   *See* ranking scale.

scale, ratio   *See* ratio scale.

scale relationship   Comparison by use of a given scale. *See also* scale.

scale, relative value   *See* relative value scale.

scale, resource-based relative-value   *See* resource-based relative-value scale.

scale, sliding   *See* sliding scale.

scalpel   A small knife with a straight handle and a thin, sharp blade used in surgery and dissection. *See also* dissect; surgery.

scan   **1.** In medicine, to examine a body or a body part with a scanning apparatus, such as a computerized axial tomography scanner. **2.** The record produced by a scanner, such as a CAT scanner. *See also* brain scan; CAT scan; PET scan.

scan, brain   *See* brain scan.

scan, CAT   *See* CAT scan.

scanner   **1.** An instrument that makes pictorial records of particular events by measuring different areas in turn and producing an integrated picture of variations over a part of the body or an organ; for example, a CAT scanner. *See also* CAT scanner; PET scanner. **2.** A device that can read or scan typed characters from paper copy and automatically transfer this information onto something else. *See also* machine readable.

scanner, CAT   *See* CAT scanner.

scanner, PET   *See* PET scanner.

scan, PET   *See* PET scan.

scar   A mark composed of new fibrous tissue that remains after the healing of a wound or other injury. *See also* keloid.

scarcity   Insufficiency of amount or supply, as in a scarcity of resources. *See also* scarcity area.

scarcity area   In health care, an area lacking an adequate supply of a particular type of health professional(s) or health service(s). *See also* medically underserved area.

SCASA   *See* Straight Chiropractic Academic Standards Association.

scatter   **1.** To cause to separate and go in different directions. *See also* scatter diagram. **2.** The diffusion or deviation of x-rays produced by a medium through which the rays pass. *See also* radiology; x-ray.

scatter diagram   A graphic representation of data depicting the possible relationship between two variables. A scatter diagram displays what happens to one variable when another variable changes in order to test a theory that the two variables are related. A scatter diagram cannot prove that one variable causes the other, but it does make clear whether a relationship exists and the strength of that relationship (positive, negative, zero). *Synonyms*: scattergram; scatterplot. *See also* confounding variable; diagram; variable.

scattergram   *See* scatter diagram.

scatterplot   *See* scatter diagram.

SCCM   *See* Society of Critical Care Medicine.

ScD   *See* Doctor of Science.

SCEH   *See* Society for Clinical and Experimental Hypnosis.

scenario building   A method of predicting the future that relies on a series of assumptions about alternative possibilities, rather than on simple extrapolation of existing trends, as in forecasting. *See also* forecasting.

schedule   **1.** A plan for performing work or achieving an objective. *See also* scheduling. **2.** A list of items in tabular form, as in a schedule of controlled substances. *See also* schedule of controlled substances.

schedule of controlled substances   A classification of five schedules of drugs based on their potential for abuse; established by the Controlled Substances Act of 1970 for the purpose of controlling the possession and use of certain drugs. *See also* controlled substances; drug abuse; schedule I substances; schedule II substances; schedule III substances; schedule IV substances; schedule V substances.

schedule I substances   Controlled substances that come under jurisdiction of the Controlled Substances Act, have no accepted medical use in the United States, and have a high abuse potential. Some examples are heroin, marijuana, LSD, peyote, mescaline, psilocybin, dihydromorphine, nicocodeine, nicomorphine, and methaqualone. *See also* controlled substances; Controlled Substances Act of 1970.

schedule II substances Controlled substances that come under jurisdiction of the Controlled Substances Act because they have a high abuse potential with severe psychic or physical dependence liability. Schedule II controlled substances consist of certain narcotic, stimulant, and depressant drugs. Some examples of Schedule II narcotic controlled substances are: opium, morphine, codeine, diphenoxylate, hydromorphone (Dilaudid), methadone (Dolophine), pantopon, meperidine (Demerol), cocaine, oxycodone (Percodan), anileridine (Leritine), and oxymorphone (Numorphan). Schedule II nonnarcotic drugs are amphetamine (Dexedrine) and methamphetamine (Desoxyn), phenmetrazine (Preludin), methylphenidate (Ritalin), amobarbital, pentobarbital, secobarbital, etorphine hydrochloride, phencyclidine, and glutethimide (Doriden). *See also* barbiturate; controlled substances; Controlled Substances Act of 1970.

schedule III substances Controlled substances that come under the jurisdiction of the Controlled Substances Act because of their abuse potential, which is less than the schedule I and schedule II substances. It includes compounds containing limited quantities of certain narcotic drugs, such as paregoric, and nonnarcotic drugs, such as derivatives of barbituric acid, except those that are listed in another schedule, mehyprylon (Noludar), chlorhexadol, nolorphine, benzphetamine, chlorphentermine, clortermine, mazindol, phendimetrazine, and anabolic steroids. *See also* anabolic steroids; controlled substances; Controlled Substances Act of 1970.

schedule IV substances Controlled substances that come under the jurisdiction of the Controlled Substances Act because of their abuse potential, which is less than those substances listed in schedule III. This group of drugs includes barbital, phenobarbital, methylphenobarbital, chloral betaine (Beta Chlor), chloral hydrate, ethchlorvynol (Placidyl), ethinamate (Valmid), meprobamate (Equanil, Miltown), paraldehyde, methohexital, fenfluramine, diethypropion, phentermine, chlordiazepoxide (Librium), diazepam (Valium), oxazepam (Serax), clorazepate (Tranxene), flurazepam (Dalmane), clonazepam (Clonopin), prazepam (Verstran), lorazepam (Ativan), mebutamate, and dextropropoxyphene (Darvon). *See also* controlled sub-

stances; Controlled Substances Act of 1970.

schedule V substances Controlled substances that come under the jurisdiction of the Controlled Substances Act because of their abuse potential, which is less than those listed in schedule IV. This group of substances consists of preparations containing limited quantities of certain narcotic drugs, generally for antitussive and antidiarrheal purposes. *See also* antidiarrheal; antitussive; controlled substances; Controlled Substances Act of 1970; cough; diarrhea; expectorant.

scheduling Devising a timetable of events to decide when, and possibly where, certain events shall occur, as in a scheduling department. *See also* schedule.

schema **1.** A diagrammatic representation. **2.** The overall organization of a database.

schematic box plot A seven-number summary of data. The median and quantiles have the same definitions as in a basic box plot. The whiskers, however, are drawn to the adjacent values. Outlier points are indicated by asterisks lying beyond the adjacent values. *See also* adjacent value, lower; adjacent value; upper; box plot; quantile.

schizoid Pertaining to a personality charactered by extreme shyness, seclusiveness, and an inability to form close relationships. *See also* schizophrenia.

schizophrenia Any of a group of psychotic disorders that may have a genetic cause, usually characterized by withdrawal from reality, illogical patterns of thinking, delusions, and hallucinations. Schizophrenia may be accompanied in varying degrees by other emotional, behavioral, or intellectual disturbances. *See also* magical thinking; paranoia; psychosis; schizophrenic.

schizophrenic **1.** Affected with or relating to schizophrenia, as in auditory hallucinations as a schizophrenic symptom. **2.** A person who is affected with schizophrenia. *See also* schizophrenia.

schmoose *See* schmooze.

schmooze To talk casually, as in the president schmoozed with the legislators. *Synonym:* schmoose.

school **1.** An institution for instruction. **2.** A group of people whose thought, work, or style demonstrate a common origin, influence, or unifying belief. *See also* culture.

school adjustment counselor *See* school social worker.

school, dental *See* dental school.

school, diploma *See* diploma school.

school health In-school program designed to protect and promote the health of students and school personnel.

School Health Association, American *See* American School Health Association.

school, medical *See* medical school.

school nurse A nurse employed at a school who specializes in promotion of the physical, dental, and mental health of children and young adults. In some states, school nurses must meet certain criteria determined by the State Board of Education, including being certified. *See also* certified nurse; registered nurse.

School Nurses, National Association of *See* National Association of School Nurses.

school of hard knocks The practical experiences of life, including hardships and disappointments, that serve to educate and temper an individual.

school psychologist A psychologist who specializes in the field of school psychology. *See also* school psychology.

School Psychologists, National Association of *See* National Association of School Psychologists.

school psychology The branch of psychology dealing with principles and techniques to help teachers understand and work more effectively with the children in their classes and to with children and their parents to help them make better adjustments to school and life. School psychologists often function as clinical psychologists in an educational setting. *See also* educational psychology; psychology.

Schools, Accrediting Bureau of Health Education *See* Accrediting Bureau of Health Education Schools.

Schools, American Association of Dental *See* American Association of Dental Schools.

Schools, Association of Minority Health Professions *See* Association of Minority Health Professions Schools.

Schools and Colleges of Acupuncture and Oriental Medicine, National Accreditation Commission for *See* National Accreditation Commission for Schools and Colleges of Acupuncture and Oriental Medicine.

Schools and Colleges, National Council of Acupuncture *See* National Council of Acupuncture Schools and Colleges.

Schools and Colleges of Optometry, Association of *See* Association of Schools and Colleges of Optometry.

Schools, Council on Accreditation of Nurse Anesthesia Educational Programs/ *See* Council on Accreditation of Nurse Anesthesia Educational Programs/Schools.

Schools, National Association of Health Career *See* National Association of Health Career Schools.

Schools of Nursing, Assembly of Hospital *See* Institute for Hospital Clinical Nursing Education.

school social worker A social worker with knowledge and skills in casework methods acquired through degrees of school social work, who aids children when they are having difficulties adapting to school life. For instance, school social workers may assist with vocational counseling or serve as a liaison between a school and community resources, such as family service agencies, child guidance clinics, protective services, physicians, and ministers. *Synonyms:* home and school visitor; school adjustment counselor; visiting teacher. *See also* school; social worker.

Schools of Public Health, Association of *See* Association of Schools of Public Health.

school, vocational *See* vocational school.

SCIA *See* Smart Card Industry Association.

sciatica Pain along the pathway of the sciatic nerve, that is, radiating from the buttock down the back and outside of the thigh and lower leg. *See also* pain.

science 1. The observation, identification, description, experimental investigation, and theoretical explanation of phenomena. *See also* scientist. **2.** The body of knowledge accumulated by such means, as in biological science or medical science. *See also* scientific method.

Science, Academy of Pharmaceutical Research and *See* Academy of Pharmaceutical Research and Science.

science, actuarial *See* actuarial science.

Science, American Association for the Advancement of *See* American Association for the Advancement of Science.

Science, American Association for Laboratory Animal *See* American Association for Laboratory Animal Science.

Science, American Society for Information *See* American Society for Information Science.

science, behavioral *See* behavioral science.

Science, Christian *See* Christian Science.

science, cognitive *See* cognitive science.

Science and Health, American Council on *See*

American Council on Science and Health.

science, information *See* information science.

Science, Joint Commission on Sports Medicine and *See* Joint Commission on Sports Medicine and Science.

science, management *See* management science.

science, materials *See* materials science.

Science and Medicine, Institute for Advanced Research in Asian *See* Institute for Advanced Research in Asian Science and Medicine.

science, neuro- *See* neuroscience.

science, physical *See* physical science.

science, political *See* political science.

Science and Protection, National Accreditation Council for Environmental Health *See* National Accreditation Council for Environmental Health Science and Protection.

Science in the Public Interest, Center for *See* Center for Science in the Public Interest.

Sciences, American Academy of Forensic *See* American Academy of Forensic Sciences.

Sciences, American Institute of Biological *See* American Institute of Biological Sciences.

Sciences, American Institutes for Research in the Behavioral *See* American Institutes for Research in the Behavioral Sciences.

Sciences, Association for Chemoreception *See* Association for Chemoreception Sciences.

Sciences, Association for Politics and the Life *See* Association for Politics and the Life Sciences.

Sciences Communications Association, Health *See* Health Sciences Communications Association.

Sciences, Federation of Behavioral, Psychological and Cognitive *See* Federation of Behavioral, Psychological and Cognitive Sciences.

sciences, forensic *See* forensic sciences.

Sciences Library Directors, Association of Academic Health *See* Association of Academic Health Sciences Library Directors.

Sciences, National Academy of *See* National Academy of Sciences.

Sciences, National Accrediting Agency for Clinical Laboratory *See* National Accrediting Agency for Clinical Laboratory Sciences.

science, social *See* social science.

Science Society, Cognitive *See* Cognitive Science Society.

scientific Using the methodology of science. *See also* science; scientific method.

scientific empiricism The philosophical view that there are no ultimate differences among the various sciences. *See also* empirical; scientific.

scientific fact *See* fact.

Scientific Investigation of Claims of the Paranormal, Committee for the *See* Committee for the Scientific Investigation of Claims of the Paranormal.

scientific method The principles and empirical processes of discovery and demonstration considered characteristic of or necessary for scientific investigation, generally involving the observation of phenomena, the formulation of a hypothesis concerning the phenomena, experimentation to demonstrate the truth or falseness of the hypothesis, and a conclusion that validates or modifies the hypothesis. *See also* empirical; method; observation; science.

scientific parsimony *See* Ockham's razor.

scientism The theory that investigational methods used in the natural sciences should be applied in all fields of inquiry. *See also* science; scientific method.

scientist An individual having expert knowledge of one or more sciences, especially a natural or physical science. *See also* science.

Scientists, American Association of Pharmaceutical *See* American Association of Pharmaceutical Scientists.

Scientists, Association of Clinical *See* Association of Clinical Scientists.

Scientists and Technical Professionals, National Organization of Gay and Lesbian *See* National Organization of Gay and Lesbian Scientists and Technical Professionals.

Sclerotherapy, American Osteopathic Academy of *See* American Osteopathic Academy of Sclerotherapy.

SCME *See* Society of Clinical and Medical Electrologists.

scoliosis Abnormal lateral curvature of the spine. *Compare* kyphosis; lordosis. *See also* orthopaedic/orthopedic surgery.

Scoliosis Research Society (SRSO) A national organization founded in 1966 composed of 445 orthopedic surgeons and other physicians interested in furthering research and education in spinal deformities, particularly scoliosis. *See also* orthopaedic/orthopedic surgery; scoliosis.

scope of care/services An inventory of processes (number, type, intensity, complexity) that make up a specified function (such as trauma care) of a health care organization (such as a hospital), including activities performed by governance, managerial, clinical, and/or support personnel. *See also* patient mix.

scope of employment   Acts performed while doing one's job duties. The phrase was adopted by the courts for the purpose of determining an employer's liability for the acts of employees. The employer is said to be vicariously liable only for those torts of the employee that are committed within the range of his or her job duties. *See also* employment.

scope of work, PRO   *See* PRO scope of work.

score   A rating, usually expressed numerically, based on the degree to which certain qualities or attributes are present, as in Apgar score and Glasgow coma score. *See also* Apgar scale; Glasgow coma scale; injury severity score; trauma score.

score, injury severity   *See* injury severity score.

scorer reliability   *See* interobserver reliability.

score, trauma   *See* trauma score.

scoring guideline   Descriptive tool that is used to assist health care organizations in their efforts to comply with standards of the Joint Commission on Accreditation of Healthcare Organizations and to determine degrees of compliance. The Joint Commission publishes scoring guidelines to correspond with each accreditation manual. *See also* guideline; Joint Commission on Accreditation of Healthcare Organizations; key items, probes, and scoring guidelines.

screen   **1.** To examine methodically in order to make a separation into different groups. **2.** To select or eliminate by a screening device. *See also* screening. **3.** An instrument used to identify opportunities for improvement or problems in processes or outcomes. *Synonym:* indicator. *See also* HCFA generic quality screens; indicator; screening. **4.** A device used for visualizing x-ray images in radiology. **5.** The visual display portion of computer monitor. *See also* computer; monitor.

screening   The identification of unrecognized occurrences or states by the application of tests, examinations, or other procedures that can be rapidly and simply applied. A screening test is not intended to be diagnostic. Individuals, groups, organizations or events identified by a screening process must be further assessed to establish a diagnosis. *See also* audiometric screening; case finding; drug screening; HCFA generic quality screens; genetic screening; screening clinic; sensitivity of a test; speci-

ficity of a test.

screening, audiometric   *See* audiometric screening.

screening clinic   A clinic in which an initial assessment of patients seeking care is performed to determine what services are needed, with what priority and, sometimes, where treatment will be performed. *See also* screening; triage.

screening criteria, occurrence   *See* occurrence criteria.

screening, drug   *See* drug screening.

screening, genetic   *See* genetic screening.

screening, occurrence   *See* occurrence screening.

screening panel   In malpractice, a fact-finding body used in the early stages of a malpractice dispute. A defense panel seeks to develop the best possible defense for a health professional accused of malpractice. An exploratory panel examines the facts for both the accused professional and the plaintiff and makes its determination on the merits of the case. *See also* panel; screening.

screening test, predictive value of a   *See* predictive value of a screening test.

screen memory   A consciously tolerable memory serving as a screen for another memory that may be disturbing or emotionally painful if recalled. *See also* memory.

screens, generic   *See* HCFA quality generic screens.

screens, HCFA generic quality   *See* HCFA generic quality screens.

screens, occurrence   *See* occurrence criteria.

scrub   To prepare to engage in surgery, as in scrubbing the hands and forearms for surgery and putting on sterile gloves, masks, hats, and operating garments. *See also* scrub nurse; scrub room.

scrub nurse   An operating room nurse who assists in surgical operations. *See also* operating room nurse; scrub.

scrub room   An area where members of a surgical team wash and scrub their hands and forearms prior to surgical operations. *See also* scrub; scrub nurse.

SCT   *See* Society for Clinical Trials.

scuttlebutt   Gossip or rumor, as in the newest hospital scuttlebutt.

scut work   Disliked, usually trivial, chores that housestaff, such as interns working in hospitals, must often perform. *See also* housestaff.

SCVIR   *See* Society of Cardiovascular and Interventional Radiology.

SD   *See* standard deviation.

SDADA *See* Seventh-Day Adventist Dietetic Association.

SDB *See* Society for Developmental Biology.

SDMS *See* Society of Diagnostic Medical Sonographers.

SE *See* Society of Ethnobiology.

seal, corporate *See* corporate seal.

search firm *See* recruitment.

search firm, physician *See* physician search firm.

searching, on-line *See* on-line searching.

Search and Rescue, National Association for *See* National Association for Search and Rescue.

seasonal affective disorder (SAD) A mild form of depression occurring at certain seasons of the year, especially during winter. It is characterized by loss of energy and sexual drive, restlessness, and often a craving for carbohydrates. *See also* affective disorder; major affective disorder.

seat-of-the-pants Use of experience and intuition rather than a plan or method, as in seat-of-the-pants management style. *See also* intuition.

sebaceous cyst A swelling of the skin due to blockage of the duct of a sebaceous gland, causing swelling with an oily secretion. Sebaceous cysts are often on the scalp, neck, and forehead. *Synonym:* wen. *See also* cyst; sebaceous gland; sebum.

sebaceous gland A small gland found in the skin in relation to hair follicles, which secretes sebum. *See also* dermis; gland; hair; sebaceous cyst; rhinophyma; sebum; smegma.

SEBM *See* Society for Experimental Biology and Medicine.

sebum Yellow, greasy semisolid secretion of sebaceous glands. *See also* sebaceous cyst; sebaceous gland.

seclusion In health care, the involuntary confinement of a patient alone in a room, which the patient is physically prevented from leaving, for any period of time. Seclusion does not include involuntary confinement for legally mandated but nonclinical purposes, such as confining a person facing serious criminal charges or serving a criminal sentence to a locked room. *See also* quiet room; restraint.

secondary Derived from what is primary or original, as in secondary care.

secondary care Services provided by medical specialists (such as a general surgeon or a dermatologist) who generally do not have first contact with patients. In the United States, however, patients often self-refer to specialists providing secondary care or even tertiary care, rather than being referred by a primary care provider. *Synonym:* specialized care. *See also* primary care; referred care; tertiary care.

secondary contact A person in contact with a primary contact; a primary contact is a person in direct contact with a communicable disease case. *See also* contact; primary contact.

secondary data Data resulting from initial analysis of primary data. *See also* data; data source; operational data; primary data.

secondary diagnosis *See* other diagnosis.

secondary negligence *See* vicarious liability.

secondary payer, Medicare *See* Medicare secondary payer.

secondary smoking *See* involuntary smoking.

secondary standards The set of standards published by the Joint Commission on Accreditation of Healthcare Organizations, or the accreditation manual that represents the majority of standards, for services/programs that do not constitute the primary clinical focus of the health care organization being surveyed. *See also* Joint Commission on Accreditation of Healthcare Organizations; primary standards; standard.

second banana An assistant or deputy who is subordinate to another. *Synonym:* second fiddle.

second-class citizen A person considered inferior in status or rights in comparison with some other people. *See also* citizen.

second fiddle *See* second banana.

second generation type I recommendation The second opportunity a health care organization has to correct a deficiency noted during a survey by the Joint Commission on Accreditation of Healthcare Organizations, either through a written progress report or through a focused survey. *See also* first generation type I recommendation; Joint Commission on Accreditation of Healthcare Organizations; type I recommendation; written progress report.

second-guess To criticize or correct a decision after an outcome is known.

secondhand smoke *See* involuntary smoking.

second opinion A consultation involving the examination of a patient by a health care provider and the rendering of an opinion by that provider as to the need for surgery or other treatment recommended by the first provider. For example, a surgeon may recommend to a patient that he or she undergo a coronary artery bypass graft procedure. A second surgeon, after examining the patient and all pertinent data, may render a second opinion that either affirms or refutes the first surgeon's opinion. A second opinion encourages individuals to seek peer review of one physician's opinion by a second physician. *See also* opinion; peer review; physician; second-opinion program.

second-opinion program   A cost-containment and quality control method in which health insurers, prepayment organizations, or practitioners advise or require a patient to obtain a second opinion from another qualified provider before deciding to undergo a procedure or treatment. *See also* opinion; program; second opinion.

second-rate   Of inferior or mediocre quality or value, as in second-rate health care.

secrecy   Keeping hidden from knowledge or view; concealment.

Secretaries, National Association of Rehabilitation   *See* National Association of Rehabilitation Secretaries.

secretary   1. A person employed to handle correspondence, keep files, and perform clerical work for another person or an organization. *See also* clerk; medical secretary; receptionist. 2. An officer who is responsible for recording minutes at meetings, maintaining records, and handling correspondence for an organization.

secretary, medical   *See* medical secretary.

section   1. An act of cutting, as in cesarean section. *See also* cesarean section. 2. A segment or subdivision of a whole, such as Section for Metropolitan Hospitals, or a functional division of an organization.

section, cesarean   *See* cesarean section.

Section for Metropolitan Hospitals (SMH)   A national organization founded in 1984 composed of institutional members of the American Hospital Association who are located within a metropolitan statistical area and/or provide a significant proportion of Medicare, Medicaid, and uncompensated care; participate in undergraduate and/or graduate medical education programs and research; provide high volumes of ambulatory care; offer specialized services; and are involved in professional and paraprofessional education and training programs. *See also* metropolitan statistical area.

section, primary cesarean   *See* primary cesarean section.

Section for Rehabilitation Hospitals and Programs (SRHP)   An organization founded in 1984 that assists hospitals in helping disabled persons reach their optimal level of functioning. It monitors and attempts to influence national standards of medical rehabilitative care and pertinent state and federal legislation and regulations. *See also* physical medicine and rehabilitation; rehabilitation hospital.

sector   1. A part of the economy, as in private sector and public sector. *See also* third sector. 2. A division of a computer diskette.

Sector, National Association of Rehabilitation Professionals in the Private   *See* National Association of Rehabilitation Professionals in the Private Sector.

sector, third   *See* third sector.

secular   Not relating specifically to religion, as in secular humanism. *See also* secular humanism; secularism.

secular humanism   A view or outlook that advocates human rather than religious values. *See also* secular; secularism.

secularism   Skepticism or indifference toward religion; the view that religion should be excluded from civil affairs or public education. *See also* secular.

secure   Free from danger or risk of loss. *See also* safety; security.

security   Freedom from danger, injury, or risk. Security often implies feelings of confidence, as in job security or health care security. *See also* job security; safety; security department; security guard; Social Security.

Security Act, Employee Retirement Income   *See* Employee Retirement Income Security Act.

Security Act, Health   *See* Health Security Act.

Security Action Council, Health   *See* Health Security Action Council.

Security Act, Social   *See* Social Security Act.

Security Administration, Social   *See* Social Security Administration.

security department   The unit of a hospital or other health care organization that provides for the security and safety of patients, employees, medical staff, visitors, and their property while in the hospital or organization or on its grounds. *See also* security; security guard.

security guard   An individual hired by a private organization, such as a hospital, to guard a physical plant and maintain order. *See also* plant; security.

security hospital A hospital controlled by, physically located within, or attached to, and providing services to, inmates of a penal institution. *Synonym*: prison hospital. *See also* hospital; security.

security income, supplemental *See* supplemental security income.

security, job *See* job security.

Security, Social *See* Social Security.

sedative A drug having a soothing, calming, or tranquilizing effect. *See also* drug; hypnotic; thalidomide.

sedentary Characterized by much sitting; idle or inactive, as in a sedentary job or a sedentary existence in front of a television set. *Compare* exercise. *See also* obesity.

seduce **1.** To lead away from duty, principles, or proper conduct. **2.** To induce one to engage in sex.

seem To give the impression of being true, as in things are not always as they seem.

SEGH *See* Society for Environmental Geochemistry and Health.

seizure *See* convulsion.

seizure disorder *See* epilepsy.

seizure, heart *See* heart seizure.

selection The act or process of taking a choice from among several choices. *See also* adverse selection; artificial selection; natural selection; selection bias.

selection, adverse *See* adverse selection.

selection, artificial *See* artificial selection.

selection bias Apparent treatment effects due to comparing groups that differed even before the treatment was administered. *See also* bias.

selection, natural *See* natural selection.

selective referral The referral or attraction of patients to physicians and hospitals with better outcomes. *See also* referral.

self-care *See* self-help.

self-care unit *See* minimal care unit.

self-employed Earning one's livelihood directly from one's own business, trade, or profession rather than as an employee of another, as in a self-employed physician versus a salaried physician. *See also* employee; salaried physician.

self-fulfilling prophecy Causing something to happen by believing it will occur. *See also* prophecy.

self-governance The act or process of governing oneself, as in a hospital medical staff is self-governing, meaning that the governing body delegates to it

certain duties and responsibilities, such as those connected with patient assessment and treatment. *See also* governance; governing body; medical staff.

self-help Pertaining to helping or improving oneself without assistance from other persons, as in personal observation and reporting of symptoms and vital signs or providing first aid to oneself and one's family. *Synonym*: self-care.

self-inflicted Imposed or inflicted on oneself, as in a self-inflicted gunshot wound.

self-insurance Insurance of oneself or one's possessions against possible loss by regularly setting aside funds; assumption of risk of loss without an insurance policy. For example, a hospital may decide to self-insure by setting aside funds to protect itself against financial loss, rather than purchasing an insurance policy from an insurance company. *See also* appropriate self-insured health plan; insurance; self-insured hospital.

self-insured health plan, appropriate *See* appropriate self-insured health plan.

self-insured hospital A hospital that assumes the risk of loss without an insurance policy. *See also* hospital; insurance; self-insurance.

self-limited Pertaining to a disease or condition that tends to end or resolve without treatment.

self-pay patient A patient who pays out of personal resources for either all or part of his or her hospital and other health care provider bills, without the assistance of insurance or other third-party benefits. *Synonym*: self-responsible patient. *See also* patient; uncompensated care.

self-responsible patient *See* self-pay patient.

seller's market A market condition characterized by a supply of commodities falling short of demand. As a result, the prices tend to rise, and the sellers can set both the prices and the terms of sale. It contrasts with a buyer's market, characterized by excess supply, low prices, and terms suited to the buyer's desires. *Compare* buyer's market. *See also* market.

sell, soft *See* soft sell.

semantic Pertaining to meaning, especially meaning in language. *See also* semantics.

semantics The science or study of the relationship between meaning and language, as in the relationship between signs and symbols and what they represent. *See also* language.

semen A white secretion of the male reproductive organs, containing spermatozoa and serving as their transporting medium. *See also* artificial insemination; onanism; spermatozoa; testis.

semiconductor Any of various solid crystalline substances, such as silicon, having electrical conductivity greater than insulators but less than good conductors. Semiconductors are used in computer circuits and act as switches in the processing of data, performing the basic actions of modern computers. Semiconductors can be tailor-made to perform special functions, such as controlling a dishwasher's action. *See also* computer; silicon.

semiconscious Partly conscious. *See also* consciousness.

seminal Highly influential in an original or creative way, providing the basis for further development, as in a seminal idea.

seminoma A malignant neoplasm of the testis. *See also* malignancy; neoplasm; testis.

semiology The study of symptoms and signs. *See also* sign; symptom.

semiprivate room A hospital room with two to four beds. *See also* private room; room accommodations; ward.

semiquantitative Denoting a test that is more specific than a qualitative test (a test that is either positive or negative, for example) but less so than a quantitative test (a test with a numerical result), usually referring to a test in which results are scored on an arbitrary scale, for example 0, +, ++, +++, ++++. *See also* qualitative; quantitative; scale.

Semmelweis, Ignaz Philipp (1818-1865) A Hungarian physician who proved that puerperal fever is a form of septicemia (blood poisoning), thus becoming the pioneer of antisepsis in obstetrics. *See also* antisepsis; obstetrics; puerperal fever.

senile Pertaining to old age.

senile dementia A progressive, abnormally accelerated deterioration of mental faculties and emotional stability in older age, occurring especially in Alzheimer's disease. *See also* dementia; senile.

senility 1. The state of being senile. *See also* senile. 2. The mental and physical deterioration characteristic of old age.

seniority 1. The condition of being older than another or higher in rank than another or others. 2. Precedence of position, especially precedence over other persons of the same rank by reason of a longer span of service. *See also* seniority system.

seniority system A system based on length of service for determining employment advantages, such as promotion and being spared layoffs. *See also* seniority.

Senior Living Industries, National Association for *See* National Association for Senior Living Industries.

Senior Physicians, American Association of *See* American Association of Senior Physicians.

senium The period of old age.

sensation An awareness of a physical experience, dependent on stimulation of sense receptors and transmission of impulses to the sensory areas of the brain. *See also* sense; sense organ; taste.

sensationalism The use of matter or methods, especially in writing, journalism, and politics, that deliberately arouses or intends to arouse strong curiosity, interest, or reaction, especially by exaggerated or lurid details. *See also* journalism; media; press.

sense 1. Any of the faculties by which stimuli from outside or inside the body are received and felt, such as the senses of hearing, sight, smell, touch, and taste. *See also* object; odor; olfaction; sensation; sense datum; sense organ; smell; taste. 2. A capacity to appreciate or understand; normal ability to think or reason soundly, as in common sense. *See also* common sense; sensible; sixth sense.

sense, common *See* common sense.

sense datum A basic, unanalyzable (at present) sensation, such as color, sound, or smell, experienced upon stimulation of a sense organ or receptor. *See also* sense; sense organ.

sense organ A specialized organ or structure, such as the nose where sensory neurons are concentrated and which functions as a receptor. *Synonym*: sensor. *See also* organ; sensation; sense; sense datum.

sense, sixth *See* sixth sense.

sensible Acting with good sense, as in a sensible choice.

sensing The use of the senses (for example, sight, hearing) and memory as the sole bases on which to form conclusions and make decisions about observed phenomena. *Synonym*: human sensing. *See also* sense.

sensitivity 1. The level of responsiveness to sensory or other stimuli. 2. Susceptible to the attitudes, feelings, or circumstances of other persons. *See also* respect and caring.

sensitivity of a test A measure of the ability of a diagnostic test, screening test, or other predictor to correctly identify the individuals or cases actually having (are positive for) the condition or occurrence for which the test is being conducted. Operationally, sensitivity is the number of true positive test results divided by the sum of true positives plus false negatives. *Synonym:* true positive rate. *Compare* predictive value of a screening test; specificity of a test. *See also* false negative; true positive.

sensitivity training Training in small groups in which people learn how to interact with each other by developing a sensitive awareness and understanding of themselves and of their relationships with other persons. *See also* training.

sensor *See* sense organ.

sensor, bio- *See* biosensor.

sensorium The nervous system apparatus involved in sensation.

sensory aphasia A condition in which a person is unable to understand spoken or written language. *Synonym:* receptive aphasia. *See also* aphasia; cerebrovascular accident; motor aphasia.

SENTAC *See* Society for Ear, Nose, and Throat Advances in Children.

sentinel event In quality and performance measurement, a serious event that triggers further investigation each time it occurs. It usually is an undesirable and rare event, such as maternal death. *See also* sentinel event indicator.

sentinel event indicator A performance measure that identifies an individual event or phenomenon that always triggers further analysis and investigation, usually occurs infrequently and is undesirable in nature. Compare aggregate data indicator. *See also* indicator; performance measure; sentinel event.

SEP *See* Society of Experimental Psychologists.

SEPI *See* Society for the Exploration of Psychotherapy Integration.

sepsis The presence of pathogenic organisms or their toxins in the blood or tissues. *See also* bacteremia; septic; septic abortion; septicemia.

septic Poisonous, toxic, especially as a result of bacterial infection or action, as in death of a septic patient. *See also* sepsis; septic abortion; septicemia.

septic abortion An abortion with serious infection of the uterus, leading to generalized infection and sometimes sepsis and death. *See also* abortion; septic.

septicemia The condition in which pathogenic organisms or their toxins are present in the bloodstream. *Synonym:* blood poisoning. *See also* bacteremia; septic; toxemia.

septum An anatomical structure that serves as a dividing wall, as in a deviated nasal septum.

sepulchre A tomb or burial place. *See also* mausoleum.

sequence A following of one thing after another; for example, a patient assessment sequence requiring that patients be seen by a physician before ordering diagnostic tests or initiating therapy. *See also* sequential.

sequential Pertaining to a sequence, as in sequential sampling of medical records for review. *See also* sequential access.

sequential access In computer science, electronic storing of records based on some sequence determinations, such as alphabetic or numeric order. Random (direct) access file processing requires a direct access device, such as a magnetic disk unit, where retrieval time can be in milliseconds as compared to several seconds or even minutes in a sequential file using a tape unit. A majority of today's computerized information systems that use the random (direct) access method also use sequential processing for some portion of the processing activities in the same information system. *See also* computer; random access.

sequential sample *See* consecutive sample.

SER *See* Society for Epidemiologic Research.

serial Arranged one after another in succession. *See also* series.

serial interface In computer science, a printer or other peripheral device connected to a computer, which transmits the bits of a byte of information sequentially, or one after another. This contrasts to a parallel interface in which a printer or other peripheral device connected to a computer transmits the bits of a byte of information all at once. *See also* interface; parallel interface.

serial transmission *See* serial interface.

series A number of events or objects arranged or coming one after the other in succession, as in a series of setbacks to the organization or a red blood cell series (the succession of morphologically distinguishable cells that are stages in red blood cell development). *See also* case series; GI series.

series, case *See* case series.

series, GI *See* GI series.

serodiagnosis Diagnosis of disease based on reactions in the blood serum, as in the reliability of serodiagnosis of syphilis or AIDS. *See also* blood serum; diagnosis; serology.

serology The science dealing with the properties and reactions of serums, especially blood serum. Blood serum contains antibodies, which represent the response of the body to exposure to certain disease-causing agents. Detection of the presence of disease-specific antibodies with various serologic tests is helpful in making diagnoses. *See also* blood serum; clinical laboratory; seronegative; seropositive.

seronegative Showing a negative test result for some disease or condition tested by using an individual's blood serum; for example, seronegative for syphilis. *Compare* seropositive. *See also* blood serum; serology.

seropositive Showing a positive test result for some disease or condition tested by using an individual's blood serum; for example, seropositive for syphilis. *Compare* seronegative. *See also* blood serum; serology.

serum *See* blood serum.

serum, blood *See* blood serum.

serum drug level Measured concentration of a medication or drug in serum or plasma, as in a serum level of an aminoglycoside. *See also* blood plasma; blood serum; drug; level.

serum hepatitis Hepatitis due to hepatitis B virus or hepatitis C (non-A non-B) virus. *See also* blood serum; hepatitis.

servant, borrowed *See* borrowed servant.

servant, fellow *See* fellow servant.

servant, master and *See* master and servant.

serve To work for; to be of assistance to promote the interests of, as in serving a customer or serving the national interest. *See also* service.

service 1. Any task performed by people to benefit other people, as in goods and services. A service, like a good, is a product of an economy. *See also* economy; health services; product; service economy. 2. A type of business that sells assistance and expertise rather than a tangible product, as in health care services. 3. A functional division of an organization, as in a pediatrics or obstetrics service of a hospital. 4. A unit of health care established largely for billing purposes, as in a brief service requires only minimal effort by a physician and lasts for only a brief period of time.

service aide, social *See* social service aide.

service, alcoholism treatment *See* alcoholism treatment service.

Service, American College Testing *See* American College Testing Service.

service area *See* catchment area.

service benefits Insurance benefits that are the health services themselves, as with Blue Cross/ Blue Shield plans or Medicare. *See also* benefits; indemnity benefits.

service, cardiology *See* cardiology service.

service caseworker, social *See* social service caseworker.

service, chaplaincy *See* chaplaincy service.

service, chief of *See* chief of service.

service, clinical *See* clinical department.

service, clipping *See* clipping service.

service-connected disability In the Department of Veterans Affairs health system, a disability incurred or aggravated in the line of duty in active military service. In this context disability includes diseases which are the primary concern of the program. *Compare* nonservice-connected disability. *See also* Department of Veterans Affairs; disability.

service corporation, dental *See* dental service corporation.

service, customer *See* customer service.

service, dental *See* dental service.

service economy An economy in which economic activity is dominated by the service sector, as opposed to manufacturing or agriculture. The United States is said to be a service economy because over 50% of the labor force is in the service sector. *See also* economy; sector; service.

service, employee health *See* employee health service.

service, fee for *See* fee for service.

service, intensity of *See* intensity of service.

service, level of *See* level of service.

service liability The onus on a producer or others to make restitution for loss related to personal injury, property damage, or other harm caused by a service. *See also* liability; personal injury; product liability; service.

service, lip *See* lip service.

service, national health *See* national health service.

service, occasion of *See* occasion of service.

service, one-to-one *See* one-to-one service.

service, outpatient *See* outpatient service.

service patient *See* ward patient.

service, patient escort *See* patient escort service.

service, physical medicine *See* physical medicine service.

service plan, fee-for- *See* fee-for-service plan.

service, public *See* public service.

service, radiology *See* radiology service.

service, rehabilitation *See* rehabilitation service.

service representative, patient *See* patient service representative.

services *See* service.

Services Administration, General *See* General Services Administration.

services for adults, foster care *See* foster care services for adults.

Services, Alcoholics Anonymous World *See* Alcoholics Anonymous World Services.

Services, American Society of Directors of Volunteer *See* American Society of Directors of Volunteer Services.

services, ancillary *See* ancillary services.

services, basic health *See* basic health services.

services, chemical dependency *See* chemical dependency services.

services for children, foster care *See* foster care services for children.

services, community health *See* community health services.

services, contract *See* contract services.

services, counseling *See* counseling services.

services, covered *See* covered services.

services, decentralized *See* decentralized services.

services, decentralized laboratory *See* decentralized laboratory services.

services, decentralized pharmaceutical *See* decentralized pharmaceutical services.

Services, Department of Health and Human *See* Department of Health and Human Services.

services, emergency *See* emergency services.

services, enteral and parenteral nutrition and infusion therapy *See* enteral and parenteral nutrition and infusion therapy services.

services, environmental *See* environmental services.

services, extended care *See* extended care services.

Services for Families and Children, Council on Accreditation of *See* Council on Accreditation of Services for Families and Children.

services, forensic mental health *See* forensic mental health services.

services, health *See* health services.

services, home equipment management *See* home equipment management services.

services, home infusion *See* home infusion services.

services, homemaker *See* homemaker services.

services, home management *See* home management services.

services, home pharmaceutical *See* home pharmaceutical services.

services, industrial health *See* industrial health services.

Services Institute, Parapsychological *See* Parapsychological Services Institute.

services, maternal and child health *See* maternal and child health services.

services, medical *See* medical services.

services, medical record *See* medical record services.

services, mental health *See* mental health services.

Services, National Association of Medical Staff *See* National Association of Medical Staff Services.

Services, National Consortium for Child Mental Health *See* National Consortium for Child Mental Health Services.

Services, National Council on Health Laboratory *See* National Council on Health Laboratory Services.

services, occupational health *See* occupational health services.

services, occupational therapy *See* occupational therapy services.

service, social *See* social service.

Services, Office of Human Development *See* Office of Human Development Services.

services, optional *See* optional services.

services, pathology and clinical laboratory *See* pathology and clinical laboratory services.

services, personal health *See* personal health services.

services, pharmaceutical *See* pharmaceutical services.

services, physical rehabilitation *See* physical rehabilitation services.

services, physical therapy *See* physical therapy services.

services, psychiatric emergency *See* psychiatric emergency services.

services, required *See* required services.

services research, health *See* health services

research.

Services Research, Association for Health *See* Association for Health Services Research.

Services, Retired Persons *See* Retired Persons Services.

services, routine *See* routine services.

services, shared *See* shared services.

Services, Special Constituency Section for Aging and Long Term Care *See* Special Constituency Section for Aging and Long Term Care Services.

services, support *See* support services.

services, transportation *See* transportation services.

services, volunteer *See* volunteer services.

service, ultrasonic diagnostic *See* ultrasonic diagnostic service.

service, urology *See* urology service.

service worker An employee who works in the service sector of the economy. As manufacturing employment declines in the United States, the service sector and its workers have grown very rapidly. *See also* service economy.

setback An unanticipated or sudden check in progress, or a change from better to worse, as in a temporary setback.

set point A target value of a controlled variable that is maintained by an automatic control system; for example, the point at which body temperature is controlled by the brain's thermostat. *See also* variable.

settle In law, to secure or assign by legal action, as in settling a malpractice suit out of court. *See also* settlement.

settlement A compromise or agreement achieved by the adverse parties in a civil suit before final judgment, whereby they agree between themselves on their respective rights and obligations, thus eliminating the necessity of judicial resolution of the controversy. *See also* negotiated settlement; structured settlement.

settlement, negotiated *See* negotiated settlement.

settlement, structured *See* structured settlement.

Seventh-Day Adventist A member of a sect of Adventism distinguished for its observance of the Sabbath on Saturday. Seventh-Day Adventists eschew meat, alcohol, tobacco, and the non-medicinal use of drugs. The sect operates over 325 medical units throughout the world. *See also* Adventist.

Seventh-Day Adventist Dentists, National Association of *See* National Association of Seventh-Day Adventist Dentists.

Seventh-Day Adventist Dietetic Association (SDADA) A national organization founded in 1956 composed of 400 Seventh-Day Adventist registered dietitians and dietitians working in Seventh-Day Adventist institutions. It strives to motivate members to attain high professional standards and to actively promote Seventh-Day Adventist health principles. *See also* dietitian; Seventh-Day Adventist.

severability clause A legal understanding in the Missouri "Living Will" in which, if other specific directions are added to the sample declaration and are found to be invalid, the validity of the remainder of the declaration would not be affected. *See also* living will.

several liability, joint and *See* joint and several liability.

severance pay An amount of money based on length of employment for which an employee is eligible upon termination. It is provided as an income bridge by some employers for employees going from employment to unemployment. *See also* pay.

severity **1.** The state of being very serious, grave, or grievous, as in severe mental illness. **2.** The criticality of an illness or disease, based on a patient's condition and ranging from mild to terminal. *See also* severity of illness.

severity adjustment The process of classifying patients by severity-of-illness data so that performance and quality across organizations and practitioners can be more meaningfully compared. Examples of systems that classify patients in this manner include Medical Illness Severity Grouping System (MedisGroups) and Apache II. *See also* adjustment; APACHE II; Medical Illness Severity Grouping System; risk adjustment; severity of illness.

severity of illness The degree or state of disease existing in a patient prior to treatment. Severity of illness is an important patient-based source of variation in organizational and practitioner performance and is an important consideration in the interpretation of performance data. For instance, a hospital that accepts the most severely injured trauma patients might be expected to have a higher trauma-related mortality rate than a hospital that does not accept this group of patients, because of the severity of illness present before patients receiving treatment. *See also* acuity; AS-SCORE index; case severity; illness; severity; trauma score.

severity score, injury   *See* injury severity score.

sewage   Liquid domestic and industrial waste, including human and animal excretions. *See also* feces; sanitation.

sex   **1.** The quality by which organisms are classified as female or male on the basis of their reproductive organs and functions. **2.** The sexual urge or instinct as it manifests itself in behavior. **3.** *See* sexual intercourse.

sex, casual   *See* casual sex.

sex change   Simulation, usually by a combination of surgical and pharmacological methods, of the secondary and external sexual characteristics of the opposite sex in patients suffering from persistent paradoxical gender identification (transsexuality). *See also* change; gender; sex; transsexuality.

Sex Educators, Counselors and Therapists, American Association of   *See* American Association of Sex Educators, Counselors and Therapists.

sex hormone   A steroid hormone responsible for sexual development and reproductive function. The main female sex hormones are estrogens and progesterone; the male sex hormones are androgens, including testosterone. *See also* anabolic steroids; estrogen; gonadotropin; hormone; testosterone.

Sex Information and Education, Council for   *See* Council for Sex Information and Education.

Sex Information and Education Council of the US (SIECUS)   A national organization founded in 1964 composed of educators, social workers, physicians, clergy, youth organizations, and parents' groups interested in human sexuality education and sexual health care. It supports the individual's right to acquire knowledge of sexuality and exercise non-exploitative sexual choices. It encourages the development of responsible standards of sexual behavior.

sexing, nuclear   *See* nuclear sexing.

sexism   Discrimination based on gender. *See also* gender.

sexologist   A specialist in the treatment of sexual disorders. *See also* sexology.

sexology   The study of sex and sexual relations and their evolutionary, physiological, developmental, sociological, and medical aspects. *See also* sexologist.

sex, safe   *See* safe sex.

sex, safer   *See* safe sex.

Sex, Society for the Scientific Study of   *See* Society for the Scientific Study of Sex.

sex therapy   The treatment of sexual dysfunction (impotence or frigidity) by methods involving counseling, psychotherapy, or behavior modification. *See also* behavior modification; counseling; frigidity; impotence; psychotherapy; sex; therapy.

Sex Therapy and Research, Society for   *See* Society for Sex Therapy and Research.

Sexual Abusers, Association for the Behavioral Treatment of   *See* Association for the Behavioral Treatment of Sexual Abusers.

sexual assault   In law, indecent conduct of a man toward another man, a woman, or a child or of a woman toward a child, accompanied by the threat or danger of physical suffering or injury or inducing fear, shame, humiliation, and mental anguish. *See also* assault; rape.

Sexual Assault, National Coalition Against   *See* National Coalition Against Sexual Assault.

sexual deviance   *See* perversion.

sexual harrassment   Unwanted and offensive verbal or physical sexual advances, as those made by an employer to an employee. Sexual harrassment often carries with it threats of employment reprisals if such advances are refused. It has been defined by the federal government and courts as illegal employment discrimination (Civil Rights Act of 1964).

sexual intercourse   In humans, sexual union, as in penetration of the vagina with the penis. Sexual intercourse usually, but not always, involves seminal emission (ejaculation of semen). *Synonym*: coitus. *See also* age of consent; coitus interruptus; frigid; impotence; masturbation; orgasm; pederasty; semen; sex therapy; sodomy; statutory rape; venereal disease.

Sexuality and Disability, Coalition on   *See* Coalition of Sexuality and Disability.

sexually-transmitted disease (STD)   Any of various diseases, including syphilis, chancroid, herpes, chlamydia, and gonorrhea, that are usually contracted through sexual intercourse or other intimate sexual contact. *Synonym*: social disease. *See also* acquired immunodeficiency syndrome; chlamydia; gonorrhea; public health field investigator; syphilis.

sexual orientation   The direction of one's sexual interest toward members of the same, opposite, or both sexes. *See also* bisexuality; heterosexuality; homosexuality.

sexual, psycho-   *See* psychosexual.

SFB   *See* Society for Biomaterials.

SFPE   *See* Society of Fire Protection Engineers.

SGI   *See* Society for Gynecologic Investigation.

SGIM   *See* Society for General Internal Medicine.

SGNA   *See* Society of Gastroenterology Nurses and Associates.

SGO   *See* Society of Gynecologic Oncologists.

SH   *See* Society for Hematopathology.

shakedown   **1.** A trial run before putting a procedure or application into production. It attempts to locate and correct all the problems before actual utilization. *See also* testing. **2.** Extortion.

shakeup   A rapid change in the management and structure of an organization. The purpose of a shakeup is to change the direction and policies of an organization undergoing some form of stress. *See also* organization.

shaman   A member of certain tribal societies who acts as a medium between the visible world and an invisible spirit world and who practices magic for purposes of healing, divination, and control over natural events. *See also* medicine man; witch doctor.

shaping   An operant conditioning technique used in behavior therapy in which new behavior is produced by providing reinforcement for progressively closer approximations of the final desired behavior. *See also* behavior therapy; operant conditioning; reinforcement.

share   To participate in, use, enjoy, or experience jointly with another or others, as in sharing credit for the outcome. *See also* risk sharing; shared decision making; shared services.

shared decision making   In health care, a principle that patients must become more involved in their health care decisions and that physicians and other health professionals must respect that development for continuous quality improvement to be effective. *Synonym*: patient empowerment. *See also* continuous quality improvement; decision maker.

shared service organization   An organization, external to a hospital, set up to provide shared services, such as group purchasing. Such an organization may or may not have been created by the organizations partaking in the shared services and may or may not be under their joint control. *See also* shared services.

shared services   Administrative, clinical, or support service functions that are common to two or more health care organizations and are used jointly or cooperatively by them in some manner for the purpose of improving service and/or containing cost through economy of scale. *Synonym*: cooperative sharing. *See also* shared service organization.

sharing, risk   *See* risk sharing.

SHC   *See* Silicones Health Council.

sheath   *See* condom.

sheltered care home   *See* residential treatment facility.

sheltered-care institution   *See* residential treatment facility.

Sherman Act   *See* Sherman Antitrust Act.

Sherman Antitrust Act   The federal statute passed in 1890 aimed at preserving free and unfettered competition. It prohibits any unreasonable interference by contract, combination, or conspiracy with the ordinary, usual, and freely competitive pricing or distribution system of the open market in interstate trade. Physicians taking advantage of exclusive service contracts with their hospitals (for example, radiologists, anesthesiologists, pathologists, and sometimes cardiologists and emergency physicians) may become the focus of Sherman Antitrust Act claims. *See also* attempt to monopolize; Clayton Act; monopoly; restraint of trade.

Shewhart cycle   *See* Plan-Do-Check-Act cycle.

Shewhart, Walter Andrew   An engineer with Western Electric Company and a member of the technical staff of Bell Telephone Laboratories who specialized in the application of statistics in engineering and the theory and practice of control of product quality. He analyzed many different processes and concluded that all manufacturing processes display variation. He then identified a steady component of variation, which appeared to be inherent in a process, and an intermittent component. Shewhart attributed inherent variation to chance and undiscoverable causes, and intermittent variation to assignable causes. He concluded that assignable causes could be economically discovered and removed with a tenacious diagnostic program, but that random causes could not be economically discovered and could not be removed without making basic changes in the process. Shewhart's original scheme for continuous quality improvement consisted of four parts: plan, do, check, and act. It has been expanded upon by other persons, notably W. Edwards Deming, who also gave it much wider exposure than it gained in Shewhart's original work. *See also* Deming, W. Edwards; Plan-Do-Check-Act cycle.

SHFCC *See* Shriners Hospitals for Crippled Children.

SHHV *See* Society for Health and Human Values.

shiatsu *See* acupressure.

shift **1.** A time period during which an employee is assigned to work, as in night shift. *See also* shift differential. **2.** To move from one place or position to another or change direction, as in paradigm shift. *See also* paradigm shift.

shift differential Extra money paid as an inducement to accept shift work, especially for shifts involving evenings and nights. *See also* shift.

shift, paradigm *See* paradigm shift.

shingles *See* herpes zoster.

shivering A physiological method of heat production by means of involuntary muscle contractions. *See also* rigor.

SHNS *See* Society of Head and Neck Surgeons.

shock **1.** A condition of profound hemodynamic and metabolic disturbance characterized by failure of the circulatory system to maintain adequate perfusion of vital organs. It may result from inadequate blood volume, such as from traumatic blood loss; inadequate cardiac function, as in cardiogenic shock after a heart attack; or inadequate vasomotor tone, as in neurogenic shock after a spinal cord injury, septic shock after severe infection, or anaphylaxis. *See also* abruptio placenta; anaphylaxis; circulatory system; toxic shock syndrome. **2.** Something that jars the mind or emotions as if it with a violent blow, as in culture shock. *See also* culture shock.

shock, anaphylactic *See* anaphylaxis.

shock, culture *See* culture shock.

Shock Society A national organization founded in 1978 composed of 450 physicians and scientists interested in shock and trauma. *See also* shock; trauma.

shock syndrome, toxic *See* toxic shock syndrome.

shock therapy *See* electroconvulsive therapy.

shortage area, physician *See* physician shortage area.

shorting Dispensing a quantity of a drug that is less than the quantity prescribed for the purpose of increasing profit by charging for the prescribed amount. *See also* drug; fraud and abuse; kiting.

short-stay hospital *See* short-term hospital.

short-term hospital A hospital in which the average length of stay for all patients is less than 30 days or in which more than 50% of all patients are admitted to units where the average length of stay is less than 30 days. *Synonym:* short-stay hospital. *See also* hospital.

short-term memory Memory that is lost within a brief period (seconds, minutes, or longer) unless reinforced. *See also* memory.

SHOT *See* Society for the History of Technology.

should A term used in standards and scoring guidelines of the Joint Commission on Accreditation of Healthcare Organizations to reflect a preferred method or way. *See also* Joint Commission on Accreditation of Healthcare Organizations; scoring guideline; standard.

showcase To display prominently to advantage, as in showcasing a young artist's talent.

show code *See* slow code.

showdown A confrontation that forces an issue to a conclusion.

SHPM *See* Society for Healthcare Planning and Marketing of the American Hospital Association.

Shriners Hospitals for Crippled Children (SHFCC) An organization of 19 orthopedic hospitals and 3 burn hospitals operated by the Imperial Council of the Ancient Arabic Order of the Nobles of the Mystic Shrine for North America. It provides no-cost orthopedic and burn care to children under 18 years of age. *See also* orthopaedic/orthopedic surgery.

SHRM *See* Society for Human Resource Management.

SHSWD *See* Society for Hospital Social Work Directors.

shunt A short-circuit or bypass, usually between blood vessels. *See also* surgery.

Siamese twins A developmental anomaly of monozygotic (identical) twins in which there is a varying degree of union of the two bodies. *Synonym:* conjoined twins. *See also* twin.

sibling A brother, sister, or litter-mate. *See also* family.

sick **1.** Suffering from a physical or a mental illness. **2.** Defective or unsound, as in a sick economy. *See also* sickness.

sick baby A baby delivered with medical complications, other than those relating to premature status. *See also* delivery; premature delivery; sick.

sick bay A place where ill and injured people receive treatment, as an a ship's sick bay. *See also* sick.

sick bed A sick person's bed. *See also* bedside; sick.

sick leave Paid absence from work allowed an

employee because of illness. *See also* employee; sick; sickness.

sickle cell   An abnormal, crescent-shaped red blood cell containing hemoglobin S, an abnormal form of hemoglobin, characterizing sickle cell anemia. *See also* cell; sickle cell anemia; sickle cell crisis; sickle cell trait.

sickle cell anemia   A hereditary hemolytic anemia seen predominantly in African-Americans and characterized by the presence of hemoglobin S and crescent-shaped red blood cells. Under conditions of reduced oxygen tension, sickle hemoglobin molecules undergo crystallization within the red blood cell, which elongates and distorts the cell. The deformed cells contribute to increased blood thickness and circulatory stasis, which leads to decreased oxygen supply to the tissues, tissue death, and organ fibrosis. People with sickle cell anemia may experience episodic pain in their joints, fever, leg ulcers, and jaundice. The disease is chronic and usually fatal. *See also* anemia; sickle cell; sickle cell crisis; sickle cell trait.

sickle cell crisis   An acute condition that occurs in individuals with sickle cell anemia. The most common crisis is a painful vaso-occlusive crisis, which results from the aggregation of misshapen red blood cells. The cells block blood vessels and cause, for example, joint pain, priapism, and headache. Other types of crises include aplastic crisis, hyperhemolytic crisis, and acute sequestration crisis. *See also* sickle cell anemia.

sickle cell disease   *See* sickle cell anemia.

sickle cell trait   An inherited condition, usually harmless and without symptoms, in which a person carries only one gene for sickle cell anemia. *See also* sickle cell anemia.

Sickle Cell Disease, National Association for   *See* National Association for Sickle Cell Disease.

sickness   Any condition or episode marked by pronounced deviation from the normal health state, as in altitude sickness or radiation sickness. *See also* disease; illness; morning sickness; radiation sickness; space sickness.

sickness, morning   *See* morning sickness.

sickness, radiation   *See* radiation sickness.

sickness, space   *See* space sickness.

SID   *See* Society for Investigative Dermatology.

side effect   *See* drug side effect.

side effect, drug   *See* drug side effect.

sidestream smoke   The stream of smoke from the burning end of a cigar, cigarette, or pipe. *See also* involuntary smoking; nicotine; smoking; tobacco.

SIDS   *See* sudden infant death syndrome.

SIECUS   *See* Sex Information and Education Council of the US.

SIGBIO   *See* Special Interest Group on Biomedical Computing.

Sight Restoration, Eye-Bank for   *See* Eye-Bank for Sight Restoration.

sigma   The Greek letter used to designate the estimated standard deviation. *See also* standard deviation.

sigmoid colon   An S-shaped section of the colon between the descending section of the intestine and the rectum. *See also* colon.

sigmoidoscope   An endoscope for viewing the sigmoid colon. *See also* endoscope; flexible sigmoidoscope; sigmoid colon; sigmoidoscopy.

sigmoidoscope, flexible   *See* flexible sigmoidoscope.

sigmoidoscopy   Inspection of the sigmoid colon with a sigmoidoscope. *See also* flexible sigmoidoscopy.

sigmoidoscopy, flexible   *See* flexible sigmoidoscopy.

sign   In medicine, objective evidence of a condition, disease, or disorder that is perceptible to an observer, as in jaundice (yellowed skin) is a sign of hepatic dysfunction. *See also* finding; pathognomonic; prodrome; semiology; symptom; vital signs.

signals, mixed   *See* mixed signals.

signs, vital   *See* vital signs.

signature   *See* prescription.

significance level   *See* level of significance.

significance, statistical   *See* statistical significance.

significant   **1.** In statistics, relating to observations or occurrences that are too closely correlated to be attributed to chance and therefore indicate some type of systematic relationship. *See also* statistics. **2.** Having meaning. *See also* meaningful.

significant compliance   *See* compliance level.

significant other   In health care, an individual with whom a patient has a close and/or formalized relationship, such as a parent, spouse, friend, caretaker, court-ordered fiduciary, or any other person so identified by the patient. *See also* family.

significant, statistically   *See* statistically significant.

signify   To denote or mean, as in the data pattern signified the need for further investigation of the process of care under study.

signing oneself out   *See* against medical advice.

signing out AMA   *See* against medical advice.

sign language   A language that uses manual movements to convey grammatical structure and meaning. *See also* deafness; language.

sign out   *See* discharge.

silent partner   An individual who makes financial investments in a business enterprise but does not participate in its management. *See also* partner.

silent treatment   Maintenance of aloof silence toward another as an expression of one's anger or disapproval.

silicon   A nonmetallic element used doped or in combination with other materials used, for example, in semiconductors. *See also* semiconductor.

silicone   Any of a group of semi-opaque polymers characterized by wide-range thermal stability, lubricity, extreme water repellence, and physiological inertness. Silicone is used in many products, including prosthetic replacements for bodily parts. *See also* plastic surgery.

Silicones Health Council (SHC)   An organization founded in 1982 composed of seven organosilicones manufacturers concerned with coordinating programs dealing with health, environmental, and safety issues of interest to the industry and to disseminate scientifically sound information about silicones. *See also* silicone.

SIM   *See* Society for Information Management.

simple random sampling   A process in which a predetermined number of cases from a population as a whole is selected for review. It is predicated on the idea that each case has a probability of being included in the sample in direct proportion to its prevalence in the population. *Synonym:* true random sampling. *Compare* stratified random sampling. *See also* random sampling; sampling.

sinew   *See* tendon.

single-blind technique   A method of studying a drug, device, or procedure in which either the subject or the investigator is kept unaware of (blind to) who is receiving what level of the treatment. This is done to reduce either subject bias or researcher bias, depending on which type of bias is more likely. *See also* bias; clinical trial; double-blind technique.

single magnetic-striped card   A smart card costing a few cents to make and containing about 250 bytes of data. The card has no internal processing capability. *See also* smart card in health care.

single-payer system   A centralized health care payment system in which one entity, such as the federal government, pays for all health care services. Canada has the best-known single-payer system. It is financed by taxes, and people go to the physician and hospital of their choice and bill the government according to a standard fee schedule. *See also* payer.

single-specialty group practice   A group practice in which all the practitioners practice the same specialty. *See also* group practice; multispecialty group practice; specialty.

sinistral   Left-handed, or on the left side of the body.

sin tax   A tax on certain items, such as cigarettes and alcohol, that are regarded as neither necessities nor luxuries. *See also* tax.

sinusoidal current   A form of low-voltage current used by podiatrists and other health professionals to stimulate muscle action.

SIS   *See* Surgical Infection Society.

situation   The combination of circumstances at a given moment, as in an opportune situation or a difficult situation. *See also* situation ethics.

situation ethics   A system of ethics that evaluates acts in light of their situational context rather than by the application of moral absolutes. *See also* ethics.

sitz bath   **1.** A bathtub shaped like a chair in which one bathes in a sitting position, immersing only the hips and buttocks. **2.** A bath taken in such a tub, especially for therapeutic reasons, such as treatment for hemorrhoids. *See also* bath.

SI units   *See* Systeme International units.

sixth sense   A power of perception seemingly independent of the five senses. *See also* parapsychology; perception; sense; telepathy.

skeleton   **1.** All the bones of the body. **2.** The bony framework of the body. *See also* bone; skull.

skiagraphy   *See* radiography.

skill   Proficiency, facility, or dexterity that is acquired or developed through training or experience. *See also* ability; proficiency.

skilled nursing care   Nursing care for patients whose professional nursing needs do not require acute hospital nursing care, but who need inpatient supervision by a registered nurse, either because of the nature of procedures that must be performed, the amount of care needed, or both. Some of the procedures and treatments generally included in skilled nursing care include injections, administration of medications, changing of dressings, and observation and monitoring of a patient's condition, including taking vital signs. *See also* extended care; home health care; intermediate care; level of care; registered nurse.

skilled nursing facility (SNF)   A facility that is primarily engaged in providing skilled nursing care. Such facilities have an organized professional staff, including physicians and registered nurses, and meet other requirements established by law. A patient may be discharged from an acute care hospital and then admitted to an SNF. Skilled nursing care may be provided in an area of an acute care hospital; this area is usually called a skilled nursing unit. Skilled nursing facilities were previously called extended care facilities. *See also* extended care facility; skilled nursing care; skilled nursing unit.

skilled nursing unit (SNU)   A unit or department of a hospital that provides skilled nursing care. To qualify as an SNU, the unit must have an organized professional staff, including medical and nursing professional, and meet other requirements established by law. A free-standing facility devoted to skilled nursing care is called a skilled nursing facility. *See also* skilled nursing care; skilled nursing facility; unit.

skim   To take away the choicest or most readily attainable parts from, as in skimming in health care. *See also* skimming in health care.

skimming in health care   The practice in health care organizations paid on a prepayment or capitation basis, and in health insurance, of seeking to enroll only the healthiest people as a way of controlling costs (since income is constant whether services are actually used). *Synonym:* creaming. *Compare* adverse selection. *See also* skimping.

skimping   The practice in health care organizations paid on a prepayment or capitation basis of denying or delaying the provision of services needed or demanded by enrolled members as a way of controlling costs. An example is the denial or delay of a cataract extraction. *See also* adverse selection; skimming in health care.

skin   The tissue, composed of epidermis and dermis, forming the external covering of a human. *See also* blister; cutaneous; cyanosis; dermatology; dermatitis; dermis; epidermis; neurodermatitis; rash; skin graft.

Skin Diseases Information Clearinghouse,

National Arthritis and Musculoskeletal and   *See* National Arthritis and Musculoskeletal and Skin Diseases Information Clearinghouse.

skin graft   A surgical graft (transplant) of healthy skin from one part of the body to another or from one individual to another in order to replace damaged or lost skin, as used for burn patients. *See also* skin; transplant.

skull   The bone that covers the brain. *Synonym:* cranium. *See also* bone; brain; trephine.

slander   Oral defamation. *See also* defamation; libel.

slant   A bias, as in the journalist's unflattering slant to the story. *See also* bias.

sleep   A natural, periodic state of rest for the mind and body, in which the eyes usually close and consciousness is completely or partially lost, so that there is a decrease in bodily movement and responsiveness to external stimuli. During sleep the brain in human beings undergoes a characteristic cycle of brain-wave activity that includes intervals of dreaming. *See also* dream; insomnia; sleep apnea; somnology.

sleep apnea   A sleep disorder in which breathing is temporarily suspended during sleep. It often affects overweight people or those having an obstruction in the respiratory tract, an abnormally small throat opening, or a neurological disorder. *See also* apnea; sleep.

Sleep Disorders Association, American   *See* American Sleep Disorders Association.

Sleep Research Society (SRS)   A national organization founded in 1961 composed of 428 physiologists, psychologists, and physicians with research interests in the study of sleep. It disseminates scientific papers on the physiological and psychological aspects of sleep. Formerly (1983) Association for the Psychophysiological Study of Sleep. *See also* polysomnographic technology; sleep; sleep apnea; somnology.

Sleep Societies, Association of Professional   *See* Association of Professional Sleep Societies.

SLHR   *See* Society for Life History Research.

slick   **1.** Deftly executed, as in a manager's slick handling of a difficult situation. **2.** Shrewd, wily, as in a slick salesman. **3.** Superficially attractive or plausible but lacking depth or soundness, as in an argument too slick to be accepted.

sliding scale   A scale in which indicated prices, taxes, or wages vary in accordance with another factor; for example; wages with the cost-of-living index or medical charges with a patient's income. *See also* scale.

slip law   In Congress, the final version of an act of Congress and its first official publication. Each public law is printed in the form of a slip law, which also lists, but does not include, the legislative history of the act, whatever earlier act may be amended by the new law, as it is amended, or any explanation or interpretation of the law. *See also* law.

slippery slope   A precarious situation. In ethics, for example, it refers to the argument that asserts that one morally questionable action or policy will set a precedent for, or lead to, other actions or policies even more morally questionable. The concern is starting a process in which classes of undesirable results grow increasingly wider and include more and more persons who are burdens to themselves and other persons. If the slope is indeed slippery and no likely stopping point exists, then avoidance of the first step may be prudent. *See also* ethics; prudence.

slogan   A phrase expressing the aims or nature of an enterprise, an organization, or a candidate. *See also* sloganeer.

sloganeer   A person who invents or uses slogans. *See also* slogan.

slow code   An intermediate course of action between full cardiopulmonary resuscitation and do-not-resuscitate orders. This option is usually inappropriate unless sound reason is known; for example, the patient requests chest compression but no intubation. *Synonyms:* limited code; partial code; show code. *See also* cardiopulmonary resuscitation; code blue; do-not-resuscitate order.

slow virus infections   Infections due to a transmissible agent that have a very long incubation period, possibly lasting many years, and are then gradually progressive. Examples are kuru and scrapie. *See also* infection; virus.

S & M   *See* sadomasochism.

SMA   *See* Society for Medical Anthropology.

small business   A private venture employing a limited number of employees (less than 100 people, according to the US Department of Commerce). For example, in health care, a private practice, nursing home, or small clinic would qualify as a small business. *See also* business.

smallpox   An infectious disease caused by a poxvirus and characterized by high fever and aches,

subsequent widespread eruption of pustules, and formation of pockmarks. The World Health Organization announced in May of 1980 that the disease had been finally eradicated in humans. The chances of smallpox recurring as a result of mutation from a related wild species is considered remote. *Synonym:* variola. *See also* infectious diseases; pox.

Small or Rural Hospitals, General Constituency Section for   *See* General Constituency Section for Small or Rural Hospitals.

small talk   Trivial or casual conversation.

smart card   A credit card-sized identification device containing an integrated circuit chip capable of storing and/or processing information. *See also* smart card in health care.

smart card in health care   A smart card that can be used to store an individual's health insurance coverage, medical information, and demographic information, such as name, address, age, and sex. There are three kinds of technologies that determine how much information a particular smart card will hold: single magnetic-striped card, optical-stripe card, and electronic-striped card. *See also* electronic-striped card; health card; optical-stripe card; single magnetic-striped card; smart card.

Smart Card Industry Association (SCIA)   A national organization founded in 1988 composed of 190 manufacturers, value-added dealers, consultants, publishers, suppliers, persons in the communications media, educational institutions, and individuals interested in promoting smart card technology and applications. *See also* smart card.

SMCAF   *See* Society of Medical Consultants to the Armed Forces.

SMCR   *See* Society for Menstrual Cycle Research.

SMDA   *See* State Medicaid Directors Association.

smear   A specimen for microscopic study prepared by spreading the material across a glass slide. *See also* microscope.

smegma   A soapy, cheesy secretion derived mainly from sebaceous glands, particularly occurring under the foreskin of the penis. *See also* sebaceous gland.

smell   The faculty of detecting odors. *See also* sense.

SMFW   *See* Society of Medical Friends of Wine.

SMH   *See* Section for Metropolitan Hospitals.

SMJ   *See* Society of Medical Jurisprudence.

SMO   *See* Society of Military Ophthalmologists.

SMO-HNS   *See* Society of Military Otolaryngologists-Head and Neck Surgeons.

smoke The vaporous system made up of small particles of carbonaceous matter in the air, resulting from, for example, the burning of tobacco. *See also* involuntary smoking; sidestream smoke; smoking; tobacco.

smoke, sidestream *See* sidestream smoke.

smoking Engaged in the process of smoking tobacco. *See also* emphysema; involuntary smoking; nicotine; sidestream smoke; smoke; tobacco.

Smoking Education Act of 1984, Comprehensive *See* Comprehensive Smoking Education Act of 1984.

Smoking or Health, Coalition on *See* Coalition on Smoking or Health.

smoking, involuntary *See* involuntary smoking.

smooth muscle *See* muscle.

SMOS *See* Society of Military Orthopaedic Surgeons.

SMRI *See* Society for Magnetic Resonance Imaging.

SN *See* Society for Neuroscience.

SNASS *See* Society of Neurosurgical Anesthesia and Critical Care.

SNACC *See* Society of Neurosurgical Anesthesia and Critical Care.

SNE *See* Society for Nutrition Education.

sneezing An abrupt expulsion of air from the nose, reflexively induced by irritation of the nasal mucous membranes. *See also* allergy; hay fever.

SNF *See* skilled nursing facility.

SNM *See* Society of Nuclear Medicine.

SNU *See* skilled nursing unit.

snuff Ground tobacco perfumed with essential oils, and taken by insertion into the nostrils. The nicotine is absorbed through the nasal mucous membranes. *See also* tobacco.

SOA *See* Society of Actuaries.

SOAP *See* Society for Obstetric Anesthesia and Perinatology.

SOAP A device for conceptualizing and recording progress notes in a problem-oriented medical record. *S* indicates subjective data obtained from the patient or a representative of the patient; *O* designates objective data obtained by observation, physical examination, and diagnostic studies; *A* refers to assessment of the patient's status based on subjective and objective data; and *P* designates the plan for patient care. *See also* medical record progress note; problem-oriented medical record; status.

sobriety Moderation in or abstinence from consumption of alcoholic beverages or use of drugs. *See*

also abstinence; alcohol; drug.

SOC *See* statement of construction.

SOCA Acronym for suffuse osmotic chemisorb asphyxiation. *See* American Podiatric Circulatory Society.

social Living together in communities.

social benefit, net *See* net social benefit.

Social Biology, Society for the Study of *See* Society for the Study of Social Biology.

social contract An agreement among the members of an organized society or between the governed and the government defining and limiting the rights and responsibilities of each; for example, the Constitution of the United States. *See also* contract; social.

social detoxification A period of enforced abstinence from a toxic substance to which one is habituated or addicted but not critically ill and whose treatment does not require intensive or comprehensive medical services. *See also* abstinence; detoxification; medical detoxification; social.

social disease *See* sexually transmitted disease.

Social Gerontology, The Center for *See* The Center for Social Gerontology.

social group worker A social worker who works with small groups of people to promote the group work concept to help members develop their own activities. Social group workers may work in community centers, neighborhood or settlement houses, youth centers, and housing projects, and they may organize groups, such as senior citizens, and develop recreational, physical education, or cultural programs. *See also* social worker.

Social Health Association, American *See* American Social Health Association.

social insurance A mechanism for the pooling of risks by their transfer to an organization, usually governmental, that is required by law to provide indemnity (cash) or service benefits to or on behalf of covered persons upon the occurrence of certain predesignated losses. Examples include social security, railroad retirement, and workers' and unemployment compensation. The purpose of social insurance is the provision of minimum standards of living for those in lower and middle wage groups. In other countries, health insurance is often a government sponsored social insurance program. *See also* insurance; national health insurance; Old Age, Survivors, Disability and Health Insurance Program; unemployment insurance.

Social Insurance, National Academy of *See* National Academy of Social Insurance.

socialism   A socioeconomic system in which government owns or controls many major industries, but may allow markets to set prices in many areas. *See also* capitalism.

Social Issues, Society for the Psychological Study of *See* Society for the Psychological Study of Social Issues.

socialized medicine   **1.** A health care system in which the organization and provision of health care services are directly controlled by the government, and health care providers are employed by or contract for the provision of services directly with the government. **2.** Any existing or proposed health care system believed to be subject to excessive governmental control. *Synonym:* state medicine. *See also* national health insurance; social insurance.

social psychiatry   The branch of psychiatry that deals with the relationship between social environment and mental illness. *See also* psychiatry; social.

Social Psychiatry, American Association for *See* American Association for Social Psychiatry.

social, psycho- *See* psychosocial.

social psychology   The branch of psychology that studies the social behavior of individuals and groups, with special emphasis on how behavior is affected by the presence or influence of other people. Social psychology deals with such processes as communication, political behavior, and the formation of attitudes. *See also* psychology; social.

Social Psychology, Society for the Advancement of *See* Society for the Advancement of Social Psychology.

Social Responsibility, Physicians for *See* Physicians for Social Responsibility.

social science   The study of human society and of individual relationships within and to society. The discipline generally includes sociology, psychology, anthropology, economics, political science, and history. *See also* anthropology; economics; history; political science; psychology; science; social; society.

Social Security   **1.** A government program that provides economic assistance to persons faced with unemployment, disability, or old age, financed by tax assessment of employers and employees. **2.** The economic assistance provided by social security, as in a social security check. *See also* Old Age, Survivors, and Disability Insurance; Social Security Act.

Social Security Act   Federal legislation signed into law by President Franklin Roosevelt in 1935 that created the Social Security Administration. The main purpose of the law was to provide protection as a matter of right for the American worker in retirement. Major provisions included "Old Age Assistance" and "Old Age Survivors Disability Insurance." *See also* Child Health Act; Federal Insurance Contribution Act; Medicaid; Medicare; Social Security Administration; supplemental security income.

Social Security Administration (SSA)   The agency of the Department of Health and Human Services under the Commissioner of Social Security that administers a national program of contributory social insurance whereby employees, employers, and the self-employed pay contributions that are pooled in special trust funds. When earnings stop or are reduced because the worker retires, dies, or becomes disabled, monthly cash benefits are paid to replace part of the earnings the person or family has lost. In addition to administering the various retirement, survivors, disability, and supplemental security income benefit programs, the SSA oversees the administrative hearing and appeals process involving benefit claims. *See also* backdoor authority; Department of Health and Human Services; Social Security Amendments of 1972.

Social Security Amendments of 1960 *See* Kerr-Mills.

Social Security Amendments of 1972   Amendments to the Social Security Act that authorized Medicare to contract with health maintenance organizations on either a cost reimbursement or risk basis; established the professional standards review organizations (PSRO) program; and defined kidney failure as a disability. *See also* professional standards review organization; Social Security Act.

Social Security Amendments of 1983   Amendments to the Social Security Act that established a comprehensive prospective payment system for hospital services provided under Medicare, using diagnosis-related groups (DRGs). *See also* diagnosis-related groups; Social Security Act.

social services   **1.** Organized efforts to advance human welfare. **2.** The services actually provided, as in free school lunches, for disadvantaged citizens.

social service aide   A person who assists social workers in interviewing applicants for social or health care services, referring persons to community services, and performing follow-up studies under the supervision of a social worker. *See also* aide; social worker.

social service caseworker   A social worker or other qualified person who counsels and helps individuals and families requiring assistance from a social service agency. *See also* caseworker; social worker.

social welfare administrator   A social worker or other qualified individual who directs the agency or the major function of a public or voluntary organization that proves services in the social welfare field. *Synonym*: social welfare director. *See also* administrator; social worker.

social welfare director   *See* social welfare administrator.

Social Welfare Organizations, National Assembly of National Voluntary Health and   *See* National Assembly of National Voluntary Health and Social Welfare Organizations.

social work   Organized work intended to advance the social conditions of a community by providing psychological counseling, guidance, and assistance, especially in the form of social services. *See also* casework; social services.

social work assistant   An individual meeting certain requirements who receives on-the-job training for specific assignments and responsibilities in the provision of social services. *See also* social services; social work.

Social Work Boards, American Association of State   *See* American Association of State Social Work Boards.

Social Work Directors, Society for Hospital   *See* Society for Hospital Social Work Directors.

social work discharge planning   The evaluation of a patient's needs by a social worker or other qualified individual, beginning on the day of admission to a health care facility. It involves assessing the family, extended family, and other resources to determine what resources are available to help the patient in returning home or if plans should be made for placement elsewhere. *See also* discharge planning; medical/hospital social worker.

Social Work Education, Council on   *See* Council on Social Work Education.

social worker   An individual qualified by education and authorized by law to practice in the field of social work. Social worker definitions vary between states. The National Association of Social Workers classifies several levels of social work positions within two groups: preprofessional and professional. A preprofessional may be classified as a social service aide or a social service technician. A professional position is one requiring a Bachelor of Social Work (BSW) degree, a Master of Social Work (MSW) degree, or more, and related experience. Social workers practice in a multitude of settings and provide a wide array of services. *See also* casework supervisor; child welfare caseworker; clinical social worker, private practice; industrial social worker; medical/hospital social worker; psychiatric social worker; public health social worker; school social worker; social group worker; social service caseworker; social welfare administrator; social worker.

social worker, clinical   *See* clinical social worker.

social worker, hospital   *See* medical/hospital social worker.

social worker, industrial   *See* industrial social worker.

social worker, licensed   *See* licensed social worker.

social worker, medical   *See* medical/hospital social worker.

social worker, medical/hospital   *See* medical/hospital social worker.

social worker, occupational   *See* industrial social worker.

social worker, private practice, clinical   *See* clinical social worker, private practice.

social worker, psychiatric   *See* psychiatric social worker.

social worker, registered   *See* registered social worker.

Social Workers, Academy of Certified   *See* Academy of Certified Social Workers.

Social Workers, American Association of Industrial   *See* American Association of Industrial Social Workers.

Social Workers, American Association of Spinal Cord Injury Psychologists and   *See* American Association of Spinal Cord Injury Psychologists and Social Workers.

Social Workers, Association of Pediatric Oncology   *See* Association of Pediatric Oncology Social Workers.

social worker, school   *See* school social worker.

Social Workers Committee on Lesbian and Gay

Issues, National Association of *See* National Association of Social Workers Committee on Lesbian and Gay Issues.

Social Workers, National Association of *See* National Association of Social Workers.

Social Workers, National Association of Black *See* National Association of Black Social Workers.

Social Workers, National Association of Oncology *See* National Association of Oncology Social Workers.

Social Work Managers, National Network for *See* National Network for Social Work Managers.

Social Work, Master of *See* Master of Social Work.

Social Work, National Federation of Societies for Clinical *See* National Federation of Societies for Clinical Social Work.

Societies for Clinical Social Work, National Federation of *See* National Federation of Societies for Clinical Social Work.

societies, specialty *See* specialty societies.

society 1. The totality of social relationships among human beings, as in human societies. *See also* social; social science. **2.** A group of human beings broadly distinguished from other groups by mutual interests, participation in characteristic relationships, shared institutions, and a common culture, as in medical societies. *See also* medical society; specialty societies; tribe.

Society for Academic Emergency Medicine (SAEM) A national organization founded in 1975 composed of 2,000 physicians teaching emergency medicine, emergency medicine residents, and non-physicians teaching emergency care. Its purposes are to educate teachers of emergency medicine and encourage its development as an academic discipline. *See also* academic; emergency medicine.

Society of Actuaries (SOA) A national organization founded in 1949 composed of 12,925 individuals trained in the application of mathematical probabilities to the design of insurance, pension, and employee benefit programs. It sponsors examinations leading to designations of fellow or associate in the society. *See also* actuarial science; actuary.

Society for Adolescent Medicine (SAM) A national organization founded in 1968 composed of 1,100 physicians, psychologists, social workers, psychiatrists, nurses, and other health professionals interested in improving the quality of health care for adolescents. *See also* adolescence; adolescent medicine; child and adolescent psychiatry.

Society for the Advancement of Ambulatory Care (SAAC) A national organization founded in 1981 composed of 508 individuals and organizations that support the advancement of primary health care programs or facilities. Its goals include furthering human welfare through the advancement of ambulatory health care and representing health centers and primary care providers before legislative and governmental bodies. *See also* ambulatory health care.

Society for Advancement of Management (SAM) A national organization founded in 1912 composed of 11,000 management executives in industry, commerce, government, and education. Its fields of interest include management education, administration, budgeting, collective bargaining, incentives, materials handling, quality control, and training. *See also* management.

Society for the Advancement of Social Psychology (SASP) A national organization founded in 1974 composed of 400 social psychologists interested in advancing social psychology as a profession by facilitating communication among social psychologists and improving dissemination and use of social psychological knowledge. *See also* social psychology.

Society of Air Force Physicians (SAFP) A national organization founded in 1958 composed of 300 Air Force internists, family practitioners, and specialists in emergency medicine, dermatology, allergy and immunology, and neurology. Its objectives are to foster advancement of the art and science of medicine in the Air Force. *See also* physician.

Society American Gastrointestinal Endoscopic Surgeons (SAGES) A national organization founded in 1980 composed of 1,500 surgeons who perform gastrointestinal endoscopy and laparoscopy. It promotes the concepts of gastrointestinal endoscopy as an integral part of surgery and establishes standards of training and practice and guidelines for privileging. *See also* endoscopy; gastrointestinal; laparoscopy.

Society for Assisted Reproductive Technology (SART) A national organization composed of 140 institutions conducting assisted reproductive procedures. It works to extend knowledge of human in-vitro fertilization techniques. *See also* noncoital reproduction; reproductive technologies.

Society of Behavioral Medicine (SBM) A national organization founded in 1978 composed of 2,500 behavioral and biomedical researchers and clinicians studying health promotion and behavior. *See also* behavioral medicine; health promotion.

Society for Behavioral Pediatrics (SBP) A national organization founded in 1983 composed of 450 pediatricians, child psychiatrists and psychologists, and other health professionals interested in improving the health care of infants, children, and adolescents by promoting research and instruction in the areas of developmental and behavioral pediatrics. *See also* behavioral medicine; pediatrics.

Society for Biomaterials (SFB) A national organization founded in 1974 composed of 1,200 bioengineers and materials scientists; dental, orthopedic, cardiac, and other surgeons and scientists interested in developing biomaterials as tissue replacements in patients; and corporations interested in the manufacture of biomaterials. *See also* bioengineer.

Society of Biomedical Equipment Technicians (SBET) A national organization founded in 1976 composed of 1,200 biomedical equipment technicians, hospital maintenance engineers, managers of hospital medical equipment departments, sales representatives, and other persons involved with the repair or installation of biomedical hospital machinery. It seeks to recognize biomedical equipment technicians and engineers as a specialty group. It supports certification programs including certified biomedical equipment technician, certified radiologic equipment specialist, and certified laboratory equipment specialist. *See also* certification; medical equipment.

Society for Cardiac Angiography and Interventions (SCA&I) A national organization founded in 1978 composed of 730 angiographers interested in the field of cardiac catheterization, especially coronary angiography and interventional angiography. *See also* angiography; cardiac catheterization; coronary angiography; invasive procedure.

Society of Cardiovascular Anesthesiologists (SCA) A national organization composed of 3,000 anesthesiologists who specialize in cardiovascular surgical conditions whose purpose is to further medical education of cardiovascular anesthesiologists. *See also* anesthesiology; cardiovascular.

Society of Cardiovascular and Interventional Radiology (SCVIR) A national organization founded in 1973 composed of 1,700 physicians who are leaders in the field of cardiovascular and inter-

ventional radiology. It facilitates exchange of new ideas and techniques and provides education courses for physicians working in the field. Formerly (1983) Society of Cardiovascular Radiology. *See also* angiography; cardiac catheterization; cardiovascular; radiology.

Society of Cardiovascular Radiology *See* Society of Cardiovascular and Interventional Radiology.

Society for Clinical and Experimental Hypnosis (SCEH) A national organization founded in 1949 composed of 1,100 physicians, dentists, doctoral level psychologists, and psychiatric social workers interested in research in hypnosis and its boundary areas as well as the therapeutic use of hypnosis in clinical practice. *See also* hypnosis.

Society of Clinical and Medical Electrologists (SCME) A national organization founded in 1985 composed of 500 electrologists. It conducts continuing education and leadership development seminars. *See also* continuing education; electrology.

Society for Clinical Trials (SCT) A national organization founded in 1978 composed of 1,450 persons with training and expertise in behavioral science, bioethics, biostatistics, computer science, dentistry, epidemiology, law, management, medicine, nursing, and pharmacology, interested in the development and dissemination of knowledge about the design and conduct of clinical trials. *See also* bioethics; biostatistics; clinical trial; computer science; dentistry; epidemiology; law; management; medicine; nursing; pharmacology.

Society of Critical Care Medicine (SCCM) A national organization founded in 1970 composed of 4,000 physicians, nurses, scientists, technicians, respiratory technicians, and engineers involved in the field of critical care medicine. *See also* critical care medicine.

Society for Cryobiology (SC) A national organization founded in 1964 composed of 450 basic and applied researchers interested in the field of low-temperature biology and medicine. It promotes an interdisciplinary approach to freezing, freeze-drying, hypothermia, hibernation, physiological effects of low environmental temperature on animals and plants, medical applications of reduced temperatures, cryosurgery, hypothermic perfusion and cryopreservation of organs, cryoprotective agents and their pharmacological action, and pertinent methodologies. *See also* cryobiology.

Society for Developmental Biology (SDB) A national organization founded in 1939 composed of 1,600 biologists interested in problems of development and growth or organisms. *See also* biology; development.

Society of Diagnostic Medical Sonographers (SDMS) A national organization founded in 1970 composed of 8,500 sonographers, physician sonologists, and other persons in medical specialties using high-frequency sound for diagnostic purposes. It developed and maintains the American Registry of Diagnostic Medical Sonographers. *See also* diagnostic medical sonographer; radiology; ultrasound imaging.

Society for Ear, Nose, and Throat Advances in Children (SENTAC) A national organization founded in 1973 composed of 350 otolaryngologists, pediatricians, audiologists, speech pathologists, and related professionals interested in evaluating the science and practice of medicine, surgery, and rehabilitation as related to diseases and disorders of the ear, nose, and throat in infants and children. *See also* audiology; otolaryngology; pediatrics; speech pathology.

Society for Environmental Geochemistry and Health (SEGH) A national organization founded in 1971 composed of 350 organizations, scientists, and students interested in furthering knowledge of the geochemical environment's effects on the health and diseases of plants and animals, including humans. *See also* environmental; geochemistry.

Society of Ethnobiology (SE) An national organization founded in 1978 composed of 450 individuals and institutions interested in ethnobiology. *See also* ethnobiology.

Society for Epidemiologic Research (SER) A national organization founded in 1967 composed of 2,500 epidemiologists, researchers, public health administrators, educators, mathematicians, statisticians, and other persons interested in epidemiologic research. *See also* epidemiology; research.

Society for Experimental Biology and Medicine (SEBM) A national organization founded in 1903 composed of 2,100 workers engaged in research in experimental biology or experimental medicine. It cultivates the experimental method of investigation in the sciences of biology and medicine. *See also* biology; experimental method; medicine; scientific method.

Society of Experimental Psychologists (SEP) A national organization founded in 1929 composed of 165 experimental psychologists in the United States and Canada. *See also* experimental psychology; psychology.

Society for the Exploration of Psychotherapy Integration (SEPI) A national organization founded in 1984 composed of 450 mental health professionals interested in the integration of theories and methods of psychotherapy. It encourages communication among members and promotes collaborative work among psychotherapists who adhere to different theories and methods. *See also* mental health professional; psychotherapy.

Society of Fire Protection Engineers (SFPE) A national organization founded in 1950 composed of 3,575 fire protection engineers. Its objectives are to advance the art and science of fire protection engineering, to maintain a high ethical standard among members, and to foster fire protection engineering education. *See also* engineer.

Society of Forensic Toxicologists (SOFT) A national organization founded in 1970 composed of 300 scientists who analyze tissue and body fluids for drugs and poisons and interpret the information for judicial purposes. Its objectives include establishing uniform qualifications and requirements for certification of forensic toxicologists and promoting support mechanisms for continued certification. *See also* certification; forensic medicine; toxicology.

Society of Gastroenterology Nurses and Associates (SGNA) A national organization founded in 1974 composed of 3,800 nurses and other health professionals engaged in the field of gastroenterology and endoscopy. It conducts national and regional educational courses and research programs and cooperates with other professional associations, hospitals, universities, industries, technical societies, research organizations, and governmental agencies. Formerly (1989) Society of Gastrointestinal Assistants. *See also* endoscopy; gastroenterology.

Society of Gastrointestinal Assistants *See* Society of Gastroenterology Nurses and Associates.

Society of General Internal Medicine (SGIM) A national organization founded in 1978 composed of 2,000 faculty members of medical schools in the United States and Canada interested in advancing primary care and general internal medicine through improved teaching, patient care, and research. *See also* internal medicine; primary care.

Society for Gynecologic Investigation (SGI) A national organization founded in 1953 composed of 600 present and former faculty members of institutions interested or engaged in gynecologic research. Its purpose is to stimulate, assist, and conduct gynecologic research. *See also* gynecology; research.

Society of Gynecologic Oncologists (SGO) A national organization founded in 1969 composed of 500 gynecologic oncologists. Its objectives include improving the care of patients with gynecological cancer, encouraging research in gynecologic oncology, advancing knowledge in the field, and upgrading standards of practice. It evaluates and addresses trends in gynecologic oncology. *See also* cancer; gynecologic oncology; gynecology.

Society for Health and Human Values (SHHV) A national organization founded in 1969 composed of 900 educators in the health professions interested in developing new understandings, concepts, and programs in the area of human values and medicine, with special emphasis on the education of health professionals. It conducts programs at national association meetings and acts as a resource service for educational institutions. *See also* health education; health professional.

Society of Head and Neck Surgeons (SHNS) A national organization founded in 1954 composed of 700 surgeons interested in advancing the art and science of surgery of disorders of the head and neck, particularly cancer. *See also* otolaryngology; surgery.

Society for Healthcare Planning and Marketing of the American Hospital Association (SHPM) A national organization composed of 3,700 employees of hospitals, allied hospital associations, multi-institutional systems, and any other direct provider of health care services; employees of consulting firms, health or hospital administration programs, government agencies, and national, state, or community health planning agencies; and other individuals interested in institutional and strategic planning and marketing policies and issues. Formerly (1987) Society for Hospital Planning and Marketing of the American Hospital Association. *See also* American Hospital Association; health planning; marketing; strategic planning.

Society for Hematopathology (SH) A national organization founded in 1981 composed of 375 physicians, doctors of science, osteopathic physicians, and dental surgeons interested in exchange of information on the hematopoietic and lymphoreticular systems. *See also* hematology; pathology.

Society for the History of Technology (SHOT) A national organization founded in 1958 composed of 2,600 academicians in science, engineering, history, sociology, economics, and anthropology interested in the study of the development of technology and its relations with society and culture. It cooperates with other societies and professional organizations in arranging educational programs on the history of technology. *See also* history; technology.

Society for Hospital Planning and Marketing of the American Hospital Association *See* Society for Healthcare Planning and Marketing of the American Hospital Association.

Society for Hospital Social Work Directors (SHSWD) A national organization founded in 1966 composed of 2,475 directors of social work departments in health care organizations. It provides a medium for the interchange of ideas and dissemination of material relative to social work administration; promotes standards and ethics for the delivery of social work in health care settings; and strengthens relationships with hospital administration and cooperates with allied hospital associations and professional social work organizations. *See also* administrator; social work.

Society for Human Resource Management (SHRM) A national organization founded in 1948 composed of 45,000 human resource, personnel, and industrial relations executives. It promotes the advancement of human resource management. Formerly (1989) American Society for Personnel Administration. *See also* human resource management.

Society for Information Management (SIM) A national organization founded in 1968 composed of 1,900 senior information systems executives with leadership capabilities in major corporations and government and nonprofit organizations. Its purposes are to serve as an exchange or marketplace for technical information about management information systems, including theory, applications, methodology, and techniques, and to enhance communication among management information systems directors and the executives responsible for management of the business enterprise. Formerly (1983) Society for Management Information Systems. *See also* management information system.

Society for Investigative Dermatology (SID) A national organization founded in 1937 composed of 2,300 members interested in research in dermatology and allied subjects. *See also* dermatology; research.

Society for Leukocyte Biology (A Reticuloendothelial Society) A national organization founded in 1954 composed of 1,025 persons holding Doctor of Medicine (MD) and/or Doctor of Philosophy (PhD) degrees who conduct research with universities; private, industrial and government institutes; hospital clinics; and members of the pharmaceutical industry, who are interested in the study of the reticuloendothelial system. Formerly (1988) Reticuloendothelial Society. *See also* reticuloendothelial system.

Society for Life History Research (SLHR) A national organization founded in 1970 composed of 700 individuals representing the disciplines of behavior genetics, medicine, statistics, psychology, psychiatry, and sociology, who are interested in psychopathology. Formerly (1984) Society for Life History Research in Psychopathology. *See also* abnormal psychology; psychiatry; statistics.

Society for Life History Research in Psychopathology *See* Society for Life History Research.

society, medical *See* medical society.

Society for Magnetic Resonance Imaging (SMRI) A national organization founded in 1982 composed of 1,700 physicians and basic scientists promoting the applications of magnetic resonance techniques to medicine and biology, with special emphasis on imaging. *See also* magnetic resonance imaging.

Society for Management Information Systems *See* Society for Information Management.

society, medical *See* medical society.

Society for Medical Anthropology (SMA) A unit of the American Anthropological Association concerned with the study of societies and cultures in relation to the practice of medicine. *See also* anthropology; medical.

Society of Medical Consultants to the Armed Forces (SMCAF) A national organization founded in 1945 composed of physicians and surgeons who have been in active military service and who have acted as consultants to the Surgeons General of the Army, Navy, or Air Force. Its purpose is to preserve and encourage the association of civilian consultants and military medical personnel and to assist in the development and maintenance of the high standards of medical practice in the Armed Forces. *See also* consultant.

Society of Medical Friends of Wine (SMFW) A national organization founded in 1939 composed of 330 physicians interested in the nutritional and therapeutic values of wine. It works to stimulate scientific research on wine.

Society of Medical Jurisprudence (SMJ) A national organization founded in 1883 composed of 300 physicians, lawyers, health professionals, chemists, and law and medical school professors interested in promoting the study and advancement of medical jurisprudence and high standards of medical expert testimony. *See also* expert witness; forensic medicine; jurisprudence.

Society for Menstrual Cycle Research (SMCR) A national organization founded in 1979 composed of 100 physicians, nurses, physiologists, psychologists, geneticists, sociologists, researchers, educators, and other individuals interested in the menstrual cycle. It identifies research priorities, recommends research strategies, and promotes interdisciplinary research on the menstrual cycle. *See also* menstruation; ovulation; premenstrual syndrome; research.

Society of Military Ophthalmologists (SMO) A national organization composed of 700 ophthalmologists on active duty in the military services or those who have retired or resigned from military service. Its purpose is to bring together ophthalmologists of the Army, Air Force, Navy, and US Public Health Service. *See also* ophthalmology.

Society of Military Orthopaedic Surgeons (SMOS) A national organization founded in 1958 composed of 600 orthopedic surgeons who have served in the active or reserve military. *See also* orthopaedic/orthopedic surgeon.

Society of Military Otolaryngologists - Head and Neck Surgeons (SMO-HNS) A national organization founded in 1952 composed of 256 otolaryngologists–head and neck surgeons of the US Army, Air Force, and Navy, and former active duty members. *See also* otolaryngologist-head and neck surgeon.

Society for Neuroscience (SN) A national organization founded in 1969 composed of 18,000 scientists who have done research relating to the nervous system. It seeks to advance understanding of the nervous system, including its relation to behavior, by bringing together scientists of various backgrounds and by facilitating integration of research directed at all levels of biological organization. It maintains a central source of information on interdisciplinary curricula and training programs in the neurosciences. *See also* nervous system; neuroscience.

Society of Neurosurgical Anesthesia and Critical Care (SNACC) A national organization founded in 1973 composed of 613 neurosurgeons and anesthesiologists interested in the care of patients with neurological disorders. *See also* anesthesiology; critical care medicine; neurological surgery.

Society of Nuclear Medicine (SNM) A national organization founded in 1954 composed of 12,000 physicians, physicists, chemists, radiopharmacists, nuclear medicine technologists, and other persons interested in nuclear medicine, nuclear magnetic resonance, and the use of radioactive isotopes in clinical practice, research, and teaching. *See also* nuclear medicine; radioisotope.

Society of Nuclear Medicine, Technologist Section of the *See* Technologist Section of the Society of Nuclear Medicine.

Society for Nutrition Education (SNE) A national organization founded in 1967 composed of 2,500 nutrition educators from the fields of dietetics, public health, home economics, medicine, industry, and education (elementary, secondary, college, university, and consumer affairs). *See also* dietetics; nutrition.

Society for Obstetric Anesthesia and Perinatology (SOAP) A national organization founded in 1969 composed of physicians and scientists interested in perinatal health care. It conducts specialized education programs and compiles statistics. *See also* anesthesia; obstetrics; perinatology.

Society for Occupational and Environmental Health (SOEH) A national organization founded in 1972 composed of 350 scientists, academicians, and industry and labor representatives interested in focusing public attention on scientific, social, and regulatory problems. It studies specific categories of hazards, methods for assessment of health effects, and diseases associated with particular jobs. It identifies hazards in the occupational and general environment and proposes actions to reduce their danger. *See also* environmental health; occupational health.

Society of Otorhinolaryngology and Head/Neck Nurses (SOHNN) A national organization found-

ed in 1976 composed of 1,000 registered nurses specializing in otorhinolaryngology and disorders of the head and neck. *See also* otolaryngology; registered nurse; rhinology.

Society for Pediatric Dermatology (SPD) A national organization founded in 1975 composed of 450 pediatricians, dermatologists, manufacturers of children's skin products, and researchers in biomedicine with studies in pediatric dermatology. *See also* dermatology; pediatrics.

Society for Pediatric Psychology (SPP) A section founded in 1968 of the American Psychological Association composed of 980 psychologists working in children's hospitals, developmental clinics, and pediatric and medical group practices. It fosters the development of theory, research, training, and professional practice in pediatric psychology and the application of psychology to medical and psychological problems of children, youths, and their families. It supports legislation benefiting children's health and welfare. *See also* American Psychological Association; pediatrics; psychology.

Society for Pediatric Radiology (SPR) A national organization founded in 1958 composed of 650 physicians working in the field of pediatric radiology. It seeks to improve pediatric imaging. *See also* pediatrics; radiology.

Society for Pediatric Research (SPR) A national organization founded in 1929 composed of 2,000 physicians and scientists under age 45 years who are engaged in research in diseases of infancy and childhood; those individuals over age 45 years are senior members. *See also* pediatrics; research.

Society for Pediatric Urology (SPU) A national organization founded in 1941 composed of 300 physicians who are specialists in urology and who have a special interest in the field of childhood urological problems. *See also* pediatrics; urology.

Society of Peripheral Vascular Nursing *See* Society for Vascular Nursing.

Society for Personality Assessment (SPA) A national organization founded in 1938 composed of 3,000 psychologists, behavioral scientists, anthropologists, and psychiatrists interested in the study and application of personality assessment. *See also* assessment; personality.

Society of Professional Business Consultants (SPBC) A national organization founded in 1956 composed of 200 persons engaged in rendering business consultant services to physicians and dentists. It provides members with educational information to upgrade their effectiveness as professionals. *See also* business; consultant.

Society of Professors of Child and Adolescent Psychiatry (SPCAP) A national organization founded in 1969 composed of 160 representatives from university psychiatric departments who meet annually to discuss issues in child and adolescent psychiatry. Formerly (1987) Society of Professors of Child Psychiatry. *See also* child and adolescent psychiatry; professor.

Society of Professors of Child Psychiatry *See* Society of Professors of Child and Adolescent Psychiatry.

Society of Prospective Medicine (SPM) A national organization founded in 1972 composed of 250 physicians, allied health professionals, scientists, and other individuals interested in extending the useful life expectancy of persons by identifying actual and potential health hazards and by developing and implementing risk assessment techniques and risk reduction programs. *See also* life expectancy; preventive medicine; risk assessment.

Society for the Psychological Study of Lesbian and Gay Issues (SPSLGI) A national organization founded in 1984 composed of 900 psychologists, graduate students in psychology, and other individuals interested in the psychological study of lesbian and gay issues and the delivery of mental health services to gay and lesbian individuals. *See also* gay; lesbianism; psychology.

Society for the Psychological Study of Social Issues (SPSSI) A national organization founded in 1936 composed of 3,000 psychologists, sociologists, anthropologists, psychiatrists, political scientists, and social workers interested in obtaining and disseminating to the public scientific knowledge about social change. *See also* psychology.

Society of Psychologists in Addictive Behaviors (SPAB) A national organization founded in 1975 composed of 600 psychologists and students in psychology interested in theoretical and clinical research, treatment, and prevention of addictive behaviors. *See also* addiction; addictive personality; behavior; psychology.

Society for Psychophysiological Research (SPR) A research organization founded in 1960 composed of 906 representatives from psychology, psychiatry,

physiology, medicine, and biomedical engineering interested in the interrelationship between behavioral and biological processes. It conducts research, including the evaluation of biofeedback in the treatment of disease states. *See also* biofeedback; physiology; psychology.

Society for Public Health Education (SOPHE) A national organization founded in 1950 composed of 1,200 professional workers in health education. It promotes and contributes to the advancement of public health by encouraging study and elevating standards of achievement in public health education. *See also* public health.

Society for Radiation Oncology Administrators (SROA) A national organization founded in 1984 composed of 500 individuals with managerial responsibilities in radiation oncology at the executive, divisional, or departmental level, whose functions include personnel, budget, and development of operational procedures and guidelines for therapeutic radiology departments. Its goals include improving the administration of the business and nonmedical management aspects of therapeutic radiology. Formerly (1985) Radiation Oncology Administrators. *See also* administrator; radiation oncology.

Society of Reproductive Endocrinologists (SRE) A national organization composed of 420 physicians with American Board of Obstetrics and Gynecology certification as reproductive endocrinologists who work to extend knowledge of human reproduction and endocrinology. *See also* American Board of Obstetrics and Gynecology; certification; endocrinology; reproduction; reproductive endocrinologist.

Society for Reproductive Surgeons (SRS) A national organization composed of 450 reproductive surgeons. It gathers and disseminates information on reproductive surgery and makes available a referrals list. *See also* reproduction; surgery.

Society for Research in Child Development (SRCD) A national organization founded in 1933 composed of 4,500 anthropologists, educators, nutritionists, pediatricians, physiologists, psychiatrists, psychologists, sociologists, and statisticians working to further research in child development. *See also* development.

Society for the Right to Die *See* Choice In Dying - The National Council for the Right to Die.

Society for the Scientific Study of Sex (SSSS) A

national organization founded in 1974 composed of 1,100 psychiatrists, psychologists, physicians, sociologists, anthropologists, social workers, demographers, criminologists, educators, attorneys, and other persons conducting sexual research. *See also* sex; research.

Society for Sex Therapy and Research (SSTAR) A national organization founded in 1974 composed of 300 university-affiliated social workers, researchers, and physicians interested in sex therapy and research. It provides a professional network for clinicians and researchers involved in the field of human sexuality and collects and disseminates information on current basic and clinical research related to human sexual matters. *See also* network; research; sex; sex therapy.

Society for the Study of Blood (SSB) A national organization founded in 1945 composed of 200 physicians and other scientists specializing in hematology, blood grouping, transfusion, and the study of physiology and pathology of blood. *See also* blood; blood transfusion; hematology.

Society for the Study of Breast Disease (SSBD) A national organization founded in 1976 composed of 250 physicians and nurses primarily engaged in the fields of obstetrics and gynecology, surgery, radiology, family practice, and medical and radiation oncology. It furthers the study of diseases of the breast and informs physicians and other health professionals of developments in the diagnosis and treatment of breast cancer and benign diseases of the breast. *See also* cancer; mammary gland.

Society for the Study of Male Psychology and Physiology (SSMPP) A national organization founded in 1975 composed of 180 psychologists, psychiatrists, biologists, and sociologists interested in the study of the behavior and physiology of men, in isolation and in relation to women. Its objectives are to conduct research and examine issues, such as social problems (crime, suicide, juvenile delinquency) and illnesses, that occur at significantly higher rates among males; factors accounting for the shorter life expectancy of males; the effects of the Y chromosome on male behavior; and male sex roles. *See also* physiology; psychology.

Society for the Study of Reproduction (SSR) A national organization founded in 1967 composed of 1,450 researchers in obstetrics and gynecology, urology, zoology, animal husbandry, and physiology,

and clinicians in human and veterinary medicine interested in promoting the study of reproduction by fostering interdisciplinary communication within the science. *See also* reproduction.

Society for the Study of Social Biology (SSSB) A national organization founded in 1926 composed of 400 geneticists, demographers, psychologists, physicians, psychiatrists, public health workers, educators, and sociologists interested in the study of heredity and populations. *See also* biology; heredity; population; social science.

Society for Surgery of the Alimentary Tract (SSAT) A national organization founded in 1960 composed of 1,117 physicians specializing in alimentary tract surgery. *See also* alimentary tract; surgery.

Society of Surgical Oncology (SSO) A national organization founded in 1940 composed of 980 physicians and scientists working in the field of cancer. It bestows an annual award to a medical resident who is performing an original research project and gives three cash awards with medals to an outstanding cancer basic scientist, clinical scientist, and contributing layman. *See also* cancer; oncology; surgery.

Society of Teachers of Family Medicine (STFM) A national organization founded in 1968 composed of 3,200 physicians involved in teaching or promoting of family medicine and other individuals in related fields. *See also* family medicine.

Society, Teratology *See* Teratology Society.

Society of Thoracic Radiology (STR) A national organization founded in 1983 composed of 200 radiologists interested in continuing medical education in thoracic radiology. *See also* radiology; thorax.

Society of Thoracic Surgeons (STS) A national organization founded in 1964 composed of 2,800 surgeons who confine their practice to the field of thoracic-cardiovascular surgery. *See also* thoracic surgery; thorax.

Society of Toxicologic Pathologists (STP) A national organization founded in 1971 composed of 500 toxicologic pathologists, veterinarians, and physicians interested in evaluating criteria and requirements applied to the interpretation of pathological changes produced by pharmacological, chemical, and environmental agents. *See also* medical toxicology; pathology.

Society of Toxicology (SOT) A national organization founded in 1961 composed of 3,000 persons who have conducted and published original investigations in some phase of toxicology and who have a continuing professional interest in this field. *See also* toxicology.

Society of United States Air Force Flight Surgeons A national organization founded in 1960 composed of 700 flight surgeons who are members of the Aerospace Medical Association and who are currently serving on active duty with, or have retired from, the United States Air Force or are serving in the Air Force Reserve or Air National Guard. It fosters advancement of aerospace medicine throughout the Air Force and encourages the clinical, laboratory, flight line, and in-flight investigation of medical problems in Air Force flying, missile, and space operations.

Society of University Otolaryngologists *See* Society of University Otolaryngologists-Head and Neck Surgeons.

Society of University Otolaryngologists - Head and Neck Surgeons (SUO-HNS) A national organization founded in 1964 composed of 380 otolaryngologists affiliated with universities through an approved residency training program, faculty appointment, or teaching or research position. It encourages basic research and clinical investigation as an integral part of university training programs. Formerly (1988) Society of University Otolaryngologists. *See also* otolaryngology; university.

Society of University Surgeons (SUS) A national organization founded in 1938 composed of 1,142 surgeons connected with university teaching. *See also* surgery; university.

Society of University Urologists (SUU) A national organization founded in 1967 composed of 400 urologists holding faculty or teaching positions in residency training programs. *See also* university; urology.

Society for Vascular Surgery (SVS) A national organization founded in 1945 composed of 500 board-certified surgeons interested in the study of and research in the circulatory system. *See also* circulatory system; vascular surgery.

Society for Vascular Nursing (SVN) A national organization founded in 1982 composed of 760 nurses and other health professionals providing care for persons with peripheral vascular disease. It seeks to educate the public about peripheral vascular dis-

ease, provides educational programs, and conducts research. Formerly (1992) Society of Peripheral Vascular Nursing. *See also* nursing; peripheral vascular disease.

Society of Vascular Technology (SVT) A national organization founded in 1977 composed of 4,300 medical technologists and other individuals in the field of noninvasive vascular technology. *See also* noninvasive vascular technology.

sociobiology The branch of theoretical biology that proposes that all human and other animals' behavior is controlled by the genes. *See also* biology; gene.

sociometry The quantitative study of interpersonal relationships in populations, especially the study and measurement of preferences. *See also* American Board of Examiners of Psychodrama, Sociometry, and Group Psychotherapy.

sociopath *See* psychopath.

Socrates (470?-399 BC) A Greek philosopher who initiated a question-and-answer method of teaching as a means of achieving self-knowledge. His theories of virtue and justice have survived through the writings of Plato, one of his pupils. *See also* Socratic irony; Socratic method.

Socratic irony The use of professing ignorance and willingness to learn when a person interrogates another person on the meaning of a term. *See also* Socrates; Socratic method.

Socratic method the use of Socratic irony in a discussion that results in either a mutual confession of ignorance with a promise of further investigation or in the elicitation of a truth assumed to be innate in all rational human beings. *See also* Socrates; Socratic irony.

sodomy Anal intercourse between one male and another, between members of opposite sexes, or between a human and an animal. *See also* sexual intercourse.

SOEH *See* Society for Occupational and Environmental Health.

SOFT *See* Society of Forensic Toxicologists.

soft sell A subtly persuasive, low-pressure method of selling or advertising, as in the pharmaceutical drug representative's soft sell of the new drugs. *Compare* hard sell. *See also* advertise.

soft market *See* buyer' market.

software *See* computer software.

software, accounting *See* accounting software.

software, communications *See* on-line searching.

software, computer *See* computer software.

software, GROUPER *See* GROUPER software.

software, speech recognition *See* speech recognition software.

software, spelling checker *See* spelling checker software.

software, system *See* system software.

SOHNN *See* Society of Otorhinolaryngology and Head/Neck Nurses.

solicitor A lawyer employed by a governmental body in the United States. *See also* barrister; lawyer; solicitor general.

solicitor general The title for a chief law officer when there is no attorney general, or for the chief assistant to the law officer when there is an attorney general. *See also* lawyer; solicitor.

solo practice Practice of a health professional as a self-employed individual. Solo practice is by definition private practice but is not necessarily a fee-for-service practice (solo practitioners may be paid by capitation, although fee for service is more common). Solo practice is common among physicians, dentists, podiatrists, optometrists, and pharmacists. *Synonym:* individual practice. *See also* private practice.

solution **1.** A homogeneous mixture of two or more substances, as in Ringer's solution. *See also* Ringer's solution. **2.** The method or process of solving a problem. *See also* problem solving. **3.** The answer to a problem.

solution, Ringer's *See* Ringer's solution.

solving, problem *See* problem solving.

somatic Pertaining to the body as contrasted to the mind, for example, a somatic complaint about abdominal pain. *Compare* mind; psychosomatic.

somatotherapy Treatment of mental illness by physical means, such as drugs, electroconvulsive (shock) therapy, or lobotomy. *See also* electroconvulsive therapy; mental illness; prefrontal lobotomy; psychosurgery.

somnolent *See* consciousness.

somnology The study of sleep and sleep disorders. *See also* sleep; sleep apnea.

Somnology, American Academy of *See* American Academy of Somnology.

sonogram An image produced by ultrasonography; for example, a sonogram of a fetus or kidney. *Synonyms:* echogram; sonograph; ultrasonogram; ultrasound image. *See also* ultrasound imaging.

sonograph *See* sonogram.

sonographer, diagnostic medical *See* diagnostic medical sonographer.

Sonographers, American Registry of Diagnostic Medical *See* American Registry of Diagnostic Medical Sonographers.

Sonographers, Society of Diagnostic Medical *See* Society of Diagnostic Medical Sonographers.

sonography *See* ultrasound imaging.

Sonography, Joint Review Committee on Education in Diagnostic Medical *See* Joint Review Committee on Education in Diagnostic Medical Sonography.

sonometer *See* audiometer.

SOPHE *See* Society for Public Health Education.

sophist An individual skilled in elaborate and plausible, but devious, argumentation. *See also* sophistry.

sophistry A seemingly plausible, but fallacious and devious, argumentation. *See also* sophist.

sore **1.** Painful to the touch. **2.** Any circumscribed area of skin or mucous membrane that is tender, injured, ulcerated, or otherwise diseased, as in canker sore, cold sore, or pressure sore. *See also* canker sore; pressure sore.

sore, canker *See* canker sore.

sore, cold *See* herpes simplex.

sore, pressure *See* pressure sore.

SOT *See* Society of Toxicology.

soul The animating and vital nature of human beings, credited with the faculties of thought, action, and emotion and often conceived as an immaterial entity. *See also* soul-searching.

soul-searching The process of examining one's motives, convictions, and attitudes. *See also* soul.

sound **1.** A physiological sensation received by the ear, generated by a vibrating source transmitted through an elastic material or a solid, liquid, or gas. *See also* noise; pitch. **2.** In linguistics, an articulation made by the vocal apparatus. *See also* voice.

sound bite A short extract from a recorded interview or speech used for maximum impact on listeners or viewer as part of a news broadcast. *See also* media.

sounding board A person or group whose reactions to an idea, opinion, or point of view will serve as a measure of its effectiveness, appropriateness, or acceptability.

sound pollution *See* noise pollution.

source The point from which something derives or

is obtained, as patient admission source. *See also* admission source; data source; source document.

source, admission *See* admission source.

source book A primary document, as of history, literature, or religion, on which secondary writings are based. *See also* source.

source, data *See* data source.

source document An original record, usually written or typed on paper and used as a data source; for example, a medical record. *See also* document.

sovereign immunity A doctrine prohibiting the institution of a lawsuit against the sovereign (government) without the sovereign's consent. The doctrine was originally based on the maxim "the king can do no wrong." The sovereign is also exempt from suit on the practical ground that there can be no legal rights against the authority that creates the laws on which rights depend. The state may nevertheless be held liable when the injurious activity was "proprietary" (commercial) rather than "governmental." *See also* governmental functions; immunity; lawsuit.

SOW *See* PRO scope of work.

spa A mineral water resort or mineral spring. *See also* massage.

SPA *See* Society for Personality Assessment.

SPAB *See* Society of Psychologists in Addictive Behaviors.

space cadet **1.** A person who has difficulty in grasping reality or in responding appropriately to it. *See also* spaced-out. **2.** A person who demonstrates immature behavior.

spaced-out Stupefied or disoriented, as if from a drug, as in she seemed spaced-out after watching television. *See also* culture shock; space cadet.

space medicine The branch of medicine that deals with the biological, physiological, and psychological effects of space flight on human beings. *See also* medicine.

space sickness Motion sickness causes by sustained weightlessness during space flight. *See also* sickness.

spasm Sustained involuntary contraction of a muscle or group of muscles, as in muscle spasm, or sustained constriction of a small vessel or other channel, as in coronary artery spasm.

SPBC *See* Society of Professional Business Consultants.

SPC *See* statistical process control.

SPCS *See* Statistical Process Control Society.

SPCAP *See* Society of Professors of Child and Adolescent Psychiatry.

SPD *See* Society for Pediatric Dermatology.

special analysis unit A special section of the department of accreditation decision processing of the Joint Commission on Accreditation of Healthcare Organizations that is responsible for analysis of survey reports requiring expeditious turnaround, including denial of accreditation reports, conditional accreditation reports, validation survey reports, follow-up survey reports, and unscheduled or unannounced survey reports. *See also* accreditation; conditional accreditation; Joint Commission on Accreditation of Healthcare Organizations; survey report.

special care unit In hospitals, an organized service area with a concentration of professional staff and supportive resources established to provide intensive care continuously on a 24-hour basis to critically ill patients. Such units include general intensive care medical/surgical units and other types of units that provide specialized intensive care (for example, burn and neonatal intensive care). *See also* intensive care unit; medical intensive care unit; neonatal intensive care unit; pediatric intensive care unit; surgical intensive care unit; unit.

special cause A factor that intermittently and unpredictably induces variation over and above that inherent in the system. It often appears as an extreme point, such as a point beyond the control limits on a control chart, or some specific, identifiable pattern in data. *Synonyms*: assignable cause; exogenous cause; extrasystemic cause. *Compare* common cause. *See also* control chart; special-cause variation; variation.

special-cause and common-cause systems of variation The collection of variables that produces both common-cause variation and special-cause variation and the interaction of those variables. *See also* common-cause variation; special-cause variation; variable; variation.

special-cause variation The variation in performance and data that results from special causes. Special-cause variation is intermittent, unpredictable, and unstable. It is not inherently present in a system; rather, it arises from causes that are not part of the system as designed. It tends to cluster by person, place, and time, and should be eliminated by an organization if it results in undesirable outcomes. *Synonyms*: assignable-cause variation; exogenous-cause variation; extrasystemic-cause variation. *Compare* common-cause variation. *See also* process variation; special cause; tampering; variation.

Special Constituency Section for Aging and Long Term Care Services A national organization founded in 1969 composed of 2,200 hospitals that are members of the American Hospital Association and have long term care units or community-based long term care and special services for the aging. Formerly (1987) Special Constituency Section on Aging and Long Term Care. *See also* American Hospital Association; long term care.

Special Constituency Section for Mental Health and Psychiatric Services *See* Special Constituency Section for Psychiatric and Substance Abuse Services.

Special Constituency Section for Psychiatric and Substance Abuse Services A division of the American Hospital Association (AHA) composed of 3,000 long-term and short-term care institutional members providing psychiatric, substance abuse, mental retardation, and other mental health services. It assists the AHA in development and implementation of policies and programs promoting hospital-based mental health and psychiatric services. Formerly (1991) Special Constituency Section for Mental Health and Psychiatric Services. *See also* substance abuse.

special damages *See* consequential damages.

special-function laboratory A laboratory not under the jurisdiction of a main laboratory in a health care organization, such as a hospital. Special-function laboratories are sometimes focused on a discrete testing procedure, such as blood gas determination. *See also* blood gas determination; clinical laboratory; hematology laboratory; laboratory.

special interest A person, a group, or an organization formed to influence legislators in favor of one particular interest or issue. *Synonym*: special-interest group. *See also* pressure group; public interest group.

special-interest group *See* special interest.

Special Interest Group, Behavioral Neuropsychology *See* Behavioral Neuropsychology Special Interest Group.

Special Interest Group on Biomedical Computing (SIGBIO) A special-interest group of the Association for Computing Machinery founded in 1967 composed of 1,006 biological, medical, behavioral, and computer scientists; hospital administrators; programmers and other individuals interested in the application of computer methods to biological, behavioral, and medical problems. *See also* Association for Computing Machinery.

specialist 1. Anyone with extensive knowledge of a small area. *Compare* generalist. **2.** In health care, a person who is devoted to a particular profession or branch of study or research, as in a physician, dentist, podiatrist, or other health professional who limits his or her practice to a certain branch of medicine, dentistry, podiatric medicine, or other health science. Specialties frequently correspond to specific services or procedures provided (for example, anesthesiology, radiology, pathology); age categories of patients (such as pediatrics); body systems (for example, gastroenterology, orthopedics, cardiology); or types of diseases (for example, allergy, periodontics). Specialists usually have special education and training relating to their practice and may or may not be certified as a specialist by the related specialty board. *Synonym*: specialty care practitioner. *Compare* generalist. *See also* board certified; board prepared; certification; clinical nurse specialist; dentist, specialist; medical specialist; podiatric specialist; subspecialist.

specialist, allied health *See* allied health professional.

specialist in blood bank technology (SBBT) An allied health professional who performs both routine and specialized tests in blood bank immunohematology in technical areas of the modern blood bank and performs transfusion services using methodology that conforms to the *Standards for Blood Banks and Transfusion Services* of the American Association of Blood Banks. Specialists in blood bank technology specifically test for blood group antigens, compatibility, and antibody identification; investigate abnormalities, such as hemolytic disease of the newborn, hemolytic anemias, and adverse responses to transfusion; support physicians in transfusion therapy, including for patients with clotting disorders or candidates for homologous organ transplant; and collect and process blood, including selecting donors, drawing and typing blood, and performing pretransfusion tests to ensure the safety of the patient. Specialists in blood bank technology are one type of allied health professional for which the Committee on Allied Health Education and

Accreditation has accredited education programs. *Synonym*: blood bank technologist. *See also* allied health professional; blood bank.

specialist, blood banking   *See* blood banking specialist.

specialist, certified coding   *See* certified coding specialist.

specialist, child life   *See* child life specialist.

specialist, clinical nurse   *See* clinical nurse specialist.

specialist, dental   *See* dentist, specialist.

specialist, dentist   *See* dentist, specialist.

specialist, maternal-fetal medicine   *See* maternal-fetal medicine specialist.

specialist, medical   *See* medical specialist.

specialist, neonatal-perinatal medicine   *See* neonatal-perinatal medicine specialist.

specialist, nurse practitioner   *See* nurse practitioner.

specialist, nurse   *See* clinical nurse specialist.

specialist, pediatric critical care   *See* pediatric critical care specialist.

specialist, pediatric infectious disease   *See* pediatric infectious disease specialist.

specialist, pediatric sports medicine   *See* pediatric sports medicine specialist.

specialist, physical medicine   *See* physiatrist.

specialist, podiatric   *See* podiatric specialist.

specialist, reimbursement   *See* reimbursement specialist.

Specialists, American Association of Osteopathic   *See* American Association of Osteopathic Specialists.

Specialists, Council of Rehabilitation   *See* Council of Rehabilitation Specialists.

specialist, sub-   *See* subspecialist.

specialize   To concentrate or pursue a special activity, profession, occupation, or field of study, as in specializing in internal medicine or surgery. *See also* specialist; specialty.

specialized care   *See* secondary care.

special survey   Any survey conducted by the Joint Commission on Accreditation of Healthcare Organizations at an accredited health care organization that is not classified as a triennial, focused, initial, follow-up, or conditional validation survey; it may be conducted anytime during the organization's accreditation cycle. *See also* accreditation survey; Joint Commission on Accreditation of Healthcare Organizations.

specialized survey   A survey conducted by the Joint Commission on Accreditation of Healthcare Organizations in which a surveyor with specific knowledge and experience is added to the core survey team for an accreditation survey of a health care organization; for example, adding a Mental Health Care Accreditation Program surveyor to survey a health care organization's alcohol and other drug dependence program. *See also* accreditation survey; Joint Commission on Accreditation of Healthcare Organizations.

Specialties, American Board of Medical   *See* American Board of Medical Specialties.

specialties, dental   *See* dental specialties.

specialties, medical   *See* medical specialties.

specialties, nursing   *See* nursing specialties.

specialties, podiatric   *See* podiatric specialties.

specialties, surgical   *See* surgical specialties.

specialty   **1.** The field or practice of a specialist, as in a branch of medicine, dentistry, podiatric medicine, nursing, or other health profession in which a doctor, dentist, podiatrist, nurse, or other health professional specializes. *See also* dental specialties; medical specialties; nursing specialties; podiatric specialties; subspecialty; surgical specialties. **2.** A special feature or characteristic, such as a specialty bed or specialty hospital. *See also* specialty boards.

specialty association   *See* specialty societies.

specialty bed   A bed regularly maintained for a specific category of patients, as in an intensive care unit bed or an inpatient pediatric bed. *See also* bed; specialty.

specialty board examination   A written and/or an oral examination given by a specialty board to prepared (eligible) professionals who wish to become certified specialists. *Synonym*: specialty boards. *See also* board certified; board prepared; certification; examination; specialty boards.

specialty boards   **1.** Private, nongovernmental, voluntary bodies that certify physicians, nurses, dentists, pharmacists, podiatrists, and other health professionals who are specialists or subspecialists in medical, nursing, dental, pharmacy, podiatric, and other health fields. The standards for certification relate to length and type of training and experience and may include written and oral examination of applicants for certification. The boards are not educational institutions and the certificate of a board is not considered a degree. Examples of specialty boards are the American Board of Emergency Medicine, American Board of Dental Public Health, American Board of Neuroscience Nursing, and American Board of Podiatric Orthopedics. *See also* board certified; board prepared; certification; medical specialty boards. **2.** *See* specialty board examination.

specialty boards, medical   *See* medical specialty boards.

specialty care practitioner   *See* specialist.

specialty group practice, single-   *See* single-specialty group practice.

specialty hospital   A type of hospital that provides services to patients with specified medical conditions (such as cancer) or special categories of patients (such as women or children). *See also* hospital; specialty.

Specialty Nursing Organizations, National Federation for   *See* National Federation for Specialty Nursing Organizations.

specialty societies   Voluntary membership organizations of physicians, administrators, dentists, nurses, physician assistants, or any other category of professionals involved in health care, including, for example, American Medical Society, American Hospital Association, and American Nurses Association. Traditional activities of specialty societies include providing public information on the field; conducting government liaison activities; conducting educational and training programs; developing standards and guidelines; and sponsoring research. *See also* medical association; medical society.

specialty, sub-   *See* subspecialty.

specification   **1.** A detailed, exact statement of particulars prescribing the requirements with which a product or service has to conform; for example, a document prescribing materials, dimensions, and quality of work for something to be built, installed, or manufactured. **2.** A requirement for judging the acceptability of a particular characteristic of a product (a good or a service). Chosen with respect to functional or customer requirements for the product, a specification may or may not be consistent with the demonstrated capability of a process. A specification should not be confused with a control limit. *See also* control limit; job specification.

specification, job   *See* job specification.

specify   To state explicitly or in detail, as in specifying the amount of medicine needed. *See also* specification.

specificity of a test   A measure of the ability of a diagnostic test, a screening test, or other predictor to correctly identify the individuals or cases *not* having the condition being tested for, who are correctly identified as negative by the test. Operationally, specificity is the number of negative test results divided by the number of individuals or cases who actually do not have the condition (true negatives divided by the sum of true negatives plus false positives). *Synonym:* true negative rate. *Compare* sensitivity of a test. *See also* false positive; test; true negative.

specified disease insurance   Insurance that provides benefits, usually in large amounts or with high maximums, toward the expense of the treatment of a specific disease or diseases named in the policy. Coverage for diseases, such as polio and end-stage renal disease under Medicare, are examples of specified disease insurance. *See also* disease; insurance; Medicare.

spectacles   Frame-mounted lenses that correct refractive errors of vision or reduce the amount of light reaching the eye. *Synonyms:* eyeglasses; glasses. *See also* lens; ophthalmology; opticianry; optometry.

speculum   An instrument used to expose the interior of a passage or cavity of the body by enlarging the opening, as in a nasal speculum, a vaginal speculum, or a speculum for an otoscope.

speech   The utterance of vocal sounds codified into meaningful language. *See also* cued speech; deaf-mute; language; phonation; speech dysfunction.

speech, cued   *See* cued speech.

speech dysfunction   Any abnormality of speech, such as aphasia (loss of expression or comprehension of speech or written language), alexia (inability to comprehend written language), stammering, stuttering, aphonia (loss of speech), and slurring. Speech problems may develop from many sources, including neurologic injury to the cerebral cortex; muscular paralysis because of trauma, disease, or cerebrovascular accident; structural abnormality of the organs of speech; emotional or psychologic tension, strain, or depression, hysteria; and severe mental retardation. *See also* dysfunction; hysteria; phonation; speech.

Speech and Hearing, Computer Users in   *See* Computer Users in Speech and Hearing.

speech and hearing therapy aide   A person who assists speech pathologists and audiologists in testing, evaluating, and treating patients or clients with speech, hearing, and language disorders. *See also* aide; audiologist; speech pathologist.

Speech-Language-Hearing Association, American *See* American Speech-Language-Hearing Association.

speech-language pathologist *See* speech pathologist.

Speech-Language Pathology and Audiology, Council on Professional Standards in *See* Council on Professional Standards in Speech-Language Pathology and Audiology.

speech pathologist A health professional who specializes in the measurement and evaluation of language abilities, auditory processes, and speech production; clinical treatment of children and adults with speech, language, and hearing disorders; and research methods in the study of communication processes. *Synonym:* speech-language pathologist. *See also* audiologist; speech therapist.

speech pathology The study or diagnosis and treatment of disturbances of articulation, phonation, and language function (for example, aphasia) or speech disturbances due to psychiatric illness. *See also* audiology; pathology; speech; speech dysfunction; speech therapy.

speech recognition software A program in which verbal commands activate the microcomputer to perform functions, such as word processing. *See also* computer software.

speech technology *See* voice input/output technology.

speech therapist A person trained in the application and use of techniques aimed at improving language and speech disorders. *See also* language; speech; speech pathology; speech therapy.

speech therapy The study, examination, appreciation, and treatment of defects and diseases of the voice, of speech and of spoken and written language, as well as the use of appropriate substitutional devices and treatment. *See also* speech pathology.

spelling checker software Software available on some word processing programs that reads through a document looking for misspelled words, stopping at words recognized as misspelled, and allowing the user to make corrections. *See also* computer software.

spend down A method by which an individual establishes eligibility for a health care program, such as Medicaid, by reducing gross income through incurring medical expenses until net income after medical expenses becomes low enough to make him or her eligible for the program. *See also* Medicaid.

sperm *See* semen; spermatozoa.

spermatozoa Male gametes or germ cells, the essential component of semen. *See also* ovum; reproduction; semen; testis.

sperm banking Storing sperm for future use to produce a child. *See also* bank; ova banking; sperm; zygote banking.

sphincter A circular muscle guarding the orifice of an organ and controlling passage through it, as in anal sphincter.

sphygmomanometer An instrument for measuring blood pressure in the arteries, especially one consisting of a pressure gauge and a rubber cuff that wraps around an extremity and is inflated to constrict the arteries. *See also* blood pressure.

spica A spiral, figure-of-eight bandage, so called because of its resemblance to an ear of barley, applied to anatomical features of differing dimensions, such as the thumb and the hand; for example, a thumb spica cast. *See also* cast; emergency medicine; orthopaedic/orthopedic surgery; splint.

spin 1. A distinctive complex of connotations or implications inherent in a point of view. 2. Interpretation promulgated to sway public opinion. *See also* spin control; spin doctor.

spinal anesthesia *See* regional anesthesia.

spinal cord The thick, whitish cord of nerve tissue that extends from the brain down through the spinal column and from which the spinal nerves branch off to various parts of the body. The cord is surrounded by three protective membranes, or meninges, called the pia mater, the arachnoid, and the dura mater. *See also* central nervous system; lumbar puncture; meninges; myelogram.

Spinal Cord Injury Nurses, American Association of *See* American Association of Spinal Cord Injury Nurses.

Spinal Cord Injury Psychologists and Social Workers, American Association of *See* American Association of Spinal Cord Injury Psychologists and Social Workers.

Spinal Injury Association, American *See* American Spinal Injury Association.

spinal meningitis *See* meningitis.

spinal puncture *See* lumbar puncture.

Spinal Stress Research Society *See* Precision Chiropractic Research Society.

Spinal Surgeons, American Academy of *See* American Academy of Spinal Surgeons.

Spinal Surgery, American Board of *See* American Board of Spinal Surgery.

spinal tap *See* lumbar puncture.

spin control Efforts made to ensure a favorable interpretation of speech and actions, as performed especially by politicians and their spin doctors. *See also* spin; spin doctor.

spin doctor A representative who publicizes favorable interpretations of another person's words or actions, as in the politician's many spin doctors. *See also* spin; spin control.

spine The spinal column (backbone), the distinguishing characteristic of vertebrates. *See also* kyphosis; lordosis; scoliosis.

spineless Lacking courage or willpower, as in a spineless leader.

Spine Society, North American *See* North American Spine Society.

spirometer An instrument for measuring the volume of air taken in and out by the lungs during breathing. *See also* asthma; emphysema; peak flow meter; pulmonary medicine.

splint Any device for immobilizing part of the body. *See also* cast; spica.

splinter **1.** A sharp, slender piece of wood, glass, metal or other material, split or broken off a main body. **2.** Any entity that has broken off a main body, as in splinter group. *See also* splinter group.

splinter group A group, such as political faction or medical faction, that has broken away from a parent group. *See also* group; splinter.

split-half reliability A technique of dividing items in a test into two parts (such as odd and even numbered items), scoring the two parts separately, calculating the coefficient of correlation between the two parts, and performing a statistical adjustment known as the Spearman-Brown correction formula. The result informs a researcher whether the two sets of items are measuring the same thing. *See also* correlation coefficient; reliability; reliability testing; statistics.

split personality *See* multiple personality.

SPM *See* Society of Prospective Medicine.

spokesman *See* spokesperson.

spokesperson A person who speaks on behalf of another person or group. *See also* person.

spokeswoman *See* spokesperson.

sponge **1.** A gauze pad used during surgery to absorb blood and other secretions. It is referred to by size, as in "four by four" (that is, four inches by four inches), or use, as in a laparotomy sponge (a sponge used during a laparotomy). **2.** Porous plastics, rubber, cellulose, or other materials used for bathing, cleaning, and other purposes. **3.** A small absorbent contraceptive pad that contains a spermicide and is placed against the cervix of the uterus before sexual intercourse. *See also* contraception; sexual intercourse.

sponge bath A bath in which the bather is washed with a wet sponge or washcloth without being immersed in water. *See also* bath; sponge.

sponge count A count conducted during a surgical operation and immediately before closure of the surgical incision that compares the number of sponges placed in the surgical field with the number of sponges (used and unused) remaining. *See also* sponge; surgery.

sponsor A person who assumes responsibility for another person or a group during a period of instruction, apprenticeship, or probation; for example, a member of an organization's leadership who serves as an advocate or champion for a process improvement, assists in securing resources, and gives guidance to the effort.

sponsored malpractice insurance A malpractice insurance plan that involves an agreement by a professional society (such as a state medical society) to sponsor a particular insurer's medical malpractice insurance coverage and to cooperate with the insurer in the administration of the coverage. The cooperation may include participation in marketing, claims review, and review of ratemaking. Until 1975, this was the predominant approach to coverage. Since then, sponsored malpractice insurance has been replaced by professional society-operated plans, joint underwriting associations, state insurance funds, and other arrangements. *See also* insurance; medical malpractice insurance.

spontaneous abortion An abortion occurring naturally; a miscarriage. *See also* abortion; miscarriage.

spontaneous delivery The birth of an infant without any mechanical, pharmacologic, or medical assistance. *See also* delivery.

spooling A process of storing computer output

before sending it to the printer, permitting the computer to be used for other purposes. *See also* computer.

sporadic Occurring at scattered, irregular, and unpredictable intervals, as in sporadic attendance at required meetings. *See also* continuous; frequent; intermittent; occasional; periodic.

Sport and Physical Activity, North American Society for the Psychology of *See* North American Society for the Psychology of Sport and Physical Activity.

Sports Dentistry, Academy for *See* Academy for Sports Dentistry.

sports medicine The branch of medicine and subspecialty of emergency medicine, family practice, internal medicine, and pediatrics dealing with promotion of wellness and the prevention of injury during physical exercise, either as an individual or in team participation. *See also* medicine; orthopaedic/orthopedic surgery; pediatric sports medicine.

Sports Medicine, American Academy of Podiatric *See* American Academy of Podiatric Sports Medicine.

Sports Medicine, American College of *See* American College of Sports Medicine.

Sports Medicine, American Orthopaedic Society for *See* American Orthopaedic Society for Sports Medicine.

Sports Medicine, American Osteopathic Academy of *See* American Osteopathic Academy of Sports Medicine.

sports medicine, pediatric *See* pediatric sports medicine.

sports medicine physician A physician specializing in sports medicine. *See also* sports medicine.

Sports Medicine and Science, Joint Commission on *See* Joint Commission on Sports Medicine and Science.

Sports Music Institute of America, Medical and *See* Medical and Sports Music Institute of America.

Sports Physicians, American Academy of *See* American Academy of Sports Physicians.

SPP *See* Society for Pediatric Psychology.

SPR *See* Society for Pediatric Radiology; Society for Pediatric Research; Society for Psychophysiological Research.

sprain A joint injury that results in partial rupture of one or more of the supporting ligaments. *See also* joint.

spread sheet **1.** An accounting or bookkeeping program for a computer. **2.** A display characterized by multiple columns and rows that a spreadsheet program allows to be printed. *See also* computer.

SPSLGI *See* Society for the Psychological Study of Lesbian and Gay Issues.

SPSSI *See* Society for Psychological Study of Social Issues.

SPU *See* Society for Pediatric Urology.

spurious Lacking authenticity or validity in origin, as in a spurious result.

sputum Matter consisting primarily of pus and mucus, ejected from the respiratory tract as a product of coughing or hawking. Expectoration of sputum indicates inflammation of the lungs, bronchi, or trachea. *See also* bronchitis; inflammation.

SQC *See* statistical quality control.

squander To spend wastefully or extravagantly, as in squandering resources. *See also* rework.

squint *See* strabismus.

SRCD *See* Society for Research in Child Development.

SRE *See* Society of Reproductive Endocrinologists; Society for Reproductive Surgeons.

SRF *See* survey report form.

SRHP *See* Section for Rehabilitation Hospitals and Programs.

SROA *See* Society for Radiation Oncology Administrators.

SRS *See* Sleep Research Society; Society for Reproductive Surgeons.

SRSO *See* Scoliosis Research Society.

SSA *See* Social Security Administration.

SSAT *See* Society for Surgery of the Alimentary Tract.

SSB *See* Society for the Study of Blood.

SSBD *See* Society for the Study of Breast Disease.

SSI *See* supplemental security income.

SSMPP *See* Society for the Study of Male Psychology and Physiology.

SSO *See* Society of Surgical Oncology.

SSR *See* Society for the Study of Reproduction.

SSRH *See* General Constituency Section for Small or Rural Hospitals.

SSSB *See* Society for the Study of Social Biology.

SSSS *See* Society for the Scientific Study of Sex.

SSTAR *See* Society for Sex Therapy and Research.

stability Constancy of purpose, steadfastness; resistance to undesired change. *See also* change.

stacked bar graph   A bar graph in which each bar is divided into several segments. The bars are classified by one variable and the segments represent the values of a second classification variable. Because the segments are placed end-to-end on top of each other, the total height of the bar represents the sum of the categories for the second variable within each category for the first variable. *See also* bar graph; variable.

staff   **1.** The personnel of an organization, as in hospital staff. **2.** Personnel who perform a specific enterprise, as in medical staff, nursing staff, or administrative staff. *See also* hospital staff; housestaff; medical staff; nursing staff.

staff of Aesculapius   A rod or staff with a snake entwined around it, commonly appearing in the ancient representations of Aesculapius, the god of medicine. It is a well-recognized symbol of medicine. *See also* Aesculapius; symbol.

staff authority   The authority to advise, but not to direct, other managers. *See also* authority; manager.

staff bylaws, medical   *See* medical staff bylaws.

staff, chief of   *See* chief of staff.

staff, closed   *See* closed staff.

staff, closed medical   *See* closed medical staff.

staff credentialing, medical   *See* credentialing.

staff development program   An ongoing educational program for improving the knowledge and skills of a health care organization's personnel. It may involve in-service training of hospital employees in areas, such as infection control and patient rights, and may also include cooperative education programs with colleges and tuition-and-books reimbursement for job-related training and education. *See also* program; staff.

staff executive committee, medical   *See* medical staff executive committee.

staff, hospital   *See* hospital staff.

staff, house-   *See* housestaff.

staffing   In health care, the analysis and identification of a health care organization's human resource requirements, recruitment of persons to meet these requirements, and initial placement of those persons to ensure adequate numbers, knowledge, and skills to perform the organization's work. *See also* human resources; staff; staffing ratio.

staffing ratio   The total number of full-time equivalent employees in a defined unit or facility divided by its average daily patient census. *See also* average daily census; full-time equivalent; ratio; staffing.

staff, medical   *See* medical staff.

staff model HMO   A health maintenance organization (HMO) that delivers health services through a physician group that is controlled by the HMO entity. *See also* health maintenance organization.

staff nurse   A registered nurse who is responsible for assessing, planning, implementing, and evaluating the care of designated patients. *Synonym*: general duty nurse. *See also* nurse; registered nurse.

staff, nursing   *See* nursing staff.

staff, open   *See* open staff.

staff, open medical   *See* open staff.

staff, organized   *See* organized professional staff.

staff, organized medical   *See* organized professional staff.

staff, organized professional   *See* organized professional staff.

staff, physician member of the medical   *See* physician member of the medical staff.

staff president, medical   *See* chief of staff; president of the medical staff.

staff, president of the medical   *See* president of the medical staff.

staff privileges   *See* admitting privileges.

Staff Services, National Association Medical   *See* National Association Medical Staff Services.

staff, support   *See* support staff.

stage   A period or distinct phase in the course of a disease or condition, as in the third stage of labor or the primary stage of cancer. *See also* staging.

staging   The determination of the distinct phases or periods in the course of a disease, the life history of an organism, or any biological process; for example, the classification of cancer according to the anatomical extent of the tumor (primary neoplasm, regional lymph nodes, metastases). Staging in cancers is important in determining both treatment and prognosis. *Synonyms*: disease staging; staging of disease. *See also* American Joint Committee on Cancer pathologic stage classification system; disease; stage.

staging of disease   *See* staging.

stain   **1.** A reagent or dye used for staining microscopic specimens, as in Gram's stain. *See also* Gram's stain. **2.** To treat specimens for the microscope with a reagent or dye that makes visible certain structures without affecting other structures. *See also* cytopathology; histochemistry.

Stain Commission, Biological   *See* Biological Stain

Commission.

stain, Gram's *See* Gram's stain.

standard A statement of expectation concerning a degree or level of requirement, excellence, or attainment in quality or performance. A standard may be used as a criterion or acknowledged measure of comparison for quantitative or qualitative value. Conformity or compliance with standards is usually a condition of licensure, accreditation, and payment for services. In health care organizations, a standard is a statement of expectation that defines the processes that must be substantially in place in a health organization to enhance the quality of care and entitle the organization, in the aggregate, to achieve accreditation, as from the Joint Commission on Accreditation of Healthcare Organizations. *See also* accreditation; benchmark; calibration; licensure; measure; outcome standard; patient-centered standards; process standard; structural standard; tolerance; yardstick.

standard-bearer An outstanding leader or representative of a movement or an organization, for example, Motorola as a standard-bearer for quality in goods and services.

standard of care The level of conduct against which one's acts are measured to determine liability; in negligence law, that degree of care which a reasonably prudent person should exercise in the same or similar circumstances. In medical malpractice cases, a standard of care is applied to measure the competence of the professional(s) providing that care. The traditional standard for physicians is that they exercise the average degree of skill, care, and diligence exercised by members of the same profession, practicing in the same or a similar locality in light of the present state of medical and surgical science. With increased specialization, however, certain courts have disregarded geographical considerations holding that in the practice of a board-certified medical specialty, the standard should be that of a reasonable specialist practicing medicine in the same specialty field. *See also* board certified; legal malpractice; liability; locality rule; malpractice; medical specialties; national standard rule; specialist.

standard, criterion *See* criterion standard.

standard deviation (SD) A measure of variability that indicates the dispersion, spread, or variation in a distribution. The standard deviation has a constant relationship with the area under a normal curve and is equal to the square root of the arithmetic mean of the squares of the deviations from the mean; denoted by the Greek letter sigma for the estimated standard deviation. *See also* coefficient of variation; distribution; sigma; variance.

standard error The standard deviations of the sample in a frequency distribution, obtained by dividing the standard deviation by the total number of cases in the frequency distribution. *See also* error; distribution; standard deviation.

standard, gold *See* gold standard.

Standard for Hospitals, Minimum *See* Minimum Standard for Hospitals.

standard, intent of *See* intent of standard.

standardization The process or act of standardizing. *See also* adjustment; standardize.

standardize To cause to conform to a standard, as in the hospital standardization movement of the early twentieth century or a standardized test. *See also* standard; standardized test.

standardized test An examination for which average levels of performance have been established and which has shown consistent results. In addition, uniform methods of administering and scoring the test must have been developed. Standardized tests are used to help measure abilities, aptitudes, interests, and personality traits. For example, most students who plan to attend medical school take a standardized test called the Medical College Admission Test during their junior or senior year in college. This test measures some of the abilities thought to contribute to a student's success in medical school. *See also* Medical College Admission Test; national board examination.

standard of living A level of material comfort as measured by the goods, services, and luxuries available to an individual, a group, or a nation, as in a declining or an improving standard of living. *See also* poverty.

standard, minimum *See* minimum standard.

standard, monetary *See* monetary standard.

standard, occupational safety and health *See* occupational safety and health standard.

standard, optimum achievable *See* optimum achievable standard.

standard, outcome *See* outcome standard.

standard, performance *See* performance standard.

standard, process *See* process standard.

standard, reasonable person *See* reasonable person standard.

standard rule, national *See* national standard rule.

Standards Administration, Employment *See* Employment Standards Administration.

Standards Association, Straight Chiropractic Academic *See* Straight Chiropractic Academic Standards Association.

standards-based quality-of-care evaluation Evaluative approach to quality of care that measures health care organizations' and practitioners' compliance with preestablished standards. *See also* evaluation; quality of care; standard.

Standards Board, Financial Accounting *See* Financial Accounting Standards Board.

standards of composition The minimum percentages of meat and poultry that the US Department of Agriculture allows in foods labeled as meat and poultry products. *See also* standard.

Standards Educators Association, National *See* National Standards Educators Association.

standards of fill of containers Food and Drug Administration requirements specifying the minimum amounts of food that a package of a given size can contain. *See also* Food and Drug Administration; standard.

standards of identity Governmental regulations stating mandatory ingredients in certain combinations for a seller to call a product, for example, "cheese" or "catsup." This allows manufacturers of some 300 foods to omit a list of ingredients.

Standards Institute, American National *See* American National Standards Institute.

Standards Laboratories, National Conference of *See* National Conference of Standards Laboratories.

standards manuals Seven publications by the Joint Commission on Accreditation of Healthcare Organizations consisting of policies and procedures relating to accreditation surveys, current standards, and scoring guidelines for ambulatory health care, health care networks, home care, hospital care, long term care, pathology and clinical laboratory services, and mental health care. The manuals are designed for use in self-assessment by organizations; the standards are the basis for the survey report forms used by surveyors during on-site surveys. The names of these manuals are: *Accreditation Manual for Ambulatory Health Care, Accreditation Manual for Health Care Networks, Accreditation Manual for Hospitals, Accreditation Manual for Home Care,*

Accreditation Manual for Long Term Care, Accreditation Manual for Mental Health, Chemical Dependency, and Mental Retardation/Developmental Disabilities Services, and *Accreditation Manual for Pathology and Clinical Laboratory Services.* Synonyms: accreditation manuals; accreditation standards manuals. *See also Accreditation Manual for Ambulatory Health Care; Accreditation Manual for Health Care Networks; Accreditation Manual for Home Care; Accreditation Manual for Hospitals; Accreditation Manual for Long Term Care; Accreditation Manual for Mental Health, Chemical Dependency, and Mental Retardation/Developmental Disabilities Services; Accreditation for Pathology and Clinical Laboratory Services;* Joint Commission on Accreditation of Healthcare Organizations.

Standards, National Committee for Clinical Laboratory *See* National Committee for Clinical Laboratory Standards.

Standards, National Conference of States on Building Codes and *See* National Conference of States on Building Codes and Standards.

standards, patient-centered *See* patient-centered standards.

standards, primary *See* primary standards.

Standards Review Council of America, Professional *See* Professional Standards Review Council of America.

standards review organization, professional *See* professional standards review organization.

standards, secondary *See* secondary standards.

Standards in Speech-Language Pathology and Audiology, Council on Professional *See* Council on Professional Standards in Speech-Language Pathology and Audiology.

Standards and Technology, National Institute of *See* National Institute of Standards and Technology.

standard, structural *See* structural standard.

standard, sub- *See* substandard.

standing **1.** Remaining in force or use indefinitely, as in a standing committee. *See also* standing committee; standing orders. **2.** The legal capacity to initiate a lawsuit.

standing committee A permanent committee, such as an executive committee or a finance committee. *Compare* ad hoc committee. *See also* committee; executive committee; standing.

standing orders Instructions for patient care under specified circumstances (such as orders for patients presenting with chest pain), which are to be followed for all patients unless the attending physician intervenes with different instructions. *See also* order; standing.

stare decisis   Latin phrase meaning "let the decision stand"; a legal doctrine that prescribes adherence to those precedents set forth in cases that have been decided. *See also* case.

starvation   Suffering from prolonged lack of food. *See also* cachexia; hunger.

stat   A medical term meaning "immediately" (as in a stat laboratory test), which has come into the common vernacular.

state   **1.** A condition of being, as in a healthy state, depressed state, or fetal state. *See also* condition. **2.** One of the more or less internally autonomous territorial and political units composing a federation under a sovereign government, as in the United States.

State Administrators of Vocational Rehabilitation, Council of   *See* Council of State Administrators of Vocational Rehabilitation.

State Alcohol and Drug Abuse Directors, National Association of   *See* National Association of State Alcohol and Drug Abuse Directors.

state of the art   The highest level of development, as of a device, technique, or scientific field, achieved at a particular time, as in the state of the art in medicine. *See also* leading edge.

state board of medical examiners   A body, established by the laws of a state, responsible for overseeing the practice of medicine within the state. The board of medical examiners, among other activities, reviews the credentials of physicians applying for licensure to practice within the state, administers examinations if required, investigates the background of applicants, and approves or denies licensure. *See also* administrative agency; licensure.

State Boards of Nursing, National Council of   *See* National Council of State Boards of Nursing.

state data initiatives   Initiatives that expand state regulatory efforts to require the public reporting and dissemination of severity-adjusted cost, quality, and utilization data by health care organizations. The Health Care Cost Containment Council in Pennsylvania, for example, has implemented state reporting requirements for MedisGroups admission severity and morbidity scores. Colorado hospitals with over 100 beds report severity-adjusted outcome data to their state's data commission. *See also* data; initiative.

state-certified health plan   According to the Health Security Act (1993), a health plan that has been certified by a state. *See also* certified; health alliance; health plan; Health Security Act; regional alliance.

State, Department of   *See* Department of State.

state disability insurance   *See* unemployment compensation disability.

State Drinking Water Administrators, Association of   *See* Association of State Drinking Water Administrators.

State Emergency Medical Services Training Coordinators, National Council of   *See* National Council of State Emergency Medical Services Training Coordinators.

State EMS Directors, National Association of   *See* National Association of State EMS Directors.

State Executive Directors, Association of Osteopathic   *See* Association of Osteopathic State Executive Directors.

state health facility licensing agency   A unit of state government legally empowered to set standards for and grant permission to operate health care organizations. *See also* Association of Health Facility Survey Agencies; health facility.

state health plan   A statement issued by a statewide health coordinating council describing goals, such as quality health services at reasonable cost, for the health systems within the state. *See also* health plan; statewide health coordinating council.

state health planning and development agency   A state government agency once required, under a federal law that has now lapsed, to develop a state health plan and administer the state's certificate of need program. Some states have perpetuated such agencies without continuing federal support. *See also* certificate of need; state health plan.

State Medicaid Directors Association (SMDA)   A national organization composed of 54 directors and senior staff of state and territorial medical assistance programs. It promotes effective Medicaid policy and program administration and works with the federal government on issues through technical advisory groups. *See also* director; Medicaid.

state medical boards   State licensing bodies and state disciplinary bodies for physicians. Each state has its own board with its own set of requirements. A license may be obtained by examination in that state, by reciprocity endorsement if the physician is licensed in another state, or by meeting the requirements of the National Board of Medical Examiners or other credentialing examinations. A license is not always required during a residency, though in some states it is necessary to have a license after the first year or two of training. All physicians must be licensed to practice whether they are certified or not. The state licensing boards belong to the Federation of State Medical Boards. *See also* Federation of State Medical Boards; licensure; National Board of Medical Examiners; reciprocity; state board of medical examiners; state medical boards' disciplinary actions.

state medical boards' disciplinary actions The penalties imposed by state medical boards on physicians who have transgressed a provision in state medical practice acts. The penalties range from revoking licenses to practice medicine through lesser penalties, such as suspension of licenses for a period of time; probation; stipulations; limitations and conditions relating to practice; reprimands; letters of censure; and letters of concern. *See also* disciplinary action; state medical boards.

State Medical Boards of the United States, Federation of *See* Federation of State Medical Boards of the United States.

state medicine *See* socialized medicine.

State Mental Health Program Directors, National Association of *See* National Association of State Mental Health Program Directors.

State Mental Retardation Program Directors, National Association of *See* National Association of State Mental Retardation Program Directors.

statement, charter *See* charter statement.

statement of construction (SOC) A document of the Joint Commission on Accreditation of Healthcare Organizations that must be completed by a health care organization before survey for most accreditation programs. A properly completed statement of construction describes and verifies the basic structural and fire protection characteristics of each building in which patients/residents are housed or services are delivered. *See also* Joint Commission on Accreditation of Healthcare Organizations.

statement, closing *See* closing statement.

statement, financial *See* financial statement.

statement, mission *See* mission statement.

statement, opening *See* opening statement.

statement, operating *See* operating statement.

statement, opportunity *See* opportunity statement.

statement, problem *See* problem statement.

State Pharmacy Association Executives, National Council of *See* National Council of State Pharmacy Association Executives.

state, present *See* present state.

States on Building Codes and Standards, National Conference of *See* National Conference of States on Building Codes and Standards.

State Social Work Boards, American Association of *See* American Association of State Social Work Boards.

State and Territorial Dental Directors, Association of *See* Association of State and Territorial Dental Directors.

State and Territorial Directors of Nursing, Association of *See* Association of State and Territorial Directors of Nursing.

State and Territorial Directors of Public Health Education, Association of *See* Association of State and Territorial Directors of Public Health Education.

State and Territorial Epidemiologists, Council of *See* Council of State and Territorial Epidemiologists.

State and Territorial Health Officials, Association of *See* Association of State and Territorial Health Officials.

state unit on aging An agency of state government designated by the governor and state legislature to administer the Older Americans Act and to serve as a focal point for all matters relating to older people. *See also* aging; National Association of State Units on Aging.

State Units on Aging, National Association of *See* National Association of State Units on Aging.

state, vegetative *See* vegetative state.

statewide health coordinating council An organizational entity established under guidelines set forth in the National Health Planning Resources and Development Act, since allowed to lapse. The entity generally supervised the work of the state health planning and development agencies and reviewed and coordinated the plans and budgets of state's health systems agencies. *See also* health systems agency; National Health Planning and Resources Development Act of 1974.

statistic A numerical datum or value, such as standard deviation or mean (average), that characterizes a sample or a population from which a sample is derived. *See also* mean; number; population; sample; standard deviation; statistics; test statistic.

statistical area, metropolitan *See* metropolitan statistical area.

Statistical Association, American *See* American Statistical Association.

statistical conclusion validity The extent to which research is sufficiently precise or powerful to enable observers to detect effects. Conclusion errors are of two types: type I is to conclude there are effects (or relationships) when there are not; type II is to conclude there are no effects (or relationships) when in fact they exist. *See also* type I error; type II error; validity.

statistical control The condition describing a process from which all special causes have been removed, evidenced on a control chart by the absence of points beyond the control limits and by the absence of nonrandom patterns or trends within the control limits. *See also* control chart; control limit; special cause.

statistical inference The process of using observations of a sample to estimate the properties of a population from which the sample is derived. *See also* inference; inferential statistics.

statistical power The probability of detecting a difference between the groups being compared when one does exist. Failure to detect an effect is called "type II error" or "beta," analogous to false negative. *See also* false negative; type II error.

statistical process control (SPC) The application of statistical techniques, such as control charts, to analyze a process or its output so as to take appropriate actions to achieve and maintain a state of statistical control and to improve the capability of the process. *See also* control chart; process capability; statistical quality control.

Statistical Process Control Society (SPCS) A national organization founded in 1987 composed of 282 individuals and companies interested in implementing statistical process control to optimize their efficiency and product quality. It seeks to establish US industry in competitive world markets. It works to enhance professionalism among members by granting certification in statistical process control. *See also* certification; statistical process control.

statistical quality control (SQC) The application of statistical techniques for measuring and improving the quality of processes. SQC includes statistical

process control, diagnostic tools, sampling plans, and other statistical techniques. *See also* quality control; statistical process control.

statistical significance The likelihood that an observed association is not due to chance. *See also* level of significance; *p* (probability) value; significant.

statistically significant A test statistic that is as large as or larger than a predetermined requirement, resulting in rejection of the null hypothesis. *See also* null hypothesis; significant.

statistical test A procedure that is used to decide whether a hypothesis about the distribution of one or more populations or variables should be rejected or accepted. Statistical tests may be parametric or nonparametric. *See also* parametric test; test; variable.

statistician A person, such as a mathematician who specializes in statistics. *See also* biostatistician; statistics.

statistician, bio- *See* biostatistician.

statistics 1. The study of ways to analyze data. **2.** The mathematics of the collection, organization, and interpretation of numerical data that are subject to random variation, especially the analysis of population characteristics by inference from sampling. **3.** Numerical data. *See also* biostatistics; descriptive statistics; inductive statistics; inferential statistics; mortality statistics; significant.

Statistics, Association for Vital Records and Health *See* Association for Vital Records and Health Statistics.

statistics, bio- *See* biostatistics.

statistics, descriptive *See* descriptive statistics.

statistics, health *See* health statistics.

statistics, inductive *See* inductive statistics.

statistics, inferential *See* inferential statistics.

Statistics, Institute of Mathematical *See* Institute of Mathematical Statistics.

statistics, mortality *See* mortality statistics.

Statistics, National Center for Health *See* National Center for Health Statistics.

statistics, sampling *See* sampling statistics.

statistics, vital *See* vital statistics.

statistic, test *See* test statistic.

status State of condition, as in the patient's improved status. *See also* condition; status quo.

status quo The existing state or condition of affairs, as in an unacceptable status quo. *See also* state; status; temporary restraining order.

statute A formal written enactment, rule, or law of a federal, state, city, or county legislative body, as in statute of limitations. *See also* statute of frauds; statute of limitations.

statute of frauds The legal requirement that certain contracts must be made in writing and cannot be enforced if they are only oral agreements. *See also* fraud and abuse; statute.

statute of limitations A statute setting time limits on legal action in certain cases. The federal government and various states set a maximum time period during which certain actions can be brought or rights enforced; after the time period set out in the applicable statute of limitations has expired, no legal action can be brought regardless of whether any cause of action ever existed. *Synonym:* limitations period. *See also* affirmative defense; discovery rule; statute.

statutorily-defined emancipation *See* emancipated minor.

statutory Stated in or complying with law. *See also* statute; statutory law.

statutory law A body of law created by state and federal legislative bodies, in contrast to law created by court decision or administrative interpretation. *See also* law; statute; statutory rape.

statutory rape The crime of having sexual intercourse with a female under an age set by statute, regardless of whether she consents to the act. The common law set the age of consent at age 10 years and the statutes of the various states ranged from ages 11 to 18 years. The trend in modern statutes is to reduce the age of consent to 12 or 14 years and require that the male actor be some years older than the female victim. *See also* age of consent; rape.

STD *See* sexually transmitted disease.

steering committee A committee that sets agendas and schedules of business, as for a health care organization or legislative body. *See also* committee.

stenosis Abnormal narrowing of an orifice or a passage, as in aortic stenosis (narrowing of the aortic heart valve). *See also* stricture.

step-down unit A specialized intensive nursing unit capable of providing the same monitoring and patient support services as an intensive care unit but which has a higher ratio of patients to nurses. *See also* intensive care unit.

Stereotactic and Functional Neurosurgery, American Society for *See* American Society for Stereo-

tactic and Functional Neurosurgery.

stereotactic surgery A technique in neurological surgery and research for locating points within the brain and inserting delicate instruments, using an external, three-dimensional frame of reference usually based on the Cartesian coordinate system. *Synonym:* stereotaxic surgery. *See also* neurological surgery; stereotaxis; surgery.

stereotaxic surgery *See* steriotactic surgery.

stereotaxis Precise positioning in space, as in stereotactic surgery. *See also* stereotactic surgery.

sterile **1.** Not capable of producing offspring. *See also* contraceptive sterilization; infertility. **2.** Free from live bacteria or other microorganisms, as in sterile instruments. *See also* aseptic; autoclave; sterile technique; sterilization.

sterile technique A method of establishing and maintaining an environment free from pathogenic and nonpathogenic microorganisms. *See also* microorganism; sterilization.

sterilization **1.** A surgical operation in which a male or female is rendered incapable of reproducing offspring; in males, the procedure is vasectomy; in females, a form of tubal ligation. *See also* contraceptive sterilization; eugenic sterilization; infertility; therapeutic sterilization; vasectomy. **2.** The process of making free from live bacteria and other microorganisms, as in sterilizing the surgical instruments. Sterilization may be accomplished by heat, certain chemicals, radiation, ultraviolet light, or other means. *See also* sterile technique.

sterilization, contraceptive *See* contraceptive sterilization.

sterilization, therapeutic *See* therapeutic sterilization.

steroid Any of numerous naturally occurring or synthetic compounds, including bile acids, adrenal hormones, and sex hormones, and certain drugs, such as digitalis compounds and the precursors of certain vitamins. *See also* anabolic steroids; cortisol; cortisone; hormone; vitamin.

steroids, anabolic *See* anabolic steroids.

stethoscope An instrument used for listening to sounds produced within the body, especially heart sounds. *See also* auscultation; physical diagnosis.

STFM *See* Society of Teachers of Family Medicine.

stillbirth The birth of a dead newborn or fetus before complete expulsion or extraction from its mother. *See also* abruptio placenta; perinatal mortality.

stillborn Dead at birth.

stimulate To rouse to activity or heightened action, as in stimulating the medical staff. *See also* stimulus.

stimulant **1.** Any agent that increases the rate of activity of a body or a body system, such as caffeine. **2.** A group of controlled substances, including cocaine, a drug extracted from the leaves of the South American coca plant, and amphetamines, synthetic drugs first developed during the late 1800s. This class of drugs stimulates the central nervous system and is used medicinally to combat depression and narcolepsy. Excessive doses may produce hyperactivity, paranoia, and other psychotic symptoms. Prolonged use and large doses are followed by fatigue and depression. Cocaine was first outlawed with narcotics in 1914; amphetamines were first regulated in 1954. *See also* amphetamines; caffeine; caffeinism; cocaine; controlled substances.

stimulation, transcutaneous electric nerve *See* transcutaneous electric nerve stimulation.

stimulus **1.** Something causing or regarded as causing a response. *See also* tropism. **2.** Something that rouses to action. *See also* conditioning; stimulate.

stipulation In court, any agreement by attorneys on opposite sides of a case on any matter pertaining to the proceedings.

stitch 1. A sharp painful sensation in the side of the lower chest due to cramping of intercostal muscles. **2.** *See* suture.

St John's Guild-The Floating Hospital *See* Floating Hospital.

stochastic **1.** In statistics, involving or containing a random variable or variables. *See also* random variable. **2.** In statistics, involving chance or probability. *See also* random variable; statistics.

stock insurance company A company owned and controlled by stockholders and operated for the purpose of making a profit. Profits take the form of stockholders' dividends, which are distributed to stockholders. *Compare* mutual insurance company. *See also* insurance company.

stoma A surgically constructed opening, especially one in the abdominal wall, that permits the passage of waste after a colostomy (opening to the large intestine) or an ileostomy (opening to the small intestine). *See also* colostomy; ileostomy; ostomy.

stomach **1.** An organ of digestion, comprising an expansion of the upper gastrointestinal tract situated in the upper abdomen, connecting the esophagus with the duodenum. It has a muscular wall, which churns a mixture of food and digestive enzymes, and then forwards the mixture to the small intestine. It secretes mucus, hydrochloric acid, pepsin, and a protein promoting vitamin B_{12} absorption. *See also* alimentary tract; gastric juice; gastric lavage; gastric ulcer; gastritis; gastroenterology; hiatal hernia. **2.** *See* abdomen.

stomachache Pain in the stomach or abdomen.

stomach pump A device with a flexible tube inserted into the stomach through the mouth and esophagus to empty the stomach in an emergency, as in a case of drug overdose.

stomatology The study of the mouth and its diseases.

stonewalling **1.** Refusing to acknowledge that a condition or situation exists despite overwhelming evidence. **2.** Engaging in obstructive debate or delaying tactics. **3.** Being uncooperative, obstructive, or evasive.

stool The feces resulting from a single bowel movement. *See also* feces.

stopwatch study *See* motion study.

storyboard A technique that uses pictures and/or diagrams and short narratives to illustrate the essential steps of a quality improvement project. *See also* quality improvement project; storybook; storytelling.

storybook A permanent record of a quality improvement team's actions and achievements and all the data generated. *See also* quality improvement project; storyboard.

storytelling A technique that uses a storybook or storyboard to demonstrate the essential steps of a quality improvement project. Storytelling can act to accelerate the process of organizationwide quality improvement by helping quality improvement teams organize their work and their presentations so other persons can more readily learn from them. Storytelling can reduce variation in the process of quality improvement so that the focus of learning is on content, not the method of telling. *See also* storyboard; storybook.

STP *See* Society of Toxicologic Pathologists.

STR *See* Society of Thoracic Radiology.

strabismus A visual defect in which one eye cannot focus with the other on an object because of imbalance of the eye muscles. *Synonym*: squint. *See* *also* ophthalmology.

Strabismus, American Association for Pediatric Ophthalmology and *See* American Association for Pediatric Ophthalmology and Strabismus.

Straight Chiropractic Academic Standards Association (SCASA) A national organization founded in 1977 composed of chiropractic colleges. It develops and adopts standards for accreditation of straight (traditional) chiropractic institutions and evaluates programs that award the Doctor of Chiropractic degree. It assists in the formation and development of chiropractic institutions. *See also* chiropractic; standard.

Straight Chiropractic Organizations, Federation of *See* Federation of Straight Chiropractic Organizations.

straightjacket A contrivance for restraining the limbs, especially the arms, of a person who requires restraint. *See also* restraint.

strain A group of organisms within a species sharing some defining characteristic, as in a strain of bacteria. *See also* bacteria.

strangury Slow, difficult, and painful discharge of urine. *See also* dysuria; urination.

strategic planning The management act of planning action(s) resulting from strategy or intended to accomplish a specific goal. *Synonym:* long-term planning. *See also* planning; strategy.

strategy A management plan or method for completing objectives, usually large, long-term objectives. *See also* strategic planning; tactics.

stratification The process of classifying data into subgroups based on one or more characteristics, variables, or other categories. *See also* stratification category; stratification variable.

stratification category The values or ranges of values for a stratification variable that are used to establish the boundaries of the groups into which data will be separated. *See also* category; stratification; stratification variable.

stratification variable A variable, the values of which are used to separate data into stratification categories. *See also* stratification; stratification category; variable.

stratified random sampling A process in which a population is divided into subgroups and cases are pulled randomly from each subgroup rather from the population as a whole. *Compare* simple random sampling. *See also* random sampling; sampling.

street smarts Intuitive intelligence or reasoning power not gained by formal education.

streptokinase A proteolytic (protein dissolving) enzyme produced by hemolytic streptococci, capable of dissolving fibrin and used medically to dissolve blood clots. *See also* anticoagulant therapy; thrombolysis; thrombosis; tissue plasminogen activator.

stress Bodily or mental tension, anxiety, or emotional distress that can contribute to disease and fatigue. Stress is the totality of the physiological reaction to an adverse or threatening stimulus, such as physical, mental, or emotional trauma. The hormones of the adrenal cortex play an   important role in the adaptation to stress. *See also* posttraumatic stress disorder; technostress.

Stress, American Institute of *See* American Institute of Stress.

stress disorder, posttraumatic *See* posttraumatic stress disorder.

stressed out Suffering from the effects of extreme stress. *See also* culture shock; stress; stress fracture; stress incontinence; stress test; technostress.

stress fracture A break in a bone caused by repeated application of a heavy load, such as constant pounding on a hard surface by runners. *See also* fracture; stress.

stress incontinence Involuntary discharge of urine due to anatomic displacement, which exerts and opening pull on the bladder orifice, as in straining or coughing. *See also* incontinence; urinary incontinence.

stress, techno- *See* technostress.

stress test A test to measure an individual's heart rate and oxygen intake while undergoing strenuous physical exercise, as on a treadmill. *See also* cardiovascular medicine; stress; test; treadmill.

stretcher A frame consisting of two poles separated by crossbars on which canvas or other material is stretched, for carrying sick or injured persons. *See also* cart; gurney; litter.

striated muscle *See* muscle.

strict isolation A category of patient isolation designed to prevent transmission of highly contagious or virulent infections that may be spread by both air and contact. The specifications include a private room and the use of masks, gowns, and gloves for all persons entering the room.   Special ventilation requirements with the room at negative pressure to surrounding areas are desirable. *See also* isolation.

stricture An abnormal constriction of a duct or other passage, as in a stricture of the biliary duct. *See also* stenosis.

stroke *See* cerebrovascular accident.

stroke, mini- *See* transient ischemic attack.

structural data Data about organizational resources in place and arranged to deliver health care. *See also* data; outcome data; process data; structure.

structural measure of quality A measure of whether organizational resources and arrangements are in place to deliver health care, such as the number, type, and distribution of medical personnel, equipment, and facilities. Underlying the use of such measures to assess quality is the assumption that such characteristics increase the likelihood that providers will perform well and, in their absence, that providers will perform poorly. This assumption in turn raises the question whether specific structural characteristics are associated with better processes or outcomes. In many instances this association has not been demonstrated. *See also* measure; quality; structure.

structural standard A statement of expectation that defines a health care organization's structural capacity to provide quality care; pertains to characteristics of organizations' resources and form, such as the organization of the medical staff body and the numbers and qualifications of medical staff members. *See also* standard; structure.

structure Something made up of a number of parts that are held or put together in a particular way, as in resources and organization of a hospital (its structure) arranged to deliver health care services. *Compare* function; outcome; process. *See also* health services research; morphology.

structure, corporate *See* corporate structure.

structured interview An interview in which the interviewer carefully controls the subjects discussed and the nature of the question-and-answer format. *Compare* unstructured interview. *See also* interview.

structured interview, un- *See* unstructured interview.

structured programming In computer science, a method of designing and writing programs in which the statements are organized in a specific manner to minimize error or misinterpretation. *See also* computer program.

structured settlement A method of paying an agreed upon amount that generally allows predetermined payments to be made periodically. *See also* settlement.

structured text Concepts and ideas that are described in text but are assigned codes so that they can be recognized and analyzed by a computer. *See also* computer.

structure, organization *See* organization structure.

STS *See* Society of Thoracic Surgeons.

student **1.** One who attends a school, college, or university. *See also* dental student; medical student; student nurse. **2.** An attentive observer.

student, dental *See* dental student.

student, medical *See* medical student.

student nurse A person enrolled in a nursing education program. *See also* nurse intern.

Studies, Christian Association for Psychological *See* Christian Association for Psychological Studies.

Study of Aging, Center for the *See* Center for the Study of Aging.

Study of Blood, Society for the *See* Society for the Study of Blood.

Study of Breast Disease, Society for the *See* Society for the Study of Breast Disease.

study, case-control *See* case-control study.

study, cohort *See* cohort study.

study, cohort analytic *See* cohort analytic study.

study, descriptive *See* descriptive study.

study, diagnostic *See* diagnostic study.

Study of Dreams, Association for the *See* Association for the Study of Dreams.

Study, Drug Efficacy *See* Drug Efficacy Study.

study, feasibility *See* feasibility study.

Study Group, Healthcare Financing *See* Healthcare Financing Study Group.

Study of Headache, American Association for the *See* American Association for the Study of Headache.

Study of Liver Diseases, American Association for the *See* American Association for the Study of Liver Diseases.

study, longitudinal *See* longitudinal study.

study, motion *See* motion study.

study, observational *See* observational study.

Study of Orthodontics, American Society for the *See* American Society for the Study of Orthodontics.

study, patient origin *See* patient origin study.

Study of Pharmacy and Therapeutics for the

Elderly, Center for the *See* Center for the Study of Pharmacy and Therapeutics for the Elderly.

study, pilot *See* pilot study.

study, prospective *See* prospective study.

study, quick *See* quick study.

Study of Reproduction, Society for the *See* Society for the Study of Reproduction.

study, retrospective *See* retrospective study.

Study of Sex, Society for the Scientific *See* Society for the Scientific Study of Sex.

Study of Social Biology, Society for the *See* Society for the Study of Social Biology.

study, stopwatch *See* motion study.

study, time-motion *See* motion study.

study, time and motion *See* motion study.

study, triple-blind *See* triple-blind study.

study, validity *See* validity study.

stupor *See* consciousness.

subacute Somewhat or moderately acute; between acute and chronic, as in subacute bacterial endocarditis. *See also* acute; chronic; subacute care.

subacute care Medical and skilled nursing services provided to patients who are not in an acute phase of illness but who require a level of care higher than that provided in a long term care setting. *See also* long term care; subacute.

Subcommittee on Health *See* Committee on Ways and Means.

subconscious The part of the mind below the level of conscious perception, or information that a person is only vaguely aware of, as in subconscious motives. *See also* consciousness; unconscious.

subculture A cultural subgroup differentiated by factors, such as status or religion, that functionally unify the group and act collectively on each member. *See also* culture; religion.

subcutaneous Located just beneath the skin, as in subcutaneous injection or subcutaneous implant. *See also* parenteral.

subdiaphragmatic abdominal thrust *See* Heimlich maneuver.

subdiscipline A field of study within a broader discipline. *See also* discipline.

subgroup A distinct group within a group, as in the committee's subgroups met. *See also* group.

subjective **1.** Taking place within a person's mind; reality as it is perceived by a person. For example, pain is subjective because only the person experiencing it can describe it. **2.** In medicine, relating to a symptom or condition perceived by the patient and not by the examiner, as in a patient's (subjective) complaint of exhaustion. *Compare* objective. *See also* subjective data; subjectivism.

subjective data Data not readily quantified or measured, such as personal opinions, values, concepts, and social relationships. *See also* data; subjective; subjectivism; subjectivity.

subjectivism In philosophy, the doctrine that all knowledge is restricted to the conscious self and its sensory states. Objectivism, by contrast, is one of several doctrines holding that all reality is objective and external to the mind and that knowledge is reliably based on observed objects and events. *Compare* objectivism. *See also* subjective; subjectivity.

subjectivity The state of being influenced by what is taking place in a person's mind, such as emotions and personal prejudices. *Compare* objectivity. *See also* subjective; subjectivism.

sublimation The replacement of a socially unacceptable means of satisfying desires by means that are socially acceptable, especially the diversion of components of the sex drive to nonsexual goals. *See also* sex.

subnormal Less than or below normal, as in a subnormal temperature. *See also* abnormal; normal.

subordinate An individual who is subject to the authority or control of another individual. *See also* associate; employee.

suborn A term in criminal law indicating the procurement of another to commit perjury. *See also* criminal law; perjury.

subpoena An order issued under authority of a court to compel the appearance of a witness at a judicial proceeding or a deposition to give testimony. *See also* summons.

subrogation **1.** Assumption of an obligation for which another is primarily liable. **2.** A provision of an insurance policy that requires an insured individual to turn over any rights he or she may have to recover damages from another party to the insurer, to the extent to which he or she has been reimbursed by the insurer. Some experts have argued that private health insurance, including Blue Cross or group insurance, should have subrogation rights similar to those in most property insurance policies. Having paid the hospital bill of a policyholder, the health insurance company could assume the right to sue the party whose negligence might have caused the hospitalization and be reimbursed for its outlay to the policyholder. *See also* insurance.

subscriber An individual who has elected to contract for, or participate in (subscribe to), an insurance or health maintenance organization plan for himself or herself and dependents, if any. *See also* beneficiary; insured; member.

subscription *See* prescription.

subsistence **1.** The state of existing, especially barely sufficient to maintain life. *See also* poverty. **2.** The minimum (as of food, shelter) necessary to support life.

subspecialist One who subspecializes, as in a hand surgeon is a subspecialist in the specialty of general surgery and a cardiologist is a subspecialist in the specialty of internal medicine. *See also* medical subspecialist; subspecialty.

subspecialist, medical *See* medical subspecialist.

subspecialties, medical *See* medical subspecialties.

subspecialty A narrow field of study within a specialty, as pediatric nephrology is a subspecialty of pediatrics (a specialty) and geriatric psychiatry is a subspecialty of psychiatry (a specialty). *See also* medical subspecialties; specialty.

substance abuse Excessive use of addictive substances, especially alcohol and narcotic drugs, such as heroin. *Synonym:* chemical abuse. *See also* addiction; drug abuse.

Substance Abuse, Association of Medical Education and Research in *See* Association of Medical Education and Research in Substance Abuse.

substance abuse facility A hospital or other facility specializing in the treatment of patients suffering from alcoholism or chemical dependency. *See also* alcoholism and other drug dependence; substance abuse.

Substance Abuse and Mental Health Services Administration A component of the US Public Health Service that coordinates activities of the Center for Substance Abuse Treatment, Center for Mental Health Services, and Center for Substance Abuse Prevention, which sponsors the National Clearinghouse for Alcohol and Drug Information. Formerly Alcohol, Drug Abuse, and Mental Health Administration. *See also* Public Health Service; substance abuse.

Substance Abuse Services, Special Constituency Section for Psychiatric and *See* Special Con-

stituency Section for Psychiatric and Substance Abuse Services.

substance, addictive *See* addictive substance.

Substances Act of 1970, Controlled *See* Controlled Substances Act of 1970.

substances, controlled *See* controlled substances.

substances, schedule of controlled *See* schedule of controlled substances.

substances, schedule I *See* schedule I substances.

substances, schedule II *See* schedule II substances.

substances, schedule III *See* schedule III substances.

substances, schedule IV *See* schedule IV substances.

substances, schedule V *See* schedule V substances.

substandard Failing to meet a standard or below a standard, as in the organization's performance in the area was substandard. *See also* standard.

substantial Considerable in importance, value, degree, amount, or extent, as in substantial compliance with the standard. *See also* substantive.

substantial compliance *See* compliance level.

substantial violation In health care, a pattern of care over a substantial number of cases that is inappropriate, unnecessary, does not meet the recognized standards of care, or is not supported by the documentation of care required by a peer review organization (PRO). PROs identify potential violations; the Office of the Inspector General of the US Department of Health and Human Services makes the final decision as to whether the violation occurred. *Compare* gross and flagrant violation. *See also* peer review organization; violation.

substantive Having a solid or firm basis, as in a substantive improvement. *See also* substantial.

substantive due process *See* due process of law.

substantive right A basic right, such as life or liberty, seen as constituting part of the order of society and considered independent of and not subordinate to the body of human law. *See also* rights; substantive.

substituted judgment doctrine A legal rule, applied by some courts, which requires a guardian or other person making treatment decisions on behalf of an incompetent person to base that decision on what the incompetent person himself or herself would want under the circumstances, as distinguished from what the decision maker believes would be in the best interest of the incompetent patients. *See also* doctrine; incompetent; standard.

substitute food   A legal labeling definition for foods nutritionally equivalent to another, more common product. *See also* food; labeling.

substitution   The act or instance of one taking the place of another, as in the practice of filling a prescription by a pharmacist with a drug product therapeutically and chemically equivalent to, but not, the one prescribed. *See also* antisubstitution laws.

subtherapeutic   Below the dosage levels used to treat disease, as in prescribing a subtherapeutic dose of antibiotic. *See also* therapeutic.

subtotal hysterectomy   *See* partial hysterectomy.

suburban   Located or residing in a residential area or community outlying a city, as in a suburban hospital. *See also* rural; urban.

success   Achievement of something desired, planned, or attempted. *Compare* failure.

successive   Following in uninterrupted order, as in 100 successive patients were interviewed. *See also* continual; continuous; frequent; intermittent; occasional; periodic; sporadic.

succor   Assistance in time of distress.

suction lipectomy   *See* liposuction surgery.

sudden infant death syndrome (SIDS)   A fatal syndrome that affects sleeping infants typically younger than age one year, characterized by a sudden cessation of breathing. *Synonym*: crib death. *See also* infant; syndrome.

Sudden Infant Death Syndrome Clearinghouse, National   *See* National Sudden Infant Death Syndrome Clearinghouse.

suffer   To feel pain or distress.

suffering, pain and   *See* pain and suffering.

sufficient   Being as much as is needed and especially not more than is needed. *See also* adequate.

sugar   *See* glucose.

sugar-free   A food label indicating that the product contains no saccharine sweetener, such as sucrose. However, the product may contain any of the sugar alcohols (sorbitol, xylitol, or mannitol), even though they contain similar calories as sugar. *Synonym*: sugarless. *See also* calorie; labeling; saccharine.

sugarless   *See* sugar-free.

suggestion   **1.** The act of offering for consideration or action, as in suggesting an improvement. **2.** A potent psychological force that can relieve physical as well as psychological pain and other discomforts. It accounts for pain relief by placebos, by hypnosis, and some of the relief from acupuncture. *See also* acupuncture; pain; placebo.

suggestion, hypnotic   *See* hypnotic suggestion.

suicidal   Causing or relating to suicide, as in suicidal behavior. *See also* depression; suicide.

suicidal gesture   *See* suicide attempt.

suicidal ideation   *See* suicide attempt.

suicide   The taking of one's own life. *See also* completed suicide; depression; outcome following suicide attempt.

suicide attempt   Deliberate, self-injurious behavior that is intended to or may result in death and that is distinguishable from either a suicidal gesture or suicidal ideation, which, while self-destructive in nature, is not intended to result in death. *See also* completed suicide; suicide.

suicide attempt, outcome following   *See* outcome following suicide attempt.

suicide, completed   *See* completed suicide.

suicidology   The study of suicide, suicide prevention, and related phenomena of self-destruction. *See also* suicide; suicide attempt.

Suicidology, American Association of   *See* American Association of Suicidology (AAS).

suit   *See* lawsuit.

sulfites   A group of sulphur-containing agents used as food preservatives, especially on salad bars in restaurants, processed potatoes, and some convenience foods. They can cause mild to severe allergy symptoms in individuals sensitive to them, particularly sulfite-sensitive asthmatics. *See also* additive; allergy; preservative.

summary   **1.** Performed speedily and without ceremony, as in summary justice. *See also* summary judgment. **2.** *See* abstract.

summary judgment   A preverdict judgment rendered by the court (judge) in response to a motion by either the plaintiff or the defendant, who claims that the absence of factual dispute on one or more issues eliminates the need to send these issues to the jury. *See also* issue of law; judgment; summary; verdict.

summation   A concluding part of something, such as a speech or an argument. *See also* summation conference.

summation conference   An optional conference held by surveyors from the Joint Commission on Accreditation of Healthcare Organizations after the chief executive officer exit conference for all organization staff and other persons, designed to convey general observations about the survey findings and, on the basis of these findings, provide preliminary information about a health care organization's strengths and weaknesses. *See also* conference; Joint Commission on Accreditation of Healthcare Organizations; summation.

summons   A mandate requiring the appearance of a defendant under penalty of having judgment entered against him or her for failure to appear. The object of a summons is to notify a defendant that he or she has been sued. *See also* subpoena.

sunshine law   A state or federal law that requires most meetings of regulatory bodies to be held in public and most of their decisions and records to be disclosed. *See also* law.

SUO-HNS   *See* Society of University Otolaryngologists-Head and Neck Surgeons.

supercomputer   A mainframe computer that is among the largest, fastest, or most powerful of those available at a given time; for example, the Cyberplus parallel processor. *See also* computer; mainframe computer.

supererogation   Doing more than is required, ordered, or expected, as in supererogatory acts. *See also* altruism.

superscription   *See* prescription.

superseding cause   In law, an intervening cause that is so substantially responsible for the ultimate injury that it acts to cut off the liability of preceding actors regardless of whether their prior negligence was a substantial factor in bringing about the injury complained of. *See also* cause.

superintendent   A person who has the authority to supervise or direct an entity, such as a department or a system, as in a school superintendent. *See also* chief executive officer.

SuperPRO   An independent organization, working under contract to the Health Care Financing Administration (HCFA), that reviews a sample of the patient records evaluated by each of 54 peer review organizations (PROs). The purpose of the SuperPRO reviews is to validate the determinations made by PROs, including the application of the HCFA generic quality screens. *See also* HCFA generic quality screens; peer review organization.

supervening cause   *See* intervening cause.

supervise   To have the charge and oversight of the performance of other persons, as in to supervise a

nursing unit. *See also* oversight; supervisor.

supervising nurse   *See* nursing supervisor.

supervisor   One who oversees the performance of other persons. *See also* casework supervisor; oversight; nursing supervisor; supervise.

supervisor, casework   *See* casework supervisor.

supervisor, nurse   *See* nursing supervisor.

supervisor, nursing   *See* nursing supervisor.

Supervisors and Administrators of Health Occupations Education, National Association of   *See* National Association of Supervisors and Administrators of Health Occupations Education.

supplemental health insurance   Insurance that covers medical expenses not covered by separate health insurance already held by the insured individual. For example, many insurance companies sell insurance to Medicare beneficiaries, which covers either the costs of cost sharing required by Medicare, services not covered, or both. *See also* cost sharing; health insurance; insurance; Medicare.

supplemental recommendation   A recommendation or group of recommendations made by the Joint Commission on Accreditation of Healthcare Organizations that encompasses a standard(s) that was scored in less than substantial compliance (that is, less than a score of 1) in the survey process, but that did not result in a type I recommendation. If not resolved, a supplemental recommendation may affect a future accreditation decision. These recommendations are contained in the "Supplemental Recommendations" section of a health care organization's accreditation decision report. Formerly called type II recommendation. *Synonym*: consultative recommendation. *See also* accreditation survey; Joint Commission on Accreditation of Healthcare Organizations; type I recommendation.

supplemental security income (SSI)   Federally sponsored supportive income for low-income aged, blind, and disabled individuals, established by Title XVI of the Social Security Act. Supplemental security income replaced state welfare programs for the aged, blind, and disabled on January 1, 1972. Receipt of federal SSI benefits or a state supplement to SSI is often used to establish Medicaid eligibility. *See also* Medicaid; Social Security Act.

Supplementary Medical Insurance Program (Part B)   The voluntary portion of Medicare in which all persons entitled to the hospital insurance program (Part A) may enroll for a monthly premium that is matched in amount from federal general revenues. Covered services include physician services, home health care services, outpatient hospital services, and laboratory, pathology and radiologic services. The name, Part B, refers to part B of Title XVIII of the Social Security Act, the legislative authority for the program. *See also* Medicare; Social Security Act.

supplement, Medicare *See* Medicare supplement.

supplier A party or entity providing an input to a process. A supplier can be, for example, a person, a department, a company, or an organization. *See also* customer; input; internal customer; rework.

supplies Materials or provisions stored and dispensed when needed. *See also* medical supplies; supplier; supply.

supplies, medical See medical supplies.

supply In economics, the quantity of services supplied as the price of the service varies, income and other factors being held constant. For most services, increases in price will induce increases in supply. Increases in demand (but not, necessarily, in need) normally will induce an increase in price. *See also* law of supply and demand; Say's Law.

supply and demand, law of *See* law of supply and demand.

supply-side economics An economic theory that increased availability of money for investment, achieved through reduction of taxes, especially in the higher tax brackets, will increase productivity, economic activity, and income throughout the economic system. This theory was championed in the late 1970s by Arthur Laffer. *See also* economics; trickledown theory.

support To provide for or maintain, by supplying with necessities; for example, advanced cardiac life support. *See also* support care; support group; support services.

support, advanced cardiac life *See* advanced cardiac life support.

support, advanced trauma life *See* advanced trauma life support.

support, basic cardiac life *See* basic cardiac life support.

support, basic trauma life *See* basic trauma life support.

support care Care provided to assist patients in activities of daily living or maintenance and management of household routines. *See also* activities of daily living.

support group A group of individuals with the same or similar problems or issues that meets periodically to share experiences and solutions to problems, in order to support each other; for example, an alcoholism support group. *See also* group; group therapy; support.

support services Services exclusive of medical, nursing, and ancillary services, that provide support in the delivery of clinical services for patient care. Examples include laundry service, housekeeping, food service, purchasing, maintenance, central supply, materials management, and security. *See also* ancillary services; environmental services; support.

support staff Employees and volunteers of a health care organization who perform clerical, housekeeping, security, record-keeping, transportation, routine laboratory, and other routine administrative and clinical activities. *See also* staff.

suppository A medicated plug of material for insertion into the rectum, vagina, or urethra, to introduce a drug into the systemic circulation by means of absorption from the mucous membrane, or to exert local action on the mucous membrane.

suppression, immuno- *See* immunosuppression.

supracervical hysterectomy *See* partial hysterectomy.

supravaginal hysterectomy *See* partial hysterectomy.

surface ambulance *See* ambulance.

surgeon A physician specializing in surgery. *See also* physician; surgery.

surgeon assistant (SA) An allied health professional who prepares patients for surgery, assists during operations, and helps care for patients after surgery. Surgeon assistants are one type of allied health professional for which the Committee on Allied Health Accreditation and Education has accredited educational programs. *See also* allied health professional; operation; surgery.

Surgeon Assistants, American Association of *See* American Association of Surgeon Assistants.

surgeon, cardiovascular *See* thoracic surgeon.

surgeon, chest *See* thoracic surgeon.

surgeon, colon and rectal *See* colon and rectal surgeon.

surgeon, foot *See* podiatrist.

surgeon general **1.** The chief general officer in the medical departments of the US Army, Navy, or Air Force. **2.** The chief medical officer in the US Public Health Service or in a state public health service. *See* *also* Public Health Service; surgeon general of the United States.

surgeon general of the United States The individual appointed by the president of the United States with the consent of the United States Senate, serving as the nation's chief health adviser. The surgeon general commissions research concerning major health concerns and issues warnings to the public about health dangers, such as the statement about the hazards of smoking that appears on packages of cigarettes. Congress created the position of surgeon general in 1870 to direct the Marine Hospital Service, which provided health care mainly to American sailors. The Marine Hospital Service eventually developed into a national public health service during the late 1800s and early 1900s. In 1912, Congress renamed it the Public Health Service (PHS). The surgeon general has a rank equivalent to that of vice admiral in the US Navy. *See also* Office of the Surgeon General; surgeon; surgeon general.

surgeon, general *See* general surgeon.

surgeon, general vascular *See* vascular surgeon.

surgeon, hand *See* hand surgeon.

surgeon, head and neck *See* otolaryngologist-head and neck surgeon.

surgeon, neurological *See* neurological surgeon.

surgeon, operating *See* operating surgeon.

surgeon, oral *See* oral and maxillofacial surgeon.

surgeon, oral and maxillofacial *See* oral and maxillofacial surgeon.

surgeon, orthopaedic/orthopedic *See* orthopaedic/orthopedic surgeon.

surgeon, otolaryngologist-head and neck *See* otolaryngologist-head and neck surgeon.

surgeon, pediatric *See* pediatric surgeon.

surgeon, plastic *See* plastic surgeon.

Surgeons, American Academy of Neurological and Orthopaedic *See* American Academy of Neurological and Orthopaedic Surgeons.

Surgeons, American Academy of Orthopaedic *See* American Academy of Orthopaedic Surgeons.

Surgeons, American Academy of Spinal *See* American Academy of Spinal Surgeons.

Surgeons, American Association of Genito-Urinary *See* American Association of Genito-Urinary Surgeons.

Surgeons, American Association of Neurological *See* American Association of Neurological Surgeons.

Surgeons, American Association of Oral and Max-illofacial *See* American Association of Oral and Maxillofacial Surgeons.

Surgeons, American Association of Plastic *See* American Association of Plastic Surgeons.

Surgeons, American Association of Podiatric Physicians and *See* American Association of Podiatric Physicians and Surgeons.

Surgeons, American Association of Railway *See* American Association of Railway Surgeons.

Surgeons, American College of *See* American College of Surgeons.

Surgeons, American College of Foot *See* American College of Foot Surgeons.

Surgeons, American College of Oral and Maxillofacial *See* American College of Oral and Maxillofacial Surgeons.

Surgeons, American College of Osteopathic *See* American College of Osteopathic Surgeons.

Surgeons, American Society of Colon and Rectal *See* American Society of Colon and Rectal Surgeons.

Surgeons, American Society of Maxillofacial *See* American Society of Maxillofacial Surgeons.

Surgeons, American Society of Outpatient *See* American Society of Outpatient Surgeons.

Surgeons, American Society of Plastic and Reconstructive *See* American Society of Plastic and Reconstructive Surgeons.

Surgeons, American Society of Transplant *See* American Society of Transplant Surgeons.

Surgeons, Association of American Physicians and *See* Association of American Physicians and Surgeons.

Surgeons, Association of Bone and Joint *See* Association of Bone and Joint Surgeons.

Surgeons, Interamerican College of Physicians and *See* Interamerican College of Physicians and Surgeons.

surgeon's knot Any of several knots, especially one similar to a square knot, used in surgery for tying ligatures or suturing incisions closed. *See also* surgery.

Surgeons, National College of Foot *See* National College of Foot Surgeons.

Surgeons, Society American Gastrointestinal Endoscopic *See* Society American Gastrointestinal Endoscopic Surgeons.

Surgeons, Society of Head and Neck *See* Society of Head and Neck Surgeons.

Surgeons, Society of Military Orthopaedic *See*

Society of Military Orthopaedic Surgeons.

Surgeons, Society of Military Otolaryngologists - Head and Neck *See* Society of Military Otolaryngologists-Head and Neck Surgeons.

Surgeons, Society for Reproductive *See* Society for Reproductive Surgeons.

Surgeons, Society of Thoracic *See* Society of Thoracic Surgeons.

Surgeons, Society of United States Air Force Flight *See* Society of United States Air Force Flight Surgeons.

Surgeons, Society of University *See* Society of University Surgeons.

Surgeons, Society of University Otolaryngologists-Head and Neck *See* Society of University Otolaryngologists-Head and Neck Surgeons.

Surgeons (of the United States of America), Royal College of Physicians and *See* Royal College of Physicians and Surgeons (of the United States of America).

Surgeons of the United States, Association of Military *See* Association of Military Surgeons of the United States.

surgeon, thoracic *See* thoracic surgeon.

surgeon, trauma *See* traumatologist.

surgeon, vascular *See* vascular surgeon.

surge, power *See* power surge.

surgery 1. Any operative or manual procedure undertaken for the diagnosis or treatment of a disease, injury, or deformity. **2.** The branch and specialty of medicine dealing with the diagnosis and treatment of injury, deformity, and disease by manual and instrumental means. *See also* abdominal surgery; ambulatory surgery; elective surgery; emergency surgery; general surgery; major surgery; minor surgery; operation; procedure.

surgery, abdominal *See* abdominal surgery.

Surgery, Academy of Ambulatory Foot *See* Academy of Ambulatory Foot Surgery.

Surgery of the Alimentary Tract, Society for *See* Society for Surgery of the Alimentary Tract.

surgery, ambulatory *See* ambulatory surgery.

Surgery, American Academy of Cosmetic *See* American Academy of Cosmetic Surgery.

Surgery, American Academy of Facial Plastic and Reconstructive *See* American Academy of Facial Plastic and Reconstructive Surgery.

Surgery, American Academy of Neurological *See* American Academy of Neurological Surgery.

Surgery, American Academy of Otolaryngology-Head and Neck *See* American Academy of Otolaryngology-Head and Neck Surgery.

Surgery, American Association for Hand *See* American Association for Hand Surgery.

Surgery, American Association for Thoracic *See* American Association for Thoracic Surgery.

Surgery, American Board of *See* American Board of Surgery.

Surgery, American Board of Abdominal *See* American Board of Abdominal Surgery.

Surgery, American Board of Colon and Rectal *See* American Board of Colon and Rectal Surgery.

Surgery, American Board of Hand *See* American Board of Hand Surgery.

Surgery, American Board of Industrial Medicine and *See* American Board of Industrial Medicine and Surgery.

Surgery, American Board of Medical-Legal Analysis in Medicine and *See* American Board of Medical-Legal Analysis in Medicine and Surgery.

Surgery, American Board of Neurological *See* American Board of Neurological Surgery.

Surgery, American Board of Neurological/ Orthopaedic Laser *See* American Board of Neurological/Orthopaedic Laser Surgery.

Surgery, American Board of Neurological and Orthopaedic Medicine and *See* American Board of Neurological and Orthopaedic Medicine and Surgery.

Surgery, American Board of Oral and Maxillofacial *See* American Board of Oral and Maxillofacial Surgery.

Surgery, American Board of Orthopedic *See* American Board of Orthopedic Surgery.

Surgery, American Board of Plastic *See* American Board of Plastic Surgery.

Surgery, American Board of Podiatric *See* American Board of Podiatric Surgery.

Surgery, American Board of Spinal *See* American Board of Spinal Surgery.

Surgery, American Board of Thoracic *See* American Board of Thoracic Surgery.

Surgery, American College of Cryo- *See* American College of Cryosurgery.

Surgery, American College of General Practitioners in Osteopathic Medicine and *See* American College of General Practitioners in Osteopathic Medicine and Surgery.

Surgery, American Society of Abdominal   *See* American Society of Abdominal Surgery.

Surgery, American Society for Aesthetic Plastic   *See* American Society for Aesthetic Plastic Surgery.

Surgery, American Society of Cataract and Refractive   *See* American Society of Cataract and Refractive Surgery.

Surgery, American Society of Contemporary Medicine and   *See* American Society of Contemporary Medicine and Surgery.

Surgery, American Society for Dermatologic   *See* American Society for Dermatologic Surgery.

Surgery, American Society for Head and Neck   *See* American Society for Head and Neck Surgery.

Surgery, American Society for Laser Medicine and   *See* American Society for Laser Medicine and Surgery.

Surgery, American Society of Lipo-Suction   *See* American Society of Lipo-Suction Surgery.

Surgery, American Society for Stereotactic and Functional   *See* American Society for Stereotactic and Functional Surgery.

Surgery, Association for Academic   *See* Association for Academic Surgery.

Surgery Association, Federated Ambulatory   *See* Federated Ambulatory Surgery Association.

Surgery, Association of Physician's Assistants in Cardio-Vascular   *See* Association of Physician's Assistants in Cardio-Vascular Surgery.

surgery, biliary tract   *See* biliary tract surgery.

surgery, cardiovascular   *See* thoracic surgery.

surgery center, ambulatory   *See* ambulatory surgical facility.

surgery, chemo-   *See* chemosurgery.

surgery, colon and rectal   *See* colon and rectal surgery.

surgery, cosmetic   *See* cosmetic surgery.

surgery, cryo-   *See* cryosurgery.

Surgery and Cutaneous Oncology, American College of Mohs Micrographic   *See* American College of Mohs Micrographic Surgery and Cutaneous Oncology.

surgery department   A department or service of a hospital that provides diagnosis and treatment of diseases, injuries, and deformities through the use of surgical procedures. *See also* department; surgery.

surgery, elective   *See* elective surgery.

surgery, emergency   *See* emergency surgery.

Surgery Facilities, American Association for

Accreditation of Ambulatory Plastic   *See* American Association for Accreditation of Ambulatory Plastic Surgery Facilities.

surgery, general   *See* general surgery.

surgery, general vascular   *See* vascular surgery.

surgery, hand   *See* hand surgery.

Surgery of the Hand, American Society for   *See* American Society for Surgery of the Hand.

surgery, in-and-out   *See* ambulatory surgery.

surgery, keyhole   *See* keyhole surgery.

surgery, liposuction   *See* liposuction surgery.

surgery, major   *See* major surgery.

surgery, micro-   *See* microsurgery.

surgery, minor   *See* minor surgery.

surgery, neurological   *See* neurological surgery.

surgery, neuro-   *See* neurological surgery.

surgery, open heart   *See* open heart surgery.

surgery, oral   *See* oral and maxillofacial surgery.

surgery, oral and maxillofacial   *See* oral and maxillofacial surgery.

surgery, orthopaedic/orthopedic   *See* orthopaedic/orthopedic surgery.

surgery, outpatient   *See* ambulatory surgery.

surgery, pediatric   *See* pediatric surgery.

surgery, pediatric otolaryngology-head and neck   *See* pediatric otolaryngology-head and neck surgery.

surgery, plastic   *See* plastic surgery.

surgery, podiatric   *See* podiatric surgery.

surgery, psycho-   *See* psychosurgery.

surgery, reconstructive   *See* plastic surgery.

surgery, same-day   *See* ambulatory surgery.

Surgery Society, Outpatient Ophthalmic   *See* Outpatient Ophthalmic Surgery Society.

Surgery, Society for Vascular   *See* Society for Vascular Surgery.

surgery, stereotactic   *See* stereotactic surgery.

surgery, thoracic   *See* thoracic surgery.

surgery, trauma   *See* traumatology.

Surgery of Trauma, American Association for the   *See* American Association for the Surgery of Trauma.

surgery, vascular   *See* vascular surgery.

surgical   Pertaining to surgery, as in surgical schedule or surgical technique. *See also* surgery.

Surgical Association, American   *See* American Surgical Association.

Surgical Association, American Pediatric   *See* American Pediatric Surgical Association.

surgical case review   A medical staff responsibility that entails measuring, assessing, and improving the quality of surgical care. *See also* medical staff; surgery.

surgical center *See* freestanding ambulatory surgical facility.

Surgical Contraception, Association for Voluntary *See* Association for Voluntary Surgical Contraception.

surgical critical care A branch of medicine and subspecialty of general surgery involving the management of the critically ill and postoperative patient, particularly the trauma victim, in the emergency department, intensive care unit, trauma unit, burn unit, and other similar settings. *See also* critical care medicine; general surgery.

Surgical Education, Association for *See* Association for Surgical Education.

surgical facility, ambulatory *See* ambulatory surgical facility.

surgical facility, freestanding ambulatory *See* freestanding ambulatory surgical facility.

Surgical Infection Society (SIS) A national organization founded in 1981 composed of 420 surgeons and surgical specialists engaged in laboratory or clinical research in the field of surgical infections. Its objective is to encourage education and research in the nature, prevention, diagnosis, and treatment of surgical infections. *See also* infection; infection control; surgery.

surgical intensive care unit An intensive care unit for postoperative high-risk inpatients. *See also* intensive care unit; special care unit; surgical critical care.

surgical intervention Any surgical action that is intended to interrupt or change events in progress; for example, an operation for appendicitis. *See also* health intervention; intervention; medical intervention; nursing intervention.

Surgical Manufacturers Association, Orthopedic *See* Orthopedic Surgical Manufacturers Association.

surgical nurse A registered nurse qualified by special education and training to provide nursing care to surgical patients before, during, and after surgery. *See also* operating room nurse; registered nurse.

Surgical Nurses, American Society of Plastic and Reconstructive *See* American Society of Plastic and Reconstructive Surgical Nurses.

Surgical Oncology, Society of *See* Society of Surgical Oncology.

surgical resident A resident physician who is undergoing training in surgery. *See also* resident; surgery.

surgical suite One or more operating rooms with scrub areas, recovery rooms, and other facilities required for performance of surgery. *See also* operating room.

surgical specialties Branches of surgery in which surgeons specialize, such as general surgery, neurological surgery, plastic surgery, and thoracic surgery. *See also* specialty; surgery.

surgical team The group of professionals including surgeons, other physicians, nurses, technicians and other skilled personnel who work together to perform surgical procedures on patients. *See also* surgery; team.

surgical technologist An allied health professional who works closely with surgeons, anesthesiologists, registered nurses, and other surgical personnel delivering patient care and assuming appropriate responsibilities before, during, and after surgery. The surgical technologist, for instance, may prepare the operating room; function as the sterile member of the surgical team who passes instruments, suture, and sponges during surgery; and hold retractors or instruments, sponge or suction the operative site, or cut suture material as directed by the surgeon. Surgical technologists are one type of allied health professional for which the Committee on Allied Health Education and Accreditation has accredited education programs. *See also* allied health professional; surgery; technologist; technology.

Surgical Technologists, Association of *See* Association of Surgical Technologists.

Surgical Technology, Accreditation Review Committee for Educational Programs in *See* Accreditation Review Committee for Educational Programs in Surgical Technology.

surgicenter *See* freestanding ambulatory surgical facility.

surprise rate The percentage of nonfrivolous claims for which a hospital's first notification was the filing of a claim. A hospital should aim for a surprise rate of zero, meaning that a hospital should have systems in place so that it knows of and can investigate an adverse patient outcome (APO) before a claim is filed. *See also* adverse patient occurrence; occurrence screening; rate.

surrogacy *See* surrogate motherhood.

surrogate An agent who acts on behalf of another person, as in surrogate mother or surrogate father. *See also* surrogate mother; surrogate motherhood.

surrogate mother A woman who carries and delivers children on behalf of infertile couples, usually for a fee, either through artificial insemination by the other woman's husband or by carrying until birth the other woman's surgically implanted fertilized egg. *See also* surrogate motherhood.

surrogate motherhood A method of noncoital reproduction in which a fertile woman is paid to bear a child for another woman, either through artificial insemination by the other woman's husband or by carrying until birth the other woman's surgically implanted fertilized egg. A number of states have outlawed surrogacy for hire. *See also* artificial insemination; noncoital reproduction; preembryo transfer.

surrogate's court A trial court responsible for hearing proceedings regarding the estates of deceased and incompetent persons. *See also* court; trial court.

surveillance Ongoing monitoring using methods distinguished by their practicability, uniformity, and rapidity, rather than by complete accuracy. The purpose of surveillance is to detect changes in trend or distribution in order to initiate investigative or control measures. *See also* monitoring; quality surveillance; surveillance of disease.

surveillance of disease The continuing scrutiny of all aspects of occurrence and spread of a disease that are pertinent to effective control. *See also* disease; surveillance.

surveillance, quality *See* quality surveillance.

survey An inquiry in which information is systematically collected but the experimental method is not used. *See also* accreditation survey; experimental method.

survey, accreditation *See* accreditation survey.

Survey Agencies, Association of Health Facility *See* Association of Health Facility Survey Agencies.

survey data, aggregate *See* aggregate survey data.

survey, extension *See* extension survey.

survey, follow-up *See* follow-up survey.

survey, full team *See* full team survey.

survey, initial *See* initial survey.

survey instrument The interview schedule, questionnaire, medical examination record form, or other instrument used in a survey. *See also* instrument; survey.

survey In health care, an on-site assessment of a health care organization by the Joint Commission on Accreditation of Healthcare Organizations or other accrediting body. *See also* accreditation survey; extension survey; focused survey; follow-up survey; full team survey; Joint Commission on Accreditation of Healthcare Organizations; modified survey process; multiorganization system survey; special survey; specialized survey; tailored survey; triennial survey; unannounced survey; validation survey.

survey, morbidity *See* morbidity survey.

survey process, modified *See* modified survey process.

survey, re- *See* resurvey.

survey report A report resulting from the on-site assessment of a health care organization by surveyors from the Joint Commission on Accreditation of Healthcare Organizations or other accrediting body. The report outlines any identified deficiencies in standards compliance; the nature of the accreditation decision, including enumeration of type I recommendations, the implementation of which are monitored by the Joint Commission through the conduct of focused surveys or requests for written progress reports; and other supplemental recommendations that are designed to assist the organization in improving its performance. *Synonym:* official accreditation decision report. *See also* accreditation survey; Joint Commission on Accreditation of Healthcare Organizations; survey report form.

survey report form (SRF) A surveyor's data collection tool in which scores and documentation are recorded during an on-site survey by the Joint Commission on Accreditation of Healthcare Organizations. *See also* accreditation survey; Joint Commission on Accreditation of Healthcare Organizations; survey report.

survey, special *See* special survey.

survey, specialized *See* specialized survey.

survey team A group of health professionals who work together to perform an accreditation survey by the Joint Commission on Accreditation of Healthcare Organizations or other accrediting body. A typical Joint Commission hospital survey team, for instance, consists of a physician, a nurse, an administrator, and a medical technologist. *See also* Joint Commission on Accreditation of Healthcare Organizations; survey; team.

survey, unannounced *See* unannounced survey.

survey validation The process performed by survey report analysts from the Joint Commission on

Accreditation of Healthcare Organizations to assess the degree to which survey reports and accompanying documentation are consistent and accurate. Each finding is assessed by comparing the scores on the survey report form with the accompanying documentation, consulting with applicable scoring guidelines, and consulting with respective accreditation services staff members and other staff experts. *See also* Joint Commission on Accreditation of Healthcare Organizations; survey; survey report; validation.

surveyor In health care, a health professional (such as a physician, a nurse, an administrator, or a laboratorian) who meets surveyor selection criteria of the Joint Commission on Accreditation of Healthcare Organizations and is appropriately trained in the evaluation of standards. He or she evaluates standards compliance and provides education and consultation regarding standards compliance to surveyed health care organizations. *See also* accreditation survey; Joint Commission on Accreditation of Healthcare Organizations; laboratorian.

survival The act or process of remaining alive. *See also* survival of the fittest.

survival of the fittest Natural selection conceived of as a struggle for life in which only those organisms best adapted to existing conditions are able to survive and reproduce. *See also* natural selection; survival.

survival, lost chance of *See* lost chance of survival.

SUS *See* Society of University Surgeons.

suture 1. The process of joining two surfaces or edges together along a line by sewing, as in suturing the wound closed. 2. The fine thread or other material used surgically to close a wound or join tissues, as in absorbable suture. *Synonym*: stitch. *See also* laceration. 3. The inflexible fibrous articulations between the component bones of the skull.

SUU *See* Society of University Urologists.

SVN *See* Society for Vascular Nursing.

SVS *See* Society for Vascular Surgery.

SVT *See* Society of Vascular Technology.

swab A wad of cotton or other absorbent material for mopping up blood or other fluids, applying antiseptics to the skin, taking bacteriological specimens, and many other uses. *See also* tampon.

Swan-Ganz catheter A soft, flow-directed catheter with a balloon at the tip for measuring pulmonary arterial pressures. It is introduced into the venous system via the basilic, internal jugular, or subclavian vein and is guided by blood flow into the superior vena cava, the right atrium and ventricle, and into the pulmonary artery. *See also* catheter.

sweat *See* perspiration.

swelling Enlargement of any part of the body.

swing bed A bed regularly maintained by a health care organization for short-term and long-term use, depending on need. *See also* bed; bed conversion.

symbol Something that represents something else by association, resemblance, or convention, especially a material object used to represent something invisible; for example, the scales as a symbol of justice and the staff of Aesculapius as a symbol for medicine. *See also* caduceus; decision symbol; staff of Aesculapius.

symbol, decision *See* decision symbol.

sympathy Intellectual and emotional sharing of another's thoughts and feelings. *Compare* empathy.

symptom 1. Specific observed evidence of something else. 2. In medicine, an indication of disorder or disease, especially when experienced by an individual as a change from normal functions, sensation, or appearance; for example, headache is a symptom of many diseases or conditions ranging from migraine to meningitis. *See also* finding; prodrome; semiology; sign; symptomatology; syndrome; withdrawal symptoms.

symptomatology 1. The science of symptoms. 2. The combined symptoms of a disease or condition, as in her symptomatology suggests appendicitis. *See also* symptom.

symptoms, withdrawal *See* withdrawal symptoms.

syncope A sudden temporary loss of consciousness. *Synonyms*: blackout; faint.

syndrome A group of symptoms that collectively indicate or characterize a disease, a psychological disorder, or another abnormal condition, as in Down syndrome. *See also* acquired immunodeficiency syndrome; adult respiratory distress syndrome; asthma; attention-deficit disorder; battered child syndrome; congestive heart failure; Down syndrome; fetal alcohol syndrome; irritable bowel syndrome; Munchausen's syndrome; sudden infant death syndrome; temporomandibular joint syndrome; toxic shock syndrome.

syndrome, acquired immunodeficiency *See* acquired immunodeficiency syndrome.

syndrome, adult respiratory distress *See* adult

respiratory distress syndrome.

syndrome, battered child   *See* battered child syndrome.

Syndrome Clearinghouse, National Sudden Infant Death   *See* National Sudden Infant Death Syndrome Clearinghouse.

syndrome, Down   *See* Down syndrome.

syndrome, fetal alcohol   *See* fetal alcohol syndrome.

syndrome, irritable bowel   *See* irritable bowel syndrome.

syndrome, Munchausen's   *See* Munchausen's syndrome.

syndrome, posttraumatic stress   *See* posttraumatic stress disorder.

syndrome, premenstrual   *See* premenstrual syndrome.

syndrome, respiratory distress   *See* respiratory distress syndrome.

syndrome, sudden infant death   *See* sudden infant death syndrome.

syndrome, temporomandibular joint   *See* temporomandibular joint syndrome.

syndrome, toxic shock   *See* toxic shock syndrome.

syphilis   An infectious disease caused by a spirochete transmitted by direct contact, usually through sexual intercourse, or passed from mother to child in utero. It progresses through three stages. *Synonym*: lues. *See also* direct contact; infectious diseases; neurosyphilis; sexual intercourse.

syphilis, neuro-   *See* neurosyphilis.

syringe   A medical instrument used to inject fluids into the body or to withdraw liquids from the body. *Synonym*: hypodermic syringe. *See also* needle.

syringe, hypodermic   *See* syringe.

system   A network of interdependent components that work together to try to accomplish the aim of the system, as in a skeletal system or an emergency medical services system. *See also* network; weakest link theory.

system, accounting   *See* accounting system.

System Act of 1993, Emergency Medical Services   *See* Emergency Medical Services System Act of 1993.

system, all-payer   *See* all-payer system.

system, alternative delivery   *See* alternative delivery system.

system, alternative dental delivery   *See* alternative dental delivery system.

system, alternative financing   *See* alternative financing system.

system, American Joint Committee on Cancer pathologic stage classification   *See* American Joint Committee on Cancer pathologic stage classification system.

system, American Society of Anesthesiologists - Physical Status classification   *See* American Society of Anesthesiologists - Physical Status classification system.

system, computer-based patient record   *See* computer-based patient record system.

systematic error   Error that often has a recognizable source, such as a faulty measurement instrument, or pattern such as it is consistently wrong in a particular direction. *See also* bias; error.

systematic sampling   A process in which one case is selected randomly, and the next cases are selected according to a fixed period or interval; for example, every fifth patient who arrives in a hospital unit becomes part of the random sample. *See also* sampling.

system audit, quality   *See* quality system audit.

system, automatic fire extinguishing   *See* automatic fire extinguishing system.

system, case-mix management information   *See* case-mix management information system.

system, central nervous   *See* central nervous system.

system, circulatory   *See* circulatory system.

system, classification   *See* classification system.

system, clinical information   *See* clinical information system.

system, coding   *See* coding system.

system, comprehensive health care delivery   *See* comprehensive health care delivery system.

system, computer-based patient record   *See* computer-based patient record system.

System, Cooperative Health Statistics   *See* Cooperative Health Statistics System.

System, Coordinated Transfer Application   *See* Coordinated Transfer Application System.

system, database management   *See* database management system.

system, diagnosis-related group reimbursement   *See* diagnosis-related group reimbursement system.

system, digestive   *See* digestive system.

system, disk operating   *See* disk operating system.

system, electrical distribution   *See* electrical distribution system.

system, emergency medical services *See* emergency medical services system.

system, executive information *See* executive information system.

system, expert *See* expert system.

system, health *See* health system.

system, health care *See* health care system.

system, hospital discharge abstract *See* hospital discharge abstract system.

system, hospital information *See* hospital information system.

systemic Pertaining to the entire body or an entire organism, as in systemic circulation or systemic illness. *See also* systemic adjuvant therapy; systemic disease; systemic problem.

systemic adjuvant therapy Chemotherapy, hormonal/steroid therapy, biological response modifier therapy, or other systemic agents in addition to primary treatment by surgical resection and/or radiation therapy for cancer. *See also* cancer; therapy.

systemic disease Disease that affects the whole body rather than a localized area or regional portion of the body. *See also* disease; systemic.

systemic problem A problem caused not by employees but by the faulty structure of a working (or non-working) system. *See also* problem; systemic.

system, immune *See* immune system.

system, indicator measurement *See* indicator measurement system.

system, indicator monitoring *See* indicator measurement system.

system, information *See* information system.

system, interactive computer *See* interactive computer system.

Système International units (SI units) An international measurement system, commonly known as the metric system. It is based on seven base units, from which all other measurements are derived. The units are length (meter), mass (kilogram), time (second), amount of substance (mole), thermodynamic temperature (kelvin), electric current (ampere), and luminous intensity (candela).

system, knowledge-based *See* knowledge-based system.

system, life support *See* life support system.

system, management information *See* management information system.

System, Medical Illness Severity Grouping *See* Medical Illness Severity Grouping System.

System, Medical Literature Analysis and Retrieval *See* Medical Literature Analysis and Retrieval System.

System, Medical Management Analysis *See* Medical Management Analysis System.

system, medication *See* medication system.

system, multihospital *See* multihospital system.

system, nervous *See* nervous system.

system, on-line *See* on-line system.

system, operating *See* operating system.

system, patient identification *See* patient identification system.

system, peripheral nervous *See* peripheral nervous system.

system, prospective payment *See* prospective payment system.

system, prospective pricing *See* prospective pricing system.

system, quality *See* quality system.

system, reticuloendothelial *See* reticuloendothelial system.

systems analysis The study of a system, an activity, or a process to determine the desired end and the most efficient method of obtaining this end. *See also* analysis; system.

systems analyst One who performs systems analysis. *See also* computer programmer.

Systems Association, Insurance Accounting and *See* Insurance Accounting and Systems Association.

system, seniority *See* seniority system.

system, single-payer *See* single-payer system.

Systems Management, Association for *See* Association for Systems Management.

system software In computer science, the programs that instruct a system how to operate its own devices. *See also* computer program; computer software.

systems programmer An individual who writes the programs needed for a computer system to function, such as operating systems, language processors and compilers, and data file management programs. *See also* computer.

systems thinking A school of thought evolving from earlier systems analysis theory, propounding that virtually all outcomes are the result of systems rather than individuals. The theory is characterized by extensive use of computer modeling to simulate the effects or changes on existing systems. *See also* computer modeling.

system survey, multiorganization   *See* multiorganization system survey.

system, turnkey   *See* turnkey system.

system, unit-dose medication   *See* unit-dose medication system.

system, value   *See* value system.

system, voucher   *See* voucher system.

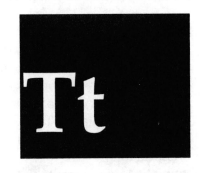

T *See* occupancy factor.

TAANA *See* The American Association of Nurse Attorneys.

table **1.** An orderly arrangement of data, especially one in which the data are arranged in columns and rows in an essentially rectangular form. *See also* data; graph. **2.** An abbreviated list, as in a table of contents. **3.** The part of the human palm framed by four lines, analyzed in palmistry. *See also* palmistry.

table, life *See* life table.

table, mortality *See* mortality table.

tablet A solid dosage form of varying weight, size, and shape, which contains a medicinal substance for oral administration. *See also* pill.

taboo **1.** Something sacred or prohibited, restricted to a particular class of person. *See also* belief; sacred. **2.** Any of the traditions and behaviors that are generally regarded as harmful to social welfare, as in the incest taboo. *See also* incest.

tactic **1.** A short-term method for resolving a particular problem or achieving a short-range objective. **2.** The means of carrying out a strategy. *See also* strategy.

tachycardia A rapid heart rate, especially one above 100 beats per minute in an adult. *Compare* bradycardia. *See also* arrhythmia.

tail coverage Insurance purchased to protect the insured after the end of a claims-made policy and to cover events that occurred during the period of the claims-made policy, but for which a claim was not made during the period. Tail coverage protects the insured in case a claim is made at a future date, after the original policy has lapsed. *See also* claims-made coverage; coverage; insurance.

tailgate pricing Pricing that responds to the demand of the market at the moment and that is not based on costs or a consistent pricing policy. *See also* prestige pricing; price; prospective pricing system.

tailored survey A survey by the Joint Commission on Accreditation of Healthcare Organizations in which standards from more than one standards manual are used in assessing compliance; it may include using specialist surveyors appropriate to the standards selected for survey. *See also* accreditation survey; compliance; Joint Commission on Accreditation of Healthcare Organizations; primary standards; standards manuals; survey.

take-charge Possessing or exhibiting strong qualities of initiative, leadership, and management, as in a take-charge manager. *See also* initiative; leadership; management.

take-home pay Amount of one's wages or salary remaining after federal, state, and often city income taxes and various other deductions have been withheld. *See also* income tax; pay.

talisman *See* amulet.

talking books Voice recordings of written material, made for the blind. *See also* book.

tamper To interfere in a harmful manner, as with the packaging of consumer goods, especially to engage in consumer terrorism. *See also* tamper evident; tamper resistant.

tamper evident Packaging that has a visible seal or other device that makes obvious any opening of the package between manufacture and sale. *See also* tamper.

tampering **1.** In data analysis, the act of taking action on some signal of variation without taking into account the difference between special-cause and common-cause variation. *See also* common-cause variation; data analysis; special-cause variation. **2.** *See* tamper.

tamper resistant A package that is constructed so

as to make tampering with the product difficult or impossible. *See also* tamper; tamper evident.

tampon A plug of cotton or other absorbent material for insertion into bodily orifices in order to control bleeding or flow of secretions. *See also* swab.

TANK *See* Floatation Tank Association.

Tank Association, Floatation *See* Floatation Tank Association.

tannin A component of tea that can irritate the digestive tract, cause constipation, and reduce iron absorption.

TAP *See* The Angel Planes.

TAPA *See* Turkish American Physicians Association.

tape The plastic medium kept on reels on which data are encoded electronically. It is used to store data and programs, to feed such data and programs into a computer, to record the computer's output, and to provide a data processing history and archives. *See also* tape drive.

tape drive A device that converts information stored on tape into signals that can be sent to a computer. *See also* computer; tape.

tarantism An epidemic form of dancing mania prevalent in parts of Italy from the fifteenth to the seventeenth centuries. It was supposed either to be caused by or to cure the effects of a spider's bite. *See also* behavioral epidemic.

target Something to be aimed at, such as a desired goal. *See also* goal; objective; milestone; target audience; target date; targeted mortality method.

target audience In advertising, a group of people to whom advertising is directed. It can be defined in terms of demographic characteristics, such as age, sex, education, income, and buying habits. *See also* advertise.

target date A date established as a goal, as for the completion of a project. *See also* goal.

targeted mortality method An approach to quality assessment in which deaths in certain types of cases are targeted for review. Examples include deaths in diagnosis-related groups (DRGs) with an average death rate of more than 5%, deaths occurring within one day of any procedure, and deaths in which burns are reported as a secondary diagnosis. *See also* mortality; target.

task The smallest measurable unit of work resulting in a predefined output. *See also* output; task force.

task force A temporary grouping of individuals

and resources assembled for the accomplishment of a specific objective, as in a task force for developing performance measures in a specified organizational area, such as medication use. A task force actively pursues the achievement of its mission, after which it is disbanded. *See also* committee; expert panel; objective.

taste The sensation produced by particular substances when they come into contact with specialized receptors scattered throughout the mucous membrane of the tongue and palate. Impulses from the taste buds are then carried to the brain. *See also* sensation; sense.

tatooing The indelible marking or designing on the skin by injecting permanent dyes through needle puncturing. Transmission of hepatitis B and other diseases is a hazard when the instruments are inadequately sterilized. *See also* hepatitis.

tax The rate or sum of money assessed on a person or property for the support of the government. A tax is commonly levied upon assets or real property (called property tax), income derived from wages and elsewhere (income tax), or upon the sale or purchase of goods (sales tax). *See also* capital gains tax; income tax; payroll tax; progressive tax; proportional tax; regressive tax; repressive tax; value added tax.

tax, capital gains *See* capital gains tax.

tax credit A reduction of tax liability for federal income tax purposes. Some national health insurance proposals allow businesses and/or individuals to reduce their taxes dollar for dollar for certain defined medical expenses. The effect of using a tax credit approach rather than a tax deduction is to give persons and businesses an equal benefit for each dollar expended on health care. *See also* tax; tax incentive.

tax deduction A reduction in the income base upon which federal income tax is calculated. Health insurance expenditures, for instance, are currently deductible by businesses as a business expense. *See also* deduction; tax.

Tax Equity and Fiscal Responsibility Act (TEFRA) Federal legislation passed in 1981 that raised tax revenue, mainly through closing various loopholes and instituting tougher enforcement procedures. It established that a Medicare prospective payment system for reimbursing hospitals must be in place by October, 1983. Because risk contracts with health maintenance organizations offered the potential to constrain Medicare costs, the Congress modified the program's health maintenance organization provision through TEFRA. *See also* Medicare; Medicare secondary payer; prospective pricing system; prospective payment system; tax.

tax-exempt Not subject to taxation, as the income of a philanthropic organization. *See also* tax.

tax expenditure Revenue losses suffered by the federal government as a result of provisions of the Internal Revenue Code, which grant special tax benefits to certain kinds of taxpayers or certain activities engaged in by taxpayers. Examples include tax credits and tax deductions. This approach recognizes that such provisions are the economic equivalent of a collection of the forgiven tax liability and a simultaneous direct budget outlay to the benefited taxpayers. An example is the subsidization of private purchase of health insurance through the federal income tax deduction for health insurance. *See also* tax expenditure budget.

tax expenditure budget In the federal budget, a listing of revenue losses resulting from tax expenditures. *See also* budget; tax expenditure.

tax incentive A feature of a taxation system that encourages or discourages certain economic activities. Common tax incentives are depreciation allowances and tax credits. *See also* incentive; tax credit.

tax, income *See* income tax.

taxonomy The science of the classification of organisms according to their resemblances and differences, with the application of names or other labels. *See also* classification of diseases; classification system; nosology.

taxpayer One that pays taxes or is subjected to taxation. *See also* tax.

tax, payroll *See* payroll tax.

tax, progressive *See* progressive tax.

tax, proportional *See* proportional tax.

tax rate, marginal *See* marginal tax rate.

tax, regressive *See* regressive tax.

tax, repressive *See* repressive tax.

tax, sin *See* sin tax.

tax, value-added *See* value-added tax.

TB *See* tuberculosis.

T & C Abbreviation for type and cross (blood). *See* blood transfusion; blood typing; crossmatching.

TCA *See* Tissue Culture Association.

T cell *See* lymphocyte.

TCSG *See* The Center for Social Gerontology.

***t*-distribution** The distribution of a quotient of independent random variables, the numerator of which is a standardized normal variate and the denominator of which is the positive square root of the quotient of a chi-square distributed variate and its number of degrees of freedom. *See also* distribution; random variable; *t*-test.

teach **1.** To impart knowledge or skill to, as in teaching allied health professionals or medical students. *See also* teacher. **2.** To cause to learn by example or experience, as in the outcome taught the medical staff an important lesson.

teacher One who teaches, especially one hired to teach. *See also* mentor; teach; teaching physician.

Teachers of Maternal and Child Health, Association of *See* Association of Teachers of Maternal and Child Health.

Teachers of Preventive Medicine, Association of *See* Association of Teachers of Preventive Medicine.

teaching hospital A medical school-affiliated or university-owned hospital with accredited programs in medical, allied health, or nursing education. Hospitals that educate nurses and other health personnel but do not train physicians, or that have only programs of continuing education for practicing professionals, are not considered to be teaching hospitals. *See also* hospital; housestaff; medical practice plan.

Teaching Hospitals, Council of *See* Council of Teaching Hospitals.

teaching physician A physician who trains and supervises medical students, interns, and residents in, for example, a teaching hospital. Teaching physicians are often salaried by the organization in which they teach. *See also* physician; salaried physician; teacher; teaching rounds.

teaching rounds A clinical instructional process in which a teaching physician takes his or her medical students, interns, and/or residents to the bedside of patients in a teaching hospital in order to review the patients' course and treatment. *Synonym:* ward rounds. *See also* rounds; teaching physician.

team A group of people organized to work together, as in an intravenous team. *See also* crossfunctional team; functional team; health care team; intravenous team; project team; quality improvement team; team building; team leader.

team building An organization development technique for improving a work group's performance and attitudes by clarifying its goals and its members' expectations of each other. *See also* team.

team, crossfunctional *See* crossfunctional team.

team, functional *See* functional team.

team, health care *See* health care team.

team, intravenous *See* intravenous team.

team leader An individual who guides or directs a team. *See also* leader; team.

team nurse A nurse who is a member of a nursing team composed of a group of registered nurses and ancillary personnel who provide nursing services under a team leader, for a designated group of patients during a single nursing shift. *See also* nursing assistant; registered nurse.

team nursing A type of organization of nursing services in which a team headed by a registered nurse, with other registered nurses and ancillary personnel, cares for a group of patients in an inpatient care unit. *See also* inpatient care unit; nursing; primary nursing; team.

team, project *See* project team.

team, quality improvement *See* quality improvement team.

team, surgical *See* surgical team.

team, survey *See* survey team.

teamwork Work performed by a team. *See also* team.

tears Watery saline secretion of the lacrimal glands. *See also* emotion; saline.

tech, high *See* high tech.

tech, low *See* low tech.

technical Having special skill or practical knowledge, especially in a mechanical or scientific field, as in a technical expert. *See also* technique.

technical aspects of medical care The application of medical science and technology to a medical problem. *See also* medical care; technical.

Technical Personnel in Ophthalmology, Association of *See* Association of Technical Personnel in Ophthalmology.

Technical Professionals, National Organization of Gay and Lesbian Scientists and *See* National Organization of Gay and Lesbian Scientists and Technical Professionals.

technician An individual having special skill or practical knowledge in an area, such as operation and maintenance of equipment or performance of laboratory procedures involving biochemical analy-

ses. Special technical qualifications are normally required, though an increasing number of technicians also possess university degrees in science, and occasionally doctorate degrees. The distinction between technician and technologist in the health care field is not always clear. *See also* technical; technologist.

technician, accredited record *See* accredited record technician.

technician, dental laboratory *See* dental laboratory technician.

technician, dermatology *See* dermatology technician.

technician, dialysis *See* dialysis technician.

technician, dietetic *See* dietetic technician.

technician, electrocardiographic *See* electrocardiographic technician.

technician, emergency medical *See* emergency medical technician.

technician, health physics *See* health physics technician.

technician, hemodialysis *See* hemodialysis technician.

technician, histologic *See* histologic technician.

technician, industrial audiometric *See* industrial audiometric technician.

technician, mental health *See* mental health technician.

technician, operating room *See* operating room technician.

technician, ophthalmic laboratory *See* ophthalmic laboratory technician.

technician, ophthalmic medical *See* ophthalmic medical technician.

technician, orthotic/prosthetic *See* orthotic/prosthetic technician.

technician-paramedic, emergency medical *See* emergency medical technician-paramedic.

technician, recreational therapy *See* recreational therapy technician.

technician, respiratory therapy *See* respiratory therapy technician.

Technicians, National Association of Air National Guard Health *See* National Association of Air National Guard Health Technicians.

Technicians, National Association of Emergency Medical *See* National Association of Emergency Medical Technicians.

Technicians, National Registry of Emergency

Medical *See* National Registry of Emergency Medical Technicians.

Technicians, Society of Biomedical Equipment *See* Society of Biomedical Equipment Technicians.

Technicians and Technologists, American Board of Certified and Registered Encephalographic *See* American Board of Certified and Registered Encephalographic Technicians and Technologists.

technique The method of procedure and the details of any process, such as techniques used in a surgical operation. *See also* method; procedure; technical.

technique, double-blind *See* double-blind technique.

technique, nominal group *See* nominal group technique.

Technique, Program Evaluation and Review *See* Program Evaluation and Review Technique.

technique, single-blind *See* single-blind technique.

technique, sterile *See* sterile technique.

technological Pertaining to the application of science, as in technological advances in radiological imaging or laser therapeutic procedures. *See also* technology.

technological obsolescence Technology becoming outdated due to technological advances. For example, word processors are making traditional typewriters obsolete. *See also* obsolescence; technology.

technologies, reproductive *See* reproductive technologies.

technologist A specialist in technology, as in radiologic technologist or medical technologist. The distinction between technician and technologist in the health care field is not always clear. *See also* technician; technology.

technologist, animal care *See* animal care technologist.

technologist, blood bank *See* specialist in blood bank technology.

technologist, cardiovascular *See* cardiovascular technologist.

technologist, chemistry *See* chemistry technologist.

technologist, circulation *See* perfusionist.

technologist, cyto- *See* cytotechnologist.

technologist, EEG *See* electroencephalographic technician/technologist.

technologist, electroneurodiagnostic *See* electroneurodiagnostic technologist.

technologist, encephalographic *See* electroen-cephalographic technician/technologist.

technologist, extracorporeal *See* perfusionist.

technologist, hematology *See* hematology technologist.

technologist, histologic *See* histologic technologist.

technologist, laboratory *See* medical technologist.

technologist, medical *See* medical technologist.

technologist, medical laboratory *See* medical technologist.

technologist, microbiology *See* microbiology technologist.

technologist, nuclear medicine *See* nuclear medicine technologist.

technologist, ophthalmic medical *See* ophthalmic medical technologist.

technologist, perfusion *See* perfusionist.

technologist, radiation therapy *See* radiation therapy technologist.

technologist, radiologic *See* radiographer.

Technologists, American Board of Certified and Registered Encephalographic Technicians and *See* American Board of Certified and Registered Encephalographic Technicians and Technologists.

Technologists, American Board of Registration of Electroencephalographic and Evoked Potentials *See* American Board of Registration of Electroencephalographic and Evoked Potentials Technologists.

Technologists, American Chiropractic Registry of Radiologic *See* American Chiropractic Registry of Radiologic Technologists.

Technologists, American Medical *See* American Medical Technologists.

Technologists, American Registry of Clinical Radiography *See* American Registry of Clinical Radiography Technologists.

Technologists, American Registry of Radiologic *See* American Registry of Radiologic Technologists.

Technologists, American Society of Electroneurodiagnostic *See* American Society of Electroneurodiagnostic Technologists.

Technologists, American Society of Radiologic *See* American Society of Radiologic Technologists.

Technologists, Association of Cytogenetic *See* Association of Cytogenetic Technologists.

Technologists, Association of Polysomnographic *See* Association of Polysomnographic Technologists.

Technologists, Association of Surgical *See* Association of Surgical Technologists.

Technologist Section of the Society of Nuclear Medicine (TSSNM) A national organization founded in 1970 composed of 4,800 members of the Society of Nuclear Medicine who have received formal or on-the-job training in nuclear medicine technology. It represents the field in areas of licensure, accreditation, and certification. *See also* accreditation; certification; licensure; nuclear medicine; nuclear medicine technologist; Society of Nuclear Medicine.

Technologists, National Association of Orthopaedic *See* National Association of Orthopaedic Technologists.

Technologists, National Board for Certification of Orthopaedic *See* National Board for Certification of Orthopaedic Technologists.

Technologists, Registered Medical Assistants of American Medical *See* Registered Medical Assistants of American Medical Technologists.

technologist, surgical *See* surgical technologist.

technology **1.** The application of science, as to industrial, commercial, or health care objectives. *See also* health care technology; high tech; low tech; reproductive technologies; technician; technologist. **2.** In anthropology, the body of knowledge available to a civilization that is of use in fashioning implements, practicing manual arts and skills, and extracting or collecting materials.

Technology, Accreditation Review Committee for Educational Programs in Surgical *See* Accreditation Review Committee for Educational Programs in Surgical Technology.

Technology, American Society for Cyto- *See* American Society for Cytotechnology.

Technology, American Society of Extra-Corporeal *See* American Society of Extra-Corporeal Technology.

Technology, American Society for Medical *See* American Society for Medical Technology.

technology assessment The process of describing and analyzing various dimensions of specific technologies, such as analyzing the effectiveness, cost, and safety of a new (or an old) therapeutic modality in health care. *See also* assessment; modality; technology.

Technology Assessment, National Center for Health Services Research and Health Care *See* National Center for Health Services Research and Health Care Technology Assessment.

Technology Assessment, Office of Health *See* Office of Health Technology Assessment.

Technology Assessment Program, Diagnostic and Therapeutic *See* Diagnostic and Therapeutic Technology Assessment Program.

technology, bio- *See* biotechnology.

Technology, Board of Nephrology Examiners-Nursing and *See* Board of Nephrology Examiners-Nursing and Technology.

Technology Certification Board, Nuclear Medicine *See* Nuclear Medicine Technology Certification Board.

technology, health care *See* health care technology.

Technology, Joint Review Committee on Education in Radiologic *See* Joint Review Committee on Education in Radiologic Technology.

Technology, National Board for Certification in Dental *See* National Board for Certification in Dental Technology.

Technology, National Institute of Standards and *See* National Institute of Standards and Technology.

Technology, National Society for Cardiovascular Technology/National Society for Pulmonary *See* National Society for Cardiovascular Technology/National Society for Pulmonary Technology.

Technology, National Society for Histo- *See* National Society for Histotechnology.

technology, noninvasive vascular *See* noninvasive vascular technology.

technology, polysomnographic *See* polysomnographic technology.

technology, reproductive *See* reproductive technologies.

technology, and safety management, plant *See* plant, technology, and safety management.

Technology, Society for Assisted Reproductive *See* Society for Assisted Reproductive Technology.

Technology, Society for the History of *See* Society for the History of Technology.

Technology, Society of Vascular *See* Society of Vascular Technology.

technology, specialist in blood bank *See* specialist in blood bank technology.

technology, voice *See* voice input/output technology.

technology, voice input/output *See* voice input/output technology.

technostress Stress arising from working in a technological environment, especially with computer technology, and being unable to adapt to the new technology. *See also* high tech; stress.

teeth *See* dentition; tooth.

teeth, permanent *See* permanent tooth.

teeth, wisdom *See* wisdom teeth.

TEFRA *See* Tax Equity and Fiscal Responsibility Act.

telecommunications The science and technology of communication at a distance by electronic transmission of impulses, as by telephone, radio, telegram, or television. *See also* communication; telecommunications companies; teleconference.

telecommunications companies In computer science, private ventures that provide a network to connect microcomputer users with remote computers. Using phone lines, the companies provide local access numbers nationwide with hourly charges that are less than charges for dialing to a remote computer directly. On-line database services may bill for telecommunications access. *See also* on-line database; network; telecommunications.

teleconference A conference held among people in different locations by means of telecommunications equipment, such as closed-circuit television. *See also* conference; telecommunications.

telefacsimile *See* fax.

telemetry The science and technology of automatic measurement and transmission of data by wire, radio, or other means from remote sources, as from mobile intensive care units (ambulances) to a receiving station, such as one located in a hospital emergency department, where the data may be recorded and analyzed. *See also* biotelemetry; data; technology.

telemetry, bio- *See* biotelemetry.

teleology The doctrine of causes, or interpretation in terms of purpose.

telepathy Extrasensory thought transference. *See also* parapsychology; perception; sixth sense.

temperament An inherent, constitutional predisposition to react to stimuli in a certain way. *See also* physiognomy.

temperature The degree of hotness or coldness of a body or an environment that can be measured on a scale. *See also* Celsius scale; clinical thermometer; Fahrenheit scale; febrile; fever; hyperpyrexia; hypothermia; Kelvin scale; measurement; scale; thermometer; vital signs.

temporary Lasting for a limited time, as in temporary disability. *See also* temporary bed; temporary disability; temporary privileges; temporary restraining order.

temporary bed A bed provided for use by patients at times when a health care organization's patient census exceeds the number of beds regularly maintained. *See also* bed; temporary.

temporary disability An illness or injury that prevents an insured individual from performing functions of his or her usual occupation or profession for an interim period of time. *See also* disability; temporary.

temporary privileges Temporary authorization granted by a hospital governing body to a licensed individual to provide patient care services in the organization for a limited period or to a specific patient for that patient's hospitalization, within limits based on the individual's professional license, education, training, experience, competence, health status, and judgment. *See also* clinical privileges; emergency privileges; temporary.

temporary restraining order A court order to do or refrain from doing some act that is of a very limited duration and is intended to maintain the status quo while additional information and evidence are gathered. *See also* restrain; status quo.

temporomandibular joint (TMJ) The joint formed by the temporal bone (skull) and the mandible (lower jaw). *See also* temporomandibular joint syndrome.

temporomandibular joint syndrome A disorder caused by faulty articulation of the temporomandibular joint and characterized by facial pain, headache, ringing ears, dizziness, and neck stiffness. *See also* American Academy of Head, Facial and Neck Pain and TMJ Orthopedics; American Equilibration Society; syndrome; temporomandibular joint.

tendon A fibrous cord, largely composed of collagen fibers, attaching a muscle to a bone. *Synonym*: sinew. *See also* bone; joint; muscle.

tenet An opinion, doctrine, or principle held as being true by a person or especially by an organization. *See also* assumption; doctrine; opinion; principle.

TENS *See* transcutaneous electric nerve stimulation.

tension *See* stress.

tenure **1.** Length of time an individual has been employed by a certain organization. **2.** An academic privilege granted to associate and full professors, allowing freedom of speech (academic freedom) and conveying implications of continued employment except in extraordinary circumstances. *See also* academic; professor.

teratogen An agent, such as a virus, a drug, or radiation, that causes malformation of an embryo or a fetus. *See also* embryo; fetal alcohol syndrome; fetus; rubella; teratology; thalidomide.

teratogenic Producing abnormal embryos. *See also* embryo; teratology.

teratology The branch of science dealing with the production, development, and classification of abnormal embryos and/or fetuses. *See also* biology; embryo; fetal alcohol syndrome; fetus; rubella; teratology; thalidomide.

Teratology Society (TS) A national organization founded in 1960 composed of 750 individuals from academia, government, private industry, and the professions concerned with exchanging ideas and information about abnormal biological development and malformations at the fundamental or clinical level. It sponsors education courses, bestows awards, and maintains a placement service. *See also* biology; teratology.

tercile *See* quantile.

term **1.** A word or group of words having a particular meaning. *See also* terminology. **2.** The end of a gestation period, as in term infant. *See also* term infant. **3.** A limited period of time, as in a term of office or an academic term.

terminable-at-will A contract that can be terminated at any time without cause. *See also* contract.

terminal **1.** Forming a limit, a boundary, or an end, as in terminal illness. **2.** *See also* computer terminal.

terminal care Care for a patient in the terminal stages of illness, as in hospice care for a dying patient. *See also* hospice.

terminal care document *See* living will.

terminal, computer *See* computer terminal.

terminal, dumb *See* dumb terminal.

terminal illness An incurable or irreversible illness. The end stage of an illness that will result in death within a short time. *See also* hopelessly ill; illness; palliative care; terminal.

terminal, interactive *See* interactive terminal.

Terminally Ill, Center for the Rights of the *See* Center for the Rights of the Terminally Ill.

termination of life support systems *See* life support system.

term infant Any neonate whose birth occurs from the beginning of the first day (260th day) of the 38th week, through the end of the last day (294th day) of the 42nd week following onset of the last menstrual period. *See also* infant; jargon; term.

terminology The vocabulary of technical terms used in a particular field, as in medical or legal terminology. *See also* term.

terms Conditions and arrangements specified in a contract. *See also* contract.

terrorism The unlawful use or threatened use of force or violence by a person or an organized group against people or property with the intention of intimidating or coercing societies or governments, often for ideological or political reasons.

tertiary Third in place, order, or degree, as in tertiary care hospital. *See also* tertiary care; tertiary care center; tertiary care hospital.

tertiary care Health services provided by highly specialized providers, such as medical subspecialists (for example, a pediatric endocrinologist or a hand surgeon). These services frequently require complex technological and support facilities. *Synonym:* tertiary health care. *See also* primary care; referred care; secondary care; tertiary care center; tertiary care hospital.

tertiary care center A medical facility that receives referrals from both primary and secondary care levels and usually offers tests, treatments, and procedures that are not available elsewhere. Most tertiary care centers offer a mixture of primary, secondary, and tertiary care services. *See also* centers of excellence; teaching hospital; tertiary care; tertiary care hospital.

tertiary care hospital A hospital specializing in severe illnesses and diseases requiring specialized resources, including personnel and technology. Most teaching hospitals are tertiary care hospitals. *See also* centers of excellence; hospital; teaching hospital; tertiary care center.

tertiary health care *See* tertiary care.

test A procedure for critical evaluation; a means of determining the presence, quality, or quantity of something. *See also* sensitivity of a test; specificity of a test; standardized test; testing; test reliability; test statistic.

test, blood *See* blood test.

test, breathalyzer *See* breathalyzer test.

test, chi-square *See* chi-square test.

test, diagnostic *See* diagnostic study.

testes *See* testis.

test, goodness-of-fit *See* goodness-of-fit test.

test hypothesis *See* null hypothesis.

testify To make a declaration of truth or fact under oath; submit testimony, as in testifying in court. *See also* oath; testimony; witness.

Testifying Physicians, American Association of *See* American Association of Testifying Physicians.

testimony A declaration by a witness under oath, as that given before a court; for example, the expert witnesses' testimony influenced the outcome. *See also* oath; testify; witness.

testing A means of determining the capability of an item to meet specified requirements by subjecting the item to a set of actions and conditions, such as physical, chemical, environmental, or operating actions and conditions. *See also* shakedown; test.

Testing, American College *See* American College Testing.

testing, conductivity *See* conductivity testing.

testing, decentralized laboratory *See* decentralized laboratory testing.

Testing and Materials, American Society for *See* ASTM.

testing, means *See* means testing.

testing process, indicator *See* indicator testing process.

testing, proficiency *See* proficiency testing.

testing, reliability *See* reliability testing.

test, inkblot *See* Rorschach test.

testis In humans, the paired reproductive organ that produces spermatozoa and the male hormones, such as testosterone. *Compare* ovary. *See also* genitalia; mumps; orchiectomy; orchitis; seminoma; spermatozoa; testosterone.

Test, Medical College Admission *See* Medical College Admission Test.

testosterone A steroid hormone produced primarily in the testes and responsible for the development and maintenance of male secondary sex characteristics. *See also* anabolic steroids; androgen; sex hormone; testis.

test, Pap *See* Pap smear.

test, parametric *See* parametric test.

test, paternity *See* paternity test.

test, predictive value of a negative *See* predictive value of a negative test.

test, predictive value of a positive *See* predictive value of a positive test.

test, predictive value of a screening *See* predictive value of a screening test.

test, pregnancy *See* pregnancy test.

test reliability In research, the dependability of a measuring tool, as reflected in the consistency of the result it provides when repeated measurements are made of the same parameter. *See also* parameter; reliability; reliability testing; test.

test, retest reliability A technique of repeating a measurement procedure on the same set of subjects to estimate reliability. The source of error assessed is that of fluctuating, temporary characteristics of the subjects. *Compare* split-half reliability. *See also* reliability; reliability testing.

test, Rorschach *See* Rorschach test.

test, sensitivity of a *See* sensitivity of a test.

test of significance *See* p (probability) value; statistical significance.

tests, liver function *See* liver function tests.

test, specificity of a *See* specificity of a test.

test, standardized *See* standardized test.

test statistic A measure calculated from data sampled from a population, used to either reject or fail to reject the null hypothesis. Rejection of the null hypothesis will take place if either the *p* (probability) value is small enough or the test statistic is larger than a predetermined requirement. *See also* null hypothesis; *p* (probability) value; statistic; two-tailed test.

test, statistical *See* statistical test.

test, stress *See* stress test.

test tube **1.** Produced or cultivated in a test tube. **2.** Conceived by or developed from artificial insemination, as in a test-tube baby. *See also* artificial insemination; test-tube baby.

test-tube baby A baby born as a result of fertilization occurring outside a mother's body. Ova are removed from a woman's body, usually via laparoscope, and mixed with sperm in a culture medium. If fertilization occurs and cleavage results, the blastocyst is then implanted in the woman's uterus and pregnancy continues. *See also* baby; in-vitro fertilization; noncoital reproduction; test tube.

test-tube baby technique *See* in-vitro fertilization.

test, two-tailed *See* two-tailed test.

tetanus An acute disease caused by the toxin of the bacteria *Clostridium tetani*, which typically gains entrance to the body through a deep puncture wound. The disease is characterized by spasmodic muscular spasms and tremors. *Synonym*: lockjaw. *See also* active immunization; bacteria; infectious diseases; trismus.

tetraplegia *See* quadriplegia.

thalidomide A drug that gained favor as a sedative and hypnotic following its introduction in Germany in 1958 but was withdrawn from use three years later when it became apparent that it caused serious congenital abnormalities, such as phocomelia (congenital deformity resulting in a missing portion of the limbs; the hands and/or feet may be attached directly to the torso), in children born of women who had taken it during pregnancy. Thalidomide was never licensed for use in the United States. *See also* hypnotic; phocomelia; pregnancy; sedative; teratogen; teratology.

thanatoid The state of being apparently dead. *See also* thanatology.

thanatology The study of death and dying, especially in their psychological and social aspects. *See also* American Institute of Life Threatening Illness and Loss (A Division of Foundation of Thanatology); Association for Death Education and Counseling; Center for Death Education and Research; death.

The Aaron Diamond Foundation, Inc An independent foundation established in 1955 in New York that provides grants primarily for medical research, including AIDS (acquired immunodeficiency syndrome) research, minority education, cultural programs, and civil and human rights. *See also* acquired immunodeficiency syndrome; foundation; private foundation.

The American Association of Nurse Attorneys (TAANA) A national organization founded in 1982 composed of 600 nurse attorneys, nurses in law school, and attorneys in nursing schools. *See also* attorney; nurse.

The Angel Planes (TAP) A national organization founded in 1985 composed of 500 volunteer pilots who fly blood to central blood banks; make emergency flights to rural hospitals to deliver special types of blood; pick up blood from mobile blood drives so that the blood can be prepared for transfusion within six hours of its donation; transport critical care (but not trauma) patients; and transport donated organs. *See also* blood; blood transfusion; organ procurement.

The Center for Social Gerontology (TCSG) A national nonmembership organization founded in 1971 that advances the well-being of older people in the United States through research, education, technical assistance, and training. It focuses primarily on legal rights, guardianship, and alternative protective services, and delivery of legal services. *See also* gerontology.

The Champlin Foundations An independent foundation with trusts established in 1932, 1947, and 1975 that supports the environment, higher education, health, hospitals, and other fields of interest. *See also* foundation; private foundation.

The Commonwealth Fund An independent foundation incorporated in 1912 that supports new opportunities to improve Americans' health and well-being and to assist specific groups of Americans who have serious and neglected problems. Its fields of interest include health, health services, hospitals, medical education, nursing, the aged, minorities, and education. Examples of its grants include support for programs for minority medical students seeking careers in academic medicine and for programs for nurses seeking to obtain advanced management training. *See also* foundation; private foundation.

The David and Lucile Packard Foundation An independent foundation established in 1964 with primary areas of interest including child development, elementary and secondary education, the environment, family planning, marine sciences, and population studies. *See also* foundation; private foundation.

The Duke Endowment An independent foundation incorporated in 1944 that supports nonprofit hospitals and child care institutions in North Carolina and South Carolina; rural United Methodist churches and retired ministers in North Carolina and their dependents; and Duke, Furman, and Johnson C. Smith universities, and Davidson College. *See also* endowment; foundation; private foundation.

The Edna McConnell Clark Foundation An independent foundation incorporated in 1950 in New York and 1969 in Delaware (the New York corporation merged into the Delaware corporation in 1974) that supports people who are least well served by the established institutions of society. The foundation seeks to identify specific programs that could make a difference in the lives of the poor. There are five areas of funding: children, disadvantaged youth, tropical disease research, homeless families, and justice. *See also* foundation; private foundation.

The Ford Foundation An independent foundation incorporated in 1936 in Michigan that supports advancement of the public well-being by identifying and contributing to the solution of problems of national and international importance. Grants are provided primarily to institutions for experimental, demonstration, and development efforts that are likely to produce significant advances within the foundation's fields of interest, which include reproductive health and population, rural poverty and resources, rights and social justice, governance and public policy, education and culture, international affairs, and urban poverty. *See also* foundation; private foundation.

The Forum for Health Care Planning (Forum) A national organization founded in 1950 composed of 500 individuals committed to planning quality health care services and facilities. It disseminates and exchanges information on hospital and health care planning. Formerly American Association for Hospital Planning. *See also* health planner.

The Healthcare Forum (THF) A national organization founded in 1927 composed of 2,000 health care executives, hospitals, and other health care providers, insurers and industry suppliers, and associations that serves as an educational and research resource for health care executives. *See also* administrator; executive.

The Henry J. Kaiser Family Foundation An independent foundation established in 1948 in California to support the efforts to make government more responsive to the health needs of the American people, to improve the health of low-income and minority groups, to help make the foundation's home state of California a leader in innovation and reform, and to develop a more equitable and effective health care system in South Africa. Its major share of resources are devoted to programs in health and medicine; its primary interests include the disadvantaged, minorities, government, health, public policy, and South Africa. *See also* foundation; private foundation.

The Information Exchange on Young Adult Chronic Patients (TIE) A national organization founded in 1983 to promote research and treatment for young adults suffering from chronic mental health problems. The organization defines a young adult chronic patient as a person aged 18 to 35 years who has a psychiatric disorder, is socially disabled, and has needed mental health services for at least two years. The psychiatric disorder may be a major mental ill-

ness or a personality disorder, or a mixture of emotional problems with substance abuse or other disabilities. *See also* adult; chronic; mental illness; personality disorder; substance abuse.

The John A. Hartford Foundation, Inc An independent foundation established in 1929 that provides support through **1.** the Aging and Health Program, to address the unique health needs of the elderly, including long term care, the use of medication in chronic health problems, increasing the nation's geriatric research and training capability, and improving hospital outcomes for frail elderly inpatients; and **2.** the Health Care Cost and Quality Program, concerned with balancing the quality and cost of medical procedures, particularly by developing systems for assessing their appropriateness, quality, and value. The Health Care Financing Program and the John A. and George L. Hartford Fellowship Program were both terminated in 1985; the Hartford Geriatric Faculty Development Award Program was terminated in 1987. *See also* foundation; private foundation.

The John D. and Catherine T. MacArthur Foundation An independent foundation established in 1970 that has seven major initiatives currently authorized: MacArthur Fellow Program, for highly talented individuals in any field of endeavor who are chosen in a foundation-initiated effort; the Health Program, for research in mental health and the psychological and behavioral aspects of health and rehabilitation (including designated programs in parasitology and aging); the Community Initiatives Program for support of cultural and community development in the Chicago metropolitan area; the Program on Peace and International Security; the World Environment and Resources Program, for support of conservation programs that protect the earth's biological diversity and work to protect tropical ecology; the Education Program, to focus on the promotion of literacy; and the Population Program, concerned with women's reproductive health, population and natural resources, communications and popular education, and leadership development. Through the General Program, the foundation makes grants for a changing array of purposes. *See also* foundation; private foundation.

The Joint Commission Journal See *The Joint Commission Journal on Quality Improvement.*

The Joint Commission Journal on Quality

Improvement A monthly journal published by the Joint Commission on Accreditation of Healthcare Organizations. *The Joint Commission Journal on Quality Improvement* is composed of clinical, research, and other articles relevant to measuring, assessing, and improving quality in health care. Also known as *The Joint Commission Journal*. Formerly (1993) *Quality Review Bulletin*. *See also* Joint Commission on Accreditation of Healthcare Organizations; journal; quality improvement.

The Kresge Foundation An independent foundation established in 1924 that primarily makes challenge grants to four-year colleges and universities; to organizations concerned with colleges and universities; and to organizations concerned with health and long term care, social services, science, the environment, public policy, and the arts. The foundation is one of the few large foundations concentrating exclusively on bricks-and-mortar campaigns, providing construction funds to recipient institutions or assisting with the renovation of existing facilities. The foundation supports only projects involving construction, renovation of facilities, purchase of major equipment or of integrated equipment systems having a capital value of not less than $75,000, and the purchase of real estate. The foundation has no predetermined grants budget by field, geography, or type of project. In 1988, the foundation began a science initiative program of offering challenge grants to upgrade and endow scientific equipment and laboratories in colleges, teaching hospitals, medical schools, and research institutions. *See also* foundation; private foundation.

The Living Bank (TLB) A registry founded in 1968 composed of 300,000 persons who, upon their deaths, wish to donate a part or parts of their bodies for transplantation, therapy, or medical research. Its primary objective is to encourage the general public to donate organs. *See also* organ donor; organ procurement; registry.

theobromine A substance (xanthine) in cocoa and chocolate that has properties similar to those of caffeine and acts as a diuretic, relaxes smooth muscles, and dilates blood vessels. *See also* caffeine; theophylline.

theophylline A xanthine central nervous system stimulant, similar to caffeine, found in tea. *See also* caffeine; central nervous system; stimulant; theobromine.

theorem An idea that is demonstrably true or is assumed to be true. *See also* assumption; idea; theory.

theoretics The theoretical part of a science or an art. *See also* science; theory.

theory **1.** A tested idea backed by data. *See also* data; idea. **2.** A set of propositions from which a large number of new observations can be deduced. Theory is one source of hypotheses. *See also* hypothesis; proposition. **3.** Abstract reasoning; speculation. *See also* deduce; force-field theory; information theory; probability theory; theorem; theory x; theory y; theory z; trickle-down theory; weakest link theory.

theory, force-field *See* force-field theory.

theory, information *See* information theory.

theory of motivation, field *See* field theory of motivation.

theory, probability *See* probability theory.

theory, trickle-down *See* trickle-down theory.

theory, weakest link *See* weakest link theory.

theory x A management theory stating that managers must coerce, cajole, threaten, and closely supervise subordinates in order to motivate them. It is an authoritarian supervisory approach to management. *See also* management; theory; theory y; theory z.

theory y A management theory stating that the right conditions and rewards will result in the average employee finding work to be a source of satisfaction, being willing to exercise self-direction toward goals to which he or she is committed, and being creative. *See also* management; theory; theory x; theory z.

theory z A management theory describing the Japanese system of management characterized by workers' involvement in management, resulting in higher productivity than the US management model, and a highly developed system of organizational and sociological rewards. *See also* management; theory; theory x; theory y.

The Pew Charitable Trusts The collective name for the seven individual charitable trusts established in 1948 by the four sons and daughters of Joseph N. Pew, the founder of the Sun Oil Company. Giving is primarily in the arts and culture, education (including theology), health and human services, conservation and the environment, public and foreign policy, religion, and the newly formed interdisciplinary fund. In each of these areas the trusts stress the importance of developing capable and committed leadership. *See also* leadership.

The Product Liability Alliance (TPLA) A national organization founded in 1981 composed of 325 trade associations, manufacturers, nonmanufacturing product sellers, and their insurers actively seeking enactment of federal product liability tort reform legislation. *See also* liability; product liability; tort.

The Proprietary Association *See* Nonprescription Drug Manufacturers Association.

therapeutic Having or exhibiting healing or curative powers, as in a therapeutic drug. *See also* modality; subtherapeutic; therapy.

therapeutic abortion A legal, induced abortion performed for medical reasons, as when the pregnancy threatens the pregnant woman's life. *See also* abortion; pregnancy.

therapeutic agent A substance, person, or activity that promotes healing. *See also* agent; therapeutic.

therapeutic equivalents Drugs that have essentially identical effects in the treatment of a disease or condition. Therapeutic equivalents are not necessarily chemical equivalents or bioequivalents. Drugs with the same treatment effect that are not chemically equivalent are called clinically equivalent. *See also* generic equivalents.

therapeutic genetics Insertion of a specific gene replacement into fertilized eggs, fetuses, or individuals to correct a genetic disorder. *See also* gene; genetic engineering.

Therapeutic Humor, American Association of *See* American Association of Therapeutic Humor.

therapeutic index The ratio between the toxic dose and the therapeutic dose of a drug, used as a measure of the relative safety of the drug for a specified treatment. *See also* therapeutic; therapeutic range.

therapeutic privilege A legal exception to the rule that an informed consent must be obtained before therapy. It generally requires that the disclosure of information would likely worsen a patient's condition or render him or her so emotionally distraught as to hinder effective therapy. It is not an excuse to omit disclosure because of a physician's concern that a competent patient will elect to forgo the care. *See also* informed consent; privilege.

therapeutic radiological physics The branch of medical physics dealing with the therapeutic applications of roentgen rays, gamma rays, electron and other charged particle beams, neutrons, and radiations from sealed radionuclide sources and the equipment associated with their production and use. *See also* radiation; radiological physics; radiology; radionuclide; x-ray.

therapeutic radiology *See* radiation oncology.

Therapeutic Radiology and Oncology, American Society for *See* American Society for Therapeutic Radiology and Oncology.

therapeutic range Dose of medication determined for specific patients, within a lowest and highest recommended amount, that is likely to produce a desired clinical response. *See also* dose; therapeutic index.

therapeutic recreation *See* recreation therapy.

Therapeutic Recreation Association, American *See* American Therapeutic Recreation Association.

Therapeutic Recreation Certification, National Council for *See* National Council for Therapeutic Recreation Certification.

Therapeutic Recreation Society, National *See* National Therapeutic Recreation Society.

therapeutic recreation specialist *See* recreational therapist.

therapeutics The science of the treatment of diseases and healing. *See also* pharmacotherapeutics.

Therapeutics, Alliance for Cannabis *See* Alliance for Cannabis Therapeutics.

Therapeutics, American Society for Clinical Pharmacology and *See* American Society for Clinical Pharmacology and Therapeutics.

Therapeutics, Council on Chiropractic Physiological *See* Council on Chiropractic Physiological Therapeutics.

Therapeutics for the Elderly, Center for the Study of Pharmacy and *See* Center for the Study of Pharmacy and Therapeutics for the Elderly.

therapeutics, pharmaco- *See* pharmacotherapeutics.

therapeutic sterilization Sterilization performed because bearing children would be harmful to an individual. *See also* sterilization.

therapeutic, sub- *See* subtherapeutic.

Therapeutic Technology Assessment Program, Diagnostic and *See* Diagnostic and Therapeutic Technology Assessment Program.

therapeutic trial *See* clinical trial.

therapeutist *See* therapist.

Therapies, Inc, Last Word: *See* Last Word: Therapies, Inc.

therapist One who specializes in the provision of a particular therapy, as in a mental health therapist, enterostomal therapist, or a physical therapist. *Synonym*: therapeutist. *See also* therapy.

therapist, enterostomal　*See* enterostomal therapist.

therapist, family　*See* family therapist.

therapist, inhalation　*See* respiratory therapist.

therapist, manual arts　*See* manual arts therapist.

therapist, occupational　*See* occupational therapist.

therapist, physical　*See* physical therapist.

therapist, poetry　*See* poetry therapist.

therapist, recreational　*See* recreational therapist.

therapist, registered respiratory　*See* registered respiratory therapist.

therapist, respiratory　*See* respiratory therapist.

Therapists, American Association of Behavioral　*See* American Association of Behavioral Therapists.

Therapists, American Association of Professional Hypno-　*See* American Association of Professional Hypnotherapists.

Therapists, American Association of Religious　*See* American Association of Religious Therapists.

Therapists, American Association of Sex Educators, Counselors and　*See* American Association of Sex Educators, Counselors and Therapists.

Therapists, American Board of Medical Psycho-　*See* American Board of Medical Psychotherapists.

Therapists, American Guild of Hypno-　*See* American Guild of Hypnotherapists.

Therapists, American Society of Hand　*See* American Society of Hand Therapists.

Therapists, Certification Board for Music　*See* Certification Board for Music Therapists.

Therapists, National Academy of Counselors and Family　*See* National Academy of Counselors and Family Therapists.

therapist, speech　*See* speech therapist.

therapy　The treatment of a disease or condition, as in speech therapy (the use of special techniques for correction of speech and language disorders), anticoagulant therapy (the use of drugs to render the blood sufficiently incoagulable to discourage thrombosis), or root canal therapy (treatment of diseases of the dental pulp through extraction of the diseased pulp, cleaning and sterilization of the empty canal, enlarging the canal to receive sealing material, and filling the canal with a nonirritating hermetic sealing agent. *See also* modality; psychotherapy; treatment.

therapy aide, speech and hearing　*See* speech and hearing therapy aide.

Therapy, American Association for Marriage and Family　*See* American Association for Marriage and Family Therapy.

Therapy, American Association for Music　*See* American Association for Music Therapy.

Therapy, American Association for Rehabilitation　*See* American Association for Rehabilitation Therapy.

Therapy, American Board of Chelation　*See* American Board of Chelation Therapy.

Therapy of the American Psychological Association, Division of Psycho-　*See* Division of Psychotherapy of the American Psychological Association.

therapy, anticoagulant　*See* anticoagulant therapy.

therapy, art　*See* art therapy.

therapy assistant, occupational　*See* occupational therapy assistant.

Therapy, Association for Advancement of Behavior　*See* Association for Advancement of Behavior Therapy.

Therapy Association, American Art　*See* American Art Therapy Association.

Therapy Association, American Dance　*See* American Dance Therapy Association.

Therapy Association, American Family　*See* American Family Therapy Association.

Therapy Association, American Group Psycho-　*See* American Group Psychotherapy Association.

Therapy Association, American Horticultural　*See* American Horticultural Therapy Association.

Therapy Association, American Kinesio-　*See* American Kinesiotherapy Association.

Therapy Association, American Massage　*See* American Massage Therapy Association.

Therapy Association, American Occupational　*See* American Occupational Therapy Association.

Therapy Association, American Oriental Bodywork　*See* American Oriental Bodywork Therapy Association.

Therapy Association, American Physical　*See* American Physical Therapy Association.

Therapy Association, National Coalition of Arts　*See* National Coalition of Arts Therapy Association.

Therapy Association, Orthopaedic Section, American Physical　*See* Orthopaedic Section, American Physical Therapy Association.

Therapy Association, Private Practice Section/ American Physical　*See* Private Practice Section/American Physical Therapy Association.

Therapy Association, US Physical *See* US Physical Therapy Association.

Therapy Associations, National Coalition of Arts *See* National Coalition of Arts Therapy Associations.

therapy, behavior *See* behavior therapy.

Therapy Certification Board, American Occupational *See* American Occupational Therapy Certification Board.

therapy, chelation *See* chelation therapy.

therapy, chemo- *See* chemotherapy.

therapy, chromo- *See* chromotherapy.

therapy, dance *See* dance therapy.

therapy, drama *See* drama therapy.

therapy, drug *See* chemotherapy.

Therapy Education, Joint Review Committee for Respiratory *See* Joint Review Committee for Respiratory Therapy Education.

therapy, electroconvulsive *See* electroconvulsive therapy.

therapy, family *See* family therapy.

therapy, gene *See* gene therapy.

therapy, gestalt *See* gestalt therapy.

therapy, group *See* group therapy.

therapy, hormone replacement *See* hormone replacement therapy.

therapy, hydro- *See* hydrotherapy.

therapy, hypno- *See* hypnotherapy.

therapy, infrared radiation *See* infrared radiation therapy.

therapy, inhalation *See* respiratory therapy.

Therapy, Institute for Rational-Emotive *See* Institute for Rational-Emotive Therapy.

Therapy, Institute for Reality *See* Institute for Reality Therapy.

therapy, intravenous *See* intravenous therapy.

therapy, kinesio- *See* kinesiotherapy.

Therapy, Laughter *See* Laughter Therapy.

therapy, maintenance *See* maintenance therapy.

therapy, manual arts *See* manual arts therapy.

therapy, music *See* music therapy.

Therapy, National Association for Drama *See* National Association for Drama Therapy.

Therapy, National Association for Music *See* National Association for Music Therapy.

Therapy, National Association for Poetry *See* National Association for Poetry Therapy.

Therapy, National Coalition of Psychiatrists Against Motorcoach *See* National Coalition of

Psychiatrists Against Motorcoach Therapy.

therapy, occupational *See* occupational therapy.

Therapy Oncology Group, Radiation *See* Radiation Therapy Oncology Group.

therapy, organo- *See* organotherapy.

therapy, orthomolecular medicine *See* orthomolecular medicine therapy.

therapy, photo- *See* phototherapy.

therapy, physical *See* physical therapy.

therapy, physio- *See* physical therapy.

therapy, play *See* play therapy.

therapy, poetry *See* poetry therapy.

therapy, psycho- *See* psychotherapy.

therapy, radiation *See* radiation therapy.

therapy, radium *See* radium therapy.

therapy, recreational *See* recreational therapy.

therapy, replacement *See* replacement therapy.

Therapy and Research, Society for Sex *See* Society for Sex Therapy and Research.

therapy, respiratory *See* respiratory therapy.

therapy, roentgeno- *See* roentgenotherapy.

therapy services, occupational *See* occupational therapy services.

therapy, sex *See* sex therapy.

therapy, shock *See* electroconvulsive therapy.

therapy, somato- *See* somatotherapy.

therapy, speech *See* speech therapy.

therapy, systemic adjuvant *See* systemic adjuvant therapy.

therapy technologist, radiation *See* radiation therapy technologist.

therapy, thrombolytic *See* thrombolytic therapy.

therapy, ultrasound physical *See* ultrasound physical therapy.

therapy, x-ray *See* x-ray therapy.

thermogenesis The production of body heat. *See also* thermography.

thermography The pictorial representation of an area in terms of its temperature and temperature differences. The most commonly used method detects and records infrared radiation from the body surface, as in detecting tumors of the breast. *See also* infrared; infrared radiation therapy; thermogenesis.

thermology *See* thermography.

Thermology, American Academy of *See* American Academy of Thermology.

thermometer An instrument for measuring temperatures. It works by using some substance with a physical property that varies in magnitude with temperature to determine a value of temperature on some defined scale. A Celsius thermometer uses the Celsius scale; a centigrade thermometer uses the centigrade scale, that is, having the interval between the two established reference points divided into 100 units; and a Fahrenheit thermometer uses the Fahrenheit scale. *See also* bioinstrumentation; Celsius scale; centigrade scale; clinical thermometer; Fahrenheit scale; scale; temperature.

The Robert Wood Johnson Foundation An independent foundation incorporated in 1936 in New Jersey (became a national philanthropy in 1972) whose purpose and activities are to identify and pursue new opportunities to address persistent health problems and to participate and respond to significant emerging problems. Its three basic goals are to ensure that Americans of all ages have access to basic health care; to improve the way services are organized and provided to people with chronic health conditions; and to promote health and prevent disease by reducing harm caused by substance abuse. It also seeks opportunities to help the nation address, effectively and fairly, the overarching problem of escalating health care expenditures. *See also* foundation; private foundation.

The William K. Warren Foundation An independent foundation established in 1945 that provides grants for local Catholic health care facilities, education, and social services and substantial support for a medical research program. Giving is done primarily in Oklahoma. *See also* foundation; private foundation.

THF *See* The Healthcare Forum.

thick-skinned **1.** Not easily offended. **2.** Insensitive.

think To formulate in the mind; to reason about or reflect on. *See also* magical thinking; mind; reason; systems thinking; thought.

thinking, magical *See* magical thinking.

thinking, systems *See* systems thinking.

third-party administrator (TPA) *See* fiscal intermediary.

third-party billing The preparation of bills, statements, and related documentation by a health care provider on behalf of a patient and their submission to a third-party payer (an insurer or a third-party administrator) for payment directly to either the health care provider or to the beneficiary. *See also* billing; third-party payer.

third-party claims administrator An individual

employed by a third-party payer, who processes insurance claims. *See also* administrator; claim; internal control number; patient service representative; third-party payer.

third-party payer A payer (usually an insurance company, a prepayment plan, or a government agency) that pays or insures health or medical expenses on behalf of beneficiaries or recipients, but does not receive or provide health care services. The payer is the third party, and the patient and the provider are the first two parties. *See also* carrier; payer.

third-party payment Payment by a private insurer or government program to a health care provider for care given to a patient. *See also* payment; third-party payer.

third sector Organizations, especially nonprofit organizations, that fit neither in the public sector (government) nor the private sector (business). *See also* sector.

thirst The urge to want to drink, mediated through osmotic and volume receptors and a thirst center, which is situated in the anterior hypothalamus of the brain. *See also* potomania.

thoracic Pertaining to the thorax or chest. *See also* thorax.

Thoracic Radiology, Society of *See* Society of Thoracic Radiology.

Thoracic Society, American *See* American Thoracic Society.

thoracic surgeon A physician who specializes in thoracic surgery. *Synonyms*: cardiothoracic surgeon; cardiovascular surgeon; chest surgeon. *See also* surgeon; thoracic surgery; thorax.

Thoracic Surgeons, Society of *See* Society of Thoracic Surgeons.

thoracic surgery The branch and specialty of medicine that encompasses the operative, perioperative, and critical care of patients with pathologic conditions within the chest. Included is the surgical care of coronary artery disease; cancers of the lung, esophagus, and chest wall; abnormalities of the great vessels and heart valves; congenital anomalies; tumors of the mediastinum; and diseases of the diaphragm. The management of the airway and injuries of the chest are also within the scope of thoracic surgery. *Synonyms*: cardiothoracic surgery; cardiovascular surgery; chest surgery. *See also* airway; critical care; perioperative; pneumothorax; surgery;

thorax.

Thoracic Surgery, American Association for *See* American Association for Thoracic Surgery.

Thoracic Surgery, American Board of *See* American Board of Thoracic Surgery.

thoracotomy Surgical incision of the chest wall. *See also* incision; surgery; thorax.

thorax The part of the human body between the neck and the diaphragm, partially encased by the ribs and containing the heart and lungs. *Synonym*: chest. *See also* thoracic; thoracic surgery.

thought 1. The product of thinking, as in a new thought or an original idea. **2.** The mental faculty of thinking or reasoning, as in he thought that he was right. *See also* mind; think; reason.

threatened abortion An abortion in which there is bloody discharge from the uterus but the loss of blood is less than in inevitable abortion and there is no dilatation of the cervix; it may proceed to actual abortion or the symptoms may subside, allowing the pregnancy to go to full term. *See also* abortion; inevitable abortion; pregnancy; term.

threshold The level or point at which a stimulus is strong enough to signal the need for response; for example, threshold of pain or threshold for review of an occurrence measured by a clinical indicator. *See also* indicator threshold; pain threshold; threshold phenomena.

threshold, indicator *See* indicator threshold.

threshold, pain *See* pain threshold.

threshold phenomena Events or changes that occur only after a certain level or point of a characteristic is reached. *See also* phenomenon; threshold.

Throat Advances in Children, Society for Ear, Nose, and *See* Society for Ear, Nose, and Throat Advances in Children.

thromboembolism A condition in which a blood vessel is blocked by an embolus carried in the bloodstream from its site of formation. *See also* embolism; embolus; thrombus.

thrombolysis Destruction or dissolution of a thrombus. *See also* streptokinase; thrombolytic therapy; thrombosis; tissue plasminogen activator.

thrombolytic therapy Administration of a pharmacological agent with the intention of causing thrombolysis of an abnormal blood clot, such as in the coronary (myocardial infarction) or pulmonary (pulmonary embolism) arteries. Available agents include streptokinase, urokinase, and tissue plas-

minogen activator. These preparations may be given either intravenously or directly into the blocked artery. *See also* anticoagulant therapy; streptokinase; thrombolysis; tissue plasminogen activator; urokinase.

thrombophlebitis Inflammation of a vein in conjunction with the formation of a blood clot (thrombus). It occurs as a result of trauma to the blood vessel, prolonged immobilization and consequent venous stasis, excessive clotting (hypercoagulability) of the blood, or infection. Pulmonary embolism is one complication of thrombophlebitis. *See also* embolism; inflammation; thrombosis.

thrombosis The formation, presence, or development of a thrombus (blood clot) in a blood vessel or chamber of the heart. Thrombosis in an artery supplying the brain results in a stroke (cerebrovascular accident); in an artery supplying the heart, a myocardial infarction; in a vein, thrombophlebitis. A thrombus may also move from its site of origin, as in an embolism. *See also* acute myocardial infarction; cerebrovascular accident; coronary thrombosis; embolism; ischemia; thrombophlebitis; thrombus.

thrombosis, coronary *See* coronary thrombosis.

thrombus An intravascular blood clot formed during the process of thrombosis. *See* blood clot; thrombosis.

throw-away journals Journals distributed free of charge to health professionals (especially physicians), which depend on revenue from advertising (chiefly of products of the pharmaceutical industry) for their income. *See also* journal.

thrush Candidiasis (a fungal infection) of the oral mucous membranes, characterized by the development of creamy, white, slightly elevated plaques made up of soft material resembling milk curds, which is easily stripped from the surface of the tissue, leaving a raw, bleeding surface. Thrush usually affects sick infants, elderly individuals in poor health, and patients with acquired immunodeficiency syndrome (AIDS). *See also* candidiasis; opportunistic infection.

Thyroid Association, American *See* American Thyroid Association.

thyroid gland An endocrine gland located in front of and on either side of the trachea (windpipe) in human beings, that produces hormones, such as thyroid hormone (thyroxine or triiodothyronine) and calcitonin. *See also* calcitonin; gland; goiter;

hyperthyroidism; hypothyroidism; iodine.

TIA *See* transient ischemic attack.

TIE *See* The Information Exchange on Young Adult Chronic Patients.

time A nonspatial continuum in which events occur in apparently irreversible succession from the past through the present to the future. *See also* access time; biological clock; chronobiology; clock; idle time; timeliness; timely.

time, access *See* access time.

time, idle *See* idle time.

timeliness In health care, a performance dimension addressing the degree to which a care/intervention is provided to a patient at the most beneficial or necessary time. *See also* care; intervention; dimensions of performance; time; timely.

timely Occurring at a suitable or an opportune time, as in timely administration of streptokinase. *See also* time; timeliness.

time-motion study *See* motion study.

time and motion study *See* motion study.

time, off *See* off time.

time plot *See* run chart.

time, real *See* real time.

tincture An alcoholic or hydroalcoholic solution prepared from animal or vegetable drugs or from chemical substances, as in benzoin tincture.

tissue A collection of structurally similar cells and associated intercellular matter acting together to perform one or more specific functions in the body. The four basic types of tissue are muscle, nerve, epidermal, and connective. An organ may be made up of several kinds of tissues. *See also* adipose tissue; connective tissue; epidermis; muscle; organ.

tissue, adipose *See* adipose tissue.

tissue bank A facility for collecting, cataloging, storing, and distributing body tissues for use in surgery (for example, corneal tissue and bone) or tissue culture. *See also* organ bank; tissue; tissue culture.

Tissue Banks, American Association of *See* American Association of Tissue Banks.

tissue committee A hospital committee that reviews and evaluates all surgery performed in the hospital on the basis of the extent of correlation among the preoperative, postoperative, and pathological diagnoses. The tissue committee also reviews the relevance and acceptability of the procedures undertaken for the diagnosis. The name derives from the use of pathologic findings from tissue

removed at surgery as a key element in the review. *See also* committee; tissue.

tissue, connective *See* connective tissue.

tissue culture The technique of keeping tissue alive and growing under artificial conditions in a culture medium, separately from the organism from which the tissue was derived. *See also* culture medium; tissue; tissue bank.

Tissue Culture Association (TCA) A national organization founded in 1946 composed of 2,500 individuals using mammalian, invertebrate, and plant cell tissue and organ cultures as research tools in medicine, chemistry, physics, radiation, physiology, nutrition, and cytogenetics. It fosters dissemination of information concerning the maintenance and experimental use of tissue cells in vitro and to establish evaluation and development procedures. *See also* in vitro; tissue culture.

tissue donor An individual who donates a body tissue, such as bone marrow, for transplantation into another human. *See also* donor; tissue; tissue transplantation.

tissue plasminogen activator (TPA) An enzyme that converts plasminogen to plasmin, used to dissolve blood clots rapidly and selectively, especially in the treatment of heart attacks. *See also* thrombolysis; thrombolytic therapy; thrombus.

tissue sample *See* biopsy.

tissue transplantation To transfer tissue from one body to another. Tissues that can be used for transplantation includes corneas, cardiac valves, bone, tendon, arteries, veins, middle ear bones, cartilage, and skin. Tissue donation can take place following death from most causes, including brain death. Tissues can be recovered up to 24 hours after death. Tissues are transplanted far more commonly than organs. *See also* organ transplantation; skin graft; transplantation.

TLB *See* The Living Bank.

T lymphocyte *See* lymphocyte.

TM *See* transcendental meditation.

TMJ *See* temporomandibular joint.

TMJ Orthopedics, American Academy of Head, Facial and Neck Pain and *See* American Academy of Head, Facial and Neck Pain and TMJ Orthopedics.

tobacco 1. Any of various plants of the genus *Nicotiana* native to tropical America and widely cultivated for its leaves, which are used primarily for smoking. **2.** Products made from these plants. *See also* involuntary smoking; nicotine; sidestream smoke; smoking; snuff.

tolerance **1.** The capacity for or the practice of recognizing and respecting the beliefs or practices of other persons. **2.** Leeway for variation from a standard. *See also* standard. **3.** Physiological resistance to a drug or poison. **4.** Acceptance of a tissue graft or transplant without immunological rejection. *See also* transplantation.

tomography A radiographic technique for making detailed x-rays of a predetermined plane section of a solid object while blurring out the images of other planes. *See also* computerized axial tomography; positron emission tomography.

tomography, computerized axial *See* computerized axial tomography.

tomography, positron emission *See* positron emission tomography.

tongue depressor A thin wooden blade for pressing down the tongue during a medical examination of the mouth and throat. *See also* gag reflex.

Tongue Depressors, Association of *See* Association of Tongue Depressors.

tonometer An instrument used to measure tension or pressure; for example, in measuring intraocular pressure to detect the existence of glaucoma. *See also* ophthalmology.

tonsillectomy Surgical removal of the tonsils. *See also* otolaryngology; pharyngitis; tonsils.

tonsils Small oval masses of lymphoid tissue embedded in both sides of the throat; their function is uncertain. *See also* fauces; pharyngitis; tonsillectomy.

tool An instrument used to perform work; for example, a measurement tool, such as a stethoscope or an outcome indicator. *See also* instrument; monitor; outcome indicator; stethoscope.

tooth A hard, bonelike structure rooted in a socket in the jaw, used for biting or chewing food or as a means of defense or attack. *See also* dentistry; dentition; odontology; permanent tooth; plaque; tooth and nail; wisdom teeth.

tooth and nail With every available resource, as in fighting tooth and nail to achieve something.

tooth, permanent *See* permanent tooth.

top banana The head person.

top-down global budgeting A total level of expenditure on health care set by government mandate.

See also global budget.

top-heavy **1.** Likely to topple because of an uneven distribution of weight, with the majority being at the top. **2.** In organizations, having a disproportionately large number of administrators, as in a top-heavy organization. *See also* administrator; organization. **3.** In accounting, overcapitalized. *See also* accounting.

topical anesthetic An local anesthetic, such as cocaine hydrochloride, applied directly to a localized area to be anesthetized, usually the mucous membranes of the skin. *See also* anesthetic.

tort In law, a private or civil (not criminal) wrongful act that is neither a crime nor a breach of contract, but that renders the perpetrator liable to the victim for damages, as in trespassing or negligence. The essential elements of a tort are the existence of a legal duty owed by a defendant to a plaintiff, breach of that duty, and a causal relation between a defendant's conduct and the resulting damage to a plaintiff. Torts generally involve personal injuries. *See also* civil law; negligence; professional negligence; tortfeasor; tort liability.

tortfeasor A person or an entity that has committed a civil wrong, other than breach of contract, resulting in loss or injury for which there is a judicial remedy. *See also* joint tortfeasors; tort.

tortfeasors, joint *See* joint tortfeasors.

tort liability Liability imposed by a court for breach of a duty implied by law, contrasted with contractual liability, which is breach of duty arising from an agreement. The tort liability system determines fault and awards compensation for civil wrongs, including medical malpractice. *See also* liability; tort.

Tort Reform Association, American *See* American Tort Reform Association.

total Pertaining to a whole quantity; an entirety, as in total quality management. *See also* total disability; total hysterectomy; total parenteral nutrition; total quality management.

total disability An illness or injury that prevents an individual from performing any duty pertaining to his or her occupation or profession or from engaging in any other type of work for remuneration. *See also* disability; total.

total hysterectomy A hysterectomy in which the uterus and cervix are completely removed. *See also* hysterectomy; total; uterus.

total parenteral alimentation *See* total parenteral nutrition.

total parenteral nutrition (TPN) The process of giving *all* nutriment within a vein (directly into the bloodstream) and not through the alimentary tract. TPN involves the continuous infusion of a hyperosmolar solution containing carbohydrates, amino acids, fats, vitamins, and other necessary nutrients through an indwelling catheter (tubing) inserted into the superior vena cava. The principle indications for TPN are found in seriously ill patients suffering from malnutrition, sepsis (blood poisoning), or surgical or accidental trauma when use of the gastrointestinal tract for feeding is not possible. *Synonym*: total parenteral alimentation. *See also* enteral and parenteral nutrition and infusion therapy services; nutritional support; parenteral nutrition; total.

total quality management (TQM) A continuous quality improvement management system directed from the top, but empowering employees and focusing on systemic, not individual, employee problems. *See also* continuous quality improvement; empower; Feigenbaum, Armand; just in time; management; quality management; transition period.

touch-and-go Dangerous and unpredictable in nature or outcome.

tough-minded Facing facts and difficulties with strength and determination. *See also* determination; mind.

touch screen In computer science, a monitor screen on which commands can be entered by pressing designated areas with a finger or other object. *See also* computer; monitor; screen.

tour de force A feat requiring great virtuosity or strength, as in reforming the American health care system.

tourniquet A constricting band encircling a limb, usually to temporarily interrupt the arterial blood supply and prevent bleeding from a site distal to the point of compression.

town meeting A legislative assembly of townspeople.

toxemia Release of toxic bacterial products into the blood stream. *See also* bacteria; septicemia; toxic; toxin.

toxemia of pregnancy *See* preeclampsia.

toxic Pertaining to a poison, as in a toxic-looking patient, or toxic waste. *See also* toxemia; toxicology; toxin.

Toxicologic Pathologists, Society of *See* Society of Toxicologic Pathologists.

Toxicologic Pathology, Department of Environmental and *See* Department of Environmental and Toxicologic Pathology.

toxicologist, medical *See* medical toxicologist.

Toxicologists, Society of Forensic *See* Society of Forensic Toxicologists.

toxicology The quantitative study of the nature, effects, and detection of materials that may or may not adversely affect the health of humans or animals. *See also* medical toxicology.

Toxicology, American Academy of Clinical *See* American Academy of Clinical Toxicology.

Toxicology, American Board of *See* American Board of Toxicology.

Toxicology, American Board of Medical *See* American Board of Medical Toxicology.

Toxicology, American College of *See* American College of Toxicology.

toxicology, clinical *See* medical toxicology.

toxicology, medical *See* medical toxicology.

Toxicology, Society of *See* Society of Toxicology.

toxic psychosis A psychosis caused by a poisonous substance; for example, lead poisoning affecting the central nervous system. *See also* organic psychosis; psychosis; toxin.

toxic shock syndrome An acute infection characterized by fever, rash, vomiting, and diarrhea, and followed in severe cases by shock. It is caused by a toxin-producing strain of the common bacterium *Staphylococcus aureus*. It typically occurs among young menstruating women using vaginal tampons. *See also* shock; syndrome.

toxin A poisonous substance produced by living cells that is capable of causing disease when introduced in the tissues of the body, as in the bacterial toxin causing toxic shock syndrome. *See also* active immunization; diphtheria; toxemia; toxic shock syndrome; toxoid.

toxoid A bacterial toxin that has been modified for the purpose of immunization, as in tetanus toxoid. *See also* bacteria; immunization; toxin.

TPA *See* third-party administrator; tissue plasminogen activator.

TPLA *See* The Product Liability Alliance.

TPN *See* total parenteral nutrition.

TQM *See* total quality management.

trace elements Elements (metals and nonmetals) found in only minute amounts in the tissues of a healthy body, which are nevertheless essential components of the human diet. Examples are copper, manganese, fluorine, chromium, selenium, molybdenum. Trace elements may be harmful if taken in excess. *See also* nutrient; nutrition; vitamin.

tracer A condition or disease chosen for appraisal in programs and organizations that seek to measure and assess performance and quality of care. The assumption is that performance and quality of care relating to the tracer condition or disease is typical or representative of the performance and quality of care provided in general.

trachea The windpipe; the tube connecting the larynx to the right and left main bronchi and forming part of the airway by which air reaches the lungs. *Synonym*: windpipe. *See also* airway; tracheotomy.

tracheotomy The act or process of cutting into the trachea through the neck to make an artificial opening for breathing, as in an emergency tracheotomy. *See also* airway; cricothyreotomy; cricothyrotomy; trachea.

track record A record of actual performance or accomplishment, as in a hospital with an excellent track record in improving the quality of care provided to patients. *See also* performance; performance assessment; record.

tract **1.** A group of organs and tissues associated with a common function or arranged serially; for example, the digestive tract or the respiratory tract. *See also* alimentary tract. **2.** A bundle of nerve fibers having a common origin, terminations, and function. *See also* nerve. **3.** A pamphlet or leaflet of political or religious propaganda.

tract, alimentary *See* alimentary tract.

traction The exertion of a pulling force on a part to maintain bone position during the healing of a fracture. *See also* fracture; orthopaedic/orthopedic surgery.

trade The business of buying and selling commodities. *See also* business; restraint of trade.

Trade Association, American Dental *See* American Dental Trade Association.

Trade Commission, Federal *See* Federal Trade Commission.

trademark A word, symbol, or other device assigned to a product by its manufacturer, registered, and legally restricted to use by the owner or manufacturer as a part of its identity. *Compare* generic name. *See also* brand name.

trade name *See* brand name.

trade-off Giving up one advantage in order to gain another.

trade, restraint of *See* restraint of trade.

trade secret A secret formula, method, or device that gives an entity an advantage over competitors. *See also* business; trade.

trailblazer An individual who leads the way in an innovative or a creative manner, as in an innovative leader in health care.

trail, paper *See* paper trail.

train To make proficient with specialized instruction and practice. In health care, training and experience are two important factors that help determine practitioner competence and level of performance. *See also* performance; practitioner; training.

trainer, athletic *See* athletic trainer.

Trainers Association and Certification Board, American Athletic *See* American Athletic Trainers Association and Certification Board.

Trainers Association, National Athletic *See* National Athletic Trainers Association.

Trainers, National Society of Pharmaceutical Sales *See* National Society of Pharmaceutical Sales Trainers.

training The process of being educated or taught, as in an arduous training period. *See also* sensitivity training; train.

Training of the American Hospital Association, American Society for Healthcare Education and *See* American Society for Healthcare Education and Training of the American Hospital Association.

training coordinator An individual in an organization who is responsible for coordinating training programs. *See also* train; training.

Training Coordinators, National Council of State Emergency Medical Services *See* National Council of State Emergency Medical Services Training Coordinators.

training, sensitivity *See* sensitivity training.

trait, sickle cell *See* sickle cell trait.

tranquilizer A drug prescribed to calm anxious or agitated people, ideally without decreasing their consciousness. Major tranquilizers, such as phenothiazines and butyrophenones, are generally used in the treatment of psychoses. Minor tranquilizers, such as chlordiazepoxide and diazepam, are usually prescribed for the treatment of anxiety, irritability, tension, insomnia, and psychoneurosis. Tranquilizers tend to induce drowsiness and have the potential for causing physical and psychologic dependence. *See also* controlled substances; drug.

transcendental meditation (TM) A technique of meditation derived from Hindu traditions that promotes deep relaxation through repetition of a mantra (a Sanskrit syllable or word). *See also* American Association of Ayurvedic Medicine; ayurvedic medicine; meditation; yoga.

transcribe To make a full written or typewritten copy of dictated material, such as transcribing an x-ray interpretation. *See also* medical transcriptionist; transcript; transcription.

transcript Something transcribed, especially a written, typewritten, or printed copy. *See also* transcribe.

transcription **1.** The act or process of making a full written or typewritten copy of dictated material, as in transcription of a dictated medical record. **2.** Something that has been transcribed, as in an accurate transcription. *See also* dictation; medical transcriptionist.

Transcription, American Association for Medical *See* American Association for Medical Transcription.

transcriptionist, medical *See* medical transcriptionist.

transcutaneous Through the skin, as in transcutaneous electric nerve stimulation or transcutaneous oxygen/carbon dioxide monitoring. *Synonym:* transdermal. *See also* nicotine patch; transcutaneous electric nerve stimulation; transcutaneous oxygen/carbon dioxide monitoring.

transcutaneous electric nerve stimulation (TENS) A noninvasive, nonaddictive method of pain control by the application of electric impulses to the nerve endings. Electrodes are placed on the skin and attached to a stimulator by wires. The electric impulses generated block transmission of pain signals to the brain. *See also* electromedicine; galvanic current; pain management; stimulate; stimulus.

transcutaneous oxygen/carbon dioxide monitoring A method of measuring the oxygen or carbon dioxide in the blood by attaching electrodes to the skin. Oxygen is commonly measured through an oximeter, which contains heating coils to raise the skin temperature and increase blood flow at the surface. Oxygen content is calculated in terms of light absorption at various wavelengths. *See also* monitor; oximeter; oximetry.

transdermal *See* transcutaneous.

transduction A technique of genetic engineering in which deoxyribonucleic acid (DNA) is exchanged between bacteria. *See also* bacteria; deoxyribonucleic acid; genetic engineering.

transfer **1.** To pass from one place, person, or thing to another, as in preembryo transfer. *See also* preembryo transfer; transmission. **2.** In health care, the formal shifting of responsibility for the care of a patient from one health professional, particularly a physician, to another; from one unit of a health care organization to another; or from one institution to another. *Synonym:* patient transfer. *See also* discharge by transfer; intrahospital transfer; transfer admission; transfer agreement.

transfer admission The formal acceptance by a health care organization of a patient by transfer from another health care facility or from another division of the hospital. *See also* admission; intrahospital transfer; transfer; transfer agreement.

transfer agreement A formal agreement between two health care organizations indicating the conditions under which there can be transfer of patients and exchange of clinical information between them. *See also* agreement; intrahospital transfer; patient dumping; transfer.

Transfer Application System, Coordinated *See* Coordinated Transfer Application System.

transfer, discharge by *See* discharge by transfer.

transference In psychotherapy, the unconscious tendency to assign to other persons in one's present environment feelings and attitudes associated with significant persons in one's early life, especially the patient's transfer to a therapist of feelings and attitudes associated with a parent. The feelings may be affectionate or hostile. *See also* psychotherapy.

transfer, intrahospital *See* intrahospital transfer.

transfer, patient *See* transfer.

transfer, preembryo *See* preembryo transfer.

transform To markedly change the form or structure of, as in transforming the culture of an organization. *See also* transformation.

transformation Change of form or structure, as in a major organizational transformation, or transformation of a normal cell to a malignant cell. *See also* transform; transition period.

transfusion *See* blood transfusion.

transfusion, auto- *See* autotransfusion.

transfusion, autologous blood *See* autologous blood transfusion.

transfusion, blood *See* blood transfusion.

transfusion, intraoperative auto- *See* intraoperative autotransfusion.

transfusion, over- *See* overtransfusion.

transfusion, postoperative auto- *See* postoperative autotransfusion.

transfusion reaction A response by the body to the administration of incompatible blood. Causes may include red cell incompatibility; or allergic sensitivity to leukocytes, platelets, or plasma protein components of the transfused blood or to the potassium or citrate preservatives in the banked blood. Transfusion reactions are variable in severity ranging from isolated fever to severe vascular collapse and death. *See also* blood transfusion; blood typing; reaction.

transient ischemic attack (TIA) An episode of temporary blockage of the blood supply to the brain (cerebrovascular insufficiency), usually associated with a partial blockage of an artery by atherosclerotic plaque or an embolism. Symptoms vary with the site and the degree of blockage and may include weakness, inability to speak normally (dysphasia), numbness, and other manifestations. *Synonym*: ministroke. *See also* cerebrovascular accident; embolism; ischemia; plaque.

transition Passage from one state, form, style, or place to another. *See also* transitional year; transition period.

transitional year The period of training, occurring after graduation from medical school and the awarding of the Doctor of Medicine (MD) degree, that is organized and sponsored by institutions or several clinical departments. PGY-1 (postgraduate year 1), by contrast, is part of a residency program in a given specialty that is organized and sponsored by a single specialty department. *See also* residency; transition.

Transition, Nurses in *See* Nurses in Transition.

transition period In total quality management, a description of the time when an organization is visibly moving from an old way toward a new way. During this time, employee attitudes and behaviors range from being excited and busy to being confused and resistant. The support for change is building. New leaders emerge, champions of the change come forward, and, with proper leadership, confusion over roles begins to clear. *See also* total quality management; transformation.

transmission **1.** Passage of nervous impulses from one nerve cell to another or to a receptor organ, as in a neurotransmitter. *See also* neurotransmitters. **2.** Transfer of communicable diseases between individuals. *See also* communicable disease; transfer. **3.** Transfer of genetically determined characteristics to and through offspring. *See also* genetics.

transplant In health care, an organ or piece of tissue removed from its native site and reestablished elsewhere, either in the same individual or to another individual of the same or another species. *Synonym*: graft. *See also* allograft; implant; multivisceral transplant; replant; skin graft; transplantation.

Transplant Act of 1984, National Organ *See* National Organ Transplant Act of 1984.

Transplant Association, American *See* American Transplant Association.

transplantation The grafting of tissues or an organ taken from a patient's own body or from another person's body to replace a diseased structure, to restore function, or to change appearance. Skin and kidneys are the most frequently transplanted structures; others include cartilage, bone, corneal tissue, portions of blood vessels and tendons, and hearts and livers. *See also* graft; histocompatibility antigen; multivisceral transplant; organ procurement; organ transplantation; rejection; tissue transplantation.

Transplantation, North American Society for Dialysis and *See* North American Society for Dialysis and Transplantation.

transplantation, organ *See* organ transplantation.

Transplantation Society (TS) A national organization founded in 1966 composed of 1,400 physicians and scientists who have made significant contributions to the advancement of knowledge in transplantation biology and medicine. *See also* transplantation.

transplantation, tissue *See* tissue transplantation.

transplant, bone marrow *See* bone marrow transplant.

Transplant Coordinators Organization, North American *See* North American Transplant Coordinators Organization.

transplant, heart *See* heart transplant.

transplant, multivisceral *See* multivisceral transplant.

Transplants, Academy for Implants and *See* Academy for Implants and Transplants.

Transplant Surgeons, American Society of *See* American Society of Transplant Surgeons.

transport To carry from one place to another, as in

transporting a patient to the operating room or transporting a patient from the mountaintop to a hospital.

Transport Association, Professional Aeromedical *See* Professional Aeromedical Transport Association.

transportation **1.** The process of carrying from one place to another. **2.** A means of conveyance, as in a mode of transportation. **3.** The business of conveying passengers or goods. *See also* transportation services.

Transportation, Department of *See* Department of Transportation.

transportation services In health care, services relating to carrying a patient from one place to another. *See also* transportation.

transsexuality The condition in which a person assumes the psychological identity of the sex opposite to his or her biological gender, occasionally undergoing sex change procedures. *See also* bisexuality; heterosexuality; homosexuality; sex change.

transvestism A compulsion to wear the clothing of the opposite sex. Transvestites are usually males who wear female clothing in order to induce sexual excitement. *See also* fetishism.

trauma **1.** Serious injury to the body, as from violence or an accident. *See also* abbreviated injury scale; blunt trauma; Glasgow coma scale; injury; injury severity score; maim; penetrating trauma; trauma center; trauma score; violence. **2.** Serious emotional injury that creates substantial, lasting damage to the psychological development or stability of a person, as in posttraumatic stress disorder. *See also* posttraumatic stress disorder.

Trauma, American Association for the Surgery of *See* American Association for the Surgery of Trauma.

trauma, birth *See* birth trauma.

trauma, blunt *See* blunt trauma.

trauma center A service providing emergency and specialized intensive care to critically ill and injured patients. *Synonym:* trauma unit. *See also* trauma; traumatology.

Trauma, Institute for Victims of *See* Institute for Victims of Trauma.

trauma life support, advanced *See* advanced trauma life support.

trauma life support, basic *See* basic trauma life support.

trauma, penetrating *See* penetrating trauma.

trauma, psychological *See* trauma.

trauma registry A repository of data on trauma patients, including causes of trauma, diagnoses, treatment, and outcome. *See also* registry; trauma.

trauma score (TS) In trauma care, a physiologic measure of injury severity developed in 1981 that provides a mechanism for predicting outcome, allocating resources, and evaluating the quality of trauma care. It evaluates seven respiratory, cardiovascular, and neurologic characteristics of trauma patients' conditions and assigns weighted point values. The total score (1 to 16, worst prognosis to best prognosis) can then be used to predict survival statistically. Patients with a trauma score of less than 13 had a mortality rate exceeding 10%. This suggests that this group of patients should be triaged to a trauma center. The trauma score was revised in 1989. Capillary refill and respiratory expansion were removed as assessment criteria and the scale range for blood pressure, respiratory rate, and Glasgow coma scale were modified. The cut-off for trauma center triage with the revised trauma score is set at 11 or less. *See also* Glasgow coma scale; severity of illness.

trauma score, revised *See* trauma score.

Trauma Society, American *See* American Trauma Society.

trauma surgeon *See* traumatologist.

trauma surgery *See* traumatology.

traumatic encephalopathy *See* encephalopathy.

traumatic injury *See* injury.

traumatic stress disorder, post- *See* posttraumatic stress disorder.

traumatize **1.** To injure a tissue, as in a surgical operation. *See also* trauma. **2.** To subject to psychological trauma. *See also* posttraumatic stress disorder.

traumatologist A physician specializing in traumatology. *Synonym:* trauma surgeon. *See also* traumatology.

traumatology The branch of medicine that deals with the treatment of serious wounds, injuries, and disabilities. *Synonym:* trauma surgery. *See also* abbreviated injury scale; advanced trauma life support; golden hour; surgery; traumatologist.

trauma unit *See* trauma center.

traveler's diarrhea Diarrhea and abdominal cramps occurring among travelers to areas where sanitation is poor, commonly caused by a toxin-producing strain of the bacterium *Esherichia coli*. *See also* diarrhea; toxin.

treadmill An exercise or test device consisting of an endlessly moving belt on which a person can walk or jog while remaining in place, as in a treadmill used for cardiac stress testing. *See also* cardiology; fitness; stress test.

Treasury, Department of the *See* Department of the Treasury.

treat To provide medical care to someone to counteract a disease or condition. *See also* treatment.

treatment **1.** The application of remedies to disease; the general management and care of illness. **2.** A substance or remedy applied, as in a costly treatment. *See also* therapy.

Treatment Association, Neurodevelopmental *See* Neurodevelopmental Treatment Association.

Treatment Centers for Children, National Association of Psychiatric *See* National Association of Psychiatric Treatment Centers for Children.

treatment, day *See* day treatment.

Treatment of Intractable Pain, National Committee on the *See* National Committee on the Treatment of Intractable Pain.

treatment, osteopathic manipulative *See* osteopathic manipulative treatment.

treatment plan, patient *See* care plan.

treatment program, residential *See* residential treatment program.

Treatment Providers, National Association of Addiction *See* National Association of Addiction Treatment Providers.

treatment, silent *See* silent treatment.

treatment, withdrawing *See* withdrawing treatment.

treatment, withholding *See* withholding treatment.

trend Any general direction of movement; for example, a trend toward improved performance in reducing unnecessary surgery. A trend, although possibly irregular in the short term, shows movement consistently in the same direction over a long term. *See also* data trend; pattern.

trend, data *See* data trend.

trend line The line that best fits the distribution of a set of values plotted on two axes. *See also* trend.

trendsetter An individual or entity initiating or popularizing a trend. *See also* pacesetter; trend; vanguard.

trephine A crown saw with a central guiding pin, designed to remove a circular disc of bone, usually from the skull. *See also* neurological surgery; skull.

triage Sorting out or screening patients seeking care to determine which service is required, with what priority, and where the service is best provided. Originally developed in military medicine and used to describe sorting out of battle casualties into groups of individuals who could wait for care, would benefit from immediate care, and were beyond care. Triage is used today on the battlefield, at disaster sites, in prehospital care of patients, in hospital emergency departments, and in any other situation when limited medical resources must be allocated. *See also* emergency medicine; overtriage; rationing; undertriage.

triage, over- *See* overtriage.

triage, under- *See* undertriage.

trial **1.** A judicial examination of issues between parties, whether they are issues of law or of fact, before a court that has jurisdiction over the cause. Trials are governed by established procedures and court rules and usually involve offering of testimony or evidence. *See also* hearing; grand jury; jury; petit jury. **2.** The act or process of testing, trying, or putting to the proof, as in a clinical trial. *See also* before-after trial; clinical trial; crossover trial; nonrandomized control trial; randomized trial.

Trial Advocacy, National Board of *See* National Board of Trial Advocacy.

Trial Advocacy, National Institute for *See* National Institute for Trial Advocacy.

Trial Advocates, American Board of *See* American Board of Trial Advocates.

trial, before-after *See* before-after trial.

trial balloon An idea or plan advanced tentatively to test public reaction, as in the president's many trial balloons. *See also* trial.

trial, clinical *See* clinical trial.

trial court A court that is responsible for receiving evidence and determining the application of the law to facts that it finds. Trial courts are usually divided into civil courts, criminal courts, matrimonial courts, and surrogate's courts. *See also* civil court; court; criminal court; matrimonial court; surrogate's court.

trial, crossover *See* crossover trial.

trial and error An empirical method of reaching a correct solution or acceptable result by trying out various means or theories until error is sufficiently reduced or eliminated. Trial and error is generally used when no theory is known. *See also* error; heuristics; trial.

trial, jury   *See* jury trial.

trial by jury   *See* jury trial.

Trial Lawyers, American College of   *See* American College of Trial Lawyers.

Trial Lawyers of America, Association of   *See* Association of Trial Lawyers of America.

trial, mis-   *See* mistrial.

trial, nonrandomized control   *See* nonrandomized control trial.

trial, randomized clinical   *See* randomized trial.

trial, randomized control   *See* randomized trial.

trial, randomized controlled   *See* randomized trial.

trial, research   *See* clinical trial.

Trials Group, AIDS Clinical   *See* AIDS Clinical Trials Group.

Trials, Society for Clinical   *See* Society for Clinical Trials.

trial, therapeutic   *See* clinical trial.

tribadism   Mutual genital friction, or more elaborate simulation of heterosexual intercourse using a prosthetic penile device, between female homosexuals. *See also* homosexuality; lesbianism.

tribe   A unit of social organization composed of a group of people sharing a common culture and leadership. *See also* society.

tribulation   Great affliction or distress, as in the tribulations of the sick.

tribunal   A seat or court of justice. *See also* court; justice.

tribute   An acknowledgement of gratitude, respect, or admiration.

trichology   The study of hair. *See also* hair; hirsutism.

trickle-down theory   An economic theory that financial benefits accorded to big business enterprises will in turn pass down to smaller businesses, consumers, and middle and lower income people. *See also* supply-side economics; theory.

triennial survey   An accreditation survey of the Joint Commission on Accreditation of Healthcare Organizations conducted every three years. *See also* accreditation survey; full team survey; Joint Commission on Accreditation of Healthcare Organizations.

trigger   To set off or initiate, as in the single undesirable outcome triggered an in-depth investigation.

Triological Society   *See* American Laryngological, Rhinological and Otological Society.

triple-blind study   A study in which subjects, investigators, and data analyzers are kept unaware of what treatment was used on which groups of individuals. *See also* clinical trial; double-blind technique.

trismus   Spasm of the jaw muscles due to many causes, including, classically, tetanus. *See also* tetanus.

trivalent live oral poliomyelitis vaccine   *See* Sabin vaccine.

trocar   A stout, sharp-pointed surgical instrument, used with a cannula to puncture a body cavity for fluid aspiration (withdrawal). *See also* needle.

troilism   The involvement of three individuals simultaneously in sexual activity. *See also* sex; sexual intercourse; voyeurism.

trolley car policy   A facetious name for an insurance policy for which benefits are so hard to collect that it is as though the policy provided benefits only for injuries resulting from being hit by a trolley car. *See also* insurance.

tropical   Pertaining to characteristics of the tropics, the region of the earth's surface lying between two parallels of latitude (Tropic of Cancer and Tropic of Capricorn) and representing the points farthest north and south at which the sun can shine directly overhead. *See also* tropical medicine.

tropical medicine   The branch of medicine concerned with the diagnosis and treatment of diseases, such as schistosomiasis, malaria, and yellow fever, found most commonly in tropical regions of the world. *See also* infectious diseases; malaria; tropical.

Tropical Medicine, American Academy of   *See* American Academy of Tropical Medicine.

Tropical Medicine, American Board of   *See* American Board of Tropical Medicine.

Tropical Medicine and Hygiene, American Society of   *See* American Society of Tropical Medicine and Hygiene.

tropism   A growth response to a stimulus, the direction of growth being either toward a stimulus (positive tropism) or away from a stimulus (negative tropism). *See also* stimulus.

trouble   A state of distress, malfunction, danger, or need, as in heart trouble or trouble in a patient care unit. *See also* problem; trouble-maker; troubleshooter, troublesome, trouble-spot.

trouble-maker   An individual who stirs up problems. *See also* trouble.

troubleshooter   An individual specializing in finding problems and solving them. Troubleshooters are

often used in organizations to clear up difficulties. *See also* problem; trouble.

troublesome Causing trouble or anxiety, as in the troublesome issue resurfaced. *See also* trouble.

trouble-spot An area of possible difficulty, as in the admissions process continued to be a trouble-spot in the organization. *See also* trouble.

true Consistent with fact or reality; not false or erroneous. *Compare* false. *See also* true negative; true positive; truth; verity.

true negative A negative result in a case that does not have the condition or characteristic for which a test is conducted; for example, a true negative result occurs when a pregnancy test is negative for a non-pregnant woman. *Compare* false positive. *See also* sensitivity of a test; specificity of a test; true positive.

true negative rate *See* specificity of a test.

true positive A positive result in a case that has the condition or characteristic for which a test is conducted; for example, a true positive result occurs when a pregnancy test is positive for a woman who is actually pregnant. *See also* sensitivity of a test; specificity of a test; true negative.

true positive rate *See* sensitivity of a test.

true random sampling *See* simple random sampling.

trunk The main undivided part of an anatomical structure, for example, the trunk of the body.

truss A device for maintaining pressure over a weak area of the abdominal wall in order to prevent a hernia from protruding. *See also* hernia.

trust, community *See* community trust.

trustee A member of a governing body, as in a hospital trustee. *See also* governing body; volunteer.

Trustees of Not-For-Profit Hospitals, Volunteer *See* Volunteer Trustees of Not-For-Profit Hospitals.

trust fund **1.** Real property or personal property held in trust for the benefit of another person or persons. **2.** In government, funds collected and used for carrying out specific purposes and programs according to terms of a trust agreement or statute, such as the social security and unemployment trust funds. Trust funds are administered by the government in a fiduciary capacity for those benefitted and are not available for the general purposes of the government. The Medicare program is financed through two trust funds: the federal Hospital Insurance Fund, which finances Part A, and the federal Supplementary Medical Insurance Trust Fund,

which finances Part B. *See also* Medicare.

Trust, Lucille P. Markey Charitable *See* Lucille P. Markey Charitable Trust.

Trusts, The Pew Charitable *See* The Pew Charitable Trusts.

truth **1.** Conformity to fact or reality. **2.** A statement proved to be or accepted as true. *See also* true; verity.

truth, moment of *See* moment of truth.

TS *See* Teratology Society; Transplantation Society; trauma score.

TSSNM *See* Technologist Section of the Society of Nuclear Medicine.

t-test A test that uses a statistic that, under the null hypothesis, has the *t*-distribution, to test whether two means differ significantly, or to test linear regression or correlation coefficients. *See also* *t*-distribution.

tubal ligation *See* ligation; sterilization.

tube Any hollow cylindrical structure, as in fallopian tube or tube feeding. *See also* tubule.

tube feeding *See* nutritional support.

tuberculosis (TB) An infectious disease of human beings and animals caused by the tubercle bacillus and characterized by the formation of tubercles in the lung and other tissues of the body. Tuberculosis of the lungs is characterized by the coughing up of bloody (sometimes) sputum, fever, night sweats, weight loss, and chest pain. *See also* consumption; infectious diseases; tuberculous isolation.

tuberculosis isolation A category of isolation for patients with pulmonary tuberculosis who have a positive sputum smear or chest x-rays that strongly suggest active tuberculosis. Specifications include use of a private room with special ventilation and a closed door. Masks are used only if the patient is coughing and does not reliably and consistently cover the mouth. Gowns are used to prevent gross contamination of clothing; gloves are not indicated. *Synonym*: AFB (acid fast bacilli) isolation. *See also* isolation; tuberculosis.

tubule Any small tube. *See also* tube.

tug of war A struggle for supremacy, as in a political tug of war between those for and those against the action.

tumor **1.** Any swelling. **2.** An abnormal growth or tissue resulting from uncontrolled, progressive multiplication of cells and serving no physiological function. *Synonym*: neoplasm. *See also* cancer; tumor registry.

Tumor Registrars Association, National *See* National Tumor Registrars Association.

tumor registry A repository of data drawn from medical records and other sources on the incidence of cancer and the personal characteristics, treatment, and treatment outcomes of cancer patients. *Synonym*: cancer registry. *See also* registry; tumor.

TUR Abbreviation for transurethral resection. *See* prostatectomy.

TURP Abbreviation for transurethral resection of the prostate. *See* prostatectomy.

Turkish American Physicians Association (TAPA) A national organization founded in 1969 composed of 1,260 Turkish-American physicians interested in developing closer relationships among physicians of Turkish origins, facilitating the exchange of information, and developing cultural and medical exchanges with physicians in Turkey. *See also* physician.

turnaround The process of, or time needed for, performing a task, as in receiving and running a laboratory test, and returning the results to the ordering physician. *See also* cycle.

turning point The point at which a meaningful change occurs, as in the turning point of the war. *See also* turn the corner.

turnkey system In computer science, a package of the hardware, software, instructions, and training sold as a unit to perform a particular application. *See also* computer.

turnoff Something that causes disinterest or distaste, as in the meeting was a turnoff for most of the attendees. *Compare* turn on.

turn on **1.** Something that causes pleasure or excitement, as in the idea of empowerment was a turn on for the employees. *Compare* turnoff. **2.** Be contingent on, as in the deal turned on their ability to provide the necessary capital.

turn the corner A turning point in a series of events. When a corner is turned, there is hope for improvement. *See also* turning point.

twerp A small, insignificant person. *See also* twit.

twin One of two offspring born at the same birth. *See also* fraternal twins; identical twins; Siamese twins.

twins, conjoined *See* Siamese twins.

twins, fraternal *See* fraternal twins.

twins, identical *See* identical twins.

twins, Siamese *See* Siamese twins.

twit A foolish person. *See also* twerp.

two-tailed test A two-sided or nondirectional test of a hypothesis. The hypothesis examines whether two estimates of parameters are equal, without caring which one is smaller or larger. The tested hypothesis is rejected if the test statistic is an extremely small or a large value. *See also* hypothesis; parameter; test; test statistic.

tying arrangement An arrangement in which one party sells a product or service (the tying product or service) only on the condition that the buyer also purchase a different (or tied) product or service. *See also* arrangement; business; trade.

type and crossmatch blood *See* blood transfusion; blood typing; crossmatching.

Type Culture Collection, American *See* American Type Culture Collection.

type I diabetes mellitus Diabetes mellitus characterized by abrupt onset of symptoms, lack of insulin, dependence on exogenous insulin to sustain life, and a tendency to develop ketoacidosis. The peak age of onset is 12 years, but onset can occur at any age. The disorder is due to lack of insulin production by the beta cells of the pancreas. The beta cell injury is associated with viral infection and autoimmune reactions and probably with genetic factors; islet cell antibodies are detectable in most patients at diagnosis. In undiagnosed or inadequately controlled type I diabetes mellitus, lack of insulin causes hyperglycemia, which leads to overflow glycosuria (excessive sugar in the urine), hyperosmolality, dehydration, diabetic ketoacidosis or hyperosmolar coma (or both), coma, and death. *Synonyms*: brittle diabetes; insulin-dependent diabetes; juvenile diabetes; juvenile-onset diabetes. *See also* diabetes mellitus; diabetic ketoacidosis; pancreas.

type II diabetes mellitus Diabetes mellitus usually characterized by a gradual onset with minimal or no symptoms of metabolic disturbance (excessive sugar in the urine and its consequences) and no requirement for exogenous insulin to prevent ketonuria and ketoacidosis. Dietary control with or without oral hypoglycemic drugs is usually effective. The peak age of onset is age 50 to 60 years. Obesity and possibly a genetic factor are usually present. Diagnosis is based on laboratory tests indicating glucose intolerance. Basal insulin secretion is maintained at normal or reduced levels, but insulin release in response to a glucose load is delayed or reduced. Defective glucose receptors on the beta cells of the pancreas may be involved. *Synonyms*: adult-onset diabetes; maturity-onset diabetes; non-insulin-dependent diabetes. *See also* diabetes mellitus.

type I error In research and statistics, a conclusion error in which the null hypothesis is rejected when it is in fact true. A conclusion is reached that there are effects (or relationships) when there are not. *Synonym*: alpha error. *See also* error; *p* (probability) value; statistical conclusion validity; statistically significant.

type II error In research and statistics, a conclusion error in which there is failure to reject the null hypothesis when it is false. In other words, a conclusion is reached that there are no effects (or relationships) when these effects (or relationships) do exist. *Synonym*: beta error. *See also* error; statistical conclusion validity; statistically significant.

type I recommendation A recommendation or group of recommendations provided by the Joint Commission on Accreditation of Healthcare Organizations that addresses insufficient or unsatisfactory standards compliance in a specific performance area. Resolution of type I recommendations must be achieved within stipulated time frames in order for a health care organization to maintain its accreditation. Resolution of type I recommendations is monitored by the Joint Commission through either focused surveys or the submission of written progress reports by the organization. *See also* accreditation; first generation type I recommendation; focused survey; Joint Commission on Accreditation of Healthcare Organizations; second generation type I recommendation; supplemental recommendation; written progress report.

type I recommendation, first generation *See* first generation type I recommendation.

type I recommendation, second generation *See* second generation type I recommendation.

type II recommendation *See* supplemental recommendation.

typhoid *See* typhoid fever.

typhoid fever An acute infectious disease caused by a bacteria (*Salmonella typhi*) transmitted chiefly by contaminated food or water and characterized by fever, headache, coughing, intestinal bleeding, and rash. *Synonyms*: enteric fever; typhoid. *See also* enteric; infectious diseases; Typhoid Mary.

Typhoid Mary An individual from whom something undesirable or deadly spreads to those nearby; named after Mary Mallon, a notorious carrier of typhoid. *See also* infectious diseases; typhoid fever.

typical Exhibiting the qualities, traits, or characteristics that identify a kind, class, group, or category, as in a typical patient case mix for a community hospital. *See also* typify.

typify To serve as a typical example, or embody the essential characteristics of, as in the situation typifies what is right with the health care system. *See also* typical.

typing, blood *See* blood typing.

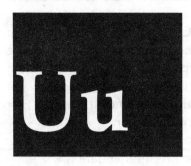

Uu

UAPD *See* Union of American Physicians and Dentists.

UAREP *See* Universities Associated for Research and Education in Pathology.

UB-92 Abbreviation for Uniform Bill-92, a uniform billing form intended to be used by major third-party payers, most hospitals (for inpatient and outpatient billing), and, at the option of individual hospitals, hospital-based skilled nursing facilities and home health agencies. The data elements and design of the form were determined by the National Uniform Billing Committee (NUBC) and subsequently approved as applicable and modified by, for example, the Illinois Uniform Billing Committee. The NUBC includes representatives of the Health Care Financing Administration, the Blue Cross Association, the Health Insurance Association of American, the Civilian Health and Medical Programs of the Uniformed Services (CHAMPUS), the Federation of American Health Systems (formerly Federation of American Hospitals), the Healthcare Financial Management Association, the American Hospital Association, and individual hospitals. The data included on the form are intended to provide a basic set of data elements needed by most third-party payers to adjudicate the greater majority of their claims. These data elements are generally available from provider records, although, in addition to the basic data elements, certain other data elements generally not as readily available are included in order to accommodate the wide-ranging needs of payers and to eliminate the need for attachments. *Synonyms*: National Uniform Billing System. *See also* billing; Health Care Financing Administration; Medicare; Uniform Hospital Discharge Data Set.

UCC *See* United Cancer Council.

UCDS *See* Uniform Clinical Data Set.

UCPA *See* United Cerebral Palsy Associations.

UCR charge *See* usual, customary, and reasonable charge.

UGME *See* undergraduate medical education.

UHDDS *See* Uniform Hospital Discharge Data Set.

UHMS *See* Undersea and Hyperbaric Medical Society.

Ukrainian Medical Association of North America (UMANA) A national organization founded in 1950 composed of 1,000 physicians, dentists, and persons in related professions who are of Ukrainian descent. It provides assistance to members, sponsors lectures, and maintains a placement service, museum, and library of 1,800 medical books and journals in Ukrainian. *See also* medical association; physician.

UL *See* Underwriters Laboratories.

ulcer A usually persistent, local defect or excavation in skin or mucous membrane; for example, duodenal ulcer. *See also* duodenal ulcer; gastric ulcer; peptic ulcer; pressure sore; ulceration.

ulceration The formation of an ulcer. *See also* ulcer.

ulcer, decubitus *See* pressure sore.

ulcer, duodenal *See* duodenal ulcer.

ulcer, gastric *See* gastric ulcer.

ulcer, peptic *See* peptic ulcer.

ulcer, pressure *See* pressure sore.

ultimate customer An entity, such as a person or unit, that receives the output from a series of processes and for whom these processes are designed. Without the ultimate customer (for example, a patient) there would be no need for intermediate processes to exist. *See also* customer.

ultrasonic Pertaining to ultrasound, as in ultrasonic cardiography. *See also* ultrasonics; ultrasound.

ultrasonic cardiography *See* echocardiography.

ultrasonic diagnostic service A unit of a hospital or other health care organization providing ultrasound imaging services. *See also* ultrasonics; ultrasound.

ultrasonic lithotripsy *See* lithotripsy.

ultrasonics The science and technology that deals with the study and application of ultrasound. *See also* ultrasound.

ultrasonogram *See* sonogram.

ultrasonograph An apparatus for producing images obtained by ultrasonography. *See also* ultrasound imaging.

ultrasonography *See* ultrasound imaging.

ultrasound **1.** Sound waves at the very high frequency of over 20,000 vibrations per second. **2.** The use of ultrasonic waves for diagnostic, therapeutic, or other purposes; for example, to monitor a developing fetus, generate localized deep heat to the tissues, or at an extremely high frequency, clean dental and surgical instruments. *See also* ultrasonics; ultrasound imaging.

ultrasound image *See* sonogram.

ultrasound imaging The use of high-frequency sound to produce an image of internal structures by the differing reflection signals produced when a beam of sound waves is projected into the body and bounces back at interfaces between those structures. Ultrasound diagnosis differs from radiologic diagnosis in that there is no ionizing radiation involved. *Synonyms*: sonography; ultrasonography. *See also* diagnostic medical sonographer; echocardiography; imaging.

Ultrasound in Medicine, American Institute of *See* American Institute of Ultrasound in Medicine.

ultrasound physical therapy A form of physical therapy employed by podiatrists and other health professionals in which tissue is stimulated by a large amount of vibration produced by sound waves. This relieves pain and inflammation of the joint structures. *See also* inflammation; joint; physical therapy; ultrasound.

ultraviolet (UV) Light beyond the range of human vision at the short end of the spectrum (wavelengths between about 4 nanometers, on the border of the x-ray region, to about 380 nanometers). It occurs naturally in sunlight and is responsible for tanning the skin and converting precursors in the skin to vitamin D. Ultraviolet lamps are used in the control of infections, the control of airborne bacteria and virus-es, and the treatment of psoriasis and other skin conditions. Ultraviolet light is a form of physical therapy used as a fungicide by some podiatrists who apply the ultraviolet light to a patient's foot by means of a machine called a fungetrol. *See also* phototherapy; physical therapy.

UMA *See* United Methodist Association of Health and Welfare Ministries.

UMANA *See* Ukrainian Medical Association of North America.

umbilical cord A cordlike structure, containing two umbilical arteries and one umbilical vein, that connects the fetal circulation with the placenta. It functions to transport nourishment to the fetus and remove its wastes. *See also* fetus; placenta; umbilical line.

umbilical line A catheter inserted into the umbilical vein or artery of a newborn infant to provide access to the bloodstream. *See also* catheter; central line; umbilical cord.

umbrella coverage Insurance coverage relating to a broad high-limit liability policy, usually requiring underlying insurance. For instance, a hospital may be insured for $1 million for general liability, $3 million dollars for professional liability, and $10 million dollars for umbrella coverage. This additional $10 million is the umbrella that picks up excess liability (not in excess of $10 million) over and above the other two policies. *Synonym*: umbrella liability insurance. *See also* coverage; insurance.

umbrella liability insurance *See* umbrella coverage.

unaccredited Not having the proper credentials, as in an unaccredited school. *See also* accreditation; accredited; not accredited.

unannounced survey A survey that is conducted without prior notification by the Joint Commission on Accreditation of Healthcare Organizations to a health care organization. It may occur *for cause*, meaning that the Joint Commission becomes aware of circumstances in an accredited organization that suggest a potentially serious standards compliance problem (for example, when there is reason to believe that an immediate threat to patient health or safety exists). Alternatively, an unannounced survey may occur *at random*. Beginning July 1, 1993, approximately 5% of all institutions accredited by the Joint Commission are surveyed by one surveyor for one day at the approximate mid-accreditation point. *See also* accreditation survey; Joint Commission on Accreditation of Healthcare Organizations; special analysis unit.

unauthorized practice A health care activity undertaken by an individual who has not been appropriately trained and certified or licensed to engage in it. *See also* practice.

unbundling **1.** The act of selling individual components of a service or product separately rather than as a package. **2.** In health care, the practice of separate pricing of goods and services that are normally billed under a single charge, resulting in a higher overall cost. **3.** Under Medicare, Part B, for nonphysician services, services that are provided to hospital inpatients and furnished to the hospital by an outside supplier or another provider. Unbundling is prohibited under the Medicare prospective pricing system, and all nonphysician services provided in an inpatient setting are paid as hospital services. *See also* billing; fractionation; Medicare, Part B; Medicare; prospective pricing system.

uncertified Not officially verified or registered, as in an uncertified nurse. *Compare* certified. *See also* certification.

uncollected revenue The amount of money billed, but not collected, for services provided. *See also* revenue.

uncompensated care Care for which no payment is expected or no charge is made. It is the sum of bad debts and charity care absorbed by a hospital or other health care organization in providing medical care for patients who are uninsured or are unable to pay. *See also* self-pay patient; underinsured.

unconscious A state of mind characterized by a loss of sensation and awareness of internal and external events. *Synonym:* falling out. *See also* blackout; consciousness; Glasgow coma scale; subconscious.

unction *See* ointment.

under the counter Refers to illegal payments made for merchandise or services, usually in excess of the stated price. Under-the-counter payments are a form of bribery and extortion.

underemployed Pertaining to people who are not fully employed according to their education, abilities, and experiences. *See also* employee.

undergraduate medical education (UGME) Medical education given before receipt of the Doctor of Medicine (MD) or equivalent degree, usually the four years of study in medical, osteopathic, dental, or podiatric school leading to a degree. *See also* con-

tinuing medical education; graduate medical education; medical education.

underground economy The part of the economy that goes largely undetected by taxing authorities. Transactions usually are barter or in cash and include illegal activities and activities that would be legal except for their unrecorded nature. *See also* economy; tax.

underinsured Pertains to people who do not have sufficient insurance coverage to compensate in the event of loss of life or property. *See also* adequacy of coverage; insurance; insured; self-pay patient; uncompensated care.

underlying cause of death *See* death certificate.

underpay Inadequate wages, as when individuals are paid less than a job or procedure is worth in market or perceived terms. *See also* pay; wage.

underreporting Failure to identify and/or count all cases, leading to reduction of the numerator of a rate, as in a (falsely) low mortality rate due to underreporting of deaths resulting from some condition. *See also* rate; report.

Undersea and Hyperbaric Medical Society (UHMS) A national organization founded in 1967 composed of 2,500 diving physiologists, physicians, biologists, and bioengineers with subsea or hyperbaric interests. Formerly (1986) Undersea Medical Society. *See also* hyperbaric chamber; hyperbaric medicine.

Undersea Medical Society *See* Undersea and Hyperbaric Medical Society.

underserved population, medically *See* medically underserved population.

understand To perceive and comprehend the nature and significance of something, as in understanding the need for self-review and self-improvement.

undertaker *See* funeral director.

undertriage In trauma care, the transportation of a patient who should have been cared for in a trauma center to a nontrauma center. This may result in increased patient morbidity or mortality. *See also* overtriage; triage.

underwrite To insure. *See also* underwriter; underwriting.

underwriter An individual or company specializing in underwriting. *Synonym:* writer. *See also* coverage; underwriting.

Underwriters Laboratories (UL) A private organization that performs a wide range of product safety tests on fire-protective equipment, electric and heating appliances, wiring, and building materials. Their certification label appears on thousands of products that have been tested successfully for their fire, shock, and casualty hazards. *See also* certification; safety; underwriter.

Underwriters, National Association of Health *See* National Association of Health Underwriters.

underwriting In insurance, the process of selecting, classifying, evaluating, and assuming risks according to their insurability. Its fundamental purpose is to make sure that the group insured has the same probability of loss and probable amount of loss, within reasonable limits, as the universe on which premium rates were based. Since premium rates are based on an expectation of loss, the underwriting process must classify risks into classes with about the same expectation of loss. *See also* insurance; risk; underwriter; underwriting profit.

underwriting association, joint *See* joint underwriting association.

underwriting profit The portion of an insurance company's earnings that comes from the function of calculating a profit factor during underwriting; the difference between incurred losses and expenses and earned premiums. *See also* insurance; profit; underwriting.

undesirable indicator A process or an outcome indicator that measures an undesirable activity or result of care; for example, patient death or failed vaginal delivery after previous cesarean section. *See also* indicator.

unearned income Support or maintenance furnished in kind or in cash; annuities, pensions, retirements, or disability benefits; prizes, gifts, and awards; proceeds from insurance policies, child support and alimony payments; inheritances; and rents, dividends, interest, and royalties. Fringe benefits of employment, such as an employer's contribution to the cost of health insurance, are often not considered as income for tax purposes, thus enhancing their real value and creating, for example, an indirect federal subsidy of group health insurance. *Compare* earned income. *See also* income.

unemployment The state of being without paid work. *Compare* employment. *See also* unemployment compensation disability; unemployment insurance.

unemployment compensation disability Insur-

ance that protects people against loss due to off-the-job injury or illness. Unemployment compensation is funded by payroll deductions, and is administered by a state agency. *Synonym*: state disability insurance. *See also* compensation; disability; unemployment.

unemployment insurance A form of social insurance that operates by means of a payroll tax, the revenues from which are used to pay calculated benefits for defined periods to people who qualify as being unemployed, as defined in the law. *See also* insurance; social insurance; payroll tax; unemployment.

unethical Not in accordance with the standards followed in a business or a profession, as in unethical conduct. *Compare* ethical. *See also* unethical conduct.

unethical conduct Actions or behavior that violate, or are not in accord with, the standards of professional practice and conduct. *See also* conduct; unethical.

unguent *See* ointment.

unified payment A payment method in which a hospital or other health care organization and a physician or other health professional are paid a single, fixed amount for each service, day, or patient case. This method usually is applied to services performed by a facility and by a physician in the facility setting. *See also* payment.

Uniform Anatomical Gift Act of 1969 A statute adopted by every state that makes it legally possible for individuals to make known their intentions, while living, to donate their organs after death. *See also* anatomical gift.

uniform basic data set *See* minimum data set.

Uniform Bill-92 *See* UB-92.

uniform capital factor A uniform percentage added onto all diagnosis-related group prices to cover hospital capital costs for pricing in prospective payment systems. *See also* diagnosis-related groups; prospective payment system.

uniform claim form A standardized claim form and a standardized format for electronic claims, which would reduce administrative costs. *See also* claim.

Uniform Clinical Data Set (UCDS) A Health Care Financing Administration (HCFA) initiative and part of the Peer Review Organization (PRO) Fourth Scope of Work that involves collection from the medical records of Medicare beneficiaries of approximately 1,800 data elements that describe patient demographic characteristics, clinical history, clinical findings, and therapeutic interventions. The purpose of this database is to assist HCFA in defining Medicare research and review samples. For instance, the UCDS will allow longitudinal analyses of large beneficiary cohorts and the identification of regional, interhospital, and intrahospital practice variations. *See also* clinical data; database; data set; Health Care Financing Administration; peer review organization.

Uniform Determination of Death　*See* death.

Uniformed Services Academy of Family Physicians (USAFP)　A national organization founded in 1973 composed of 2,000 family physicians, teachers of family medicine, medical students, and residents in the armed services, public health service, or Indian health service. *See also* family physician.

Uniform Hospital Discharge Data Set (UHDDS)　The data element set required by the federal government as the medical content of a patient's bill under Medicare and Medicaid. Assignment to a diagnosis-related group is made from this data set by a fiscal intermediary. UHDDS contains, for instance, patient age, sex, and diagnoses and procedures expressed in the category codes of *International Classification of Diseases, Ninth Revision, Clinical Modification (ICD-9-CM)*. The Uniform Hospital Discharge Abstract used to collect the Uniform Hospital Discharge Data Set is an example of a discharge abstract. *See also* data set; diagnosis-related groups; discharge abstract; fiscal intermediary; GROUPER software; *International Classification of Diseases, Ninth Revision, Clinical Modification.*

uniform reporting　Reporting of financial and service data in conformance with prescribed standardized definitions to permit accurate and meaningful comparisons among providers, such as physicians and hospitals. *See also* data.

unilateral　Affecting one side only, as in a governing body taking a unilateral action to modify the medical staff bylaws or unilateral paralysis after stroke. *Compare* bilateral; lateral; medial.

union, labor　*See* labor union.

Union of American Physicians and Dentists (UAPD)　An independent national labor organization founded in 1972 composed of state federations made up of 10,000 physicians and dentists, self-employed or employed by hospitals, teaching institutions, counties, and municipalities. Its activities include ensuring reasonable compensation for physicians commensurate with their training, skill, and the responsibility they bear for their patients. *See also* dentist; labor union; physician.

Union, Independent Hospital Workers　*See* Independent Hospital Workers Union.

unit　**1.** A single thing, as in unit-dose medication system. **2.** A quantity assumed as a standard of measurement. *See also* unit of measure. **3.** An area of a hospital or other health care organization that is staffed and equipped for care of patients with common characteristics; for example, emergency unit, special care unit.

unit, ALS　*See* ALS unit.

unit, BLS　*See* BLS unit.

unit, burn　*See* burn unit.

unit, cardiac care　*See* cardiac care unit.

unit, central processing　*See* central processing unit.

unit clerk　*See* health unit coordinator.

unit clerk, health　*See* health unit coordinator.

unit coordinator, health　*See* health unit coordinator.

unit, coronary care　*See* cardiac care unit.

unit, critical care　*See* special care unit.

unit, dental　*See* dental unit.

unit-dose medication system　A method of providing medications to hospitalized patients whereby all medications to be given a particular patient at a specific time are packaged together in the exact dosage required for that time. *See also* dose; medication.

United Cancer Council (UCC)　A federation founded in 1963 composed of 39 independent cancer agencies receiving their support from the United Way of America. It promotes programs of direct service to cancer patients and their families. *See also* cancer.

United Cerebral Palsy Associations (UCPA)　A national voluntary federation founded in 1948 composed of 180 state and local affiliates aiding persons with cerebral palsy. Its goals are to prevent cerebral palsy, minimize its effects, and involve individuals with cerebral palsy and their families in the mainstream of society. *See also* cerebral palsy.

United Methodist Association of Health and Welfare Ministries (UMA)　A national organization founded in 1940 composed of 355 individual, staff, and board members of United Methodist-affiliated hospitals, retirement homes, and children's homes. It offers communications and church relations guidance, and provides leadership development training for health and welfare professionals in the United Methodist Church. It develops ethical and theological statements on institutional care and operates Educational Assessment Guidelines Leading Toward Excellence, a self-assessment and peer review program. Formerly (1983) National Association of Health and Welfare Ministries of the United Methodist Church.

United Network for Organ Sharing (UNOS) A national network founded in 1984 composed of 377 transplant and organ procurement centers, tissue-typing laboratories, and health care professionals engaged in organ transplant operations. It was established by law as the clearinghouse for organs used in US transplant operations. It operates the Organ Center, which matches patients in need of transplants with donated organs and arranges transport of organs to transplant sites. It formulates and implements national policies on equitable access and organ allocation, AIDS testing, and organ procurement standards. *See also* network; organ procurement; organ transplantation.

United States Adopted Names (USAN) A nonproprietary designation for any compound used as a drug, established by negotiation between the manufacturer of the compound used as drug and a nomenclature committee known as the USAN Council, which is sponsored jointly by the American Medical Association, the American Pharmaceutical Association, and the United States Pharmacopeial Convention. *See also* drug.

United States of America), Royal College of Physicians and Surgeons (of the *See* Royal College of Physicians and Surgeons (of the United States of America).

United States Air Force Flight Surgeons, Society of *See* Society of United States Air Force Flight Surgeons.

United States Association of Physicians *See* American Association of Ayurvedic Medicine.

United States Civil Defense Council *See* National Coordinating Council on Emergency Management.

United States Conference of City Health Officers *See* United States Conference of Local Health Officers.

United States Conference of Local Health Officers (USCLHO) A national organization founded in 1960 composed of chief health officers, commissioners, directors, and other officials representing city,

county, or city-county health departments. It promotes cooperation and exchange of ideas to assist in the improvement of local public health administration. Formerly (1983) United States Conference of City Health Officers. *See also* public health.

United States foreign medical graduate (USFMG) *See* foreign medical graduate.

United States medical graduate (USMG) A graduate of a medical school in the United States, Puerto Rico, or Canada. *See also* foreign medical graduate; graduate.

United States - Mexico Border Health Association (USMBHA) An organization founded in 1943 composed of 2,300 physicians, public health administrators, nurses, sanitary engineers, veterinarians, scientists, laboratory workers, and other health officers from the four American and six Mexican states bordering the two countries. It seeks to make easier and more efficient the improvement of public health along both sides of the border. *See also* public health.

United States and Mexico, Medical Society of the *See* Medical Society of the United States and Mexico.

United States, National Catholic Pharmacists Guild of the *See* National Catholic Pharmacists Guild of the United States.

United States Pharmacopeia (USP) A compendium of standards for drugs, published by the United States Pharmacopeial Convention, and revised periodically; it includes assays and tests for the determination of drug strength, quality, and purity. One of the three official compendia of drugs and medications in the United States recognized in the federal Food, Drug, and Cosmetic Act. The other two are the *Homeopathic Pharmacopeia of the United States* and the *National Formulary*. *See also* compendium; *Homeopathic Pharmacopeia of the United States*; *National Formulary*; pharmacopeia; United States Pharmacopeial Convention.

United States Pharmacopeial Convention (USP) A convention founded in 1820 composed of 391 recognized authorities in medicine, pharmacy, and allied sciences. It revises and publishes legally recognized compendia of drug standards. *See also* compendium; drug; pharmacopeia; standard; *United States Pharmacopeia*.

unit, emergency *See* emergency department.
unit, extended care *See* extended care unit.
unit, government relations *See* government relations unit.

unit, inpatient care   *See* inpatient care unit.

unit, intensive care   *See* intensive care unit.

unit, intermediate care   *See* intermediate care unit.

unit, living-in   *See* living-in unit.

unit manager   An individual who supervises and coordinates administrative management functions for one or more inpatient care units. The scope of the supervision may include the unit nursing staff, unit clerks, and technical staff temporarily or permanently assigned to the unit. *Synonyms:* charge nurse; nursing supervisor; unit supervisor; ward manager; ward service manager. *See also* manager; unit.

unit, maximum security   *See* maximum security unit.

unit of measure   A defined amount of an attribute of a person, an activity, or a thing (such as an event, an object, or a phenomenon). For example, a Fahrenheit degree (a unit of measure) is a defined amount of the heat (an attribute) of an oven (an object). *See also* measure; unit.

unit, medical intensive care   *See* medical intensive care unit.

unit, minimal care   *See* minimal care unit.

unit, mobile health   *See* mobile health unit.

unit, mobile intensive care   *See* mobile intensive care unit.

unit, neonatal   *See* newborn nursery.

unit, neonatal intensive care   *See* neonatal intensive care unit.

unit, nursing care   *See* nursing care unit.

unit, organization   *See* organization unit.

unit, patient care   *See* inpatient care unit.

unit, pediatric intensive care   *See* pediatric intensive care unit.

unit price   The price per unit (a quart, for example) of a product. *See also* price; unit.

unit, psychiatric inpatient   *See* psychiatric inpatient unit.

unit, rehabilitation   *See* rehabilitation unit.

unit, relative value   *See* relative value unit.

unit, respiratory diseases   *See* respiratory diseases unit.

unit secretary   *See* health unit coordinator.

unit, self-care   *See* minimal care unit.

unit, skilled nursing   *See* skilled nursing unit.

unit, special analysis   *See* special analysis unit.

unit, special care   *See* special care unit.

units, Systeme International   *See* Systeme International units.

unit, step-down   *See* step-down unit.

unit supervisor   *See* unit manager.

unit, surgical intensive care   *See* surgical intensive care unit.

Universities Associated for Research and Education in Pathology (UAREP)   A national organization founded in 1964 composed of 23 university pathology departments, including faculty members, residents, and research fellows. It provides core material in convenient form for updating and enriching teaching and researching of pathology, with special emphasis on toxicology and chemical carcinogens. *See also* pathology; toxicology; university.

university   An institution for higher learning with teaching and research facilities constituting a graduate school and professional schools that award master's degrees and doctorates and an undergraduate division that awards bachelor's degrees. *See also* bachelor's degree; doctorate; master's degree.

University Affiliated Programs for Persons with Developmental Disabilities, American Association of   *See* American Association of University Affiliated Programs for Persons with Developmental Disabilities.

University Anesthesiologists, Association of   *See* Association of University Anesthesiologists.

University Environmental Health/Sciences Centers, Association of   *See* Association of University Environmental Health/Sciences Centers.

university hospital   A hospital that is owned by or affiliated with a medical school and used in the education of physicians. *See also* medical school; physician; teaching hospital; university.

University Otolaryngologists-Head and Neck Surgeons, Society of   *See* Society of University Otolaryngologists-Head and Neck Surgeons.

University Professors of Ophthalmology, Association of   *See* Association of University Professors of Ophthalmology.

University Programs in Health Administration, Association of   *See* Association of University Programs in Health Administration.

University Programs in Occupational Health and Safety, Association of   *See* Association of University Programs in Occupational Health and Safety.

University Radiologists, Association of   *See* Association of University Radiologists.

University Surgeons, Society of   *See* Society of University Surgeons.

University Urologists, Society of *See* Society of University Urologists.

UNOS *See* United Network for Organ Sharing.

unprofessional **1.** Not a qualified member of a professional group. **2.** Not conforming to the standards of a profession, as in unprofessional conduct. *Compare* professional.

unrestricted fund Money donated to an organization that can be expended at the discretion of the administration of the governing board. *Compare* restricted fund. *See also* fund.

unstructured interview An interview in which the interviewer does not determine the format or subject to be discussed. Rather, the interviewee has major control of the conversation. *Compare* structured interview. *See also* interview.

update To provide current information to an individual or group of persons or revise printed information according to the most current information available.

upload **1.** To transfer user data to a remote computer system. **2.** To transfer data from a disk or other storage device to a computer. *Compare* download. *See also* computer; data.

upper adjacent value *See* adjacent value, upper.

upper control limit *See* control limit.

UR *See* utilization review.

URAC *See* Utilization Review Accreditation Commission.

urban Pertaining to or characteristic of a city or an intensively developed area. *See also* rural; rurban; suburban; urban renewal; urban sprawl.

urban renewal The process of rehabilitating impoverished urban neighborhoods by large-scale renovation or reconstruction of housing and public works. *See also* urban.

urban sprawl The unplanned, uncontrolled spreading of urban development into areas adjoining the edge of a city. *See also* urban.

urgent A degree of severity of illness or injury that is less severe than immediately life-threatening (emergency), but requiring care more quickly than elective care. *Compare* nonurgent. *See also* acuity level; elective; emergency; severity of illness; urgent admission.

urgent admission The formal acceptance by a health care organization of a patient who requires immediate attention for the care and treatment of a physical or mental disorder. Generally, such a patient is admitted to the first available and suitable accommodation. *Compare* elective admission. *See also* admission; elective admission; emergency admission; urgent.

urgent care center *See* freestanding urgent care center.

urgent care center, freestanding *See* freestanding urgent care center.

urgicenter *See* freestanding urgent care center.

urinary incontinence Failure of voluntary control of the vesical and urethral sphincters, with constant or frequent involuntary passage of urine. *See also* stress incontinence; urination.

Urinary Surgeons, American Association of Genito- *See* American Association of Genito-Urinary Surgeons.

urination The act of voiding urine. *Synonym:* micturition. *See also* strangury; urinary incontinence.

urokinase An enzyme in human urine that catalyzes the conversion of plasminogen to plasmin and is used in medicine to dissolve blood clots. *See also* blood clot; thrombolytic therapy; thrombosis.

Urological Association Allied, American *See* American Urological Association Allied.

Urological Association, American *See* American Urological Association.

Urologic Allied Health Professionals, American Board of *See* American Board of Urologic Allied Health Professionals.

Urologic Diseases Information Clearinghouse, National Kidney and *See* National Kidney and Urologic Diseases Information Clearinghouse.

urologist A physician who specializes in urology. *See also* urology.

Urologists, American Association of Clinical *See* American Association of Clinical Urologists.

Urologists, Society of University *See* Society of University Urologists.

urology The branch and specialty of medicine dealing with the management of benign and malignant medical and surgical disorders of the adrenal gland and of the reproductive and urinary systems and their adjoining structures. *See also* medical specialties.

Urology, American Board of *See* American Board of Urology.

urology service A service providing study, diagnosis, care, and treatment of patients with diseases and dysfunctions of the urinary tract in females and the genitourinary tract in males. *See also* urology.

Urology, Society for Pediatric *See* Society for Pediatric Urology.

USAFP *See* Uniformed Services Academy of Family Physicians.

usage The customary practice or established use, as in medication usage; usage here refers to the way in which medications are used. *See also* blood usage review; use; user.

usage review, blood *See* blood usage review.

USAN *See* United States Adopted Names.

USCLHO *See* United States Conference of Local Health Officers.

use 1. To apply or implement for a purpose, as in using a hearing aid. *See also* useful. 2. The act of using, as in skilled in the use of statistics. *See also* user.

Use of Antibiotics, Alliance for the Prudent *See* Alliance for the Prudent Use of Antibiotics.

use-by date A date marked on a food package or other perishable goods to show the latest time by which the contents should be used to avoid risk of deterioration. *See also* best-before date.

useful Having a beneficial and practical use, as in a useful invention. *See also* use; utility.

useful many The remaining factors in Pareto analysis after the vital few have been identified; the relatively large set of factors that account for only a small minority of any problem. *See also* Pareto analysis.

user A person who uses something, as in designing a product or service with the user in mind. *See also* use; user-friendly; user-unfriendly.

user-friendly Easy to use or operate, or learn to use or operate, as in a user-friendly computer system. *Compare* user-unfriendly. *See also* user.

user-unfriendly Unhelpful to a user or difficult to use or learn to operate, as in user-unfriendly computer software. *Compare* user-friendly. *See also* user.

USFCC *See* US Federation for Culture Collections.

US Federation for Culture Collections (USFCC) A federation founded in 1970 composed of 260 persons interested in culture collections, particularly those involved in collecting, maintaining, and preserving microbial cultures. It encourages research, finds means of preserving collections of microorganisms, and encourages establishment of microbial strain data services. It sponsors workshops on the preservation of microbial cultures and the operation of culture collections. *See also* culture; microorganism.

US General Accounting Office (GAO) The independent congressional agency established in 1921 that reviews federal financial transactions. It examines the expenditures of appropriations of federal agencies and reports directly to Congress. The head of the agency is the Comptroller General of the United States who is appointed by the president with the advice and consent of the Senate for a nonrenewable 15-year term of office. Some of its activities include conducting on-site monitoring of federal agencies and performing special studies requested by members and committees of Congress. Reports are issued by the GAO to the Congress and are often made available to the public. Its Human Resources Division conducts health-related studies; its Audit Operations Group conducts audits on health care programs. One example of a GAO activity is the one it recently conducted (1991) on behalf of the Agency for Health Care Policy and Research to study the experience of medical societies in developing, disseminating, updating, implementing, and evaluating the impact of clinical practice guidelines (GAO/PEMD-91-11, Feb 1991). The GAO Study found that no two societies had produced similar guidelines for similar reasons using similar methods. *See also* Agency for Health Care Policy and Research; practice guideline.

USFMG Abbreviation for US foreign medical graduate. *See* foreign medical graduate.

USMBHA *See* United States - Mexico Border Health Association.

USMG *See* United States medical graduate.

USP *See United States Pharmacopeia.*

USPC *See* United States Pharmacopeial Convention.

US Pharmacopeial Convention *See* United States Pharmacopeial Convention.

US Physical Therapy Association (USPT) A national organization founded in 1970 composed of 12,700 physical therapists and assistants. It maintains the US Physical Therapy Academy, which, among other activities, accredits hospital and nursing home physical therapy departments, universities and colleges of physical therapy, and certifies physical therapists through board examinations. *See also* certification; physical therapy.

US Public Health Service *See* Public Health Service.

USPT *See* US Physical Therapy Association.

usual Commonly encountered, experienced, or observed, as in the usual fee or the usual way of diagnosing the condition.

usual, customary, and reasonable (UCR) charge A method used by health insurance plans for determining payment for services and procedures rendered by an individual health care provider. A reimbursement is based on allowing the provider's full charge if it does not exceed his or her usual charge; it does not exceed the amount customarily charged for the service by other physicians in the area (often defined as the 90th or 95th percentile of all charges in the community); or it is justified in the specific circumstances of a given patient (otherwise reasonable). *See also* charge.

uterus A hollow muscular organ located in the pelvis of female mammals in which the fertilized egg implants and develops. *Synonym:* womb. *See also* curettage; endometriosis; endometritis; hysterectomy; obstetrics and gynecology; pessary; procidentia; puerperal fever; total hysterectomy; vagina.

utilitarianism An ethical theory stating that an action is judged in terms of its consequences, that the value of an action is determined by its utility, and that all action should be directed toward achieving the greatest happiness for the greatest number of people. *Synonyms*: axiological ethics; consequential ethics. *Compare* deontological ethics. *See also* ethics.

utilities management A component of a health care organization's plant, technology, and safety management program designed to ensure the operational reliability, assess the special risks, and respond to failures of utility systems that support the patient care environment. *See also* management; utility; utility systems.

utility **1.** The condition or quality of being useful. For example, in decision analysis theory, utility is the usefulness or desirability of an outcome resulting from a decision. *See also* decision analysis; marginal utility. **2.** A commodity or service, such as electricity, water, or public transportation, that is provided by a public utility.

utility, marginal *See* marginal utility.

utility systems In health care organizations, systems for life support, infection control, environment support, and equipment support. *See also* infection control; utility.

utilization The use, patterns of use, or rates of use of a specified health care service, as in utilization of diagnostic tests, hospital beds, or medications. *See also* hospital utilization; utilization management.

utilization, hospital *See* hospital utilization.

utilization and quality control peer review organization (PRO) *See* peer review organization.

utilization management The planning, organizing, directing, and controlling of resource use relating to patient care by a health care organization. Utilization management programs are generally required by third-party payers, such as Medicare and Blue Cross, who may deny payment for services deemed inappropriate. *See also* management; utilization; utilization review.

utilization review (UR) The examination and evaluation of the necessity, appropriateness, and efficiency of the use of health care services, procedures, and facilities. In a hospital this includes review of the appropriateness of admissions, services ordered and provided, length of stay, and discharge practices, both on a concurrent and retrospective basis. Utilization review is typically performed by a utilization review committee, peer review group, or public agency. *See also* external review; internal review; managed indemnity plan; medical review; private review; utilization; utilization management.

Utilization Review Accreditation Commission (URAC) A body founded in 1990 that evaluates and accredits utilization review programs and organizations. It develops and promulgates minimum industry standards, which serve as a basis for a voluntary accreditation process. Its Board of Directors includes representatives from the American Medical Association, American Hospital Association, American Nurses Association, American Psychiatric Association, Washington Business Group on Health, National Association of Insurance Commissioners, International Union of United Auto Workers, National Association of Manufacturers, American Managed Care & Review Association; Blue Cross/Blue Shield Association, and Health Insurance Association of America. Its goal is to continually improve the quality and efficiency of the interaction between the providers, payers, and purchasers of health care. *See also* accreditation; utilization review.

utilization review, drug *See* drug usage evaluation.

Utilization Review Physicians, American Board of Quality Assurance and *See* American Board of

Quality Assurance and Utilization Review Physicians.

utilization review committee A committee of a health care organization or a group outside the organization responsible for conducting utilization review activities for that organization. Medicare and Medicaid require as a condition of participation that hospitals perform utilization review. *See also* committee; utilization review.

utilization review coordinator An individual who coordinates a health care organization's utilization review activities. A coordinator's activities may include providing staff support to an organization's utilization review committee and acting as a liaison with community agencies (such as visiting nurse associations, social services, and rehabilitation centers) and external review bodies concerned with utilization review matters. *See also* utilization review.

utopia A perfect place, especially in its social, political, and moral aspects.

UV *See* ultraviolet.

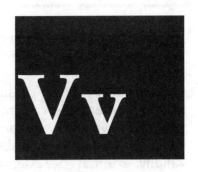

VA *See* Department of Veterans Affairs.

vacate When a court sets aside a previously entered order or decision; to render void. *See also* court.

vaccinate To inoculate with a vaccine in order to produce immunity to an infectious disease, such as diphtheria or tetanus. *Synonym*: immunize. *See also* active immunization; vaccine.

vaccine **1.** A suspension of an attenuated (weakened) or a killed microorganism, such as a bacteria or virus, administered for the prevention, amelioration, or treatment of infectious diseases. *See also* active immunization; DPT; infectious diseases; Sabin vaccine; Salk vaccine. **2.** A program that protects a computer system against being attacked by malicious software, such as a virus or worm. *See also* computer virus; worm.

vaccine, oral poliovirus *See* Sabin vaccine.

vaccine, Sabin *See* Sabin vaccine.

vaccine, Salk *See* Salk vaccine.

vaccine, trivalent live oral poliomyelitis *See* trivalent live oral poliomyelitis vaccine.

vague Not clearly expressed, as in a vague plan.

vagina The passage leading from the opening of the vulva to the cervix of the uterus in female mammals. *See also* pessary; uterus; vaginal birth after cesarean section; vaginal delivery.

vaginal birth *See* vaginal delivery.

vaginal birth after cesarean section (VBAC) A trial of labor in a patient with a history of cesarean section or uterine scar from previous surgery as documented in the medical record, resulting in vaginal delivery. An *attempted vaginal birth after cesarean section* is a trial of labor in a patient with a history of cesarean section or uterine scar from previous surgery as documented in the medical record. A *failed vaginal birth after cesarean section* is a trial of

labor in a patient with a history of cesarean section or uterine scar from previous surgery as documented in the medical record, resulting in delivery by repeat cesarean section. *See also* birth; cesarean section; labor; vagina.

vaginal birth after cesarean section, attempted *See* vaginal birth after cesarean section.

vaginal birth after cesarean section, failed *See* vaginal birth after cesarean section.

vaginal delivery Delivery of an infant through the normal openings of the uterus and vagina. *See also* birth; delivery; vagina.

vaginal hysterectomy *See* hysterectomy.

vaginitis Inflammation of the vagina with, for example, *Candida* or trichomonas. *See also Candida*; inflammation; vagina.

valid **1.** Containing premises from which a conclusion may logically be derived, as in a valid argument. **2.** Correctly inferred or deduced from a premise, as in a valid conclusion. *See also* validation; validity.

validation The process of establishing that a given method is sound; for example, that proper procedures are used to collect data and that the data are a reasonable representation of the phenomenon they are collected to measure. *See also* survey validation; validity; validity study.

validation, survey *See* survey validation.

validity **1.** The degree to which an observed situation reflects the true situation. **2.** In performance measurement, the degree to which an indicator or other measure identifies an event that merits further review by various individuals or groups providing or affecting the process or outcome defined by the indicator or other measure. *See also* construct validity; content validity; convergent validity; discriminant validity; external validity; face validity; indicator; internal validity; predictive validity; statistical conclusion validity.

validity, construct *See* construct validity.

validity, content *See* content validity.

validity, convergent *See* convergency validity.

validity, discriminant *See* discriminant validity.

validity, external *See* external validity.

validity, face *See* face validity.

validity, faith *See* face validity.

validity, indicator *See* indicator validity.

validity, internal *See* internal validity.

validity, predictive *See* predictive validity.

validity, statistical conclusion *See* statistical conclusion validity.

validity study The degree to which an inference drawn from an inquiry, especially generalizations extending beyond the study sample, is warranted when account is taken of the study methods, the representativeness of the study sample, and the nature of the population from which it is drawn.   There are two varieties of study validity: internal validity and external validity. *See also* internal validity; external validity; validity.

valid value All of the possible data elements that could be assigned to a particular category of information; for instance, if the category is "month," the valid values would be January through December. *See also* data element; valid; value.

value **1.** An amount, as of goods, services, or money, considered to be a fair and suitable equivalent for something else. **2.** In health care, a judgment based on the inverse relationship between the perceived quality of an organization's service and the cost of that service. *See also* cost; quality; value-added; worth.

value-added Relating to the estimated value that is added to a product or material at each stage of its manufacture or distribution. *See also* value; value-added tax.

value-added tax (VAT) A tax on the estimated market value added to a product or material at each stage of its manufacture or distribution, ultimately passed on to the consumer. *Synonym*: ad valorem tax. *See also* tax; value-added.

value judgment A decision reflecting values and opinions; a subjective evaluation. *See also* evaluation; judgment; subjective.

value, p (probability) *See* p (probability) value.

value system A system of "goods" cherished by an individual. The most commonly cited "goods" are life, happiness, pursuit of beauty, excellence, money, power, and opportunities. *See also* life-style.

value, valid *See* valid value.

vanguard The foremost or leading position in a trend or movement. *See also* pacesetter; trendsetter.

VA Physicians and Dentists, National Association of *See* National Association of VA Physicians and Dentists.

variable **1.** Any item, such as a quantity, attribute, phenomenon, or event, that can have different values. Examples are length in millimeters, time in minutes, and temperature in degrees. *See also* attribute; dependent variable; independent variable; unit of measure. **2.** Something that varies, as in a variable number of factors.

variable, confounding *See* confounding variable.

variable, continuous *See* continuous variable.

variable cost A cost that changes directly with the amount of production or use, such as direct labor needed to provide a service. *See also* cost; variable.

variable, dependent *See* dependent variable.

variable, discrete *See* discrete variable.

variable, independent *See* independent variable.

variable indicator, continuous *See* continuous variable indicator.

variable indicator, discrete *See* rate-based indicator.

variable, key process *See* key process variable.

variable, random *See* random variable.

variables data Data that arise from the measurement of a characteristic of a product, service, or process; and from the computation of a numerical value from two or more measurements of variables data. For instance, the number of minutes a patient waits to see a practitioner is variables data. Attribute data, by contrast, would be whether the patient waited to see the practitioner for more than *or* less than 20 minutes. *Compare* attribute data. *See also* data; variable.

variable, stratification *See* stratification variable.

variance **1.** The state or quality of being variant or variable; the difference between what is expected and what actually occurs or is observed. **2.** In statistics, a measure of variability that indicates how far all of the scores in a distribution vary from the mean. Variance is equal to the square of the standard deviation. *See also* precision; standard deviation; statistics.

variant Exhibiting variation, as in deviating from a standard, usually by only a slight difference. *See also* deviation; standard; variation.

variate A variable that may assume any of a set of values, each with a preassigned probability (known as its distribution). *See also* random variable; variable.

variation The inevitable difference among individual outputs of a process; excessive variation frequently leads to waste and loss, such as the occurrence of undesirable patient health outcomes and increased cost of health services. The sources of variation can be grouped into two major classes: common causes and special causes. *See also* calibration; common-cause variation; indicator underlying factors; output; practice pattern analysis; process variation; special-cause variation; variant.

variation, coefficient of *See* coefficient of variation.

variation, common-cause *See* common-cause variation.

variation, process *See* process variation.

variation, special-cause *See* special-cause variation.

varicella *See* chickenpox.

varices *See* varicose veins.

varicose veins Abnormally dilated and tortuous veins associated with conditions or circumstances resulting in persistently high venous pressure and with defective venous valves allowing retrograde flow. They are commonly seen in the subcutaneous tissue of the legs. *Synonym*: varices (singular, varix). *See also* vein.

variety The condition of being various or varied; diversity.

variola *See* smallpox.

varix *See* varicose veins.

vary To undergo change, as in attributes or qualities; for example, a patient's varying temperature.

vascular Characterized by or containing vessels that carry or circulate fluids, such as blood or lymph, as in vascular surgeon or vascular bed. *See also* blood vessel; cardiovascular; peripheral vascular disease; vascular surgery.

Vascular Credentialing International, Cardio- *See* Cardiovascular Credentialing International.

vascular disease, peripheral *See* peripheral vascular disease.

Vascular Nursing, Society for *See* Society for Vascular Nursing.

Vascular and Pulmonary Rehabilitation, American Association of Cardio- *See* American Association of Cardiovascular and Pulmonary Rehabilitation.

vascular surgeon A general surgeon who specializes in general vascular surgery. *Synonym*: general vascular surgeon. *See also* surgeon; vascular surgery.

vascular surgery The branch of medicine and subspecialty of general surgery dealing with the management of surgical disorders of the blood vessels, excluding those immediately adjacent to the heart, lungs, or brain. *Synonym*: general vascular surgery. *See also* blood vessel; general surgery.

Vascular Surgery, Association of Physician's Assistants in Cardio- *See* Association of Physician's Assistants in Cardiovascular Surgery.

vascular surgery, general *See* general vascular surgery.

Vascular Surgery, Society for *See* Society for Vascular Surgery.

Vascular Technology/National Society for Pulmonary Technology, National Society for Cardio- *See* National Society for Cardiovascular Technology/National Society for Pulmonary Technology.

vascular technology, noninvasive *See* noninvasive vascular technology.

Vascular Technology, Society of *See* Society of Vascular Technology.

vasectomy *See* sterilization.

VAT *See* value-added tax.

VBAC *See* vaginal birth after cesarean section.

vector A person, animal, or microorganism that carries and transmits disease. Mosquitoes carrying disease-producing parasites, for example, are vectors of malaria and yellow fever. *Compare* carrier. *See also* epidemiology; indirect contact; *Phlebotomus*; microorganism; rickettsiae.

vegans Strict vegetarians who use no animal products. They eat no animal protein at all, including eggs and other dairy products, and wear no leather. *See also* vegetarian.

vegetarian An individual who subsists on a diet composed primarily or wholly of vegetables, grains, fruits, nuts, and seeds, with or without eggs and dairy products. *See also* diet; lactovegetarian; ovolactovegetarian; vegans.

vegetarian, lacto- *See* lactovegetarian.

vegetarian, ovolacto- *See* ovolactovegetarian.

vegetative state A condition in a patient in which

there is no evidence of cortical (cerebral) functioning but the patient continues to have sustained capacity for spontaneous breathing and heart beat. A patient in a vegetative state specifically shows no evidence of verbal or nonverbal communication, demonstrates no purposeful movement or motor ability, is unable to interact purposefully with stimulation provided by his or her environment, is unable to provide for his or her basic needs, and demonstrates all these findings for longer than three months. *Synonyms*: cerebral death; persistent vegetative state. *See also* brain death.

vegetative state, persistent   *See* vegetative state.

vehicle   *See* excipient.

vein   A vessel through which blood passes from various organs or parts back to the heart. All veins except the pulmonary veins carry blood low in oxygen. *Compare* artery. *See also* blood vessel; phlebitis; varicose veins; venipuncture.

veins, varicose   *See* varicose veins.

venereal   Transmitted by sexual intercourse, as in venereal wart or venereal disease. *See also* sexual intercourse; venereal disease.

venereal disease   Any of several sexually transmitted diseases. *See also* disease; gonorrhea; sexually transmitted disease.

Venereal Disease Association, American   *See* American Venereal Disease Association.

venereology   The study of sexually transmitted diseases. *See also* sexually transmitted disease.

venipuncture   Puncture of a vein, as with a needle. *See also* phlebotomy; vein.

ventilation   The process of exchange of air between the lungs and the ambient air. *See also* breathing; mechanical ventilation; respiration; ventilator.

ventilation, mechanical   *See* mechanical ventilation.

ventilator   An apparatus designed to assist or control pulmonary ventilation, either intermittently or continuously. *See also* mechanical ventilation; ventilation.

ventricular fibrillation   An often fatal arrhythmia characterized by rapid, irregular fibrillar twitching of the ventricles of the heart in place of normal contractions. It results in loss of pulse and loss of perfusion of blood to the brain and rest of the body. *See also* arrhythmia; demand pacemaker; defibrillation; fibrillation.

venture, joint   *See* joint venture.

venue   The locale in which a court with authority over the persons and subject matter may hear cases. It is the geographical area within which an action may be brought. *See also* action; court.

verbiage   An excess of words for the purpose. *See also* verbose.

verbose   Using or containing a great and usually an excessive number of words, as in the verbose report. *See also* verbiage.

verdict   The finding of a jury, or of a judge when there is no jury, on a question of fact. A verdict differs from a judgment in that a verdict is not a judicial determination, but rather a finding of fact that the trial court may accept or reject and use in formulating its judgment. *See also* apportionment of damages; directed verdict; jury; summary judgment; trial.

verdict, directed   *See* directed verdict.

verification   The act of reviewing, inspecting, testing, checking, auditing, or otherwise establishing and documenting whether items, processes, services, or documents conform to specified requirements. *See also* data verification process; verify.

verification process, data   *See* data verification process.

verify   To prove the truth of by presentation of evidence or testimony; to substantiate, as in verifying the physician's credentials. *See also* verification.

verity   The condition or state of being true. *See also* true; truth.

vernacular   **1.** The native language of a country or locality. **2.** The everyday language spoken by a people as distinguished from the literary language. **3.** The idiom of a trade or profession, as in medical vernacular.

verrucae   Warts caused by the virus of the papovavirus group. *Plantar verrucae* are warts on the bottom of the foot. *Needling of verrucae* is one method of destroying plantar warts by multiple punctures of the lesion under local anesthesia. *Synonym*: warts. *See also* dermatology; hyfrecator; podiatric medicine; virus.

vertical integration   Organizing a range of facilities or programs in a general field, such as health care, so that business services are brought under one management to increase efficiency and profitability; for example, the establishment of a system of health care facilities ranging from nursing homes to clinics to hospitals under one management. *Compare* horizontal integration. *See also* integration; management.

vessel, blood   *See* blood vessel.

veteran   **1.** A person who has served in the armed forces, as in a Vietnam veteran. *See also* disabled veteran. **2.** A person long experienced or practiced in an activity or a capacity, as in a veteran of the health care system.

veteran, disabled   *See* disabled veteran.

Veterans Administration   *See* Department of Veterans Affairs.

Veterans' Affairs, Committee on   *See* Committee on Veterans' Affairs.

Veterans Affairs, Department of   *See* Department of Veterans Affairs.

Veterans Affairs, Nurses Organization of   *See* Nurses Organization of Veterans Affairs.

Veterans Writing Project, Hospitalized   *See* Hospitalized Veterans Writing Project.

VHA   *See* Voluntary Hospitals of America.

viable   **1.** Capable of success or continuing effectiveness, as in a viable plan. **2.** Capable of living outside the uterus, as in a viable fetus. *See also* fetus.

vibromassage   A method of massage using an electrically powered vibrating instrument. *See also* massage.

VICA   *See* Vision Council of America.

vicarious liability   One person's liability due to the actions of another; for example, an employer's liability for an employee's negligence while the employee is performing work at the place of employment. In tort law, if an employee, such as a nurse, while in the scope of his or her employment for his or her employer, such as a hospital, injures a patient, the hospital may be vicariously liable for the injuries sustained by the patient, under the doctrine of respondeat superior. *Synonyms:* passive negligence; secondary negligence. *See also* liability; respondeat superior.

vice president   A corporate officer, subordinate to the president (or chief executive officer), often having responsibility over a functional department, such as the vice president of nursing services or marketing. *See also* chief executive officer.

vice president of buildings and grounds   *See* administrative engineer.

vice president of facilities   *See* administrative engineer.

vice president of medical affairs   *See* medical director.

vice president for/of nursing services   *See* chief of nursing; nurse executive.

vice president of professional services   *See* medical director.

victim   **1.** One who is harmed by another. **2.** One who is harmed by an act, circumstance, agency, or condition, as in a trauma victim.

Victims, National Committee for Radiation   *See* National Committee for Radiation Victims.

Victims of Trauma, Institute for   *See* Institute for Victims of Trauma.

violation   The act or process of breaking or disregarding, for example, a law or promise. *See also* gross and flagrant violation; per se violation; substantial violation.

violation, gross and flagrant   *See* gross and flagrant violation.

violation, per se   *See* per se violation.

violation, substantial   *See* substantial violation.

violence   Physical force exerted for the purpose of violating, damaging, or abusing people or things. *See also* maim; trauma.

Violence Information, Clearinghouse on Family   *See* Clearinghouse on Family Violence Information.

Violence, National Coalition Against Domestic   *See* National Coalition Against Domestic Violence.

Violence, National Council on Child Abuse and Family   *See* National Council on Child Abuse and Family Violence.

Virchow-Pirquet Medical Society (VPMS)   A national organization founded in 1975 composed of 250 physicians practicing in the United States who are graduates of German, Austrian, Hungarian, Czechoslovakian, and Swiss medical schools. It promotes the continuation of medical education and cultivates the tradition of the Central European clinical approach to medicine.

virology   The branch of microbiology that deals with viruses. *See also* microbiology; virus.

virulence   Degree of pathogenicity, as in the bacterial strain's virulence. *See also* pathogenicity.

virus   Simple submicroscopic parasites of plants, animals, and bacteria that often cause disease and that consist essentially of a core of ribonucleic acid (RNA) or deoxyribonucleic acid (DNA) surrounded by a protein coat. Unable to replicate without a host cell, viruses are not considered living organisms. Viruses are responsible for a large number of diseases, including the common cold, herpes, influenza, measles, mumps, and acquired immunodeficiency syndrome (AIDS). *See also* cold; computer virus; deoxyribonucleic acid; germ; herpes simplex; herpes zoster; measles; microorganism; oncogene; parasite; poliovirus; ribonucleic acid; verrucae.

virus, computer *See* computer virus.

virus infections, slow *See* slow virus infections.

virus, polio- *See* poliovirus.

virus, retro- *See* retrovirus.

viscus *See* viscera.

viscera The soft internal organs of the body, for example, heart, liver, pancreas. A single organ is called a viscus. *See also* multivisceral transplant; organ.

visceral transplant, multi- *See* multivisceral transplant.

visible patient care function A goal-directed interrelated series of processes that has an immediate and tangible effect on the patient and his or her family; for example, nursing care. *Compare* invisible patient care function. *See also* function.

vision **1.** Ability to see; perception of things through the action of light on the eyes and optic centers in the brain. *See also* blindness; ophthalmology; optometry; visual acuity. **2.** Unusual competence in discernment or perception, as in a leader with vision. **3.** A mental image produced by the imagination, as in a vision for the organization.

Vision Council of America (VICA) A national organization founded in 1985 composed of 450 optical industry companies that sponsor exhibits at industry trade shows. Formerly (1990) Vision Industry Council of America. *See also* vision.

Vision Development, College of Optometrists in *See* College of Optometrists in Vision Development.

Vision Industry Council of America *See* Vision Council of America.

Vision and Ophthalmology, Association for Research in *See* Association for Research in Vision and Ophthalmology.

Vision Professionals, National Association of *See* National Association of Vision Professionals.

visit In health care, an encounter between a patient or client and a health professional. *See also* friendly visit; house call; office visit; outpatient visit.

visit, friendly *See* friendly visit.

visit group, ambulatory *See* ambulatory visit group.

visit, office *See* office visit.

visit, outpatient *See* outpatient visit.

visiting nurse association (VNA) A private, nonprofit health care agency that provides nursing services in the home. Visiting nurse associations employ nurses and other personnel, such as home health aides, who are trained to perform specific tasks of personal bedside care. *Synonym:* visiting nurse service. *See also* home health agency; home health aide; nurse.

Visiting Nurse Associations of America (VNAA) A national organization founded in 1983 composed of 150 voluntary, nonprofit home health care agencies. It develops competitive strength among voluntary nonprofit health care agencies and works to strengthen business resources and economic programs through marketing and contracting. *See also* visiting nurse association.

visiting nurse service (VNS) *See* visiting nurse association.

visiting teacher *See* school social worker.

visual acuity Sharpness of vision, typically measured by standardized vision charts. *See also* acuity; vision.

visually impaired **1.** Pertaining to a diminished or defective sense of sight, although not blind from birth, to such an extent as to have to relay on aids. **2.** A blind person. *See also* blind; blindness; hearing impaired.

vital **1.** Pertaining to life, as in vital records. *See also* vital records; vital signs; vital statistics. **2.** Necessary to continued existence or effectiveness; essential. *See also* vital few.

vital few The very limited set of factors identified by a Pareto analysis as being associated with the great majority of a problem. *See also* Pareto analysis; useful many; vital.

vital records Certificates of birth, death, marriage, and divorce required for legal and demographic purposes. *See also* birth certificate; death certificate; record; vital.

Vital Records and Health Statistics, Association for *See* Association for Vital Records and Health Statistics.

vital signs Signs that show the overall condition of a person, changes in which are often clues to disease or signs of alteration in a person's health. Vital signs typically include temperature, pulse, respiration, and blood pressure. *See also* blood pressure; pulse; respiration; sign; temperature; vital.

vital statistics   Tabulated data concerning births, marriages, divorces, separations, diseases, and deaths based on registrations of these vital events in vital records. *See also* birth certificate; epidemiology; health statistics; statistics; vital.

vitamin   Any of various fat-soluble or water-soluble organic substances essential in minute amounts for normal growth and activity of the body and obtained naturally from plant and animal foods. *See also* fat-soluble vitamin; trace elements; vitamin A; vitamin B complex; vitamin C; vitamin D; vitamin E; vitamin K; vitamin P; water-soluble vitamin.

vitamin A   A fat-soluble vitamin necessary for vision, reproduction, and the formation and maintenance of skin, mucous membranes, bones, and teeth. Megadoses can produce birth defects. Good sources include liver, eggs, and butter. A precursor, beta carotene, is found in yellow, orange, and dark green vegetables and fruit. *See also* bile; fat-soluble vitamin; vitamin.

vitamin B complex   A group of water-soluble vitamins including thiamine, riboflavin, niacin, pantothenic acid, biotin, pyridoxine, folic acid, inositol, and vitamin B_{12} and occurring in yeast, liver, eggs, and some vegetables. *Synonym*: B complex. *See also* vitamin; water-soluble vitamin.

vitamin C   A water-soluble vitamin that is important in the production of collagen and the maintenance of capillaries, cartilage, bones, and teeth. It promotes healing and helps the body fight infection. Good sources include citrus fruits and juices, green or leafy vegetables, potatoes, cabbage, and cauliflower. *Synonym*: ascorbic acid. *See also* vitamin; water-soluble vitamin.

vitamin D   A fat-soluble vitamin necessary for the body's absorption and metabolism of calcium and phosphorus and important for the maintenance of teeth and bones. Good sources include egg yolks, fish, cod liver oil, fortified milk, and butter. The body can also derive it from exposure to sunlight. Megadoses are toxic. *See also* bile; fat-soluble vitamin; vitamin.

vitamin E   A fat-soluble vitamin found chiefly in plant leaves, wheat germ oil, and milk and used to treat sterility and various abnormalities of the muscles, red blood cells, liver, and brain. *See also* fat-soluble vitamin; vitamin.

vitamin, fat-soluble   *See* fat-soluble vitamin.

vitamin K   A fat-soluble vitamin that enables the liver to manufacture prothrombin and other proteins that bind calcium and are necessary for normal blood clotting and bone crystal formation. Intestinal bacteria manufacture it to provide part of the body's requirement. Dietary sources, such as spinach and other green leafy vegetables, milk products, meats, eggs, cereals, fruits, and vegetables, provide the remainder. *See also* bile; coagulation; fat-soluble vitamin; vitamin.

vitamin P   A water-soluble vitamin found in citrus juices that promotes capillary resistance to hemorrhaging. *See also* capillary; vitamin; water-soluble vitamin.

vitamin, water-soluble   *See* water-soluble vitamin.

vivisection   The act or practice of cutting into or otherwise injuring living animals, especially for the purpose of scientific research. *Compare* antivivisectionist. *See also* animal experimentation.

VNA   *See* visiting nurse association.

VNAA   *See* Visiting Nurse Associations of America.

VNS   Abbreviation for visiting nurse service. *See* visiting nurse association.

vocabulary   All the words of a language. *See also* language.

vocation   A regular occupation, especially one for which a person is suited or qualified, as in a vocational nurse. *See also* occupation; vocational assessment; vocational habilitation; vocational rehabilitation; work.

vocational assessment   In health care, the process of evaluating a patient's work experiences and attitudes toward work, current motivations and areas of interest, and possibilities for future training, education, and employment. *See also* assessment; vocation.

vocational habilitation   The development of persons born with limited functional capability to the fullest physical, mental, social, vocational, and economic usefulness of which they are capable. *See also* habilitation; vocational rehabilitation.

vocational nurse   *See* licensed vocational nurse.

vocational rehabilitation   The restoration of persons with limited functioning to the fullest physical, mental, social, vocational, and economic usefulness of which they are capable. *See also* rehabilitation; vocation.

Vocational Rehabilitation, Council of State Administrators of   *See* Council of State Administrators of Vocational Rehabilitation.

vocational rehabilitation counselor   *See* rehabilitation counselor.

vocational school   A school, especially one on a secondary level, that offers instruction and practical introductory experience in skilled trades, such as mechanics, carpentry, plumbing, and construction. *See also* school; vocation.

voice   The sound produced by the vocal organs. *See also* sound; voice input/output technology.

voice input/output technology   Applications of voice recognition and synthesis with and through computers. *Synonyms:* automated speech technology; voice technology. *See also* computer; technology; voice recognition.

voice recognition   Direct conversion of spoken data into computer language. *See also* computer; voice; voice input/output technology.

voice technology   *See* voice input/output technology.

voir dire   French phrase meaning "to speak the truth." This is the procedure whereby prospective jurors are questioned before determining who will sit in judgment on a case. Depending on the court, the questioning may be conducted by the judge, counsel for the parties, or both. *See also* jury; trial.

volume   Amount or quantity, as in the number of cases with a specific procedure, diagnosis, or condition treated in a hospital or by a physician. *See also* high-volume function; hospital volume; physician volume.

volume function, high-   *See* high-volume function.

volume, hospital   *See* hospital volume.

volume, physician   *See* physician volume.

volume process, high-   *See* high-volume process.

voluntary   Acting, serving, or doing willingly and without constraint or expectation of reward, as in voluntary hospital work. *See also* voluntary blood donor; voluntary health agency; voluntary hospital.

voluntary blood donor   A blood donor who does not receive payment for donating his or her blood. *Compare* professional blood donor. *See also* blood donor; donor; voluntary.

voluntary demotion   A demotion usually resulting from a reduction in work force. *See also* demotion; RIF; voluntary.

Voluntary Health Agencies, National   *See* National Voluntary Health Agencies.

voluntary health agency   Any nonprofit, nongovernmental agency, governed by lay and/or professional individuals, whose primary purpose relates to health care; for example, the American Cancer Society. *Synonyms:* private health agency; voluntary organization. *See also* agency; voluntary.

Voluntary Health and Social Welfare Organizations, National Assembly of National   *See* National Assembly of National Voluntary Health and Social Welfare Organizations.

voluntary hospital   A private, not-for-profit hospital that is autonomous, self-established, and self-supported, as in a facility owned and operated by a fraternal, religious, or not-for-profit community organization. *See also* hospital; voluntary.

Voluntary Hospitals of America (VHA)   A national organization founded in 1977 composed of 834 members. It manages the health insurance plans of 662 US not-for-profit hospitals, their affiliates (172), and 250,000 physicians. It offers programs and services to improve members' competitive position. *See also* health insurance; voluntary hospital.

voluntary muscle   *See* muscle.

voluntary organization   *See* voluntary health agency.

Voluntary Surgical Contraception, Association for   *See* Association for Voluntary Surgical Contraception.

volunteer   An individual who provides a service without compulsion or requirement, and typically without compensation, as in a hospital trustee serving a hospital or other health care organization without pay. *See also* auxilian; auxiliary; candy striper; trustee; voluntary.

volunteer services   Organizations of persons who donate their time and energy to providing nonmedical assistance in support of a health care organization's operations. Volunteers, for example, may operate a gift shop, escort and transport family members and patients, deliver flowers, or staff clerical desks. *See also* volunteer.

Volunteer Services, American Society of Directors of   *See* American Society of Directors of Volunteer Services.

Volunteer Trustees of Not-For-Profit Hospitals   A national organization founded in 1980 composed of representatives of 155 not-for-profit hospitals and their voluntary governing boards. Its objectives include providing a trustee voice in policy-making and legislative activities and developing a communications network among trustees in order to provide the highest quality medical care at the lowest possible price. Areas of concern include Medicare, controlling hospital costs, and strategic planning for the not-for-profit hospital community. *See also* not-for-profit hospital; trustee; voluntary.

volvulus Twisting of a loop of intestine and its mesenteric attachment, causing intestinal ischemia (decreased blood supply) and obstruction. *See also* intestine; ischemia; surgery.

vomit To eject part or all of the contents of the stomach through the mouth, usually in a series of involuntary spasmic movements. *See also* antiemetic; bulimia nervosa; emetic; gastroenteritis; indigestion; nausea.

voucher A certificate that may be exchanged for a contract for services for a given period of time under a prepayment plant. *See also* certificate; voucher system.

voucher system A system in which Medicare beneficiaries use vouchers issued by the federal government to enroll in health care plans of their choice. Under the voucher system, the beneficiary enrolls in a federally qualified health care plan, and payment is made directly to the care-providing organization in a predetermined, fixed amount in exchange for the beneficiary's voucher. *See also* beneficiary; Medicare; voucher.

voyeurism A sexual proclivity in which vicarious pleasure is obtained from observation of the sexual activity of other persons. It includes troilism and the peeping-tom syndrome. *See also* troilism.

VPMS *See* Virchow-Pirquet Medical Society.

vulnerable **1.** Susceptible to physical injury or attack. **2.** Liable to succumb, as to temptation or infection.

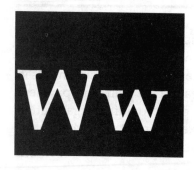

WA *See* Wellness Associates.

wage A form of earnings based on hourly, daily, weekly, or piecework performance. *See also* area wage adjustment; minimum wage; salary.

wage adjustment, area *See* area wage adjustment.

wage, minimum *See* minimum wage.

Wagner-Murray-Dingell Bill One of the original national health insurance proposals first introduced by Congressmen Wagner, Murray, and Dingell in the 1940s. It is still updated and introduced in each Congress by Congressman John Dingell of Michigan, who succeeded his father, the original sponsor, in office. *See also* national health insurance.

waiting period In health insurance, a period of time an individual must wait either to become eligible for insurance coverage or to become eligible for a given benefit after overall coverage has commenced. Some insurance policies, for instance, will not pay maternity benefits until nine months after the policy has been in force, and insurance coverage under other policies may not begin until an employee has been with an organization over 30 days. *See also* eligible; health insurance.

waiver An agreement attached to an insurance policy that exempts from coverage certain disabilities or injuries normally covered by the policy. *See also* coverage; exclusions.

walker A light metal apparatus, about waist high with four legs, used as an aid in walking. *See also* cane; crutch; wheelchair.

WAN *See* wide area network.

ward **1.** A hospital room set up to accommodate more than four patients. *See also* private room; semiprivate room. **2.** An inpatient care unit of a hospital, as in maternity ward. *See also* inpatient care unit; maternity ward. **3.** An individual for whom a guardian or conservator has been appointed by a court, to care for and make decisions concerning the ward's person, property, or both. A ward is legally incompetent to act on his or her behalf, usually because of immaturity or lack of mental capacity. *See also* incompetent.

ward clerk *See* health unit coordinator.

ward manager *See* unit manager.

ward, maternity *See* maternity ward.

ward patient A patient whose care is the financial responsibility of a health program or institution. *Synonyms*: public patient; service patient. *Compare* private patient. *See also* patient; ward.

ward rounds *See* teaching rounds.

warfare, biological *See* biological warfare.

warfarin An oral anticoagulant used in the prevention and treatment of venous thrombosis and its complications and in other situations when blood coagulation inhibition is desired. *See also* anticoagulant; coagulation; thrombosis.

Warren Foundation, The William K. *See* The William K. Warren Foundation.

warts **1.** Imperfections or flaws, as in admiring him, warts and all. **2.** *See* verrucae.

waste An undesired result of a process. *See also* hazardous waste; rework.

waste, hazardous *See* hazardous waste.

Water Administrators, Association of State Drinking *See* Association of State Drinking Water Administrators.

water bed A water-filled rubber mattress sometimes used for patients whose weight needs to be distributed evenly. *See also* bed.

water-soluble vitamin The B complex, C, and P vitamins, which are soluble in water. *Compare* fat-soluble vitamin. *See also* vitamin; vitamin B complex;

vitamin C; vitamin P.

wave A periodic disturbance in a medium or in space that involves the elastic displacement of material particles or a periodic change in some physical quantity, as in a pressure wave or pulse. *See also* pulse; wavelength.

wavelength The distance between one peak or crest of a wave of light, heat, or other energy and the next corresponding peak or crest. *See also* wave.

Ways and Means, Committee on *See* Committee on Ways and Means.

WBC *See* white blood cell.

WC *See* workers' compensation.

WE *See* Women's Caucus of the Endocrine Society.

weakest link theory A system in which components of the system are dependent on the support of the whole, and the whole is only as reliable as the weakest member or link in the system. *See also* link; linkage; system; theory.

weakness Lack of strength; feebleness or ill health. *See also* illness.

weekend hospitalization A type of partial hospitalization in which a patient spends weekends in a health care facility and functions in the community during the rest of each week. *See also* hospitalization; partial hospitalization.

weeping Pertaining to a wound or surface that is discharging clear serous fluid.

WEHAC *See* Wills Eye Hospital Annual Conference.

Weibull distribution *See* probability distribution.

weight 1. A measure of the heaviness of an object, as in birth weight. *See also* anorexia nervosa; birth weight; desirable weight; height; low birth weight; measurement; obesity. 2. The force with which a body is attracted to earth or another celestial body, equal to the product of the object's mass and the acceleration of gravity. 3. In statistics, a factor assigned to a number in a computation, as in determining a mean, to make the number's effect on the computation reflect its importance; for example, DRG (diagnosis-related group) weight. *See also* DRG weight; statistics.

weight, birth *See* birth weight.

weight, desirable *See* desirable weight.

weight, DRG *See* DRG weight.

weight, low birth *See* low birth weight.

welfare Public financial assistance to certain categories of poor persons. *See also* poor; public welfare.

welfare administrator, social *See* social welfare administrator.

Welfare Administrators, National Association of Public Child *See* National Association of Public Child Welfare Administrators.

Welfare Association, American Public *See* American Public Welfare Association.

Welfare Association, Presbyterian Health, Education and *See* Presbyterian Health, Education and Welfare Association.

welfare caseworker, child *See* child welfare caseworker.

Welfare Institute, Child *See* Child Welfare Institute.

Welfare League of America, Child *See* Child Welfare League of America.

Welfare Ministries, United Methodist Association of Health and *See* United Methodist Association of Health and Welfare Ministries.

welfare, public *See* public welfare.

Well-Being of Health Professionals, Center for the *See* Center for the Well-Being of Health Professionals.

well-defined Accurately and unambiguously stated or described, as in a well-defined argument.

wellness Good physical and mental health, especially when maintained by proper diet, exercise, and habits. *Compare* illness. *See also* fitness; physical fitness program; wellness program.

Wellness Associates (WA) A national organization founded in 1975 that provides high quality resource materials for life-style improvement integrating the major components of wellness: self-responsibility, stress management, nutrition, and physical awareness. It provides consultation for wellness centers, individuals, universities, agencies, hospitals, and government groups. *See also* preventive medicine; wellness.

Wellness Association, National *See* National Wellness Association.

Wellness and Health Activation Networks (WHAN) A national organization founded in 1980 composed of 5,000 individuals interested in health activation, that is, the process of maintaining good health and preventing illness. It concentrates on programs designed to increase awareness of health rights and responsibilities and serves as a clearinghouse for the Wellness and Health Activation program, which designs and acts as national distributor of trainers' course guides, planning guides, program texts, home health care equipment, and other health activation materials. *See also* network; preventive medicine; wellness.

Wellness Institute, National *See* National Wellness Institute.

wellness program A program that encourages improved health status and a healthful life-style through health education, exercise, nutrition, and health promotion. A wellness program may focus on, for example, weight reduction, smoking cessation, cholesterol reduction, and stress reduction. *See also* health promotion; physical fitness program; wellness.

wen *See* sebaceous cyst.

wet nurse A woman who breastfeeds another woman's child. *See also* nurse.

WHAN *See* Wellness and Health Activation Networks.

wheelchair A chair mounted on wheels for the use of ill or disabled persons. *See also* cane; crutch; walker.

whiplash A colloquial term for an injury to the neck vertebrae and their associated ligaments and muscles, causing pain and stiffness in the neck. It is often the result of rapid acceleration or deceleration, as in a motor vehicle accident.

whistleblower An individual who reveals wrongdoing within a organization to the public or those in positions of authority. *See also* muckraker.

white blood cell (WBC) Any of five types of elements of the circulating blood system including: lymphocytes, monocytes, neutrophils, basophils, and eosinophils. The white blood cell's functions include ingestion of bacteria, fungi, and viruses; detoxification of toxic proteins; and development of immunities. Normal blood usually contains 5,000 to 10,000 leukocytes per cubic millimeter. *Synonyms*: granulocyte; leukocyte; WBC; white cell; white corpuscle. *See also* blood cell; lymphocyte.

white cell *See* white blood cell.

white corpuscle *See* white blood cell.

whitlow *See* paronychia.

WHO *See* World Health Organization.

whole blood Blood drawn from the body from which no component, such as plasma or platelets, has been removed. *See also* blood.

Wholesale Druggists' Association, National *See* National Wholesale Druggists' Association.

wholistic health *See* holistic health.

WHR *See* Women and Health Roundtable.

wide area network (WAN) A computer network in which computers over a wide area are enabled to communicate and share resources. *See also* local area network; network.

Wilderness Medical Society (WMS) A national organization founded in 1983 composed of 2,500 persons with advanced degrees in the biomedical or life sciences with an interest in the medical, behavioral, and life sciences aspects of wilderness environments. Its objectives are to promote research and educational activities that increase scientific knowledge about human activities in wilderness environments and stimulate interest and research in health consequences of wilderness activities. Areas of interest include treatment of victims of bites and stings, exotic infectious diseases and toxic plants, desert survival, avalanche control, and search and rescue.

will **1.** The mental faculty by which one deliberately chooses or decides upon a course of action. **2.** The act of exercising one's determination, as in the will to win or the will to change. *See also* mind. **3.** A legal document declaring how a person wishes his or her possessions to be disposed of after death. *See also* living will.

will, living *See* living will.

William K. Warren Foundation, The *See* The William K. Warren Foundation.

Williams-Steiger Act *See* Occupational Safety and Health Act of 1970.

Wills Eye Hospital Society *See* Wills Eye Hospital Annual Conference.

Wills Eye Hospital Annual Conference (WEHAC) An organization founded in 1932 composed of 1,256 ophthalmologists interested in disseminating information and research findings relating to the field of ophthalmology. Formerly (1991) Wills Eye Society of Ex-Residents; (1992) Wills Eye Hospital Society. *See also* ophthalmology.

Wills Eye Society of Ex-Residents *See* Wills Eye Hospital Annual Conference.

windbag A talkative person who communicates nothing of substance or interest. *See also* wordy.

window **1.** A limited time during which an opportunity should be seized, or it will be lost, as in a window of opportunity. **2.** A portion of a computer display screen. Computer programs sometimes allow the user to divide the screen into two or more windows, making it possible to work on two different tasks at once. *See also* computer.

windpipe   *See* trachea.

Wine, Society of Medical Friends of   *See* Society of Medical Friends of Wine.

wisdom teeth   The third molar teeth, the last of the permanent teeth to erupt. They often do not appear until early adult life and sometimes do not appear at all. *See also* permanent tooth; tooth.

wit   **1.** The natural ability to perceive and understand. **2.** Keenness and quickness of perception or discernment. *See also* perception.

witch doctor   **1.** One who professes to cure disease by magic arts. **2.** One who professes to detect witches and to counteract the effects of their magic, especially among African peoples. *See also* doctor; medicine man; shaman.

withdrawal symptoms   Symptoms experienced by drug and alcohol addicts during the early stages of abstinence from the addictive substance. *See also* addiction; detoxification; medical detoxification.

withdrawing treatment   Termination or removal of a particular treatment without termination of care. There is no necessary difference (moral or legal) between withdrawing or withholding the same treatment, for example, stopping mechanical ventilation versus not starting mechanical ventilation. *See also* omission; treatment; withholding treatment.

withholding treatment   Omission of treatment. *See also* omission; treatment; withdrawing treatment.

witness   An individual who can give a firsthand account of something seen, heard, or experienced, as in one who is called to testify before a court. *See also* cross-examination; expert witness; impeachment; leading question; testify; testimonial; witness stand.

witness, expert   *See* expert witness.

witness stand   A raised or an enclosed area in a courtroom from which a witness presents testimony. *See also* court; witness.

WMAFPH   *See* American Association of Ayurvedic Medicine.

WM Keck Foundation   A private foundation established in 1954 whose purpose is to strengthen studies and programs in the areas of earth science, involving the development of natural resources; engineering; medical research and education; and, to some extent, other sciences, liberal arts, and law/legal administration. Eligible institutions in these fields are accredited colleges and universities, medical schools, and major independent medical research institutions. *See also* foundation; private foundation.

WK Kellogg Foundation   A private foundation established in 1930 whose purpose is to aid programs concerned with the application of existing knowledge rather than research. It supports pilot projects, which, if successful, can be continued by the initiating organization and emulated by other communities or organizations with similar problems. Its current funding priorities include projects designed to improve human well-being with a focus on youth; higher education; leadership; community-based, problem-focused health services; food systems; rural development philanthropy; volunteerism; and groundwater resources. *See also* foundation; private foundation.

WMS   *See* Wilderness Medical Society.

womb   *See* uterus.

Women Attorneys, National Association of Black   *See* National Association of Black Women Attorneys.

Women Dentists, American Association of   *See* American Association of Women Dentists.

Women Lawyers, National Association of   *See* National Association of Women Lawyers.

Women Physician's Association, National Osteopathic   *See* National Osteopathic Women Physician's Association.

Women in Psychology, Association for   *See* Association for Women in Psychology.

Women Radiologists, American Association for   *See* American Association for Women Radiologists.

Women's Association, American Medical   *See* American Medical Women's Association.

Women's Caucus of the Endocrine Society (WE)   An organization founded in 1975 composed of 850 members interested in promoting the professional advancement of women and younger members of the Endocrine Society. *See also* Endocrine Society; endocrinology.

Women's Health Network, National   *See* National Women's Health Network.

Women's Health, Obstetric, and Neonatal Nurses, Association of   *See* Association of Women's Health, Obstetric, and Neonatal Nurses.

Women's Health Project, National Black   *See* National Black Women's Health Project.

Women's Health Research, Melpomene Institute for   *See* Melpomene Institute for Women's Health Research.

Women's Health Resource Center, National   *See*

National Women's Health Resource Center.

Women and Health Roundtable (WHR)   A monthly forum founded in 1976 on women's health issues for representatives of health-related and women's organizations, consumer groups, and federal agencies. It monitors and attempts to improve federal and state health policies' responsiveness to women's health priorities.

women's rights   Socioeconomic, political, and legal rights for all women equal to those of men. *See also* rights.

wonder drug   *See* miracle drug.

Woodruff Foundation, Inc, Robert W.   *See* Robert W. Woodruff Foundation, Inc.

word processing   In computer science, the creation, input, editing, and production of documents and texts by means of computer systems. *See also* computer; footer; header; word processor; word wrapping.

word processor   A programmable typewriter or computer program used to compose, format, sort, and rearrange text upon command and sometimes perform other related functions, such as correcting misspelled words. *See also* computer; footer; header; word processing.

word salad   Words combined in a way that has no or little meaning.

word wrapping   A word processing technique that automatically moves a word to the next line if it does not fit at the end of the original line. *See also* word processing.

wordy   Tending to use, using, or expressed in more words than are necessary to convey meaning. *See also* windbag.

work   **1.** Mental or physical effort or activity directed toward the production or accomplishment of something. *See also* rework. **2.** A job, profession, occupation, or means of livelihood. *See also* job; occupation; profession; vocation.

worker   One who performs work. *See also* work.

worker, community organization   *See* community organization worker.

worker, eligibility   *See* eligibility worker.

worker, full-time   *See* full-time worker.

worker, part-time   *See* part-time worker.

worker, sanitation   *See* sanitation worker.

workers' compensation (WC)   A system, required by law, of compensating workers injured or disabled in connection with work. *Synonym*: workmens' compensation. *See also* workers' compensation acts;

workers' compensation insurance; workers' compensation programs.

workers' compensation acts   Statutes that, in general, establish the liability of an employer for injuries or sickness that arise over and in the course of employment. The liability is created without regard to the fault or negligence of the employer. Benefits generally include hospital and other medical payments and compensation for loss of income. If the injury is covered by the statute, compensation will be the employee's only remedy against his or her employer. These statutes have had the effect of abolishing the notion that the hazards of a particular job or workplace are voluntarily encountered by the employee by virtue of his or her agreement to work there, and thus could not give rise to liability for negligence on the part of the employer. *See also* personal injury; workers' compensation.

workers' compensation insurance   Insurance contract paid by an employer for all employees and providing protection against loss due to injury or illness at the workplace. *See also* insurance; workers' compensation.

workers' compensation programs   State social insurance programs that provide cash benefits to workers or their dependents injured, disabled, or deceased in the course, and as a result, of employment. The employee is also entitled to benefits for some or all of the health services necessary for treatment and restoration to a useful life and, possibly, a productive job. These programs are mandatory under state laws in all states. *See also* workers' compensation.

worker, service   *See* service worker.

worker, social   *See* social worker.

worker, social group   *See* social group worker.

workforce   **1.** The workers employed in a specific project or activity. **2.** All the people working or available to work, as in a company or an industry.

workhorse   A person who works tirelessly, especially at difficult or time-consuming tasks.

working poor   People who are economically disadvantaged despite being fully employed. *See also* poor.

workload   The amount of work assigned to or expected from a worker in a specified time period. *See also* work; worker.

workmens' compensation   *See* workers' compensation.

workout 1. A session of exercise or practice to improve fitness, as for athletic competition. *See also* aerobics; exercise; fitness. **2.** A strenuous test of ability and endurance.

work, piece- *See* piecework.

work, piece of *See* piece of work.

workplace A place, such as a physician's office, a laboratory, or an operating room, where people are employed and perform work. *See also* work.

work, re- *See* rework.

work, scut *See* scut work.

work, social *See* social work.

workstation A configuration of computer equipment and peripheral devices that are intended for use by a single person. *See also* computer.

World Health, American Association for *See* American Association for World Health.

World Health Organization (WHO) A division of the United Nations founded in 1948 and based in Geneva that serves to coordinate and improve health activities worldwide. *See also* health.

World Health Organization, Committee for the *See* American Association for World Health.

World Medical Association for Perfect Health *See* American Association of Ayurvedic Medicine.

worldview The overall perspective from which one sees and interprets the world. *See also* culture; religion.

worm 1. In pathology, infestation of the intestine or other parts of the body with worms or wormlike parasites. *See also* infestation; intestine; parasite. **2.** A computer program that, like a computer virus, replicates itself and interferes with software function or destroys stored information. It is designed to sabotage a computer or network of computers. *See also* computer virus; network.

worn-out Thoroughly exhausted or spent. *See also* burnout.

worry To feel uneasy or be concerned about something. *See also* anxiety; worrywart.

worrywart One who worries excessively and needlessly. *See also* worry.

worst-case The most unfavorable; being or involving the worst possibility, as in a worst-case scenario.

worth The inherent value of a commodity, good, service, or other economic factor. *See also* value; worthy.

worthy Useful or valuable; honorable or admirable. *See also* worth.

wound A lesion produced by external mechanical force involving damage to the normal continuity of tissues. Types of wounds include bruises (contusions), cuts (incisions), tears (lacerations), stabs (punctures), and breaks (fractures). *See also* wound infection.

wound ballistics *See* ballistics.

wound infection A postoperative infection that varies in incidence and type with the nature of a surgical procedure, degree of surgical skill, and adequacy of aseptic technique before, during, and after an operation. *See also* infection; operation; postoperative care; postpartum care; surgery; wound.

WPR *See* written progress report.

writ In law, a written order issued by a court, commanding the party to whom it is addressed to perform or cease performing a specified act. *See also* court; writ of certiorari.

writ of certiorari A writ that commands a lower court to certify proceedings for review by a higher court. The writ is issued in order that the higher court may inspect the proceedings and establish if any legal irregularities have occurred. This is a common method of obtaining review of a case by the US Supreme Court. *See also* case; court; writ.

writer 1. One who writes, especially as an occupation. *See also* occupation; writer's cramp. **2.** *See* underwriter.

Writers Association, American Medical *See* American Medical Writers Association.

writer's cramp An occupational disorder consisting of spasm or cramps of the muscles of the fingers, hand, and forearm during writing. *See also* writer.

Writing Project, Hospitalized Veterans *See* Hospitalized Veterans Writing Project.

written progress report (WPR) A postsurvey activity of the Joint Commission on Accreditation of Healthcare Organizations that involves a surveyed organization preparing a report documenting evidence that correction of a compliance problem(s) is complete. Preparing a written progress report involves summarizing, documenting, and collecting facts and other evidence that prove an organization's current compliance with the standards that caused the type I recommendation. *See also* accreditation decision processing; first generation type I recommendation; Joint Commission on Accreditation of Healthcare Organizations; type I recommendation.

wrongful birth   A tort action concerning a child who would not have been born but for legally liable contraceptive failure, unsuccessful sterilization, failure to diagnose a pregnancy, unsuccessful abortion, failure to warn the parent(s) of genetic risks, or failure to timely diagnose (or inform the parents about) a birth defect or disease of the fetus. A wrongful birth action is brought by the parents on their own behalf, as opposed to a wrongful life action. *See also* birth; tort; wrongful life.

wrongful death   A tort action concerning a death for which there is legal liability; for example, a death caused by professional negligence. Deaths are treated differently than injuries in the legal system. For example, a different statute of limitations may apply to a wrongful death action than to a negligence action, even though negligence may have been the cause of the wrongful death, and the amount of recovery for wrongful death may be limited to a specific dollar amount. Wrongful death actions are ordinarily governed by state statutes. *See also* death; tort; wrongful life.

wrongful life   A tort action brought by or on behalf of a baby who is suffering from a birth or genetic defect or other disease, and who would not have been born but for professional negligence concerning the same matters as identified with wrongful birth. *See also* action; life; tort; wrongful birth.

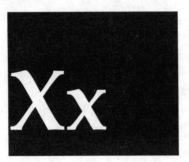 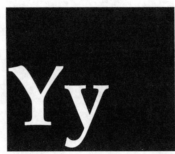 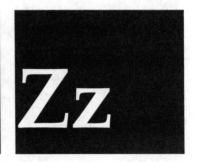

x-axis On a graph, the x-axis runs horizontally across the page. *See also* axis; graph; y-axis.

xenophobia A pathological fear of strangers or a dislike of foreigners. *See also* phobia.

x-ray 1. A relatively high-energy photon with a wavelength in the approximate range from 0.01 to 10 nanometers, used in a stream for its penetrating power in radiology, radiotherapy, and scientific research. *Synonym:* roentgen ray. *See also* radiation; ray; scatter. **2.** The process of exposing a person or an object to x-rays for the purpose of making an image on a sensitized surface, as in x-raying a patient. **3.** An image created by the transmission of x-rays through a person or object onto a sensitized surface. *See also* radiograph; roentgenogram.

x-ray technologist *See* radiographer.

x-ray therapy Medical therapy using controlled doses of x-ray radiation. *See also* radiation therapy; x-ray.

yardstick A test or standard used in measurement, comparison, or judgment. *See also* benchmark; standard.

yawn A semivoluntary wide opening of the mouth, which may be associated with deep breathing and sometimes with stretching of the limbs. It is a manifestation of fatigue, anxiety, or boredom.

y-axis On a graph, the y-axis runs vertically down the page. *See also* axis; graph; x-axis.

year, calendar *See* calendar year.

year, fiscal *See* fiscal year.

year, transitional *See* transitional year.

yield To produced a return for effort or investment, as in performance measures that yield useful information.

yoga A system of mental concentration, abstract meditation, asceticism, and physical discipline derived from Hindu philosophy and practices. The object of yoga is to emancipate the soul and achieve union with a supreme spirit. *See also* meditation; transcendental meditation.

Young Adult Chronic Patients, The Information Exchange on *See* The Information Exchange on Young Adult Chronic Patients.

zero defects Having no flaws or errors; for example, zero defects as a primary goal for all total quality management organizations. *See also* Crosby, Philip B.; defect.

Zero to Three/NCCIP An organization founded in 1977 composed of professionals in mental health, pediatrics, psychology, social work, nursing, and education who are interested in improving the health, mental health, and development of infants, toddlers, and their families. It facilitates development through preventive clinical approaches in the earliest years of life. Formerly (1992) National Center for Clinical Infant Programs. *See also* infant.

zoophilism Abnormal fondness for animals.

zoophobia Irrational fear of animals. *See also* phobia.

zygote banking Storing a cell formed by the union of an ovum and a sperm for future use in producing a child. *See also* ova banking; sperm banking.